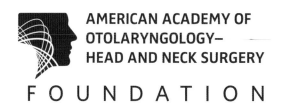

AMERICAN ACADEMY OF
OTOLARYNGOLOGY–
HEAD AND NECK SURGERY

FOUNDATION

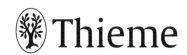

Otolaryngology Lifelong Learning Manual

3rd Edition

American Academy of Otolaryngology—Head and Neck Surgery Foundation

Sonya Malekzadeh, MD, FACS, Editor in Chief
Professor
Georgetown University Medical Center
Washington, DC

Section Editors

The Business of Medicine
Brendan C. Stack Jr., MD, FACS, FACE

Clinical Fundamentals
Brendan C. Stack Jr., MD, FACS, FACE and Karen T. Pitman, MD, FACS

General Otolaryngology
Karen T. Pitman, MD, FACS

Head and Neck Surgery
Richard V. Smith, MD, FACS

Laryngology and Bronchoesophagology
Catherine Rees Lintzenich, MD, FACS

Otology and Neurotology
Brad W. Kesser, MD

Pediatric Otolaryngology
Kenny H. Chan, MD

Rhinology and Allergy
Brent A. Senior, MD, FACS, FARS

Facial Plastic and Reconstructive Surgery
James Randall Jordan, MD, FACS and Fred G. Fedok, MD, FACS

Trauma
Joseph A. Brennan, MD, FACS, Colonel, MC, USAF

210 illustrations

Thieme
New York • Stuttgart • Delhi • Rio de Janeiro

Executive Editor: Timothy Hiscock
Managing Editor: J. Owen Zurhellen IV
Editorial Assistant: Kate Barron
Production Editor: Kenneth L. Chumbley
International Production Director: Andreas Schabert
Senior Vice President, Editorial and E-Product
    Development: Cornelia Schulze
International Marketing Director: Fiona Henderson
International Sales Director: Louisa Turrell
Director of Sales, North America: Mike Roseman
Senior Vice President and Chief Operating Officer:
    Sarah Vanderbilt
President: Brian D. Scanlan

Library of Congress Cataloging-in-Publication Data

Otolaryngology lifelong learning manual / American Academy
of Otolaryngology, Head and Neck Surgery Foundation. — Third
edition.
    p. ; cm.
    Preceded by: Maintenance manual for lifelong learning /
editor-in-chief, Jonas T. Johnson. 2nd ed. c2002.
    Includes bibliographical references.
    ISBN 978-1-62623-975-3 (alk. paper) —
    ISBN 978-1-60406-646-3 (e-book)
I. American Academy of Otolaryngology—Head and Neck
Surgery, issuing body.
[DNLM: 1. Otolaryngology. 2. Otorhinolaryngologic
Diseases. WV 100]
RF56
617.5′1—dc23

                                            2014033911

© 2015 Thieme Medical Publishers, Inc., and
American Academy of Otolaryngology–Head and
Neck Surgery Foundation
Thieme Publishers New York
333 Seventh Avenue, New York, NY 10001 USA
+1 800 782 3488, customerservice@thieme.com

Thieme Publishers Stuttgart
Rüdigerstrasse 14, 70469 Stuttgart, Germany
+49 [0]711 8931 421, customerservice@thieme.de

Thieme Publishers Delhi
A-12, Second Floor, Sector-2, Noida-201301
Uttar Pradesh, India
+91 120 45 566 00, customerservice@thieme.in

Thieme Publishers Rio, Thieme Publicações Ltda.
Argentina Building 16th floor, Ala A, 228 Praia do Botafogo
Rio de Janeiro 22250-040 Brazil
+55 21 3736-3631

Cover design: Thieme Publishing Group
Typesetting by Prairie Papers, Rantoul, Illinois

Printed in China by Everbest Printing Ltd   5 4 3 2 1

ISBN 978-1-62623-975-3

Also available as an e-book:
eISBN 978-1-62623-976-0

Important note: Medicine is an ever-changing science undergoing continual development. Research and clinical experience are continually expanding our knowledge, in particular our knowledge of proper treatment and drug therapy. Insofar as this book mentions any dosage or application, readers may rest assured that the authors, editors, and publishers have made every effort to ensure that such references are in accordance with the state of knowledge at the time of production of the book.

Nevertheless, this does not involve, imply, or express any guarantee or responsibility on the part of the publishers in respect to any dosage instructions and forms of applications stated in the book. Every user is requested to examine carefully the manufacturers' leaflets accompanying each drug and to check, if necessary in consultation with a physician or specialist, whether the dosage schedules mentioned therein or the contraindications stated by the manufacturers differ from the statements made in the present book. Such examination is particularly important with drugs that are either rarely used or have been newly released on the market. Every dosage schedule or every form of application used is entirely at the user's own risk and responsibility. The authors and publishers request every user to report to the publishers any discrepancies or inaccuracies noticed. If errors in this work are found after publication, errata will be posted at www.thieme.com on the product description page.

Some of the product names, patents, and registered designs referred to in this book are in fact registered trademarks or proprietary names even though specific reference to this fact is not always made in the text. Therefore, the appearance of a name without designation as proprietary is not to be construed as a representation by the publisher that it is in the public domain.

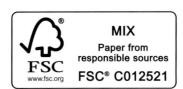

Contents

IX Facial Plastic and Reconstructive Surgery

X Trauma

Foreword

There is a native curiosity and unquenchable desire for knowledge that characterizes the medical profession. Every student who begins the journey to become a physician accepts the premise that continuing professional development (CPD) and lifelong learning will be an integral part of his or her professional life forever. The purpose of the *Otolaryngology Lifelong Learning Manual* is to assist otolaryngologists–head and neck surgeons and other clinicians—to engage in a practical approach to continuing professional development and learning in a systematic and integrated manner.

While essential, a work such as this must be accompanied by other elements to ensure that what is learned is applied, tested, improved, implemented, and the results measured and reported. Only when unbiased analysis at the appropriate level (individual, group, patient care, system, and global levels) of the total process is applied can we assure that our commitment to lifelong learning pays off in improved patient outcomes. Combining this process with identifying and filling gaps in knowledge and care leads to the most effective use of education resources.

The systematic approach to effective continuous education and professional development includes:

- knowledge-based learning of many types of unbiased and validated content
- methodology for applying or implementing what is learned
- methodology for documenting and reporting of learning and application
- methods for measuring the effect of applying knowledge to clinical care, reporting on improvement, and the results of care at patient level, system level, and global population level
- methods for increasing timely access to relevant information, including real-time, point-of-care access to clinical information
- decision support systems and methods
- links to evidence-based guidelines (EBG) and validated, relevant performance measures (PM)

- simulation, testing, and benchmarking where appropriate and data are available
- documenting the links between learnings, application to clinical care, improved patient outcomes, and improved population health
- CPD accreditation systems, including methods for developing and recognizing excellent education programming and CPD
- appropriate links to related clinical care accelerators, such as administrative, cost, capacity, structure, care coordination, communications, and team-based elements of care that require physician education, skill development, and integration for optimal clinical outcomes

The expectations of the physician of the future will be significantly different from today. At the American Board of Medical Specialties (ABMS) National Policy Conference in May 2014, Dr. George Thibault, president of the Josiah Macy Foundation, addressed how the changes in health care delivery will affect the need for interdisciplinary integrated education to match the requirements for integrated team-based collaborative care.

What physicians *know* will no longer be their distinguishing characteristic, but how they access information, work in teams, how resilient they are, and how effectively they can mobilize the right resources at the right time. Dr. Thibault describes the following ten elements of next generation medical skills:

Critical thinking skills. Physicians of the future will acquire exceptional analytical skills and the ability to use and sort information more effectively. This will allow them to generate hypotheses with greater accuracy and focus, with a more holistic approach to the health of the patient and the community.

Teamwork skills. The collaborative team-based care model of health care delivery may still include, but will increasingly replace the centuries-old tradition of the more intimate and private doctor-patient relationship. Interprofessional and interdisciplinary teams, along with interdisciplinary training models, will improve patient care but require new approaches to maintaining privacy and confidentiality, while sharing necessary clinical information across disciplines and care sites.

Leading skills. Understanding and utilizing the unique professional skills of team members, physician and nonphysician alike, will be required. Leadership development will be part of the training and experience of successful physicians.

Following skills. Physicians will need to know when and whom to follow. Not only clinical, but administrative and systems support personnel will provide essential services to patients through teams. Knowing when critical expertise is missing, appreciating what others know, do, and offer, and knowing when to endorse the leadership of others is key.

Quality Improvement skills. Experience in and an understanding of the science of quality improvement (QI), patient safety (PS), and medical error reduction principles and protocols will characterize successful physicians.

Communication skills. Learning to excel in eliciting and sharing information and appropriately communicating necessary data with patients and family, with other caregivers, and with data systems, while respecting cultural sensitivity, eliciting patient preferences, and showing sincere empathy will be essential for the physician of the future.

Partnering skills. Tomorrow's clinicians will use individual and systems approaches to optimize care. Partnering in system design, implementation, and evaluation with patients, with family, with the community, and understanding community resources will foster more effective care, as well as improve population health through preventive services and lifestyle practices.

Advocacy skills. While physicians have traditionally seen and behaved themselves as patient advocates in a private sense, participation in legislative, regulatory, and other formal forms of advocacy have not been strengths of the medical profession. Skills in additional forms of advocacy for patients with other disciplines and in health care reform will grow.

Informatics skills. Much of the progress in health care reform in the future will depend on optimizing data management. Future physicians will play a leadership role in designing and implementing improved systems for getting and storing information, facilitating communication with colleagues, patients, and other data systems and optimizing resource allocation using that data.

Change management skills. This includes the ability to learn about, embrace, and lead change in the areas listed above, as well as others, including the use of social media, telemedicine, and new device and drug technological developments. Throughout the process of managing and facilitating necessary change, the skill of understanding one's limitations and a healthy dose of self-awareness and emotional intelligence will be required.

As a profession, physicians have been well respected for their flexibility. Every patient is different, and each clinical challenge is nuanced. In addressing lifelong learning, each physician will determine how to preserve the best of traditional values that should never change, while having the flexibility to lead needed change and improvement. As can be seen, continuous learning involves far more than accumulating new information or technical skills.

The concept of professionalism can serve as a foundation supporting lifelong learning. As defined by the Council of Medical Specialty Societies, professionalism entails: (1) altruism— putting the needs of the patient and public health ahead of personal interests; (2) voluntary self-regulation— educating, improving, and managing our patients' health care interests because it is the right thing to do, not because of externally imposed requirements; and (3) transparency—honestly and openly sharing what we know, being accountable to each individual patient and the public for our charge to reduce disease and suffering.

As you use the *Otolaryngology Lifelong Learning Manual*, recognize its place as a critical element in continuous learning, but commit to linking what you learn to implementing, measuring, and reporting outcomes to ensure that what we know is effectively being applied to improve the individual patient and population health.

David R. Nielsen, MD
Chief Executive Officer and Executive Vice President,
June 2002–January 2015
American Academy of Otolaryngology–Head and
Neck Surgery

Preface

Otolaryngology–head and neck surgery continues to evolve and advance at an outstanding rate. In order to keep pace with these changes, we all must remain current by engaging in ongoing personal and professional development strategies. For physicians with hectic schedules in an increasingly strained and demanding healthcare environment, lifelong learning remains one of our greatest challenges. The American Academy of Otolaryngology–Head and Neck Surgery Foundation (AAO-HNS/F) supports otolaryngologists throughout their careers by providing timely educational opportunities and resources designed to foster knowledge growth, skills advancement, and maintenance of competency in our field.

The aims of this third edition are no different from those of the first, published in 1998. The first edition's chief editor, Dr. Jonas Johnson, visionary in his understanding of continuous professional development, challenged otolaryngologists to keep abreast of the ongoing changes in our field. The *Maintenance Manual for Lifelong Learning* was intended to "address issues of practical importance for otolaryngologists in improving patient care."

In response to the recent advances in the field of otolaryngology-head and neck surgery, this manual contains substantial revision and additions to the content carried forward from the first edition. The format and contents have been thoroughly analyzed. The chapters have been restructured to cover topics by subspecialty area, while also including the business of medicine and clinical fundamentals. Our goal has been to provide an efficient and easy-to-read, comprehensive reference manual to meet the needs of the practicing surgeon, and simultaneously serve the needs of the maturing resident.

The publication of this manual would not have been possible without the collective efforts of numerous individuals: the original contributors who formed a remarkable blend of experts and provided us with a truly broad perspective on our specialty and the current contributors who are members of the AAO-HNS Education Committees and actively involved in the advancement of otolaryngology. This latter group enthusiastically embraced the enormous task of reviewing, revising, and updating the content. Each offered expertise and numerous suggestions, enhancing the value and quality for the resident and practitioner. Finally, a resounding appreciation goes to Audrey Shively, who devoted countless hours and tireless support to this project.

Sonya Malekzadeh, MD
AAO-HNS/F Coordinator for Education

Contributors

The Business of Medicine

Brendan C. Stack Jr., MD, FACS, FACE
Professor
Department of Otolaryngology–Head and Neck Surgery
University of Arkansas for Medical Sciences Thyroid Center
Little Rock, Arkansas

David M. Jakubowicz, MD, FACS
Chairman
Department of Otolaryngology
Bronx Lebanon Hospital Center
Bronx, New York

Michael E. McCormick, MD
Assistant Professor
Medical College of Wisconsin
Milwaukee, Wisconsin

John S. Rhee, MD, MPH
Professor and Chairman
Medical College of Wisconsin
Milwaukee, Wisconsin

Lawrence M. Simon, MD, FAAP
Pediatric and General Otolaryngology
Hebert Medical Group
Eunice, Louisiana

Michael E. Stadler, MD
Assistant Professor
Department of Otolaryngology and Communication
  Services
Medical College of Wisconsin
Milwaukee, Wisconsin

Richard W. Waguespack, MD, FACS
Clinical Professor
Department of Surgery
Division of Otolaryngology–Head and Neck Surgery
University of Alabama at Birmingham
Birmingham, Alabama

Clinical Fundamentals

Brendan C. Stack Jr., MD, FACS, FACE
Professor
Department of Otolaryngology–Head and Neck Surgery
University of Arkansas for Medical Sciences Thyroid Center
Little Rock, Arkansas

Karen T. Pitman, MD, FACS
Division of Surgical Oncology
Banner MD Anderson Cancer Center
Gilbert, Arizona

Scott E. Brietzke, MD, MPH
Associate Professor of Surgery
Department of Otolaryngology
Walter Reed National Military Medical Center
Bethesda, Maryland

Vasu Divi, MD, FACS
Assistant Professor
Department of Otolaryngology
Stanford University Medical Center
Stanford, California

Daniel J. Gallagher, MD, LTC, MC
Assistant Professor
Chief
Uniformed Services University of Health Sciences
Fort Belvoir Community Hospital
Fort Belvoir, Virginia

Eric M. Gessler, MD, FAAOA, Capt, MC
Assistant Professor of Clinical Otolaryngology
Uniformed Services
University of the Health Sciences
Eastern Virginia Medical School
Virginia Beach, Virginia

Ashutosh Kacker, MBBS, MS, MD, FACS
Professor of Clinical Otorhinolaryngology
Weill Cornell Medical Center
New York, New York

Esther Kim, MD, Maj, MC
Assistant Professor
Director of Rhinology/Anterior Skullbase Surgery
Department of Otolaryngology
Walter Reed National Military Medical Center
Uniformed Services University of the Health Sciences
Bethesda, Maryland

Philip E. Zapanta, MD, FACS
Assistant Professor of Surgery
Otolaryngology Residency Program Director
Division of Otolaryngology–Head and Neck Surgery
George Washington University School of Medicine
   and Health Sciences
Washington, DC

General Otolaryngology

Karen T. Pitman, MD, FACS
Division of Surgical Oncology
Banner MD Anderson Cancer Center
Gilbert, Arizona

James A. Burns, MD, FACS
Assistant Professor
Division of Laryngeal Surgery
Massachusetts General Hospital
Boston, Massachusetts

James I. Cohen, MD, PhD
Professor
Oregon Health and Science University
Portland, Oregon

Mehul J. Desai, MD, MPH
Director
Spine, Pain Medicine, and Research
Metro Orthopedics and Sports Therapy
Silver Spring, Maryland

Ashutosh Kacker, MBBS, MS, MD, FACS
Professor of Clinical Otorhinolaryngology
Weill Cornell Medical Center
New York, New York

Ian K. McLeod, MD, FACS, LTC(P), MC
Assistant Professor
Department of Surgery
Fort Belvoir Community Hospital
Uniformed Services University of the Health Sciences
Fort Belvoir, Virginia

Max D. Pusz, MD
Walter Reed National Military Medical Center
Bethesda, Maryland

Christopher H. Rassekh, MD, FACS
Associate Professor
Department of Otorhinolaryngology–Head and Neck
  Surgery
University of Pennsylvania
Philadelphia, Pennsylvania

Elie E. Rebeiz, MD, FACS
Professor and Chair
Tufts Medical Center
Boston, Massachusetts

P. Daniel Ward, MD, MS
Assistant Professor
University of Utah School of Medicine
Salt Lake City, Utah

Robert A. Weatherly, MD
Chief
Section of Otolaryngology
Children's Mercy Hospitals and Clinics
Associate Professor
University of Missouri–Kansas City School of
  Medicine
Kansas City, Missouri

Philip E. Zapanta, MD, FACS
Assistant Professor of Surgery
Otolaryngology Residency Program Director
Division of Otolaryngology–Head and Neck Surgery
George Washington University School of Medicine
  and Health Sciences
Washington, DC

Head and Neck Surgery

Richard V. Smith, MD, FACS
Professor and Vice-Chair
Department of Otorhinolaryngology–Head and Neck Surgery
Professor
Departments of Surgery and Pathology
Albert Einstein College of Medicine
Montefiore Medical Center
Program Director
Head and Neck Cancer
Montefiore-Einstein Center for Cancer Care
Bronx, New York

Neil N. Chheda, MD
Assistant Professor
University of Florida
Gainesville, Florida

Julie A. Goddard, MD
Assistant Professor
University of California–Irvine
Orange, California

Neil D. Gross, MD, FACS
Associate Professor
Director of Clinical Research
Head and Neck Surgery
MD Anderson Cancer Center
Houston, Texas

Stephen Y. Lai, MD, PhD, FACS
Associate Professor
Department of Head and Neck Surgery
University of Texas MD Anderson Cancer Center
Houston, Texas

Derrick T. Lin, MD, FACS
Associate Professor
Harvard Medical School
Boston, Massachusetts

Kelly Michele Malloy, MD, FACS
Assistant Professor
University of Michigan
Ann Arbor, Michigan

Matthew C. Miller, MD
Assistant Professor
University of Rochester Medical Center
Rochester, New York

Michael G. Moore, MD, FACS
Assistant Professor, Chief
Division of Head and Neck Surgery
Indiana University School of Medicine
Indianapolis, Indiana

Matthew O. Old, MD, FACS
Assistant Professor
The Ohio State University
Columbus, Ohio

Yash J. Patil, MD
Associate Professor
University of Cincinnati
Cincinnati, Ohio

Bradley A. Schiff, MD
Associate Professor
Montefiore Medical Center
Albert Einstein College of Medicine
Bronx, New York

Alfred A. Simental Jr., MD, FACS
Chair
Loma Linda University School of Medicine
Loma Linda, California

Rodney J. Taylor, MD, MSPH
Associate Professor, Director
University of Maryland School of Medicine
Baltimore, Maryland

John W. Werning, MD, DMD, FACS
Associate Professor
University of Florida
Gainesville, Florida

Jeffrey S. Wolf, MD, FACS
Associate Professor
Associate Chair of Clinical Practice
University of Maryland School of Medicine
Baltimore, Maryland

Laryngology and Bronchoesophagology

Catherine Rees Lintzenich, MD, FACS
Riverside ENT Physicians and Surgeons
Williamsburg, Virginia

James A. Burns, MD, FACS
Assistant Professor
Division of Laryngeal Surgery
Massachusetts General Hospital
Boston, Massachusetts

Neil N. Chheda, MD
Assistant Professor
University of Florida
Gainesville, Florida

C. Michael Haben, MD, MSc
Center for the Care of the Professional Voice
Haben Practice for Voice and Laryngeal Laser
   Surgery, PLLC
Rochester, New York

Priya D. Krishna, MD, MS, FACS
Assistant Professor and Director
Department of Otolaryngology
Loma Linda University
Loma Linda University Voice and Swallow Center
Loma Linda, California

Diego Preciado, MD, PhD
Associate Professor
Children's National Medical Center
Washington, DC

Otology and Neurotology

Bradley W. Kesser, MD
Associate Professor
University of Virginia Health System
Charlottesville, Virginia

Seilesh C. Babu, MD
Chief Financial Officer
Michigan Ear Institute
Assistant Professor
Department of Otolaryngology
Wayne State University
Detroit, Michigan

Marc L. Bennett, MD, FASC
Assistant Professor
Vanderbilt University School of Medicine
Nashville, Tennessee

Matthew L. Carlson, MD
Assistant Professor
Department of Otolaryngology
Mayo College of Medicine
Rochester, Minnesota

John C. Goddard, MD
Northwest Permanente
Clackamas, Oregon

Richard K. Gurgel, MD
Assistant Professor
University of Utah School of Medicine
Salt Lake City, Utah

David S. Haynes, MD, FACS
Professor, Vice Chair
Vanderbilt University Hospital
Nashville, Tennessee

David M. Kaylie, MD, FACS
Associate Professor, Director
Duke University Medical Center
Durham, North Carolina

Lawrence R. Lustig, MD
Professor
University of California–San Francisco
San Francisco, California

Alan G. Micco, MD
Associate Professor
Program Director
Chief of Otology/Neurotology
Northwestern University
Chicago, Illinois

Ahn Nguyen-Huynh, MD, PhD
Assistant Professor
Oregon Health and Science University
Portland, Oregon

Bradley Pickett, MD
Associate Professor
Department of Surgery
University of New Mexico School of Medicine
Albuquerque, New Mexico

Pediatric Otolaryngology

Kenny H. Chan, MD
Professor
Department of Otolaryngology
University of Colorado School of Medicine
Aurora, Colorado

Eunice Y. Chen, MD, PhD
Assistant Professor
Dartmouth-Hitchcock Medical Center
Children's Hospital at Dartmouth
Lebanon, New Hampshire

Stacey L. Ishman, MD, MPH
Associate Professor
Cincinnati Children's Hospital Medical Center
University of Cincinnati College of Medicine
Cincinnati, Ohio

Shelby C. Leuin, MD
Assistant Professor
University of California–San Diego
San Diego, California

Anna H. Messner, MD, FACS
Professor and Vice-Chair
Residency Program Director
Stanford University
Stanford, California

Diego Preciado, MD, PhD
Associate Professor
Children's National Medical Center
Washington, DC

Jeffrey C. Rastatter, MD, FACS, FAAP
Assistant Professor/Attending Physician
Northwestern University
Ann and Robert Lurie Children's Hospital
Chicago, Illinois

James E. Saunders, MD
Associate Professor
Dartmouth-Hitchcock Medical Center
Lebanon, New Hampshire

Rhinology and Allergy

Brent A. Senior, MD, FACS, FARS
Professor and Vice Chair
Department of Otolaryngology–Head and Neck Surgery
University of North Carolina Hospitals
Chapel Hill, North Carolina

Benjamin S. Bleier, MD
Assistant Professor
Massachusetts Eye and Ear Infirmary
Harvard Medical School
Boston, Massachusetts

Peter C. Bondy, MD, FACS
Attending Surgeon
Conway Medical Center
Conway, South Carolina

Ashutosh Kacker, MBBS, MS, MD, FACS
Professor of Clinical Otorhinolaryngology
Weill Cornell Medical Center
New York, New York

Devyani Lal, MD
Assistant Professor
Mayo Clinic College of Medicine
Consultant
Department of Otorhinolaryngology
Mayo Clinic
Phoenix, Arizona

Amber U. Luong, MD, PhD, FACS
Associate Professor and Director of Research
Department of Otorhinolaryngology–Head and Neck
    Surgery
Center of Immunology and Autoimmune Diseases at
    the Institute of Molecular Medicine
University of Texas Medical School
Houston, Texas

R. Peter Manes, MD, FACS
Assistant Professor
Yale University School of Medicine
New Haven, Connecticut

Maria T. Peña, MD, FACS, FAAP
Associate Professor
Children's National Medical Center
Washington, DC

Facial Plastic and Reconstructive Surgery

James Randall Jordan, MD, FACS
Professor and Vice-Chair
University of Mississippi Medical Center
Jackson, Mississippi

Fred G. Fedok, MD, FACS
Professor
Facial Plastic Surgery, Otolaryngology/Head and Neck Surgery
Department of Surgery
Hershey Medical Center
Pennsylvania State University
Hershey, Pennsylvania
The McCollough Plastic Surgery Clinic
Gulf Shores, Alabama
Adjunct Professor
Department of Surgery
University of South Alabama
Mobile, Alabama

Anthony E. Brissett, MD, FACS
Director of Facial, Plastic, and Reconstructive Surgery
Department of Otolaryngology
Baylor College of Medicine
Houston, Texas

C. W. David Chang, MD
Jerry W. Templer Associate Clinical Professor
University of Missouri
Columbia, Missouri

Robert W. Dolan, MD, MMM, FACS
Chairman
Department of Otolaryngology
Lahey Hospital and Medical Center
Burlington, Massachusetts

Harley S. Dresner, MD
Assistant Professor
Health Partners Clinic
St. Paul, Minnesota

Jill A. Foster, MD
Clinical Associate Professor
The Ohio State University
Columbus, Ohio

Jonathan R. Grant, MD, FACS
Surgeon
Cascade Medical Group
Mt. Vernon, Washington

W. Marshall Guy, MD
Baylor College of Medicine
Houston, Texas

Clinton D. Humphrey, MD, FACS
Assistant Professor
University of Kansas Medical Center
Kansas City, Kansas

Carlos J. Puig, DO, FAACS, ABHRS
Instructor
Baylor Facial Plastic Surgery Center
Houston, Texas

Jonathan M. Sykes, MD, FACS
Professor, Director
University of California–Davis Medical Center
Davis, California

Trauma

Joseph A. Brennan, MD, FACS, Colonel, MC, USAF
Chief
Department of Surgery
San Antonio Military Medical Center
San Antonio, Texas

Jose E. Barrera, MD, FACS
Associate Professor and Chair
San Antonio Uniformed Services Consortium and
  Joint Base
Department of Otolaryngology
Chief, Division of Facial Plastic and Reconstructive
  Surgery
San Antonio Military Medical Health System
San Antonio, Texas

Jeffrey A. Faulkner, MD, DDS
Chief
Division of Surgery
Landstuhl Regional Medical Center
Kaiserslautern, Germany

Mitchell Jay Ramsey, MD
Director
Department of Otology/Neurotology
Landstuhl Regional Medical Center
Kaiserslautern, Germany

Nathan L. Salinas, MD
Chief
Department of Otolaryngology
Bassett Army Community Hospital
Fort Wainwright, Alaska

Contributors, 2nd Edition

Peter A. Adamson, MD
Robert M. Arnold, MD
Jonathan E. Aviv, MD
Shan R. Baker, MD
Thomas J. Balkany, MD
Daniel G. Becker, MD
Michael S. Benninger, MD
William J. Binder, MD
Andrew Blitzer, MD
Michael Broniatowski, MD
Eugenie Brunner, MD
Brian Burkey, MD
Michael P. Cannito, PhD
C. Ron Cannon, MD
Roy R. Casiano, MD
John Casler, MD
Mack L. Cheney, MD
Richard A. Chole, MD
James M. Chow, MD
Gary L. Clayman, MD, DDS
Dean M. Clerico, MD
James I. Cohen, MD, PhD
Wayne B. Colin, DMD, MD
Marc D. Coltrera, MD
Jacquelynne P. Corey, MD
Robin T. Cotton, MD
William S. Crysdale, MD
Hugh D. Curtin, MD
Lianne de Serres, MD
James C. Denneny III, MD
Amelia F. Drake, MD
David W. Eisele, MD
Adel El-Naggar, MD
Joseph Eskridge, MD
Johannes J. Fagan, MD
Stephan A. Falk, MD
Joseph G. Febhali, MD
Fred G. Fedok, MD
John Fornadley, MD
Jill Foster, MD
Jeremy C. Freeman, MD

Marvin P. Fried, MD
Ellen M. Friedman, MD
Neal D. Futran, MD, DMD
Bruce J. Gantz, MD
Rebecca N. Gaughan, MD
Lyon L. Gleich, MD
Jack L. Gluckman, MD
George S. Goding Jr., MD
Joel A. Goebel, MD
Charles W. Gross, MD
Patrick J. Gullane, MD
Ehab Hanna, MD
Gady Har-El, MD
Robert A. Hillman, MD
Barry E. Hirsch, MD
Marcelo Hochman, MD
Lauren D. Holinger, MD
G. Richard Holt, MD
David B. Hom, MD
Martin L. Hopp, MD
John W. House, MD
Gordon B. Hughes, MD
Darrell H. Hunsaker, MD
Andrew F. Inglish Jr, MD
Robert K. Jackler, MD
C. Gary Jackson, MD
Jonas T. Johnson, MD
Gary D. Josephson, MD
Charles A. Jungreis, MD
Haskins K. Kashima, MD
David Keith, BDS, DMD
George G. Kitchens, MD
Raymond J. Konior, MD
David E. Kraus, MD
Frederick A. Kuhn, MD
Paul R. Lambert, MD
Wayne F. Larrabee, MD
Lorenz F. Lassen, MD
Pierre Lavertu, MD
K. J. Lee, MD
Joseph E. Leonard, MD

Donald A. Leopold, MD
Paul A. Levine, MD
Denis P. Lynch, DDS, PhD
Corey S. Maas, MD
Robert H. Maisel, MD
Scott C. Manning, MD
Mark A. Marunick, DDS, MS
W. Frederick McGuirt, MD
Jesus E. Medina, MD
Richard T. Miyamoto, MD
Willard B. Moran Jr., MD
Brett Mullin, MD
Charles M. Myer III, MD
Eugene N. Myers, MD
James L. Netterville, MD
Lisa Newman, MD
David R. Nielsen, MD
Mark Ochs, MD
Robert H. Ossoff, DMD, MD
Ira D. Papel, MD
Norman J. Pastorek, MD
Dennis Patin, MD
Phillip K. Pellitteri, DO
Myles L. Pensak, MD
Stephen W. Perkins, MD
Jay F. Piccirillo, MD
Karen T. Pitman, MD
Michael Poole, MD, PhD
J. Christopher Post, MD
Gregory W. Randolph, MD
James S. Reilly, MD
Lou Reinisch, PhD
Gregory J. Renner, MD
Mark A. Richardson, MD
Russell Ries, MD
K. Thomas Robbins, MD
Peter S. Roland, MD
Steven D. Schaefer, MD
Gary L. Schechter, MD
Richard L. Scher, MD
Larry D. Schoenrock, MD
Mitchell K. Schwaber, MD
Vanessa Schweitzer, MD

Steven J. Scrivani, DDS
Robert W. Seibert, MD
Allen M. Seiden, MD
Michael Setzen, MD
Jo A. Shapiro, MD
Stanley M. Shapshay, MD
Clough Shelton, MD
Maisie L. Shindo, MD
William W. Shockley, MD
Thomas Shpitzer, MD
Kevin A. Shumrick, MD
Sol Silverman, MA, DDS
Aristides Sismanis, MD
Richard J. H. Smith, MD
Robert A. Sofferman, MD
Joon K. Song, MD
F. Thomas Sporck, MD
Scott Stringer, MD
Jonathan M. Sykes, MD
Thomas A. Tami, MD
M. Eugene Tardy Jr., MD
Dean M. Toriumi, MD
Katherine Verdolini, PhD, CCC-SLP
Richard W. Waguespack, MD
Regina P. Walker, MD
Randal S. Weber, MD
Gregory S. Weinstein, MD
Mark C. Weissler, MD
Ralph F. Wetmore, MD
Ernest A. Weymuller Jr., MD
J. Paul Willging, MD
Paul J. Wills, MD
Welby I. Winstead, MD
Gregory J. Wolf, MD
Peak Woo, MD
Rebecca Woods, CPC
Audie L. Woolley, MD
Robert Yellon, MD
Bevan Yueh, MD
Kathryn S. Yung, BA
Steven M. Zeitels, MD
S. James Zinreich, MD

I

The Business of Medicine

1 The Quality Landscape

■ Introduction

In the last few decades, otolaryngologists, along with other medical providers, have become increasingly cognizant of health care concepts, such as quality improvement, patient safety, meaningful use, value-based purchasing, best practices, and a multitude of other buzzwords and acronyms (**Tables 1.1** and **1.2**).

With changes in health care progressing at a rapid pace, these previously abstract ideas are now quickly becoming realities, necessitating clear understanding, swift adaptation, and incorporation into daily practices. Although much of the current health care legislation deals with increased access to care, the focus on quality and value is also being aggressively addressed. It is of paramount importance for the modern-day practitioner to be aware of the increased focus on these issues.

Created in 1970, the Institute of Medicine (IOM) of the National Academies has been committed to improving the quality of health care in the United States by providing unbiased and authoritative information regarding our nation's health care delivery system. The IOM defines *quality* as "the degree to which health services for individuals and populations increase the likelihood of desired health outcomes and are consistent with current professional knowledge." Other institutions, such as the Agency for Healthcare Research and Quality (AHRQ), describe quality care in broader terms, stating that it entails "doing the right thing, at the right time, in the right way, for the right person, and having the best possible results." Regardless of the precise definition, most practitioners would agree that providing quality medical care should represent treatment that is appropriate and efficient and allows for the best possible clinical outcomes, while also minimizing medical error and maximizing value through the limitation of unnecessary and wasteful care.

Avedis Donabedian, often thought of as one of the primary architects within the field of health care quality and clinical outcomes research, helped better define the approach to measuring and quantifying quality in health care. The "Donabedian Triad" divides quality measures into three main components: structure, process, and outcome:

- *Structure* refers to a health care system's characteristics, focusing on how a care system is organized.
- *Process* focuses on what providers within this health care system actively do and how they carry out these actions.
- *Outcome* describes what actually happens to the patient as the end result.

These three pillars form the basis of how health care quality is analyzed today. Yet measuring the quality of care through a combination of outcomes, processes, and structures can be a difficult task. Although outcomes are the end result of the care that physicians provide, most health care practitioners would agree that outcomes alone should not represent the sole metric used to evaluate, compare, and reward providers. The complexities involved in patient care outcomes must include appropriate quality measures that take into account both process and structure.

■ The Recent History of Quality Care

In 1996, the IOM's Committee on Quality of Health Care in America launched a concerted effort focused on assessing and improving the quality of health care in the United States. It aimed to close the gap between what was known to be good-quality health care and what actually existed in practice. The committee's first report, *To Err Is Human: Building a Safer Health System*, was released in 1999 and focused mainly on patient safety and its relationship to overall health care quality. This report used a wealth of data from the landmark Harvard Medical Practice Study, as

3

Table 1.1 Health care organizations, institutions, programs, and laws that deal with health care quality and safety (representative sample only)

ACA (PPACA)	The Patient Protection and Affordable Care Act (Affordable Care Act) of 2010—A federal statute that represents the largest regulatory overhaul of the U.S. health care system since the inception of Medicare and Medicaid and aims to increase affordability and accessibility of health care for all Americans
ACS–NSQIP	American College of Surgeons National Surgical Quality Improvement Program—A large, nationally validated, risk-adjusted, outcomes-based program to measure the quality of surgical care and promote quality improvement
AHRQ	Agency for Healthcare Research and Quality (formerly the Agency for Health Care Policy and Research)—A federal organization focused on health care quality improvement and patient safety and outcomes research. AHRQ is a division of the U.S. Department of Health and Human Services (DHHS).
CMS	Centers for Medicare and Medicaid Services—Established in 1965, CMS is a division of DHHS that is responsible for the administration of Medicare, Medicaid, and several other key health-related programs, such as the Health Insurance Portability and Accountability Act.
DHHS	U.S. Department of Health and Human Services—A cabinet of the U.S. government whose goal is to protect the health of all citizens and to ensure proper human services. DHHS consists of 12 agencies, including the AHRQ, CMS, U.S. Food and Drug Administration, and Centers for Disease Control and Prevention.
HQA	Hospital Quality Alliance—A public–private collaboration of various stakeholders that is committed to making meaningful and easily understood information about hospital performance accessible to the public. Hospital Compare, a Web-based tool for consumers, is one such project of the HQA.
IHI	Institute for Healthcare Improvement—An independent, nonprofit organization focused on health care improvement, education, and innovation
IOM	Institute of Medicine—A nonprofit, private organization that provides unbiased, evidence-based guidance to lawmakers, health care professionals and societies, and the American public on a variety of health- and science-related topics
JCO	Joint Commission Observer—Founded in 1951 with the aim to improve health care for the public, JCO is an independent, nonprofit standards-setting and accrediting body for health care organizations and programs. JCO has become a symbol of organizational quality and safety.
NQF	National Quality Forum—A nonprofit, nonpartisan, public service organization committed to the transformation of the U.S. health care system. NQF serves as a quality measure clearinghouse; it reviews, endorses, and recommends the use of various standardized health care performance measures.
PCPI	Physician Consortium for Performance Improvement—Convened by the American Medical Association, the PCPI is committed to the development, testing, and maintenance of evidence-based clinical performance measures and measurement resources for physicians.
QASC	Quality Alliance Steering Committee—A collaborative effort among existing quality alliances, providers, institutions, and accrediting agencies that work to improve the quality of health care. QASC works to ensure that quality measures are constructed and reported clearly and consistently to inform both consumer and practitioner decision making.
WHO	World Health Organization—A division of the United Nations responsible for providing leadership on global health matters. In 2007–2008, WHO demonstrated that surgical safety checklists can lower the incidence of surgery-related deaths and complications by one-third during major operations.

well as behavioral concepts and research related to human decision making, and latent conditions and errors. Although this report was by no means the beginning of the quality and patient safety movement in this country, it gained vast attention after it estimated that up to 98,000 people die each year due to medical errors. Furthermore, the report suggested that the majority of these errors resulted from a flawed health care system and medical culture, rather than individual careless or poorly trained providers. In our own field of otolaryngology–head and neck surgery (OHNS), it has been estimated that up

to 2,600 episodes of major morbidity and 165 deaths occur annually due to avoidable medical errors.

In a subsequent 2001 IOM report, *Crossing the Quality Chasm: A New Health System for the 21st Century*, six aims for health care system quality improvement were proposed: patient safety, timeliness, effectiveness, efficiency, equity, and patient-centeredness (**Table 1.3**). These six components were the framework for the report that called for an urgent and drastic change in the way health care was provided in the United States. Beyond the overarching concept of improved quality, the report

Table 1.2 Terms and acronyms commonly used in health care quality and safety (representative sample only)

ACO	Accountable Care Organization—endorsed by Centers for Medicare and Medicaid Services (CMS) and the Patient Protection and Affordable Care Act, ACOs are groups of providers and care delivery centers that voluntarily join together to give patients coordinated high-quality care with the goal of avoiding unnecessary duplication of services and preventing medical errors. Newly designed CMS reimbursement programs, such as the Medicare Shared Savings Program, are possible through ACOs.
CER	Comparative Effectiveness Research—Designed to inform health care decision making, CER aims to develop, expand, and use various data sources to provide evidence on the potential benefits and risks of various treatment options.
EBM	Evidence-Based Medicine—The conscientious use and application of current best evidence (based on relevant and valid research) when making decisions about individual patient care
EHR	Electronic Health Record—The systematic and unified collection of health information about patients and populations. An EHR is also known as an electronic medical record (EMR).
FFS	Fee-for-Service—The dominant physician payment method in the United States. Most FFS services are unbundled and paid for individually, and their cost is often related to the quantity of care, rather than the quality of care.
Lean	Lean—Coined in the late 1980s to describe Toyota's business and production model, this term has now been adopted in the health care industry to represent quality improvement and the concept of efficiency through maximizing patient/consumer value while minimizing waste.
MU	Meaningful Use—A set of standards from CMS pertaining to EHR use by providers and institutions, whereby incentives are provided for meeting specific criteria (e.g., electronic prescribing (eRx), maintaining an updated problem list for individual patients)
PCMH	Patient-Centered Medical Home—Also referred to as the primary care medical home, PCMHs represent a promising model for transforming the organization and delivery of primary care by focusing on comprehensive, patient-centered, coordinated, accessible, safe, and high-quality care.
P4P	Pay-for-Performance—An increasingly popular reimbursement model whereby providers and institutions are incentivized according to preestablished performance measures, with the goal of rewarding high-quality care. Performance targets are often tied to delivery of quality care, cost of care, and patient satisfaction scores.
Six Sigma	Six Sigma—Similar to lean principles, six sigma is a more statistical/data-driven philosophy of quality improvement that places a high value on defect prevention and limiting variation in processes.
VBP	Value-Based Purchasing—Similar to P4P, VBP is a method for reimbursement that aims to reward for the quality of delivered care through the use of transparency and incentives. Providers and institutions are held accountable for the quality and cost of care that is provided.

addressed the following issues: defined performance benchmarks, enhanced patient–clinician relationships, expanded information systems, revamped alignment for incentives, and increased accountability. A systems approach to closing the quality gap, or chasm, that was detailed in the report was proposed, further acknowledging the inherent complexities in executing this change.

These high-profile reports served as catalysts for the reevaluation of the current U.S. system of health care delivery, and have subsequently led to a refined and vigorous focus on quality as it relates to the medical system in which we work. Since their release, extensive efforts have been established to monitor, measure, and reward practices consistent with these six quality and patient safety aims. In examining these efforts, it is important for clinicians to recognize that quality care is not simply synonymous with the provision of evidence-based medicine, but also

includes much broader issues, such as timeliness, equity, and patient-centeredness. This broader, comprehensive, systems-based approach to the analysis of health care delivery is new to many, but will continue to be the basis for ongoing evaluation of this complex system.

Originally created as the Agency for Health Care Policy and Research in 1989, the renamed AHRQ now exists as one of 12 agencies within the U.S. Department of Health and Human Services (DHHS). AHRQ represents the health service arm of DHHS and complements the biomedical research mission of its better-known sister agency, the National Institutes of Health (NIH). The AHRQ mission focuses on quality improvement and patient safety research, as well as outcomes and comparative effectiveness research. Another AHRQ goal is to encourage research efforts tied to clinical practice, technology assessment, and health care delivery systems.

Table 1.3 Crossing the Quality Chasm: A New Health System for the 21st Century

Safe	Avoiding injuries to patients from the care that is intended to help them
Timely	Reducing waits and harmful delays for providers and patients
Effective	Providing services based on scientific knowledge to all who could benefit and refraining from providing services to those not likely to benefit
Efficient	Avoiding waste (equipment, supplies, ideas, and energy)
Equitable	Providing care that doesn't vary in quality due to personal characteristics (gender, ethnicity, location, socioeconomic status)
Patient-centered	Providing care that is respectful of and responsive to individual patient preferences, needs, and values

Data from National Research Council. Crossing the Quality Chasm: A New Health System for the 21st Century. Washington, DC: National Academies Press; 2001.

The increased focus on research related to outcomes, value, and quality is in line with the legislative, policy, and cultural shifts recently observed in the U.S. health care system. Over the last 2 decades, AHRQ has been leading the way in generating effective research strategies, meaningful knowledge, and useful tools required for long-term improvement to the U.S. health care system, with 80% of its budget dedicated to grants and contracts in these areas.

■ A Changing Health Care Landscape

With various stakeholders focusing on the delivery of quality care, policy makers have taken notice and enacted legislation that is closely tied to these issues. Legislative reform efforts have been ongoing over the last decade; the most prominent has been the 2010 Patient Protection and Affordable Care Act (PPACA). In the PPACA, quality measures are defined as a "standard for measuring the performance and improvement of population health or of health plans, providers, and other clinicians." It is clear that the PPACA focuses on the delivery of quality health care because two of the nine categories of the bill deal directly with quality care: "Quality, affordable health care for all Americans" and "Improving the quality and efficiency of health care."

A section of the PPACA is also devoted to the development, collection, and public reporting of quality measures, and multiple groups, such as the National Quality Forum (NQF) and the Centers for Medicare and Medicaid Services (CMS), are working toward these goals. The quality measures that are currently being used and developed must reflect a multitude of complex metrics, including patient outcomes, processes of care, efficiency, perceptions of care and patient satisfaction, costs, and value. It is imperative that health care providers play an active role in defining and guiding implementation of appropriate, meaningful quality metrics and performance measures that will be increasingly transparent to the general public.

The traditional fee-for-service (FFS) reimbursement model has been shown by many to be unsustainable in its current structure; health care spending is one of the fastest-growing components of our expanding national debt and is projected to soon represent over 20% of the U.S. gross domestic product. The basic FFS payment model links reimbursement to the quantity and volume of services provided, thus providing no financial incentive for necessary investments toward health care quality, efficiency, and value. Data have shown that "doing more" (interventions, diagnostics, etc.) does not necessarily lead to improved outcomes. Yet, FFS payment models are based on the premise that doing more leads to greater financial incentives for providers.

One strategy being used to counteract this phenomenon, and thus promote improved quality care for patients, is the Pay for Performance (P4P) reimbursement model. In this model, incentivized payments are tied to transparent performance measures closely aligned with the provision of quality patient care. The PPACA payment reform provisions, such as value-based purchasing (VBP), bundled payments, medical homes, meaningful use, and other various quality-based incentive programs, are just a few of the efforts tied to the P4P model.

In relation to cost, the concept of health care "value" is becoming more central to the discussion of health care quality. Most simply defined, value represents quality divided by cost, or the output achieved relative to the cost incurred. Providers of care are continually being encouraged to improve both the numerator (quality) and the denominator (cost) of the value equation. With the term *value* being mentioned in the PPACA a total of 214 times, a cost-conscious focus is now embedded into the fabric of our health care system and will continue to be a central focus of future health care delivery.

As part of the Medicare Improvements for Patients and Providers Act of 2008 and the PPACA of 2010, CMS has recently instituted numerous quality-reporting initiatives. The Electronic Health Record (EHR) Meaningful Use (MU), the Electronic Prescribing (eRx), and the Physician Quality Reporting System (PQRS) incentive programs are all part of the PPACA's increased focus on improved efficiency and quality care. Although many of these programs are currently incentive-based programs, most will eventually convert to penalty-based programs, cutting provider reimbursements up to 1 to 5% if certain measures are not met.

Nationwide quality improvement efforts are also focused on increased transparency and improved patient access to provider performance information. The CMS Physician Compare Website was developed in 2011, and the PPACA required physician data to be reported starting in 2013. Although very limited data are currently reported, increased breadth and volume of physician performance metrics will soon be made available to the general public. CMS is required to ensure that the data are statistically valid, reliable, risk adjusted, and physician reviewed. Multiple physician-advocacy groups are actively engaged in the ongoing development and expansion of the Physician Compare Website.

■ Otolaryngology–Head and Neck Surgery's Involvement and Efforts

Maintenance of Certification

Quality performance and patient outcome measures will also be used in the Maintenance of Certification (MOC) process, and there will likely be indirect financial consequences as a result. CMS and other payer entities may use participation in MOC programs as another quality measure of provider performance and tie this into physician reimbursement.

The American Board of Otolaryngology has instituted a four-part process for maintaining board certification for its members. The fourth part will consist of Performance Improvement Modules (PIMs). These PIMs will require physicians to submit data on a series of patients to an online database, and the data will then be compared with existing guidelines and quality/outcome measures. The physicians will then receive feedback on areas to improve their practice and will subsequently have the opportunity to submit data on new patients to demonstrate improvement. PIMs will typically need to be completed every 3 to 5 years.

Treatment Guidelines, Best Practices, and Clinical Consensus Statements

The IOM has identified guideline development as one of the three crucial tasks for a highly effective national health care system. In its simplest form, an effective clinical guideline is one that synthesizes the best evidence on a topic and generates recommendations whose aims are to promote best practice for the audience. The American Head and Neck Society created the Quality of Care Committee in 2007, and the group has systematically reviewed the literature to develop treatment guidelines and quality measures for laryngeal and oral cancers. Since 2006, the American Academy of Otolaryngology–Head and Neck Surgery (AAO-HNS) has published nine guidelines and has collaborated on other guidelines published through other medical societies as well. In 2013, Rosenfeld et al published a revised manual to help convey the importance behind effective clinical guideline development, stating that "a well-crafted guideline promotes quality by reducing health care variations, improving diagnostic accuracy, promoting effective therapy, and discouraging ineffective—or potentially harmful—interventions."

Similar to treatment guidelines, "best practices" represent recommendations to practitioners to address the value of diagnostic and therapeutic interventions for various disease processes. The evaluation of potential benefits, risks, and value of interventions is usually addressed through the synthesis of best available evidence and is provided in a succinct "usable" format for clinicians.

Clinical consensus statements serve a similar purpose as practice guidelines, but they have several key differences. While still promoting quality practice, they typically have a narrower scope and often have a limited quality of evidence available for analysis and incorporation. Clinical consensus statements are products of organized expert opinions and evaluation of best evidence that are reviewed and refined in a standardized manner to converge on the "best" recommendations. In OHNS, clinical consensus statements exist on such topics as tracheostomy care, computed tomography for paranasal sinus disease, and diagnosis and management of nasal valve compromise. These tools represent necessary steps in the process of translating best evidence into best practices, as well as performance measurement and assessment (**Fig. 1.1**).

Quality Measures, Checklists, and Clinical Care Pathways

It was not until 2010 that the first report of a quality of care project in a primarily surgical patient group was published in the OHNS literature. The project

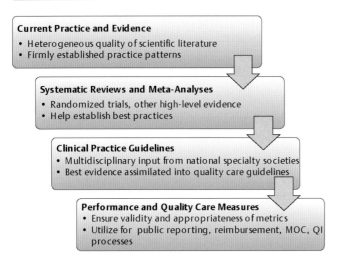

Fig. 1.1 Processes for translating evidence into practice and performance measurement.

Table 1.4 The AAO–HNS Choosing Wisely list

Don't order computed tomography (CT) scan of the head/brain for sudden hearing loss.
Don't prescribe oral antibiotics for uncomplicated acute tympanostomy tube otorrhea.
Don't prescribe oral antibiotics for uncomplicated acute otitis externa.
Don't routinely obtain radiographic imaging for patients who meet diagnostic criteria for uncomplicated acute rhinosinusitis.
Don't obtain computed tomography (CT) or magnetic resonance imaging (MRI) in patients with a primary complaint of hoarseness prior to examining the larynx.

involved patients with early-stage oral tongue cancer and had the objective of identifying measurable quality metrics for assessing how well cancer care adhered to accepted treatment guidelines. In a subsequent study, the same institution aimed to create a method for assessing surgeon performance and care outcomes that were risk-adjusted for procedure acuity and patient comorbidity. These progressive efforts have helped lay the foundation for other institutions to participate in self-assessment and analysis, and will certainly help identify and interpret meaningful quality measurements for OHNS in the future.

Checklists are increasingly used as quality tools in the health care setting to reduce variability, decrease human error, and improve patient outcomes. In a multinational study at eight hospitals in diverse economic settings, the use of the World Health Organization's Surgical Safety Checklist reduced major perioperative complications by 36% and mortality by 47%. In OHNS, multi-institutional application of an endoscopic sinus surgery safety and quality checklist was performed and was found to have standardized disparate practices and significantly increased the likelihood that individual safety tasks were performed during surgery.

A clinical care pathway is another quality care tool used to help streamline the sequence of perioperative care of patients. Aimed at reducing variation and, therefore, minimizing chances for adverse events, clinical care pathways have found their place in quality improvement processes. In OHNS, these pathways have been found to improve intraoperative work flow through the reduction of anesthesia and operative time, hospital costs, and length of stay in certain complex procedures.

Choosing Wisely Campaign

Initially conceived by the National Physicians Alliance, the Choosing Wisely Campaign has to date yielded lists of "Five Things Physicians and Patients Should Question" from more than 25 medical and surgical societies, including the AAO–HNS. The goals of this campaign have been to promote awareness and conversation about proper use of certain tests, procedures, and other treatments in an effort to promote overall improved quality of care. The items in each list are not necessarily intended to be used as a metric or to determine coverage by health plan carriers. The final items on the list from the AAO–HNS were determined by reviewing candidate items and by assessing the clinical evidence as well as the frequency of use of each test, procedure, or treatment (**Table 1.4**).

■ Conclusion

As health care continues to rapidly evolve in the 21st century, many established practices and systems of care have become stagnant and antiquated. New legislation has made the provision of high-value, high-quality health care a clear priority for the U.S. health care system. Innovative programs are being developed to help ensure effective processes are implemented into the evolving U.S. health care delivery system that both improve patient care and contain cost. The rapid changes that are ongoing can be overwhelming for everyday practitioners, yet it is imperative that we remain well informed about and receptive to this dynamic process. Providers and institutions will be required to continue to adapt at a rapid pace, so that ongoing quality improvement efforts can become firmly established within quality patient care.

■ Suggested Reading

Albright HW, Moreno M, Feeley TW, et al. The implications of the 2010 Patient Protection and Affordable Care Act and the Health Care and Education Reconciliation Act on cancer care delivery. Cancer 2011;117(8):1564–1574

American Academy of Otolaryngology—Head and Neck Surgery Foundation. Clinical Consensus Statement Manual. http://www.entnet.org/Practice/upload/Clinical-Consensus-Statement_June08-2.pdf. Accessed May 28, 2013

America COQOHCI, Institute of Medicine. To Err Is Human: Building a Safer Health System. Washington, DC: National Academies Press; 2000

America COQOHCI, Institute of Medicine. Crossing the Quality Chasm. Washington, DC: National Academies Press; 2001

Baugh RF, Archer SM, Mitchell RB, et al; American Academy of Otolaryngology-Head and Neck Surgery Foundation. Clinical practice guideline: tonsillectomy in children. Otolaryngol Head Neck Surg 2011;144(1, Suppl):S1–S30

Bhattacharyya N, Baugh RF, Orvidas L, et al; American Academy of Otolaryngology-Head and Neck Surgery Foundation. Clinical practice guideline: benign paroxysmal positional vertigo. Otolaryngol Head Neck Surg 2008;139(5, Suppl 4):S47–S81

Borchard A, Schwappach DLB, Barbir A, Bezzola P. A systematic review of the effectiveness, compliance, and critical factors for implementation of safety checklists in surgery. Ann Surg 2012;256(6):925–933

Brennan TA, Leape LL, Laird NM, et al; Harvard Medical Practice Study I. Incidence of adverse events and negligence in hospitalized patients: results of the Harvard Medical Practice Study I. 1991. Qual Saf Health Care 2004;13(2):145–151, discussion 151–152

Chalian AA, Kagan SH, Goldberg AN, et al. Design and impact of intraoperative pathways for head and neck resection and reconstruction. Arch Otolaryngol Head Neck Surg 2002;128(8):892–896

Chen AY. Quality initiatives in head and neck cancer. Curr Oncol Rep 2010;12(2):109–114

Cylus J, Anderson GF. Multinational Comparisons of Health Systems Data 2006. New York, NY: The Commonwealth Fund; 2007

Donabedian A. The quality of care. How can it be assessed? JAMA 1988;260(12):1743–1748

Gornick M, Lubitz J, Riley G. U.S. initiatives and approaches for outcomes and effectiveness research. Health Policy 1991;17(3):209–225

Haynes AB, Weiser TG, Berry WR, et al; Safe Surgery Saves Lives Study Group. A surgical safety checklist to reduce morbidity and mortality in a global population. N Engl J Med 2009;360(5):491–499

Hessel AC, Moreno MA, Hanna EY, et al. Compliance with quality assurance measures in patients treated for early oral tongue cancer. Cancer 2010;116(14):3408–3416

Hewitt ME, Simone JV; National Cancer Policy Board (U.S.). Ensuring Quality Cancer Care. Washington, DC: National Academies Press; 1999

Hilger PA, Weber RS. American Board of Otolaryngology (ABOto) Maintenance of Certification (MOC) Newsletter. 2012. http://www.aboto.org/pub/ABOto%20MOC%20Newsletter%202012.pdf. Accessed May 20, 2013

Mitchell RB, Hussey HM, Setzen G, et al. Clinical consensus statement: tracheostomy care. Otolaryngol Head Neck Surg 2013;148(1):6–20

Porter ME. What is value in health care? N Engl J Med 2010;363(26):2477–2481

Reason J. Understanding adverse events: human factors. Qual Health Care 1995;4(2):80–89

Rhee JS, Weaver EM, Park SS, et al. Clinical consensus statement: diagnosis and management of nasal valve compromise. Otolaryngol Head Neck Surg 2010;143(1):48–59

Robertson PJ, Brereton JM, Roberson DW, Shah RK, Nielsen DR. Choosing wisely: our list. Otolaryngol Head Neck Surg 2013;148(4):534–536

Roland PS, Rosenfeld RM, Brooks LJ, et al; American Academy of Otolaryngology—Head and Neck Surgery Foundation. Clinical practice guideline: Polysomnography for sleep-disordered breathing prior to tonsillectomy in children. Otolaryngol Head Neck Surg 2011;145(1, Suppl):S1–S15

Roland PS, Smith TL, Schwartz SR, et al. Clinical practice guideline: cerumen impaction. Otolaryngol Head Neck Surg 2008;139(3, Suppl 2):S1–S21

Rosenfeld RM, Andes D, Bhattacharyya N, et al. Clinical practice guideline: adult sinusitis. Otolaryngol Head Neck Surg 2007;137(3, Suppl):S1–S31

Rosenfeld RM, Brown L, Cannon CR, et al; American Academy of Otolaryngology—Head and Neck Surgery Foundation. Clinical practice guideline: acute otitis externa. Otolaryngol Head Neck Surg 2006;134(4, Suppl):S4–S23

Rosenfeld RM, Shiffman RN, Robertson P. Clinical practice guideline development manual, third edition: a quality-driven approach for translating evidence into action. Otolaryngol Head Neck Surg 2012;148(1 Suppl):S1–S55

Schwartz SR, Cohen SM, Dailey SH, et al. Clinical practice guideline: hoarseness (dysphonia). Otolaryngol Head Neck Surg 2009;141(3, Suppl 2):S1–S31

Setzen G, Ferguson BJ, Han JK, et al. Clinical consensus statement: appropriate use of computed tomography for paranasal sinus disease. Otolaryngol Head Neck Surg 2012;147(5):808–816

Shah RK, Kentala E, Healy GB, Roberson DW. Classification and consequences of errors in otolaryngology. Laryngoscope 2004;114(8):1322–1335

Soler ZM, Poetker DA, Rudmik L, et al. Multi-institutional evaluation of a sinus surgery checklist. Laryngoscope 2012;122(10):2132–2136

Stachler RJ, Chandrasekhar SS, Archer SM, et al; American Academy of Otolaryngology-Head and Neck Surgery. Clinical practice guideline: sudden hearing loss. Otolaryngol Head Neck Surg 2012;146(3, Suppl):S1–S35

The Laryngoscope. Author Guidelines. http://onlinelibrarywiley.com/journal/101002/%28ISSN%291531-4995/homepage/ForAuthorshtml

U.S. Department of Health & Human Services, Agency for Healthcare Research and Quality. About Us. September 2012. http://www.ahrq.gov/about/index.html

U.S. Department of Health & Human Services, Agency for Healthcare Research and Quality. Your Guide to Choosing Quality Health Care. Memphis, TN: Books LLC, Reference Series; 2011

Weber RS, Lewis CM, Eastman SD, et al. Quality and performance indicators in an academic department of head and neck surgery. Arch Otolaryngol Head Neck Surg 2010;136(12):1212–1218

2 Health Policy

■ Introduction

Health policy encompasses a wide range of issues that affect the daily practice and business of medicine. Most commonly, *health policy* refers to the study and analysis of rules and regulations from the federal government and private insurers who regulate policies, guidelines, and reimbursement for medical services and procedures. This chapter discusses the role of health policy regulation, who is responsible for developing and implementing specific health policy regulations and initiatives, and the basics of payment policy.

■ Role of Health Policy Regulation

Health care is a highly regulated industry in the United States. Numerous congressional committees and federal agencies hold jurisdiction over different parts of the industry, both public and private. Everything from insurance coverage, to the quality of health care administered by health professionals, to their scope of practice is regulated in some fashion by federal and state governments. Therefore, it is important to understand not only the role that regulatory bodies play in health care but also how regulations are developed. In many cases, before federal and state agencies can issue regulations designed to govern the practice and business of medicine, federal or state congressional committees must draft legislation that becomes health policy once passed and enacted into law.

From Legislation to Regulation

At a federal and state level, multiple congressional committees hold jurisdiction over specific portions of the health care industry, ranging from Medicare and Medicaid to insurance regulations and health-specific taxes. These committees often hold hearings and draft legislation that has a direct effect on the practice of medicine in the United States. For draft legislation (a "bill") to become law at the federal level, both the U.S. House of Representatives and the U.S. Senate must approve it. Once passed, the bill is sent to the president to be signed. This is the political process most often seen covered in the news. However, once a bill has been passed and becomes law, the process for developing health policy regulation has just begun.

Federal Administrative Agencies

Laws passed by Congress are sent to federal administrative agencies to undergo a process called rulemaking. In the rulemaking process, experts from different federal agencies turn the legal language of a law into regulations and policies designed to implement the legislative intent of the law in a practical manner that can be clearly understood by the public.

Numerous federal agencies are tasked with implementing federal laws relating to health care. The U.S. Department of Health and Human Services (HHS) is the principal department charged with health administration. HHS includes several agencies, such as the Centers for Medicare and Medicaid Services (CMS), the U.S. Food and Drug Administration (FDA), the Agency for Healthcare Research and Quality (AHRQ), the Health Resources and Services Administration (HRSA), and the Centers for Disease Control and Prevention (CDC). These agencies issue regulations to carry out the requirements of enacted laws. If a law charges an agency with the implementation of a regulation, the agency has broad administrative authority to interpret the regulation and developing specific guidelines for its implementation.

The rulemaking process can take months, or even years. Many regulations undergo a proposed rulemaking phase and a final rule, both of which allow the general public and interested stakeholders to comment on proposed and final regulations. This public comment period allows input that can affect final regulation and rulemaking. Once this process has been finalized, agencies begin the implementation process.

■ Implementation of Health Policy Legislation

In the last few years, HHS and its agencies have been implementing several landmark pieces of health care legislation. These include the Patient Protection and Affordable Care Act (PPACA) and the Health Information Technology for Economic and Clinical Health (HITECH) Act. The scope of these laws has had a broad impact on both the business and the practice of medicine, including the implementation of extensive insurance reforms under PPACA, the creation and funding for delivery system reforms, and the enactment of incentive and penalty programs for the adoption of health information technology systems under the HITECH Act.

The Patient Protection and Affordable Care Act

Enacted in 2010, PPACA is the most extensive piece of health legislation passed since the creation of Medicare in the 1960s. The scope of the legislation ranges from extensive insurance reforms and regulations, designed to drastically decrease the number of uninsured individuals, to the expansion of Medicaid and the creation of many new delivery systems intended to decrease the rising cost of health care and increase the quality of services provided.

Insurance Coverage Reforms

PPACA provides for extensive insurance reforms, including the removal of lifetime limits on insurance coverage, the ability for dependents to stay on their parents' insurance plans until age 26, and the elimination of denial of coverage by insurers based on preexisting conditions. Along with these reforms, PPACA created state-based insurance exchanges that had to be operational by 2014 and required states to have minimal insurance coverage by 2014 or pay a penalty. Along with insurance reforms, PPACA expanded Medicaid and Children's Health Insurance Plan (CHIP) eligibility. The combined effect of the insurance reforms and increased Medicaid and CHIP eligibility is an expected decrease in the number of uninsured Americans starting in 2014.

Delivery System Reform

To address the rapidly rising cost of health care, PPACA also implemented several delivery system reforms. The Medicare Shared Savings Program, also known as accountable care organizations, was created to allow physicians to earn incentive pay-

ments from Medicare for achieving a minimum level of savings and quality. PPACA also created a 5-year bundled payment program, starting January 1, 2013, that provides a single payment for bundled services during hospital stays.

Another program created by PPACA, slated for implementation for all physicians by 2017, was the Hospital Value-Based Purchasing (VBP) Program, which requires CMS to create a value-based payment modifier (which is an incentive payment or penalty) for specific physicians and groups of physicians, based on their reporting of quality and cost metrics as compared with other physicians.

These are only a few of the programs designed to help slow the growth of health costs by working to gradually shift Medicare, and health care generally, from a fee-for-service system that pays per service provided, to a more quality-based, episode-of-care reimbursement system.

Other Provisions

PPACA also created, and provided funding for, several other programs, including the Patient Centered Outcomes Research Institute, which is designed to compare the health outcomes and clinical effectiveness, risks, and benefits of two or more medical treatments, services, or items; and the Independent Payment Advisory Board, which is charged with developing proposals, starting in 2014, to reduce Medicare spending by targeted amounts. Other provisions in PPACA included a bonus payment for primary care physicians and a redistribution of Medicare graduate medical education residency slots.

American Recovery and Reinvestment Act and Health Information Technology for Economic and Clinical Health Act

Another important piece of legislation that has had an impact on health policy regulations was the American Recovery and Reinvestment Act of 2009 (ARRA), which contained the HITECH Act. This legislation created incentive programs designed to spur the development of, and investments in, electronic health records (EHRs) by physicians and hospitals. The EHR Incentive Program is designed to encourage providers and hospitals to adopt EHRs and demonstrate "meaningful use" through the reporting of specific core and quality measures with incentive payments and payment penalties. The program uses a staged approach to gradually increase the number of measures participants must report using their EHR system. Along with the increased measures, incentive payments are reduced over time, while penalties for participants who fail to meet "meaningful use" criteria will increase.

Other Recent Key Health Policy Legislation

Several other programs are having a profound impact on the business and practice of medicine, including the Physician Quality Reporting System (PQRS), formerly known as the Physician Quality Reporting Initiative and created by the Tax Relief and Health Care Act in 2006; and the Electronic Prescribing (eRx) Incentive Program, created by the Medicare Improvements for Patients and Providers Act.

PQRS is a program that uses incentive payments and payment penalties to require eligible professionals (EPs), including physicians, nurse practitioners, and physician assistants, to report key quality measures to CMS through several reporting mechanisms, including registries, claims forms, and EHRs. The eRx Incentive Program uses a combination of incentive payments and payment penalties to encourage EPs to electronically write prescriptions.

Many of the initiatives implemented since 2006 are designed to gradually shift the health care system to one based on quality and preventative care, rather than the traditional fee-for-service model that Medicare has relied on since its inception. CMS is currently linking many of these quality initiatives, such as the EHR Incentive Program, PQRS, eRx Incentive Program, and the VBP modifier, in hopes of increasing participation, the quality of health care, and reducing costs.

◾ Payment Policy

One of the most important aspects of health policy is to understand regulations issued by the government and private payers. According to CMS, the federal government financed 29% of total health spending in 2010, whereas private businesses financed 21%. This section explains the basics of how payment policy is developed for many public and private payers.

Medicare/Medicaid

Medicare is the federal program that provides health care insurance to individuals over 65 and to some disabled individuals, meeting certain criteria, under the age of 65. Medicare is divided into four parts:

- Part A: includes inpatient hospital, hospice, nursing home, and home health services
- Part B: includes physician services, laboratory and diagnostic tests, durable medical equipment, and hospital outpatient services
- Part C: includes Medicare benefits received through a managed care plan
- Part D: includes prescription drugs

The Medicare Physician Fee Schedule (MPFS) is published annually by CMS. It dictates payment for physician services with a formula consisting of the sum of the three components (physician work, practice expense, and malpractice expense), an adjustment for geographic location, and multiplication by a conversion factor. As mentioned previously, the MPFS goes through the annual rulemaking process with time for comments from the public and is finalized in November of the calendar year before it is enacted.

Medicare provides physicians three options for participation in Medicare: participating, nonparticipating, and private contracting. Participating physicians receive 100% of the Medicare reimbursement rate, while nonparticipating providers only receive 95% if they choose to accept assignment of Medicare claims. A private contract is an agreement between a Medicare beneficiary and a nonparticipating physician, in which the beneficiary agrees to pay fully out-of-pocket for a Medicare-covered service; in this case, a physician cannot bill Medicare for 2 years after opting out of the program.

Medicaid is a jointly funded federal and state program that provides coverage to low-income individuals and children. Unlike Medicare, Medicaid payment rates can be established by states within federal requirements. Providers who accept Medicaid patients are paid on a monthly capitation payment rate. Payment rates for participating providers are often updated based on specific trending factors, such as the Medicare Economic Index or a Medicaid-specific trend factor that uses a state-determined inflation adjustment rate.

Hospital Outpatient Prospective Payment System (HOPPS) and Ambulatory Surgical Centers (ASCs)

Hospital Outpatient Prospective Payment System (HOPPS) payments cover facility resources, including equipment, supplies, and hospital staff, but do not pay for the services of physicians and nonphysician practitioners, who are paid separately under the MPFS. All services under the HOPPS are technical and are classified into groups called Ambulatory Payment Classifications (APCs). A payment rate is established for each APC using 2-year-old hospital claims data adjusted by individual hospitals' cost-to-charge ratios. APC national payment rates are adjusted for geographic cost differences, and payment rates and policies are updated annually through the rulemaking process.

Payments for covered surgical procedures and ancillary services in an ambulatory surgical center

(ASC) setting are also updated through the rulemaking process. CMS performs an annual review of the legislative history and regulatory policies regarding changes to the lists of codes and payment rates in an ASC. CMS reviews the ASC payment system to implement applicable statutory requirements and changes arising from continuing experience with this system and annually proposes relative payment weights and payment amounts for services furnished in ASCs.

Inpatient Prospective Payment System (IPPS)

Medicare uses the Inpatient Prospective Payment System (IPPS) to establish payment rates for the inpatient care of beneficiaries. Through the annual rulemaking process, CMS establishes payment rates for different diagnosis-related groups, which cover all associated costs for inpatient care. Payment rates are updated annually to reflect changes in the markets, including technological advances and hospital costs.

Medicare Administrative Contractors (MACs)

The administration of Medicare, including claims processing, provider and beneficiary services, appeals, and audits, is contracted out to Medicare Administrative Contractors (MACs). Each MAC is responsible for a specific jurisdiction throughout the country and handles the local responsibilities for the administration of all Medicare services. Although CMS provides national guidance through transmittals, policy manuals, and National Coverage Determinations, the majority of all Medicare functions are handled through the MACs' own local coverage policies.

Carrier Advisory Committees (CACs)

Every MAC is required to have a Contractor Medical Director (CMD) to aid in the development of local medical policies. Along with these medical directors, MACs also have Carrier Advisory Committees (CACs) composed of physicians from different specialties, beneficiary representatives, and representatives of other medical organizations. These CACs advise the CMD and MACs on the development of local coverage policies and allow physicians to work with MACs on key policy issues.

National Coverage Determinations (NCDs) and Local Coverage Determinations (LCDs)

Medicare uses the standard of "reasonable and necessary" to determine coverage for medical services. Medicare coverage for different services is dictated through national and local coverage determinations. CMS issues a limited number of National Coverage Determinations (NCDs) that dictate coverage to all MACs for a specific service. If no NCD exists, MACs are allowed to issue Local Coverage Determinations (LCDs), which dictate coverage for that specific jurisdiction only. These LCDs are developed by the CMDs with the help of CACs and are regularly reviewed.

Private Payer Policy and Insurance Coverage

Private insurance coverage and plans (also commonly referred to as private payers or third-party payers) can have large degrees of variation among their coverage policies. There are services required by PPACA, such as access to free annual preventive services. However, private insurers are not required to provide coverage for most services, or to follow Medicare coverage policies, although many do. Private insurers also have a wide degree of variation regarding their requirements for documentation, billing, and appeals.

Individual private insurers often follow a coverage policy development process that involves a task force, team, or office led by a CMD. The task force reviews available literature and existing policies and works with medical specialty societies to develop coverage policies. These policies list what services are covered, how medical necessity is defined, and what the documentation requirements are for those services. Because this process can vary from insurer to insurer, there can often be differences in these policies among private payers.

Under the Health Insurance Portability and Accountability Act of 1996 (HIPAA), private insurers, along with Medicare, are required to use the same national code set (Current Procedural Terminology Category I, II, III or Health Care Financing Administration Common Procedural Coding System Level II codes) to ensure some level of continuity for reporting and billing medical services among all payers. HIPAA also regulates the protection of personal and confidential patient information, including patients' medical history and all personal information. The HIPAA privacy requirements regulate the communication of this confidential health and personal information and its disposal.

■ Suggested Reading

The Henry J. Kaiser Family Foundation. Summary of New Health Reform Law [Patient Protection and Affordable Care Act]. http://www.kff.org/healthreform/upload/8061.pdf

U.S. Department of Health and Human Services. Centers for Medicare & Medicaid Services. Acute Care Hospital Inpatient Prospective Payment System. Payment System Fact Sheet Series. http://www.cms.gov/Outreach-and-Education/Medicare-Learning-Network-MLN/MLNProducts/downloads/AcutePaymtSysfctsht.pdf

U.S. Department of Health and Human Services. Centers for Medicare & Medicaid Services. CMS National Health Expenditures 2010 Highlights. http://www.cms.gov/Research-Statistics-Data-and-Systems/Statistics-Trends-and-Reports/NationalHealth ExpendData/Downloads/highlights.pdf.

U.S. Department of Health and Human Services. Centers for Medicare & Medicaid Services. EHR Incentive Programs. http://www.cms.gov/Regulations-and-Guidance/Legislation/EHRIncentive Programs/index.html?redirect=/ehrincentiveprograms/

U.S. Department of Health and Human Services. Centers for Medicare & Medicaid Services. Electronic Prescribing (eRx) Incentive Program. http://www.cms.gov/Medicare/Quality-Initiatives-Patient-Assessment-Instruments/ERxIncentive/index.html?redirect=/erxincentive

U.S. Department of Health and Human Services. The Health Insurance Portability and Accountability Act of 1996 (HIPAA) Privacy and Security Rules. http://www.hhs.gov/ocr/privacy/

U.S. Department of Health and Human Services. Centers for Medicare & Medicaid Services. Hospital Outpatient PPS (Prospective Payment System). http://www.cms.gov/Medicare/Medicare-Fee-for-Service-Payment/HospitalOutpatientPPS/index.html?redirect=/HospitalOutpatientPPS/

U.S. Department of Health and Human Services. Centers for Medicare & Medicaid Services. Part A/Part B Medicare Administrative Contractor. http://www.cms.gov/Medicare/Medicare-Contracting/MedicareContractingReform/PartAandPartBMedicare AdministrativeContractor.html

U.S. Department of Health and Human Services. Centers for Medicare & Medicaid Services. Physician Fee Schedule. http://www.cms.gov/Medicare/Medicare-Fee-for-Service-Payment/PhysicianFeeSched/index.html?redirect=/PhysicianFeeSched/

U.S. Department of Health and Human Services. Centers for Medicare & Medicaid Services. Physician Quality Reporting System. http://www.cms.gov/Medicare/Quality-Initiatives-Patient-Assessment-Instruments/PQRS/index.html?redirect=/pqrs

3 Coding and Reimbursement

■ Introduction

Establishing diagnostic and Current Procedural Terminology (CPT) codes, and allocating a value to a given physician service is a complex process. For diagnoses, the end point is the creation of an International Classification of Disease (ICD-9 or ICD-10) code. Codes for procedures and physician work begin with the creation of a CPT code and then proceed to the assignment of Relative Value Units (RVUs), which determine payment. This chapter has the following objectives:

- Define the key regulatory terms of coding and reimbursement
- Outline the system used for creating codes and RVUs

International Classification of Disease, Ninth Revision

The ICD system was first devised by the World Health Organization in 1900 to aid in the statistical reporting of mortality. The current iteration used in the United States is the 9th edition, or ICD-9. These are four- or five-digit numerical codes used to specify a certain disease entity or, in some instances, a procedure. There are ~ 17,000 codes in ICD-9. Familiarity with them is important, because all billable patient encounters, ordered tests, and medications must be associated with a diagnosis code as a criterion for reimbursement.

International Classification of Disease, Tenth Revision

The 10th edition of the codes (ICD-10) was finalized in 1992 and put into use in 1999 in Europe. The United States is mandated to switch to ICD-10 in 2015. ICD-10 codes are alphanumeric and far more specific than ICD-9 codes. Consequently, there are many more ICD-10 codes, totaling ~ 155,000 diagnostic and procedural codes.

Current Procedural Terminology Codes

CPT codes are a system of numerical identifiers used for reporting medical services and procedures. They represent the most widely used and accepted system for communicating with both public and private health insurance programs and are maintained and copyrighted by the American Medical Association (AMA).

When an individual wishes to generate a code for a new service, the request must pass through several evaluations before it comes to fruition. The first step involves submitting a request/proposal to either the AMA CPT Editorial Panel or the CPT/RVU Committee of the American Academy of Otolaryngology–Head and Neck Surgery (AAO-HNS). Many requests from industry are made directly to the CPT Editorial Panel. The CPT Editorial Panel will then post the proposals on the publicly available CPT Web site and invite impacted specialties to comment on the code change proposals. After allowing time for public comment, the CPT Editorial Panel will review the code change proposals during an in-person meeting. These meetings are convened three times per year, in the winter, spring, and fall. The CPT Editorial Panel makes the final determination on whether to issue a code, or allow proposed revisions to an existing code, requested by the code change proposal.

Most otolaryngologists will begin by submitting a code change request at the AAO-HNS level. In this case, the Academy's CPT/RVU Committee evaluates the proposal and determines whether to refer the request to the Physician Payment Policy Workgroup (3P) for review and final approval. If approved by 3P, a formal AAO-HNS code change proposal is submitted to the AMA CPT Editorial Panel.

The CPT Editorial Panel is authorized by the AMA Board of Trustees to revise, update, or modify CPT codes, descriptors, rules, and guidelines. The Panel is made up of 17 member physicians, 11 nominated by the National Medical Specialty Societies. One of the 11 is reserved for expertise in performance measurement. One physician is also nominated from each of the following: the Blue Cross/Blue Shield Association, Americas Health Insurance Plans, the Centers for Medicare and Medicaid Services (CMS), and the American Hospital Association. The remaining two seats are reserved for members of the CPT Health Care Professionals Advisory Committee (HCPAC). Once the CPT Editorial Panel assigns a code for a procedure or service, the code may be used for billing. However, the existence of a code does not guarantee payment.

Supporting the CPT Editorial Panel is a larger body of advisors, the CPT Advisory Committee. The members of this committee are primarily physicians nominated by the national medical specialty societies represented in the AMA House of Delegates. Currently, the Advisory Committee is limited to national medical specialty societies seated in the AMA House of Delegates and to the AMA HCPAC organizations. Additionally, the Performance Measures Advisory Group (PMAG), who represents various organizations concerned with performance measures, also provides expertise. The Academy currently holds a seat on the House of Delegates, and therefore, has a standing CPT Advisor and Alternate Advisor to represent our specialty at the annual CPT Editorial Panel meetings.

The Advisory Committee's primary objectives are to serve as a resource to the CPT Editorial Panel by giving advice on procedure coding and appropriate nomenclature as relevant to the member's specialty; provide documentation to staff and the CPT Editorial Panel regarding the medical appropriateness of various medical and surgical procedures under consideration for inclusion in CPT; suggest revisions to CPT; assist in the review and further development of relevant coding issues and in the preparation of technical education material and articles pertaining to CPT; and promote and educate its membership on the use and benefits of CPT.

■ Relative Value Units

The AMA first developed and published the CPT code set in 1966 in conjunction with the initiation of the Medicare program. During the early phases of Medicare, payment was based on a system of "customary, prevailing, and reasonable (CPR)" fees, typically referred to as "usual and customary." It was recognized that there was wide variation in the amount that Medicare paid for similar services due to this system. By the mid-1980s, physicians' dissatisfaction with CPR-based payment resulted in government overhaul of the system.

One of the key changes made was the landmark Harvard "Resource Based Relative Value System" (RBRVS) study. Initially, 12 specialties were involved in the study: anesthesia, family practice, general surgery, internal medicine, obstetrics and gynecology, ophthalmology, orthopedics, otolaryngology, pathology, radiology, thoracic and cardiovascular surgery, and urology. Later, allergy and immunology, dermatology, oral maxillofacial surgery, pediatrics, psychiatry, and rheumatology joined the study.

The intent of the Harvard study was to scale all services and procedures relative to each other. As a standard, the repair of an inguinal hernia was rated at 100. All other services and procedures were then assigned "relative values" according to their work in comparison to this standard (inguinal hernia). As such, in the RBRVS system, payments are determined by the "resource cost" of a particular service. This cost is derived from three components: physician work, practice expense, and professional liability insurance. Payments are calculated by multiplying the combined cost of the service by a conversion factor—a monetary amount that is determined annually by CMS based on fluctuations in the Medicare Sustainable Growth Rate. Adjustments are also made for geographical differences in resource costs.

Initial physician work relative values were based on the results of the Harvard studies. The factors used to determine physician work under the current system include the time it takes to perform the service, the technical skill and physical effort, the required mental effort in judgment, and stress due to the potential risk to the patient. Legislation enacting the RBRVS (Section 1448 of the Social Security Act, "payment for physician services") requires CMS to review relative value units established under the fee schedule at least every 5 years.

There are typically two different classifications of "practice expense" RVUs—a Facility RVU, which is used if the procedure is performed in a hospital inpatient or outpatient setting, and a nonfacility RVU, which is used if the procedure is performed in the physician's office. Until recently, practice expense relative values were based on a formula using average Medicare-approved charges from 1991 (the year before RBRVS was implemented), and the proportion of each specialty's revenues were attributable to the practice expense. However, in January 1999, CMS began a transition to resource-based practice expense RVUs for each CPT code, which differ based on the site of service (facility or nonfacility).

The third component of the RBRVS is professional liability or malpractice insurance. Malpractice RVUs are resource based and were implemented in the 1999 final Medicare Physician Fee Schedule rule. They are based on malpractice insurance premium data collected from commercial and physician-owned insurers.

Correct Coding Initiative (CCI) Edits

Correct Coding Initiative (CCI) is a program devised by Medicare to promote correct coding of services and prevent Medicare overpayment. The "edits" actually refer to rules governing which CPT codes may or may not be billed together and which modifiers must be used when certain codes are billed for the same patient during the same encounter. The edits can be found at http://www.cms.gov/Medicare/Coding.

American Medical Association's Relative Value Scale Update Committee (RUC)

AMA formed its specialty society Relative Value Scale Update Committee (RUC) in November 1991 to provide RVU recommendations to CMS for new or revised CPT codes. As a committee of the AMA and national medical specialty societies, the RUC makes recommendations to CMS regarding updates to the physician work and direct practice expense components of medical services under the Medicare physician fee schedule. The RUC represents the entire medical profession, with 21 of its 31 members nominated by major national medical specialty societies, including those recognized by the American Board of Medical Specialties, those with a large percentage of physicians in patient care, and those that account for high percentages of Medicare expenditures. Four seats rotate on a 2-year basis, with two reserved for an internal medicine subspecialty, one for a primary care representative, and one for any other specialty. The RUC chair, the co-chair of the HCPAC, representatives of the AMA and the American Osteopathic Association, the chair of the Practice Expense Advisory Committee (PEAC), and CPT Editorial Panel hold the remaining six seats.

In our original scenario, when a code is passed through the CPT Editorial Panel and given a CPT code, it is then referred to the RUC for determination of its physician work RVUs. When the code arrives at the RUC, it must be surveyed, using a very strict process to obtain information regarding how the code's work (based on time and intensity) relates to other already established codes. The members of the specialty society who are most familiar with, and frequently provide, the service serve as an important support group because these surveys are distributed to them for completion. These surveys are quite detailed and take some time and effort to complete. Despite this, it is critical that members participate in these surveys, when requested by the Academy, and provide robust and accurate data to the Academy's RUC Advisors, as that data will be used to develop the Academy's physician work RVU recommendations to the AMA RUC.

To pass through the RUC successfully, a two-thirds majority must vote positively for a recommended RVU. This takes skill and negotiation on the parts of the RUC Advisors representing their societies, as well as cooperation with other societies. At times, in the case of a surgical code, there may be multiple specialties that perform this procedure. It then becomes a combined effort of these societies to survey the code and reach a consensus to obtain the most accurate RVU possible. When a new code is presented at the RUC, the physician work, clinical staff time, and direct practice expenses are determined.

Practice Expense Advisory Committee

In 1999, Congress mandated that the practice expense component of each RVU also become resource based. The original assignments of practice expense were made by the Clinical Practice Expert Panels (CPEPs). To continuously update and validate the expense data originally provided by the CPEPs, the RUC developed a Practice Expense Advisory Committee (PEAC) subcommittee. This committee meets three times a year, during the RUC meetings, and is responsible for recommendations regarding the direct practice expense and clinical staff time components for both new and existing CPT codes.

The RUC's annual cycle for developing recommendations is closely coordinated with both the CPT Editorial Panel's schedule for annual code revisions and the CMS's schedule for annual updates in the Medicare physician fee schedule final rule. Once a code has successfully been passed through the RUC, it is referred to CMS for final approval. At present, CMS's acceptance rate of RUC values is in the mid-90% range. Once CMS has accepted these values, they are printed in the *Federal Register*, and a 60-day period for public comment follows. Absent a technical error within the final rule by CMS, the values assigned to physician services that were reviewed by the RUC in the previous year are assigned interim values for the coming calendar year (e.g., codes reviewed in 2012 are assigned an interim value for the 2013 physician fee schedule). The public may comment to CMS on areas of disagreement or concerns regarding the assignment of relative values for physician services; however, modifications to contested interim values are not made until the following year's physician fee schedule final rule.

Because CMS operates on a fixed-dollar budget, which only allows increments for increasing the number of Medicare patients, RVU and code payment assignment is a budget-neutral process. Another way to think about the process is to understand that the Medicare budget is fixed. No new money comes into the system when a new code is authorized. Thus the only way money can be allocated to a new code is by decreasing the money given to existing codes. This fiscal reality is what creates a fair amount of discussion and confusion among physicians because payment for services fluctuates from year to year as a result of budget neutrality. Additionally, many third-party payers typically adopt reimbursement rates similar to the Medicare fee schedule.

■ Suggested Reading

American Medical Association. CPT—Current Procedural Terminology. http://www.ama-assn.org/ama/pub/physician-resources/solutions-managing-your-practice/coding-billing-insurance/cpt.page

American Medical Association. The Medicare Physician Payment Schedule.http://www.ama-assn.org/ama/pub/physician-resources/solutions-managing-your-practice/coding-billing-insurance/medicare/the-medicare-physician-payment-schedule.page

American Medical Association. The RVS Update Committee. http://www.ama-assn.org/ama/pub/physician-resources/solutions-managing-your-practice/coding-billing-insurance/medicare/the-resource-based-relative-value-scale/the-rvs-update-committee.page

Centers for Medicare and Medicaid Services. National Correct Coding Initiative Edits. http://www.cms.gov/Medicare/Coding/NationalCorrectCodInitEd/index.html?redirect=/NationalCorrectCodInitEd/

Centers for Medicare and Medicaid Services. Physician Fee Schedule. https://www.cms.gov/PhysicianFeeSched/PFSRVF/list.asp

4 Critical Steps for Successfully Managing Revenue and Expenses

■ Introduction

This chapter is written for the otolaryngologist who realizes that successfully managing the continually evolving health care marketplace requires more than superior clinical skills. It also requires a core understanding of business and management principles. In these increasingly competitive and complex times, the proper application of these principles is important to both private and academic practices. This chapter provides a concise and practical introduction to many of these principles. All practices seeking to maintain long-term viability must preserve and monitor the existing revenue stream, create new revenue streams, and control overhead or expenses.

■ Step 1: Form a Single Legal Multiphysician Business Entity

A vital first step in successfully managing revenues and overhead is the formation of a single legal multiphysician business entity. Without this first step, tackling many of the challenges facing physicians today or managing revenue and overhead becomes nearly impossible. By forming a single entity, a group of formerly isolated and disparate physicians may form a more coordinated voice in interactions with other parties in and outside the health care system. This group is now in a better position to negotiate contracts with patients, landlords, suppliers and vendors, the government, the media, hospitals, and insurance companies. The group practice can pool its clinical outcomes data to determine its own best practice guidelines and informatics platform and communicate them to professional associations, the news media, or government regulatory agencies.

On a practical level, a coordinated physician voice can enable your practice to provide better patient care by negotiating more reasonable working conditions. One example involves reducing the degree to which insurance companies restrict your clinical decision-making abilities. Negotiation with insurance companies can also help to preserve your revenue stream by maintaining fair and reasonable reimbursement rates. Honest, transparent negotiation can ensure adequate revenue, leading to a sustainable business model for better patient care. This collective negotiation must be conducted within the proper legal framework, and engagement of reputable health care and antitrust attorneys early in the process will ensure an optimal outcome.

Many incarnations of "group practices" have sprung up in the recent past, such as independent practice associations (IPAs), physician–hospital organizations (PHOs), physician organizations (POs), physician provider organizations (PPOs), accountable care organizations (ACOs), and medical homes. The long-term viability of each model has been suspect. For the most part, these models have not succeeded because they are group practices only in name; in reality they are still a collection of disparate solo practitioners with decentralized operations and interests that may conflict with each other. They are competitors, rather than members of a single business entity working for a common corporate mission statement and goals.

At its core, the concept of a physician group practice as a single business entity is all about a collection of *providers* coming to work together for a common purpose. Because of this human element, it is imperative to lay the foundation for a successful enterprise by finding the right people to join the group. As with consulting firms, large national law firms, and other industries that offer the services of highly skilled professionals, the quality of the physicians (i.e., the human capital) is your practice's most important asset. Aside from possessing high-quality clinical skills, subjective qualities in the member physicians can be just as important in determining the success or failure of your group endeavor. Such "intangibles" include good chemistry with other members of the practice, a sense of camaraderie, good teamwork skills, and a positive attitude.

The specific traits that promise success in one group may not work for another. It all depends on achieving the right fit with the unique atmosphere of the specific practice in question.

A practice must meet certain legal and operational criteria to be considered a "real" group practice:

- It must be a real business—a for-profit company with a formal legal structure. One can choose from among several different alternative structures—limited liability corporation (LLC), limited liability partnership (LLP), or professional corporation (PC), just to name a few. Physician organizations or networks, such as IPAs, PPOs, and PHOs, do not qualify. Consultation with a health law/business attorney will allow a proper match between corporate and legal structure.
- It must operate under a single federal tax identification number (TIN). Under this umbrella, individual physicians have separate provider identification numbers (PINs), national provider identifier (NPI) numbers, as well as individual TINs. These allow individual tracking of utilization, productivity, and revenue stream, as well as filing of individual tax returns.
- It must have a group entity in the public eye—(e.g., to patients, to other physicians, and to insurers). Official letterhead, business cards, prescription pads, and so forth, should state, along with the name of the individual physician, that he or she is a member of the group practice.
- It should, in the interests of efficiency, centralize some office functions and devote certain staff members specifically to these tasks. However, some functions become inefficient if centralized and therefore should be conducted individually. Depending on geographical constraints, the physicians' offices may be grouped in one location or may occupy several locations in the interests of capturing market share. Regardless of the arrangement, the practice should designate one central location as the home base where "back office" functions are performed. Following are some suggestions for the most efficient ways to centralize back office functions:
  - *Accounts receivable—billing and insurance claims processing.* All charges, payment, and encounter information are posted from the site of service into a centralized computer system in real time. Retrieval of records for checking the status of a patient account or a claim should be accessible from all practice sites. The claims should be "scrubbed" to ensure completeness and accuracy by dedicated, trained staff members.
  - *Payment processing.* Claim payments need to be tracked and deposited by dedicated staff members into the corporate accounts. Distributions should be made to the providers according to contracted terms that comply with state and federal statutes. A centralized staff can also monitor Explanation of Benefits (EOB) statements, post payments into patients' records, conduct follow-up for error detection/correction, and refile claims. These dedicated staff members are devoted to these crucial functions to gain continued expertise and efficiency in these tasks. Write-offs, whether due to a professional, friendship, or hardship courtesy for patients, or due to the discrepancy between the physician's full *office fee* and the insurance companies' *contractual fee* (refer to Step 3: Monitor Fee-for-Service Insurance Claim Payments) should be entered by these staffers.
  - *Payroll.* The central office will administer payroll out of a central account through an agency, which is both efficient and cost-effective. Wages for centralized back office staff are often shared by all the physicians in the group. Staff members who cater to individual physicians are allocated in accordance with the bylaws of the company. This should be done in a manner that promotes cost-effectiveness in each practice, thus reducing overhead and helping the group to be more competitive. It is advisable to make benefits packages and other human resources policies uniform across the company. Sometimes exceptions in the case of employees employed prior to the creation of the business entity are helpful to retain critical personnel.
  - *Accounts payable.* A coordinated system and staff will administer the purchasing of supplies and track payment to vendors (see the Accounts Payable section under Step 5). This group should have an incentive structure to encourage frugal spending and use of supplies. One way to do this is to make each location accountable for expenditures. Costs that can be tracked individually include rent, labor, supplies, utilities, and equipment. Communal costs (e.g., the wages of employees who perform the centralized back office functions, or capital equipment that will be used by all the physicians) should be allocated in accordance with the bylaws of the business entity.

Centralization can be a means to increase the efficiency and productivity of the group practice. If done properly, it should enhance the productivity and satisfaction of physicians. Hence, the practice should encourage that sense of ownership in how each physician manages patients and monitors clinical assistants and back office support staff. Under this system, each physician is compensated according to a productivity incentive, a system similar to the commission system on which real estate agents or sales people operate. Again, the exact formulation of the system can be customized for the specific group practice in question, so long as it is in compliance with federal and state statutes.

Centralized operations are meant merely to streamline and increase the efficiency of the administrative, accounting, and clerical tasks that support the practice. This is done to enhance the practice's goal to provide high-quality medical care with excellent customer service at a competitive price.

The care itself must be local and individualized. If the group practice has multiple sites, care can be customized to the patient. Illness frequency, requested treatments, and cultural norms may vary by location. So long as certain quality standards are met, then the individual practitioner can customize care to practice circumstances, in the interests of providing the best patient care at the most cost-effective price possible.

Another rationale for organizing into a single business entity is that grouped physicians can offer convenient, on-the-spot ancillary services to their patients at a lower per-physician cost. For example, a 20-member physician group can offer diagnostic tests (such as sleep laboratories, computed tomographic scans, or magnetic resonance imaging scans) or surgical facilities. This one-stop-shopping approach offers convenience and cost savings. Furthermore, because of the close proximity, doctors can better monitor the quality of the ancillary services, detect errors, and coordinate care. This total continuum of care is financially possible only in the group practice situation, because more doctors can share the capital equipment costs to build the facilities and the overhead costs to run them. Also, only a group of multiple physicians will have enough patient volume to use such facilities at their full capacity. Ultimately, the cost efficiency will allow the group to offer these needed services to patients on a higher-quality, more convenient, and more cost-competitive basis.

■ Step 2: Negotiate Salient Points of Contracts

When negotiating with vendors, landlords, or insurance companies, your goal is to negotiate for fair and equitable terms of contract in accordance with common business practices. General principles include the importance of including explicit billing procedures, specifying recourse for delinquent accounts, preventing unilateral changes to the contract, and making provisions for renewal and termination of the contract. These principles should be applied any time your practice negotiates a contract with outside parties. The services of a trusted health law attorney may ensure proper protection when negotiating with entities, such as health care consultants or providers of computer information systems.

Practice Guidelines, Clinical Indicators, and Fee Schedules

Practice guidelines, clinical indicators, and fee schedules (corresponding to Current Procedural Terminology [CPT] codes) should be explicitly and unambiguously stated and attached as an exhibit of the agreement. For example, it should be explicitly stated what, if any, and how many pre- or postoperative visits are covered by a fee for a surgical procedure. All agreement documents should be attached and reviewed. Practice guidelines, clinical indicators, and fee schedules should also be developed collaboratively between the insurance company and the physician group.

Precertification and Utilization

Precertification and utilization review should be performed by practicing physicians in the same specialty, not by insurance company administrators or representatives who do not hold board certification to practice in that specialty. Insurance companies may only accept board-certified or eligible physicians to take care of patients. It is only reasonable that utilization reviews and precertification be performed by similarly qualified individuals.

Explanation of Insurance Benefits

It is the responsibility of the insurance company to explain to the patient subscribers covered and noncovered services under their health plans and the rationale for the decision. The physician should not have to shoulder that burden. After all, it is the insurance company that sells the health plan and collects the revenues from the insurance premiums, revenues that include a margin for administrative overhead, sales commissions, and profit. Thus it is the responsibility of the insurance company to also provide customer service for its product. This customer service should include explaining to its subscribers the extent of coverage and benefits under the plan, as well as what services are not covered.

Primary Care Practitioner Referrals

In the event a primary care practitioner (PCP) referral is needed, the agreement should allow for a "universal referral," such that the specialist has free rein to do what is medically necessary for the patient and is not constrained to doing only certain procedure(s) that have been prespecified by the PCP on the referral form. After all, if the PCP knew what tests to order to diagnose the condition or what therapeutic course to initiate, the PCP would not need to refer the patient in the first place. It is below the standard of care to refer a patient to a specialist and then "gag" the specialist by limiting his or her ability to render quality care, as is medically necessary, to the patient.

Claims Filing

The following procedures are recommended for filing claims:

- The procedure for filling out and submitting a claim form should be clearly described within the agreement, explicitly stating what constitutes a "clean" claim with all required information.
- The responsibilities of the physician and the insurance company with regard to procedures for submitting claims and processing payments should be clearly and explicitly stated.
- The agreement should clearly and explicitly state how multiple, related procedures performed on the same patient should be billed, so as to prevent inappropriate bundling of claims by the insurance companies or inappropriate unbundling of claims by the physician. Bundling refers to grouping several independent procedures into a single CPT code, whereas unbundling imparts describing a procedure by its component parts. Both terms have negative context when used to describe unfair or deceitful business practices.

Payment Provisions

The following provisions are recommended to ensure timely payment by insurance companies:

- The insurance company has an obligation to pay the claim within a window of time from the date of submission.
- The insurance company must notify the physician within that window of time if there is any reason not to pay the claim.
- There must not be any retroactive denial of claims, except for arithmetical errors.

- If payment is not received by the deadline, the insurer must pay interest on the amount of the claim for each day that the payment exceeds the deadline, until the payment is received.

Recourse or Delinquent Claims

- If the claim is still unpaid after a certain number of days (which should be negotiated and stated clearly in the agreement), the claim will be marked delinquent, and the physician has the right to refer the matter to a collection agency or an attorney for immediate action.
- It is the responsibility of the insurance company to pay for any attorney's or collection agency's fees required to collect the debts.

Termination and Renewal of Contracts

The agreement should contain the following clauses regarding termination and renewal of contract:

- The duration of the term of the agreement, and the procedure for renewal of the agreement should be agreed upon and stated explicitly within the contract.
- In the event that the agreement is terminated, the patients who are subscribers to the health plan should be notified in neutral language that the particular physician or physician group has elected not to participate in the plan, without casting any negative implications on either the insurance company or the providers.
- If an agreement is terminated, the physician must be paid through to the date of termination, in accordance with the terms of the agreement.
- Furthermore, if the insurance company requires the physician to treat its subscribers after the termination of the contract, then the physician will be compensated for those services in accordance with the terms of the original, terminated agreement. In the interests of providing quality care, the physician will not refuse to treat a current patient who has an emergent, acute need for care during the transition period but after the crisis is resolved, it is the responsibility of the insurance company to find a replacement physician.
- If the physician decides to terminate the contract "for cause" (e.g., unilateral changes to the agreement or breach of contract by the insurance company), the physician is entitled to full reimbursement of fees for services

rendered up to that point of termination, as well as a separation compensation to be stated in the agreement. A physician who decides to terminate "without cause" will not be entitled to separation compensation.

Step 3: Monitor Fee-for-Service Insurance Claim Payments

Perhaps the most common billing system is the third-party payer system, in which a third party (someone other than the patient) is responsible for reimbursing you for your professional fees. Usually, this third party will be an insurance company, a health maintenance organization (HMO), a health care cooperative, or a governmental payer (Medicaid or Medicare). This situation does involve some loss of control over your income stream because you cannot bill the patient for the remainder, even if the third party does not reimburse you or if it reimburses you inadequately.

Many otolaryngologists are probably all too familiar with insurance companies' frequent delays in payment, arbitrarily rejected claims, bundled claims, and reduced reimbursement rates. In addition, errors in payment processing are very common, such that insurers often reimburse otolaryngologists less than what they are entitled to under the contract terms by using vastly discounted fee schedules.

Develop and Update a Computer Monitoring System

The best way you can protect your income stream is by employing a systematic, efficient, and timely computer monitoring system to quickly identify and address claims processing errors. Once this monitoring system is set in place, it should be updated regularly and analyzed at least weekly. Timely identification of errors is key to allowing the physician's office staff to query the insurance company and resolve the problem. Any errors need to be resolved in a proactive, timely manner, through a combination of calling, writing, and persistent follow-up with the insurer. This is particularly true, because many insurance companies have a filing time limit—a window of time beyond which claims or refiling of claims cannot be submitted.

This system enables otolaryngologists to track what is owed and actually being paid and to discover any discrepancies. Physicians should ensure full receipt of payment for their professional services. The terms of contract are often austere. You should at least ensure that the health plans are under compensating you out contractually required reimburse-

ment. It may require additional initial effort to set up the monitoring system and persistence to check and update the system regularly, but it will greatly improve the efficiency of your claims processing and accounts receivables department and better ensure financial health.

In setting up such a monitoring system and resolving errors with the insurance companies, a few practical guidelines should be kept in mind.

Develop a Fee Schedule and Data Collection Database

Otolaryngologists should compile a list of their practice's most commonly performed procedures, the respective CPT codes, and the undiscounted fee for each—that is, the full amount that the physician charges to indemnity plans and self-paying patients, also known as an *office fee*. Some practices set this rate as a percentage of the Medicare fee schedule (e.g., 250%, 300%). When submitting claims, make sure the CPT codes correspond to the correct International Classification of Diseases 9th edition (ICD-9) diagnostic code. The insurer will pay only a percentage of the full *office fee*, based on a negotiated discounted rate stipulated in its contract with the physician—this is called the *contractual fee*. This contractual fee for each CPT code will differ from plan to plan and from year to year as contracts are renegotiated. A list of the plan's contractual fees should also be compiled by CPT code.

The database should also track copayments and risk pool contributions. Each patient usually has to pay the physician a copayment or an out-of-pocket expenditure for each office visit or procedure. This copayment to the physician either will be *in addition to* the contractual fee received from the insurer or will be *deducted from* the insurer's contractual fee, depending on the contract between the physician and the insurer, and even depending on the rendered service. This may vary from contract to contract, so the specifics should be entered in the database.

A risk pool contribution is the amount deducted from the contractual fee for each service (usually 10–20%). Some insurers do this as a way of making the physician share in the risks of overutilization. Risk pool withholding does not apply to all procedures or all contracts, so any such withholdings should be clearly noted by procedure (i.e., CPT code) when posting each claim into the computer. If the insurance company experiences a profitable year, then that withheld amount will be returned to the physician. But all too often, even if the company has been successful, it seldom returns all the risk pool funds. Tracking how much has been withheld for the risk pool by patient, by CPT code, by procedure, by date of service, and by insurance company will ensure your practice knows how much it can expect to be refunded. In the event of a dispute, you will have the data to substantiate your case.

Analyze Database Results

Now that all these categories have been tracked, it is possible to compute the amount owed:

$$\text{Amount owed} = [(\text{contractual fee}) \pm (\text{copay}) - (\text{risk pool})].$$

The system can then track the amount of reimbursement that has been received (amount paid) from the insurer, to make sure that it matches the negotiated amount owed. If not, the amount of the discrepancy should be noted so that the insurance company can be queried and the error resolved. The discrepancy between the amount paid and the amount owed should not be written off. It should be duly noted as a discrepancy and pursued.

Recommended Office Procedures

Keep a log in the patient file whenever you or your office staff communicates with an insurance company regarding a claim. Maintaining this paper trail will make it easier to resolve a dispute in the event an appeal must be made. Keep proof of submission of claims, in case the insurance company refuses to pay on the grounds that the filing limit (usually 90 days) has been exceeded.

Making sure claims are accurate, complete, and in compliance with insurance requirements prior to submission is a critical first step in ensuring timely and accurate reimbursement. Errors, omissions, and inconsistencies are some more common reasons for claim rejection or payment delay. Check the following categories:

- CPT code(s)
- Corresponding ICD-9 code(s)—make sure they match the CPT codes
- Referring physician and physician number, if needed
- Insurance ID and group numbers
- Patient demographic information
- Multiple tests or procedures—make sure correct units are entered and that each respective CPT code corresponds to the correct ICD-9 code
- Modifiers—check for any that are needed
- NPI number

The EOB is either a paper or an electronic form sent by the insurance company that breaks out the various components of each claim. A preemptive check of the various components on the EOB, even before they are entered or received into the computer monitoring system, can help quickly identify errors and ensure that possible refiling or appeals fall within contractually specified timeframes. Put the process of resolving the problem into motion by verifying the following items:

- *Billed amount (office fee)* Does the billed amount on the EOB match the physician's standard charge (the amount that a self-paying patient would be charged) for that CPT code?
- *Allowed amount (contractual fee)* Does this match the allowed amount for the billed CPT code on the fee schedule for that particular insurance plan? Sometimes an insurance contract does not include a comprehensive fee schedule for all CPT codes. Or, an insurer may simply pay a percentage (which usually exceeds 100%) of Medicare reimbursement rates for the same CPT code. If the reimbursement rate is not listed, then call the insurer to clarify the allowed amount. If a fee schedule lists a CPT code multiple times with different allowed rates, call the insurance company to clarify the matter in writing.
- *Copayment amount* Does the copay amount fall within the normal range? It varies from plan to plan, but usually ranges from $5 to $25 for each office visit or is a percentage of the billed amount for surgical procedures. Make sure that the copay amount is noted correctly as either "in addition to" or "deducted from" the allowable fee, in accordance with the terms of the insurance contract.
- *Coinsurance amount* Sometimes a patient will have secondary or tertiary coverage from another insurance plan. In such cases, make sure the payment amount from coinsurance is correct. Sometimes, an insurer will reject a claim on the grounds that it is the responsibility of the secondary insurer to pay. If that is the case then the claim must be researched and, if correct, submitted to the secondary insurer.
- *Risk pool withholdings* Check that these figures are correct. They should typically be 10 to 20% of the allowable amount.
- *Net payment/amount paid* This is the actual amount of payment sent with the EOB. Check that it matches the *amount owed*, which is the allowed amount, net of copay, deductibles, coinsurance, and risk pool with holdings.
- *Improperly bundled procedures* Check that payments for multiple, related procedures have not been bundled. These procedures should be reimbursed fully and separately.

At least once a month, proactively check for aged accounts (> 45 days) that have not been settled to identify claims that need to be resolved before the filing deadline is exceeded. Reviewing an account may reveal that the outstanding balance is the responsibility of the secondary insurer. In such cases, the secondary plan should be billed as soon as possible. Keep proof of previous submission in the case of a refile, in the event an insurer denies payment on the grounds that the claim is past the filing limit.

■ Step 4: Understand Capitation Plans for Professional Services

Capitation differs fundamentally from the traditional fee-for-service or discounted-fee-for-service payment method. Instead of reimbursing the otolaryngologist after each service or office visit, each month the insurance company or capitated health plan pays the otolaryngology physician group a fee up front for each patient enrolled in the plan with that group. This fee is also known as a per member per month (PMPM) fee, which is the entire sum that the group will receive from the health plan for that month.

For example, if otolaryngology physician group X in New York City has 1,000 patients who are members of its capitated health plan, and the PMPM is $2, then for that month, the group will receive $2,000. In return for that $2,000, the group must provide those 1,000 patients with all the otolaryngology professional services they need, provided that those services (as listed by their corresponding CPT codes) are covered in the prenegotiated capitated plan. Because of the structuring and provisions of capitated health plans, it is crucial to have a clear definition, by CPT code, of which services and procedures will be covered under the capitated contract. For financial or risk management reasons, it may be desirable to exclude certain procedures from the contract, a practice known as a carve-out.

As another example, if an acoustic neuroma is not covered under the contract and an enrolled patient has an acoustic neuroma, the otolaryngologist can still treat this condition and can charge extra fees. It is wise, if possible, to prenegotiate these carved-out fees beforehand. On the other hand, if a tympanoplasty is covered under the plan, the otolaryngologist cannot charge an additional fee to perform this service. Carve-outs protect the otolaryngology physician group from having to bear the burden of very costly professional fees (such as acoustic neuromas and cochlear implants) out of the capitated fee. Although carving out more procedures may increase the number of additional fees that the otolaryngology physician group can charge and also reduce financial risk,

it will also lower the up-front PMPM, because that PMPM fee covers fewer services. So it is important to carefully weigh the pros and cons before deciding on which CPT codes to include in the contract.

Terms of Contract and Other Forms of Risk Mitigation

Analyze Your Patient Pool

Before negotiating the PMPM, make sure to do a thorough analysis of the demographic and health risk profiles of your patient pool. It is also beneficial to do an analysis of expected incidence rates for various illnesses and the professional fees associated with each. Doing so will allow you to better predict what level of professional services you can expect to provide from month to month and will help set an appropriate "target" PMPM fee for negotiations with the capitated health plan. This is because demographic characteristics, such as age, gender, race, and occupation, are fairly good predictors for risk of various illnesses. Other factors to consider include the patient's preexisting health conditions, chronic diseases, past medical history, and family history of heritable diseases. As a demographic group, the elderly and the very young tend to require more care than other age groups, on a per-patient basis.

Purchase Stop-Loss Insurance

It is wise not only to negotiate an appropriate PMPM but also to purchase stop-loss insurance to limit the financial liabilities the group would have to face in reimbursing for services out of the PMPM fee pool. Even one or two patients with very serious illnesses could threaten the financial viability of your group and the wisdom of the contract. The stop-loss insurance ensures that after a threshold of professional fees (paid out for a particular patient in a particular time frame) has been exceeded, the stop-loss insurance will pay the rest, protecting the group from financial ruin. Another stop-loss threshold is invoked if the total amount spent in professional fees for all the covered individuals for a given month exceeds the threshold. In this case, the stop-loss insurance will cover the rest. This type of stop-loss policy is particularly useful in the event that an otolaryngology physician group simultaneously has large numbers of patients who become ill, perhaps individually at a subcatastrophic level, but when taken as an aggregate require a great deal of care and thus incur a high level of professional fees. Of course, one must remember that, for a given month, many of the group's 1,000 patients may not need your services at all, and yet the group will still retain the $2,000 in PMPM fees.

Specify Who Pays for Professional Services

The terms of the capitated contract should also specify who pays for professional services rendered when a patient goes out of the geographic area covered by your otolaryngology physician group, or if the patient sees an otolaryngologist who is outside of your group but in the same geographic area. For example, your otolaryngology physician group covers New York City, but while your patient is traveling in California, he needs to have an emergency myringotomy. This qualifies as an out-of-area procedure. You need to negotiate with the insurer who will pay for those services, though in such a case it is common for the patient's home otolaryngology physician group to pay usual and customary fees to the provider in California. If your patient goes to see another otolaryngology physician who is not in your group, but is in New York City, this qualifies as an "in area but out-of-network" service. Again, the specific terms of the capitation contract are negotiable, but it is common practice for the home otolaryngology physician group to pay usual and customary fees to the out-of-network otolaryngology physician, provided that an in-network otolaryngologist makes the referral. If, however, the patient decides to independently seek the opinion of an out-of-network otolaryngologist, then this is not covered under the capitated plan, and the patient will have to pay out of pocket for those services.

Proper Utilization

Proper utilization is based on the efficient, economical, and needful use of patient visits, procedures, and other ancillaries, as gauged by a utilization committee composed of members of the group using standard practice guidelines. The inclusion of this category counterbalances any incentive that an individual otolaryngologist might have to artificially inflate the number of procedures performed, thereby boosting his or her compensation based on productivity. Because the member otolaryngologists all work together, the decisions of such a utilization committee will be based on dialogue among clinical peers. Peer pressure can then guide behavior. This is more effective than utilization review by a remote case manager pronouncing judgment on proper usage.

■ Step 5: Control Expenditures and Overhead

After monitoring and preserving its revenue stream, the group should strive to maximize the efficiency of the medical office's day-to-day operations, and thus minimize operational expenditures or overhead. Some physicians concentrate on patient care and try to delegate this step, leaving all administrative and managerial tasks to an office manager. This approach usually fails because clinicians understand the practice requirements for efficiently conducting patient care better than any office manager. On the other hand, physicians should not micromanage all the clerical and administrative tasks, but instead should broadly establish a systematic approach for staff to follow, and then audit their performance. Office managers should have input, but decision making should be ultimately controlled by an otolaryngologist.

Following are clear, step-by-step guidelines to the most important principles and procedures to run a successful practice organized into several main categories.

Accounts Payable

This refers to all outgoing monies or funds owed to other businesses for services and goods it requires to run its own operations. As it applies to a group practice, accounts payable essentially amounts to a purchase order system that keeps track of orders and payments for office and medical supplies and equipment. Other suggestions include the following:

- Maintain a centralized inventory.
- Dedicate a staff member for first-round approval of purchases.
- Specify physicians for final approval of purchases.
- Stock a 3-month supply of inventory.
- Make payment on invoices, not packing slips.
- Institute internal checks and balances.
- Consider a computerized purchase order system.

Other Office Procedure Guidelines

Institute uniform office protocols on all standard tasks that staff members may have to perform. Collect these protocols into a "procedure book" so that all staff can refer to them as necessary. In addition, train all new staff in the standard protocol for performing these procedures before they begin their duties.

Ensure Accountability

Have your staff initial any documents or messages that they handle, so that if something goes wrong, it will be possible to identify the person to speak to about the problem; on the flip side, the practice is then also able to compliment a staff member responsible for an outstanding performance.

Perform Medical Audits

Every month, select approximately five patient cases at random from the appointment book to spot check. Trace the handling of each case from the beginning to the end to make sure it was handled correctly. Did the patient show up? If not, determine the reason. Was patient and insurance information entered into the charts completely and correctly? Were all ancillary services (as designated by CPT codes) posted correctly and correlated with the appropriate diagnoses (as designated by ICD-9 codes)? Were all laboratory results and diagnostic tests handled correctly and then filed into the chart? Were insurance claim forms submitted promptly and correctly? Has payment been received and posted? Is the payment accurate and timely?

■ Conclusion

Given recent developments transforming health care delivery and payment, the prudent reader will realize that physicians have to adapt to survive in this constantly changing environment. Physicians should view this period as an *opportunity* for the profession to evolve. Savvy management of revenue and overhead can lead to more efficient and higher-quality patient care. Clinical skills that physicians devote their lives to mastering and maintaining can be enhanced by effective practice management. Careful attention to changing state and federal policies and programs with focusing on how these changes will affect your practice is vital to maintaining long-term success. Proper application of the presented principles of revenue/overhead and operational management will lead to a more efficient and profitable practice.

■ Suggested Reading

Centers for Medicare & Medicaid Services. Accountable Care Organizations (ACOs). https://www.cms.gov/Medicare/Medicare-Fee-for-Service-Payment/ACO/index.html?redirect=/ACO.

Centers for Medicare & Medicaid Services. Bundled Payments for Care Improvement. http://innovations.cms.gov/initiatives/bundled-payments/index.html

Centers for Medicare & Medicaid Services. Legislative Update. http://www.cms.gov/regulations-and-guidance/legislation/legislativeupdate/downloads/ppaca.pdf

Lee KJ, Lee ME. Universal healthcare: a bold proposal. Conn Med 2000;64(8):485–491

Mujtaba F, Sullivan E, Lee KJ. A method for detecting errors in discounted fee-for-service payments by insurance companies. Ear Nose Throat J 2000;79(3):148–149, 152

National Committee for Quality Assurance. Patient-Centered Medical Home. http://www.ncqa.org/tabid/631/Default.aspx

Read the law. http://www.healthcare.gov/law/full/index.html

Terry K. ACOs forging the links. Hospitals & Health Networks. January 2011. http://www.hhnmag.com/hhnmag_app/jsp/articledisplay.jsp?dcrpath=HHNMAG/Article/data/01JAN2011/0111HHN_Coverstory&domain=HHNMAG

United Hospital Fund. The Patient-Centered Medical Home: Taking a Model to Scale in New York State. http://www.uhfnyc.org/publications/880791

II

Clinical Fundamentals

5 Ethics for the Otolaryngologist

■ Introduction

"Ethics gives you a compass, not an itinerary. But I will suggest that this means that you and all your patients will be well served if, in all of your clinical decision making, your ultimate value is always the good of the patient."
—*Daniel P. Sulmasy, OFM, MD, PhD,*
The John J. Conley Department of Ethics

Thousands of bright, optimistic, and enthusiastic medical school graduates raise their right hand each May and affirm the oath by which we practice our healing craft. The meaning of the Hippocratic oath is simple. We are entrusted with the responsibility of placing our patients' needs above all else. With busier offices, diminishing reimbursements, daunting medicolegal claims, and declining social status, we threaten to lose sight of this promise. While preparing to study the latest advances in otolaryngic diagnosis and treatment found in this textbook, take this opportunity to review and reaffirm that oath you took on your medical school graduation day. Read the Hippocratic Oath and be reminded of why we are members of such a coveted profession:

I swear to fulfill, to the best of my ability and judgment, this covenant:

I will respect the hard-won scientific gains of those physicians in whose steps I walk, and gladly share such knowledge as is mine with those who are to follow.

I will apply, for the benefit of the sick, all measures [that] are required, avoiding those twin traps of overtreatment and therapeutic nihilism.

I will remember that there is art to medicine as well as science, and that warmth, sympathy, and understanding may outweigh the surgeon's knife or the chemist's drug.

I will not be ashamed to say "I know not," nor will I fail to call in my colleagues when the skills of another are needed for a patient's recovery.

■ American Academy of Otolaryngology–Head and Neck Surgery Code of Ethics

The American Academy of Otolaryngology–Head and Neck Surgery published its Code of Ethics in 2010, providing a framework of honorable behavior among the Academy's fellows and members. Similar to the Oath of Hippocrates, this code emphasizes the principles of acting in the patient's best interest; treating patients with competence, dignity, and respect; and maintaining proficiency and academic inquiry. Unique from the time of Hippocrates, the code further defines ethical behavior in areas of commercial interests, prescribing and referral practices, and fees and advertising.

Preamble

The following Statement of Principles and Code of Ethics articulate principles of conduct that are deemed appropriate and acceptable by the American Academy of Otolaryngology–Head and Neck Surgery Foundation, Inc. The statements and principles contained herein are not laws, but rather guidelines for honorable behavior. They are voluntary and nonbinding. However, we believe that these ethical principles should be aspired to by all Fellows and Members of the Academy. They should serve to bring clarity and definition to areas where confusion might occur in the course of contemporary otolaryngology practice.

The Academy further endorses the current opinions of the Council on Ethical and Judicial Affairs of the American Medical Association. Adhering to these principles should help otolaryngologists to act honorably and professionally toward their patients.

Principles

1. The best interest of the patient must be the foremost concern of the physician in all circumstances.
2. The patient must be treated with competence, respect, dignity, and honesty. Confidences shall be kept except as required by law.
3. The physician must maintain proficiency and competence through continuing study and be diligent in the administration of patient care.
4. Fees must be commensurate with the service rendered.
5. The impaired physician must withdraw from that part of the practice that is affected by the impairment.
6. Academy members should assist fellow members in complying with these principles.

The Physician–Patient Relationship

Each patient must be treated with respect, dignity, compassion, and honesty. The patient's right to participate in the treatment process must be recognized and promulgated by the otolaryngologist. The otolaryngologist shall be free to choose whom to serve; however, discrimination against a patient on the basis of race, color, gender, age, sexual orientation, socioeconomic status, religion, or national origin is inappropriate. Confidentiality of patient information is to be maintained, within the constraints of the law and the obligation to protect the welfare of the individual and the community. The otolaryngologist must establish and maintain appropriate relational boundaries, avoiding exploitation of patient vulnerability and specifically avoiding sexual misconduct with patients.

The otolaryngologist must disclose actual or potential conflicts of interest to patients, including but not limited to, fee arrangements and professionally related commercial interests. If a conflict of interest cannot be resolved, the otolaryngologist should withdraw from the relationship in a timely, appropriate manner. After having accepted a patient for care, the otolaryngologist may not neglect that patient.

Colleague Interactions

Interactions with colleagues should be based on mutual respect and a desire to improve patient care. Otolaryngologists must recognize their own professional limitations and expertise. Consultation and referral must be sought when appropriate. Communication with colleagues must be truthful and forthright. Disparagement of any kind is to be discouraged.

Commercial Interests

This Code of Ethics does not seek to restrict legal trade practices. However, a physician's commercial or financial interests should never be placed ahead of the interests and welfare of patients. Conflicts of interest undermine the trust that patients place in their physician. For this reason, physicians should endeavor to avoid any venture that creates a conflict between personal financial interests and the best interests of the patient. Conflicts that develop between a physician's financial interests and the physician's responsibilities to the patient should be to the benefit of the patient.

Referral Practices

All decisions regarding patient referral should be based primarily upon consideration of the needs and best interests of the patient. A physician's referral practice should never lead to exploitation of patients or third-party payers. Referral to a health facility in which a physician has a financial interest is not in and of itself unethical. However, such referrals are best when the referring physician will be directly involved in providing care to the patient at the facility. In cases where it is not possible or feasible to provide direct care, disclosure of financial interests should be made.

Prescribing Practices

Financial interests that the physician might have in the company supplying the product should not influence a physician in the prescribing of drugs, devices, appliances, or treatments. Neither should a physician's referral or admission patterns be constructed so as to enhance the physician's financial interests in any health facility. Physicians should not accept gifts from industries that would influence their prescribing patterns or practices.

Patents

Physicians should be allowed to patent devices, but the use of these devices must be in accordance with the patient's best medical interests, without regard to the physician's financial interests. Although it is currently lawful in the United States to patent medical and surgical procedures, such patents issued after October 1, 1996, may not be lawfully enforced against physicians or their affiliated health care institutions. This law is consistent with established principles of medical ethics. Medical and surgical procedures contribute to a universal body of medical knowledge. Unrestricted access to that knowledge is one of the defining characteristics of the medical and surgical profession. Enforcing patent restrictions on medical and surgical procedures limits access to medical knowledge, denies potential benefit to patients, and thus is unethical. Physicians should be allowed to charge a reasonable fee for instructional courses that describe and teach techniques and procedures to other physicians.

Advertising

It is ethical for otolaryngologists to advertise their services. Advertisement must be truthful and not misleading. An otolaryngologist should not misrepresent his/her qualifications and/or training, and should not exaggerate the efficacy or uniqueness of treatments rendered. Advertisements should also conform to local legal and commercial requirements with regard to format and content.

Research

Otolaryngologists–head and neck surgeons must conduct biomedical research according to ethical, moral, medical, and legal guidelines. All research should respect the dignity and sanctity of human life. The goal of research should be the betterment of humankind, the alleviation of suffering, and the ultimate improvement of medical practice. Anything that knowingly and unnecessarily jeopardizes the health, safety, or longevity of human subjects is unethical.

Biomedical research projects should be approved by institutional animal research boards, or human subject boards when appropriate. When possible, animal studies should precede the use of new and experimental techniques in humans. All human research subjects should be fully informed of the benefits and risks of the research being conducted and should give their informed consent prior to participating as a subject in any prospective trial. Further, any subject should be allowed to withdraw from a research protocol at any time without penalty. Research protocols should not be designed in a manner such that the research subject would receive a treatment that knowingly provides less benefit than the currently accepted standard of care.

The patient's right to privacy must be observed. Communications to the public must not convey false, untrue, deceptive, or misleading information. In addition, these communications should not misrepresent a surgeon's credentials, training, experience, or ability. Otolaryngologists should seek to avoid conflicts of interest in research. When unavoidable, such conflicts should be publicized.

Credit should be given to all investigators who contribute in a material way to a project. Conversely, coauthorship should not be assigned to individuals who do not participate in the project.

Character Issues

Patients and society at large place a high level of trust in physicians. Physicians are held to the highest moral standards in the community. This level of trust is based on an assumption that the physician maintains a high degree of personal integrity and adheres to a professional code of ethics. Physicians are expected to be truthful and honest. Otolaryngologists should conduct themselves morally and ethically so as to merit the confidence placed in them. Anything that detracts from the ability of an otolaryngologist to conduct himself or herself in such a fashion should be avoided. Otolaryngologists have an obligation to their colleagues to assist them in avoiding or eliminating behavior that is not conducive to maintaining personal integrity.

Impairment

Physician impairment represents a potential hazard to patients and to the affected physician. Otolaryngologists should make every effort to recognize the signs of physician impairment in themselves and in their colleagues. The otolaryngologist who suspects impairment in a colleague has an ethical obligation to the impaired physician and his/her patients. Self-referral for appropriate treatment should be advised and encouraged. The physician should withdraw from any component of practice that adequate assessment deems impaired. Appropriate management, including counseling, should follow. Should a physician refuse to self-refer when presented with evidence of impairment, otolaryngologists have an obligation to report the suspected physician to their supervisor or medical licensing authorities, particularly if the impairment is a threat to safe patient care. Confidentiality should be maintained for physicians undergoing evaluation and treatment for impairment. Physicians who have completed rehabilitation for impairment should not be restricted from practice provided that proper postrehabilitation monitoring shows no evidence of relapse.

Illegal Activity

Otolaryngologists should realize that they are subject to all civil and criminal statutes applicable to the region in which they practice. They are further subject to federal regulations governing medical practice. Illegal activity by an otolaryngologist compromises his or her personal integrity and casts aspersions on the medical profession at large. Otolaryngologists who knowingly participate in illegal or fraudulent behavior should be reported to the appropriate local authorities.

Fees

Fees must be commensurate with the service(s) rendered. It is unethical for a physician to charge an illegal or excessive fee. Illegal fee arrangements include charges for services not rendered, fee-splitting in exchange for referrals, and repeated up coding (i.e., submitting with higher codes than is appropriate for the services rendered). Fee collection efforts should take into account the ability of the patient to pay. Physicians should not withhold vital and emergent treatment to patients because of their inability to pay. Physicians should not abandon a patient in a postoperative period because of that patient's inability to pay.

Community Relations

Physicians have been bestowed by society with trust and respect that no other profession can claim. Physicians in turn have a responsibility to their communities that goes beyond that of other commercial enterprises. Physicians must preserve their role as health advocates within the community. This may involve participation in health education programs. It also may involve the physician adopting a protective role when the health and safety of a community is threatened. Academy members should refuse to cooperate in policies that violate the patients' interests and should become advocates for the sick whenever economics, organizations, or regulations threaten the good and welfare of our patients. Physicians may be called upon to act in other roles as civic leaders within the community. Each physician must respond within the scope of his or her abilities. Activities that promote the health and well-being of the community in a cost-effective way should be supported.

Otolaryngologists should not abandon the underprivileged segments of our society and should be encouraged to devote some time in caring for patients who are unable to pay.

Otolaryngologists should work hard to preserve their good reputation within the community and should avoid activities that undermine the trust and high regard society places in them.

Disciplinary Actions

Otolaryngologists have an ethical duty to report colleagues to state licensing authorities when documentary evidence exists of illegal activity. The Academy's board of directors shall have the power to censure, suspend, or expel any member who violates the Academy's Code of Ethics, as amended from time to time, including violations of the ethical guidelines of expert witness qualifications and testimony as stated in this code. The board shall follow the procedures set forth in Section 2.23 of the Academy Bylaws and other procedures that it establishes before taking any disciplinary action based on violation of the Code of Ethics.

Expert Witness Testimony and Qualifications

The Academy believes it is important for otolaryngologists to serve as expert witnesses in legal proceedings to assist in the administration of justice. The otolaryngologist, as a medical expert witness, shall be appropriately qualified and shall be thoroughly prepared with relevant facts so that he or she can, to the best of his or her ability, provide the court with opinions that are accurate and capable of substantiation with respect to the matters at hand. Physicians serving as expert witnesses must provide informed, objective, and truthful testimony without adopting a position of advocacy, and serve as spokespersons for the field of special knowledge the medical expert witness represents. It is unethical for physicians to accept compensation for expert witness testimony that is linked to the outcome of the case. Academy members must follow the "Statement on Qualifications and Guidelines for the Physician Expert Witness."

Code for Interactions with Companies

In September 2011, the American Academy of Otolaryngology–Head and Neck Surgery (AAO-HNS/F) adopted this code to reinforce the core principles that help maintain actual and perceived independence. Adopting this code helps to ensure that AAO-HNS/F's interactions with companies will be for the benefit of patients and members and for the improvement of care in the field of otolaryngology.

Gender Equity Policy and Procedural Guidelines

The AAO-HNS Code of Ethics endorses the current opinions of the Council on Ethical and Judicial Affairs of the American Medical Association. Opinion

E-9.035 sets forth the American Medical Association's (AMA's) position against gender discrimination in the medical profession. The AAO-HNS Ethics Committee will receive and review complaints about such discrimination in accordance with the procedures, as elaborated in this document.

■ Informed Consent

Educating our patients regarding their illness and its treatment is a crucial component to the physician–patient relationship and serves multiple ends. Fully informed patients are involved in the medical decision-making process, better understand their disease, and can more easily be willing participants in their treatment. This enhanced relationship and education can reduce discontent and litigation when complications occur, especially if they were discussed and agreed upon in detail prior to intervention. In order for consent to be valid, it must be given voluntarily and by a competent patient. The patient must have the mental capacity to understand problems, make decisions, and accept or reject the offered medical treatment. Competence is always presumed except when obvious clinical or judicial reasons are encountered. Another key component of informed consent that can easily be overlooked is disclosure.

■ Disclosure

Disclosure plays an important role in the informed consent process and is vital to the health of the patient relationship. A physician should truthfully answer when a patient inquires about his or her success rate and experience with a particular procedure. Furthermore, the law presumes that financial conflicts of interest could affect medical judgment and thus must be disclosed. This includes, for example, referral to a laboratory, ambulatory surgical center, or radiology service in which a physician has ownership or use of a new device or technique for which a physician has commercial interest. Failure to disclose these potential conflicts can both undermine the patient's trust and leave the physician open to legal claims of fraud, misrepresentation, or negligent nondisclosure.

■ Controversies in Otolaryngology

Ethical debates are common in specialties with particularly polarizing issues, such as organ transplant priority, premature infant delivery, and life-sustain-

ment procedures in terminal diseases. Although these situations are uncommon in otolaryngology, we are not immune to ethical controversy. Our awareness of community issues will aid in our understanding and sensitivity.

Cochlear Implantation

Otolaryngologists have the ability to restore hearing in the deaf with cochlear implantation. Although this is professionally satisfying, there exists considerable opposition to this procedure among the Deaf World. The cochlear implant community perceives deafness as a disability, seriously impacting the patient's ability to communicate and function in mainstream society. The Deaf World contends that deafness is a culturally defining condition, and implanting deaf children dilutes an entire minority class. It further contends that cochlear implants are ineffective, restrict ability to participate in sports, and delay patients' contact with their natural Deaf World culture. Last, they believe hearing parents are imposing their beliefs on their nonconsenting deaf children.

The cochlear implant community counters that people are not culturally defined by a physical defect, but rather by customs, values, and language, and that cochlear implants have been shown to be effective, especially when implanted early in life. In addition, ethical and legal history supports parents' being best equipped to make decisions in the best interest of their children.

As experts in the field of otolaryngology, we must remain open to philosophical discussion and be sensitive to the conflict between the cultural and disability viewpoints, eventually bridging the ethical divide.

New Devices and Technologies

New devices and technologies are introduced and marketed to physicians at an alarming rate. The first we hear of a new device may be from patients who present with Internet advertisements for a new device marketed to treat their specific ailment. It is therefore crucial for otolaryngologists to understand the development background, cost, and efficacy of these rapidly emerging technologies.

Although the device may have Food and Drug Administration (FDA) approval, otolaryngologists should know that more than 95% of medical devices received their FDA approval as a result of the expedited 510(k) process, given to devices with claims of being "substantially equivalent" to an existing device. As such, devices may not have demonstrated clinical efficacy prior to patient use. Physician consultants may be offered compensation for their expert guidance in product development. Although this is crucial to the appropriate development of a new technology and helps establish its efficacy, this may lead to unexpected bias in the literature or practice. Disclosure of these relationships in academics and patient consent maintains transparency. It is incumbent upon each of us to weigh the risks and benefits of using new technology, recognizing the potential for added cost and unproven efficacy. Innovation prior to proven efficacy, however, has produced now standard technologies, such as powered instrumentation and endoscopy.

Ethical Publication Standards

In an era of academic scholarly productivity, journals are flooded with publication requests. Authors should maintain ethical integrity and avoid these several common pitfalls. Ensure original information is truly original. Avoid duplicate publications from simultaneous manuscript submission, or disclose this to the editors. Be wary of digital enhancement of photos or illustrations because these could be misleading. Ensure data are presented accurately and unbiased, and maintain supporting data for a minimum of 5 to 7 years. Last, avoid "preliminary reporting" by leaking original research to the media or industry prior to publication, unless agreed upon by the editor. In 2006, the editors of many of our specialty's journals undertook a consortium approach and agreed to communicate any of the foregoing violations to each other in an effort to improve ethical publication standards.

■ Summary

We fortunately participate in one of the most respected professions in society. This responsibility cannot be taken lightly. Practice your craft with the utmost professionalism and moral character, and avoid those ethical traps inherent to careers with the allure of money and power. Many people believe the status of physicians in society has plummeted, and the reasons are elusive. Possibly the commercialization of medicine, loss of control of the physician-patient relationship to insurance companies and business entities, increasing cost of delivering health care, or overwhelming patient volume with less time to spend with patients is to blame. We must continue to live by our Code of Ethics and the words of the Hippocratic oath we once swore; may we enjoy life and art, be respected while we live and remembered with affection thereafter, may we always act so as to preserve the finest traditions of our calling, and may we long experience the joy of healing those who seek our help.

■ Suggested Reading

American Academy of Otolaryngology—Head and Neck Surgery. Code of Ethics. http://www.entnet.org/aboutus/Ethics.cfm

Cantrell RW. Medical professionalism. Arch Otolaryngol Head Neck Surg 2008;134(3):237–240

Davis DS. Cochlear implants and the claims of culture? A response to Lane and Grodin. Kennedy Inst Ethics J 1997;7(3):253–258

Gonsoulin TP. Cochlear implant/Deaf World dispute: different bottom elephants. Otolaryngol Head Neck Surg 2001;125(5):552–556

Johnson JT, Niparko JK, Levine PA, et al. Standards for ethical publication. Ear Nose Throat J 2006;85(12):792–795

Orlandi RR, Marple BF. Developing, regulating, and ethically evaluating new technologies in otolaryngology-head and neck surgery. Otolaryngol Clin North Am 2009;42(5):739–745, vii

Ryan M, Sinha M. Informed consent. In: Sanfrey H, ed. UpToDate. Waltham, MA: 2013

Sulmasy DP. Appearance and morality: ethics and otolaryngology-head and neck surgery. Otolaryngol Head Neck Surg 2002;126(1):4–7

WGBH Educational Foundation. The Hippocratic Oath: Modern Version. Doctors' Diaries

6 Pain Management

■ Introduction

The practicing otolaryngologist is confronted daily with patients experiencing acute, chronic, or cancer-related pain. Optimal management of these patients requires knowledge about the evaluation and treatment of pain and familiarity with advances in the field of pain management. Such knowledge allows clinicians to provide pain relief to their patients more effectively and to recognize those patients who would benefit from referral to a pain management specialist.

■ Evaluation

Pain is a subjective phenomenon. It is defined as an unpleasant sensory and emotional experience that is (1) associated with actual or potential tissue damage, or (2) described in terms of such damage. Evaluation begins with a medical history, a physical exam, and diagnostic studies. The pain-specific assessment includes inquiry into location, onset, description, temporal course, severity, associated symptoms, alleviating and aggravating factors, and previous treatments. On the basis of this initial evaluation, the type or classification of pain may be ascertained and treatment begun.

Pain may be classified broadly in terms of a temporal relationship as in acute pain versus chronic pain. Pain is also classified in terms of the etiology of the pain. In this classification, the pain may be acute nonmalignant pain, chronic nonmalignant pain, or malignant pain. A final useful classification is based on the pathophysiology of the pain and is described as nociceptive pain or neuropathic pain. Nociceptive pain arises from activation of peripheral pain receptors. In contrast, neuropathic pain is caused by injury to or dysfunction of the nervous system.

Nociceptive Pain

Nociceptive pain is produced by stimulation of specific sensory receptors located in tissues. With this type of pain, the neural pathways are normal and intact. In fact, nociceptive pain requires an intact sensory nervous system and involves the processes of transduction, transmission, modulation, and perception. Advances in the understanding of the neuroanatomy and neuropharmacology of these pathways have led to effective treatments targeting individual processes. Examples include the use of nonsteroidal anti-inflammatory agents to reduce the sensitivity of peripheral pain receptors, local anesthetics to block the transmission of painful impulses, and opioids to inhibit the transmission or modulate the processing of painful impulses at the central nervous system level. Nociceptive pain may be "somatic" and involve the skin and superficial structures, or it may be "visceral" and involve deep-seated structures.

Neuropathic Pain

Neuropathic pain has also been a subject of increased understanding. Neuropathic pain is caused by injury to the central or peripheral nervous system (CNS, PNS). Pain is caused when the injured nerves react abnormally to stimuli or discharge spontaneously. Neuropathic pain is described as burning, stinging, or feeling like pins and needles. Neuropathic pain is also described as shooting and lancinating. A new concept, which increases our understanding of neuropathic pain, is that the nervous system is not static; it is dynamic, with peripheral events inducing changes in the spinal cord and CNS, which in turn induce changes in the PNS. This concept would explain the various pain syndromes that persist even when there appears to be no ongoing tissue injury.

■ Pain Management

Acute and Postoperative Pain

Acute pain is not an isolated clinical event, but rather a symptom accompanying a variety of traumatic, infectious, medical, and surgical conditions. In 2012, the American Society of Anesthesiologists (ASA) published updated guidelines for acute pain management in the perioperative setting. These guidelines were developed to help clinicians assess and treat pain according to the latest knowledge, technology, and state of practice. They emphasize the assessment and prevention of pain when possible and use a health care team approach. Key points in the guidelines include the need to educate all providers, monitor and document all outcomes, and establish a dedicated acute pain service.

When pain cannot be prevented, treatment of the disease or condition responsible for the pain may reduce or eliminate the pain as a symptom. Analgesics may be indicated as an adjunct and are often a necessity in the postoperative setting. Acute pain analgesics might be broadly classified as either nonopioid, such as the nonsteroidal anti-inflammatory drugs (NSAIDs) and acetaminophen, or opioid. There are drugs that combine nonopioid agents with opioids, but these drugs are discouraged because one drug may have a dosage limitation (acetaminophen), or a ceiling of effect (e.g., nonsteroidal anti-inflammatory agents), whereas an opioid may have no ceiling. To use each drug to its maximum potential, it is better to prescribe combinations of drugs rather than the combined drugs.

Nonsteroidal Anti-inflammatory Drugs

NSAIDS provide analgesia through their effect on prostaglandin synthesis. Prostaglandins are found in most tissues and organs and they act on platelets, endothelium, and uterine and mast cells. Prostaglandins can mediate everyday physiological "housekeeping" functions, such as aiding in platelet aggregation, increasing glomerular filtration rate, and inhibiting acid secretion in the stomach, but they can also be produced in response to inflammatory stimuli, and then they can produce fever, pain, and an increased inflammatory response. Prostaglandins are synthesized via the arachidonic acid pathway and rely on the enzymatic action of cyclooxygenase isoenzymes (COX-1 and COX-2) for their synthesis. The COX-1 enzyme is produced constitutively and is responsible for the synthesis of prostaglandins important in the everyday physiological housekeeping functions. The COX-2 isoenzymes are produced in response to inflammatory stimuli; these prostaglandins induce fever, increase the inflammatory response, and can cause pain by sensitizing peripheral nociceptors. Aspirin and nonselective NSAIDs inhibit both the COX-1 and COX-2 enzymes and therefore can decrease the level of both types of prostaglandins. However, selective COX-2 inhibitors (e.g., celecoxib) selectively decrease the production of those prostaglandins associated with pain, fever, and inflammation. Acetaminophen may also be grouped under the nonopioid category. Acetaminophen has primarily central effects; it lacks peripheral anti-inflammatory effects. This means that acetaminophen lacks the NSAID gastrointestinal (GI), hepatic, renal, hematologic, and hypersensitivity side effects. Many NSAIDs are available by prescription and over the counter (OTC).

NSAIDs all have the same mechanism of action, so choice should be influenced by pharmacological parameters, such as dose and frequency, available dosage forms, side-effect profile, previous patient experience with the drug, and practitioner familiarity with the agent. Dosage forms are immediate- or sustained-release tablets and capsules, with some agents available in liquid or suppository form. Of the true NSAIDs, the nonacetylated salicylates, such as choline magnesium trisalicylate (Trilisate), salsalate (Disalcid), and diflunisal (Dolobid, Merck, Whitehouse Station, NJ) have the lowest incidence of gastric irritation and platelet dysfunction. (Note that choline magnesium trisalicylate and salsalate are no longer available in the United States.) NSAIDs that are available OTC differ from their prescription forms only in dose and, in general, represent those agents of proven analgesic efficacy and favorable side-effect profile. NSAIDs may be used in combination with opioid analgesics for additive or synergistic benefit. As a class, they do not possess opioid side effects, but they do have a limit or ceiling to their analgesic efficacy. It is advantageous to prescribe the opioid separately from the NSAID because, unlike the NSAIDs, the opioids do not have a ceiling to their analgesic efficacy. When the drugs are given as a single formulation, they cannot be titrated to effect.

Until ketorolac was introduced to the United States, postoperative use of NSAIDs was limited based on the lack of a parenteral dosage form. Ketorolac has subsequently proven useful, especially in the perioperative setting, because it does not have the cardiovascular, respiratory, or CNS depression associated with opioids, and its use in combination with opioids has an opioid-sparing effect. Ketorolac 2 mg intramuscular (IM) is approximately equianalgesic to morphine 1 mg IM. Ketorolac is usually given by the intravenous (IV) route. The IM administration is painful to the patient. Ketorolac is also available in 10 mg tablet form. The loading dose is 30 mg IV, with 30 mg IV every 6 hours. The maximum dose is 120 mg given parenterally or 40 mg orally per day. In patients over 65 years of age who weigh less than 110 pounds or have renal impairment, the foregoing parenteral doses should be reduced by half. Oral use is indicated only as a continuation therapy to parenteral therapy, and the combined use is not recommended to exceed 5 days.

Because most NSAIDs will inhibit platelet function, the surgeon needs to consider the increased risk of postoperative bleeding. However, in 2005, the Cochrane Database published a systematic review that stated NSAID use in postoperative pediatric tonsillectomies resulted in no increase in bleeding and an improvement in nausea and vomiting. The AAO-HNS tonsillectomy guideline (2011) concluded, based on this review and other supporting evidence, that NSAIDs, with the exception of ketorolac, can be safely used for the postoperative treatment of pain following tonsillectomy. In contrast, the FDA advised in 2012 that codeine should not be used after pediatric tonsillectomy because some children are ultra-rapid metabolizers who may experience death or breathing problems.

NSAIDS, which are selective COX-2 inhibitors, are sometimes recommended because they can specifically inhibit the COX-2 enzyme and decrease synthesis of the prostaglandins associated with pain, fever, and inflammation without the worry of bleeding and GI side effects that may occur when COX-1 enzymes are inhibited. If the COX-1 enzyme is inhibited, so is the synthesis of prostaglandins that promote platelet aggregation, renal glomerular filtration rate (GFR), and maintain the gastric mucosa. Celecoxib (Celebrex, Pfizer, New York, NY), which is a selective COX-2 inhibitor, has been shown to be an effective pain medication in the postoperative period and can decrease overall total opioid consumption.

In the ASA guidelines, the committee agrees that multimodal pain management should include the use of NSAIDS, selective COX-2 inhibitors, and acetaminophen used in combination with opioids. If possible, the aforementioned three medications should be used around the clock. Administration of pain medications around the clock, rather than on an as-needed basis, is preferable for the management of pain. However, one must be careful to respect the toxicity or dose limits for each drug—particularly for acetaminophen. There have been occurrences of providers giving patients combination drugs (hydrocodone 5 mg/acetaminophen 500 mg) and prescribing the combination drug every 4 hours, around the clock. Such dosing may have been acceptable for the opioid but not for the acetaminophen over several days. If acetaminophen is taken every 4 hours at 500 mg per dose, the patient may experience liver failure in 2 days. It is better to prescribe the two drugs independently.

Opioids

The term *opioid* refers to all compounds that bind to opiate receptors. Opioids used for pain are often described as "mu agonists," because their effects are mediated primarily by binding to mu receptors.

Opioids are usually necessary to treat moderate to severe postoperative pain. They may be classified as either agonists (activate receptor fully) or partial agonists/mixed agonists–antagonists. Clinical drugs that act as pure agonists are morphine, meperidine, and fentanyl/remifentanil. Naloxone is a pure antagonist, blocking the action of agonist drugs.

Partial agonists/mixed agonists–antagonists incompletely activate their receptors and thus have a limit to their analgesic efficacy. Their use may complicate the previous or subsequent administration of a pure agonist by either precipitating withdrawal or limiting the analgesic effect of the agonist. Dysphoria is a potential side effect. Nevertheless, these opioids remain a useful class in mild to moderate pain or when avoidance of opioid side effects is desirable. Examples include butorphanol, nalbuphine (Nubain, Endo Pharmaceuticals, Inc., Chadds Ford, PA), pentazocine, and dezocine (Dalgan). Currently, these drugs are rarely used and their commercial availability is mixed.

Tramadol (Ultram, Janssen Pharmaceuticals, Titusville, NJ) is a recently introduced drug that is classified as a weak or partial μ-opioid receptor agonist and may also inhibit norepinephrine and serotonin reuptake. Compared with other opioids, it has less potential for respiratory depression and the development of tolerance. Although it is indicated for the management of moderate to moderately severe pain, its role in acute pain management remains to be seen.

Pure agonists are the opioids historically and currently used in the treatment of severe acute pain, postoperative pain, and cancer pain. There is no limit (or ceiling) to their analgesic efficacy in appropriate and sufficient dosage. Significant improvements in their use reflect increased understanding of pharmacokinetics, pharmacodynamics, and advances in delivery systems. The role of pure agonists in cancer pain management is discussed separately in this chapter.

In the postoperative setting, if enteral delivery of opioids is not a viable option, the parenteral route is chosen. IM injection is strongly discouraged but may be used in select circumstances. The disadvantages of IM injection are (1) delayed onset of action, (2) unpredictable availability, (3) difficulty in titration, and (4) pain on injection. IV administration avoids these disadvantages. Patient-controlled analgesia (PCA), which allows patients to titrate their own IV opioid administration through the use of a microprocessor-controlled pump, has revolutionized postoperative pain relief. Compared with IM injections, PCA use results in (1) decreased analgesic requirements, (2) decreased sedation, (3) improved pain relief, and (4) increased patient satisfaction. Although PCA use may be perceived as a costly modality, its cost must be weighed against its many advantages. Under the direction of the acute pain service, drug, concentration, bolus amount, frequency or lockout interval, basal rate, and maximal hourly doses are determined. Supplemental orders include provision for monitoring of vital signs, the patient's level of sedation, pain intensity, and the need for adjuvant medications, as well as medications that may mitigate potential side effects, such as nausea and sedation.

Combination Drugs

Combination drugs are enteral fixed-ratio combinations of either aspirin or acetaminophen with weak- to moderate-potency opioids. They are the most widely prescribed opioid drugs for acute and postoperative pain when the patient is able to tolerate oral intake. Examples by opioid content are codeine (Tylenol No. 3), hydrocodone (Vicodin, Abbott Pharmaceuticals, North Chicago, IL; Lortab, Amneal Pharmaceuticals, Hauppauge, NY), oxycodone (Percodan, Endo Pharmaceuticals, Inc., Chadds Ford, PA: Percocet, Tylox). It should be pointed out that hydrocodone is less potent than oxycodone. To limit hepatic toxicity, the daily doses are limited according to acetaminophen content. The typical recommendation is a maximum daily dose of 4,000 mg for the nonelderly and 2,500 mg for the elderly. As a class of drugs, opioids are associated with nausea and vomiting. Probably the opioid that causes the most nausea is codeine. Many believe its use should be reserved for cough suppressants. Also, morphine releases histamine and has active metabolites. This limits its usefulness in patients with reactive airway disease or bronchospasm due to asthma, smoking, or history of COPD. In addition, morphine has active metabolites that may accumulate in patients with decreased urine output or decreased renal function, as often occurs in the perioperative period. Because fentanyl and hydromorphone do not have active metabolites, these drugs are often used preferentially over morphine to treat acute postoperative pain. The rapid onset of fentanyl makes it a favorable choice when the patient is in acute pain and rapid titration of analgesic properties is desired. Once the pain has been controlled and a longer-acting agent is desired for maintenance of pain relief, hydromorphone (Dilaudid, Purdue Pharma) is often the choice.

Chronic Pain Management

Headache and Facial Pain

Headache and facial pain are common symptoms in otolaryngological practice. These symptoms may be the result of an underlying otolaryngological disorder, or they may be caused by a disorder in which the clinician provides initial consultation prior to definitive referral. Familiarity with the latest developments in diagnosis and therapy for these conditions ultimately ensures the best patient outcome.

Headache Pain

Evaluation

Headache is the most common symptom in all clinical practice and is frequently encountered by the otolaryngologist in acute, chronic, or postoperative settings. Because the list of differential diagnoses of headache is one of the longest in medicine, a systematic approach to the diagnosis is essential. The first priority is to discern the causes of headache that are acute medical emergencies from the chronic, less emergent causes of headache. Next one must determine whether the headache represents a primary headache disorder or is associated with a concomitant medical or surgical condition.

The correct diagnosis can usually be obtained from a patient's history. Headaches that are described as the "first or worst" headache that the patient has experienced may signal that the patient has an acute subarachnoid hemorrhage. Headaches associated with neurological deficits, systemic illness, infection, exertion, Valsalva maneuver, or nocturnal or morning occurrence, may represent intracranial mass lesions, or infections, such as meningitis. Urgent neurological consultation is warranted in this small subset of patients. Key elements of a headache history, especially in a nonurgent patient, include frequency, duration, chronicity, temporal pattern, character, location, age at onset, precipitating factors, premonitory symptoms, accompanying symptoms, and previous tests and treatments. Environmental, occupational, social, allergic, drug, medical, and surgical histories complete the questioning.

Subsequent to the history, a general physical and neurological examination is performed. Laboratory tests include a complete blood count and blood chemistries. An erythrocyte sedimentation rate is ordered if there is suspicion of temporal arteritis in the elderly patient. Neuroimaging with computed tomography or magnetic resonance imaging (MRI) is indicated only if there is an abnormality in the neurological exam, because the yield in the patient with a normal exam is less than 3%. Except in rare circumstances, an electroencephalogram is not indicated.

Treatment

Common headache classifications are tension, migraine or vascular, cluster, and those due to secondary organic disorders. Regardless of the type, all headaches are mediated by the trigeminocervical nucleus and its nociceptive system. Treatment may use nonpharmacological measures, such as physical modalities, acupuncture, biofeedback, and transcutaneous electrical nerve stimulation, as well as abortive or prophylactic pharmacotherapy.

Several new developments in the understanding of the pathophysiology of headaches deserve mention. One is the increased use of NSAIDs in vascular headaches. Another is the discovery that the neurotransmitter serotonin plays an important role in the development and maintenance of these headaches. This discovery has led to the introduction of the 5-hydroxytryptamine-1D serotonin receptor agonist sumatriptan (Imitrex, GlaxoSmithKline, Philadelphia, PA). Sumatriptan, as a serotonin-1 agonist, can bind to receptors and constrict dural and pial vessels. This drug, available in IM or tablet form, has revolutionized the treatment of migraine. Contraindications to its use include complicated migraine, ischemic and uncontrolled hypertensive cardiac disease, and peripheral vascular disease.

Otolaryngological disease may specifically be involved in the pathogenesis of headache symptoms. There is now a greater awareness of the role of the nose and paranasal sinuses in headache symptoms, with up to 83% of patients improved or cured of their pain after therapy. Allergies and sleep apnea should be considered in the etiology of chronic or recurrent headache. Postoperative headaches can also be a problem, especially in acoustic neuroma surgery. The incidence of postoperative headaches is higher with the suboccipital approach, whereas bone flaps or reconstruction of the defects reduce the frequency and intensity of these headaches.

Facial Pain

Neuropathic facial pain may be a primary disorder, or it may result from trauma, surgery, infection, neoplasm, or antineoplastic chemotherapy. The common denominator in these neuralgic conditions is dysfunction of, or injury to, a sensory nerve, usually the trigeminal or glossopharyngeal, and rarely the vagus.

Trigeminal Neuralgia

Trigeminal neuralgia, or tic douloureux, is a distinctive unilateral, lancinating facial pain in the distribution of the fifth cranial nerve, most commonly the second or third division or both. Although trigeminal neuralgia is a primary disorder not associated with trauma or surgery, MRI often shows vascular compression of the nerve as it exits the pons in the posterior fossa. The treatment of choice is pharmacological, and the drug of choice is carbamazepine (Tegretol, Novartis, New York, NY). Other effective drugs include anticonvulsants, such as diphenylhydantoin (Dilantin) and gabapentin (Neurontin), and the skeletal muscle relaxant baclofen (Lioresal). For patients whose pharmacological therapy fails or is accompanied by adverse side effects, anesthetic and neurosurgical procedures are indicated.

Percutaneous gasserian gangliolysis has been the procedure of choice for trigeminal neuralgia. Initially performed with chemical neurolytic agents, the procedure is now more commonly performed by radiofrequency thermal ablation. This technique avoids the anesthesia, dysesthesia, and short-lived relief of peripheral branch procedures. The most recent advance is intracranial microvascular decompression (Jannetta procedure), which is the procedure of choice in patients in whom nerve compression has been demonstrated by MRI or in those who have failed gasserian gangliolysis. The reported success rate is in excess of 80%.

Pain may also occur in the distribution of the trigeminal nerve because of trauma, surgery, infection, neoplasia, and other causes. This pain is different from that of classic trigeminal neuralgia. It tends to be more constant and is often accompanied by anesthesia and dysesthesia in the affected sensory distribution. Treatment begins with antidepressants and progresses to anticonvulsants and other neuropathic pain drugs.

Herpes Zoster and Postherpetic Neuralgia

Herpes zoster, postherpetic neuralgia, and sympathetically mediated pain may also occur in the distribution of the trigeminal nerve.

Chickenpox, which usually occurs in children and young adults, is caused by infection with varicella zoster virus. However, once the short-lived chickenpox episode has resolved, the virus is not eliminated from the body. In fact, herpes zoster is the reactivation of the latent varicella zoster or chickenpox virus. Involvement of the trigeminal ganglion may occur, and the most worrisome finding is the involvement of the ophthalmic division that supplies the cornea. Ptosis and Argyll Robertson pupil (a pupil that accommodates but does not react to light) may also be seen. Involvement of the geniculate ganglion can cause Ramsay Hunt syndrome, symptoms of which include Bell palsy, vestibulocochlear dysfunction, and vesicular rash of the external auditory canal. Antivirals such as acyclovir and valacyclovir shorten the acute episode, decrease pain, promote healing, and reduce the incidence of postherpetic neuralgia. Combination therapy of gabapentin and nortriptyline are efficacious in treating the neuropathic pain. Antidepressants, anticonvulsants, steroids, and nerve blocks are also useful for symptom control. Capsaicin (Zostrix, Qutenza) is also useful because it depletes substance P, a neuropeptide neurotransmitter involved in the transmission of painful stimuli.

Glossopharyngeal Neuralgia

Glossopharyngeal neuralgia presents with otalgia and odynophagia and may be triggered by actions such as swallowing. It is much less common than trigeminal neuralgia, with a relative frequency of 0.2 to 1.3%. Trauma, surgery, neoplasia, and an elongated styloid process (Eagle syndrome) are some of the causes.

Glossopharyngeal neuralgia has received greater attention recently due to the concomitant occurrence of the carotid sinus syndrome and the glossopharyngeal neuralgia asystole syndrome. In these syndromes, abnormal afferent activity in the glossopharyngeal nerve triggers reflex efferent activity in the vagus nerve, resulting in bradycardia or asystole in the extreme. Pain may be absent. Initial treatment involves administration of carbamazepine (Tegretol). In refractory patients, neurodestructive procedures, such as neurectomy or microvascular decompression, would be appropriate.

Complex Regional Pain Syndrome (CRPS)

This group of chronic pain conditions was once called reflex sympathetic dystrophy. Complex regional pain syndrome (CRPS) is thought to be due to dysfunction in the central or peripheral nervous system. After the syndrome has been triggered, high levels of nerve impulses are sent to an affected site. CRPS is rare in the head and neck, and instead typically occurs in the limbs following an injury. In addition to pain, symptoms may include other disturbances, such as sensory (hyperalgesia, hyperesthenia), motor (paresis, tremor, dystonia, tremor), and autonomic (skin color and temperature, sweating) problems. It may by clinically impossible to predict which facial pain of patients has a sympathetic component. A high index of suspicion is warranted, because delayed treatment has a worse prognosis. Stellate ganglion block is diagnostic and may be therapeutic. Patients with suspected CRPS are best managed by a neurologist.

Management of Head and Neck Cancer Pain

Along with the potential functional limitations and changes in appearance that accompany head and neck cancer, the prospect of suffering from unrelieved pain is one of the most feared aspects of a cancer diagnosis. According to 1994 American Cancer Society statistics, 75% of patients with advanced disease have pain; of those, 50% experience moderate to severe pain, and 25% experience very severe pain.

Because worldwide cancer pain has been underrecognized and undertreated, the World Health Organization (WHO) in 1986 released the three-step analgesic ladder pain relief guidelines. Subsequently, in 1994 the Agency for Health Care Policy and Research (AHCPR) (now the Agency for Healthcare Research and Quality [AHRQ]) of the U.S. Department of Health and Human Services released guidelines for cancer pain management that amplify the WHO guidelines. Since then, WHO has released additional updates, which can be accessed via the Web site http://www.who.int/cancer/palliative/en/. For the physician treating head and neck cancer, review of these clinical practice guidelines will assist in pain assessment, pain treatment, understanding barriers to effective pain management, and indications for referral to a pain management specialist.

Pain-Specific Assessment

Assessment is the most important component of cancer pain management because failure to comprehensively evaluate the patient is the most common reason for unrelieved pain. A pain-specific assessment should be performed in addition to the history, physical examination, and diagnostic workup. The pain-specific assessment involves inquiry into the location, onset and pattern, description, severity, alleviating and aggravating factors, associated symptoms, previous treatments, and effect of the pain upon the patient. The goals of assessment are to ascertain the type of pain, determine its etiology, consider the possible presence of a specific pain syndrome, and formulate a management plan.

Pain accompanies both disease and therapy and may have multiple simultaneous causes. Soft tissue, neural, and osseous invasion is responsible for disease-related pain, with chemotherapy, radiotherapy, and surgery responsible for therapy-related pain. Specific pain syndromes can be found in each category.

Pain Management Options

Pain management options include chemotherapy, radiotherapy, surgery, pharmacological therapy, invasive techniques, physical interventions, and psychosocial interventions. Curative treatment of disease is paramount, but palliative therapy is indicated at any point. Some pain management options are both curative and palliative. Pharmacological therapy is the main focus of the WHO and AHCPR guidelines, because 80 to 90% of pain can be adequately relieved by using the three-step analgesic ladder as the framework for an individualized regimen.

Nonsteroidal Anti-inflammatory Drugs and Weak and Strong Opioids

The first step of the conceptual ladder is the use of NSAIDs, unless their use is contraindicated. Second and third steps on the ladder are the use of weak opioids and then strong opioids in addition to the NSAIDs, with adjuvant drugs being added at any step. Examples of weak opioids are codeine (Tylenol No. 3), hydrocodone (Vicodin, Lortab), oxycodone (Percocet, Tylox), and tapentadol (Nucynta). Many of the weak opioids are formulated as fixed-dose combinations with acetaminophen or aspirin. Strong opioids include morphine, hydromorphone (Dilaudid, Exalgo), oxymorphone (Opana), methadone (Dolophine), and fentanyl (Duragesic, Actiq, Onsolis, Fentora). Adjuvant drugs may be used to treat specific types of pain or to treat side effects of other medications or treatment modalities.

Opioid Analgesics

Opioid analgesics are the cornerstone of pharmacological therapy. Their effective use requires individualization of the route, dosage, and schedule of administration. The oral route is preferable because it is convenient, simple, and cost-effective. Tablet, capsule, and liquid preparations are available. Alternative routes are transmucosal, rectal, transdermal, subcutaneous, IV, epidural, and intrathecal. Constant blood levels are desirable to maximize pain relief and minimize side effects. This may be achieved by the frequent administration of a short-acting agent, but it is more conveniently accomplished, once the initial pain has been controlled, by use of a long-acting or time-release preparation.

Over the past decade oxycodone (OxyContin) and fentanyl (Duragesic) have joined morphine sulfate (MSContin) as long-acting preparations. Additionally hydromorphone (Exalgo), oxymorphone (Opana), and tapentadol (Nucynta ER) have been introduced to the U.S. market. However, long-acting drugs should not be used for breakthrough pain because of the delays associated with their absorption and the attainment of steady-state concentrations.

Breakthrough pain should be treated with immediate-release preparations. Partial agonists and mixed agonists-antagonists, such as buprenorphine, dezocine, pentazocine, butorphanol, and nalbuphine, are not recommended because they have a limit to their analgesic efficacy. In contrast, the pure agonists have no ceiling or maximum dose so immediate-release morphine 15 to 60 mg given orally or oral transmucosal fentanyl citrate, in addition to the usual pain regimen, is usually effective for breakthrough pain. Meperidine (Demerol) is also not recommended, because it has an active metabolite, normeperidine, which can behave as a neurotoxic metabolite, causing seizures with prolonged use. If one agent is ineffective or is accompanied by adverse side effects, another should be substituted because of the phenomenon of incomplete cross-tolerance. Side effects seen classwide with all opioid agents include respiratory depression, sedation, constipation, nausea and vomiting, pruritus, and urinary retention; these should be anticipated and treated.

Analgesic Adjuvants

Analgesic adjuvants include antidepressants, anticonvulsants, steroids, stimulants, antiemetics, and miscellaneous other agents. Antidepressants are useful in neuropathic pain, with the newer serotonin norepinephrine reuptake inhibitors, such as duloxetine (Cymbalta) and milnacipran (Savella) gaining popularity. Selective serotonin reuptake inhibitors have no role in pain management. Gabapentin (Neurontin) is joined by pregabalin (Lyrica) as the newest anticonvulsant used in pain management. Their advantages include lack of toxicity and no requirement for laboratory testing during use. Ondansetron (Zofran), a 5-hydroxytriptamine antagonist, is a new antiemetic used in the perioperative setting, during chemotherapy, and in pain management. Its advantage is its efficacy and lack of side effects, specifically the extrapyramidal reactions that may be seen with prochlorperazine (Compazine) or metoclopramide (Reglan).

Invasive Options

In the 10 to 20% of patients who do not obtain satisfactory relief of pain by conventional therapy, invasive options, such as neurodestructive procedures, nerve blocks, and epidural and intrathecal opioids may be indicated. Neurodestructive procedures, most commonly performed in the head and neck cancer patient, are trigeminal and glossopharyngeal nerve ablations by radiofrequency or by the use of neurolytic agents. However, overlapping innervation, adjacent vital anatomical structures, and the distortion of normal anatomy due to surgery and radiotherapy limit the application of these procedures.

Nerve blocks may be classified as diagnostic, therapeutic, and prognostic. Diagnostic blocks determine the etiology of the pain and may be classified as somatic, visceral, or sympathetic. Examples of therapeutic blocks are trigger-point injections for myofascial pain, subcutaneous infiltration for herpes zoster, and stellate ganglion blocks for CRPS. Prognostic blocks are performed prior to neurolytic procedures. Intraspinal (epidural and intrathecal) opioids may be indicated in pain unrelieved by conventional techniques or accompanied by intractable side effects. Multiple systems are available to deliver opioids epidurally or intrathecally. The most sophisticated is the totally implantable computer-programmable infusion pump.

Multifactorial Pain

In the head and neck cancer patient, pain is often multifactorial, with soft tissue, osseous, and neural invasion. Normal anatomy and physiological processes are distorted, and pain is often aggravated by movement or speaking and swallowing. For the various skull base metastasis syndromes that may occur, diagnosis depends on a high index of suspicion and appropriate diagnostic imaging. The trigeminal, facial, glossopharyngeal, vagus, spinal accessory, and hypoglossal nerves may also be affected, along with branches of the cervical plexus.

Pain may be chemotherapy related (such as mucositis), radiation related (such as mucositis, trismus, and osteoradionecrosis), and postsurgically related (such as in the post radical neck dissection syndrome). In intractable pain, a trial of antibiotics may be considered because of unrecognized local infection.

An excellent review of pain syndromes in head and neck cancer is that of Greenslade and Portenoy.

■ Summary

Barriers to effective acute, chronic, and cancer pain management include (1) those unique to the health care system, (2) those related to patients (such as failure to report pain, and poor compliance with medication), and (3) those related to health care professionals. Health care professional problems primarily relate to inadequate assessment, inadequate treatment, the need for further education, and failure to refer patients to a pain management specialist when indicated.

Assessment is such a key element to the proper management of pain that the American Pain Society, as part of its quality improvement guidelines, has recommended the charting and display of patients' self-report of pain intensity as an additional vital sign. These data should alert clinicians to consider further analgesic modalities or referral for specialized pain management consultation.

The following are indications for referral:

- Uncertainty regarding type of pain or syndrome
- Inadequate pain relief or adverse side effects
- Desire of patient or physician
- Complex or difficult cases
- Specific pain syndromes
- Desirability of multidisciplinary consultation

Educational issues are continually being addressed by various organizations. The inclusion of this chapter in a recertification study guide demonstrates the importance of pain management in today's health care environment.

■ Controversies

- Concerns about side effects, long-term efficacy, functional outcomes, and the potential for drug abuse in patients taking opioids can lead to controversies in prescribing opioids.
- Perceived and real risks associated with regulatory and legal scrutiny can result in hesitance to prescribe opioids.
- The use of opioids for chronic pain in patients with non-cancer-related pain is controversial.
- Safe driving recommendations. Opioid drugs have the highest incidence of medication-related patient harm of any kind.
- The distinction between physical dependence and addiction.

■ Practice Guidelines, Consensus Statements, and Measures

Agency for Health Care Policy Research. Clinical Practice Guideline. Acute Pain Management: Operative or Medical Procedures and Trauma. Washington, DC: U.S. Department of Health and Human Services, AHCPR; 1992

Agency for Health Care Policy Research. Clinical Practice Guideline. Management of Cancer Pain. Washington, DC: U.S. Department of Health and Human Services, AHCPR; 1994

American Society of Anesthesiologists Task Force on Acute Pain Management. Practice guidelines for acute pain management in the perioperative setting: an updated report by the American Society of Anesthesiologists Task Force on Acute Pain Management. Anesthesiology 2012;116(2):248–273

World Health Organization. Cancer: Palliative Care. http://www.who.int/cancer/palliative/en/

■ Suggested Reading

American Pain Society Quality of Care Committee. Quality improvement guidelines for the treatment of acute pain and cancer pain. JAMA 1995;274(23):1874–1880

Bogduk N. Anatomy and physiology of headache. Biomed Pharmacother 1995;49(10):435–445

Cardwell M, Siviter G, Smith A. Non-steroidal anti-inflammatory drugs and perioperative bleeding in paediatric tonsillectomy. Cochrane Database Syst Rev 2005;18(2):CD003591

Chow JM. Rhinologic headaches. Otolaryngol Head Neck Surg 1994;111(3 Pt 1):211–218

Derry S, Moore RA. Single dose oral celecoxib for acute postoperative pain in adults. Cochrane Database Syst Rev 2012;3:CD004233

Evans RW. Diagnostic testing for the evaluation of headaches. Neurol Clin 1996;14(1):1–26

Ferrante FM, Ostheimer GW, Covino BG, eds. Patient-Controlled Analgesia. Chicago, IL: Blackwell; 1990

FitzGerald GA, Patrono C. The coxibs, selective inhibitors of cyclooxygenase-2. N Engl J Med 2001;345(6):433–442

Gilron I, Bailey JM, Tu D, Holden RR, Jackson AC, Houlden RL. Nortriptyline and gabapentin, alone and in combination for neuropathic pain: a double-blind, randomised controlled crossover trial. Lancet 2009;374(9697):1252–1261

Laghmari M, El Ouahabi A, Arkha Y, Derraz S, El Khamlichi A. Are the destructive neurosurgical techniques as effective as microvascular decompression in the management of trigeminal neuralgia? Surg Neurol 2007;68(5):505–512

Marcus DA. Serotonin and its role in headache pathogenesis and treatment. Clin J Pain 1993;9(3):159–167

Pedrosa CA, Ahern DK, McKenna MJ, Ojemann RG, Acquadro MA. Determinants and impact of headache after acoustic neuroma surgery. Am J Otol 1994;15(6):793–797

Poceta JS, Dalessio DJ. Identification and treatment of sleep apnea in patients with chronic headache. Headache 1995;35(10):586–589

Schuller DE, Cadman TE, Jeffreys WH. Recurrent headaches: what every allergist should know. Ann Allergy Asthma Immunol 1996;76(3):219–226, quiz 226–230

Yaksh TL, Luo DZ. Dynamics of the pain processing system. In: Waldman SD, ed. Waldman: Pain Management. Philadelphia, PA: Elsevier; 2011:19–30

7 Blood Transfusion Medicine and Coagulation Disorders

■ Introduction

The first successful transfusion of human blood was performed in 1818 by British obstetrician James Blundell for the treatment of postpartum hemorrhage. Many of the inherent risks at that time were unknown, since the type ABO blood groups and many infectious agents were not yet discovered. Red blood cells (RBCs) are used to improve oxygen delivery to tissues in situations of hemorrhage and anemia. Surgeons must weigh the life-saving benefits of blood transfusion against the risks of adverse reaction and transmitted infectious disease, while considering appropriate resource allocation and alternatives to transfusion.

■ Evaluation and Screening

Risks of Transfusion

Blood transfusion has the potential to transmit viruses, such as human immunodeficiency virus (HIV), hepatitis B virus (HBV), hepatitis C virus (HCV), and human T-lymphotropic virus (HTLV). Infected donors can transmit malaria, parasites, and prion disease as well. Bacterial infections and sepsis can also occur with RBC transfusion, although this risk is higher in platelet transfusion due to higher storage temperatures.

The World Health Organization recommends that all blood donations be screened for HIV, HBV, HCV and syphilis prior to use. Each unit of donated blood in the United States undergoes the following tests:

1. HBV surface antigen
2. Antibody to HBV core
3. Antibody to HCV
4. Antibody to HIV type 1 and 2
5. Antibody to HTLV type I and II
6. Syphilis testing
7. Nucleic acid testing (NAT) for HIV 1 and HCV

NAT was implemented for blood donation screening in the United States in 1999; it provides a more direct assay by testing for viral ribonucleic acid (RNA), rather than host antibodies to the virus. NAT decreases the testing window period, or the time between infection and the time a test detects a change (period for a false-negative test result), for HIV 1 and HCV in the blood supply. Statistics stated herein will be specific for the United States.

Human Immunodeficiency Virus Infection

The risk of being infected by HIV from a blood transfusion is estimated at ~ 1 in 1.5 million. The window period of infectivity for newly infected individuals to transmit the virus before it is detectable by NAT is ~ 11 days, down from 56 days by the first-generation enzyme-linked immunosorbent assay (ELISA) anti-HIV antibody testing in the 1980s, and 33 and 22 days, respectively, for second- and third-generation tests.

Hepatitis B Infection

Public health agencies estimate that 1.25 million people in the United States are infected with HBV, and 2 billion people are infected worldwide. Approximately 10% of these cases will result in chronic HBV infection, with increased incidence of cirrhosis and liver cancer. The window period for HBV surface antigen (HBsAg) and HBV core antibody (anti-HBc) is roughly 30 to 38 days. Risk for HBV infection from a blood transfusion is estimated to range from 1 to 8 in 1 million. Although this risk is higher than the risk of HIV or HCV transmission, the widespread vaccination for HBV in donors and recipients in the United States has resulted in the prevention of clinical disease in some of the cases of HBV transmission. Since ultrasensitive HBV surface antigen screening was implemented, no documented cases of HBV transmission through transfusion in the United States have occurred from 2006 through 2011.

Hepatitis C Infection

Blood transfusion recipients have a 1 in 1,150,000 risk of being infected with HCV, a causative agent for cirrhosis and hepatocellular carcinoma. Anti-HCV antibody testing alone leaves an infectious window period of 70 days. This has been reduced to 12 days with the implementation of HCV NAT. Because no effective HCV vaccine currently exists, thorough pre-donation screening questionnaires and continued advances in laboratory detection are critical.

Human T-Lymphotropic Virus Infection

HTLV is estimated to infect 15 to 20 million people worldwide. Of these, 2 to 10% will develop an associated disease, such as adult T cell leukemia/lymphoma, or tropical spastic paraparesis/HTLV-1-associated myelopathy. There is very limited literature concerning transfusion- or transplant-related HTLV transmission resulting in one of these diseases. One study showed that in 15 HTLV-1-infected renal transplant patients, no myelopathy or adult T cell lymphoma developed during follow-up for 1 to 10 years.

Posttransfusion Bacterial Infections and Sepsis

Posttransfusion bacterial infections and sepsis are complications of blood product usage worldwide. These are the predominant areas for improvement in Western countries, where modern laboratory screening has already significantly diminished rates of viral infection. Bacterial contamination is more prevalent in platelets, which are stored at 24°C, compared with RBCs stored at 4°C.

Pathogen Inactivation

Recent efforts to reduce the incidence of transfusion-transmitted infections have also focused on pathogen inactivation (PI) after blood is donated. HBV transmission risk has been reported to be nearly 100% eliminated from platelets and plasma in the nations where PI has been implemented, although this has not yet been developed for whole blood and RBCs. Similar results for PI for HCV transmission have been seen in vitro. In the future, effective PI through a variety of methods currently under investigation has the potential to reduce the costs of testing in developing countries and to significantly impact worldwide health.

ABO Incompatibility

ABO incompatibility is a very rare complication of blood transfusion, thanks to multiple layers of safety implemented by blood banks and clinical staff. Of more than 23 million U.S. blood component transfusions (RBCs, platelets, plasma, and cryoprecipitate) in 2008, 39 acute ABO incompatibility reactions occurred, making the risk of an ABO incompatibility/acute hemolysis ~ 1 in 600,000.

Cost of a Blood Transfusion

The cost of a blood transfusion is not insignificant. Although the payment for a single unit of packed RBCs has been estimated at $233, the total cost incurred with collection, storage, and administration derived from four U.S. and European hospitals is on the order of $761 per unit.

■ Management

Guidelines for Transfusion

Historically, the widely accepted clinical standard was to transfuse patients when the hemoglobin level dropped below 10 g/dL or the hematocrit fell below 30%. This "10/30 rule" was first proposed by Adams and Lundy in 1942 and served as an RBC transfusion trigger for decades. In the 1970s, cardiac surgery for coronary artery disease drastically increased demand for blood resources and prompted consideration of more restrictive thresholds for transfusion of RBCs. Liberal transfusion triggers, such as the 10/30 rule, have not been shown to improve outcomes over more restrictive triggers, which decrease demand on blood resources, risk of infection, and adverse events.

In 2009, a U.S. practice management guideline was developed by a joint taskforce of the Eastern Association for Surgery of Trauma and the American College of Critical Care Medicine. This comprehensive literature review of data, published in the United States, Canada, western Europe, and the United Kingdom from 1980 through 2006, performed a scientific grading of evidence and recommendations. Level 1 recommendations supported transfusion in patients with hemorrhagic shock, and for those with acute hemorrhage and hemodynamic instability or inadequate oxygen delivery. The study also supported a "restrictive" strategy of RBC transfusion (transfuse when hemoglobin [Hb] < 7 g/dL), which is as effective as a "liberal" transfusion strategy (transfuse when Hb < 10 g/dL) in critically ill patients with hemodynamically stable anemia. This was not applicable to patients with evidence of myocardial ischemia. In addition, a level 2 recommendation was made to transfuse RBC one unit at a time in the absence of acute hemorrhage.

A Cochrane review comparing clinical outcomes in patients randomized to restrictive versus liberal transfusion thresholds was published in 2012. Available data were pooled from 19 studies with 6,264 patients over a 55-year period ending in 2011. There was considerable variability between studies, with some published restrictive strategies using an Hb trigger of 7 to 9 g/dL, whereas some of the liberal strategies targeted an Hb of 12 g/dL, or "normal." The authors concluded that, in patients who do not have acute coronary artery disease, blood transfusion can probably be withheld in the presence of hemoglobin levels as low as 7 to 8 g/dL as long as there is no notable bleeding. In the setting of acute coronary syndrome, there was no evidence to guide treatment. This study also reported that the benefits of minimizing allogeneic RBC transfusion are likely to be greatest in underdeveloped regions where there is doubt about the safety of the blood supply.

Limiting Blood Transfusion

Alternatives to blood transfusion offer another avenue for decreasing demand for blood products, transmitted infection, and adverse events. Minimizing intraoperative blood loss, preserving normothermia with warming blankets, and using pediatric tubes for phlebotomy can all contribute to lowering rates of transfusion. Stimulating increased RBC production with recombinant human erythropoietin has been shown to decrease transfusion requirements in intensive care unit patients in multiple well-designed prospective trials. Use of crystalloid and colloid products, such as albumin and hetastarch, can effectively expand the circulating blood volume and in most cases should be implemented before considering blood products.

Preoperative Autologous Blood Donation

Preoperative autologous blood donation (PABD) was recommended in the early 1980s due to concerns about transmission of HIV. The current very low risk of transfusion-transmitted infection from allogeneic blood in the United States makes PABD not cost-effective. PABD patients have been shown to be transfused more often with their own blood and banked blood products. The risk of hemolytic transfusion reaction with PABD is not reduced, given that clerical error rates are similar for autologous and allogeneic transfusion. The cost of PABD is significantly higher than with using allogeneic blood because more than 50% of PABD units are never used. PABD is still used in orthopedic total joint surgery and cardiovascular surgery, and it still has a role in patients with rare blood groups, or those who will not consent to allogeneic blood.

Normovolemic Hemodilution

Normovolemic hemodilution (NH) is an autotransfusion procedure that was introduced in the 1970s. Three or four units of blood are removed from the patient after induction of anesthesia and are replaced with colloid or crystalloid. After a large intraoperative blood loss, the units are returned to circulation. Multiple meta-analyses in the past 15 years have shown that NH does not significantly reduce the need for allogeneic transfusion and has led to increased bleeding in cardiac, liver, and thoracic surgery. Currently one of the only roles for NH is in the management of Jehovah's Witnesses, who find it acceptable that the blood removed remains in a closed circuit with their own circulation.

Cell Saver

Use of a cell saver to recover blood during surgery is another method of reducing the need for allogeneic blood transfusion. This method has traditionally been avoided in oncological surgery because of concern for reinfusing malignant cells into circulation. Through the use of leucodepletion filters and radiation of the RBCs (25 gray [Gy]) prior to reinfusion, multiple studies in urological surgery have shown no increased risk of cancer recurrence. Leucodepletion filters have also been shown to significantly reduce bacterial contamination in salvaged blood.

Topical Fibrin Sealant

Topical fibrin sealant has been employed in surgery for more than 20 years. In January 2012, the U.S. Food and Drug Administration approved fibrin sealant to include general hemostasis in surgery when control of bleeding by standard surgical techniques is ineffective or impractical. The main components of fibrin sealant are calcium chloride, fibrinogen, factor XIII, and thrombin. Pooled human plasma is the source of the fibrinogen and thrombin. The final phase of the coagulation cascade is reproduced during application of this product when thrombin activates fibrinogen to create a fibrin clot. Fibrin sealant can minimize the use of blood transfusion by controlling bleeding in select cases. It is also used in head and neck surgery to aid in repair of skull base defects and chylous fistula, among other uses.

Hemoglobin-Based Oxygen Carriers

On the frontier of transfusion medicine are RBC substitutes. Hemoglobin-based oxygen carriers (HBOCs) are currently in phase 3 clinical trials in the United States. This latest generation of HBOCs is polymerized hemoglobin solutions, made from either bovine RBCs or outdated human RBCs. Among the potential benefits of HBOCs are prolonged shelf life at room temperature, universal compatibility, no disease transmission or antigenic reaction, and abundant supply.

Preoperative Coagulation Screening

Routine use of laboratory coagulation screening, such as prothrombin time (PT) and activated partial thromboplastin time (aPTT), to predict postoperative bleeding risk in unselected patients has not been shown to be clinically useful. The American Academy of Otolaryngology–Head and Neck Surgery's clinical indicators have suggested that a preoperative coagulation workup is necessary only "if an abnormality is suspected by history or genetic information is not available." The 2008 British Committee for Standards in Hematology recommended against universal screening but suggested that a structured bleeding history be obtained prior to surgery. Most published bleeding questionnaires acquire information on easy bleeding or bruising of the patient; family history of severe bleeding, coagulopathy, or blood transfusions; and drugs that affect coagulation. In an Austrian multicenter prospective observational study of more than 3,000 adult tonsillectomies, a positive history of coagulopathy on a standardized questionnaire doubled the risk of postoperative bleeding. Similar results have been seen in pediatric adenotonsillectomy patients when standardized bleeding questionnaires were obtained preoperatively. Tailoring laboratory testing to only those patients at highest risk for postoperative bleeding affords the clinician a higher yield in detecting clinically relevant coagulopathy and initiating further hematologic evaluation.

Postoperative Deep Venous Thromboembolism Prophylaxis

Approximately 900,000 cases of deep venous thromboembolism (DVT) and pulmonary embolism (PE) occur annually in the United States. This leads to longer hospital stays, increased costs, and higher mortality. Evidence-based clinical practice guidelines have been created for procedures in several surgical specialties that have the highest risk of DVT and PE. The American College of Chest Physicians (ACCP) published its updated thromboprophylaxis guidelines in February 2012. These guidelines apply specifically to orthopedic surgery procedures. To date no specific guidelines have been developed for head and neck surgical procedures. The incidence of DVT and PE is significantly lower in head and neck surgical patients, and the risk of postoperative bleeding, neck hematoma, and resulting airway compromise has been estimated to be 10-fold higher than the risk of DVT in one review of 16,000 thyroidectomy and parathyroidectomy patients in the American College of Surgeons NSQIP database.

Otolaryngologists must assess each of their surgical patients and formulate a postoperative thromboprophylaxis plan. Intermittent pneumatic compression devices (IPCDs) and early ambulation make up a common strategy. The goal for IPCD should be 18 hours per day of compliance. The addition of a pharmacological agent, such as low molecular weight heparin, should be considered in those patients deemed to be at higher risk for DVT and PE. Individual risk factors to be considered include previous DVT/PE, body mass index > 25, cardiovascular disease, and age > 85 years. These must be weighed against the risk of surgical site bleeding complications.

■ Practice Guidelines, Consensus Statements, and Measures

American Academy of Otolaryngology-Head and Neck Surgery. Clinical indicators: tonsillectomy, adenoidectomy, adenotonsillectomy in childhood. http://www.entnet.org/Practice/upload/TA_Adenotonsillectomy-CI_May-2012-2.pdf

Falck-Ytter Y, Francis CW, Johanson NA, et al; American College of Chest Physicians. Prevention of VTE in orthopedic surgery patients: Antithrombotic Therapy and Prevention of Thrombosis, 9th ed: American College of Chest Physicians Evidence-Based Clinical Practice Guidelines. Chest 2012;141(2 Suppl):e278S–e325S

Napolitano LM, Kurek S, Luchette FA, et al; American College of Critical Care Medicine of the Society of Critical Care Medicine; Eastern Association for the Surgery of Trauma Practice Management Workgroup. Clinical practice guideline: red blood cell transfusion in adult trauma and critical care. Crit Care Med 2009;37(12):3124–3157

■ Suggested Reading

Advancing Transfusion and Cellular Therapies Worldwide (AABB). http://www.aabb.org/resources/bct/Pages/bloodfaq.aspx

Candotti D, Allain JP. Transfusion-transmitted hepatitis B virus infection. J Hepatol 2009;51(4):798–809

Carless P, Moxey A, O'Connell D, Henry D. Autologous transfusion techniques: a systematic review of their efficacy. Transfus Med 2004;14(2):123–144

Carson JL, Carless PA, Hebert PC. Transfusion thresholds and other strategies for guiding allogeneic red blood cell transfusion. Cochrane Database Syst Rev 2012;4:CD002042

Chee YL, Crawford JC, Watson HG, Greaves M; British Committee for Standards in Haematology. Guidelines on the assessment of bleeding risk prior to surgery or invasive procedures. Br J Haematol 2008;140(5):496–504

Dwyre DM, Fernando LP, Holland PV. Hepatitis B, hepatitis C and HIV transfusion-transmitted infections in the 21st century. Vox Sang 2011;100(1):92–98

Food and Drug Administration. http://www.fda.gov/downloads/BiologicsBloodVaccines/BloodBloodProducts/ApprovedProducts/LicensedProductsBLAs/FractionatedPlasmaProducts

Heit JA. The epidemiology of venous thromboembolism in the community. Arterioscler Thromb Vasc Biol 2008;28(3):370–372

Licameli GR, Jones DT, Santosuosso J, Lapp C, Brugnara C, Kenna MA. Use of a preoperative bleeding questionnaire in pediatric patients who undergo adenotonsillectomy. Otolaryngol Head Neck Surg 2008;139(4):546–550

Liumbruno GM, Bennardello F, Lattanzio A, Piccoli P, Rossetti G; Italian Society of Transfusion Medicine and Immunohaematology (SIMTI) Working Party. Recommendations for the transfusion management of patients in the peri-operative period. I. The pre-operative period. Blood Transfus 2011;9(1):19–40

Liumbruno GM, Bennardello F, Lattanzio A, Piccoli P, Rossetti G; Italian Society of Transfusion Medicine and Immunohaematology (SIMTI) Working Party. Recommendations for the transfusion management of patients in the peri-operative period. II. The intra-operative period. Blood Transfus 2011;9(2):189–217

Madjdpour C, Spahn DR. Allogeneic red blood cell transfusions: efficacy, risks, alternatives and indications. Br J Anaesth 2005;95(1):33–42

Moore EE, Johnson JL, Moore FA, Moore HB. The USA Multicenter Prehosptial Hemoglobin-based Oxygen Carrier Resuscitation Trial: scientific rationale, study design, and results. Crit Care Clin 2009;25(2):325–356

Pape A, Habler O. Alternatives to allogeneic blood transfusions. Best Pract Res Clin Anaesthesiol 2007;21(2):221–239

Roy M, Rajamanickam V, Chen H, Sippel R. Is DVT prophylaxis necessary for thyroidectomy and parathyroidectomy? Surgery 2010;148(6):1163–1168, discussion 1168–1169

Sarny S, Ossimitz G, Habermann W, Stammberger H. Preoperative coagulation screening prior to tonsillectomy in adults: current practice and recommendations. Eur Arch Otorhinolaryngol 2013;270(3):1099–1104

Segal JB, Dzik WH; Transfusion Medicine/Hemostasis Clinical Trials Network. Paucity of studies to support that abnormal coagulation test results predict bleeding in the setting of invasive procedures: an evidence-based review. Transfusion 2005;45(9):1413–1425

Srámek A, Eikenboom JC, Briët E, Vandenbroucke JP, Rosendaal FR. Usefulness of patient interview in bleeding disorders. Arch Intern Med 1995;155(13):1409–1415

Stramer SL, Wend U, Candotti D, et al. Nucleic acid testing to detect HBV infection in blood donors. N Engl J Med 2011;364(3): 236–247

Vaiman M, Eviatar E. Lymphatic fistulae after neck dissection: the fibrin sealant treatment. J Surg Oncol 2008;98(6):467–471

Waters JH. Red blood cell recovery and reinfusion. Anesthesiol Clin North America 2005;23(2):283–294, vi

Whitaker BJ, Schlumpf K, Schulman J, Green J. The 2009 National Blood Collection and Utilization Survey Report. Washington, DC: U.S. Department of Health and Human Services, Office of the Assistant Secretary for Health; 2011

World Health Organization. Blood safety and availability. Fact sheet No. 279. June 2012. http://www.who.int/mediacentre/factsheets/fs279/en/

World Health Organization. Hepatitis B Fact sheet No. 204. July 2012. http://www.who.int/mediacentre/factsheets/fs204/en/index.html

Zou S, Dorsey KA, Notari EP, et al. Prevalence, incidence, and residual risk of human immunodeficiency virus and hepatitis C virus infections among United States blood donors since the introduction of nucleic acid testing. Transfusion 2010;50(7):1495–1504

8 Universal Precautions

■ Introduction

The concept of universal precautions became a new reality in the mid-1980s with the rise of the human immunodeficiency virus (HIV) epidemic. In 1987, the Centers for Disease Control (CDC) released an article that emphasized "the need for health-care workers to consider all patients as potentially infected with HIV and/or other blood-borne pathogens and to adhere rigorously to infection-control precautions for minimizing the risk of exposure to blood and body fluids of all patients." The precautions were initially designed to prevent the spread of bloodborne pathogens (i.e., HIV, hepatitis B virus (HBV), and hepatitis C virus (HCV) from patients to health care providers. The precautions require that health care providers "use appropriate barrier precautions to prevent skin and mucous-membrane exposure when contact with blood or other body fluids of any patient is anticipated." Barriers include medical gloves, protective eyewear, masks, bodily gowns, and shoe covers as necessary based on risk of exposure. Double gloving with latex gloves provides an even greater degree of protection from accidental exposure during surgical procedures. Eye protection should include lenses and side shields to prevent lateral splashes from entry into the eye.

The recommendations also included disposing of all needles and sharps in appropriately labeled and secured containers. Appropriate management and care when using sharps in the office as well as in the operating room environment help decrease the risk of inadvertent exposure. Simple measures include (1) avoiding the recapping of hypodermic needles; (2) using a Mayo stand or kidney basin between the surgeon and scrub nurse for passing of sharp instruments; and (3) locating sharps disposal units appropriately and conveniently, and using them to provide a quick, easy, and safe repository for used disposable sharps.

In 1992, the Occupational Safety and Health Administration (OSHA) established regulations for the prevention of occupational exposure to blood-borne pathogens. In its guidelines, OSHA emphasized that universal precautions should be a part of the workplace environment and that engineering controls should be developed and instituted to minimize exposure. Engineering controls might include such items as puncture-resistant sharp instrument containers and splash guards. OSHA also recommended practice controls that would result in alteration of task performance to reduce exposures. These included washing hands after removing gloves, removing personal protective equipment after leaving the work area, not resheathing needles or other sharp instruments, and performing procedures in such a fashion as to minimize splashing and spraying. The guidelines also recommended personal protective equipment and further stated that the employer would provide appropriate protective equipment, including gloves, gowns, head and foot coverings, face shields or masks, eye protection, and fluid-resistant aprons when indicated. According to the OSHA policy, HBV vaccination must be provided at no cost to all employees at risk of exposure. Finally, when exposures occur, postexposure evaluation must be available to employees, including a confidential medical evaluation and follow-up. Employers must offer exposed workers serological testing for HIV and HBV as soon as possible after the exposure, with repeat testing at 6 weeks, 12 weeks, and 6 months. In addition, they should offer medical evaluation and postexposure therapy to all employees according to standard medical practice.

Standard Precautions

In 1996, the CDC broadened its approach to infection control to prevent transmission of any infectious agent to providers, patients, and visitors of hospitals. The concept of standard precautions was born, and it came to supersede Universal Precautions as an all-encompassing approach. "*Standard Precautions* apply to (1) blood; (2) all body fluids, secretions, and excretions, *except sweat*, regardless of whether or not they contain visible blood; (3) non-intact skin; and (4) mucous membranes. Standard precautions are designed to reduce the risk of transmission of microorganisms from both recognized and unrecognized sources of infection in hospitals." This may include respiratory precautions for patients with a known or potential infectious source that is transmitted by respiratory means.

Occupational Exposure to Human Immunodeficiency Virus, Hepatitis B, and Hepatitis C

A factor always of concern among physicians who manage patients with HIV, HBV, and HCV infection is the possibility of becoming infected themselves. In fact, according to the CDC, only 57 health care workers had been infected by HIV due to occupational exposure as of December 2001. None of those infected included physicians who practiced surgical specialties. Nevertheless, it is well understood that the risk to the health care provider is real, and certain precautions must be taken to prevent infection with this virus.

Body fluids known to contain HIV include, in order of viral concentration: cerebrospinal fluid, serum, semen, vaginal secretions, urine, tears, and middle ear secretions. HIV transmission, however, has been documented only from serum, semen, and vaginal secretions. Currently, the risk of acquiring HIV from a percutaneous injury is ~ 0.3%. The risk from mucous membrane exposure is ~ 0.09%. Risk of transmission depends on the type and severity of exposure. In general, deeper injuries, injuries involving visible contamination with blood, injury with an object previously in a patient's artery or vein, and higher viral titers lead to an increased risk of transmission.

The transmission methods for HBV and HCV are similar to those for HIV, although the risks of transmission are higher. Following needlestick or cut injuries, the transmission rate of HCV is ~ 1.8%. The transmission rate for HBV if the source blood was both hepatitis B surface antigen and hepatitis B e-antigen positive was 22 to 31%, although this drops to 1 to 6% if they are hepatitis B e-antigen negative.

Postexposure Prophylaxis

When considering postexposure prophylaxis for HIV, it must be kept in mind that the risk of exposure is small, even after a contaminated injury. Nevertheless, the CDC has published recommended guidelines for chemoprophylaxis following exposure. These recommendations may continue to change as

new medications are introduced. The most up-to-date guidelines are available at the CDC Morbidity and Mortality Weekly Report's Updated U.S. Public Health Service Guidelines for the Management of Occupational Exposure to HIV. Treatment must be started within hours of exposure, so if there is any delay in confirming the HIV status of a patient, with high-risk exposures, consider the risks and benefits of starting prophylaxis empirically. Rapid testing for HIV should provide results within this window to more accurately determine the need for prophylaxis. Although efficacy data are limited, postexposure prophylaxis has been shown, in a case control study of health care workers, to decrease seroconversion by as much as 79%.

For HBV exposure, postexposure prophylaxis includes hepatitis B immune globulin (HBIG) and hepatitis B vaccine series (depending on vaccine status of the injured worker). There is no prophylaxis given for HCV exposure. Immune globulin and antivirals (e.g., ribavirin) are not recommended for HCV exposure per CDC guidelines.

There are five classes of drugs available for postexposure prophylaxis for HIV: nucleoside reverse transcriptase inhibitors (NRTIs), nucleotide reverse transcriptase inhibitors (NtRTIs), nonnucleoside reverse transcriptase inhibitors (NNRTIs), protease inhibitors (PIs), and a single fusion inhibitor. Treatment involves two or more drugs for a full 4 weeks, although often side effects limit full treatment. Use of two or more drugs theoretically inhibits the virus at multiple stages of replication to enhance effectiveness.

There are numerous drug combinations and schedules recommended based on the clinical scenario. Although zidovudine (AZT) is the only agent with data to support its efficacy, additional NRTIs and potentially a protease inhibitor can be added. Basic regimens include the following:

- Zidovudine (AZT) + lamivudine (3TC) available as Combivir (ViiV Healthcare, Research Triangle Park, NC)
- Zidovudine (AZT) + emtricitabine (FTC)
- Tenofovir DF (TDF) + lamivudine (3TC)
- Tenofovir DF (TDF) + emtricitabine (FTC) available as Truvada (Gilead Sciences, Foster City, CA)

■ Treatment of Medical Devices And Instruments

In 1987, the CDC stated that "devices or items that contact intact mucous membranes should be sterilized or receive high-level disinfection, a procedure that kills vegetative organisms and viruses but not necessarily large numbers of bacterial spores. Medical devices or instruments that require sterilization or disinfection should be thoroughly cleaned before being exposed to the germicide, and the manufacturer's instructions for the use of the germicide should be followed." This policy is largely applicable today, although more thorough descriptions of processes required for medical devices have been instituted.

When discussing processing of reusable medical devices, it is important to delineate three different processes: cleaning, disinfection, and sterilization. Cleaning is the process of removing gross visible contaminants, both organic and inorganic material, from an instrument. This first step is critical for the subsequent disinfection or sterilization to be effective. This can include manual washing or using an ultrasonic cleaner with an enzymatic solution. This process is not designed to kill microorganisms.

Disinfection is a relative term that is categorized into levels by the particular types of microorganisms that are reliably killed. The three types of disinfection are high-level, intermediate-level, and low-level. Disinfection does not eliminate microbacterial spores, although high-level disinfection does have some limited sporicidal activity. The spores not killed by high-level disinfection either are not pathogenic or have not been shown to cause infections in endoscopic transmission. Intermediate-level disinfection does not have any sporicidal activity, but it is effective against tuberculosis. Low-level disinfection does not have any tuberculocidal activity.

Sterilization is a process that destroys or eliminates all forms of microbial life, including bacterial spores. This is an absolute term and is the most thorough way of preventing any possible disease transmission for reusable instruments. The primary methods for sterilization used include pressurized steam, dry heat, ethylene oxide gas, hydrogen peroxide gas plasma, and liquid chemicals.

The level of processing required for reusable medical equipment is readily understood if items are separated by their risk for causing infection. Although this categorization has some limitations, most equipment can be separated into categories of critical, semicritical, and noncritical. Critical items are devices that enter sterile tissue or the vascular system. Therefore, they have a high risk for infectious transmission. Any invasive surgical device would fall into this category.

Semicritical items are devices that contact mucosal membranes or nonintact skin. These items include laryngoscopes, flexible endoscopes, rigid endoscopes, or noninvasive instruments for the oral cavity. The CDC recommends that these instruments be free of all microorganisms, although small amounts of bacterial spores are permissible. Therefore, semicritical items require high-level disinfection by such products as glutaraldehyde, hydrogen peroxide, ortho-phthalaldehyde, or peracetic acid with hydro-gen peroxide. The U.S. Food and Drug Administration (FDA) maintains a list of chemicals suitable for high-level disinfection on its Web site. Practitioners must check with the device guidelines to see which products are compatible with their instruments and scopes to avoid damage.

Noncritical items come into contact with intact skin. Therefore, low-level disinfectants can be used to clean these items. This category includes such items as bedside tables, computers, stethoscopes, or blood pressure cuffs.

Processing of Endoscopes

Flexible and rigid endoscopes in otolaryngology fall into the semicritical category, therefore requiring high-level disinfection. Sterilization is not necessary for scopes that are not entering sterile cavities (e.g., arthroscopes used in orthopedic surgery), although some institutions have local policies that require complete sterilization. High-level disinfection is a multistep process that requires a protocol that office staff both understands and adheres to.

The area used to perform these tasks should be large enough to allow for separation of clean and soiled areas. In addition, staff performing these tasks should use protective barriers as appropriate to safeguard themselves from both infectious material and the cleaning products used for disinfection. The first step is to do a leak test of the scope to ensure that the mechanical integrity and watertight construction of the scope have not been compromised. The specifics on how to perform this step can be found in the instruction manual from each scope manufacturer.

The next step is to properly clean the scope, which involves removing all debris and gross contamination. This cleaning can be done with an enzymatic detergent in a sink or basin. The external components of the scope should be brushed or sponged completely. All accessories should be removed from the scope and cleaned separately. If applicable, the instrument channel or suction port of the scope should be opened and cleaned with a brush to remove any debris. After brushing, the channel should be flushed with detergent using a syringe until the irrigant is clear, and then air should be forced down the channel to remove excess detergent. This process should be completed immediately following scope use to prevent drying of organic material on the scope, which makes it harder to remove. After cleaning, rinse the scope of any residual detergent.

The next step is disinfection. For selection of a high-level disinfectant or chemical sterilant, check the FDA-approved list of disinfectants, as well as the manufacturer's care instructions, to avoid damage to the scope. Again, immerse the scope in the disinfectant, and flush the instrument channel and suction ports with the disinfectant. After soaking the scope for the recommended period of time, rinse it thoroughly to wash off any residual disinfectant and thus avoid contact of these chemicals with patient mucosal membranes. The rinse solution should be either sterile or high-quality potable water and should not be reused between scopes. Any accessory channels again need to be flushed to remove any residual within them.

Following disinfection, the scopes must be carefully dried to avoid creating a moist environment that could promote bacterial growth. To dry scopes, flush the instrument channel with 70% alcohol and then with forced air to remove any remaining moisture. Wipe the external scope with a cloth moistened with 70% alcohol, and then with a dry, lint-free cloth. Store scopes in a way that prevents recontamination and promotes drying (e.g., hang them vertically). Do not curl scopes for storage and do not store them in a carrying case. A contaminated scope should never be placed back into a carrying case, unless that case can undergo the same high-level disinfection.

The processing of scopes needs frequent monitoring to ensure that protocols are followed. Some institutions require maintaining a log that includes the procedure, date, time, patient-identifying information, physician performing procedure, a means of identifying the scope, and the name of the staff member processing the scope. These logs can then be used to identify people at risk if a break in protocol is discovered or to trace a potential source if an infectious outbreak occurs.

The CDC has acknowledged the role of endoscopic sheaths in the infection control process. However, it falls short of fully recommending a protocol or guidelines for their use. The CDC states that "endoscopes employing disposable components (e.g., protective barrier devices or sheaths) might provide an alternative to conventional liquid chemical high-level disinfection/sterilization." Two studies in the otolaryngology literature validate that an endosheath followed by cleaning and intermediate-level disinfection can be used instead of high-level disinfection, based on cultures of scopes after processing.

As part of its approval for endoscopic sheaths, the FDA endorsed this protocol, with intermediate-level disinfection to replace high-level disinfection. Given the simplicity of sheath use and intermediate-level disinfection, this may be a more effective way of sterilizing scopes due to the complexity of high-level disinfection processes. It would also protect staff and patients from harmful cleaning products. This would not apply to invasive transnasal esophagoscopy (TNE) scopes with a procedural lumen.

Processing of Other Office Equipment

The CDC does not address every instrument used in an otolaryngology practice, but it does give additional guidance when it discusses processing of dental instruments. The CDC and the American Dental Association classify any instrument that penetrates bone or soft tissue within the oral cavity to be a critical instrument that requires sterilization after each use. Nonpenetrating instruments that contact oral cavity tissues are semicritical. In these instances, high-level disinfection is adequate; however, sterilization is preferred, if possible.

Another area not discussed in the CDC recommendations is the use of equipment for spraying topical medications intranasally. There exist multiple methods for intranasal delivery in otolaryngology practices. A few studies have examined the risk of disease transmission between patients for reusable delivery systems. It is difficult to compare the results between studies because each study uses a slightly different delivery device. In addition, clinically relevant outcomes measures have not been identified. The results are likely highly technique and instrument dependent. The use of long disposable tips, which provide a maximal distance from the contacting surface to the nondisposable portion of the delivery device, is most likely an optimal strategy. Single-use disposable devices and high-level disinfection following each use are two resource- and cost-intensive options that have not been shown to provide any clinical benefit to date.

■ Practice Guidelines, Consensus Statements, and Measures

http://www.cdc.gov/niosh/topics/bbp/universal.html

■ Suggested Reading

Alvarado CJ, Anderson AG, Maki DG. Microbiologic assessment of disposable sterile endoscopic sheaths to replace high-level disinfection in reprocessing: a prospective clinical trial with nasopharyngoscopes. Am J Infect Control 2009;37(5):408–413

Aydin E, Hizal E, Akkuzu B, Azap O. Risk of contamination of nasal sprays in otolaryngologic practice. BMC Ear Nose Throat Disord 2007;7:2

Centers for Disease Control and Prevention (CDC). Updated U.S. Public Health Service guidelines for the management of occupational exposures to HIV and recommendations for post-exposure prophylaxis. MMWR Morb Mortal Wkly Rep 2005;54(RR09):1–17

Cleaning Equipment in Today's ENT Office. AAO-HNS Bulletin. 2005 May:40-41. http://www.entnet.org/press/bulletin/upload/Cleaning-Equipment-in-Today-s-ENT-Office.pdf

Collins WO. A review of reprocessing techniques of flexible nasopharyngoscopes. Otolaryngol Head Neck Surg 2009;141(3):307–310

Elackattu A, Zoccoli M, Spiegel JH, Grundfast KM. A comparison of two methods for preventing cross-contamination when using flexible fiberoptic endoscopes in an otolaryngology clinic: disposable sterile sheaths versus immersion in germicidal liquid. Laryngoscope 2010;120(12):2410–2416

Muscarella LF. Prevention of disease transmission during flexible laryngoscopy. Am J Infect Control 2007;35(8):536–544 Association for Professionals in Infection Control and Epidemiology, Inc.

Rashid M, Karagama YG. Study of microbial spread when using multiple-use nasal anaesthetic spray. Rhinology 2011;49(3):281–285

Rizzi M, Batra PS, Hall G, Citardi MJ, Lanza DC. An assessment for the presence of bacterial contamination of Venturi principle atomizers in a clinical setting. Am J Rhinol 2005;19(1):21–23

Rutala WA, Weber DJ; Healthcare Infection Control Practices Advisory Committee. Guideline for Disinfection and Sterilization in Healthcare Facilities, 2008. Atlanta, GA: Centers for Disease Control and Prevention; 2008

Siegel JD, Rhinehart E, Jackson M, Chiarello L; Healthcare Infection Control Practices Advisory Committee. 2007 Guideline for Isolation Precautions: Preventing Transmission of Infectious Agents in Healthcare Settings. Atlanta, GA: Centers for Disease Control and Prevention; 2007. http://www.cdc.gov/ncidod/dhqp/pdf/isolation2007.pdf

Silberman HD. Non-inflatable sterile sheath for introduction of the flexible nasopharyngolaryngoscope. Ann Otol Rhinol Laryngol 2001;110(4):385–387

U.S. Department of Labor, Occupational Safety & Health Administration. Healthcare Wide Hazards: (Lack of) Universal Precautions. http://www.osha.gov/SLTC/etools/hospital/hazards/univprec/univ.html

U.S. Food and Drug Administration. FDA-Cleared Sterilants and High Level Disinfectants with General Claims for Processing Reusable Medical and Dental Devices. March 2009. http://www.fda.gov/MedicalDevices/DeviceRegulationandGuidance/ReprocessingofSingle-UseDevices/ucm133514.htm

9 Anaphylaxis

■ Introduction

Anaphylaxis is an amplified, harmful, immunological reaction that occurs after reexposure to an antigen to which an organism has become sensitive. It is also a condition caused by an immunoglobulin E (IgE)-mediated reaction that is often life threatening and almost always unanticipated. It involves the antigen-specific crosslinking of IgE molecules on complement proteins on the surface of tissue mast cells and peripheral blood basophils, resulting in immediate release of potent mediators.

Richet first coined the term *anaphylaxis* in 1902 when he observed dogs dying within minutes of receiving a second injection of the fluid from the sea anemone in which he had anticipated the injection to be a protective "antitoxic" immunization. Though this was the first documented study of anaphylaxis, it was not the first documented case; Pharaoh Menes died of a wasp sting in 2640 BC, which was likely the first documented case in written history.

Epidemiology

The overall lifetime prevalence of anaphylaxis is 0.05 to 2%. The reasons for the wide range are the general belief that there is underreporting and that some events are partially treated but are not accounted for in these studies. The incidence of a fatal event is ~ 0.002%, or 600 to 1,000 people in the United States. The average time in which a fatal cardiopulmonary arrest occurred after food anaphylaxis symptoms was 25 to 35 minutes, 10 to 15 minutes with insect stings, and 5 minutes for drug-related anaphylaxis. Fatalities can be from asphyxiation from laryngeal or oropharyngeal swelling, collapse from hypotensive shock, cardiac arrest, or acute severe bronchoconstriction causing respiratory failure and arrest. Anaphylaxis is more common in males than females up to age 15, whereas it is more common in females than males after age 15. Patients who have a history of atopy and asthma are predisposed to more severe anaphylaxis.

Pathogenesis

Anaphylaxis can be categorized by four general categories based on the triggers, which include food, insect stings, medication, and other/unknown. In a study of 179 patients who had anaphylaxis, Yocum and Kahn reported that 33% of cases were triggered by food, 14% by insect stings, 13% by medication, 7% by exercise, and 19% by an unidentified trigger.

Approximately 2% of the U.S. population has an allergy to food. Food is the leading single known cause of anaphylaxis treated in U.S. hospital emergency departments; a change that many clinicians believe has come about in the last 10 to 20 years. A U.S. survey reports an annual incidence of food anaphylaxis of 7.6 cases per 100,000 person-years. Foods that have commonly caused anaphylaxis are tree nuts, fish, milk, eggs, and foods containing bisulfites. **Table 9.1** lists the most common foods that are implicated in food-related anaphylaxis. Hymenoptera venom is found in honey bees, hornets, wasps, yellow jackets, and fire ants. An estimated 0.5 to 3% of the U.S. population has anaphylactic reactions to this venom. Valentine reported that 0.5 to 5% have reactions to Hymenoptera stings.

Antibiotics, particularly penicillins, nonsteroidal anti-inflammatory drugs, opioids, and aspirin are the most common triggers of anaphylaxis. Of the 2 to 3% of hospital patients who experience a drug reaction, 1 in 2,700 of them will have a severe reaction. Approximately 75% of drug-related fatal anaphylactic reactions are penicillin related. Penicillins cause a reaction in 1 to 5 patients per 10,000 courses of treatment and fatalities in 1 patient per 50,000 to 100,000 courses of treatment. The rate of vaccine-associated anaphylaxis is approximately 0.65 per 1 million shots.

Other triggers of anaphylaxis include exercise and latex. Vigorous anaerobic activity is more likely to trigger anaphylaxis than less strenuous activities. The incidence of exercise triggers tends to decrease over time. There is also a relationship between food ingestion and exercise-induced anaphylaxis. The onset will generally occur 2 to 4 hours after ingestion and is more common in females. Latex sensitivity was first reported in 1933 in the form of contact dermatitis to *Hevea brasiliensis*. Latex is found in as many as 40,000 household products. Patients at risk of a latex reaction include patients with spina bifida, congenital urinary tract abnormalities, multiple surgeries, and health care workers. The incidence of latex sensitivity is 6% in the general populations.

Anaphylaxis has been described in several mechanisms, with the most common being the IgE-mediated response (**Fig. 9.1**). Immune aggregates, the complement system, the coagulation system, and autoimmune-related disorders are other mechanisms. Anaphylaxis triggered by cold, exercise, and some medications is fully understood. The releases of both immediate and late mediators ultimately cause the sometimes catastrophic event(s) within the body. These immediate mediators include histamine, tryptase, chymase, heparin, and chondroitin. Late-phase mediators include prostaglandins, leukotrienes, and platelet-activating factor. **Fig. 9.2** depicts a summary of the pathogenesis of anaphylaxis.

■ Evaluation

A typical patient who presents with anaphylaxis has dizziness, weakness, flushing, angioedema, urticaria, nausea, and emesis. Severe symptoms include respiratory tract obstruction, hypotension, and vascular collapse. When evaluating a patient for anaphylaxis,

Table 9.1 Common foods in food-related anaphylaxis

Peanut	
Tree nuts	Walnut, hazelnut, Brazil nuts, pistachios, pecans, pine nuts, cashews, almonds, macadamia nuts
Fish	Salmon, cod, tuna
Shellfish	Shrimp, crab, lobster, oyster, scallop
Milk	Cow, goat, sheep
Eggs	Chicken
Seeds	Sesame, mustard, psyllium, cotton seed
Fruits	Kiwi

it is important to establish a temporal relationship between the onset of symptoms and exposure to the trigger. The sooner the symptoms present, the more severe the reaction is likely to be. Although a grading system has yet to be adopted for universal use, several have been described. **Table 9.2** separates anaphylaxis into mild, moderate, and severe reactions by symptoms. **Table 9.3** further categorizes symptoms by organ system and delineates absolute indications for administration of epinephrine.

Sampson et al reported diagnostic criteria that would make the diagnosis of anaphylaxis highly likely when one of the following three criteria is present:

1. Acute onset of an illness (over minutes to hours) involving skin (generalized hives), mucosal tissue (swollen lips–tongue–uvula), or both and at least one of the following: (a) respiratory compromise or (b) reduced blood pressure or associated symptoms of end-organ dysfunction (collapse, syncope, or incontinence).
2. Two or more of the following that occur rapidly after exposure to a likely allergen (minutes to several hours): (a) involvement of the skin–mucosal tissue (generalized hives, swollen lips, tongue, or uvula; (b) respiratory compromise (acute dyspnea, wheezing, stridor, or hypoxemia); (c) reduced blood pressure or associated symptoms (collapse or syncope); and (d) persistent gastrointestinal symptoms (abdominal cramping or vomiting).
3. Reduced blood pressure after exposure to a known allergen for that patient (minutes to several hours), for infants age-specific decline or > 30% decrease in blood pressure; for adults, systolic blood pressure < 90 mm of hemoglobin (mm Hg) or > 30 decrease from a patient's baseline.

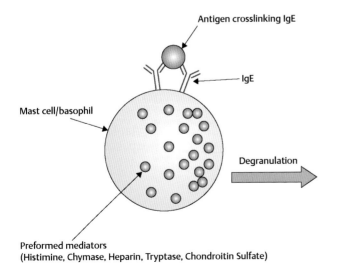

Fig. 9.1 Antigen crosslinking with immunoglobulin E (IgE).

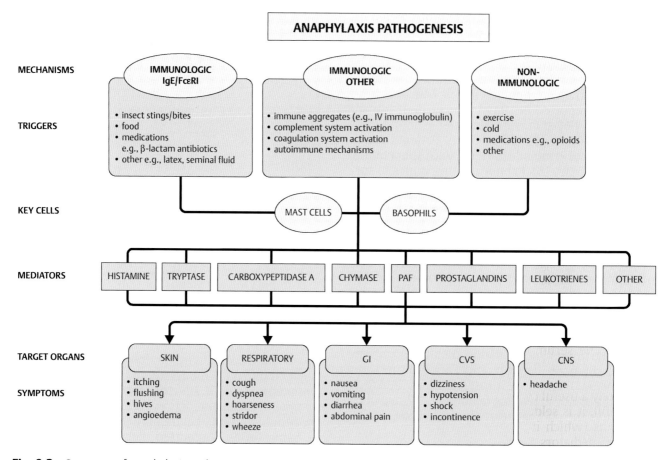

Fig. 9.2 Summary of anaphylaxis pathogenesis.

Table 9.2 Signs and symptoms of anaphylaxis by severity

Severity	Onset	Symptoms
Mild	Up to 1 hour, local	Major wheal and flare at cutaneous side, pruritus, rhinorrhea, sneezing, flushing, sweating, globus, "uneasy" feeling, tachycardia
Moderate	Within 30 minutes	Mild symptoms above, mild wheeze, cough, urticaria, angioedema with hoarseness
Severe	Within 20 minutes	Symptoms above plus some of the following: pulmonary symptoms with status asthmaticus; cutaneous with angioedema from lips to larynx—stridor, massive urticaria; gastrointestinal with nausea, vomiting, cramps, diarrhea; genitourinary with cramps or incontinence; cardiovascular with hypotension, arrhythmia, signs of shock; central nervous system with feeling of impending doom, loss of consciousness

Adapted with permission from Noone MC, Osguthorpe JD. Anaphylaxis. Otolaryngol Clin North Am 2003;36(5):1009–1020, ix.

When these criteria are met, treatment must be initiated immediately.

Though most episodes are uniphasic, there is a need to recognize biphasic episodes and protracted episodes. Biphasic episodes occur after the apparent resolution of initial symptoms, usually ~ 8 hours. A biphasic episode can occur in 1 to 20% of all cases. Because of the potential for recurrence of life-threatening symptoms, it is necessary to observe patients with clinical findings consistent with anaphylaxis.

Protracted episodes are symptoms that persist for hours or days following the initial reaction.

The pediatric population often poses a diagnostic challenge due to the nature of children's inability to describe their symptoms. In addition, there is a lack of cutaneous symptoms in 18% of cases. The primary symptom in children is respiratory in nature, such as wheezing and shortness of breath.

Tryptase and histamine are currently the only blood markers regularly used for evaluating ana-

Table 9.3 Signs and symptoms of anaphylaxis by organ system

Skin	Respiratory	GI	CVS	CNS
Itching-localized or generalized	Cough	Nausea	Tachycardia	Headache
Flushing	Rhinorrhea	Vomiting	**Dysrhythmia**	Feeling of doom
Hives	**Throat tightness or**	Diarrhea	**Hypotension**	**Loss of consciousness**
Angioedema	**pruritus**	Abdominal pain	**Severe bradycardia**	
	Hoarseness		**Cardiac arrest**	
	Barky cough		**Shock**	
	Stridor			
	Wheezing			
	Cyanosis			
	Respiratory arrest			

Abbreviations: CNS, central nervous system; CVS, cardiovascular system; GI, gastrointestinal.

Note: **Boldface symptoms** are absolute indications for the use of epinephrine; use of epinephrine with other symptoms will depend on the patient's history.

Data from Neugut AI, Ghatak AT, Miller RL. Anaphylaxis in the United States: an investigation into its epidemiology. Arch Intern Med 2001;161(1):15–21; and Oswalt ML, Kemp SF. Anaphylaxis: office management and prevention. Immunol Allergy Clin North Am 2007;27(2):177–191, vi.

phylaxis. Tryptase is preferred because it has a longer half-life and is released by mast cells on antigen exposure. The serum levels peak around 60 to 90 minutes after antigen exposure, and the half-life is ~ 90 minutes. Histamine has a very short half-life and is rarely a useful clinical test. Though tryptase is most useful, it is seldom elevated in food-triggered anaphylaxis (which is most common) because the release of mediators from basophils is much more prominent than that from mast cells. Currently, research is being done in markers to include mature B tryptase, mast cell carboxypeptidase A3, chymase, and platelet-aggregating factor.

Diagnosis is essentially clinical, and treatment must not be delayed. Some conditions share clinical features with anaphylaxis, such as an acute asthma attack, vasovagal reaction, systemic mast cell disorders, myocardial dysfunction, hereditary angioedema, pulmonary embolism, foreign body aspiration, acute poisoning, hypoglycemia, hysteria, anxiety attack, and seizure disorder. Complement factor C4 is a helpful screening test that can exclude hereditary angioedema and acquired C1 inhibitor deficiency syndrome.

■ Management

Management begins with recruiting help, calling 911; supporting the airway, breathing, and circulation; and reducing or eliminating exposure to the trigger, if possible. Using a tourniquet or ice can help reduce the trigger burden. If the reaction is severe, epinephrine must be administered. The ideal dose is 0.01 mg/kg of epinephrine 1:1,000 administered intramuscularly. Commercially available prefilled, spring-loaded syringes come in doses of 0.3 mg and 0.15 mg (EpiPen, Mylan, Cannonsburg, PA), which

are ideal doses for a 30 kg and 15 kg patient, respectively. Repeat dosing is often necessary to fully treat the patient. Although the auto injectors are designed to penetrate through clothing, it is prudent to understand the needle lengths are 1.27 cm and 1.58 cm for the 0.15 mg and 0.3 mg doses, respectively. This may not penetrate the subcutaneous tissue to achieve an intramuscular injection in overweight individuals. Most reports suggest that the earlier epinephrine is administered in the course of anaphylaxis, the better the chance of a favorable outcome. The reluctance to inject epinephrine because of fear of adverse cardiac effects should be tempered by the awareness that the heart is a potential target in anaphylaxis, and that myocardial ischemia and dysrhythmia can occur even if epinephrine is not given. Other therapies include H1 antihistamines (diphenhydramine, 1 mg/kg up to 75 mg) and H2 antihistamines (cimetidine, 4 mg/kg up to 300 mg), prednisone (1 mg/kg), and β-adrenergic agonists. **Table 9.4** lists the pharmacotherapy and the dosage for each medication. It is important to understand that H1 antihistamines and β-adrenergic agonists cannot be substituted for epinephrine. Supplemental oxygen and intravenous fluids are important steps in management, as well as positioning the patient. Adult fatalities have been reported within seconds if the patient stands or sits suddenly. Vasopressors, such as dopamine or norepinephrine, should be administered if the patient's cardiovascular system fails to respond to the first-line therapies. **Fig. 9.3** depicts a summary of management.

One pertinent clinical condition where a provider may hesitate on the administration of epinephrine is if a patient is taking a β-blocker. Beta-blockers will competitively inhibit the β-adrenergic receptors. Beta-blockers relax the smooth muscles in blood vessels, bronchi, gastrointestinal tract, and genito-

Table 9.4 Medications and dosages for anaphylaxis

Medication	Adult Dosing	Pediatric Dosing
Epinephrine	0.3–0.5 mg IM Repeat every 5–10 min Adult EpiPen (Mylan) (0.3 mg)	0.01 mg/kg IM Repeat every 5–10 min Peds EpiPen (0.15 mg)
Diphenhydramine	1 mg/kg IV/IM up to 75 mg	1 mg/kg IV/IM up to 50 mg
Ranitidine	1 mg/kg IV/IM	1 mg/kg IV/IM
Cimetidine	4 mg/kg IV/IM up to 300 mg	4 mg/kg IV/IM up to 150 mg
Albuterol	2 puffs Nebulized 0.25–0.5 mL in 2 mL	2 puffs
Prednisone	1 mg/kg up to 75 mg	1 mg/kg
Hydrocortisone	250–500 mg IV/IM	10–100 mg IV/IM
Methylprednisolone	125 mg IV	1–2 mg/kg IV up to 125 mg
Glucagon	5–15 µg/min	5–15 µg/min
Dopamine	5–20 µg/kg/min	

Abbreviations: IM, intramuscular; IV, intravenous; kg, kilogram; mL, milliliter; mg, milligram; min, minute; µg, microgram.
Data from Blatman KH, Ditto AM. Chapter 25: Idiopathic anaphylaxis. Allergy Asthma Proc 2012;33(Suppl 1):S84–S87; and Oswalt ML, Kemp SF. Anaphylaxis: office management and prevention. Immunol Allergy Clin North Am 2007;27(2):177–191, vi.

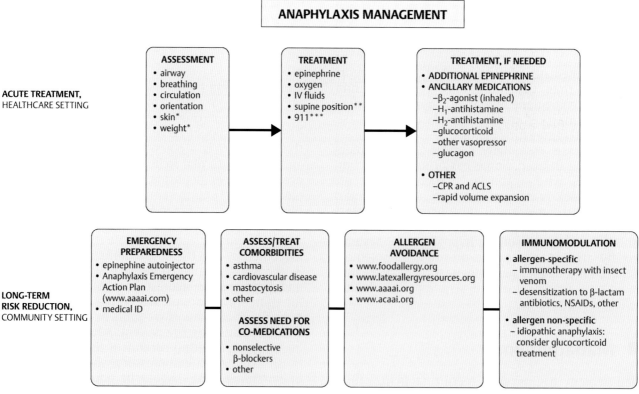

Fig. 9.3 Summary of anaphylaxis management. Acute treatment is the same regardless of the mechanism or trigger involved in anaphylaxis. In contrast, for long-term risk reduction, avoidance measures and immunomodulation are trigger-specific; currently, immunomodulation is available only for a minority of individuals with anaphylaxis. All at-risk individuals need to have comorbidities and comedications assessed, to be taught the importance of emergency preparedness, and to be instructed in the use of self-injectable epinephrine. *The skin should be inspected, and weight estimation is important, especially in infants and children, and also in overweight and obese teens and adults, in order to calculate an optimal dose of epinephrine and other medications needed in treatment and resuscitation. **Supine position, as tolerated, to prevent empty ventricle syndrome. ***Call 911/emergency medical services for anaphylaxis occurring in community healthcare facilities such as medical, dental, or infusion clinics, where optimal backup might not be available for resuscitation. ACLS, Advanced cardiac life support; CPR, cardiopulmonary resuscitation; CVS, cardiovascular; GI, gastrointestinal; ID, identification (e.g., bracelet, wallet card); IV, intrintravenous. (Used with permission from Simons FE. Anaphylaxis. Journal of Allergy Clinical Immunology 2008;121: S402–S407.)

urinary tract. The effect on patients who have an anaphylactic reaction while on β-blockers is severe bronchospasm, paradoxical bradycardia, and profound hypotension. Because epinephrine is an α- and β-agonist, when epinephrine is administered to a patient on β-blockers, it will result in unopposed α-adrenergic response. The patient would ultimately have vasoconstriction and severe and potentially life-threatening hypertension. Glucagon can be administered to reverse the hypotension and bronchospasm. This is also why a patient who is undergoing allergy immunotherapy must not be on a β-blocker for the remote chance of a shot reaction.

Prevention and education are the mainstays of management once an individual has been identified as having had anaphylaxis. Action plans must be implemented for patients who have a history of anaphylaxis. Children especially must have an emergency action plan because their events may not always occur in the home. Medical identification jewelry and identification cards within a wallet are useful for first responders. Premedication with antihistamines and steroids if an individual comes knowingly close to a trigger can help reduce the risk. Most patients who undergo immunotherapy can be cured from reaction to future Hymenoptera stings. An estimated 98% of patients with anaphylaxis from bee stings who undergo a course of venom immunotherapy will have a reduced risk of anaphylaxis from subsequent stings.

Food allergies are generally managed by avoiding the foods once they are identified. If a trigger is not clearly identified, a physician-directed oral challenge can be performed to precisely identify the trigger. This must be performed in a well-controlled environment. IgE levels to specific foods can also be measured and followed. After an extended period of food elimination on the order of 2 years, patients can outgrow the food allergy. However, clinical reactivity to peanuts, tree nuts, fish, and shellfish are less likely to diminish over time. Currently, the risk of desensitizing patients' food is unacceptably too high, and new strategies are under way, such has anti-IgE therapy.

When a patient's history does not reveal a precipitating trigger or event, it is still treatable with a good prognosis. These patients are generally managed with prednisone (40–60 mg) for 1 to 2 weeks, which is then tapered, and an antihistamine until the symptoms resolve. The patients are maintained on an antihistamine for at least 1 year.

■ Controversial Issues

Administering epinephrine will often present a treatment dilemma to providers and first responders alike. There is often a hesitation in giving the very medication that will save a person with anaphylaxis but can cause harm if given to a person who does not have anaphylaxis. Education to understand the importance of early delivery must be emphasized because this will affect the outcome of the individual in distress. Of the fatalities that occur as a result of anaphylaxis, 86% had symptoms within 20 minutes of exposure to the trigger.

■ Practice Guidelines, Consensus Statements, and Measures

Currently there are no practice guidelines or consensus statements regarding anaphylaxis from the American Academy of Otolaryngology–Head and Neck Surgery. The American Academy of Allergy, Asthma, and Immunology; the American College of Allergy, Asthma, and Immunology; and the Joint Council on Allergy, Asthma, and Immunology formed a task force developing practice parameters on the diagnosis and management of anaphylaxis, as well as management of stinging insect hypersensitivity. A comprehensive practice parameter is also available for food and drug allergies. These documents are great reference materials for otolaryngologists who may encounter specific situations. A comprehensive review of literature with classification of the data with recommendations makes these resources particularly helpful.

■ Suggested Reading

Blatman KH, Ditto AM. Chapter 25: Idiopathic anaphylaxis. Allergy Asthma Proc 2012;33(Suppl 1):S84–S87

Bock SA. The incidence of severe adverse reactions to food in Colorado. J Allergy Clin Immunol 1992;90(4 Pt 1):683–685

Bock SA, Muñoz-Furlong A, Sampson HA. Further fatalities caused by anaphylactic reactions to food, 2001-2006. J Allergy Clin Immunol 2007;119(4):1016–1018

Burks AW, Jones SM, Boyce JA, et al. NIAID-sponsored 2010 guidelines for managing food allergy: applications in the pediatric population. Pediatrics 2011;128(5):955–965

Chapman JA, Bernstein IL, Lee RE, et al; American College of Allergy, Asthma, & Immunology. Food allergy: a practice parameter. Ann Allergy Asthma Immunol 2006;96(3, Suppl 2):S1–S68

Dinakar C. Anaphylaxis in children: current understanding and key issues in diagnosis and treatment. Curr Allergy Asthma Rep 2012;12(6):641–649

Georgy MS, Pongracic JA. Chapter 22: Hereditary and acquired angioedema. Allergy Asthma Proc 2012;33(Suppl 1):S73–S76

Golden DBK. Insect sting allergy and venom immunotherapy: a model and a mystery. J Allergy Clin Immunol 2005;115(3):439–447, quiz 448

Golden DB, Moffitt J, Nicklas RA, et al; Joint Task Force on Practice Parameters; American Academy of Allergy, Asthma & Immunology (AAAAI); American College of Allergy, Asthma & Immunology (ACAAI); Joint Council of Allergy, Asthma and Immunology. Stinging insect hypersensitivity: a practice parameter update 2011. J Allergy Clin Immunol 2011;127(4):852–854, e1–e23

Greenberger PA, Rotskoff BD, Lifschultz B. Fatal anaphylaxis: postmortem findings and associated comorbid diseases. Ann Allergy Asthma Immunol 2007;98(3):252–257

Gupta R, Sheikh A, Strachan DP, Anderson HR. Burden of allergic disease in the UK: secondary analyses of national databases. Clin Exp Allergy 2004;34(4):520–526

Kelly KJ, Kurup VP, Reijula KE, Fink JN. The diagnosis of natural rubber latex allergy. J Allergy Clin Immunol 1994;93(5):813–816

Kemp SF, Lockey RF, Wolf BL, Lieberman P. Anaphylaxis. A review of 266 cases. Arch Intern Med 1995;155(16):1749–1754

Kounis NG. Kounis syndrome (allergic angina and allergic myocardial infarction): a natural paradigm? Int J Cardiol 2006;110(1):7–14

Laroche D, Vergnaud MC, Sillard B, Soufarapis H, Bricard H. Biochemical markers of anaphylactoid reactions to drugs. Comparison of plasma histamine and tryptase. Anesthesiology 1991;75(6):945–949

Lieberman P. Biphasic anaphylactic reactions. Ann Allergy Asthma Immunol 2005;95(3):217–226, quiz 226, 258

Lieberman P, Camargo CA Jr, Bohlke K, et al. Epidemiology of anaphylaxis: findings of the American College of Allergy, Asthma and Immunology Epidemiology of Anaphylaxis Working Group. Ann Allergy Asthma Immunol 2006;97(5):596–602

Lieberman P, Nicklas RA, Oppenheimer J, et al. The diagnosis and management of anaphylaxis practice parameter: 2010 update. J Allergy Clin Immunol 2010;126(3):477–480, e1–e42

Neugut AI, Ghatak AT, Miller RL. Anaphylaxis in the United States: an investigation into its epidemiology. Arch Intern Med 2001;161(1):15–21

Noone MC, Osguthorpe JD. Anaphylaxis. Otolaryngol Clin North Am 2003;36(5):1009–1020, ix

Oswalt ML, Kemp SF. Anaphylaxis: office management and prevention. Immunol Allergy Clin North Am 2007;27(2):177–191, vi

Pumphrey R. Anaphylaxis: can we tell who is at risk of a fatal reaction? Curr Opin Allergy Clin Immunol 2004;4(4):285–290

Pumphrey RSH, Gowland MH. Further fatal allergic reactions to food in the United Kingdom, 1999-2006. J Allergy Clin Immunol 2007;119(4):1018–1019

Rusznak C, Peebles RS Jr. Anaphylaxis and anaphylactoid reactions. A guide to prevention, recognition, and emergent treatment. Postgrad Med 2002;111(5):101–104, 107–108, 111–114

Sampson HA. Anaphylaxis and emergency treatment. Pediatrics 2003;111(6 Pt 3):1601–1608

Sampson HA. Food anaphylaxis. Br Med Bull 2000;56(4):925–935

Sampson HA, Muñoz-Furlong A, Bock SA, et al. Symposium on the definition and management of anaphylaxis: summary report. J Allergy Clin Immunol 2005;115(3):584–591

Sampson HA, Muñoz-Furlong A, Campbell RL, et al. Second symposium on the definition and management of anaphylaxis: summary report—Second National Institute of Allergy and Infectious Disease/Food Allergy and Anaphylaxis Network symposium. J Allergy Clin Immunol 2006;117(2):391–397

Sicherer SH, Muñoz-Furlong A, Burks AW, Sampson HA. Prevalence of peanut and tree nut allergy in the US determined by a random digit dial telephone survey. J Allergy Clin Immunol 1999;103(4):559–562

Simons FE. 9. Anaphylaxis. J Allergy Clin Immunol 2008;121(2, Suppl):S402–S407, quiz S420

Solensky R, Khan DA, Bernstein IL, et al; Joint Task Force on Practice Parameters; American Academy of Allergy, Asthma and Immunology; American College of Allergy, Asthma and Immunology; Joint Council of Allergy, Asthma and Immunology. Drug allergy: an updated practice parameter. Ann Allergy Asthma Immunol 2010;105(4):259–273

Thomas M, Crawford I. Best evidence topic report. Glucagon infusion in refractory anaphylactic shock in patients on beta-blockers. Emerg Med J 2005;22(4):272–273

Valentine MD. Anaphylaxis and stinging insect hypersensitivity. JAMA 1992;268(20):2830–2833

Weiler JM. Anaphylaxis in the general population: A frequent and occasionally fatal disorder that is underrecognized. J Allergy Clin Immunol 1999;104(2 Pt 1):271–273

Yocum MW, Khan DA. Assessment of patients who have experienced anaphylaxis: a 3-year survey. Mayo Clin Proc 1994;69(1):16–23

Yunginger JW, Nelson DR, Squillace DL, et al. Laboratory investigation of deaths due to anaphylaxis. J Forensic Sci 1991;36(3):857–865

10 Outcomes Research

■ Introduction

Outcomes research is the scientific analysis of treatment effectiveness. With methods from epidemiology, biostatistics, economics, management, and psychometrics, clinical investigators in this field seek the bottom line: does the health intervention under study achieve a satisfactory outcome?

This simple question becomes complex due to the lack of universally accepted standards for each component of the analysis. Which population of patients is being addressed? How do we account for the quality of an intervention? What are the aspects of treatment? What is a satisfactory outcome? Who defines satisfaction? How do we measure effectiveness?

■ History

In 1900, Ernest Codman proposed the study of what he termed the "end results" of therapy at Massachusetts General Hospital. He asked his fellow surgeons to report the success and failure of each operation and developed a classification scheme by which failures could be further detailed. His efforts over 2 decades included the construction of a hospital committed to his methods. However, his emphasis on outcomes was scorned by the medical establishment, and the study of end results gradually faded.

With the integration of the scientific method and its reliance on experimentation in American medicine, the randomized clinical trial (RCT) became the dominant method for evaluating treatment effectiveness. By the 1960s, the authority of the RCT was rarely questioned, reducing the need for subjective reports of outcomes. Nonrandomized techniques were therefore used less often to study outcomes and more often to study the process and delivery of care.

In 1973, Wennberg and Gittelsohn published a landmark study that reported on significant geographic variations in health care delivery. These investigators found, for example, that tonsillectomy rates in 13 Vermont regions varied from 13 to 151 per 10,000 people. Without evidence of variation in the prevalence of tonsillitis, they suggested that the variations in utilization were more likely from differing physician beliefs regarding the indications and efficacy of the procedure.

Therefore, the next step was to investigate the appropriateness of surgical indications. Robert Brook and other investigators at the RAND Corporation led the effort. Criteria for appropriate indications were developed by combining data from existing literature with expert opinion from consensus conferences. When these criteria were used, rates of inappropriateness seemed high. However, utilization rates were not correlated with rates of inappropriateness, and therefore did not explain the variation in surgical rates. To some investigators, this suggested that the practice of medicine was anecdotal and inadequately scientific.

The national emphasis on cost containment and the rapid growth of the managed care industry intensified the effort to evaluate the link between medical treatments and their outcomes. Realizing that most treatment outcomes cannot be studied in a randomized fashion, Congress created the Agency for Health Care Policy and Research (AHCPR) in 1989 (now the Agency for Healthcare Research and Quality), which was charged with "systematically studying the relationships between health care and its outcomes." One of the AHCPR's early vehicles were Patient Outcomes Research Teams (PORTs). Fourteen PORTs were established to study a variety of diseases, such as low-back pain, diabetes mellitus, and cataracts. Second-generation PORT II centers are now under way; however, no otolaryngological diseases have been included.

Concomitant with the rising emphasis on outcomes, increased attention has been given to quality assurance. The National Committee for Quality Assurance was created by an alliance of employers, consumers, organized medicine, and the managed care industry to serve as the accrediting organization for managed care. The Health Plan Employer Data and Information Set (HEDIS) incorporates outcomes measures, such as patient satisfaction, along with traditional process measures. In addition, the Joint Commission on Accreditation of Healthcare Organizations has also adopted outcomes measures. The increasing application of outcomes information accentuates the importance of appreciating some of its basic principles.

No discussion of the development and evolution of outcomes research would be complete without mention of the Cochrane Collaboration. The Cochrane Collaboration was named in honor of Scottish physician Archie Cochrane, who championed the development of evidence-based medicine in the 1970s to 1990s. Based in Oxford, England, the Cochrane Collaboration organizes study groups to critically investigate the current published evidence regarding myriad medical and surgical treatments using systematic review and meta-analysis methodology. Any inquiry into the effectiveness of any treatment should start here.

■ Methodology

Concepts

Several concepts must first be discussed to better understand the methodology of outcomes research.

Clinical Efficacy and Effectiveness

The distinction between efficacy and effectiveness illustrates one of the fundamental differences between traditional clinical research and outcomes research. *Efficacy* refers to whether a health intervention, in a controlled environment, achieves better outcomes than placebo does. Two aspects of this definition bear mention. First, efficacy is a comparison: is the intervention better than placebo? As long as the intervention is better, it is efficacious. Second, controlled, experimental environments may shelter patients and physicians from unexpected factors that might be encountered in an actual clinical setting. Thus an "efficacious" antibiotic may lose its advantage in real patients who are not reminded and not monitored.

Effectiveness refers to whether a treatment is useful under usual clinical circumstances. However, the lack of randomization introduces myriad potentially confounding variables, so outcomes investigators need to determine which factors truly affect outcome. For example, the severity of the disease, the compliance of the patient, or the abilities of the surgeon may have as much impact on an outcome

as treatment does. For these reasons, the RCT will always be prominent. Nonetheless, because clinicians now recognize that for ethical or practical reasons it is frequently difficult to randomize therapy (e.g., how does one blind a patient to endoscopic sinus surgery or antibiotics?), researchers must learn to account for the effects of variables that that they cannot control.

Bias and Confounding

Bias occurs when "compared components are not sufficiently similar." The compared components may involve any aspect of the study. For example, *selection* bias exists if, in comparing an operation to chemotherapy, we avoid operating on patients who are too ill. This is an unfair comparison because the surgical cohort will then on average have healthier patients. *Performance* bias occurs if we attempt to compare the results of two operations, but one is performed by a surgeon with 40 years of experience, and the other is performed by resident staff.

Similar to bias, *confounding* also has the potential to distort the results. However, confounding refers to specific variables. Confounding occurs when a variable thought to cause an outcome is actually not responsible for the outcome because of the unseen effects of another variable. Consider a hypothetical case where an investigator postulates that nicotine-stained teeth cause laryngeal cancer. Despite a strong statistical association, this relationship is not causal, because the relationship of another variable—cigarette smoking—is responsible. Cigarette smoking is confounding because it is associated with both the outcome (laryngeal cancer) and the supposed exposure (stained teeth).

Comorbidity

Comorbidity refers to the presence of concomitant disease unrelated to the "index disease" (the disease under consideration), which may affect the diagnosis, treatment, and prognosis for the patient. The failure to identify comorbid conditions, such as renal, liver, or congestive heart failure, may result in inaccurately attributing poor outcomes to the index disease being studied.

Principles in Research Design

Some of the basic requirements of an outcomes study are (1) the establishment of the pretreatment baseline state, (2) the development of a format to collect treatment data, and (3) the description of the post-treatment outcome.

Baseline State

To establish the baseline state, the disease under investigation must be carefully defined, and the patients to be studied must be characterized. Without this information, the results of a study are difficult to interpret and impossible to reproduce.

Diagnostic criteria need to be established. For instance, in a study of the treatment of head and neck cancer recurrences, investigators must detail the sites of tumor and histological patterns that are being studied. In addition, the way tumors were identified has significance: were they diagnosed after becoming symptomatic, or detected through routine cancer surveillance? Are any referral patterns present that might make these tumors atypical? Another difficult issue is how investigators handle persistent tumors. What are the objective criteria that distinguish between persistence and recurrence, or even a second primary site that is close to the original site of tumor?

It is also important to consider the severity of disease. Although it is almost inconceivable that the oncology literature would fail to stratify 5-year survival results by primary tumor, regional nodes, and metastasis (TNM) stage, the study of other diseases, such as sinusitis and otitis, frequently overlooks this important notion. Several patient issues that may confound impact on the outcome must also be characterized. Inclusion criteria (or lack thereof) for entrance into a study should be detailed. Are the patients in a tertiary care practice, or are these community patients? Most important, such factors as comorbidity, compliance, and socioeconomic and educational levels must also be considered.

Data Collection and Types of Study Designs

Primary Data

Data gathered about patients from direct observation are called primary data. Four popular methods for collecting primary data are randomized trials, observational trials, case-control studies, and cross-sectional surveys. Each has advantages and disadvantages that should be considered when interpreting results (see **Table 10.1**).

RCTs have already been discussed. They involve assembling a group of patients, assigning therapy randomly, and observing outcomes prospectively. *Cohort studies* are a form of *observational trial*; they assign patients to treatment based on routine criteria in clinical practice (see efficacy vs. effectiveness). Placebos are absent, and adjustments for bias are made with epidemiological or statistical techniques. These disadvantages are offset by the relative ease of enrollment of patients and avoidance of operational obstacles, such as the maintenance of double blind-

ing. Observational trials are not necessarily prospective; retrospective cohorts of patients can also be assembled, and observations can be made from subsequent records, such as medical charts, X-rays, and tumor registry data.

Both observational and randomized studies identify patients before they are "exposed" to a treatment (or a pathogen), and then follow them forward in time to see what happens (the outcome). In contrast, *case-control studies* select patients based on an identified outcome, and then look backward in time to determine rates of exposure. Whereas a prospective study seeking to establish an association between cigarette use and cancer of the pyriform sinus would require numerous patients and decades of observation, a case-control study could be conducted relatively quickly and inexpensively. The premise of such a study would be to identify patients with and without pyriform sinus cancer (the cases and controls, respectively), and then to compare the percentages of smokers in each group.

Cross-sectional studies gather information about a patient population at a single point in time. The studies are relatively simple to execute and can be used to collect a variety of data, such as health status and satisfaction information, or laboratory values in a clinical disease. However, these studies are unable to establish temporal and, therefore, causal relationships.

Secondary Data

Data that have been previously collected for another purpose are called secondary data. The Medicare database or datasets from insurance or managed care organizations are examples of secondary data. These large collections of data allow a quick examination of clinical associations, utilization review, or readmission or morbidity rates. However, these largely administrative datasets have significant clinical limitations, and investigators must guard against missing, inaccurate, and biased information.

A relatively new research format, meta-analysis, also makes use of previously collected data. The purpose of these systematic literature reviews is to elucidate areas of clinical practice in which conflicting data exist. In theory, by assembling data from relevant individual studies, the larger, combined body of evidence permits insights that may not otherwise be possible. Again, investigators must be aware of potential sources of bias and subjectivity.

Outcomes Measures

Traditional outcomes in clinical studies make use of mortality and morbidity rates, or of other "hard" end points, which can be "objectively" described

Table 10.1 Advantages and disadvantages of various study designs

Study design	Advantages	Disadvantages
Primary data		
Randomized clinical trial	Highest level of evidence possible, least prone to bias and error	Costly, time consuming; can be ethical concerns for randomization in certain scenarios (i.e., surgery)
Cohort study	Can directly observe outcomes in association with risk factors or exposures; can directly measure risk	Costly, time consuming; patients who are lost to follow-up can be a major source of bias
Case-control study	Can estimate outcomes associated with exposure/risk factors in a much less costly and time-consuming approach than a cohort study	Can be very difficult to identify the appropriate control group, which can lead to bias, error, and wrong conclusions
Cross-sectional study	Can rapidly obtain data comparing exposures/risk factors to outcomes at one point in time (prevalence)	Only gives data from one time point, cannot assess risk over time (incidence)
Secondary data		
Case report/case series	Easy, inexpensive; can rapidly explore hypothesis and associations between exposures/risk factors and an outcome	Very prone to selection bias, retrospective design can impact data quality, lack of a control group can make conclusions uncertain
Meta-analysis/systematic review	Can compile all available data in one place for complete analysis and thorough evaluation of weakness and limitations of existing data	Prone to publication bias; garbage in, garbage out principle; complex mathematics can make conclusions difficult to interpret

by laboratory methods or their like. These include documentable changes in physiological states, such as elevated white cell counts, opacified paranasal sinuses, or even jitter and shimmer. Yet in practice, clinicians use "soft" data to determine whether patients are improving. Because it has been difficult to quantify skin erythema, periorbital pain, or voice quality, however, these outcome variables have been ignored, with few exceptions.

The prototype of a clinical scale is the Apgar score for the condition of a newborn baby. The House grading system for facial paresis has also found acceptance, despite its "soft" nature. Opponents of clinimetric scales argue that they are unreliable because of high interobserver variability. However, this problem is minimized if the scales can be clearly defined, as with the Apgar score or the Glasgow Coma Scale. Furthermore, proponents of clinimetrics point out that rates of interobserver variability of accepted "hard" outcomes, such as chest X-ray findings and histological reports, remain distressingly high.

In addition to clinimetric variables, psychometric techniques are used to construct composite variables that measure abstract concepts, such as satisfaction or quality of life. These "instruments" quantify responses to a series of questions and combine them in a predetermined way to produce an overall score, or a profile of scores, for an otherwise qualitative concept. Such instruments must meet rigorous standards of sensitivity, reliability, and validity, and of course must also make basic clinical sense ("face validity"). Although instruments measuring general

concepts of satisfaction and quality of life provide a useful barometer for the overall status of a population of patients, disease-specific instruments are also needed because they are often much more sensitive to a change in a specific patient's condition. Examples of such instruments are widespread and include multiple instruments developed for specific clinical entities within otolaryngology. A matrix of the high-quality, existing instruments is maintained on the American Academy of Otolaryngology–Head and Neck Surgery (AAO-HNS) Web site, https://www.entnet.org.

Finally, an increasingly popular outcome is monetary cost. Outcomes may be expressed in actual dollars or, more often, as the cost of an expected benefit, such as the cost to achieve an extra quality-adjusted life-year. It is important to distinguish between costs and charges in these analyses, and also to specify whose cost is involved—that of the individual, the institution, or the society. Without statistical tests to determine the stability of the results, properly conducted decision and cost analyses make liberal use of sensitivity analyses, which systematically vary the assumptions in a financial model to determine if and how outcomes are affected.

One important subtype of cost outcome studies is decision analysis/cost analysis studies. Decision analyses organize information about treatment options so that the options can be ranked in order of their expected benefit. For example, in a hypothetical study of treatment for head and neck cancer, investigators would list all treatment options, determine the probabilities of success or failure with each option, and anticipate the costs and benefits of every possible outcome. These data would then be combined to provide the best possible choice "on average." Decision analyses have been used primarily in head and neck cancer to systematically evaluate complicated decisions.

Cost-Based Studies Can Also Be Partitioned into Three Categories

- *Cost-identification studies* simply aim to document the costs (or charges) of services and equipment. When the outcomes for alternative outcomes are not equivalent, these studies are unable to provide valid comparisons.
- *Cost-effectiveness* (or *cost-utility*) *analyses*, on the other hand, are more sophisticated, because costs are assigned to a measure of health. These health measures are generally nonmonetary, such as an added year of health or the prevention of a nosocomial infection. Because the "price" of an arbitrary health measure has only relative meaning, these results need to be compared with other alternatives.
- *Cost-benefit analyses* can be the most complex type of study, because both costs and benefits are expressed in units of currency. This necessitates a conversion of abstract health measures into dollars.

Outcomes Projects

The scope and scale of outcomes projects continue to evolve as researchers adapt to the changing health care environment. The borders between projects once classified as clinical epidemiology and others traditionally from the arena of health services research are becoming less apparent. Otolaryngological efforts from these fields are categorized next.

Outcomes Measurement

AAO–HNS has begun a nationwide study of treatment effectiveness for otitis media and sinusitis. Similar to an effort of the American Academy of Ophthalmology and the cataract PORT, practicing otolaryngologists will be asked to pool their results in a national database for analysis. A separate study has documented improvements in quality of life and income for recipients of cochlear implants.

Analogous to established "instruments," such as the Short-Form General Health Survey (SF-36) and the Sickness Impact Profile, which assess *general*

health status, investigators have designed instruments for *disease-specific* outcomes. These validated tools provide an objective measure of function or quality of life as they relate specifically to diseases, such as sinusitis (Sino-Nasal Outcome Test [SNOT-20], Chronic Sinusitis Survey); hearing loss (Hearing Evaluation and Auditory Rehabilitation [HEAR-14] test, Hearing Device Satisfaction Scale); obstructive sleep apnea (Symptoms of Nocturnal Obstruction and Related Events [SNORE-25]); and head and neck cancer (University of Washington Quality of Life scale, Head and Neck Radiotherapy Questionnaire).

Prognosis/Staging

One of the foundations of clinical epidemiology is the establishment of prognostic models. The TNM staging system is a prime example. The integration of clinical symptoms and other patient factors, such as comorbidity, with TNM information can improve predictive ability. The combined clinical severity staging system significantly improved the differentiation of survival rates between stages.

Prognostic factors for successful outcomes in patients with sinusitis have been identified and have led to the development of staging systems. Several staging systems based primarily on radiographic appearance have been proposed, and efforts to combine elements from patient history and clinical examination into a more comprehensive model are ongoing.

Improving Methodology

Another aspect of clinical epidemiology is the emphasis on improving the methods of research. Evaluations of the methods used to describe outcomes, or of the quality of the literature on a particular topic, such as sleep apnea, point out the limitations of what is known. Other investigators have discussed the inconsistency in head and neck cancer data and have proposed methods for improving their reliability.

■ Meta-Analyses

The use of meta-analysis has gained popularity for obtaining insight into controversial topics. Although the treatment of acute otitis media and otitis media with effusion (OME) has been controversial, meta-analyses have demonstrated the utility of steroid therapy for OME and antibiotic therapy for both disorders. Meta-analyses have also been used to examine the utility of adjuvant therapy in the treatment of head and neck cancer.

Cost Analyses

Cost analysis studies are distinct from cost-effectiveness analyses and cost-utility studies but can be frequently confused in the literature. In some instances, "cost-effective" is incorrectly substituted for "inexpensive."

Quality-of-Care Studies

Quality of care includes appropriateness studies, quality improvement and assurance, and treatment guidelines. Treatment guidelines have increasing visibility in many hospitals and have taken on many forms. Critical pathways represent guidelines for inpatient care that some clinicians hope may reduce oversights and improve uniformity and, therefore, quality of care.

Summary

Outcomes research is the scientific analysis of treatment effectiveness and has evolved with the changing health care environment. Clinical investigators in this field use a variety of techniques to answer questions, not only about outcomes and treatment effectiveness but also about prognosis, methodology, cost-effectiveness, and quality of care. It behooves the practicing clinician to become familiar with some of these basic principles to better understand the increasing application of outcomes research.

Suggested Reading

Agency for Healthcare Research and Quality. www.ahrq.org

American Academy of Otolaryngology–Head and Neck Surgery Outcomes Research. www.entnet.org

Cochrane Collaboration. www.cochrane.org

Codman EA. The product of a hospital. Surg Gynecol Obstet 1914;18:491–496

Hollenbeak CS, Stack BC Jr, Daley SM, Piccirillo JF. Using comorbidity indexes to predict costs for head and neck cancer. Arch Otolaryngol Head Neck Surg 2007;133(1):24–27

Khalid AN, Hollenbeak CS, Quraishi SA, Fan CY, Stack BC Jr. The cost-effectiveness of iodine 131 scintigraphy, ultrasonography, and fine-needle aspiration biopsy in the initial diagnosis of solitary thyroid nodules. Arch Otolaryngol Head Neck Surg 2006;132(3):244–250

Khalid AN, Quraishi SA, Hollenbeak CS, Stack BC Jr. Fine-needle aspiration biopsy versus ultrasound-guided fine-needle aspiration biopsy: cost-effectiveness as a frontline diagnostic modality for solitary thyroid nodules. Head Neck 2008;30(8):1035–1039

Lowe VJ, Hollenbeak CS, Stack BC Jr. Decision tree analysis in the treatment of the N0 neck. Cancer 2001;92:2341–2348

National Committee for Quality Assurance. www.ncqa.org

Rosenfeld RM. How to systematically review the medical literature. Otolaryngol Head Neck Surg 1996;115(1):53–63

Ruda JM, Hollenbeak CS, Stack BC Jr. A systematic review of the diagnosis and treatment of primary hyperparathyroidism from 1995 to 2003. Otolaryngol Head Neck Surg 2005;132(3):359–372

Ruda J, Stack BC Jr, Hollenbeak CS. The cost-effectiveness of additional preoperative ultrasonography or sestamibi-SPECT in patients with primary hyperparathyroidism and negative findings on sestamibi scan. Arch Otolaryngol Head Neck Surg 2006;132(1):46–53

Stack BC Jr, Spencer HJ, Lee CE, Medvedev S, Hohmann SF, Bodenner DL. Characteristics of inpatient thyroid surgery at US academic and affiliated medical centers. Otolaryngol Head Neck Surg 2012;146(2):210–219

Stack BC Jr, Spencer H, Moore E, Medvedev S, Bodenner D. Outpatient parathyroid surgery data from the University Health System Consortium. Otolaryngol Head Neck Surg 2012;147(3):438–443

Wineland AM, Stack BC Jr. Modern methods to predict costs for the treatment and management of head and neck cancer patients: examples of methods used in the current literature. Curr Opin Otolaryngol Head Neck Surg 2008;16(2):113–116

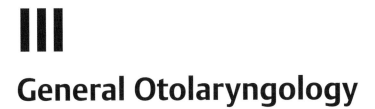

III

General Otolaryngology

11 Core Competencies

■ Introduction

In 2007, the Accreditation Council for Graduate Medical Education (ACGME) initiated the concept of the "core competencies" for residents in training. ACGME's Outcome Project was designed to support programs in their implementation of the competencies in their curricula, as well as the valid and reliable assessment of performance based on these competencies. Since then, hospitals and other health care institutions have adopted these core competencies in their evaluation of physicians and their credentialing criteria.

■ Accreditation Council for Graduate Medical Education's Core Competencies

Residents are expected to obtain competency in the following six areas to the level expected of a new practitioner:

- Patient Care
- Medical Knowledge
- Interpersonal and Communication Skills
- Professionalism
- Practice-Based Learning and Improvement
- Systems-Based Practice

Patient Care

Programs need to integrate improvement activities with patient care and other competencies. In addition, they should have a standardized Core Assessment System that facilitates evaluating and improving resident performance. Residents must demonstrate compassion, pertinence, and effectiveness for the treatment of health problems and the promotion of health. They are expected to do the following:

- Communicate effectively and demonstrate compassionate, caring, and respectful behaviors when interacting with patients and their families
- Gather essential and accurate information about their patients
- Make informed decisions about diagnostic and therapeutic interventions based on patient information and preferences, up-to-date scientific evidence, and clinical judgment
- Develop and carry out appropriate patient management plans
- Counsel and educate patients and their families
- Use information technology to support patient care decisions and patient education
- Perform competently all medical and invasive procedures considered essential for the area of practice
- Provide health care services aimed at preventing health problems or maintaining health
- Work with health care professionals, including those from other disciplines, to provide patient-focused care

Medical Knowledge

Residents must demonstrate knowledge about established and evolving biomedical, clinical, epidemiological, and social-behavioral sciences and the application of this knowledge to patient care. They are expected to demonstrate an investigatory and analytical thinking approach to clinical situations, and to know and apply the basic and clinically supportive sciences that are appropriate to their discipline.

Programs must require residents to acquire competence in medical knowledge and should define knowledge, skills, and behaviors required, as provided educational experiences. Residents of the program should be aware of this definition and of the resources available to achieve this competency. Departmental improvement activities must ensure full integration of this and other competencies with learning and clinical care.

Interpersonal and Communication Skills

Residents must be able to demonstrate interpersonal and communication skills that result in effective information exchange and teaming with patients, patients' families, and professional associates, and communication as related to medical recordkeeping. Programs should define the specific knowledge, skills, behaviors, and attitudes required, and provide educational experiences to permit their residents to acquire competency in interpersonal and communication skills.

Residents are expected to do the following:

- Communicate effectively with patients, families, and the public, and maintain a medically and ethically sound relationship with patients
- Use effective listening skills and elicit and provide information using effective nonverbal, explanatory, questioning, and writing skills
- Work and communicate effectively with other physicians, health care team members, and other professional groups, and act as a health care leader
- Effectively consult other physicians, other health professionals, and health-related agencies
- Maintain comprehensive, timely, and legible medical records, if applicable
- Exchange information, collaborate, and communicate with patients, families, the public, physicians, other health professionals, and health-related agencies

Training programs should have clear instruction in communication with patients and families, such as clinical teaching, case-based teaching, role modeling, and interactive workshops. Instructions in Communication with Colleagues include standardized patient handoff, clinical teaching, medical record-keeping, role modeling, and interactive workshops.

The Institute for Healthcare Improvement has various resources available to improve communications. The Situation-Background-Assessment-Recommendation (SBAR) technique is an example. It provides a framework for communication between members of the health care team about a patient's condition. SBAR is an effective and useful means of communication, especially for emergency or critical situations, and facilitates immediate attention and action.

The ACGME requires full integration of the competencies and their assessment with learning and clinical care. Program improvement activities can occur as part of educational retreats and departmental clinical competency committees, as well as feedback from internal review reports. Programs must now document the framework for program improvement. Such programs include internal program evaluations looking at in-training examinations and board certification performance, residents' evaluations of the educational program, and surveys by alumni and patients. External program evaluations are also necessary and may include National Clinical Practice Indicators and improvement plans resulting from internal review and/or site review.

Professionalism

Residents should commit to professional qualities by upholding ethical principles and giving respect to patients regardless of ethnicity, age, gender, orientation, or disabilities. They should thus demonstrate compassion; integrity; responsiveness to patient needs that supersedes self-interest; respect for patient privacy and autonomy; accountability to patients, society, and the profession; and sensitivity and responsiveness to a diverse patient population, including but not limited to diversity in gender, age, culture, race, religion, disabilities, and sexual orientation.

It is important for programs to define the specific knowledge, skills, behaviors, and attitudes required for professionalism. They must also provide educational experiences in order for their residents and fellows to demonstrate their professional competency. As for other competencies, several instructions and evaluation methods can be used, such as clinical and case-based teaching, mentoring, role modeling, and role playing with clinical cases where aspects of respect, integrity, honesty, compassion, and empathy can be discussed. Other venues include retreats and workshops. Web-based, self-directed learning activities are valuable and allow residents to view case studies involving patients from diverse cultural and racial backgrounds and with various disabilities, all of which can affect patient care and its delivery. Tufts University School of Medicine performs training courses on the Ethics of Clinical Investigation, aimed to increase awareness of research ethics and their practical application to medical practitioners and researchers.

ACGME has developed a guide to provide an educational resource for program directors and other medical educators, Advancing Education in Medical Professionalism, to aid teaching and assessing professionalism. The American Medical Association also has a valuable free online resource for ethics education with a new topic presented each month.

Practice-Based Learning and Improvement (PBLI)

The ACGME requires residents to investigate and evaluate their care of patients, appraise and assimilate scientific evidence, and continuously improve patient care based on constant self-evaluation and lifelong learning. Residents and fellows are expected to develop skills and habits so they can do the following:

- Identify strengths, deficiencies, and limits in their knowledge and expertise
- Set learning and improvement goals
- Identify and perform appropriate learning activities
- Systematically analyze practice, using quality improvement methods, and implement changes with the goal of practice improvement
- Incorporate formative evaluation feedback into daily practice
- Locate, appraise, and assimilate evidence from scientific studies related to their patients' health problems
- Use information technology to optimize learning
- Participate in the education of patients, families, students, residents, and other health professionals, as documented by evaluations of residents' teaching abilities by faculty and/or learners

The following are key components of the Practice-Based Learning and Improvement (PBLI) competency:

- *Lifelong learning and practice improvement*
  Residents and fellows must regularly evaluate their own practice and determine improvement. They must assess lifelong learning annually.
- *Appraisal and assimilation of scientific literature (evidence-based medicine)*
  This component helps ensure that residents obtain and evaluate scientific evidence in its application to patient care. Such methods include lectures, seminars, journal clubs, research projects, and clinical teaching.
- *Implementation of quality improvement*
  This component also includes lectures, seminars, conferences, or a quality improvement project.
- *Active participation in the education of others*
  The concept of residents as teachers includes such activities as clinical teaching, role modeling, and interactive workshops. Program directors must document inclusion of a formal teaching curriculum and assessment of resident and fellow performance in the semiannual evaluation of resident and fellow performance.

- *Teaching in the continuing education of physicians*
  Ideal clinical teachers exhibit many attributes that will make them effective teachers. Program directors should ensure that their curricula and evaluation mechanisms can document these attributes.

Systems-Based Practice (SBP)

Residents are expected to learn how to work within the larger context of health care. Programs must require residents to obtain competence in Systems-Based Practice (SBP). These programs must define the specific knowledge, skills, behaviors, and attitudes required to acquire this competency and must provide the necessary educational support for their residents to demonstrate this competency. Residents should be willing and able to call effectively and appropriately on other resources in the system to provide optimal health care.

Residents must be aware of and responsive to the larger context of the health care system. They are expected to work effectively in various health care delivery settings and systems relevant to their clinical specialty. They should be able to coordinate patient care within the health care system relevant to their clinical specialty, and they should be aware of cost and the risk–benefit analysis in patient care. They must act as advocates for quality patient care and optimal patient care systems, demonstrate their ability to work in interprofessional teams to enhance patient safety and improve patient care quality, and participate in identifying system errors and implementing potential systems solutions.

Programs should offer instructions on topics of health care delivery systems and patient safety and advocacy. These instructions may include clinical teaching, patient safety projects, lectures, workshops, seminars, and working with interdisciplinary teams. Mortality–morbidity conferences should be directed toward a systems-based approach. Topics of discussion should include different types of medical practice and delivery systems; system resources; reduction of error, including root cause analysis; and tools and techniques for controlling costs and allocating resources.

■ Methods for Evaluating Competencies

Programs must have clear and measurable means of assessing the competency skills. These methods can include the following:

- Global clinical performance ratings
- Focused observation evaluation
- Multirater/360-degree evaluation

- Performance on cognitive tests: in-training examinations, internal quizzes, and board exam first-time pass rate
- Case log review

- Portfolios: documents that highlight residents' efforts, progress, and achievements in multiple areas of the curriculum

■ Suggested Reading

Accreditation Council for Graduate Medical Education. Program Director Guide to the Common Program Requirements. Chicago, IL: ACGME; September 2012. http://www.acgme.org/acgmeweb/Portals/0/PDFs/commonguide/CompleteGuide_v2%20.pdf

American Medical Association. Virtual Mentor. http://virtualmentor.ama-assn.org/

The Institute for Healthcare for Improvement. http://www.ihi.org/knowledge/Pages/Tools/SBARTechniqueforCommunicationASituationalBriefingModel.aspx

Tufts University Sackler School of Graduate Biomedical Sciences. http://sackler.tufts.edu/Academics/Non-Degree-Programs/Certificate-in-Clinical-and-Translational-Science

12 Head and Neck Manifestations of Acquired Immunodeficiency Syndrome

■ Introduction

The human immunodeficiency virus (HIV) has had a major impact on the practice of medicine worldwide. Since its initial description in this country in 1981, the HIV epidemic has expanded dramatically. Globally, the number of people living with HIV has become relatively stable since 2007, after reaching its current peak prevalence of ~ 34,000 cases, with ~ 2.7 million new cases worldwide in 2010. Approximately 10% of all cases are in children, but the percentage of newly diagnosed cases is now disproportionately large in children (~ 15%). The epidemic affects approximately equal numbers of males and females. Approximately 1.8 million deaths from HIV infection were reported in 2010, and more than 30 million people have died of acquired immunodeficiency syndrome (AIDS)-related diseases since it was first described. Nearly 70% of all people living with HIV reside in sub-Saharan Africa. Epidemics in Asia have remained relatively stable and are still largely concentrated among high-risk groups. Conversely, the number of people living with HIV in eastern Europe and Central Asia has more than tripled since 2000.

In the United States, the initial sites of concentration of AIDS cases were major coastal metropolitan areas, such as New York, San Francisco, Los Angeles, and Miami. However, the epidemic has spread throughout mid-America, leaving essentially no major metropolitan area unaffected. Because up to 70% of patients infected with HIV have signs and symptoms of illnesses in the head and neck areas at some time during their illness, otolaryngologists should be prepared to safely and effectively deal with this patient population.

Human Immunodeficiency Virus Virology

The retrovirus HIV contains a ribonucleic acid (RNA) genetic core that must be translated into a deoxyribonucleic acid (DNA) analogue to be effective. The glycoprotein surface receptors of HIV have a high affinity for CD4 receptors, which are found primarily on the surface of T cell–helper lymphocytes. After attaching to a T-helper lymphocyte, the virus injects its RNA core into the host cell. Accompanying this RNA is the enzyme reverse transcriptase, which uses the RNA as a template to make a strand of DNA. This DNA migrates to the host cell nucleus, where it is incorporated into the host cell DNA as a provirus. At some future time, this provirus begins to direct the host cellular machinery to produce HIV viral particles. These are then assembled and cause cell lysis and the release of free HIV particles. These can then infect other cells, thus completing the cell cycle.

Since the T-helper lymphocyte is the primary human cell affected by HIV (although other cells, such as macrophages and glial cells, can be infected given that they possess a low concentration of surface CD4 receptors), the serial evaluation of peripheral CD4 cell count is used as a surrogate marker for progression of HIV disease. HIV disease can be staged based on the CD4 cell count. Patients with CD4 cell counts greater than 500 cells per deciliter are generally healthy. When the CD4 cell count drops below 500 but is greater than 200, the symptomatic stage of HIV disease begins. Patients develop opportunistic infections and symptoms secondary to systemic HIV infection. As the CD4 cell count drops below 200, severe immunodeficiency results in serious opportunistic infections as well as HIV-associated malignancies.

The CD4 cell count has become a well-accepted monitor of HIV disease progression. In 1993, the Centers for Disease Control and Prevention modified its definition of AIDS to include a CD4 count of less than 200. Currently, even in the absence of other significant HIV-associated diseases, a patient who is HIV infected and has a CD4 count of less than 200 has AIDS by definition.

The CD4 cell count is often used as an indicator to begin various AIDS therapies. Currently, two classes of AIDS drugs have been effective in altering the disease.

The first class of drugs used extensively in patients with AIDS consisted of inhibitors of reverse transcriptase. Drugs, such as azidothymidine (AZT) or zidovudine, dideoxyinosine (DDI), and lamivudine (3TC), all were initially used with great optimism and enthusiasm; however, over the last 5 years their ability to provide long-term survival benefit has been disappointing. Recently, a new class of drugs, the protease inhibitors, has been introduced. These drugs—indinavir, saquinavir, and ritonavir—have shown remarkable short-term ability to both reduce viral burden in HIV-infected patients and provide tremendous symptomatic improvement because of improved immune response. They act by inhibiting HIV protease activity, an enzyme critical for the final intracellular production of virus particles. Although the long-term efficacy of the latter class of drugs has not been established, AIDS specialists are cautiously enthusiastic that when used in combination with the older drugs, the protease inhibitors may convert what was previously a universally fatal disease into a chronic illness.

The natural history of HIV infection clinically includes three phases: an initial acute phase lasting ~ 4 months; a second latent phase, which may last for more than 10 years without retroviral treatment; and finally AIDS, diagnosed by one or more AIDS-defining illnesses and a reduction of the CD4 count to less than 200 cells per cubic millimeter. Many of the ear, nose, and throat (ENT) manifestations, as well as the AIDS-defining illnesses, respond to antiretroviral therapy, but because some of these manifestations occur prior to the CD4 count being below 200, other approaches to treatment are necessary.

■ Ear, Nose and Throat Manifestations

As the CD4 cell count decreases, systemic infections and illnesses, as well as localized diseases, become prominent features. The head and neck area is commonly involved with these various manifestations (**Table 12.1**).

Ears

Acute Otitis Media

One of the most common head and neck manifestations of HIV infection is acute otitis media and serous otitis media. Patients often present with hearing loss, aural pressure, or acute infection secondary to immune dysfunction. Although a course of antibiotics can often produce a successful remedy in patients who have CD4 counts of over 200, patients with low CD4 counts are often resistant to antibiotic therapy. The placement of a tympanostomy tube can provide tremendous symptomatic relief for these patients.

Otitis Externa

Otitis externa is also a common problem. Because these patients often experience underlying dermatitis, superinfection and inflammation in the external auditory canals are common. If this infection progresses to involve the conchal bowl or pinna, the possibility of herpes simplex infection must be considered. In these cases, treatment with acyclovir as well as local wound care can usually produce a dramatic clinical response.

Sensorineural Hearing Loss

Sensorineural hearing loss has often been described in patients with HIV. Even when there are no overt clinical symptoms or audiometric findings, abnormalities of auditory brainstem response are frequently detectable. These changes may be secondary to primary cochlear effects of either the virus or ototoxic drugs, or they may be due to demyelination in the auditory tract.

Table 12.1 Most common head and neck manifestations of HIV and AIDS and treatment

Affected Areas	Manifestations	Treatments
Ears	Otitis media	Medical and PE tubes
Nose and paranasal sinuses	Sinusitis	Quinolones and clindamycin Rule out invasive fungus
Oral cavity	Candidiasis	Topical and systemic antifungals
Pharynx and larynx	Viral and other infection	Organism-specific
Neck	Lymphadenopathy	FNAB guides management
Salivary glands	Benign lymphoepithelial cysts	FNAB/sclerotherapy

Abbreviations: FNAB, fine-needle aspiration biopsy; PE, pressure equalization.

Skin

Seborrheic Dermatitis

Seborrheic dermatitis is common in HIV-infected patients. In many instances, this condition can become secondarily infected, most commonly with *Staphylococcus aureus*. Local treatment with topical steroids, topical antibiotics, and occasionally systemic antibodies can effectively manage this problem.

Herpes Zoster and Herpes Simplex

Herpes zoster and herpes simplex are also common findings. Herpes zoster is often more resistant to therapy, more prolonged, and associated with greater posttherapeutic neuralgia than in non-HIV-infected patients. Herpes simplex is also a common problem that requires early culture for diagnosis and that usually responds very well to oral therapy with acyclovir.

Molluscum contagiosum

Molluscum contagiosum is a skin disease caused by a pox virus. Although it also occurs in non-HIV-infected patients, patients who are immunosuppressed due to HIV often develop crops of these molluscum bodies. They are often much larger and more difficult to manage in this patient population. These lesions are predisposed to develop in the periorbital and eyelid areas, often producing functional as well as cosmetic disturbances.

Nose and Paranasal Sinuses

Herpes Simplex

As on the skin, herpes simplex can often be seen in the nasal vestibule. This infection usually starts as a chronic nonhealing inflammatory process that extends onto the septum, the nasal alae, and ultimately to the upper lip and face. Appropriate diagnosis and treatment usually result in a dramatic response.

Allergic Rhinitis

Allergic rhinitis is more frequent in the HIV patient population. Symptoms of allergic rhinitis increase as do eosinophilia and IGE levels, as the underlying disease process progresses. Treatment with topical nasal steroids and second-generation antihistamines can often ameliorate these rhinitis symptoms. High-dose guaifenesin has also been effective for these symptoms.

Sinusitis occurs with increasing frequency as the CD4 cell count decreases. When the CD4 cell count drops below 200, sinusitis often becomes a chronic problem. Besides the obvious immunodeficiency that contributes to this problem, other etiologies include atopic disease, which is increased in these patients, and abnormal mucosal inflammation, which contributes to the production of mucus with abnormally thick, tenacious characteristics.

Acute Sinusitis

Acute sinusitis in patients with a CD4 count higher than 200 is usually caused by bacteria similar to those found in non-HIV-infected patients. On the other hand, chronic sinusitis in patients with low CD4 cell counts has *Pseudomonas aeruginosa* as an etiologic agent in up to 20% of cases. *Staphylococcus aureas* and coagulase-negative staphylococcus are also prominent features of chronic sinusitis in these patients. Treatment should take into account this high preponderance of pseudomonal and staphylococcal organisms. Empirical therapy with ciprofloxacin and clindamycin is often an effective combination for these patients, though it can be fraught with a high rate of diarrhea.

Fungal Sinusitis

Patients with suspected fungal sinusitis should be carefully evaluated for the invasive forms of the disease because HIV is a risk factor. Although most patients with invasive fungal sinusitis have neutropenia, patients with HIV, particularly those with hematologic malignancy of lymphoma, may develop life-threatening invasive fungal sinusitis.

Oral Cavity

Oral Candidiasis

One of the most common head and neck problems in this patient population is oral candidiasis. This is often the first manifestations of HIV disease in an otherwise healthy individual. Thrush usually takes on the typical cottage cheese inflammatory appearance. On the other hand, flat atrophic lesions on the oral and oropharyngeal mucosa representing atrophic thrush can also appear in this patient population. Treatment is usually effective with topical agents; however, when immunodeficiency becomes profound, systemic therapy with such drugs as fluconazole and occasionally amphotericin may be indicated. If patients develop severe sore throat and odynophagia that do not respond immediately to topical agents, the possibility of esophageal candidiasis should be investigated.

Aphthous Stomatitis

Aphthous stomatitis is another serious and potentially life-threatening problem in this population. These oral ulcers are common and can often attain sizes up to 2 to 3 cm. Because of the severe pain and anorexia that can accompany these lesions, they can be a terminal event if untreated. Topical steroids, as well as systemic antibiotics, can occasionally be effective; however, in severe cases systemic steroids are usually necessary.

Herpes Simplex

Herpes simplex is also a common problem in the oral cavity. Since it is often difficult to differentiate these lesions from aphthous stomatitis, cultures are usually indicated prior to instituting therapy with acyclovir.

Papilloma

Papilloma of the oral cavity are also fairly common. These can present as single lesions on the soft palate, buccal mucosa, lips, or tongue, and can occasionally occur as crops of papillomata throughout the oral cavity and oropharynx. Papillomas are usually amenable to laser therapy when they become symptomatic.

Hairy Leukoplakia

Hairy leukoplakia, a condition of the lateral tongue, was initially described early in the AIDS epidemic. Although it is usually asymptomatic and consists of a vertically correlated, whitish plaque along the lateral surface of the tongue, it was initially considered as a productive guide to the development of AIDS in patients at risk for HIV. The etiology is felt to be an Epstein-Barr virus. Because it is asymptomatic, it does not usually require treatment.

Periodontal Disease and Necrotizing Gingivitis

Periodontal disease and necrotizing gingivitis can produce substantial morbidity in AIDS patients. Gingival atrophy is a very common condition, and necrotizing infections of the periodontal region can occur despite aggressive local and systemic therapy. For this reason, HIV-infected patients should develop good oral hygiene habits and should be seen and evaluated by a dentist on a regular basis to help provide good oral hygiene and prevent gingival atrophy.

Pharynx and Larynx

As already mentioned, aphthous stomatitis, as well as fungal and viral infections that can occur in the oral cavity, can also be found in the oropharynx and hypopharynx. The treatment of these infections is essentially the same as for the oral cavity.

The larynx is an often difficult area to evaluate and accurately diagnose. Viral infections, including herpes virus and cytomegalovirus, have been described in the larynx of HIV-infected patients. Also, various fungal infections, including histoplasmosis, coccidiomycosis, aspergillosis, and candidiasis, have all also been reported in these patients. Bacterial epiglottitis may be more common in these patients, although the etiology and treatment are similar to those for non-HIV-infected populations. Treatment of yeast infections involves the use of both systemic antifungals, such as fluconazole, and topical treatment with nystatin.

Neck

Neck masses are common in HIV-infected patients. The most common etiology is the generalized AIDS-related lymphadenopathy, which is frequently seen in the early stages of HIV disease. This generalized lymph node enlargement occurs throughout the lymphatic system and is not confined to the neck. When the lymphadenopathy is symmetrical and otherwise asymptomatic, there is usually no indication for open or fine-needle aspiration biopsy. On the other hand, if a lymph node begins to enlarge out of proportion with the other lymph nodes of the neck, or when associated with other systemic symptoms suggesting an underlying illness other than HIV disease, biopsy is indicated. In such cases, fine-needle aspiration biopsy (FNAB) is useful to confirm the lymphoid nature of the neck mass (and to exclude other malignant conditions, such as squamous cell carcinoma, which may arise from both the skin of the head and neck and the upper aerodigestive tract and is sometimes associated with viral etiology). Indication for open biopsy is guided by the cytology report. Otolaryngologists should consult with the patient's primary care or infectious disease specialist in equivocal cases to determine the need for and timing of open biopsy.

Salivary Glands

Xerostomia

The salivary glands, especially the parotid, are also often affected by HIV infection. Xerostomia, secondary to a Sjögren type illness, is often described and appears to result from a lymphocytic infiltration of the salivary glands. In sub-Saharan Africa, HIV pathology is perhaps the most common pathology of the parotid gland. Up to 50% of patients with HIV will be affected by salivary gland pathology. The variety of pathology seen in the parotid is shown in **Table 12.2**, and the differential diagnosis of parotid cysts is shown in **Table 12.3**.

Benign Lymphoepithelial Cysts

Benign lymphoepithelial cysts of the parotid glands are one of the most common problems with HIV-infected patients and often occur in the latent phase of the disease. These cysts are best evaluated with imaging studies, which are often diagnostic. Ultrasonography and computed tomography (CT) are both useful in this regard.

Benign lymphoepithelial cysts are bilateral in ~ 80% of patients and are multiple in up to 90% of patients. As the name suggests, these cysts are not associated with malignancy, but they may become very disfiguring. Patients are often disturbed by these cysts as being visible stigmata of their disease. Repeated needle aspiration is usually ineffective, radiotherapy has significant side effects and risk of secondary malignancy, and parotidectomy is risky to health care personnel and to the patient's facial nerve and poses different cosmetic considerations in the treatment of a primarily cosmetic problem. Injections with tetracycline have been shown to be effective, but injectable tetracycline is no longer available. Injection with doxycycline or bleomycin has been reported as effective, but in Africa, ethanol has been used for economic reasons.

◼ Neoplasms

Kaposi Sarcoma

Kaposi sarcoma (KS) is the most common malignancy associated with HIV and AIDS. These lesions typically present as red-to-violaceous discolorations over the skin or mucous membranes. AIDS-related KS lesions occur in almost all areas of the body, compared with the classic non-AIDS-related KS, which usually involves the lower extremities. Of interest, KS appears to be a disease primarily of the homosexual population. Nearly 40% of gay men with AIDS will develop KS. A much smaller percentage of intravenous drug abusers develop this malignancy, and essentially no hemophiliacs with AIDS develop KS. This interesting association initially raised the possibility that KS may be caused by a secondary virus that uses a sexual-transmission mode of spread. Recent studies have uncovered a herpes-type virus

Table 12.2   Salivary gland manifestations of HIV infection and AIDS

Xerostomia
Benign lymphoepithelial cysts
Infectious sialadenitis
Sjögren-type illness with lymphocytic infiltration
Other "cysts"
Neoplasms

associated with the KS tumor, which appears to suggest such a relationship.

In the head and neck area, KS appears to have a predisposition for the mucous membranes, as well as for facial skin. Treatment for KS is usually palliative. Patients rarely die of KS; instead, they succumb to some other generalized AIDS-related medical condition.

The primary treatment for KS has been radiation therapy. This is usually conducted effectively at fairly low doses ranging from 1,500 to 2,500 centigray. The disadvantage of radiation therapy is that many HIV-infected patients respond adversely to radiation therapy to the upper aerodigestive tract mucous membranes by developing severe mucositis. For individual symptomatic lesions, other local treatment options include laser therapy, cryotherapy, and, more recently, intralesional injection of vinblastine. When KS becomes widespread, chemotherapy is often used and has been shown to have some effect in managing this disease.

Table 12.3   Differential diagnosis of cystic masses in the parotid gland and neck in HIV and AIDS

Benign lymphoepithelial cysts
Branchial cleft cysts
Salivary duct cysts
Traumatic sialoceles
Sjögren syndrome
Lymphangiomas
Cryptococcus
Polycystic parotid disease
Warthin tumor
Malignant primary tumors (mucoepidermoid carcinoma, adenoid cystic carcinoma, lymphoma)
Mycobacterial infections/tuberculosis
Cystic metastases (carcinoma, melanoma)

Non-Hodgkin Lymphoma

Non-Hodgkin lymphoma (NHL) is the second-most-common malignancy seen in HIV-infected patients. NHL tends to present in extranodal locations compared with non-HIV-infected patients, where nodal lymphoma is usually the rule. These tumors are usually of B cell origin and can be fairly aggressive, with rapid onset and progression.

T cell Lymphomas and Burkitt Lymphoma

T cell lymphomas and Burkitt lymphoma have also been reported with HIV. These malignancies are often treated with a combination of chemotherapy and radiation therapy; however, in cases with widespread disease the outcome is usually disappointing.

Squamous Cell Carcinoma

There is increasing evidence that the occurrence of squamous cell carcinoma of the upper aerodigestive tract may be slightly increased in this patient population. Tobacco and alcohol use both seem to play significant contributing roles in the development of this malignancy. However, these tumors are often more advanced at presentation, seem to be somewhat more aggressive, and occur in a younger population. Human papilloma virus may be a risk factor for both mucosal and cutaneous squamous cell carcinomas in patients with HIV. The decision regarding treatment should always take into account the poor and often adverse response that HIV-infected patients can have to radiation therapy. Surgical management should be considered, based on the underlying health and immune status of the patient.

■ Controversial Issues

Whether to operate on patients with AIDS or patients who are HIV positive was considered controversial. Fears of disease transmission to the medical staff and short patient life expectancies were the principle issues driving the controversy. With universal precautions, a very low rate of transmission of the disease to health care workers, anti-HIV drugs available for prophylaxis, and a longer-living and healthier HIV-positive population, this controversy has subsided.

■ Practice Guidelines, Consensus Statements, and Measures

Surgery on HIV/AIDS patients. www.cmej.org.za/index.php/cmej/article/download/1853/1564

■ Suggested Reading

Bayraktar UD, Ramos JC, Petrich A, et al. Outcome of patients with relapsed/refractory acquired immune deficiency syndrome-related lymphoma diagnosed 1999-2008 and treated with curative intent in the AIDS Malignancy Consortium. Leuk Lymphoma 2012;53(12):2383–2389 [e-pub ahead of print]

Hunt SM, Miyamoto RC, Cornelius RS, Tami TA. Invasive fungal sinusitis in the acquired immunodeficiency syndrome. Otolaryngol Clin North Am 2000;33(2):335–347

Marsot-Dupuch K, Quillard J, Meyohas MC. Head and neck lesions in the immunocompromised host. Eur Radiol 2004;14(Suppl 3): E155–E167

Meyer E, Lubbe DE, Fagan JJ. Alcohol sclerotherapy of human immunodeficiency virus related parotid lymphoepithelial cysts. J Laryngol Otol 2009;123(4):422–425 [e-pub 2008 Jul 1]

Shiels MS, Engels EA. Increased risk of histologically defined cancer subtypes in human immunodeficiency virus-infected individuals: clues for possible immunosuppression-related or infectious etiology. Cancer 2012;118(19):4869–4876 10.1002/cncr.27454 [e-pub ahead of print]

13 Physics and Uses of Lasers in Otolaryngology

■ Introduction

Laser Physics

The three essential elements to a laser are (1) the lasing medium, (2) an excitation source, and (3) two mirrors to provide the optical feedback. In the first laser made, the lasing medium was a ruby crystal and the excitation source was a flash lamp, similar to the flash from a camera.

A laser is distinguished from an ordinary lamp by four basic characteristics:

1. *Monochromatic* Individual wavelengths or a single color of light is emitted. This is used to target blood vessels for hemostasis and in selective photothermolysis to treat vascular lesions.
2. *Coherence* The wavelengths all rise and fall together. The coherence of laser light is not widely used in medicine.
3. *Collimated* A parallel beam of light is emitted. This permits focusing the laser to the smallest possible point and is essential for tissue ablation.
4. *High power* With focusing, a high power can be delivered to a small area.

When dealing with power, one should always remember to use power density or irradiance, which is the intensity of the laser divided by the area of the beam. The normal units for irradiance are watts per square centimeter (cm^2). Besides the irradiance, one needs to know the energy density or the laser fluence. The fluence is the irradiance multiplied by the exposure time. The units of fluence are typically watts times seconds per cm^2, or equivalently, joules (J) per cm^2.

Irradiance = intensity → watts area cm^2

Fluence = intensity × time → watts × sec = J area cm^2 cm^2

Laser Light Delivery

Articulated Arms

The articulated arm is a simple but elegant device. Mirrors placed at 45 degrees to tubes carry the laser light. The tubes can rotate about the optical axis of the mirrors. The result is a tremendous amount of flexibility in the arm and in delivering the laser light. The articulated arm is typically used with the carbon dioxide (CO_2) laser, but it works with all wavelengths and intensities of light. It preserves the coherence and the collimated characteristics of the laser light.

Optical Fibers

Optical fibers are frequently used with near-infrared and visible lasers but cannot work for the very short pulsed laser with high peak intensities. Light is trapped in the glass and propagates down through the fiber in a process called total internal reflection. Optical fibers can be tens of micrometers in diameter or greater than hundreds of micrometers in diameter. They can transmit light with almost no loss. The beam is no longer coherent or collimated when emitted from the fiber.

Beam Profiles

Most commercial lasers produce a beam with a Gaussian profile. This profile is called the fundamental mode or the transverse electromagnetic mode $(TEM)_{00}$ of the laser. A laser beam does not have a constant intensity across the beam diameter; instead, the intensity peaks at the center of the beam. The peak intensity then falls off with a normal (or Gaussian) type of distribution. This particular mode of lasing gives the smallest focal point when the beam is focused through a lens.

One can work both in and out of the focal plane of the laser beam. Working with the light in focus, one gets a more direct incision. Working out of the focal plane, one has more of a surface removal of tissue. In diagrams of light being focused by the lens, one frequently sees pictures of a cone of light focused down to an infinitely small spot. In fact, light does not do this, but instead focuses to a minimum size, or what is called a beamwaist.

The beamwaist is determined by the focal length of the lens, f, the laser beam diameter, D, and the wavelength of green light, gl. For large focal length lenses, such as the $f = 400$ mm on the surgical microscope for microlaryngeal surgery, the beamwaist is quite large. When one uses a handpiece with an $f = 100$ mm focal length, there is a much smaller spot size, or beamwaist. There is a tradeoff between the depth of field and how large of a range the beam remains in focus with the beamwaist. With a very large beamwaist, the beam is in focus for a relatively large distance.

Light and Tissue Interactions

Light can interact with tissue in four different mechanisms: transmission, reflection, scatter, and absorption. The *reflection* off the surface of tissue is minimal when the laser is delivered perpendicular to the surface. *Scattering* not only spreads out a focused spot but limits the depth of penetration; the shorter the wavelength of the laser, the more it is scattered by the tissue. *Absorption* can cause three different processes:

1. *Photothermal* The laser energy can be absorbed by chromophores within the tissue. The resulting effect can be the production of heat. This is the thermal effect seen in most conventional laser systems in use today.
2. *Photochemical* The radiant energy of a laser can stimulate or react with specific molecules within a cell. This reaction can cause a chemical change to occur within the cell. An example is the reaction that occurs with injection of a photosensitizing drug into tissue and the biochemical effect that is produced when the drug is activated by the stimulating effect of radiant laser energy.
3. *Photoacoustic* The use of short pulses of high-wattage laser energy can disrupt cellular architecture because of the production of sound waves or photoacoustic shock waves.

Penetration Depth

The interaction of light with tissue is a complicated process. **Table 13.1** lists the more common surgical lasers and the distance each of these lasers pen-

Table 13.1 Commonly used surgical lasers with depth of penetration

Laser	Wavelength (mm)	Typical tissue penetration depth (mm)
Argon	514 and 488	0.8
KTP	532	0.9
Flashlamp pumped dye laser	585	0.9
Argon pumped dye laser	630	1.0
Nd:YAG	1,064	4.0
Ho:YAG	2,150	0.4
Er:YAG	2,940	0.002
Carbon dioxide	10,600	0.03

Abbreviations: Er:YAG, erbium:yttrium-aluminum-garnet; Ho:YAG, holmium:yttrium-aluminum-garnet; KTP, potassium-titanyl-phosphate; Nd:YAG, neodymium:yttrium-aluminum-garnet.

etrates into tissues. These general numbers do not represent any particular tissue; instead, they represent an average of several tissues.

Ablation Process

Photothermal ablation, the most common mechanism of laser incisions, is a straightforward process. The energy of the laser is absorbed by the tissue and changed to heat energy. The tissue heats, and once the temperature passes above 100°C, the water in the tissue starts to vaporize. Once sufficient energy has been added to change the water from liquid to steam, the tissue is torn open by the expansion of the steam.

The ablation crater can be left with lateral tissue damage. This damage might include charred debris on the bottom of the crater, additional damage near the bottom of the crater from forward-scattered light, damage around the mouth of the crater from the edges of the focused beam with subablation fluence, and nearly isotropic damage from thermal diffusion. In addition, blood vessels can transport heat away from the ablation site, creating cooler locations or locations with less thermal damage.

■ Laser Types and Applications

The potential clinical applications of surgical lasers are determined by the wavelength, the output pulse length, and the specific tissue absorption characteristics. Therefore, the surgeon should consider the properties of each wavelength and time structure when choosing a particular laser (**Table 13.2**). Doing so will allow the surgical objectives to be met with minimal morbidity and maximal efficiency. **Table 13.3** lists common lasers used in otolaryngology and their applications. Patently, a procedure can be accomplished with different lasers, and the skills of the surgeon can often affect outcome as much as wavelength selection.

Carbon Dioxide Laser

Laryngeal Disease

The CO_2 laser functions primarily as a hemostatic scalpel when the beam is focused. When the beam is defocused, the CO_2 laser can also be used effectively to ablate and cytoreduce epithelial disease, such as diffuse papillomatosis. Operating at a wavelength 10.6 μm (μm) in the infrared region, CO_2 lasers deliver nonionizing electromagnetic radiation that is well absorbed by water, which is ubiquitous in the laryngeal soft tissues. Care must be taken near phonatory membranes, because thermal energy can result in fibrosis of the delicate superficial lamina propria (SLP), which is the primary oscillator responsible for voice production. It is reasonable to use the CO_2 laser on the vibratory membranes when (1) there is no functional SLP present, as may be encountered in patients who have had previous surgery; and (2) cancer has already invaded and replaced the SLP.

The aiming beam (line-of-sight) delivery system using a joystick and foot pedal offers surgeons greater ease in performing precise bimanual surgery. However, the enhanced manual dexterity of the joystick is offset by the vaporization and ablation of varied amounts of the phonatory membranes. The CO_2 laser is also valuable in treating selected posterior glottal disorders that require arytenoidectomy or dissection of subepithelial stenosis. The microspot CO_2 laser is ill suited to treat benign subepithelial masses of the phonatory vocal fold, such as nodules, polyps, and cysts. These lesions are optimally resected by cold-instrument tangential dissection, with maximal preservation of underlying SLP and complete preservation of overlying epithelium.

Facial Skin Resurfacing

Resurfacing of photoaged skin with laser is a well-established tool for treatment of facial rhytids. The use of CO_2 laser in skin resurfacing is advantageous because the thermal damage to the surrounding tissue causes an insult that prompts fibroblasts to increase collagen production and results in the observed clinical effects. The three treatment modalities for facial skin resurfacing are ablative skin resurfacing (ASR), nonablative dermal remodeling (NDR), and fractional photothermolysis (FP).

The most effective laser treatment option for repair of most photodamaged skin has been ASR with the pulsed CO_2 laser; however, the side effects are significant. In the first week following treatment there is oozing, edema, crusting, and a burning discomfort. Adverse effects include acneiform eruption, herpes simplex outbreak, bacterial infections, and hyperpigmentation. Therefore, ASR with erbium:yttrium-aluminum-garnet (Er:YAG) laser was introduced, because at 2,940 nanometers (nm) its wavelength is much closer to an absorption maximum of water (3,000 nm); therefore, there is shallower absorption depth, leading to less residual thermal damage.

Table 13.2 Wavelength, pulse length, and chromophore in tissue by type of laser

Laser	Wavelength (nm)	Chromophore in tissue	Pulse length
Argon	514 and 488	Hemoglobin and melanin	Cw
KTP	532	Hemoglobin and melanin	Quasi-cw
Flashlamp pumped dye laser	585	Hemoglobin	$4 \times 10^{/n/4}$s
Argon pumped dye laser	630	Photoactive dyes	Cw
Ruby (Q-switched)	694	Tattoo dyes, pigments	10^{-8}s
Nd:YAG	1,064	Pigments	Cw
Nd:YAG (Q-switched)	1,064	Tattoo dyes, pigments	10^{-8}s
Ho:YAG	2,150	Water	1×10^{-3}s
Er:YAG	2,940	Water	2.5×10^{-4}s
Carbon dioxide	10,600	Water	Cw

Abbreviations: cw, continuous wave; Er:YAG, erbium:yttrium-aluminum-garnet; Ho:YAG; holmium:yttrium-aluminum-garnet; KTP, potassium-titanyl-phosphate; Nd:YAG, neodymium:yttrium-aluminum-garnet; s, seconds.

Table 13.3 Lasers and their use in otolaryngology–head and neck surgery.

Laser	Anatomical site	Therapy	Reason
Argon	Ear	Lysis of middle ear adhesions Stapedotomy	
Argon	Lips, tongue, and oral cavity	Telangiectatic vessels	Hemoglobin absorption
Argon pumped dye laser		PDT	Able to tune the laser to maximum absorption of photosensitizer
CO_2	Ear	Stapedotomy	
CO_2	Glottis	Bilateral vocal cord paralysis Polyps Reinke edema T1 midcordal SCC with no anterior commissure involvement	Laser arytenoidectomy, coagulation Microspot, precision Microspot, precision Microspot, precision, microflap Excisional biopsy
CO_2	Larynx	Laryngoceles, cysts, granulomas Laryngomalacia Stenoses (glottic, posterior, and subglottic) Suprahyoid supraglottic T1 SCC Recurrent respiratory papilloma	Coagulation, hands-off technique Aryepiglottic fold division, coagulation Microtrapdoor techniques Excision with frozen section control Hands-off technique, less scarring precision
CO_2	Lingual tonsils	Recurrent tonsillitis, hypertrophy	Minimal edema with complete vaporization
CO_2	Nose	Turbinate hypertrophy	Coagulation, less scabbing, and scarring
CO_2	Oral cavity	Carcinoma (verrucous, superficial T1) Lymphangioma Premalignant (leukoplakia, erythroplakia) Tongue T1 and limited T2	Less pain and edema, covers a large area Minimal edema, coagulation Vaporization, excision, can cover a large area Less pain and edema, precise cutting, coagulation
CO_2	Oropharynx	T1 and T2 squamous cell carcinoma Laser assisted uvulopalatoplasty	Precision, coagulation, less edema
CO_2	Subglottis	Hemangioma	Defocused beam, shrinkage, coagulation
CO_2	Trachea	Papilloma Stenoses	
Flashlamp pumped dye laser		Port wine stains	Selective photothermolysis
KTP	Ear	Stapedotomies Cholesteatoma	Fiber delivery
KTP	Larynx	Obstructing SCC	Debulking airway, staging, coagulation
KTP	Nose	Epistaxis Polyps, concha bullosa	Fiber delivery, coagulation, debulking for visualization, coagulation
KTP	Oropharynx	Sleep apnea, UPPP	Coagulation
KTP	Palatine tonsils	Recurrent tonsillitis, obstructive apnea	Coagulation
Nd:YAG	Esophagus	Obstructing malignant lesions	Debulking, coagulation fiber delivery
Nd:YAG	Nose	Osler-Weber-Rendu (HHT)	Coagulation, hands-off technique
Nd:YAG	Trachea	Obstructing malignant lesions	Debulking, coagulation, fiber delivery
Solid state diode laser	Larynx, traches, esophagus, bronchi, oral cavity, skin	Head and neck cancer	Tunable laser to maximize absorption of photosensitizer drug
Thulium	Larynx, trachea, oral cavity, oropharynx, hypopharynx		Head and neck cancer, ablation, cutting, coagulation

Abbreviations: HHT, hereditary hemorrhagic telangiectasia; KTP, potassium-titanyl-phosphate; Nd:YAG, neodymium:yttrium-aluminum-garnet; PDT, photodynamic therapy; SCC, squamous cell carcinoma; UPPP, uvulopalatopharyngoplasty for obstructive sleep apna.

In 2004, Manstein introduced the concept of FP for cutaneous remodeling to overcome the problems with ASR and NDR. FP creates microscopic thermal wound zones (MTZs) and specifically spares tissue surrounding each wound. Each MTZ allows fast epidermal repair and short migratory paths for keratinocytes. The density of MTZs and the amount of space between them can be varied for a given energy level. The FP modality is currently used for treatment of photoaging, acne scarring, and skin laxity, among others. Few complications have been reported with FP, and the neck-banding and ectropion seen following treatments with the FP CO_2 laser are much less than what is seen with traditional CO_2 lasers and dermabrasion. Therefore, fractional resurfacing through FP has resulted in a dependable skin rejuvenation system with minimal downtime and predictable results.

Photoangiolytic Lasers

Pulsed-Dye Laser (PDL, 585 nm)

Anderson's development of the concept of selective photothermolysis for the treatment of dermatologic vascular malformations led to the development of the 585 nm pulsed-dye laser (PDL), because its wavelength is precisely selected to target an absorbance peak of oxyhemoglobin (~ 571 nm) and to fully penetrate the intralumenal blood, thereby depositing heat uniformly into the vessel. The laser pulse width (0.5 ms) is precisely selected to contain the heat to the vessel without causing collateral damage to the extravascular soft tissue from heat conduction.

Pilot studies were performed using the 585 nm PDL for laryngeal papillomatosis by Bower and McMillan. Shortly thereafter, large-scale investigations in the treatment of a spectrum of laryngeal lesions, including vocal fold dysplasia, papillomatosis, and ectasias/varices were reported. The aberrant and/or abundant microvasculature present in each of the aforementioned lesions is a key feature when considering photoangiolysis for surgical management. The microcirculation could be targeted to involute laryngeal lesions (dysplasia, cancer, papilloma, and varices) or to facilitate cold-instrument resection (ectasias and polyps), while minimizing thermal trauma to the surrounding soft tissue, SLP, and epithelium. In theory, this would be ideal for maintaining the pliability of the vocal folds' layered microstructure (SLP and epithelium) and glottal sound production.

The PDL has been effective in treating papillomatosis and dysplasia without the associated clinically observed soft tissue complications associated with the CO_2 laser (thermal damage, tissue necrosis, superficial lamina propria scarring, and anterior commissure web formation). The presumed mechanism of disease regression is the selective destruction of the subepithelial microvasculature and separation of the epithelium from the underlying SLP by denaturing the basement membrane zone-linking proteins. This results in ischemia to the diseased mucosa, albeit not permanently. This microvascular "angiolysis" approach restricts survival and growth of neoplastic epithelium, while minimizing cytotoxicity to the delicate layered microstructure (SLP) of the vocal fold.

A potential disadvantage of PDL treatment is that it can be difficult to accurately quantify the energy delivery and real-time tissue effects, despite the fact that this laser is unlikely to cause substantial soft tissue injury to the vocal folds. Furthermore, given the extremely short pulse width (~ 0.5 millisecondsec), it is not unusual for the vessel walls of the microcirculation to rupture, resulting in extravasation of blood into the surrounding tissue. In laryngeal lesions, such as papillomatosis, the extravasated blood diverts the laser energy in the form of a heat sink, which diminishes the effectiveness and selectivity of the laser.

Potassium-Titanyl-Phosphate Laser (KTP, 532 nm)

The potassium-titanyl-phosphate (KTP) laser is a green light laser with a wavelength of 532 nm, which coincides with one of the absorbance peaks of oxyhemoglobin. Similar to the PDL, this laser has a fiber-based delivery system. It has been used to treat papilloma, dysplasia, and vascular lesions within the larynx and as a new surgical strategy in the management of early vocal fold cancer.

Comparative experiments between the KTP and PDL lasers using the chick chorioallantoic membrane to simulate vocal fold microvasculature reveal several advantages of the KTP laser over the PDL. The longer pulse width of the KTP laser (15 millisecondsec) as compared with the PDL (0.1 millisecondsec) creates better coagulation and diminishes vessel rupture, which had been experienced clinically with the PDL. The longer pulse width of the KTP laser also takes advantage of the fact that the energy delivery time is less than the thermal relaxation time of the tissue. Consequently, there is minimal collateral extravascular thermal soft tissue trauma, compared with using the same laser in a continuous mode. The KTP laser has been used clinically to treat papilloma and dysplasia. There has been less blood extravasation into the surrounding tissue, and the cytology of overlying diseased (papilloma and dysplasia) epithelium has been virtually unaltered by the subepithelial photoangiolysis.

Office-Based Applications of the KTP Laser

Photoangiolytic lasers are now used routinely in office-based laryngeal surgery to involute premalignant laryngeal disease and papilloma without resection. The selectivity of photoangiolytic lasers leads to improved vocal outcomes by allowing for aggressive treatment of dysplasia and papilloma with maximum preservation of the layered microstructure of the vocal fold, including the SLP. Current treatment strategies using office-based laryngeal laser surgery are limited to treatment of dysplasia and papilloma, although the use of office-based techniques in the management of microvascular angiomata; benign phonotraumatic lesions, such as polyps; or chronic inflammatory conditions, such as polypoid corditis, has been reported.

Office-based laryngeal laser surgery sacrifices a certain degree of precision due to the loss of binocular visualization, high-powered magnification, and an immobile and insensate operative field that exist when surgery is performed on patients who are under general anesthesia. Due to the avoidance of multiple general anesthetics and the ability to treat regrowth of disease more often with less recovery time, office-based laryngeal laser surgery is advantageous in cases of recurrent dysplasia and papilloma.

Dysplasia and papillomatosis are the two most common indications for photoangiolysis using the pulsed KTP laser, both in the operating room and in the office. Current strategy involves treating patients initially in the operating room, where the extent of epithelial disease and the prior surgically induced soft tissue changes can be adequately assessed. The KTP laser has proven its utility in ablating disease, with maximum preservation of the underlying SLP, and this laser is used in almost every patient with dysplasia or papilloma.

Neodymium:YAG Laser

Rhinology—Turbinate Hypertrophy

The neodymium:yttrium-aluminum-garnet (Nd:YAG) laser emits light at a 1,064 nm wavelength, making it the longest penetration depth (4 mm) of any of the surgical lasers. Within the subspecialty of rhinology in the head and neck, the Nd:YAG laser has been mainly used to reduce hyperplastic inferior nasal turbinates. A review article looking at more than 2,000 cases of laser treatment of hyperplastic inferior nasal turbinates concludes that, irrespective of laser type, laser treatment can be considered a useful, cost-effective modality to treat turbinates, and it had comparable or better results than most traditional conventional techniques, such as electrocautery, cryotherapy, or conchotomy. Although various lasers have been used in this treatment, the solid-state Nd:YAG laser can be described as an effective tool for the reduction of hyperplastic inferior nasal turbinates. By penetrating into the soft tissues to coagulate zones of the turbinate's venous plexus with

relative preservation of superficial epithelial layers, the Nd:YAG laser can cause less postoperative nasal crusting compared with other lasers.

Rhinology—Hereditary Hemorrhagic Telangiectasia (HHT)

The vascular malformations of inferior turbinates and nasal septum that characterize HHT and lead to intractable nosebleeds can be effectively managed with the Nd:YAG laser. The Nd:YAG laser can coagulate these large vessels readily and can be delivered on a fiber that can bend within the nasal cavity for optimal delivery. However, again one must consider the significant depth of penetration with this laser, which may be problematic if one is delivering treatment to areas near the lamina papyracea, because the medial rectus muscle adjacent to it is dark in color and can readily absorb the laser's thermal effect. Therefore, the Nd:YAG should be used only on the septum and inferior turbinates, where there is less risk of injury, given their further distance from any vital adjacent structures.

Argon Laser

The argon laser operates in the visible range (488–514 nm, blue-green light) in a continuous mode. Its small spot size is ideal during otologic surgery in the small confines of the middle ear. In the head and neck, the argon laser has most often been used in otologic surgery for stapedotomy, or middle ear adhesions, but has also been used in treating cutaneous lesions, such as rhinophyma, and in eustachian tuboplasty. During stapedectomy the small spot size of the argon laser facilitates precise placement of a control hole prior to removal of the small stapes footplate. The argon laser has a shallow depth of penetration, thereby minimizing the thermal effect to the facial nerve or the saccule of the inner ear (both of which lie in close proximity to the stapes footplate).

Because the argon laser is strongly absorbed by hemoglobin and melanin, it can also be used to treat vascular cutaneous lesions of the head and neck. Rhinophyma is a benign inflammatory growth of the caudal one-third of the nose. This disease process, which most commonly affects men in their fifth to seventh decades, can be both cosmetically and functionally impairing. The increased vascularity at the caudal aspect of the nose from the proliferation of sebaceous glands allows for multiple treatment modalities, including the use of either argon or CO_2 laser. The argon laser's advantage is that there is selective coagulation of blood capillaries. Both the argon and the CO_2 lasers provide effective hemostasis during sculpting of the nasal tip, but can cause dermal necrosis due to uncontrolled depth of tissue destruction and scar contraction.

Thulium:YAG 2 μm Continuous-Wave Laser

Laryngeal Disease

The thulium laser is a diode-pumped, solid-state laser with a thulium-doped YAG laser rod that produces a continuous-wave beam with a wavelength of 2.013 μm. This wavelength has a target chromophore of water and therefore simulates the hemostatic cutting properties of the CO_2 laser. Its fiber-based delivery system offers a distinct advantage in laryngeal surgery during three-dimensional and tangential cutting needed during endoscopic partial laryngectomy.

The authors of this chapter have used the thulium laser to perform several endoscopic partial laryngectomy procedures in both the glottis and the supraglottis. The most remarkable observation during a reported series of endoscopic partial laryngectomies involving the glottis and supraglottis was that the procedure was never halted to stop bleeding from laser dissection during any case. Although preliminary observations suggest that there is increased thermal damage on the soft tissues at the margin of the cancerous section compared with damage from the CO_2 laser, ex vivo studies indicate that the increased thermal effect is not excessive.

The thulium laser can also be used in an office-based setting with topical anesthesia through the side-port working channel of a flexible laryngoscope to ablate a variety of benign and malignant epithelial lesions of the larynx. The clinical indication for this use of the thulium laser can damage the delicate layered microstructure of phonatory membranes, so care must be taken to properly select patients who require less selective debulking of their disease. The optimal clinical scenarios are still evolving for the thulium laser, but the overall positive preliminary clinical experience thus far warrants further prospective investigations to determine its optimal application in laryngeal surgery.

■ Safety Considerations

Lasers are precise but potentially dangerous surgical instruments that must be used with extreme caution. Distinct advantages are associated with the use of lasers in the management of selected benign and malignant diseases of the head and neck; yet these advantages must be balanced against the possible risks of complication associated with laser surgery.

Smoke Evacuation

Thermal destruction of tissues during laser surgery results in a smoke by-product. Carbon monoxide, polyaromatic hydrocarbons, and a variety of trace toxic gases can be found in smoke plumes, leading to upper respiratory irritation. Surgical plumes have the potential for generating infectious viral fragments, although there has been no documented transmission of infectious disease through surgical smoke.

Although there are no specific Occupational Safety and Health Administration (OSHA) standards for laser plume hazards, laser cases should be equipped with local smoke evacuation systems. Constant suctioning is required to remove laser-induced smoke from the operative field when performing laser surgery with a closed anesthetic system. Suctioning should be limited to an intermittent basis to maintain the oxygen at a safe level when working with an open anesthetic system or with a jet ventilation system. Laryngoscopes, bronchoscopes, operating platforms, mirrors, and anterior commissure and ventricle retractors with built-in smoke evacuating channels simplify removal of smoke from the operative field.

Eye Protection

Certain precautions must be followed to reduce the risk of ocular damage during cases involving the laser. A sign must be placed on the operating room door warning all persons entering the room to wear the appropriate protective glasses because the laser is in use. The doors to the operating room should remain closed during laser surgery. Protection of the eyes of the patient, surgeon, and operating room personnel must be provided for with the actual protective device varying according to the wavelength of the laser used.

Although it may appear that the beam direction and point of interaction of the laser and tissue are confined within the endoscope and optical fiber, inadvertent deflection of the beam may occur because of a faulty contact, a break in the fiber, or accidental disconnection between the fiber and endoscope. Therefore, strict compliance with this portion of the safety protocol is necessary. A detailed radiometric analysis of the output from a frosted tip surgical probe of a 30W Nd:YAG laser shows that a "nominal hazard zone" extends 1.3 m in all directions from the frosted probe. All personnel within the 1.3 m range must wear standard protective eye wear.

Skin Protection

A double layer of saline-saturated surgical sponges, towels, or lap pads are used to protect the patient's exposed skin and mucous membranes outside the surgical field. Because it is possible for the beam to reflect off the proximal rim of the laryngoscope when performing microlaryngeal laser surgery, the patient's face is completely draped with saline-saturated surgical towels, exposing only the proximal lumen of the laryngoscope. For all laser cases, the meticulous attention that is paid to the protective draping procedures at the beginning of the case should be displayed throughout the case.

Anesthetic Considerations

Anesthetic management of the patient undergoing laser surgery of the head and neck must include attention to the safety of the patient, the hazards of the equipment, and the requirements of the surgeon. Most patients will require general anesthesia, and any of the nonflammable anesthetic agents is suitable; halothane and enflurane are most often used. Mixtures of helium plus oxygen should be used to maintain the oxygen level around but not above 40% and to insure that the patient is adequately oxygenated. Nitrous oxide should not be used in the anesthetic mixture. Muscle relaxation is required to prevent movement of the vocal cords when working in the larynx.

The most frequent laser-related complication is airway fire. Laser-resistant endotracheal tubes should be used to prevent airway fires during airway laser surgery. Initially, fires are located on the surface of the endotracheal tube, resulting in thermal injury to tissues. Should the fire burn through an endo-

tracheal tube carrying oxygen, ignition of the tube creates a catastrophic, intraluminal, blowtorch type endotracheal tube fire. Oxygen and positive pressure ventilation lead to blowing heat and toxic products down into the lungs.

Cuff puncture allowing O_2 enriched atmosphere can also increase the chance of fire after a laser burst. The cuff should be inflated with methylene blue–colored saline, and saline-saturated cottonoids need to be placed above the cuff in the subglottic larynx to protect the cuff. These cottonoids must be moistened frequently during the procedure. Should the cuff become deflated from an errant hit of the laser beam, the already saturated cottonoids turn blue to warn the surgeon of impending danger.

For a fire in the airway or breathing circuit, The Practice Advisory for the Prevention and Management of Operating Room Fires recommends that the tracheal tube and all flammable and burning materials be removed from the airway. The delivery of all airway gases should stop, and saline should be poured into the patient's airway to extinguish any residual embers and cool the tissues.

After a fire has been extinguished, the patient's status should be assessed, and a plan should be devised for ongoing care of the patient. Ventilation should be reestablished, avoiding supplemental oxygen and nitrous oxide, if possible. The tracheal tube should be examined to assess whether fragments have been left behind in the airway. Rigid bronchoscopy should be considered to assess thermal injury, look for tracheal tube fragments, and aid in the removal of residual materials.

■ Practice Guidelines, Consensus Statements, and Measures

Practice Advisory for the Prevention and Management of Operating Room Fires. Anesthesiology 2008;108(5):786–801

■ Suggested Readings

Broadhurst MS, Akst LM, Burns JA, et al. Effects of 532 nm pulsed-KTP laser parameters on vessel ablation in the avian chorioallantoic membrane: implications for vocal fold mucosa. Laryngoscope 2007;117(2):220–225

Burns JA, Friedman AD, Lutch MJ, Hillman RE, Zeitels SM. Value and utility of 532 nanometre pulsed potassium-titanyl-phosphate laser in endoscopic laryngeal surgery. J Laryngol Otol 2010;124(4):407–411

Burns JA, Kobler JB, Heaton JT, Anderson RR, Zeitels SM. Predicting clinical efficacy of photoangiolytic and cutting/ablating lasers using the chick chorioallantoic membrane model: implications for endoscopic voice surgery. Laryngoscope 2008;118(6):1109–1124

Burns JA, Kobler JB, Heaton JT, Lopez-Guerra G, Anderson RR, Zeitels SM. Thermal damage during thulium laser dissection of laryngeal soft tissue is reduced with air cooling: ex vivo calf model study. Ann Otol Rhinol Laryngol 2007;116(11):853–857

Burns JA, Zeitels SM, Akst LM, Broadhurst MS, Hillman RE, Anderson RR. 523 nm pulsed potassium-titanyl-phosphate laser treatment of laryngeal papillomatosis under general anesthesia. Laryngoscope 2007;117(8):1500–1504

Collawn SS. Fraxel skin resurfacing. Ann Plast Surg 2007;58(3):237–240

DiBartolomeo JR, Ellis M. The argon laser in otology. Laryngoscope 1980;90(11 Pt 1):1786–1796

Fife DJ, Fitzpatrick RE, Zachary CB. Complications of fractional CO2 laser resurfacing: four cases. Lasers Surg Med 2009;41(3):179–184

Franco RA Jr, Zeitels SM, Farinelli WA, Anderson RR. 585-nm pulsed dye laser treatment of glottal papillomatosis. Ann Otol Rhinol Laryngol 2002;111(6):486–492

Franco RA Jr, Zeitels SM, Farinelli WA, Faquin W, Anderson RR. 585-nm pulsed dye laser treatment of glottal dysplasia. Ann Otol Rhinol Laryngol 2003;112(9 Pt 1):751–758

Grant DG, Repanos C, Malpas G, Salassa JR, Hinni ML. Transoral laser microsurgery for early laryngeal cancer. Expert Rev Anticancer Ther 2010;10(3):331–338

Janda P, Sroka R, Baumgartner R, Grevers G, Leunig A. Laser treatment of hyperplastic inferior nasal turbinates: a review. Lasers Surg Med 2001;28(5):404–413

Manstein D, Herron GS, Sink RK, Tanner H, Anderson RR. Fractional photothermolysis: a new concept for cutaneous remodeling using microscopic patterns of thermal injury. Lasers Surg Med 2004;34(5):426–438

Poe DS, Metson RB, Kujawski O. Laser eustachian tuboplasty: a preliminary report. Laryngoscope 2003;113(4):583–591

Rees CJ, Halum SL, Wijewickrama RC, Koufman JA, Postma GN. Patient tolerance of in-office pulsed dye laser treatments to the upper aerodigestive tract. Otolaryngol Head Neck Surg 2006;134(6):1023–1027

Sadick H, Goepel B, Bersch C, Goessler U, Hoermann K, Riedel F. Rhinophyma: diagnosis and treatment options for a disfiguring tumor of the nose. Ann Plast Surg 2008;61(1):114–120

Shamsaldeen O, Peterson JD, Goldman MP. The adverse events of deep fractional CO(2): a retrospective study of 490 treatments in 374 patients. Lasers Surg Med 2011;43(6):453–456

United States Department of Labor. https://www.osha.gov/SLTC/laserelectrosurgeryplume/index.html. Accessed July 30, 2013

Ward PD, Baker SR. Long-term results of carbon dioxide laser resurfacing of the face. Arch Facial Plast Surg 2008;10(4):238–243, discussion 244–245

Zeitels SM, Akst LM, Burns JA, Hillman RE, Broadhurst MS, Anderson RR. Office-based 532-nm pulsed KTP laser treatment of glottal papillomatosis and dysplasia. Ann Otol Rhinol Laryngol 2006;115(9):679–685

Zeitels SM, Akst LM, Bums JA, Hillman RE, Broadhurst MS, Anderson RR. Pulsed angiolytic laser treatment of ectasias and varices in singers. Ann Otol Rhinol Laryngol 2006;115(8):571–580

Zeitels SM, Barbu AM, Landau-Zemer T, et al. Local injection of bevacizumab (Avastin) and angiolytic KTP laser treatment of recurrent respiratory papillomatosis of the vocal folds: a prospective study. Ann Otol Rhinol Laryngol 2011;120(10):627–634

Zeitels SM, Burns JA. Office-based laryngeal laser surgery with local anesthesia. Curr Opin Otolaryngol Head Neck Surg 2007;15(3):141–147

Zeitels SM, Burns JA. Office-based laryngeal laser surgery with the 532-nm pulsed-potassium-titanyl-phosphate laser. Curr Opin Otolaryngol Head Neck Surg 2007;15(6):394–400

Zeitels SM, Burns JA, Akst LM, Hillman RE, Broadhurst MS, Anderson RR. Office-based and microlaryngeal applications of a fiber-based thulium laser. Ann Otol Rhinol Laryngol 2006;115(12):891–896

Zeitels SM, Burns JA, Lopez-Guerra G, Anderson RR, Hillman RE. Photoangiolytic laser treatment of early glottic cancer: a new management strategy. Ann Otol Rhinol Laryngol Suppl 2008;199:3–24

Zeitels SM, Franco RA Jr, Dailey SH, Burns JA, Hillman RE, Anderson RR. Office-based treatment of glottal dysplasia and papillomatosis with the 585-nm pulsed dye laser and local anesthesia. Ann Otol Rhinol Laryngol 2004;113(4):265–276

Zeitels SM, Lopez-Guerra G, Burns JA, Lutch M, Friedman AM, Hillman RE. Microlaryngoscopic and office-based injection of bevacizumab (Avastin) to enhance 532-nm pulsed KTP laser treatment of glottal papillomatosis. Ann Otol Rhinol Laryngol Suppl 2009;201(9 Pt 2):1–13

14 Diagnosis and Management of Deep Neck Infections

■ Introduction

Sepsis in the deep fascial spaces of the neck was reported in ancient medical literature. In the pre-antibiotic era, therapy was limited to incision and drainage. Understandably, morbidity and mortality were high. Since the introduction of antibiotics to our therapeutic armamentarium, physicians are better able to successfully treat these conditions. Today, suppuration in the deep fascial spaces in the neck is relatively unusual, and a physician may have limited experience with diagnosis and treatment. Modern imaging techniques, such as computed tomography (CT), magnetic resonance imaging (MRI), and otolaryngologist-performed ultrasonography, facilitate diagnosis and offer the potential for nonoperative therapy where the diagnosis is made early. The modern head and neck surgeon should be familiar with the changing spectrum of bacterial antibiotic resistance, an increasing number of immunocompromised individuals in the community, and the potential to encounter iatrogenic disease.

Anatomy

The deep fascial spaces of the neck are defined by condensations of connective tissue. These spaces are defined by planes of greater resistance and are all potentially connected when the pressure associated with virulent infection exceeds the ability of the soft tissues to resist.

The prevertebral space is defined by the densely adherent fascial layers overlying the vertebral column. Infection here may arise from osteomyelitis of the spine (in prior times most commonly due to tuberculosis) or may be secondary to trauma or surgery involving the cervical spine. The retropharyngeal space is continuous inferiorly into the posterior mediastinum, whereas the parapharyngeal space is perforated at its apex by the carotid sheath (termed the Lincoln Highway of the neck), which offers a potential avenue for transmission of infection into the superior mediastinum. The soft tissue surrounding the visceral structures lower in the neck, such as the esophagus, larynx, and trachea, may also become sites of infection. This is most commonly associated with perforation of a hollow organ.

Etiology and Incidence

Deep neck infection may develop from suppurative lymphadenitis secondary to a focus of infection somewhere in the upper aerodigestive tract. Odontogenic infection is reportedly the most common identifiable source; however, more than 50% of patients developing deep neck abscess have no clearly identifiable primary site of infection. A recent study also suggests that substance abuse plays a big role in the development of a deep neck space infection. If deep neck infection is identified prior to actual suppuration and abscess formation, patients can theoretically be treated and cured with antibiotic administration alone. Most reports indicate that ~ 15% of adults and perhaps as many as 50% of children fall into this category. Once abscess formation develops, surgical intervention is almost always required.

Perforation of a mucosal surface in the upper aerodigestive tract may allow introduction of saliva, with its concomitant high bacterial count, and may result in a cervical infection. Accordingly, ingestion of foreign bodies (fish bones, sharp objects) or iatrogenic perforation during intubation or diagnostic endoscopy has been associated with deep neck infection.

Modern society must recognize that a significant percentage of deep neck infections may be associated with intravenous drug abuse when direct cervical injection is employed.

Pathology

The organisms most commonly identified in deep neck infections are streptococcus and staphylococcus; however, a wide spectrum of pathogens may be encountered. The most commonly identified pathogens include *Streptococcus viridans, Streptococcus pyogenes* (group A β-hemolytic *Streptococcus*), *Staphylococcus epidermidis, Staphylococcus aureus, Bacteroides, Fusobacterium, Peptostreptococcus, Neisseria, Pseudomonas, Escherichia,* and *Haemophilus.* The astute reader will note these flora are representative of the flora of odontogenic infections. Some reviews note that community-acquired methicillin-resistant *Staphylococcus aureus* (MRSA) is increasing in incidence, especially in the pediatric population.

The severity of these infections associated with an immunocompromised host requires prompt and accurate characterization of the offending organism. Material obtained from deep neck infection should routinely be submitted to the laboratory for appropriate processing, which includes Gram stain, culture, and antibiotic sensitivity testing. As previously mentioned, various organisms, including gram-negative enterics and anaerobic bacteria, are reported in sporadic cases.

Necrotizing cervical fasciitis characterizes an especially virulent form of deep neck infection. This infection is most commonly associated with concomitant dental infection. Almost invariably, the infection is polymicrobial, with a significant role played by anaerobic bacteria. Nonclostridial gas-forming organisms are often encountered. The presence of gas in the neck on physical examination or identified radiographically should alert the clinician to this diagnosis.

■ Evaluation

Clinical Findings

Common symptoms of deep neck space infections include dysphagia, odynophagia, drooling, extreme sore throat, muffled or "hot potato" voice, dysphonia, dyspnea, trismus, meningismus, and referred otalgia. Otolaryngologists must be aware of these relationships and should not be misled in thinking a stiff neck and fever are necessarily indications of meningitis.

Physical examination may show pharyngeal pooling of secretions, displacement of the lateral pharyngeal wall toward the midline, or tongue swelling. Trismus may indicate parapharyngeal, pterygoid, or masseteric space irritation or inflammation. The dentition should be closely examined; poor dental health could be the cause of the deep neck space infection. Brawny induration of the neck may be commonly encountered with parapharyngeal space infection, but palpable fluctuance is almost never described, due to the thickness of the overlying cervical musculature.

Any workup of a deep neck space infection requires an evaluation of the airway. If the patient has any complaints or signs of hoarseness, dysphagia, shortness of breath, or stridor, the otolaryngologist must assess the airway with a flexible fiberoptic laryngoscope. Airway obstruction is a not uncommon complication of a deep neck space infection. If the airway is a concern during the evaluation, this should be secured first before the completion of the workup. Classic Ludwig angina is associated with airway obstruction secondary to floor mouth and submental swelling and displacement of the tongue (**Fig. 14.1**). Up to 75% will need a surgical airway. The awake tracheotomy is the preferred surgical airway.

Review of the past medical history should include an inquiry on the patient's immunity status, human immunodeficiency virus (HIV) status, history of diabetes, history of malignancy and possible use of chemotherapy, use of steroids or intravenous drug abuse, and history of collagen vascular disease. These patients will be more at risk for aggressive disease and atypical bacterium.

Special Investigations

Laboratory work should include a complete blood count with a differential, basic chemistries, possibly prothrombin time/partial thromboplastin time testing, HIV screening as indicated, and cultures. The cultures should be checked for the classic aerobic and anaerobic pathogens, as well as fungal and acid-fast bacilli cultures.

When a deep neck space infection is suspected, CT scanning with intravenous (IV) contrast is an appropriate initial investigation (**Fig. 14.2**). The presence of free gas in the neck should alert the clinician

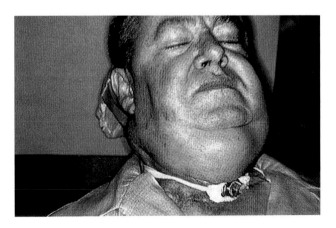

Fig. 14.1   Clinical appearance of Ludwig angina.

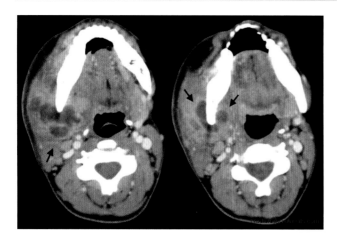

Fig. 14.2 Contrast-enhanced axial computed tomography of the neck shows inflammation of the right muscles of mastication and a fluid collection with septations and enhancing margins posterior to the right angle of the mandible (*arrows*), involving the submandibular space.

to the possibility of necrotizing fasciitis. Abscess formation may be distinguished from cellulitis, based on a mass with a lytic center and a thick rim. However, the sensitivity and specificity are no better than 85 to 90%, and therapeutic decision making should reflect clinical judgment. Miller et al demonstrate that a contrast CT of the neck showing a hypodensity greater than 2 mL in volume is much more predictive of an abscess than a CT scan showing a hypodensity with rim enhancement.

Although MRI scans of the neck may show soft tissue definition better than a neck CT scan, MRI is not commonly employed. MRI is expensive, time consuming, and troublesome for a patient who is in pain or showing signs of airway problems. As a secondary imaging tool, it can definitely provide better information about complications, such as thromboses, emboli, or intracranial involvement. Clinician-performed ultrasonography may help distinguish abscess from cellulitis and can accurately guide needle aspiration of a suspected abscess. Ultrasonography may expedite radiographic imaging in pediatric patients because general anesthesia or sedation is not required; additional benefits are cost, no requirement for IV contrast, and lack of exposure to radiation compared with CT scanning.

Needle aspiration may result in a specimen that can be forwarded to the laboratory and potentially offers some symptomatic relief from the infection. The deep cervical spaces and the proximity to vital structures may limit the usefulness of needle aspiration, and image-guided needle aspiration (CT-guided or ultrasound-guided) can assist avoidance of critical structures.

■ Management

When a diagnosis of deep neck suppuration is made, the patient should be hospitalized for close monitoring, fluid replacement, pain control, and IV antibiotic administration. IV hydration may be required if severe odynophagia, dysphagia, and trismus have limited oral intake and there is clinical evidence of dehydration. Prior to identification of the offending organism, it is appropriate to use a broad-spectrum antibiotic with activity against β-lactamase-resistant organisms and anaerobic bacteria. MRSA is commonly encountered in patients whose deep neck infection is secondary to IV drug abuse and increasingly in community-acquired pediatric neck abscess. Vancomycin administration should be considered under these circumstances, especially if there is no improvement clinically with more standard antibiotics. Airway compromise due to the deep neck space infection requires early intervention with tracheotomy and incision and drainage. If cellulitis is suspected, careful airway monitoring should accompany the administration of IV antibiotics. Failure to defervesce and rapidly improve clinically is generally considered an indication to proceed with appropriate imaging studies, neck exploration, and drainage.

The diagnosis of cervical necrotizing fasciitis requires early aggressive intervention. Necrotic tissue should be debrided and all the involved spaces of the neck left widely open. The surgeon should not depend on drains; rather, cervical flaps must be left open and the cervical spaces widely exposed and drained. Cosmetic considerations must be deferred until all evidence of infection has been eradicated. Failure to recognize this principle may be associated with unnecessary death.

Well localized retropharyngeal, parapharyngeal, or prevertebral abscess may occasionally be successfully drained using a transoral approach. However, the transcervical approach is more conservative, which allows the surgeon to identify and avoid vital neurovascular structures and to more securely place drains.

Despite some reports of needle aspiration being inadequate in deep neck space infections, it can be effective in the management of this disease. It may avoid the risks associated with general anesthesia and is sometimes effective as the sole treatment of an abscess and in establishing the bacterial pathogens in the suspected abscesses.

Complications

Despite widespread use of antibiotics, various complications continue to be reported in association with deep neck infection. These most commonly involve erosion of associated neurovascular structures or the spread to contiguous sites.

The most common site of complicated deep neck space infections is the mediastinum. Mediastinitis requires aggressive intervention and consultation with thoracic surgery and infectious disease. Tracheotomy, thoracotomy, or pericardiotomy may be required, in conjunction with IV antibiotics and systemic support of hypotension and sepsis.

Septic thrombophlebitis of the internal jugular vein (Lemierre syndrome) is rare, but must be suspected with a history of peritonsillar abscess or IV drug abuse, extreme lethargy, rigors, bacteremia, and a spiking febrile course, and it may be confirmed with CT. Septic emboli to the pulmonary vasculature and dural sinus thrombosis may be encountered. The most conservative therapy is probably antibiotic administration effective against *Fusobacterium necrophorum*, cervical exploration, and ligation and excision of the involved jugular vein. The use of anticoagulation is controversial. Consultation with other specialists in accordance with the accompanying clinical picture should be considered given the measurable mortality still associated with Lemierre syndrome.

Pseudoaneurysm or erosion of the carotid artery or one of its branches is rare but may occur. Diagnosis should be suspected if hematoma or spontaneous bleeding is encountered with a sentinel bleeding episode from the ear, nose, or mouth. Treatment requires proximal and distal vessel control and may require vascular ligation. Failure to recognize this complication is associated with 24 to 40% mortality.

■ Conclusion

Infections of the deep neck spaces present a challenging problem for otolaryngologists for the following reasons:

1. Complex anatomy makes the precise localization of infections in this region difficult.
2. Deep location makes the diagnosis challenging because the infected spaces are covered by unaffected superficial soft tissue and can be difficult to palpate and visualize externally.
3. Access is difficult because superficial tissues are traversed to gain surgical access to the deep neck spaces.
4. Proximity to important neural, vascular, and bony structures increases risks.
5. There is possible communication with and potential spread of infection to adjacent spaces.

In the absence of airway compromise, bleeding, or evidence of gas formation, surgical therapy is usually reserved for patients whose symptoms do not respond to aggressive medical management within 24 to 48 hours. However, there are no absolute rules, and keen clinical judgment and a low index of suspicion for associated complications must be used for each patient based on clinical and radiographic evaluation.

■ Suggested Reading

Brook I, Frazier EH. Clinical and microbiological features of necrotizing fasciitis. J Clin Microbiol 1995;33(9):2382–2387

Broughton RA. Nonsurgical management of deep neck infections in children. Pediatr Infect Dis J 1992;11(1):14–18

Daramola OO, Flanagan CE, Maisel RH, Odland RM. Diagnosis and treatment of deep neck space abscesses. Otolaryngol Head Neck Surg 2009;141(1):123–130

Henrich DE, Smith TL, Shockley WW. Fatal craniocervical necrotizing fasciitis in an immunocompetent patient: a case report and literature review. Head Neck 1995;17(4):351–357

Langford FP, Moon RE, Stolp BW, Scher RL. Treatment of cervical necrotizing fasciitis with hyperbaric oxygen therapy. Otolaryngol Head Neck Surg 1995;112(2):274–278

Lazor JB, Cunningham MJ, Eavey RD, Weber AL. Comparison of computed tomography and surgical findings in deep neck infections. Otolaryngol Head Neck Surg 1994;111(6):746–750

Lustig LR, Cusick BC, Cheung SW, Lee KC. Lemierre's syndrome: two cases of postanginal sepsis. Otolaryngol Head Neck Surg 1995;112(6):767–772

Mathieu D, Neviere R, Teillon C, Chagnon JL, Lebleu N, Wattel F. Cervical necrotizing fasciitis: clinical manifestations and management. Clin Infect Dis 1995;21(1):51–56

Miller WD, Furst IM, Sàndor GK, Keller MA. A prospective, blinded comparison of clinical examination and computed tomography in deep neck infections. Laryngoscope 1999;109(11):1873–1879

Oliver ER, Gillespie MB. Deep neck space infections. In: Flint PW, Haughey BH, Lund VJ, et al., eds. Cummings Otolaryngology–Head and Neck Surgery. Philadelphia, PA: Mosby Elsevier; 2010:201–208

Ossowski K, Chun RH, Suskind D, Baroody FM. Increased isolation of methicillin-resistant *Staphylococcus aureus* in pediatric head and neck abscesses. Arch Otolaryngol Head Neck Surg 2006;132(11):1176–1181

Rabuzzi DD, Johnson JT, Weissman JL. Diagnosis and Management of Deep Neck Infections. Self-Instructional Package. 3rd ed. Alexandria, VA: American Academy of Otolaryngology–Head and Neck Surgery; 1993

Thomason TS, Brenski A, McClay J, Ehmer D. The rising incidence of methicillin-resistant *Staphylococcus aureus* in pediatric neck abscesses. Otolaryngol Head Neck Surg 2007;137(3):459–464

Tovi F, Fliss DM, Noyek AM. Septic internal jugular vein thrombosis. J Otolaryngol 1993;22(6):415–420

Vieira F, Allen SM, Stocks RMS, Thompson JW. Deep neck infection. Otolaryngol Clin North Am 2008;41(3):459–483, vii

15 Stomatitis

■ Introduction

Stomatitis is inflammation of the oral mucosa due to physical, chemical, infectious, or immunologically mediated processes. Stomatitis can present as a single oral manifestation or a combination of clinical signs. The most common appearance is that of mucosal erythema, which may be associated with hyperkeratosis, ulceration, and pseudomembrane formation. Stomatitis is almost always symptomatic.

Physical, chemical, infectious, and immunologic reactions can all induce stomatitis. The most common etiologies include allergies (erythema multiforme); immunologic and autoimmune mucocutaneous diseases (lichen planus, pemphigoid, and pemphigus); human herpesvirus, type 1 (HHV-1) infection (primary and recurrent); fungal infections (*Candida albicans*); bacterial overgrowth; stomatitis secondary to chemotherapy and radiation therapy; xerostomia (drug induced and disease related); hypersensitivity to dental materials (denture acrylic and cast metal restorations) and therapeutic agents (toothpastes and mouthwashes); blood dyscrasias (leukemia); aphthous ulcers; and malnutrition. **Table 15.1** summarizes the more "classic" etiologies where the cause is not easily determined by history, along with important pathophysiological factors and exam findings.

■ Evaluation

The constellation of clinical signs and symptoms in most patients with stomatitis varies to such an extent that characteristic changes are not always associated with specific etiologic conditions or diseases. A well-constructed differential diagnosis that prioritizes potential etiologies is essential in developing organized and rational diagnostic and therapeutic approaches. The patient history and physical exam are to be supplemented by diagnostic testing, as required. Treatment is often based on a presumptive diagnosis, and the response to treatment is closely followed.

■ Management

Erythema Multiforme

Erythema multiforme (EM) and related conditions (e.g., Stevens-Johnson syndrome and toxic epidermal necrolysis) are disorders that represent an immune response to a variety of antigens (e.g., HHV-1; *Mycoplasma pneumoniae,* and medications). These disorders are diagnosed primarily on the basis of clinical signs and symptoms. Pathognomonic "bull's eye," "iris," or "target" lesions on the skin are frequently absent; however, the oral lesions are characteristic in their presentation. Large, serosanguinous vesicles and bullae affecting the vermilion borders of the lips are accompanied by similar widespread oral lesions that rapidly rupture. Routine histopathological staining of biopsies of oral lesions does not reveal any disease-specific findings. Direct immunofluorescence may be useful in ruling out clinically similar entities, especially in the absence of cutaneous or nonoral mucosal manifestations.

Of greatest importance is ruling out the possibility of primary herpetic gingivostomatitis in patients who cannot provide a compelling history of exposure to HHV-1 (see Human Herpesvirus, Type 1 section). That is because the lesions of EM are normally treated with high-dose (60–80 mg daily), short-term (10–14 days) systemic corticosteroids, often supplemented with topical corticosteroids (fluocinonide, clobetasol, or halobetasol). Levamisole, an immunomodulating agent, has also been used in the treatment of EM. If prior HHV-1 (recurrent herpes labialis) infection has been present, dosing with antiviral drugs at less than full therapeutic doses has reduced the chances of recurrence of EM. Topical

Table 15.1 Important features of the more common etiologies of stomatitis, when a causative factor cannot be determined by history

Diagnosis	Cause	Key features
Erythema multiforme	Immune response	Target lesions on skin, serosanguinous vesicles and bullae beginning on the lips
Lichen planus	Idiopathic	Occasional Wickham striae, may be erosive or atrophic, biopsy recommended
Pemphigus vulgaris/cicatricial pemphigoid	Immune mediated	Nikolsky sign is rare, nonspecific erosive lesions, biopsy recommended
Human herpesvirus, type 1	Infectious	Ulcerations often involving the gingiva and hard palate, unlike aphthous ulcers, Tzanck test recommended
Candidiasis	Infectious	Immunocompetent and immunocompromised individuals; potassium hydroxide (KOH) smear is usually diagnostic
Mucositis	Chemical/physical	Typically erythematous, painful, diffusely ulcerated mucosa; requires a multimodal approach to therapy; self-limited

anesthetics (2% viscous lidocaine), occlusive mucosal dressings (Orabase with benzocaine, Colgate Oral Pharmaceuticals, New York, NY; and Zilactin-B, Blairex Laboratories, Inc., Columbus, IN), and palliative mouth rinses containing anesthetic agents (diphenhydramine, promethazine, or Xylocaine), coating agents (Kaopectate, Chattem, Inc., Chattanooga, TN; milk of magnesia, or sucralfate), and topical corticosteroid rinses (dexamethasone) are all useful in alleviating discomfort.

Lichen Planus

Lichen planus is a common mucocutaneous disease affecting up to 2% of the population. Oral lesions are often found in the absence of cutaneous manifestations. Oral lichen planus is a disease of immunologic origin that is mediated by a T cell lymphocytic reaction to antigenic components within the surface epithelial layer, leading to increased inflammation in the submucosa, along with lymphocyte deposition. When Wickham striae are present, lichen planus is clinically recognizable; however, the erosive and atrophic forms may not have these pathognomonic striations. Because of the clinical similarities between reticular lichen planus and other diseases (e.g., discoid lupus erythematosus and lichenoid stomatitis, and the relationship with liver disease and oral cancer), it is advisable to biopsy representative lesions, to both confirm the diagnosis and rule out other entities. Gingival lichen planus may mimic inflammatory periodontal disease, as well as mucocutaneous disease (e.g., cicatricial pemphigoid); therefore, a confirmatory biopsy is indicated in such cases as well. Direct immunofluorescence may be useful in cases that are equivocal by light microscopy.

Asymptomatic lichen planus requires no treatment. Mildly symptomatic lesions are best treated with intermediate-strength topical corticosteroids (fluocinonide gel), often in conjunction with occlusive dressings (Orabase or Zilactin-B) or, in the case of gingival lesions, a vinyl stent. More severe cases respond to super-potent topical corticosteroids (clobetasol or halobetasol) or systemic prednisone (40–60 mg daily), often in conjunction with azathioprine (50 mg twice a day). Solitary lesions that do not resolve following application of topical corticosteroids can be treated with intralesional injection of triamcinolone, 5 mg. Other medications used with some success include dapsone, hydroxychloroquine, cyclosporine, vitamin A analogues, tacrolimus, pimecrolimus, and etanercept. There is a small but definite risk of progression of oral lichen planus to oral squamous cell carcinoma, so close follow-up is recommended for lesions that do not readily respond to treatment.

Cicatricial Pemphigoid and Pemphigus Vulgaris

Cicatricial pemphigoid and pemphigus vulgaris both have a great propensity for oral involvement. In fact, oral lesions of pemphigus vulgaris often precede the onset of cutaneous involvement, and cicatricial pemphigoid often exists solely as an oral mucosal condition. Unfortunately, none of the vesiculoerosive diseases is characteristic in its presentation. Nikolsky sign is variable but is more commonly reported in pemphigus vulgaris. Although all of the vesiculoerosive diseases are characterized by variably symptomatic erosions, intact vesicles and bullae are rare, and cutaneous or nonoral mucosal involvement is a late-stage phenomenon.

For these reasons, histopathological confirmation is essential for diagnosis. A 3 to 4 mm biopsy punch is adequate to obtain sufficient tissue. Routine histology reveals characteristic clefting; however, direct immunofluorescence is frequently done to rule out other blistering diseases. Indirect immunofluorescence, while inconsistent in cicatricial pemphigoid, is useful in both the diagnosis and the management of pemphigus vulgaris. Antigen/antibody complexes to the adhesion molecule desmoglein 3 in mucosal epithelium are almost always present in pemphigus vulgaris, and to a lesser extent the presence of antigen/antibody complexes to what could be a variety of basement membrane molecules in cicatricial pemphigoid is not as easily demonstrated.

Oral lesions of cicatricial pemphigoid may often be treated with topical corticosteroids of varying strengths (fluocinonide, clobetasol, or halobetasol); however, occasional flares may require high-dose (60–80 mg daily), short-term (10–14 days) corticosteroids (prednisone). In patients who cannot tolerate systemic corticosteroids or where such treatment is contraindicated, systemic dapsone (50–150 mg daily) is an acceptable alternative drug. Because of the potential eye involvement, an ophthalmology consultation is essential in patients with cicatricial pemphigoid.

Oral lesions of pemphigus vulgaris may be quite severe and frequently require systemic therapy with prednisone or other corticosteroids, often in combination with azathioprine or mycophenolate mofetil. For systemic treatment, prednisone in doses of 40 to 80 mg daily for up to 10 days will usually give considerable, if not complete, relief. Because of the concern for recurrence and the potential for side effects, either periodic pulse courses or potent topical corticosteroids (fluocinonide, clobetasol, or halobetasol) can be used. These have excellent local effects with minimal or no significant systemic absorption. These topical corticosteroids can be prepared by mixing equal parts Orabase and the 0.05% ointment, or they can be prescribed without mixing as the 0.05% gel. The advantage of the mixture is the adhesive property for longer mucosal contact. Occlusion of the gel form with Zilactin-B provides both mucosal protection and prolonged corticosteroid effect.

Antimetabolites (cyclophosphamide), cyclosporine, gold, plasmapheresis, and rituximab have all been used in severe cases of pemphigus vulgaris with variable success. Eventual cutaneous involvement is to be expected, and the oral lesions often benefit from systemic therapy used to treat widespread skin disease. Interestingly, patients with pemphigus will often undergo spontaneous remission of their disease, lasting from months to years. Because there is no cure for any of the mucocutaneous diseases, the end point of treatment is patient satisfaction, at whatever level of remission can be obtained without significant side effects.

Human Herpesvirus, Type 1

Primary herpetic gingivostomatitis due to HHV-1 is accompanied by acute fever, pain, malaise, and cervical lymphadenopathy, in addition to a vesiculoerosive stomatitis. Although this is normally an infection of childhood, it can occur in adults and be confused with EM. Therefore, a history of clinically similar episodes casts doubt on the diagnosis of a primary HHV-1 infection. The vermilion borders of the lips may also be involved, in addition to oral mucosa. During the first week of infection, the patient is contagious. Viral shedding is significant only until the vesicles rupture and begin to heal. This initial infection usually resolves within 10 days and is forced into remission by the host's own immune system within 2 weeks.

Recurrent herpes labialis and intraoral herpes are localized, vesiculoerosive lesions that recur with varying frequency following initial exposure to HHV-1. Vermilion border lesions may extend to involve the perioral skin. In contrast to recurrent aphthous ulcers, recurrent intraoral HHV-1 lesions are limited to keratinized mucosa (i.e., attached gingiva and hard palate). Intact vesicles are rare intraorally and usually appear as clusters of pseudomembranous ulcers surrounded by erythema.

The diagnosis of HHV-1 infections is most frequently made on the basis of clinical signs and symptoms, although several diagnostic techniques are available. The Tzanck test may be useful as an in-office procedure; however, a microscope is required. Although cultures are useful to confirm atypical cases of recurrent HHV infection, they are expensive and time consuming. Other tests are available and may be helpful if the clinical presentation is unusual.

Herpes Culture

A sample of fluid is collected from an open sore, is incubated, and will grow the virus if present. This test is sensitive and specific, but it takes 2 or more days to complete. Fresh lesions are the best for this test. Viral shedding decreases over time and can lead to a false-negative result. Once the virus is grown in culture, it is possible to determine if it is HSV-1 or HSV-2.

Herpes Simplex Virus DNA Testing

DNA testing is usually done only if the culture is negative but the physician still suspects herpes or if the patient is being treated for herpes. This method can detect the virus as well as identify the type and is good in circumstances where the virus is present in low numbers (such as viral encephalitis) or if the lesion is several days old. This is the best method to detect HSV meningitis, encephalitis, or keratitis because this method is more sensitive.

Herpes Simplex Virus Antibody Testing

HSV immunoglobulin M (IgM) antibody production begins several days after a primary HSV infection and may be detectable in the blood for several weeks. HSV IgG antibody production begins after HSV IgM production. Once someone has been infected with HSV, they will continue to produce small quantities of HSV IgG. Antibody testing can detect both viral types (HSV-1 and HSV-2), and tests are available that can detect the early IgM antibodies as well as the IgG antibodies.

Rapid laboratory tests for HHV using immuno-fluorescence, immunoperoxidase, and polymerase chain-reaction techniques are also available.

Most recurrent HHV-1 infections are self-limiting in immunocompetent patients and do not require antiviral therapy. Severe, protracted episodes of recurrent HHV-1 infections are common in immuno-suppressed patients, including those with leukemia, receiving chemotherapy, and receiving bone marrow transplants.

If HHV-1 is suspected, especially in an immuno-compromised patient, it is appropriate to empirically prescribe systemic acyclovir (200 mg, five times daily). Topical acyclovir has limited usefulness in treating herpes labialis, although it can be effective if applied very early in the prodromal stage of recurrent infection. Penciclovir cream has also been reported to be effective in reducing the clinical signs and symptoms of herpes labialis. Ionotophoresis has been used successfully with a variety of antiviral agents to treat recurrent herpes labialis. Newer anti-viral drugs (valacyclovir, famciclovir) have been used with some success in treating herpetic infections in immunosuppressed patients; however, the appropri-ateness of their use in uncomplicated HHV-1 infec-tions in immunocompetent patients has not been well established.

Candidiasis

Oral mucosal yeast infection, most frequently due to C. albicans, is common in both immunocompe-tent and, especially, immunosuppressed patients. It is especially common in patients with radiation- or chemotherapy-related stomatitis and those who wear dentures and have poor oral hygiene.

The infection is usually symptomatic and pres-ents as red and/or white mucosal changes. Pseudo-membranous candidiasis is characterized by white plaques that can be dislodged to reveal an erythema-tous, often eroded, mucosa. Erythematous candidia-sis exhibits no visible superficial fungal colonization, whereas hyperplastic candidiasis is characterized by superficial fungal invasion of the epithelium with subsequent hyperkeratosis (candidal leukoplakia).

A potassium hydroxide–digested smear is usually sufficient to reveal candidal hyphae and/or spores, although Gram-stained smears are equally satis-factory for rapid identification. Occasionally, other diagnostic methods, such as silver-based staining of smears, culture, fluorescence microscopy, latex agglutination, and biopsy, may also be employed.

Drug selection and administration are depen-dent on the type of candidiasis present and the health status of the patient. Topical or systemic antifungals (nystatin, clotrimazole, ketoconazole, fluconazole) are effective; however, resistant strains to the systemic antifungal drug, itraconazole, have been reported. This newest azole is currently used to treat fungal infections of the nails and has not been extensively evaluated for use in treating oral candidiasis. Identifying and treating precipitat-ing factors (e.g., hyperglycemia, xerostomia, drugs, and poor denture hygiene) are important, due to the propensity for frequent recurrences. Continued therapy after clinical clearing of signs and symp-toms has no documented benefit; however, prophy-laxis with chlorhexidine-containing mouth rinses may be of benefit in individuals who are at high risk for recurrent infection (e.g., immunosuppressed individuals).

Bacterial Infections

Bacterial infections are usually associated with mucosal erythema, pain, and fever, often with atten-dant edema and lymphadenopathy. Mucosal cultures often give a mixed oral flora; therefore, the use of cultures is normally limited to suppurative lesions. However, even in those situations, a pure culture is difficult to obtain. Aerobic gram-positive cocci (*Streptococcus viridans*) and anaerobic gram-neg-ative bacilli (*Porphyromonas, Prevotella,* and *Fuso-bacterium* species) are the most commonly cultured organisms in odontogenic infections.

Various antibiotics have been found to be suc-cessful in treating oral bacterial infections. Peni-cillin remains the drug of choice in treating most odontogenic infections; however, other antibiotics have well-defined roles in specific clinical situations. Erythromycin is a useful alternative for mild infec-tions, but it cannot be used in high doses. Tetracy-clines are also effective for mild infections because they have a broad spectrum; however, there is a high incidence of bacterial resistance. Clindamycin is an acceptable antibiotic alternative, especially for penicillin-resistant anaerobic infections. First-generation cephalosporins are excellent for use in penicillin-allergic patients or when atypical flora are suspected. Metronidazole is useful in treating anaerobic oral bacterial infections, especially in HIV-positive patients.

Chemotherapy and Radiation Therapy

Chemotherapy for the treatment of malignancies has its greatest side effects on cells and tissues with rapid turnover rates, including oral mucosa. Iatrogenic stomatitis secondary to chemotherapy is characterized by widespread mucosal ulceration, with attendant dysphagia and oral discomfort. Alterations of taste are also common in patients undergoing chemotherapy and contribute to decreased appetite, food intake, and negative nutritional balance.

Radiation therapy can cause stomatitis both directly and indirectly. Direct effects are seen in mucosa within the primary path of the radiation beam. Affected mucosa is erythematous, tender, and occasionally ulcerated. Indirect effects are usually due to radiation-induced xerostomia, dental caries, and secondary candidiasis.

Fortunately, the side effects of chemotherapy- and radiation therapy–induced stomatitis are transient, whereas the resultant xerostomia may be permanent. During therapy, it is best to prevent the possible side effects by encouraging patients to stay well hydrated and to keep the oral mucosa moist. As treatment continues it is important to identify the attendant complications and deal directly with them, if possible (e.g., leukopenia and toxicity). Infections normally respond to appropriate antimicrobial agents, although they are often prescribed empirically, based on the acute nature of the patient's symptoms and the delay in obtaining microbial culture and sensitivity. Usually an analgesic must also be used to allow the patient to maintain an appropriate caloric and fluid intake and avoid weight loss and dehydration.

Hypersensitivity

Contact stomatitis due to hypersensitivity to various dental materials (acrylic, base metals, dental amalgam) and therapeutic agents (mouthwashes and toothpastes) can present a diagnostic challenge because the clinical signs and symptoms are not diagnostic. Acrylic allergy is rare, and suspected cases are more often due to localized candidal infections or irritation due to incompletely cured acrylic. Base metal allergies to partial denture frameworks or porcelain fused to metal crowns are also not common, and diagnosis is complicated because of the variety of formulations used in such materials. The most common metal allergen is nickel. Allergy to dental amalgam has been reported and appears as a lichenoid hyperkeratosis with associated erythema.

Allergies to various mouthwashes and toothpastes have been reported. Sodium lauryl sulfate, a commonly used detergent compound in toothpastes, can cause a widespread, symptomatic stomatitis, characterized by intense erythema, burning, and mucosal ulceration. Flavoring agents in mouthwashes and other oral therapeutic agents (e.g., cinnamaldehyde) can also result in a nonspecific inflammation of the oral mucosa.

Symptomatic treatment of true allergies with antihistamines or anti-inflammatory agents is not effective. In the case of dental materials, the diagnosis is often made by removing the appliance or dental restoration and finding that the lesion resolves. Cutaneous patch testing may reveal the offending substance; such testing is appropriate if replacement with a similar appliance or restoration is anticipated. The diagnosis of contact stomatitis from toothpastes and mouthwashes is usually one of exclusion in which the patient either discontinues the use of the product altogether or changes brands until one is found that is well tolerated.

Leukemia and Other Blood Dyscrasias

Leukemias and other blood dyscrasias are often manifested by oral signs and symptoms. Acute monocytic leukemia is the most common leukemia to manifest such changes. Mucosal atrophy of the tongue with depapillation is frequently seen. Gingival involvement is also common and is characterized initially by pallor, followed by enlargement, often with widespread purpura and spontaneous hemorrhage secondary to thrombocytopenia.

Although management of the underlying hematologic problem is of prime importance, adjunctive oral hygiene measures, including antiseptic mouthwashes, are essential to prevent secondary oral infections. Oral candidiasis is common and, while responding well to antifungal therapy, frequently recurs.

Aphthous Ulcers

Aphthous ulcers are the most commonly reported oral ulcer, occurring in ~ 25% of the population. They can occur as minor or major aphthae and as single or multiple lesions.

They are usually seen in adults; however, they can occur in children. Minor aphthous ulcers are much more common, accounting for ~ 85% of cases. Minor aphthae are generally located on labial or buccal mucosa, the soft palate, and the floor of the mouth. They can be singular or multiple, and tend to be small (less than 1 cm in diameter) and shallow and heal within 10 days without scarring. The lesions arise as de novo ulcers on nonkeratinized mucosa; therefore, their lack of occurrence on the attached gingiva and hard palate helps distinguish them from recurrent intraoral HHV-1 lesions.

Major aphthae are larger, involve deeper ulceration, and take longer to heal. Major aphthae may also be more likely to scar with healing. Patients with benign aphthous ulcers should have no other findings such as fever, adenopathy, gastrointestinal symptoms, or other skin or mucous-membrane symptoms.

Solitary or infrequent aphthous ulcers are treated similarly to other inflammatory ulcers, with topical corticosteroids (fluocinonide, clobetasol, halobetasol) being the drugs of first choice, either applied directly on the lesions, often in combination with an adhesive paste (Orabase), or applied with occlusive dressing (Zilactin-B). Intralesional triamcinolone (5 mg) is useful in treating refractory major aphthous ulcers. Palliative mouth rinses are also beneficial, as are topical anesthetics.

Severe lesions can be treated with systemic prednisone, usually in daily dosages of 40 to 60 mg. Dosage adjustments for mg/kg of body weight have not been found to be clinically significant. Frequently recurrent lesions are most effectively treated with pulse therapy, rather than topical application of corticosteroids. The use of systemic corticosteroid therapy is primarily based on the history of the attacks, severity of symptoms, and any contraindications for corticosteroid therapy (e.g., diabetes mellitus, ulcers, significant hypertension, glaucoma). High-dose, short-course regimens are preferred, and tapering is not necessary for systemic therapy of fewer than 14 days. Colchicine and dapsone have also been reported as effective in treating refractory oral aphthae.

Malnutrition

Malnutrition can result in a constellation of oral signs and symptoms that are frequently complicated by other oral diseases (e.g., severe periodontal disease and oral candidiasis). Vitamin B complex deficiency is a frequent finding in patients who abuse alcohol. The oral manifestations are characterized by angular cheilitis, which is often secondarily infected with *C. albicans,* and a nonspecific, erythematous, occasionally ulcerative mucositis. The tongue mucosa is often atrophic and depapillated, and stomatopyrosis is a common symptom. Other less common nutritional deficiencies that cause stomatitis include niacin, biotin, folic acid, pantothenic acid, zinc, and ascorbic acid.

The diagnosis of specific nutritional deficiencies can often be elusive. Once the diagnosis is made, the clinical signs and symptoms resolve following the institution of a normal diet with appropriate supplementation of deficient nutrients.

■ Practice Guidelines, Consensus Statements, and Measures

National Cancer Institute. Statement on Oral Complications of Chemotherapy and Head/Neck Radiation (Physician Data Query). www.cancer.gov/cancertopics/pdq/supportivecare/oralcomplications/HealthProfessional

■ Suggested Reading

Eusterman VD, Meyers A. Preface: Oral disease. Otolaryngol Clin North Am 2011;44(1):ix–x

Langlais RP, Miller CS, Nield-Gehrig JS. Color Atlas of Common Oral Diseases. 4th ed. Philadelphia, PA: Lippincott Williams & Wilkins; 2009

Little JW, Falace DA, Miller CS, Rhodus NL. Dental Management of the Medically Compromised Patient. 6th ed. St. Louis: Mosby-Year Book; 2002

Neville BW, Damm DD, Allen C, Bouquot JE. Oral and Maxillofacial Pathology. 3rd ed. St. Louis, MO: Saunders/Elsevier; 2009

Silverman S Jr. Oral Cancer. 4th ed. Philadelphia, PA: BC Decker; 1998

Topazian RG, Goldberg MH, Hupp JR. Oral and Maxillofacial Infections. 4th ed. Philadelphia, PA: WB Saunders; 2002

16 Diseases of the Temporomandibular Joint

■ Introduction

Temporomandibular disorders (TMDs) are a subgroup of orofacial pain conditions that involve the temporomandibular joint (TMJ), the masticatory muscles, and associated head and neck musculature. TMDs most frequently present with pain, limited or asymmetric mandibular motion, occlusal abnormalities, and TMJ sounds. The discomfort is primarily around the jaw, TMJ, and/or muscles of the head, face, and neck. Common associated symptoms include earache, dizziness, tinnitus, and headache. Many TMDs are of acute onset, have mild symptoms, and are usually self-limiting. However, some TMDs can become chronic. Chronic TMD pain syndromes present with persistent pain and TMD-associated symptoms that often last for months and even years. These symptoms are thought to be associated with a complex of physical, behavioral, psychological, and psychosocial factors similar to those of other chronic pain syndromes.

Anatomy

The TMJ is a diarthrotic synovial joint (specifically a ginglymoarthrodial joint) consisting of the mandibular condyle, the glenoid fossa portion of the temporal bone, and a meniscus (the "disk"). The TMJ disk maintains attachments to the joint capsule and moves in unison with the mandibular condyle. The joint undergoes both hinge and gliding motions. Initial jaw opening occurs when the articular surface of the mandibular condyle pivots on the undersurface of the disk. Full jaw opening occurs only with additional pivoting and forward displacement of the disk as it slides along the undersurface of the zygomatic process of the temporal bone. The innervation of the joint is provided by branches of the third division of the trigeminal nerve, which can allow for referred pain to and from other similarly innervated structures, and radiate to areas innervated by the other divisions of the nerve.

Demographics

An estimated 75% of the U.S. adult population has at one time or another experienced one or more of the signs and symptoms of TMD. Epidemiological studies show a prevalence of 40 to 75% of adults having at least one sign of joint dysfunction and ~ 33% of the population having at least one symptom of TMD. Some signs appear to be relatively common in the general population: TMJ sounds and deviation on opening occur in ~ 50% of healthy people. Other signs are relatively rare: limited mouth opening and occlusal changes occur in less than 5% of healthy people. TMDs are disorders of middle-aged adults (age 30–50), with a significant female preponderance of those seeking care (female-to-male ratio of 3:1–9:1). Despite large numbers of people experiencing signs and symptoms of TMD over their lifetime, only 5 to 10% of these individuals are estimated to be in need of treatment.

Etiological Studies

When considering the etiology of TMD, a historical review should begin with Costen's 1934 paper, in which he observed that patients with pain in or near the ear, tinnitus, dizziness, a sensation of ear fullness, and difficulty in swallowing seemed to improve by altering the vertical dimension of their occlusion. Malocclusion and improper jaw position were perceived to be the causes of this disorder, and the emphasis of treatment was on altering the occlusion. With continued research in the areas of joint biomechanics, neuromuscular physiology, rheumatology, musculoskeletal disorders, and pain mechanisms, a considerable change came about with regard to the etiology of TMD. It is now thought of as a musculoskeletal disorder in the realm of medical orthopedics.

Currently, there is no single proven causal factor for TMD, but numerous events are associated with its development. Contributing events are generally grouped into predisposing factors, initiating factors, and perpetuating factors. Any or all of these can be involved in the development of TMD for a given patient. In addition, numerous other structural, functional, and psychological abnormalities can influence the etiologic mechanisms involved in causing and prolonging TMD.

◼ Evaluation

Although TMD is a common cause of craniofacial pain, it is imperative that a comprehensive history, a clinical examination, and additional appropriate diagnostic studies be performed to exclude other potentially more serious disorders. A detailed history of the pain problem should be taken, along with a complete medical history, family history, and psychosocial history. Clinical examination should include (1) palpation of the muscles of mastication (masseter, temporalis, medial, and lateral pterygoids) and the cervical musculature; (2) observation of mandibular motion (opening, closing, lateral movement, and protrusion); (3) palpation and/or auscultation of the TMJ; (4) examination of the oral cavity, dentition, occlusion, and salivary glands; and (5) cranial nerve examination, with special attention to the trigeminal nerve. Additional diagnostic modalities may include imaging studies of the maxillofacial region, TMJs, salivary glands, brain, and brainstem with plain film radiography, computed tomography (CT), magnetic resonance imaging (MRI), nuclear medicine scintigraphy, and ultrasonography. Diagnostic nerve blocks, muscle injections, and electromyography may also prove helpful.

To assist in consistency of diagnosis and treatment, an established classification of related disorders provides general guidelines for grouping specific signs and symptoms with common etiologies and treatment strategies. In 2004, the International Headache Society published the second edition of its International Classification of Headache Disorders (**Table 16.1**). TMDs are listed under the 11th major group of this diagnostic classification. To be attributed to TMD (group 11.7), a headache must meet specific criteria (**Table 16.2**).

TMD can be divided into masticatory muscular disorders, such as myofascial pain dysfunction (MPD) syndrome, true intracapsular TMJ disorders, and other disorders that affect the TMJ structures. **Table 16.3** shows a further breakdown of these groups of disorders. As outlined by several organizations in their policy statements, such as the

National Institutes of Health, the American Society of TMJ Surgeons, and the American Association for Dental Research, the level of evidence for each treatment modality varies widely. In general, not all TMD patients are surgical candidates. In fact, patients with MPD syndrome do not benefit from surgical intervention. Many TMD patients benefit greatly from minimally invasive measures, which should generally be attempted before more aggressive therapy is recommended.

◼ Management

Masticatory Muscle Spasm (Myofascial Pain Dysfunction Syndrome)

Masticatory muscle spasm (MPD syndrome) is the most common of all TMDs. It is generally agreed that patients will exhibit one or more of the following signs:

1. Decreased range of mandibular motion
2. Impaired jaw function (e.g., deviation, TMJ sounds, sticking, or locking)
3. Pain on palpation of the masticatory muscles or TMJs, or on movement of the mandible

They may also have one or more of the following symptoms:

1. TMJ sounds
2. Fatigue or stiffness of the jaws
3. Pain in the face or jaws
4. Pain on opening the mouth widely
5. Jaw locking
6. Imaging studies of the TMJs will show no evidence of disease

The etiology of this clinical complex is multifactorial. The factors most commonly cited are structural, functional, and psychological. It is important to understand that for any individual patient, one clear etiologic component is rarely apparent, and more often several possible components will be identified as contributing factors. Basic treatment goals should be formulated, bearing in mind the combination of etiologic factors.

Treatment of Myofascial Pain Dysfunction

The vast majority of MPD patients will respond to simple, noninvasive treatments. These should include (but need not necessarily be limited to) reassurance, rest, heat, medication, occlusal therapy, behavioral interventions, and physical medicine concepts. It is important that patients understand the problem and that they are not alone with their symptoms. They

Table 16.1 Classification of headache disorders

Group	Classification
1.	Migraine
2.	Tension-type headache (TTH)
3.	Trigeminal autonomic cephalalgias (TACs)
4.	Other primary headache disorders
5.	Headache attributed to trauma or injury to the head and/or neck
6.	Headache attributed to cranial or cervical vascular disorder
7.	Headache attributed to nonvascular intracranial disorder
8.	Headache attributed to substance or its withdrawal
9.	Headache attributed to infection
10.	Headache attributed to disorder of homeostasis
11.	Headache or facial pain attributed to disorder of cranium, neck, eyes, ears, nose, sinuses, teeth, mouth, or other facial or cervical structure
	11.1. Headache attributed to disorder of cranial bone
	11.2. Headache attributed to disorder of neck
	11.3. Headache attributed to disorder of eyes
	11.4. Headache attributed to disorder of ears
	11.5. Headache attributed to disorder of the nose or paranasal sinuses
	11.6. Headache attributed to disorder of the teeth or jaw
	11.7. Headache attributed to temporomandibular disorder (TMD)
	11.8. Head or facial pain attributed to inflammation of the stylohyoid ligament
	11.9. Headache or facial pain attributed to other disorder of cranium, neck, eyes, ears, nose, sinuses, teeth, mouth or other facial or cervical structure
12.	Headache attributed to psychiatric disorder
13.	Painful cranial neuropathies and other facial pains
14.	Other headache disorders

Adapted with permission from Headache Classification Committee of the International Headache Society (IHS). The International Classification of Headache Disorders, 3rd edition (beta version). Cephalalgia. 2013;33(9):629-808.

Table 16.2 Headache attributable to temporomandibular disorder (TMD)

IHS	Diagnosis	Diagnosis criteria	Comment

11.7	Headache caused by a disorder involving structures in the temporo-mandibular region	A. Any headache fulfilling criterion C
		B. Clinical and/or imaging evidence of a pathological process affecting the temporomandibular joint (TMJ), muscles of mastication and/or associated structures
		C. Evidence of causation demonstrated by at least two of the following:
		  1. headache has developed in temporal relation to the onset of temporomandibular disorder
		  2. either or both of the following:
		    a) headache has significantly worsened in parallel with progression of the temporomandibular disorder
		    b) headache has significantly improved or resolved in parallel with improvement in or resolution of the temporomandibular disorder
		  3. the headache is produced or exacerbated by active jaw movements, passive movements through the range of motion of the jaw and/or provocative manoeuvres applied to temporomandibular structures such as pressure on the TMJ and surrounding muscles of mastication
		  4. headache, when unilateral, is ipsilateral to the side of the temporomandibular disorder
		D. Not better accounted for by another ICHD-3 diagnosis
			Usually most prominent in the preauricular areas of the face, masseter muscles and/or temporal regions. Pain generators include disk displacements, joint osteoarthritis, joint hypermobility and regional myofascial pain. Tends to be unilateral when the tempormandibular complex is the generator of pain, but may be bilateral when muscular involvement is present. Pain referral to the face is common.

Adapted with permission from Headache Classification Committee of the International Headache Society (IHS). The International Classification of Headache Disorders, 3rd edition (beta version). Cephalalgia. 2013;33(9):629-808.

Table 16.3 Categories of disorders causing temporomandibular joint (TMJ)

Symptoms	Diagnoses with symptoms referred to the TMJ	True TMJ Disorders
Myofascial pain dysfunction syndrome	Dental infections Parotitis Trigeminal neuralgia Tetanus Eagle syndrome	Congenital anomalies Trauma Neoplasms Arthritis Ankylosis Disc derangement

should also understand the role of muscle spasm in this disorder, its benign nature, that it is usually self-limiting, and that no joint disease exists. Although it is not prudent to immobilize the mandible entirely, patients should be instructed to have a mechanically soft diet for ~ 2 weeks, and to avoid yawning and laughing with the mouth opened widely. Habits with the jaw, such as chewing gum and biting fingernails, should be resisted.

Heat

The application of heat to the sides of the face by means of a heating pad, hot towel, or hot water bottle will be comforting and will help to relieve muscle spasm. More vigorous treatment can be achieved with ultrasound or short-wave diathermy heat treatments, which are widely available in physical therapy offices.

Medication

MPD syndrome patients often benefit from appropriate medication use. *Nonsteroidal anti-inflammatory agents* are often of value in the acute stage. An appropriate agent can be prescribed for 10 to 14 days at an anti-inflammatory dose. *Muscle relaxants* are widely used but have yet to be proven efficacious. They are contraindicated for a chronic problem. *Narcotic analgesics* should be avoided if at all possible. *Antidepressants* have a long history of effectiveness in the treatment of chronic pain, and in view of the strong association between TMD and psychological factors, their use is often justified, especially when the dysfunction is part of the complex of generalized muscle pain with other signs and symptoms of depression. Tricyclic antidepressants are the most widely used, and a bedtime-only schedule of 25 to 100 mg (mg) of nortriptyline, desipramine, or doxepin can be expected to alleviate symptoms in 2 to 4 weeks. Treatment is maintained for 2 to 4 months and tapered to a low-maintenance dose.

Recently, some of the *serotonin selective reuptake inhibitors* have also been used as part of the treatment regimen. Some of these agents (fluoxetine and paroxetine) have unfortunately been implicated in producing increased masticatory muscle spasms (bruxism), especially during sleep. *Anxiolytic agents*, such as the benzodiazepines, are also commonly used. Several agents and regimens exist, and dosing should be individualized. It is important that this treatment be limited and that patients are monitored because of potential for dependency.

Interocclusal Appliances

There are many types of interocclusal appliances for the treatment of TMD, and their multiplicity suggests that the optimum design has yet to be found. These devices are usually made of processed, hard acrylic and are designed to serve the following functions: (1) improve TMJ function; (2) improve the function of the masticatory motor system while reducing abnormal muscle function; and (3) protect the teeth from attrition and adverse occlusal loading.

A full-arch occlusal stabilization appliance has proven to be the most effective type of appliance. Partial occlusal coverage appliances tend to produce significant and often irreversible changes in the dentition. In some patients an appropriately designed appliance can be effective and will both reduce masticatory muscle pain and control attrition and adverse tooth loading. Referral to a dentist or maxillofacial prosthodontist is initiated for these devices.

There have been numerous reports that occlusal interferences of various types are the chief cause of masticatory muscle pain and that their elimination will result in improvement. The negative influence of malocclusion, loss of teeth, and occlusal interferences on masticatory function is not well supported by the evidence. However, on general principle, occlusal disharmony (including premature contacts) should be eliminated, and missing teeth should be replaced in an effort to achieve optimum occlusion and masticatory function. In addition, the long-term efficacy of repositioning adult nongrowing jaws with occlusal splints or functional appliances has not been proven satisfactorily.

Behavioral Modalities

Because of psychological factors often present in MPD syndrome patients, attempts to lower patient stress are important. Relaxation techniques, stress management, work pacing, imaging, biofeedback, cognitive therapy, and other behavioral modalities have all been shown to be advantageous. A 1996 National Institutes of Health Consensus Conference on Behavioral Medicine in the Management of Chronic Pain began the process of outlining techniques that have been found to be effective and indications for such treatment modalities. Unfortunately, many of these techniques still have relatively little research-based support. The most important factor is undoubtedly the therapeutic interaction of the practitioner with the patient. Physical therapy techniques are helpful in reconditioning and retraining muscles and the musculoskeletal apparatus. These techniques are applicable to the masticatory muscles, as well as to the other craniocervical muscles that can be involved in TMD. Passive motion is an additional physical modality that has been shown to be effective in rehabilitating the adverse morphological, biochemical, and biomechanical changes that can occur in injured synovial joints, muscles, and periarticular tissues. Several commercial passive-motion devices are currently in use for rehabilitation of the TMJ, and clinical trials on efficacy are ongoing.

Complementary Therapy

Recent literature supports the use of complementary treatment in masticatory muscle spasm. Consideration may be given to acupuncture, manual therapy, massage, and cognitive and behavioral therapy. Clinical research supports the use of acupuncture and manipulation showing a statistically significant improvement in pain and jaw opening. A full discussion of complementary treatments is outside of the scope of this review. Given the policy statements of several professional societies to treat initially with conservative measures, complementary treatments seem a viable first step.

Internal Temporomandibular Joint Derangement

Internal derangement of the TMJ is another cause of TMD. The techniques of arthrography, MRI, and diagnostic arthroscopy have demonstrated that the TMJ meniscus (disc) can be displaced or deformed and may account for a patient's symptoms of pain and limitation. The two main categories of internal derangement are anterior displacement with and without reduction.

Anterior Displacement with Reduction

Anterior displacement with reduction occurs when the disc is displaced in the closed-mouth position and reduces (with a click) to the normal relationship at some time during opening. In these circumstances, the patient complains of the click, with a variable amount of pain on opening. Also, on opening, the mandible deviates to the affected side, until the click occurs and then returns to the midline. Preventing the mouth from fully closing with a splint, tongue blade, or dental mirror handle eliminates the click. An arthrogram or MRI will demonstrate the displaced disc, which reduces on opening. This situation may worsen and include intermittent locking, which can then finally progress to the second category of internal derangement, closed lock.

Anterior Displacement without Reduction

In anterior displacement without reduction (closed lock), patients may have a variable amount of pain. If muscle spasm has been adequately relieved, they may be pain free. However, patients often feel that something in the joint is preventing it from fully opening. Opening may be limited to 25 to 30 mm (mm) with restricted movement of the contralateral side. There may also be a history of clicking with intermittent locking. An arthrogram or MRI will demonstrate a displacement of the disc without reduction on opening (closed lock), and may also demonstrate degenerative changes. In such cases, the signs and symptoms of degenerative joint disease may also be present.

Initial Treatment

Initial treatment for internal derangement of either type consists of the same noninvasive therapies used for myofascial pain dysfunction syndrome. In the patient who has an anterior displacement with reduction (intermittent locking), these strategies are often successful. In the patient with a closed lock, especially one that is long-standing, these treatments may reduce muscle spasm and pain and restore some motion, but the underlying displacement may remain. When noninvasive treatments have been attempted and the patient remains restricted, interventions, such as arthrocentesis or arthroscopy, should be considered.

Chronic Hypomobility (Ankylosis)

Chronic hypomobility (ankylosis) is an uncommon but important cause of TMD. Ankylosis is the persistent inability to open the mouth. It may be caused by pathological involvement of the joint structures (true ankylosis) or limitation produced by extra-articular causes (false ankylosis). Infection and trauma (including previous surgery) are the primary causes of true ankylosis. The finding is severe limitation of opening, possible with mandibular retrognathism, if mandibular growth has been restricted.

False ankylosis may be caused by a variety of disorders that can be categorized as (1) myogenic (e.g., contracture of the masticatory muscles); (2) neurogenic (e.g., tetanus, dystonia); (3) psychogenic (e.g., conversion disorders); (4) osteogenic (e.g., impingement of an enlarged coronoid process); (5) histiogenic (e.g., following TMJ surgery, temporalis muscle flaps, trauma); and (6) neoplastic (e.g., nasopharyngeal carcinoma). Imaging studies show destruction of the joint surfaces, loss of joint space, and in extreme cases, ossification across the joint. The key to successful management is identifying the cause of the hypomobility and addressing that as aggressively as possible. However, true ankylosis with fibrosis and calcification can be recalcitrant to treatment.

Trauma to the Jaw

Trauma to the jaw can sprain the TMJ, cause a joint effusion, or fracture the neck of the mandibular condyle. In the acute sprain, the joint is painful, and there is limitation of movement caused by the pain and muscle spasm. Heat, rest, and nonsteroidal anti-inflammatory medications will resolve the acute symptoms, but other forms of treatment may be necessary to alleviate the residual muscle spasm and pain.

In the case of a joint effusion, in addition to pain and limitation, patients will be unable to close their teeth together on the affected side. In a more severe injury, a hemarthrosis may develop, with damage to the disc. Active physical therapy is required to restore range of motion and prevent the development of ankylosis.

A fracture of the neck of the condyle is a common maxillofacial injury, and if undisplaced, it requires analgesics and a soft diet for a few days. In a unilateral displacement or dislocated variety, a patient will have a premature bite on the affected side and deviation to that side on opening. Maxillomandibular fixation for 7 to 10 days may be required, with active physical therapy thereafter to restore function. Patients with bilateral fractures will have an anterior open bite and posterior displacement of the mandible. Depending on the position of the displaced fragment, it may interfere with mandibular motion. More aggressive surgical treatment will be required to restore the occlusion and normal function.

Degenerative Disease (Osteoarthritis) of the Temporomandibular Joint

Degenerative disease (osteoarthritis) of the TMJ may be the end point of several different insults to the joint structures, exceeding the TMJ's capacity to remodel and repair. The insults may be trau-

matic (acute or chronic), chemical injury, infection metabolic disturbances, and previous joint surgery. The patient complains of pain on moving the mandible, and of limited movement with deviation to the affected side. There may be acute tenderness over the joint itself. Joint sounds are described as grating, grinding, or crunching, but not as clicking or popping. Imaging studies typically reveal degenerative changes and remodeling, and a loss of joint space.

The features of degenerative disease of the TMJ are different from those of most of the other joints in the body in that it most commonly occurs in women in their third or fourth decade. Rarely is it part of a generalized osteoarthritis. The natural course of the disease suggests that the pain and limitation may "burn themselves out" after several months in some individuals. The majority of patients can be kept comfortable until remission with the noninvasive techniques already outlined. Some patients require injection of corticosteroid into the joint. This treatment is generally reserved for older patients and is limited to two or three injections. For patients who do not respond to these techniques, surgery may be indicated to remove the loose fragments of bone (so-called joint mice) and reshape the condyle. Attention should also be directed toward the disc because its displacement may be a primary reason for the degenerative changes.

Rheumatoid Arthritis

Rheumatoid arthritis can also affect the TMJ in individuals of any age. In young patients, an associated micrognathia may be noted; in older patients with advanced cases, ankylosis may be the presenting complaint. Imaging findings are of joint destruction possibly involving both the condyle and the articular eminence of the temporal bone. Other stigmata of rheumatoid arthritis will be evident. If medical management is ineffective, treatment of the degenerative joint disease or the ankylosis, as already outlined, may be necessary.

Congenital Abnormalities

Studies on facial growth have demonstrated the major contributions made by the mandibular condyle to the adaptive growth of the mandible within the functional soft tissue matrix. Several abnormalities can reduce this normal growth, which can manifest as TMD, including hypothyroidism, hypopituitarism, and nutritional deficiency (e.g., vitamin D deficiency). In gigantism, all the skeletal structures are enlarged, and in acromegaly, a marked mandibular prognathism is produced. Several local conditions, such as trauma, infection, rheumatoid arthritis, exposure to radiation, and scarring from burns or surgery, are other causes of reduced postnatal growth.

In congenital abnormalities, the complex and coordinated growth of facial structures necessary for the achievement of normal form and function are altered, and craniofacial malformations can occur. It is beyond the scope of this chapter to review all the craniofacial anomalies that can occur; suffice it to say that most abnormalities of the TMJ occur in conjunction with recognized syndromes (e.g., hemifacial microsomia, Treacher Collins syndrome). A full clinical and radiological workup is necessary for evaluation of the deformity and the planned multidisciplinary treatment.

Temporomandibular Joint Infections

Infections of the TMJ can occur and are most often due to an open wound or to direct extension from adjacent structures (e.g., osteomyelitis of the mandible, suppurative otitis media). More rarely, an infection may be due to hematogenous spread from a distant site. With improved medical care, better nutrition, and antibiotics, infections of the TMJ have diminished in frequency. Septic arthritis usually affects one joint, which becomes acutely painful, warm, and swollen. Characteristically, the swelling of the joint causes difficulty in opening, and prevents the posterior teeth from meeting properly. Diagnostic features are the systemic indications of an infection and bacteria in the joint fluid. Imaging studies may show an increased joint space, bony destruction, and sclerosis in the chronic stage. As sequelae of acute infections, arthritis with ankylosis and growth retardation may develop. Treatment is directed at the underlying cause with drainage, debridement, and appropriate antimicrobial therapy.

Temporomandibular Joint Tumors

Tumors of the TMJ are rare, but clinicians need to maintain a high index of suspicion, because the signs and symptoms of neoplastic disease can mimic those of other, more common TMD. Tumors may arise from the native cell line of the tissues of the joint and invade the adjacent structures, or they may metastasize from distant primary sites. Benign connective tissue tumors (e.g., osteoma, chondroma, osteochondroma) are most common. They present with pain and limitation of opening and an open bite on the affected side. In osteoma, a globular expansion of the condyle (as opposed to an elongation or overall enlargement seen in condylar hyperplasia) is noted on imaging. In synovial chondromatosis, foci of cartilage develop in the synovial membrane, and

occasionally radiopaque masses are seen within the joint. Malignant tumors are rare, and may be indicated by pain, swelling, numbness, and hearing loss. Tumors may spread from surrounding structures or metastasize from distant sites. Radiographic changes are osteolytic or osteoblastic, depending on the tumor type. Treatment of these tumors follows the same principles of treatment as other head and neck neoplasia.

◼ Conclusion

Management of TMD integrates several medical disciplines: otolaryngology, dentistry, oral maxillofacial surgery, neurology, and rheumatology, and among these specialists there is no unified strategy for the management of this disease. Most cases of TMD respond to conservative treatment, and the prognosis is good. In cases of secondary TMJ involvement, the prognosis depends on the primary disease. It is important to diagnose the specific condition and provide definitive treatment or appropriate referral. In some cases consultation of a dentist, oral maxillofacial surgeon, neurologist, or rheumatologist is needed.

In a recent policy statement from the American Association of Dental Research, it was recommended that treatment of TMD patients be initially based on the use of conservative, reversible, and evidence-based therapeutic modalities. Studies of the natural history of many TMDs suggest that they tend to improve or resolve over time. Although no specific therapies have been proven to be uniformly effective, many of the conservative modalities have proven to be at least as effective in providing symptomatic relief as most forms of invasive treatment. Because those modalities do not produce irreversible changes, they present much less risk of producing harm. Professional treatment should be augmented with a home care program, in which patients are taught about their disorder and how to manage their symptoms.

◼ Controversial Issues

- The best test(s) to use to help in making a specific diagnosis when a patient presents with TMJ complaints
- Second-line medications to consider if nonsteroidal anti-inflammatory drugs have been ineffective
- Actual indications for TMJ arthroscopy and other surgical interventions
- Methods to help patients modify their bite and other factors to prevent future episodes of TMJ pain

■ Practice Guidelines, Consensus Statements, and Measures

American Association for Dental Research. Policy Statement on Temporomandibular Disorders. Revised 2010. http://www.aadronline.org/i4a/pages/index.cfm?pageid=3465

American Society of TMJ Surgeons. Guidelines for Diagnosis and Management of Disorders Involving the Temporomandibular Joint and Related Musculoskeletal Structures. 2001. www.astmjs.org/guidelines.html

American Association of Oral and Maxillofacial Surgeons. Guidelines to the Evaluation of Impairment of the Oral and Maxillofacial Region. 2008. www.astmjs.org/impairment.html

International Headache Society. IHS Classification ICHD-III (beta version). 2013. http://www.ihs-classification.org/en/

NIH Technology Assessment Panel on Integration of Behavioral and Relaxation Approaches into the Treatment of Chronic Pain and Insomnia. Integration of behavioral and relaxation approaches into the treatment of chronic pain and insomnia. JAMA 1996;276(4):313–318

■ Suggested Reading

Balasubramaniam R, Klasser GD. Orofacial pain and dysfunction: Preface. Oral Maxillofac Surg Clin North Am 2008;20(2):ix–x

Bell WE. Temporomandibular Disorders: Classification, Diagnosis, Management. 3rd ed. Chicago, IL: Year Book Medical Publishers; 1990

Dworkin SF, Burgess JA. Orofacial pain of psychogenic origin: current concepts and classification. J Am Dent Assoc 1987;115(4):565–571

Dworkin SF, Huggins KH, LeResche L, et al. Epidemiology of signs and symptoms in temporomandibular disorders: clinical signs in cases and controls. J Am Dent Assoc 1990;120(3):273–281

Dym H, Israel H. Diagnosis and treatment of temporomandibular disorders. Dent Clin North Am 2012;56(1):149–161, ix

Flint PW, Haughey BH, Lund VJ et al, eds. Cummings Otolaryngology—Head and Neck Surgery. 5th ed. Philadelphia, PA: Mosby Elsevier; 2010

Fordyce WE. Pain and suffering: a reappraisal. Am Psychol 1988;43(4):276–283

Fricton JR, Kroening RJ, Hathaway KM, eds. TM Disorders and Craniofacial Pain: Diagnosis and Management. St. Louis, MO: Ishiro Euro America; 1988

Huber MA, Hall EH. A comparison of the signs of temporomandibular joint dysfunction and occlusal discrepancies in a symptom-free population of men and women. Oral Surg Oral Med Oral Pathol 1990;70(2):180–183

Levitt SR, McKinney MW. Validating the TMJ scale in a national sample of 10,000 patients: demographic and epidemiologic characteristics. J Orofac Pain 1994;8(1):25–35

McNeill C, Danzig WM, Farrar WB, et al. Position paper of the American Academy of Craniomandibular Disorders. Craniomandibular (TMJ) disorders—the state of the art. Position paper of the American Association of Craniomandibular Disorders. J Prosthet Dent 1980;44:434–437

Michael LA. Jaws revisited: Costen's syndrome. Ann Otol Rhinol Laryngol 1997;106(10 Pt 1):820–822

Okeson JP. Bell's Orofacial Pains. 5th ed. Chicago, IL: Quintessence; 1995:123–133

Okeson JP. Management of Temporomandibular Disorders and Occlusion. 7th ed. St. Louis, MO: Elsevier Mosby; 2013

Parker MW, Holmes EK, Terezhalmy GT. Personality characteristics of patients with temporomandibular disorders: diagnostic and therapeutic implications. J Orofac Pain 1993;7(4):337–344

Sarnat BG, Laskin DM. The Temporomandibular Joint: A Biological Basis for Clinical Practice. 4th ed. Philadelphia, PA: WB Saunders; 1992

Schiffman E, Fricton JR. Epidemiology of TMJ and craniofacial pains. In: Friction JR, Kroening RJ, Hathaway KM, eds. TMJ and Craniofacial Pain. St. Louis, MO: Ishiro Euro America; 1988:1–10

Scrivani SJ, Keith DA, Kaban LB. Temporomandibular disorders. N Engl J Med 2008;359(25):2693–2705

Solberg WK. Epidemiology, incidence and prevalence of temporomandibular disorders: a review. In: Report of the President's Conference on the Examination, Diagnosis and Management of Temporomandibular Disorders. Chicago, IL: American Dental Association; 1983:30–39

Wabeke KB, Spruijt RJ. On temporomandibular joint sounds: dental and psychological studies [thesis]. Amsterdam, the Netherlands: University of Amsterdam; 1994:91–103

17 Xerostomia

■ Evaluation

Xerostomia is a dry mouth related to decrease or lack of saliva. Although a dry mouth may be indicative of an existing or past medical condition, it is considered a subjective complaint, rather than a disease.

Physiology

Saliva is a dilute aqueous solution containing both organic and inorganic components. Under stimulated conditions, 90% of saliva by volume is produced by the three paired major salivary glands—parotid, submandibular, and sublingual—which are serous, mixed serous and mucous, and mucous-secreting, respectively. The remaining 10% of saliva by volume is produced by the minor salivary glands located beneath the lingual, palatal, buccal, and labial mucosa, which are all primarily mucous-secreting glands. The submandibular, sublingual, and minor salivary glands are responsible for most salivary production during nonstimulated periods. The parotid is the major producer under stimulated conditions. At moderate flow rates, it accounts for half of the salivary output, and at higher flow rates it can account for two-thirds of the output.

The major functions of saliva include lubrication, digestion, solvent action, antibacterial and antifungal activity, buffering action, and remineralization. Saliva plays a key role in mastication for bolus formation and in lubrication for swallowing and speech. The importance of saliva is generally appreciated when it is significantly reduced or absent, affecting the hard and soft tissues within the oral cavity, thereby altering function and diminishing quality of life.

Normal salivation is controlled by the nervous system and is dependent on peripheral receptors, such as mechanoreceptors and visual, gustatory, and olfactory receptors, to stimulate central neurons. The neurons then send excitatory signals to the salivary glands, resulting in salivary secretions. The parasympathetic nerves supply the mucin-secreting cells and

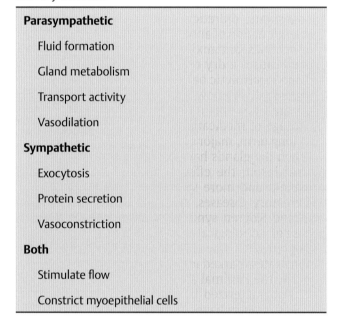

Table 17.1 Autonomic nervous system effect on salivary function

Parasympathetic
Fluid formation
Gland metabolism
Transport activity
Vasodilation
Sympathetic
Exocytosis
Protein secretion
Vasoconstriction
Both
Stimulate flow
Constrict myoepithelial cells

the intralobular duct cells. The sympathetic nerves control the serous cells and the myoepithelial cells (**Table 17.1**).

These cells are considered to be responsible for the contractile action that promotes salivary secretion. Compromise of the nerve supply to the glands, including interference with neurotransmitters and receptors, can result in altered gland function and salivary output.

Incidence

Twenty-five percent of the geriatric population and as many as 10% of the general population suffer from xerostomia.

Between 2010 and 2050, the U.S. population is projected to grow from 310 million to 439 million, an increase of 42%. The population is expected to become much older, with nearly one in five U.S.

residents aged 65 and older in 2030. Although xerostomia is not related to aging itself, the geriatric population consumes a large array of medications for various conditions that can induce a dry mouth.

Etiology

There are many causes of temporary or permanent reductions in salivary flow. Use of certain drugs, viral infections, dehydration, and psychogenic causes may temporarily inhibit saliva production to varying degrees in patients who have healthy functioning glands.

More than 400 common prescription drugs list dry mouth as a side effect. Some of these are drugs to prevent motion sickness. Other types include antihistamines, antidepressants, antipsychotics, antianxiety agents, anti-Parkinsonism drugs, antihypertensives, decongestants, diuretics, and analgesics. The anticholinergic action of antihistamines, antidepressants, antipsychotics, antianxiety medications, and decongestants causes a dry mouth. Other drugs affect the fluid and electrolytic balance in a way that results in decreased salivary flow. Usually the symptoms of dry mouth are transient and are related to length of time and dosage of medications. If these medications are taken long term, major effects can be observed.

When the glands have been altered by disease or external insult, the effects on salivary flow can be permanent and more severe in magnitude. Chronic inflammatory diseases, such as sarcoidosis, amyloidosis, and Sjögren syndrome, can cause xerostomia because of pathological changes in the salivary glands.

Sjögren syndrome is an autoimmune disease that demonstrates marked infiltration of exocrine glands, primarily the lacrimal and salivary glands. The infiltrate is characterized by CD4 lymphocytes, plasma cells, and macrophages replacing the parenchymal gland tissue. The disease occurs in two forms: primary Sjögren syndrome, which affects the salivary and lacrimal glands, and secondary Sjögren syndrome, which is associated with rheumatoid arthritis and other autoimmune diseases.

Sarcoidosis involves granulomatous inflammation with Langerhans-type giant cells and epithelioid macrophages resulting in noncaseating granulomas. When the salivary glands are involved, xerostomia can occur. In amyloidosis, deposits of amyloid can occur in the salivary glands, causing decreased salivary output.

The effects of radiation therapy for head and neck cancer on salivary gland function and xerostomia are well documented. These effects are both immediate and delayed. The immediate effects are related to direct damage inflicted on the end organ structures during treatment. The delayed effect is ischemic in nature. The functioning glandular tissue is replaced with fibrotic tissue. The severity of the xerostomia is related to total volume of gland exposure and total dose delivered to the glands. The xerostomia can include minimal to no changes following irradiation of a T1 laryngeal lesion to over 90% permanent reduction in salivary flow for treatment of an unknown primary or nasopharyngeal lesion. These changes are usually permanent, with either minimum or no recovery in glandular function.

Xerostomia can be observed in graft-versus-host disease. This is caused by donor lymphocytes infiltrating salivary gland tissue. This pattern and clinical presentation are similar to those of Sjögren syndrome. Some human immunodeficiency virus (HIV) patients can demonstrate enlarged salivary glands and xerostomia. The T-lymphocyte infiltration is primarily CD8 cells. Xerostomia is also observed in patients with uncontrolled diabetes, dialysis for chronic renal failure, interferon therapy, and cystic fibrosis.

■ Evaluation

Symptoms

Patients with xerostomia will complain of an uncomfortably dry mouth. They may report difficulty eating, swallowing, or speaking. Complaints may also include a burning sensation involving the oral mucosa and tongue, alterations in taste, intolerance to spicy or acidic foods or liquids, awakening at night to sip water and replenish oral moisture, and difficulty wearing removable dentures.

Signs

Clinical findings with a dry mouth may include any or all of the following features in varying degrees, depending on the severity of the xerostomia. Examination of the oral cavity reveals a decrease or absence of saliva pooled on the floor of the mouth or coating the soft tissues. The dry mucosa may feel sticky on palpation. Saliva, if present, may appear thick and viscous, ropey, or foamy. The soft tissues will appear thin and fragile with atrophic changes, including atrophy of the dorsal surface of the tongue.

Significant decreases in the volume of saliva, and alterations in the organic and inorganic constituents result in a decreased buffering capacity and a lower pH, which is conducive to significant shifts in the microbial oral flora. There is an increase in microorganisms that are associated with dental caries (*Streptococcus mutans, Lactobacillus*) and periodontal disease (*Actinomyces*), with fungal populations (*Candida albicans*) increasing dramatically. These factors are the major reasons for often-observed rampant caries and fungal infections. Teeth, if present, may demonstrate dental caries at the gingival margins, and at atypical sites, such as on cusp tips or incisal edges. Fungal infections may be seen on the soft tissue as patches of white plaque that, when removed, have a red or bleeding base, or as erythematous areas involving the oral mucosa. If the commissures of the mouth are involved, angular cheilitis may be observed. Edentulous patients may have areas of irritation or trauma associated with denture function in a desiccated environment. Enlarged parotid and submandibular glands can be observed in patients with Sjögren syndrome or HIV infection. Patients with severe xerostomia will carry a water or fluid container to replenish oral moisture as needed.

Assessment

A correlation of signs and symptoms can establish a clinical diagnosis of xerostomia. An actual assessment of salivary flow (sialometry) provides an objective measure to grade the severity of the xerostomia. It also provides a quantitative assessment to determine the efficacy of a prescribed intervention to alleviate the xerostomia. Standardized techniques must be used to ensure reproducible results. Resting or unstimulated saliva is usually measured by collecting whole saliva. Flow rates are expressed in milliliters per minute (mL/min). Normal resting flow rates are around 0.3 to 0.4 mL/min. Reductions of 50% or more in resting whole salivary flow rates are usually associated with the complaint of dry mouth and xerostomia. Stimulated whole salivary flow rates can be assessed using mechanical stimulation (chewing) or citric acid. Normal stimulated whole salivary flow rates are reported to be ~ 2 mL/min.

Based on these reports and the fact that virtually no saliva is produced during sleep, the estimated total daily flow of whole saliva is 600 to 700 mL.

Flow rates for the parotid, submandibular, and sublingual glands can be assessed by placing collection devices over the duct orifices. The mean resting flow rate for the parotid gland is 0.04 mL/min per gland. For the submandibular and sublingual glands, it is 0.12 mL/min.

The stimulated flow rate for the parotid, submandibular, and sublingual gland is ~ 0.5 to 0.8 mL/min per gland. Reduced stimulated salivary flow rates may not be associated with the complaint of a dry mouth.

Secretions from the minor salivary glands can be collected on absorbent paper strips and assayed with a device that measures small volumes of fluids. The flow rates for the minor salivary glands from the lip, cheek, and palate are reported to be 0.96, 2.64, and 0.74 mL/min per centimeter (cm), respectively. There are no differences between resting and stimulated flow rates for the minor salivary glands. Though the minor salivary glands contribute 10% or less of the total volume of saliva, they account for ~ 70% of the mucous secreted.

Function of the major salivary glands can also be assessed using scintigraphy. Salivary scintigraphy is performed using technetium pertechnetate, a gamma-emitting radionuclide with affinity for salivary glands. Tracer movement can be scanned in a resting or stimulated state. Technetium, which is transported by salivary acinar cells, is a good indicator of functional tissues. Consequently, it can be used to assess the extent of residual functional parenchyma that may respond to treatment aimed at increasing salivary production.

◼ Management

Rational management of xerostomia is dependent on establishing the diagnosis and cause. A history of previous radiation therapy for head and neck cancer, current medications, or reported medical conditions that can cause a dry mouth are indicative of the cause of the xerostomia. Xerostomia, in the absence of such a history, warrants appropriate investigation and medical workup to rule out underlying medical conditions that could be causing the dry mouth, and may require medical treatment. Drug-induced xerostomia may be managed by consulting with the treating doctor and changing or reducing the doses of medication if the patient's condition permits. Strategies for management include treatment and prevention of the side effects of xerostomia. Preventive measures include staying well hydrated by taking regular sips of water and/or sugar-free liquids, avoiding oral irritants (e.g., coffee, alcohol, and nicotine) and acidic drinks (e.g., carbonated beverages and juices). Maintenance of open nasal passages to avoid mouth breathing helps to minimize xerostomia.

If teeth are present and have caries, appropriate dental referral is in order. A strict oral hygiene regimen consisting of frequent rinsing with baking soda solutions and application of topical fluorides with custom fluoride carriers for patients postirradiation for head and neck cancer is indicated for all dentate patients with xerostomia. Patients having difficulty with dentures should be referred to a prosthodontist for specialty care.

Fungal infections can be managed with the appropriate diagnosis and intervention. This would include microscopic examination of smears and cultures. The use of salty rinses, such as baking soda or saline, can provide some degree of protection against fungal overgrowth. Patients are instructed to keep dental prostheses and teeth scrupulously clean and to soak prostheses overnight in an appropriate cleansing solution. Nystatin, ketoconazole, and fluconazole are routinely used to treat these infections.

Various commercial saliva substitutes are available for symptomatic treatment. These solutions are generally most useful during the night or prior to eating. Patient acceptance of these solutions is generally poor. Water alone remains the most frequently used mouth-wetting agent.

Inert chewing gum or sugarless gum is recommended to stimulate residual salivary flow. Sucking on sugared candy mints or citrus mints to stimulate flow is not recommended for dentate patients, because it can lead to rampant dental caries with sugared candy and dissolution of enamel with citrus mints. Water-based gels can provide moisture to dry oral tissues and lips. A humidifier in the room, especially at night in dry environments, may be helpful.

Patients should avoid over-the-counter mouthwashes that are high in alcohol content because they can be drying and irritating to the tissues. Alcohol-free mouthwashes are available. Regular use of alcohol and tobacco is discouraged.

Management can also include consulting a dietitian to make diet plans and recommendations for proper nutrition, caloric intake, and food preparation. In other approaches, drugs (sialagogues) have been used to stimulate residual gland activity and alleviate xerostomia, and anetholetrithione has been used to treat xerostomia, with differing reports regarding its efficacy. Some reports indicate improvement for drug-induced xerostomia. Studies in people with Sjögren syndrome are inconsistent.

Pilocarpine has been partially successful in stimulating additional secretions in patients with residual salivary gland parenchyma. It stimulates the salivary tissue by its muscarinic-cholinergic agonist properties. Stimulated secretions are similar to normal salivary secretions. With severe xerostomia, although little objective increase in salivary output is noted, subjective improvement is often noted by the patient. On the other hand, impressive increases of residual saliva in a moderately dry mouth may provide little or no subjective gain. It should be noted that maximum salivary flow may not be realized until after 90 days of treatment with pilocarpine. The most common side effect of the drug is sweating, which is transient and dose related. The drug is contraindicated in patients with bowel obstruction, asthma, and chronic obstructive lung disease. Dosage levels above 20 mg a day may precipitate toxic side effects. Thus, for a patient who is properly informed and has reasonable expectations regarding possible benefits, pilocarpine may help diminish some of the signs and symptoms associated with xerostomia.

Another drug used for xerostomia is cevimeline, which is in a class of medications called cholinergic agonists. Cevimeline works by increasing the amount of saliva in the mouth. Cevimeline can cause side effects, which include sweating, nausea, and a runny nose.

◼ Summary

Otolaryngologists, by the nature of the specialty, will frequently encounter patients with xerostomia. A thorough understanding of this complaint and condition as it relates to past and present medical conditions is essential for its correct diagnosis and appropriate management. Interaction with other physicians, medical specialists, dentists, and dental specialists is required for the comprehensive management of this problem. The otolaryngologist's knowledge in this area should direct the patient in the care of this condition and in possible diagnosis and treatment of any underlying causes.

◼ Suggested Reading

Aghemo A, Rumi MG, Monico S, et al. Ribavirin impairs salivary gland function during combination treatment with pegylated interferon alfa-2a in hepatitis C patients. Hepat Mon 2011;11(11):918–924

Beumer J, Curtis T, Marunick M. Maxillofacial rehabilitation, prosthodontic and surgical considerations. In: Radiation Therapy of Head and Neck Tumors: Oral Effects Dental Manifestations and Dental Treatment. St. Louis, MO: Ishiyaku Euroamerica Inc.; 1996:43–112

Bradley RM. Salivary secretion. In: Bradley RM, ed. Essentials of Oral Physiology. St. Louis, MO: Mosby-Year Book; 1994:161–186

Furness S, Worthington HV, Bryan G, Birchenough S, McMillan R. Interventions for the management of dry mouth: topical therapies. Cochrane Database Syst Rev 2011;12(12):CD008934

Garg AK, Kirsh ER. Xerostomia: recognition and management of hypofunction of the salivary glands. Compend Contin Educ Dent 1995;16(6):574–584, 576–584, quiz 586

Greenspan D. Xerostomia: diagnosis and management. Oncology (Williston Park) 1996;10(3, Suppl):7–11

Mandel ID, Sreebny L, Izutsu KT, Fox PC, Ferguson MM. A symposium on the endogenous benefits of saliva in oral health. Compend Contin Educ Dent 1989;13:S5450–S5481

Marunick MT, Seyedsadr M, Ahmad K, Klein B. The effect of head and neck cancer treatment on whole salivary flow. J Surg Oncol 1991;48(2):81–86

National Institute of Dental and Craniofacial Research—National Institute of Health. Dry Mouth—Xerostomia. 2011. http://www.nidcr.nih.gov/OralHealth/Topics/DryMouth/DryMouth.html

Noce CW, Gomes A, Copello A, et al. Oral involvement of chronic graft-versus-host disease in hematopoietic stem cell transplant recipients. Gen Dent 2011;59(6):458–462, quiz 463–464

Onelmis H, Sener S, Sasmaz S, Ozer A. Cutaneous changes in patients with chronic renal failure on hemodialysis. Cutan Ocul Toxicol 2012;31(4):286–291

Oral Cancer Foundation. Xerostomia. 2011. http://www.oralcancerfoundation.org/treatment/xerostomia.html

Rousseau P. Pilocarpine in radiation-induced xerostomia. Am J Hosp Palliat Care 1995;12(2):38–39

Van Dongen CA. Management of Oral Complications of Cancer Therapy. Providence, RI: Miriam Hospital Department of Dentistry; 1995

Wind DA. Management of xerostomia: an overview. J Prac Hygiene 1996;5:23–27

18 Sleep-Disordered Breathing

■ Introduction

Sleep-disordered breathing (SDB) comprises a spectrum of sleep-related breathing abnormalities that range from snoring and upper airway resistance syndrome (UARS) to obstructive sleep apnea–hypopnea syndrome (OSAHS). The American Academy of Sleep Medicine's *International Classification of Sleep Disorders: Diagnostic and Coding Manual* defines Primary Snoring (ICSD 786.09) as "loud upper airway breathing sounds in sleep, without episodes of apnea or hypoventilation." UARS is characterized by snoring and frequent microarousals in the absence of oxygen desaturations that result in fragmented sleep architecture and daytime somnolence. OSAHS is a disease of upper airway obstruction that manifests as recurring episodes of either partial or complete upper airway collapse, necessitating frequent awakenings or arousals to reestablish airway patency. Understanding this spectrum of disorders, whether upper airway obstruction is occurring and at what level, and the different treatment modalities available for each is essential to the armamentarium of the otolaryngologist.

Obstructive apneas are commonly defined as a 90% or greater drop in airflow for at least 10 seconds, despite continuing ventilatory effort. Hypopneas are events with only a 30 to 90% decrease in airflow for 10 or more seconds and a desaturation of 4% or greater from baseline. Some patients may exhibit episodes of enhanced upper airway resistance, characterized by an arousal from sleep to enhance breathing, yet airflow measurement devices detect only brief changes in airflow with no significant reduction in oxyhemoglobin saturation. These events are called respiratory effort–related arousals (RERAs).

The apnea index (AI) is defined as the number of apneas per hour of sleep. The apnea/hypopnea index (AHI) is the number of apneas and hypopneas per hour of sleep. The respiratory disturbance index (RDI) is defined as the number of apneas, hypopneas, and RERAs divided by the total sleep time, usually expressed as events per hour. Most clinicians and researchers use the AHI when discussing treatment options and describing OSAHS severity. RDI is being used more frequently and should not be overlooked in the event of a low AHI and a high RDI. Many centers use RDI and AHI interchangeably when reporting the results of polysomnograms (PSGs), and incorrectly use RDI in place of AHI without including RERAs.

Epidemiology

Epidemiological studies suggest that OSAHS is a relatively common disorder in the general population. A large U.S. epidemiological study demonstrated that 4% of middle-aged males and 2% of middle-aged females have an AHI of 5 or more and suffer from daytime somnolence severe enough for the diagnosis of OSAHS. In addition, 24% of males and 9% of females have an AHI of 5 or more. It is estimated that 82% of males and 93% of females with moderate to severe OSAHS remain undiagnosed.

Specialists have estimated that the prevalence of pediatric SDB may be as high as 5 to 6%. In some studies, these rates increase up to 10-fold in the elderly population. In people 30 to 60 years old, major risk factors have been found to be obesity, male sex, and large neck diameter. Modified Mallampati grade, tonsil size, and increased body mass index (BMI) are all clinical indicators that are associated with an increased RDI. Anomalies associated with mandibular maldevelopment, such as Treacher Collins syndrome and Pierre Robin syndrome, often lead to OSAHS. Unfortunately, the majority of people with OSAHS do not receive appropriate treatment for their disease.

Daytime somnolence has been found to be a significant risk factor for automobile and truck accidents. Patients with obstructive sleep apnea (OSA) have been shown to have seven times as many motor vehicle accidents as the general population, and a disturbing proportion of truck drivers have been shown to have OSA. It has been estimated that at least one-third of fatal car accidents may be sleep-disorder related. Patients with severe OSA have been shown to have a threefold increase in all-cause mortality, independent of age, sex, BMI, and other potential confounders.

Pathophysiology

Pharyngeal occlusion during OSAHS occurs at the velopharyngeal, oropharyngeal, and hypopharyngeal levels. Oropharyngeal collapse with tongue prolapse is due to diminished neuromuscular activity in the genioglossus muscle during rapid eye movement (REM) sleep. Hypopharyngeal collapse depends primarily on the muscles that insert on the hyoid arch, which include the hyoglossus, middle constrictor, geniohyoid, mylohyoid, anterior digastric, sternohyoid, and thyrohyoid muscles. Nasopharynx and oropharynx dilatation requires tensor veli palatini and masseter muscle activity.

During sleep, the parapharyngeal muscles are phasically active with inspiration, causing dilation and stiffening of the airway. With the onset of sleep, there is a reduced phasic input to these pharyngeal constrictors, a reduced gain for reflexes that protect the pharynx from collapsing, and a reduction in load compensation. With non-REM sleep, the chemoreceptor "set point" is increased, and the sensitive hypocapnia-induced apneic threshold is revealed.

Even in normal individuals, sleep is associated with pharyngeal narrowing and a substantial increase in inspiratory resistance. Part of the narrowing is due to the reduced atmospheric pressure caused by an expanding thorax during inspiration. An abnormal pharynx can be kept open during wakefulness by an appropriate compensatory increase in pharyngeal dilator muscle activity, but with sleep apnea, this compensation fails and the airway collapses. Partial collapse results in snoring, hypopneas, and, in some cases, prolonged obstructive hypoventilation, and complete closure results in apnea. A change in the sleep state or arousal is required for the return of sufficient pharyngeal dilator activity and adequate airflow. With the elevated sleep stage and relief of obstruction, there is ventilatory overcompensation. This resets the "set point" and sets the stage for a return to the apneic stage.

Excessive daytime sleepiness (or hypersomnolence) results from the fragmented sleep and microarousals associated with these apneic events. The resulting impaired cognition and memory loss cause poor work performance and emotional distress. Patients with OSAHS have an increased risk of diurnal hypertension, nocturnal dysrhythmias, pulmonary hypertension, right and left ventricular failure, myocardial infarction, and stroke. It is worth noting that the incidence of hypertension in OSAHS patients is independent of obesity, age, sex, and cigarette and alcohol use. Retrospective studies indicate that there

is an association of sleep apnea with cardiovascular- and cerebrovascular-related morbidity and mortality. This association appears to be mediated by the repetitive upper airway closure and its effect on the autonomic nervous system. Sleep fragmentation as well as nocturnal desaturation cause daytime sleepiness, fatigue, irritability, and personality changes.

■ Evaluation

OSAHS Predictors

Questionnaires to evaluate for severity of OSAHS are available but are not used widely. The Epworth Sleepiness Scale has a high correlation with daytime somnolence caused by OSAHS. Increasing neck size (circumference) has a linear relationship to a high probability for OSAHS. When ascertaining neck size with (1) the presence or absence of hypertension, (2) heroic snoring, and (3) observed nocturnal choking or gasping, physicians can reliably tell patients whether they need any further evaluation. Severity can be scored and a high probability for apnea predicted, though these scores do not substitute for physical examination and polysomnography.

There have been several inconclusive studies objectively evaluating uvular size, oropharyngeal volume, and tongue size as independent predictors of OSAHS. However, an examination of the awake patient does not directly correlate with the complex physiological mechanism revolving around pharyngeal closure pressure, coordination of muscle contraction, and pharyngeal atmospheric pressure production. Even large tonsils can be found in patients who have no difficulty with breathing during sleep. Nonetheless, staging systems for the clinical evaluation of patients with SDB, such as Friedman Palate Position and Stage, are helpful in stratifying groups of patients with similar anatomical findings to assess treatment effects.

Testing

Polysomnography is the gold standard for OSAHS diagnosis. The simultaneous measurement of electroencephalography (EEG), electrooculography, electromyography (EMG) for the chin, airflow (nasal), respiratory effort (abdominal and thoracic), oxygen saturation, leg movement, and electrocardiography is performed. The most complete PSG also includes measurement of esophageal pressures. Abbreviated full-night studies or split-night studies can incorporate diagnosis and then effect continuous positive airway pressure (CPAP) titration to avoid the cost of a second night of testing. This technique, however, may result in an incomplete diagnosis of the severity of disease.

Home study assessment has been perfected, which allows a less costly and a less stressful and unencumbered examination. The validated systems subtract and modify the recording parameters of a full PSG, yet have been shown to be reliable in the diagnosis of OSAHS. Less sophisticated systems do not measure airflow, ventilatory effort, or arousals; significant episodes of apnea, hypopnea, and upper airway resistance events are missed. More rigorous systems have increased sensitivity, yet the diagnosis of OSA by oximetry alone is often as accurate as electrophysiological monitoring with esophageal manometry. "Screening studies" have been shown to miss clinically significant sleep disorders and can be a disservice to the sleep-disturbed patients who may be falsely led to believe that they have no SDB problems. There is no more reliable evaluation than a comprehensive history, physical exam, and complete sleep evaluation.

In 2011 the American Academy of Sleep Medicine published a revision of sleep scoring rules that had not undergone a significant change since the original sleep scoring manual by Rechtschaffen and Kales in 1968. The revisions are as follows: Sleep epochs were kept at 30 second intervals. EMG derivation is from EMG electrodes placed above and below the chin. The stages of sleep were divided into Stage W (wakefulness), Stage N1 (NREM 1 sleep), Stage N2 (NREM 2 sleep), Stage N3 (NREM 3 sleep), and Stage R (REM sleep).

Stage N1 is the transition between wakefulness and sleep and presents with slow eye movement and low amplitude activity (4–7 Hz) with a and theta waves on EEG. Stage N2 is defined as low amplitude activity with distinct waveforms known as K complexes and sleep spindles. Stage N3, or slow-wave sleep, is defined with characteristic delta waves, with 20% of the epoch having slow wave (0.5–2 Hz) activity. Stage N3 combines the previous sleep stages 3 and 4. Stage R, or REM sleep, is defined by the presence of three phenomena: low-amplitude mixed-frequency EEG background, REM, and low-chin EMG tone. Sawtooth waves on EEG and transient muscle activity are also features commonly seen in Stage R sleep.

OSA severity is classified as mild if the AHI is between 5 and 15, moderate if between 16 and 30, and severe if greater than 30. The severity of oxygen desaturation, sleep fragmentation, arousals, and other monitored factors are included when evaluating a PSG.

■ Management

Nonsurgical Treatment

Behavioral Therapy

The mainstay of behavioral therapy is dietary modification for weight loss and restriction of body position during sleep. Obesity is strongly associated with worsening sleep apnea. Weight reduction of 10% has been shown to reduce the RDI up to 26%, as well as lower blood pressure, reduce snoring, and improve sleep architecture. Computed tomographic (CT) scans of the posterior airway space in overweight patients reveal increased fat deposits that encroach on the airway, presumably enhancing the closing pressure of the pharynx. Although several epidemiological studies have demonstrated that increasing neck circumference is a definite risk factor in OSA, its relationship to fatty pharyngeal deposits is not known.

Behavioral therapy can be directed to affect the upper airway muscle activity during sleep. Avoidance of sedatives and alcohol before sleep has a demonstrable positive effect on the AI because they increase the incidence of SDB and have been shown to decrease airway muscle activity in animals. Pharmacologically decreasing pharyngeal muscle activity can effectively negate other treatments to decrease airway-collapsing pressure, such as pharyngeal soft tissue surgery. General anesthetics also suppress upper airway muscle activity and reduce airway patency in OSAHS patients. Most hospitals and anesthesia departments require routine overnight observation for high-risk OSA patients who are administered general anesthesia.

Pharmacological Treatment

Various medications have been used to enhance upper airway muscle activity during sleep, but they have met with limited success. Neuroactive drugs, such as nicotine, strychnine, and protriptyline, are effective in reducing OSA, but their side effects are too extensive for widespread use. Drugs such as decongestants and steroids that reduce mucosal swelling with the potential to enhance airway dimensions are not effective. Supplemental oxygen may have an indirect effect on muscle activity, possibly through alterations in the hypoxic or hypercapneic drive cycle, but such therapy has been restricted to people who sleep in high altitudes. Newer analeptic drugs, such as modafinil (Provigil, Teva Pharmaceuticals, Frazer, PA) and armodafinil (Nuvigil, Teva Pharmaceuticals), are effective in improving symptoms of excessive sleepiness caused by OSA and are useful adjunctive treatments, but they do not actually treat the disorder.

Continuous Positive Airway Pressure

CPAP has become the mainstay of the nonsurgical mechanical treatment of OSA and is the initial treatment of choice in clinically significant OSA. CPAP is administered through a nasal mask, nasal prongs, or a mask covering the mouth and nose. In some laboratories, CPAP titration can be performed during PSG.

In these split-night studies, essentially half of the night is spent in diagnosis. In obvious cases, the technician will proceed with a CPAP trial and adjustment for the second half of the night study. CPAP is titrated in each patient to raise the pharyngeal intraluminal pressure above the pharyngeal closure pressure, eliminating pharyngeal soft tissue collapse. Most patients require pressures of 5 to 10 cm of water to create a pneumatic splint. This increased pressure may also reduce the upper airway muscle activity.

Alternate systems include the use of bilevel positive airway pressure (BiPAP), which allows the separate adjustment of inspiratory and expiratory airway pressure. Lower expiratory pressures often reduce the claustrophobic feeling, as well as the sensation of too much pressure in the nose. BiPAP machines are usually more costly than routine CPAP devices, but they may be a more comfortable option for patients who have high CPAP requirements.

Efficacy is excellent for both machines, ranging up to 100% in selected patients. Recent data suggest a significant reduction in all-cause mortality in OSA patients who use CPAP for more than 6 hours per day, and even for just 1 to 6 hours per day. Whereas obesity is sometimes a contraindication for a surgical procedure, obese patients with severe apnea are excellent candidates for CPAP therapy. However, CPAP compliance can often be a problem. Use of the machine for more than 4 hours per night for more than 70% of the observed nights was found to be slightly less than 50%. Compliance appears to be related more to the degree of relief of daytime symptoms and the return of neuropsychiatric function, rather than to objective reduction in the AI. (Again, this raises questions as to the validity of the AI in measuring clinical disease.)

Patients successfully treated with CPAP exhibit improved control of diurnal hypertension, ventilatory-related arousals, pulmonary hypertension, and right-sided heart failure, similar to the improvement seen in patients treated with tracheotomy. Side effects include mask irritation of the paranasal tissue, nasal congestion, hypertrophy of turbinates, rhinitis sicca, and excessive rhinorrhea. Topical nasal steroids, saline sprays, humidification of the CPAP air, and antihistamines have shown some effectiveness in relieving these symptoms.

Oral Devices and Appliances

Oral appliances modify the position of the mandible, tongue, and related oropharyngeal soft tissue to enlarge the pharyngeal airway or otherwise reduce the collapsing pressure of the pharyngeal tissue. Evaluation of patients for these devices should include a cephalometric analysis for true or relative retrognathia. Success with these devices is variable but appears to be greatest in patients with mild, rather than sever, OSA. Initial use is for a portion of the night until patient adaptation occurs. Compliance with the device for the first year tends to be very good, but drops to 50% as treatment time increases. Side effects include excessive salivation and transient discomfort with awakening. Long-term noncompliance results from temporomandibular joint pain and perceptive changes in occlusal alignment.

■ Surgery

Preoperative Evaluation

Evaluation of the upper airway is mandatory in all snoring and sleep apnea patients. Space-occupying lesions that can result in sleep-related upper-airway obstruction have been found in 2% of OSA patients. In the awake patient, the examination seeks to identify disproportionate and abnormal anatomy of the upper airway and its supporting structures. Nasal obstruction can result from bony and cartilaginous anatomical abnormalities (e.g., deviated nasal septum and turbinate hypertrophy), as well as from reactive soft tissue obstruction, to include nasal polyposis, turbinate hypertrophy, and adenoid hypertrophy.

The dimensions and spatial relationships of the pharynx are determined by the following:

1. Soft tissue structures (e.g., tonsils) that directly abut the air column
2. The underlying foundation of muscles comprised by the pharynx, the orientation of which affects the dimensions, configuration, and activity of the pharyngeal closure pressures
3. The location of the bony insertions and origins of these muscles in the bones of the craniofacial skeleton
4. Known (and unknown) craniofacial anomalies, which can be assessed by lateral cephalometric X-rays

Awake fiberoptic endoscopy can aid in identification of the site of pharyngeal collapse during apnea. The fiberoptic endoscope is passed transnasally for evaluation of the velopharyngeal inlet and the hypopharynx. A Müller maneuver is performed with the patient sitting upright and in the supine position. The patient makes a strong inspiratory effort while the mouth has been closed and the nose pinched shut around the endoscope. The percentage of airway collapse is noted in each position.

Limited success has been achieved in using asleep fluoroscopy, static and dynamic CT and magnetic resonance imaging (MRI), and manometry to differentiate patients whose primary site of obstruction is retropalatal or retropharyngeal. Drug-induced sleep endoscopy (DISE) has recently been accepted as a useful technique that can aid in defining the specific location(s) in the upper airway that are collapsing. Surgical treatment plans can then be individualized for each patient. DISE provides a dynamic evaluation of the upper airway under unconscious sedation with propofol and/or midazolam. Interrater reliability is moderate to substantial, and the study may be useful in determining the location of residual upper airway obstruction in patients who have failed previous pharyngeal surgery.

With the evaluation of all data, as well as the remainder of the head and neck exam, most patients can be categorized into three general groups, commonly known as the Fujita classification, based on the area of obstruction. Use of these groupings or other classification systems can help in the decision-making process for the choice of surgical procedure:

- *Type I* patients represent narrowing or collapse of the upper pharyngeal region at the retropalatal or velopharyngeal level.
- *Type II* patients demonstrate significant collapse in both the oropharynx and the hypopharynx; this is the most common.
- *Type III* patients have predominant narrowing or collapse in the hypopharynx; this occurs in 10 to 20% of patients.

Traditionally, surgical success rates are defined as at least a 50% reduction in postoperative AHI and a postoperative AHI of < 20. Surgical cure rates are defined as an AHI of < 5. This definition is important in comparing the variety of surgical techniques available in the treatment of OSAHS patients. The majority of OSAHS patients have obstruction at more than one level; in these patients it has been demonstrated that multilevel surgery can lead to better surgical outcomes.

Nasal Surgery

Nasal surgery is often performed to reduce nasal airway resistance in patients with SDB. Abnormally high resistance through the nasal cavity can promote pharyngeal closure by increasing transmission of subatmospheric intrathoracic pressure into the pharyngeal airway. Deviated nasal septum, hypertrophied turbinates, nasal polyps, chronic rhinitis, and adenoidal hypertrophy are conditions often associated with snoring and apnea. Simple surgery to correct these is effective in decreasing nasal airway resistance. However, the subatmospheric pharyngeal pressure during inspiration often remains unchanged, and there is no effect on the closing pressure of the pharynx.

A recent study demonstrated only a 15.8% success rate when performing septoplasty alone in patients with OSA. Surgical corrections of these nasal conditions have shown significant reduction in the AHI only when done in conjunction with procedures that address other sites of upper airway collapse and obstruction.

Soft Palate Surgery

Numerous procedures to modify the soft palate and address collapse in this location have been developed over the last 30 years. These include uvulopalatopharyngoplasty (UPPP) and its various modifications, laser-assisted uvuloplasty, cautery-assisted palatal stiffening operation, pillar implants, lateral pharyngoplasty, Z-palatoplasty, transpalatal advancement pharyngoplasty, and expansion sphincter pharyngoplasty. It is beyond the scope of this chapter to address each of these individually, so only the more traditional procedures are described. Overall success for these procedures ranges from 22 to 83%, with the best success rates occurring in patients with Fujita type I or type II anatomy. Readers are referred to the Suggested Reading section for more information regarding these procedures.

Uvulopalatopharyngoplasty

Fujita introduced the UPPP as a surgical procedure to treat OSA in 1981, attempting to decrease the upper airway closure pressure through resection of soft tissue structures in the nasopharynx and oropharynx. The classic UPPP involves resection of the tonsils and adenoids if present, uvula, rim of the soft palate, and excess soft tissue of the pharyngeal walls. Before surgery, the patient is asked to elevate the palate; the palatal dimple, caused by contraction of the levator veli palatini muscle, is then marked. Complications, including severe pharyngeal stenosis, have resulted in multiple modifications of the classic procedure. These emphasize judicious, directed tissue removal and meticulous surgical technique.

In a patient who has had a tonsillectomy, the mucosa of the tonsillar fossa is excised; otherwise a tonsillectomy is performed. An incision is made in the soft palate, several millimeters lateral to the medial margin of the glossopalatal arch. The incision is extended from the inferior pole of the tonsillar fossa to an area just below the palatal dimple, ~ 2 cm below the posterior margin of the hard palate. The incision continues along the pharyngopalatal arch to the inferior pole of the tonsillar fossa. A nasopharyngeal mucosa advancement flap is then anastomosed to the oropharyngeal mucosa flap. Multiple modifications of this procedure have been advocated, including less tissue resection and greater definition of palate and pharyngeal flaps, with generally the same result in treatment of snoring and OSAHS.

The results of UPPP treatment for snoring and OSAHS vary. In patients whose clinical symptoms are predominantly disruptive snoring with minimal daytime somnolence, the definition of cure is subjective, and high cure rates are reported (up to 90%). When comparing preoperative and postoperative PSGs and the AHI, the results are not as good. Several recent studies demonstrate a success rate ranging from 51 to 68%. It is very clear that judicious selection of patients makes for better results. If patients are evaluated as Fujita type II or type III collapse or are ill defined, the response rate to surgery can fall to 6 to 8%. High success rates (up to 81%) are much more common in patients with an AHI of less than 30 and a type I pattern of pharyngeal collapse or Friedman stage I classification.

A higher AHI is often associated with low success rates after UPPP and can result in higher incidence of postoperative complications, some fatal. In these patients, UPPP should be considered part of an overall treatment plan that includes nasal surgery, genioglossal advancement, hyoid suspension, bimaxillary advancement, more effective CPAP administration modalities, and weight loss.

Complications from UPPP include velopharyngeal insufficiency, nasopharyngeal stenosis, voice changes, postoperative bleeding, vague foreign-body sensations, and a dry throat, the latter two being the most common. Clinically significant velopharyngeal reflux appears in ~ 3% of postoperative patients, most commonly when they bend over to drink from a fountain. Uvular fricatives can be changed to alveolar or dental sound creation in 5% of patients. Significant complaints of hypernasality are less frequent.

Laser-Assisted Uvuloplasty

Laser-assisted uvuloplasty (LAUP) enlarges the oropharyngeal air space by resection of the uvula, free edge of the soft palate, and pharyngeal pillars. It is effective in treatment of snoring. Pharyngeal stiffness and reduced upper airway closing pressure are obtained by varying degrees of surgically induced scarring, while avoiding potential complications from general anesthesia.

In the classic operation, full-thickness vertical incisions are made on either side of the uvula with a carbon dioxide (CO_2) laser. The uvula itself is then shortened and thinned. Snoring is significantly reduced or eliminated in up to 90% of patients. Success rates in patients with OSAHS vary from 20 to 60%. Type I patients with a low AHI benefit the most from LAUP. A large number of patients experience significant postoperative pain, temporary palatal incompetence, and a persistent vague feeling of dryness or foreign body sensation in the posterior oropharynx.

Tongue Base Surgery

Much like other surgical options for OSAHS, tongue base surgery is rarely performed alone. More often, it is performed either simultaneously or as a staged procedure. If lingual tonsil hypertrophy is present, reduction via direct visualization using coblation or microdebrider resection can be performed.

Radiofrequency base of tongue (RFBOT) ablation for the treatment of OSAHS was first described by Powell in 1997. Radiofrequency ablation works by transmitting low-frequency radio waves through electrodes, which denature proteins through relative low-temperature coagulation necrosis, leading to inflammation and fibrosis. There is a rapid drop in energy from the site of the source, which allows the procedure to take place in proximity to vital structures without damage. An average reduction of 31% in both postoperative RDI and Epworth sleepiness scale has been shown in short-term follow-up.

Submucosal minimally invasive lingual excision (SMILE) was first described in 2006 by Maturo and Mair. The procedure is performed through a midline tongue incision 2 cm posterior to the tip of the tongue. Blunt dissection is then performed, and a coblation wand is inserted under bimanual guidance and directed posterior and inferior. A 0 degree endoscope can be inserted through the incision periodically to assess the created cavity. SMILE has been shown to have a statistically significant higher success rate than RFBOT but also has the potential for increased morbidity.

The Repose bone screw system (Influence Inc., San Francisco, CA) uses a bone screw that is anchored to the inner table of the mandible. The screw has monofilament suture crimped to the base, which is passed through the base of the tongue and used to perform the suture tongue base suspension procedure. This procedure has shown high success rates in the surgical treatment of OSAHS, especially when performed concomitantly with other procedures, such as UPPP.

Recently, due to improved technology, hypoglossal nerve stimulation has been gaining interest in the treatment of OSAHS. An implantable neurostimulator transmits electrical signals to a cuff implanted on the hypoglossal nerve. The device has respiratory leads that sense respirations to deliver stimulation during the respiratory phase. Initial studies have demonstrated favorable safety, efficacy, and compliance.

Midline Glossectomy

Laser midline glossectomy was pioneered by Fujita in 1991 and was developed for the treatment of type III collapse in patients whose preoperative evaluation demonstrates a small posterior air space and increased tongue size. In this procedure, the CO_2 laser is used for excision of a significant portion of the midline tongue, lingual tonsils, and redundant epiglottis. Temporary tracheotomy is required in many cases for airway management. Postoperative success is reported between 42 and 83%, with volumetric reduction of the tongue base limited by inadequate visualization. Open transcervical approaches offer improved visualization but are associated with increased morbidity.

With the recent paradigm shift toward minimally invasive surgery and the advent of surgical robotics, current investigations are exploring transoral robotic midline glossectomy and other procedures with reasonable success. Use of such technology has the potential advantages of improved visualization and surgical dexterity in the narrow confines of the pharynx, possibly allowing more aggressive volumetric reduction of the tongue base, without the expected increased morbidity associated with previous techniques. Further research is necessary before these techniques can be recommended.

Mandibular and Maxilla Surgery

Surgical correction of patients with types II and III collapsing patterns is effective. Riley and Powell have developed a treatment plan that involves procedures to decrease pharyngeal closure pressure by increasing the pharyngeal size and/or stiffness of the oropharyngeal and hypopharyngeal airway. In patients who have already had a UPPP, a mandibular osteotomy with genioglossus advancement performed in conjunction with hyoid myotomy is recommended.

A rectangular osteotomy of the genial tubercle that includes the attachments of the genioglossus and geniohyoid muscles is performed through an intraoral approach. The genial tubercle is advanced forward, so the lingual cortex reaches the facial cortex of the mandible. The segment is then fixed with a miniplate or other prefabricated securing device. In the hyoid myotomy, a skin incision similar to that made for a Sistrunk procedure is made, and dissection is carried down to the hyoid musculature. After identifying the midportion of the hyoid, the inferior

body is dissected free, and the inferior musculature is detached. The strap muscles are divided in the midline, and the thyroid cartilage is exposed. Large nonabsorbable sutures are placed through the thyroid cartilage rim and around the hyoid bone. The hyoid is suspended anteroinferiorly over the thyroid cartilage by tying the suture, and the anterior wall of the pharynx is displaced ventrally.

The short-term success rate varies from 42 to 78% depending on BMI and severity of OSAHS. Long-term results (more than 3 years) have been shown to be 64%. Complications can include fractures of the mandible, tooth root injury, temporary chin and tooth numbness, and temporary dysphagia. Patients with type II or III collapse with a small pharyngeal inlet, as detected by preoperative endoscopy, cephalometrics, CT and/or MRI, benefit from this surgery.

Maxillomandibular advancement (MMA) is one of the most successful surgeries for OSAHS. It is often considered after failure from prior procedures, but it should not be overlooked as a first-line therapy for patients who are morbidly obese or who have severe OSAHS with an AHI of > 50. A meta-analysis of 22 studies showed a success rate of 86% and a cure rate of 43.2%. MMA is generally described as a Le Fort I maxillary osteotomy, bilateral sagittal split osteotomy of the mandible, and genioglossal advancement.

Tracheotomy

Tracheotomy represents the gold standard surgical procedure for treatment of OSAHS. It bypasses the pharyngeal collapse during sleep. The intraluminal pharyngeal pressure is not a factor because tracheal closing pressure is much less than the subatmospheric intraluminal airway pressure created by the thorax during inspiration. Tracheotomy is indicated (1) for patients with severe OSAHS who are unable to tolerate CPAP, (2) as a temporary airway for patients undergoing extensive upper airway surgery, and (3) for patients with life-threatening cardiac arrhythmias and severe chronic heart failure. Long-term conversion of the routine tracheotomy tube to a Montgomery cannula is common.

■ Suggested Reading

American Academy of Sleep Medicine. International Classification of Sleep Disorders, Revised: Diagnostic and Coding Manual. Chicago, IL: American Academy of Sleep Medicine; 2001:195. www.esst.org/adds/ICSD.pdf. Accessed March 2, 2012

Babademez MA, Yorubulut M, Yurekli MF, et al. Comparison of minimally invasive techniques in tongue base surgery in patients with obstructive sleep apnea. Otolaryngol Head Neck Surg 2011;145(5):858–864

Black JE, Hull SG, Tiller J, Yang R, Harsh JR. The long-term tolerability and efficacy of armodafinil in patients with excessive sleepi-

ness associated with treated obstructive sleep apnea, shift work disorder, or narcolepsy: an open-label extension study. J Clin Sleep Med 2010;6(5):458–466

Cahali MB. Lateral pharyngoplasty: a new treatment for obstructive sleep apnea hypopnea syndrome. Laryngoscope 2003; 113(11):1961–1968

Campos-Rodriguez F, Peña-Griñan N, Reyes-Nuñez N, et al. Mortality in obstructive sleep apnea-hypopnea patients treated with positive airway pressure. Chest 2005;128(2):624–633 deBerry-Borowiecki B, Kukwa A, Blanks RHI. Cephalometric analysis for diagnosis and treatment of obstructive sleep apnea. Laryngoscope 1988;98(2):226–234

Eastwood PR, Barnes M, Walsh JH, et al. Treating obstructive sleep apnea with hypoglossal nerve stimulation. Sleep 2011;34(11):1479–1486

Farrar J, Ryan J, Oliver E, Gillespie MB. Radiofrequency ablation for the treatment of obstructive sleep apnea: a meta-analysis. Laryngoscope 2008;118(10):1878–1883

Friedman M, Hamilton C, Samuelson CG, et al. Transoral robotic glossectomy for the treatment of obstructive sleep apnea-hypopnea syndrome. Otolaryngol Head Neck Surg 2012;146(5):854–862 [Epub ahead of print]

Friedman M, Ibrahim HZ, Vidyasagar R, Pomeranz J, Joseph NJ. Z-palatoplasty (ZPP): a technique for patients without tonsils. Otolaryngol Head Neck Surg 2004;131(1):89–100

Friedman M, Soans R, Gurpinar B, Lin HC, Joseph N. Evaluation of submucosal minimally invasive lingual excision technique for treatment of obstructive sleep apnea/hypopnea syndrome. Otolaryngol Head Neck Surg 2008;139(3):378–384, discussion 385

Friedman M, Tanyeri H, La Rosa M, et al. Clinical predictors of obstructive sleep apnea. Laryngoscope 1999;109(12):1901–1907

Fujita S, Woodson BT, Clark JL, Wittig R. Laser midline glossectomy as a treatment for obstructive sleep apnea. Laryngoscope 1991;101(8):805–809

Guilleminault C, Lee JH, Chan A. Pediatric obstructive sleep apnea syndrome. Arch Pediatr Adolesc Med 2005;159(8):775–785

Holty JE, Guilleminault C. Maxillomandibular advancement for the treatment of obstructive sleep apnea: a systematic review and meta-analysis. Sleep Med Rev 2010;14(5):287–297

Johns MW. A new method for measuring daytime sleepiness: the Epworth sleepiness scale. Sleep 1991;14(6):540–545

Kao YH, Shnayder Y, Lee KC. The efficacy of anatomically based multilevel surgery for obstructive sleep apnea. Otolaryngol Head Neck Surg 2003;129(4):327–335

Kezirian EJ. Nonresponders to pharyngeal surgery for obstructive sleep apnea: insights from drug-induced sleep endoscopy. Laryngoscope 2011;121(6):1320–1326 doi: 10.1002/lary.21749

Kezirian EJ, White DP, Malhotra A, Ma W, McCulloch CE, Goldberg AN. Interrater reliability of drug-induced sleep endoscopy. Arch Otolaryngol Head Neck Surg 2010;136(4):393–397

Khan A, Ramar K, Maddirala S, Friedman O, Pallanch JF, Olson EJ. Uvulopalatopharyngoplasty in the management of obstructive sleep apnea: the Mayo Clinic experience. Mayo Clin Proc 2009;84(9):795–800

Kuna ST, Sant'Ambrogio G. Pathophysiology of upper airway closure during sleep. JAMA 1991;266(10):1384–1389

Li HY, Li KK, Chen NH, Wang PC. Modified uvulopalatopharyngoplasty: the extended uvulopalatal flap. Am J Otolaryngol 2003;24(5):311–316

Li HY, Wang PC, Hsu CY, Chen NH, Lee LA, Fang TJ. Same-stage palatopharyngeal and hypopharyngeal surgery for severe obstructive sleep apnea. Acta Otolaryngol 2004;124(7):820–826

Maturo SC, Mair EA. Submucosal minimally invasive lingual excision: an effective, novel surgery for pediatric tongue base reduction. Ann Otol Rhinol Laryngol 2006;115(8):624–630

Neruntarat C. Genioglossus advancement and hyoid myotomy: short-term and long-term results. J Laryngol Otol 2003;117(6):482–486

Pang KP, Woodson BT. Expansion sphincter pharyngoplasty: a new technique for the treatment of obstructive sleep apnea. Otolaryngol Head Neck Surg 2007;137(1):110–114

Ravesloot MJ, de Vries N. One hundred consecutive patients undergoing drug-induced sleep endoscopy: results and evaluation. Laryngoscope 2011;121(12):2710–2716

Riley RW, Powell NB, Guilleminault C. Obstructive sleep apnea and the hyoid: a revised surgical procedure. Otolaryngol Head Neck Surg 1994;111(6):717–721

Riley RW, Powell NB, Guilleminault C. Obstructive sleep apnea syndrome: a review of 306 consecutively treated surgical patients. Otolaryngol Head Neck Surg 1993;108(2):117–125

Shepard JW Jr, Gefter WB, Guilleminault C, et al. Evaluation of the upper airway in patients with obstructive sleep apnea. Sleep 1991;14(4):361–371

Sher AE, Schechtman KB, Piccirillo JF. The efficacy of surgical modifications of the upper airway in adults with obstructive sleep apnea syndrome. Sleep 1996;19(2):156–177

Shine, Lewis RH. Transpalatal advancement pharyngoplasty for obstructive sleep apnea syndrome: results and analysis of failures. Arch Otolaryngol Head Neck Surg 2009;135(5):434–438

Silber MH, Ancoli-Israel S, Bonnet MH, et al. The visual scoring of sleep in adults. J Clin Sleep Med 2007;3(2):121–131

Steward DL, Huntley TC, Woodson BT, Surdulescu V. Palate implants for obstructive sleep apnea: multi-institution, randomized, placebo-controlled study. Otolaryngol Head Neck Surg 2008;139(4):506–510

Verse T, Maurer JT, Pirsig W. Effect of nasal surgery on sleep-related breathing disorders. Laryngoscope 2002;112(1):64–68

Vicini C, Dallan I, Canzi P, et al. Transoral robotic surgery of the tongue base in obstructive sleep Apnea-Hypopnea syndrome: anatomic considerations and clinical experience. Head Neck 2012;34(1):15–22

Woodson BT. A tongue suspension suture for obstructive sleep apnea and snorers. Otolaryngol Head Neck Surg 2001;124(3):297–303

Woodson BT. Transpalatal advancement pharyngoplasty. Operative Techniques in Otolaryngology-HNS 2007;18(1):11–16

Woodson BT, Robinson S, Lim HJ. Transpalatal advancement pharyngoplasty outcomes compared with uvulopalatopharygoplasty. Otolaryngol Head Neck Surg 2005;133(2):211–217

Young T, Finn L, Peppard PE, et al. Sleep disordered breathing and mortality: eighteen-year follow-up of the Wisconsin sleep cohort. Sleep 2008;31(8):1071–1078

19 Acute and Chronic Sialadenitis

■ Introduction

Overview

Sialadenitis is an *inflammation* of the salivary gland(s) typically causing redness, pain, tenderness, and swelling. Sialadenitis can be classified as acute, chronic, or recurrent, with the most common etiologies being bacterial, viral, and autoimmune. Sialadenitis differs from sialadenosis, which is a nonneoplastic and noninflammatory disorder causing bilateral, non painful enlargement of the major salivary glands. It occurs secondary to systemic diseases, including diabetes, hypothyroidism, alcoholism, malabsorption, malnutrition, hepatic cirrhosis, and some medications. Pathologically sialadenosis is characterized by acinar cell hypertrophy, atrophy of striated ducts with parenchymal edema, and, in the final stages, fatty infiltrates. Treatment is best directed at the underlying medical problem because there is effective primary treatment, and surgery is not recommended.

Anatomy and Physiology Considerations

The three paired major salivary glands (parotid, submandibular, and sublingual) are responsible for the stimulated secretion of saliva during the oral phase of swallowing. The numerous minor salivary glands are responsible for maintaining the resting levels of moisture and oral lubrication. Various functions of saliva include moisturizing, lubrication, cleansing, immunologic protection, buffering, mineralization of dentition, and digestion.

The water content of saliva obviously contributes to moisturizing; proteins, lipids, and mucins act as lubricants. Buffers and phosphorproteins help regulate the oral cavity pH and the calcium and phosphate concentration of the teeth. Given that several mineral salts remain at a saturated state in saliva, it is perhaps surprising that sialolithiasis is not more common than it is. Saliva contributes antimicrobial activity by its cleansing activity and the presence of immunoglobulin and antimicrobial factors. The major digestive enzyme in saliva is α-amylase (explaining why elevated amylase levels may be seen in pancreatitis or sialadenitis), whereas minor enzymes include phosphatases, esterases, kallikreins, and nucleases. Saliva typically contains no intact cells; therefore, it is a relatively inefficient vehicle for transmitting infections mediated by strictly intracellular pathogens (such as human immunodeficiency virus [HIV]).

The Stensen duct, after leaving the parotid at the anterior border, crosses lateral to the masseter muscle, passes through the buccinator muscle, and enters the oral cavity opposite the second maxillary molar. The submandibular duct, after leaving the hilum of the gland, passes anteriorly and superiorly over the mylohyoid muscle. The relatively dependent position of the submandibular gland may contribute to an increased rate of stasis and sialolith formation.

Disorders of secretion of saliva may result in excessive or inadequate amounts of saliva. Hypersecretion may be associated with inflammation or irritation (pharyngitis, teething), rabies, mercury poisoning, or anticholinesterase exposure. Hyposecretion is commonly iatrogenically caused by antihistamines, anticholinergic agents (thiazides, antiemetics), chemotherapeutic agents, radiation therapy, and diuretics. Pathological conditions associated with hyposecretion include Sjögren syndrome, HIV infection, diabetes, bulemia, and most commonly dehydration. Causes of hyposecretion of saliva are important because they are often the critical factor in the development of acute, chronic, or relapsing salivary gland infections.

▪ Evaluation and Management

Viral Sialadenitis

Mumps, or epidemic parotitis, is caused by paramyxo-virus and remains one of the most common causes of acute salivary inflammation, despite widespread childhood immunization protocols. Young children (age 4–10) are most commonly affected. Mumps is usually a bilateral process: infection follows exposure by 2 to 3 weeks, and symptoms last 7 to 10 days. Acute and convalescent antiviral titers are diagnostic, although the diagnosis is usually made clinically and does not require the use of laboratory testing. The infection is self-limiting, requiring only symptomatic treatment, which includes hydration and pain control. Rarely, complications can occur and include menin-goencephalitis, profound hearing loss, and orchiitis/oophoritis in postpubescent patients. Infection or adequate immunization confers lifelong immunity.

Cytomegalovirus is probably the next most common cause of acute viral sialadenitis and may be associated with a mononucleosis-type clinical and hematological picture. Epstein-Barr virus, coxsacki-evirus, influenza A, and parainfluenza viruses are less common etiologies. When an infection does not resolve with appropriate treatment, unusual organisms, such as opportunistic organisms in HIV-infected patients and atypical tuberculosis (TB) should be considered.

Acute Bacterial Sialadenitis

Acute bacterial sialadenitis may develop without obvious inciting events, but it is most commonly associated with hyposecretion, stasis, or obstruction. Poor oral hygiene and exacerbation of chronic low-grade sialadenitis are also contributing factors. Up to 40% of cases occur in postoperative patients, probably a result of dehydration. Another clinical setting is the older patient whose risk factors include dehydration or diuretic use. The presenting symptoms are fever and painful diffuse enlargement of the gland, with erythema and tenderness. As opposed to a partially obstructed and noninfected gland, the swelling lasts well beyond mealtimes. Purulent saliva can be seen exuding from the parotid or submandibular ducts, and can usually be expressed with massage of the affected gland. The exudate can be sent for Gram stain, culture and sensitivity tests. In the typical acute case, imaging studies are of value only if one suspects a parotid abscess.

The most common organism, especially prevalent in parotitis, is *Staphylococcus aureus.* Other organisms include streptococci, coliforms (e.g., *Escherichia coli*), and various anaerobic bacteria. The traditional antibiotic selection has been an antistaphylococcal penicillin, such as a first-generation cephalosporin (cephalothin, cephalexin) or cloxacillin/dicloxacillin. Alternatives have been clindamycin or erythromycin. However, changing susceptibilities are forcing clinicians to be alert to the possibility of multidrug resistance. In particular, methicillin-resistant *S. aureus* (MRSA) and drug-resistant *Streptococcus pneumoniae* are rapidly increasing in prevalence. MRSA is especially common in long-term care facilities, and resistant pneumococci are more likely present in patients who have been on multiple oral antimicrobials. Vancomycin is the only consistently active agent against those two organisms.

Because of the rapid rise in antibiotic resistance, it may become increasingly prudent to obtain material for culture from the duct papilla intraorally or by transcu-taneous fine-needle aspiration of the parotid. Culture seems particularly useful in patients who are immuno-compromised by medical problems (neutropenia, diabetes), medications, or prolonged hospitalization, because the likelihood of atypical organisms is increased.

Important adjunctive measures for parotid infections include adequate hydration, sialogogues, warm compresses, and gland massage. In the case of sub-mandibular sialadenitis, if a stone is suspected at or near the duct orifice based on palpation, or obstruction of the duct orifice is suspected, dilation of the duct orifice by lacrimal probes or incision and mar-supialization of the duct in this location can be helpful. Patients can usually be treated on an outpatient basis, with the administration of an appropriate oral antibiotic for a period of 7 to 10 days and adjunctive measures. Patients who exhibit significant morbidity, are significantly dehydrated, or are septic should be admitted to the hospital. In this latter group of patients, computed tomographic (CT) scanning of the area should be performed.

Abscess formation may be suspected in persistent painful infections, in infections where glandular enlargement seems more focal than diffuse, and when there is overlying skin erythema. Overt fluctuance is unusual because of the dense fibrous capsule that invests the parotid. CT or ultrasonography will confirm the diagnosis. Once diagnosis has been established, incision and drainage should be performed; however, on rare occasions needle aspiration may suffice.

Chronic Sialadenitis

Chronic sialadenitis is characterized by recurrent, mildly tender, unilateral parotid enlargement that is exacerbated with salivation, and most often during eating. In contrast to acute disease, massaging the gland produces scant amounts of saliva. The occasional patient with chronic or relapsing sialadenitis represents a diagnostic and therapeutic challenge. Salivary gland stones and strictures are a common etiology of chronic salivary gland infections, especially in the submandibular gland. Strictures can happen from prior salivary gland infections, including mumps. In the case of stricture or sialolith formation, when the obstruction cannot be alleviated by conservative means (including dilation and/or ductoplasty of the duct orifice) and the patient remains symptomatic, excision of the affected gland has traditionally been regarded as the only therapy likely to produce long-term symptom control. The absolute threshold for surgical intervention has not been defined, although the typical surgical case would have several years of symptoms, with persistent painful enlargement for months, despite appropriate antimicrobial therapy. The role of intensive antibiotic therapy is less clear, unless persistent infection is known or suspected. There is no single oral antibiotic that will be effective for all cases of chronic or acute bacterial sialadenitis, and the increasing problem of multidrug resistance makes the case for pretreatment culture even stronger. Reasonable choices for empirical antibiotic treatment of chronic disease include amoxicillin-clavulanate or clindamycin (alone or with gram-negative coverage, such as third-generation cephalosporin or a fluoroquinolone).

Imaging in these cases has significant limitations in terms of this decision. Sialograms have been ordered over the years, but their predictive value is not as great as once assumed. Some patients with relatively severe radiological patterns of sialoectasia do well without surgical treatment. Plain film radiographs or CT may show sialoliths, although 20 to 40% of calculi are radiolucent on plain films. The submental vertex occlusal view is appropriate for radiographic evaluation of the submandibular gland. In short, the decision to operate on a chronically affected salivary gland remains largely a clinical issue.

For many patients with chronic parotitis, a superficial parotidectomy will be therapeutic, although several surgeons would remove additional deeper parotid tissue, especially if such tissue appears abnormal at the time of surgery. Facial nerve dissection through the dense, chronically infected, and inflamed gland is usually substantially more difficult and tedious than in noninfected glands. Because the problem is the relative density and vascularity of the tissue, some physicians would advocate intraoperative facial nerve monitoring to facilitate dissection.

Recent advances in instrumentation have made sialoendoscopy a technically feasible procedure for both diagnosis and management of salivary gland disease caused by a salivary stone or ductal stricture. A small endoscope is introduced to the gland's ductal system transorally, and the appropriate instrumentation can be used to remove a stone or dilate a stricture. This technology can be used to access more proximal portions of the affected gland.

The resulting renewed interest in nonneoplastic salivary gland disease has also focused attention on the use of ultrasonography in the diagnosis of salivary gland diseases and, in Europe, on the use of lithotripsy for selected instances of sialolithiasis. As experience with these modalities is increasing, the traditional algorithms for diagnosis and treatment are being redefined, with a move away from sialadectomy as a first-line treatment if medical management alone fails.

Autoimmune Sialadenitis

Autoimmune sialadenitis is characterized by persistent, indolent, and usually asymptomatic swelling of the parotid gland of unpredictable duration. Both childhood and adult forms occur, with the childhood form 10 times less common and resolution of symptoms by puberty. Autoimmune sialadenitis may be the first manifestation of more widespread systemic autoimmune disease; Sjögren syndrome is a familiar form of this entity and is covered in Chapter 20. The autoimmune diseases of the parotid gland have a unifying histological pattern of an early lymphocytic infiltrate, followed by thinning and fragmentation of the connective tissue in the terminal or intercalated duct walls with destruction of the acini. The larger ducts are usually uninvolved unless there is a superimposed infection. The sialographic appearance of the autoimmune forms is also similar. It consists of a diffuse pattern of globular collections of contrast material.

Noninfectious Related Conditions

Radioiodine related (RAI) sialadenitis can occur from day 1 to several months after receiving therapy with radioiodine. Symptoms are dose related, and usually the patient has received at least 100 millicurie (mCi). Sialadenitis has also been reported in patients receiving iodinated contrast for nuclear imaging studies. Patients who receive radioiodine therapy should be informed that the salivary glands normally excrete and clear iodine from the body, as well as instructions to help clear the tracer including hydration, massage of the glands, and eating "tart" foods to stimulate salivary secretions. The salivary pain and swelling are usually resolved with conservative treatment.

Miscellaneous causes of parotid enlargement include sarcoidosis and the lymphoepithelial cysts that occur in HIV patients. Radiographically and cytologically confirmed cysts can be followed. Surgical excision is rarely recommended given the high incidence of multiple cysts and recurrences; it is reserved for unclear diagnoses, rapid enlargement, or disfiguring masses. Sclerosis is an option for large painful or disfiguring cysts. Because of the increased risk for atypical pathogens in parotitis in patients positive for human immunodeficiency virus, culture is important, but initial therapy as provided for immunocompetent patients is probably reasonable.

■ Suggested Reading

Blitzer A, Lawson W, Reino A. Sialadenitis. In: Johnson JT, Yu VL, eds. Infectious Diseases and Antimicrobial Therapy of the Ears, Nose, and Throat. Philadelphia, PA: WB Saunders; 1997:471–480

Capaccio P, Torretta S, Pignataro L. The role of adenectomy for salivary gland obstructions in the era of sialendoscopy and lithotripsy. Otolaryngol Clin North Am 2009;42(6):1161–1171

Katz P, Hartl DM, Guerre A. Clinical ultrasound of the salivary glands. Otolaryngol Clin North Am 2009;42(6):973–1000

Koch M, Zenk J, Iro H. Algorithms for treatment of salivary gland obstructions. Otolaryngol Clin North Am 2009;42(6): 1173–1192

Lamey PJ, Felix D, Nolan A. Sialectasis and HIV infection. Dentomaxillofac Radiol 1993;22(3):159–160

Maresh A, Kutler DI, Kacker A. Sialoendoscopy in the diagnosis and management of obstructive sialadenitis. Laryngoscope 2011;121(3):495–500

Seifert G, Miehlke A, Haubrich J, Chila R. Physiology and biochemistry. In: Seifert G. Diseases of the Salivary Glands. New York, NY: Thieme; 1986:27–43

20 Sjögren Syndrome

■ Introduction

In the late 1800s Mikulicz described the simultaneous existence of keratoconjunctivitis sicca and xerostomia in the same patient. Later, in 1933, Sjögren recognized the association of these symptoms with polyarthritis. The combination of dry eyes and dry mouth alone is referred to as sicca syndrome. When the etiology of these symptoms is a systemic autoimmune disorder it is called primary Sjögren syndrome (pSS). If another connective tissue disorder is present, it is referred to as secondary Sjögren syndrome. Women in middle age are most likely to be affected, the condition being nine times more common in females than males.

It is characterized by lymphocytic infiltration and chronic inflammation of the exocrine glands, most commonly salivary and lacrimal glands. Extraglandular manifestations are seen in some patients and may involve almost any organ (e.g., Hashimoto thyroiditis, lymphadenopathy, interstitial pulmonary or lymphocytic alveolitis, vasculitis, neuropathy, and Raynaud phenomenon).

B-lymphocyte hyperactivity in pSS is reflected by the presence of anti-SS-A and anti-SS-B antibodies, rheumatoid factor, type 2 cryoglobulins, and hypergammaglobulinemia. Prolonged B cell survival and excessive B cell activity may lead to mucosa-associated lymphoid tissue lymphoma occurring in 5% of pSS patients. The etiology is not well understood.

■ Evaluation

Signs and Symptoms

Ocular

Keratoconjunctivitis sicca manifests as burning, pain, photophobia, or persistent foreign body sensation. Physical examination may reveal diffuse erythema of the conjunctiva. Insufficient tearing may eventually result in corneal ulceration.

Oral

Xerostomia, the most common symptom of the syndrome, may result in soreness, increased thirst, altered taste, and difficult speech that negatively impacts quality of life. Persistently decreased salivation in patients with Sjögren syndrome results in significant changes in oral physiology and microbiology, leading ultimately to dental caries and demineralization. These physiological changes are reviewed in Chapters 17 and 19 on xerostomia and sialadenitis. Dental caries, fissured tongue with atrophy, and parotid hypertrophy are possible sequelae and are more common in the primary rather than in the secondary form of the syndrome.

Gland-Specific Changes

Systemic B cell hyperactivity is a dominant feature of pSS, whereas T lymphocytes targeting glandular epithelial cells are involved in the chronic changes seen in the salivary and lacrimal glands. The majority of the T cells are CD4-positive and express cytokines, such as interferon-g (IFN-g) and tumor necrosis factor-a (TNF-a) and are considered characteristic for Th1 cells. Involved glandular tissue also shows B cell activity and formation of ectopic germinal center–like structures. Th2 cytokines, such as interleukin (IL)-6 and IL-10, are also present. Furthermore, local IFN-a production has been demonstrated that may ultimately underlie B cell hyperactivity and prolonged B cell survival.

Involvement of other exocrine glands may result in nasal crusting, hyposomia, dyspareunia, dry skin, decreased sweating, and pancreatitis. Some patients may complain of otalgia, tinnitus, and decreased hearing.

Systemic

The remaining symptoms of Sjögren syndrome depend on the associated autoimmune connective tissue. The most commonly associated disorder is rheumatoid arthritis, which occurs in ~ 50% of patients with the syndrome.

Various other diseases have been associated with the secondary syndrome, including systemic lupus erythematosus, scleroderma, dermatomyositis, vasculitis, parotid malignancies, leukemia, lymphosarcoma, Waldenström macroglobulinemia, and psoriatic arthritis among others. Systemic symptoms, such as fatigue and malaise, are not uncommon. Other possible systemic manifestations include cough, dysphagia, gastric atrophy, glomerulonephritis, and Raynaud phenomenon.

The risk of developing non-Hodgkin lymphoma is significantly increased in patients with pSS, especially in the presence of parotid enlargement, splenomegaly, lymphadenopathy, prior radiotherapy, and immunosuppressive therapy. A persistently enlarged diffuse parotid swelling should raise suspicion, as should the development of one or more focal parotid masses. Computed tomographic (CT) scanning may clarify the physical examination. If an experienced cytopathologist is available, fine-needle aspiration (FNA) may yield sufficient tissue to confirm the diagnosis of lymphoma. If the FNA is nondiagnostic or local expertise is not available, an open biopsy is indicated.

Differential Diagnosis

Other causes of xerophthalmia include autonomic dysfunction, vitamin A deficiency, conjunctivitis, ocular pemphigus, aging, and facial nerve disorders. Sarcoidosis, diabetes, and hypothyroidism are other potential causes of xerostomia. A variety of medications, including anticholinergics, sympathomimetics, ergotamine, opiates, and digoxin, may result in sicca syndrome. The numerous conditions associated with chronic parotid swelling include hyperlipoproteinemias, malnutrition, diabetes, cirrhosis, tuberculosis, and sarcoidosis. *Mikulicz syndrome* is a term used to describe all causes of recurrent parotid swelling that are not autoimmune in origin.

Classification Criteria

Several classification criteria for Sjögren syndrome were designed primarily for clinical research studies but are also used to guide the clinical diagnoses.

The American–European Consensus Group's (AECG's) criteria for the classification of Sjögren syndrome were proposed in 2002 and are the most commonly used criteria for the diagnosis of Sjögren syndrome.

American–European Consensus Group Classification

The AECG criteria for the classification of Sjögren syndrome are outlined here. These criteria allow a diagnosis of Sjögren syndrome in patients without sicca symptoms or who have not undergone a biopsy.

According to the American–European classification system (as modified by Tzioufas and Voulgarelis), diagnosis of pSS requires 4 of 6 of the following criteria; in addition, either criterion number 5 or criterion number 6 must be included. Sjögren syndrome can be diagnosed in patients who have no sicca symptoms if 3 of 4 objective criteria are fulfilled.

1. *Ocular symptoms* Dry eyes for more than 3 months, foreign-body sensation, use of tear substitutes more than 3 times daily
2. *Oral symptoms* Feeling of dry mouth, recurrently swollen salivary glands, frequent use of liquids to aid swallowing
3. *Ocular signs* Schirmer test performed without anesthesia (< 5 mm in 5 min), positive vital dye staining results
4. *Oral signs* Abnormal salivary scintigraphy findings, abnormal parotid sialography findings, abnormal sialometry findings (unstimulated salivary flow < 1.5 mL in 15 min)
5. Positive minor salivary gland biopsy findings
6. Positive anti-SSA or anti-SSB antibody results

Secondary Sjögren syndrome is diagnosed when, in the presence of a connective-tissue disease, symptoms of oral or ocular dryness exist in addition to criterion 3, 4, or 5.

Application of these criteria has yielded a sensitivity of 97.2% and a specificity of 48.6% for the diagnosis of pSS. For secondary Sjögren syndrome, the specificity is 97.2% and the sensitivity is 64.7%.

Exclusion criteria include past head-and-neck irradiation, hepatitis C infection, acquired immunodeficiency syndrome (AIDS), prior lymphoma, sarcoidosis, graft versus host disease, and the use of anticholinergic drugs.

The American College of Rheumatology Classification Criteria for Sjögren Syndrome

A new set of classification criteria was developed by the Sjögren International Collaborative Clinical Alliance (SICCA) of the American College of Rheumatology (ACR) in 2012.

These classification criteria were developed by SICCA investigators in an effort to improve specificity of criteria used for entry into clinical trials, especially in light of the emergence of biologic agents as potential treatments for Sjögren syndrome and their associated comorbidities. This high specificity makes the

ACR criteria more suitable for application in situations in which misclassification may present a health risk. They were accepted by the ACR as a provisional criteria set in 2012.

In comparison with commonly used AECG criteria, the ACR criteria are based entirely on a combination of objective tests that assess the three main components of Sjögren syndrome (serologic, ocular, and salivary) and do not include criteria based on subjective symptoms of ocular and oral dryness.

Application of these criteria has yielded a sensitivity of 93% and a specificity of 95% for the diagnosis of Sjögren syndrome. These criteria do not distinguish between primary and secondary forms of Sjögren syndrome.

According to the ACR criteria, the diagnosis of Sjögren syndrome requires at least two of the following three findings:

1. Positive serum anti-SSA and/or anti-SSB antibodies or positive rheumatoid factor and antinuclear antibody titer of at least 1:320
2. Ocular staining score of at least 3
3. Presence of focal lymphocytic sialadenitis with a focus score of at least 1 focus/4 mm^2 in labial salivary gland biopsy samples

Diagnostic Tests

Laboratory

The use of laboratory tests helps to confirm the diagnosis. SS-A and SS-B are autoantibodies found in patients with pSS. The corresponding antigens may be found in a variety of epithelial and hematologic cells. The autoantibodies react with both ductal and acinar elements of the salivary glands. A positive test is helpful, but a negative test does not rule out Sjögren syndrome. Antinuclear antibodies and rheumatoid factor are frequently present in both forms of the syndrome. The erythrocyte sedimentation rate is typically elevated, and polyclonal hypergammaglobulinemia may be present.

Ocular Staining

Objective criteria for ocular staining in the diagnosis of Sjögren syndrome is done with both fluorescein staining of the cornea and lissamine green staining of the conjunctiva by an ophthalmologist. The total score for both tests is computed, and, based on the severity of objective findings, a grade is assigned; a grade of 3 or more is reflective of Sjögren syndrome.

Histopathology

Biopsy of salivary tissue has been the most commonly employed method for diagnosing Sjögren syndrome. The tissue is most commonly obtained from the oral vestibule (usually the lower lip) due to ease of accessing the minor salivary glands and minimal complications. Many pathologists prefer to sample at least four minor salivary glands to ensure that representative tissue is obtained. Autoimmune diseases of the salivary glands display a histology featuring focal lymphocytic infiltrates, thinning and fragmentation of the connective tissue in the terminal or intercalated duct walls, and destruction of the acini.

Histopathological diagnosis of Sjögren syndrome is based on the presence of more than one cluster of > 50 lymphocytes per 4 square mm, which is referred to as a focus score of > 1. The focal clusters of lymphocytes are most commonly around the ducts. Atrophy, fibrosis, and fatty changes in the minor salivary gland specimens may represent the end stage of Sjögren syndrome or may simply be age-related changes. Failure to detect lymphocytic infiltration could be due to sampling error or disease fluctuation. The sensitivity range is 58 to 100%. The specificity is greater than 95% and is highly dependent on the expertise of the pathologist. Parotid and sublingual gland biopsies have been reported to be more sensitive than labial biopsies but are more complicated to obtain. Myoepithelial islands are easier to find in parotid specimens. These islands consist of metaplastic ductal epithelium accompanied by associated myoepithelial cells.

Other tests can be used, but the diagnosis can be made based on the results of ocular staining, histopathology, and antibody testing. The following are some of the ancillary tests.

Schirmer Testing

A Schirmer test resulting in less than 5 mm of moisture on the filter paper is considered to be representative of significantly dry eyes. Rose bengal dye application, along with slit lamp examination, will identify filiform keratosis and early corneal ulcerations.

Salivary Flow

Salivary flow can be directly measured and compared with standards to assess xerostomia. However, sialometry is of limited practical use for the otolaryngologist because of the difficulty in testing and the variations in methodology and results.

Radiology

Historically, many radiological tests have been used in an effort to diagnose Sjögren syndrome. CT or plain film parotid sialography may demonstrate dilation and truncation of the parotid ducts. Because it is not specific to Sjögren syndrome and only late changes are detectable, this test is rarely used today. Salivary scintigraphy with technetium-pertechnetate may reveal decreased uptake in the parotid gland and can be used with the AECG criteria.

◼ Management and Treatment

Treatment is primarily supportive in the management of the sicca side effects, rather than management of the underlying autoimmune exocrinopathy. Treatment of xerostomia and xerophthalmia is primarily directed at preventing associated complications. Artificial saliva and good dental hygiene including dental referral for ongoing care are keys to preventing dental caries. Methylcellulose drops and ointments are effective in preventing corneal ulcerations, with patients best served by ophthalmology referral. Patients should be counseled to avoid decongestants, antihistamines, diuretics, and some cardiovascular and psychiatric agents that may accentuate the dry mouth. Oral steroids or steroid eye drops are usually reserved for severe cases. The use of pilocarpine and cevimeline (muscarinic agonists) to stimulate lacrimation and salivary flow in patients with Sjögren syndrome is currently being investigated and may benefit some patients. Any systemic pharmacological treatment is best managed by a rheumatologist. A discrete parotid mass should be thoroughly investigated because patients with Sjögren syndrome have a 7.5-fold increased risk of developing lymphoma.

Parotidectomy is rarely indicated in the management of Sjögren syndrome because most patients develop atrophic sialadenitis, as opposed to recurrent bacterial parotitis. A rare patient with recurrent or chronic parotitis may benefit from a total parotidectomy, sparing the facial nerve, if antimicrobial therapy fails.

◼ Suggested Reading

Ariji Y, Ohki M, Eguchi K, et al. Texture analysis of sonographic features of the parotid gland in Sjögren's syndrome. AJR Am J Roentgenol 1996;166(4):935–941

Bayetto K, Logan RM. Sjögren's syndrome: a review of aetiology, pathogenesis, diagnosis and management. Aust Dent J 2010; 55(Suppl 1):39–47

Fox RI. Sjögren's syndrome. Lancet 2005;366(9482):321–331

Izumi M, Eguchi K, Ohki M, et al. MR imaging of the parotid gland in Sjögren's syndrome: a proposal for new diagnostic criteria. AJR Am J Roentgenol 1996;166(6):1483–1487

Marx RE, Hartman KS, Rethman KV. A prospective study comparing incisional labial to incisional parotid biopsies in the detection and confirmation of sarcoidosis, Sjögren's disease, sialosis and lymphoma. J Rheumatol 1988;15(4):621–629

Pennec YL, Leroy JP, Jouquan J, Lelong A, Katsikis P, Youinou P. Comparison of labial and sublingual salivary gland biopsies in the diagnosis of Sjögren's syndrome. Ann Rheum Dis 1990;49(1): 37–39

Rothschild BM. Sjögren's syndrome. Compr Ther 1996;22(1): 39–43

Ramos-Casals M, Tzioufas AG, Stone JH, Sisó A, Bosch X. Treatment of primary Sjögren syndrome: a systematic review. JAMA 2010;304(4):452–460

Shiboski SC, Shiboski CH, Criswell L, et al; Sjögren's International Collaborative Clinical Alliance (SICCA) Research Groups. American College of Rheumatology classification criteria for Sjögren's syndrome: a data-driven, expert consensus approach in the Sjögren's International Collaborative Clinical Alliance cohort. Arthritis Care Res (Hoboken) 2012;64(4):475–487

Vitali C, Bombardieri S, Jonsson R, et al; European Study Group on Classification Criteria for Sjögren's Syndrome. Classification criteria for Sjögren's syndrome: a revised version of the European criteria proposed by the American-European Consensus Group. Ann Rheum Dis 2002;61(6):554–558

Whitcher JP, Shiboski CH, Shiboski SC, et al; Sjögren's International Collaborative Clinical Alliance Research Groups. A simplified quantitative method for assessing keratoconjunctivitis sicca from the Sjögren's Syndrome International Registry. Am J Ophthalmol 2010;149(3):405–415

21 Concepts in New Imaging Techniques

■ Introduction

This chapter summarizes the basic principles of imaging as they apply to problems in otolaryngology and provides the otolaryngologist with a minimum foundation necessary for using imaging as an effective tool for evaluating patients.

■ Strengths and Weaknesses of New Techniques

Plain films, fluoroscopy, computed tomography (CT), magnetic resonance imaging (MRI), ultrasonography, and nuclear medicine can all be applied in an otolaryngology practice. Each has strengths and weaknesses that must be considered in defining appropriate imaging strategies.

Plain Films

Plain films provide a survey, but they present problems of superimposition. For instance, multiple projections have been used to project important structures away from the confusing shadows of the skull base. An example of this principle in practice today is the difficulty in adequately assessing the ethmoid sinuses using plain films. Although an air-fluid level or complete opacification of the maxillary sinuses can be evaluated by plain films, the ethmoids are difficult to assess because the cells are superimposed on the deeper skull base and even on themselves.

Plain films provide very little information about soft tissues. Only when a structure is projected completely away from confusing bone structures can one hope to distinguish even fat from muscle density. Contrast agents can be used to improve visibility of some structures, such as the salivary ducts during sialography, because the contrast agent is dense enough that visualization is possible even when the structure is projected over bone.

Fluoroscopy

Fluoroscopy provides the same information as a plain film and poses the same projection problems, but it adds a dynamic element. The radiologist can watch as a column of barium passes through the pharynx and esophagus, following the pliability of the wall or the movement of the larynx.

Computed Tomography

CT uses X-rays to create sectional images. It clearly separates materials with large density differences. Thin, cortical plates of bone show very well. Air and soft tissue are clearly differentiated. Fat has a very characteristic density; as a result, any other soft tissues, such as tumor or muscle, that are bordered by a fat plane are easily seen. However, the density difference between muscle and tumor is not great enough to allow routine confident separation.

A CT scan of the neck, sinus, or temporal bone can be obtained much more quickly than an MRI scan. The entire neck scan takes only 45 seconds when spiral CT is used.

Iodine-based radiopaque contrast can be given intravenously and, because of various degrees of differentiated enhancement, some lesions become more conspicuous. Contrast enhancement can differentiate vascularized tissue from nonvascularized spaces, such as a cyst, an obstructed sinus, or a petrous air cell.

Magnetic Resonance Imaging

MRI uses radio waves rather than ionizing X-rays. The radio waves are generated by stimulation of nuclei and their subsequent relaxation. This relaxation process gives off signals that depend on various characteristics of the tissues. High signal is shown on most images as white, low signal as black.

Many different sequences can be applied, so tissues can be "given" many different appearances.

For instance, on standard T1-weighted images, fat is bright and fluid, such as cerebrospinal fluid (CSF), is dark. On T2-weighted images, fluid is bright (high signal) and fat is darker (low signal). Pulse sequences, such as fast spin-echo and fat suppression, alter some of these characteristics, but routine fluid remains dark on T1 and bright on T2. Air gives almost no signal (black) on any sequence. Cortical bone gives almost no signal, but the soft tissues within a medullary cavity will give a signal. Rapidly flowing blood carries stimulated nuclei out of the plane before the relaxation process, so these vessels appear as black signal voids.

Contrast (gadolinium) can be given to reflect vascularization of tissues and to accentuate differences between tissues. This generally causes increased signal in tissues when viewed on a T1-weighted image.

MRI is considered to hold an advantage over CT in discriminating among various soft tissues. This effect is particularly obvious in demonstrating interfaces of tumor against muscle. In areas of interface between tumor and fat, MRI and CT are equivalent.

MRI can be very sensitive to motion. This sensitivity is particularly problematic in patients with airway disease or respiratory distress. This "problem" has been molded into a new technology where the artifact becomes the basis of a new image, as in magnetic resonance angiography (MRA). MRA performed without intravenous (IV) contrast is sensitive to flow in major veins and arteries. Most sequences on MRI take several minutes, resulting in longer examination times and dependence on patient compliance. This is a disadvantage compared with CT, which creates a high-resolution image in seconds.

On the other hand, MRI creates an image in any plane, without having to reposition the patient, and does not expose patients to ionizing radiation. Recent progress, such as with spiral CT, allows reformatting of axially collected data into high-quality images in other planes, such as coronal and sagittal. Very believable three-dimensional images can also be created. The reformatted images are not quite as good as directly acquired scans, but the resolution is very close.

Kidney function can be affected by the contrast agents used for both CT and MRI, necessitating an evaluation estimated glomerular filtration rate (eGFR) in at-risk patients prior to the administration of either agent. Iodinated CT contrast is associated with contrast-induced nephropathy (CIN) in patients with significantly reduced renal function. Gadolinium contrast has been implicated in nephrogenic systemic fibrosis (NSF) in patients with severely impaired renal function. The physician ordering the study is usually responsible for ordering laboratory tests prior to imaging and may be called upon to make a decision about the risk–benefit ratio of contrast administration in borderline cases.

Ultrasonography

Ultrasonography uses noninvasive sound waves to "interrogate" the deeper soft tissues. Sound is blocked by bone or air, but in unobscured regions such as the neck or parotid gland, ultrasound provides a high-resolution, dynamic (or real-time) evaluation. One could think of ultrasonography essentially as an extension of the physical exam of the neck. The anatomy of a lesion is defined. Cystic lesions can be separated from solid. Calcifications can at times be detected. Biopsy can be performed under ultrasound guidance more easily than with CT or MRI. Recent improvements in ultrasound resolution and in the affordability and portability of these machines have led to increasing use among otolaryngologists in the office setting to improve diagnostic accuracy and efficiency of care. Advantages of ultrasonography include the lack of radiation exposure, the fact that no contrast is required, and it is a real-time study that can be performed quickly and in a moving patient. Accordingly, it should be given consideration in pediatric patients.

Nuclear Medicine

Nuclear medicine is a physiological technique that can be used to assess the function of tissues or organs. Various tissues take up isotopes reflecting the metabolism of that tissue. For instance, in the thyroid, functioning tissue can be separated from nonfunctioning thyroid tissue with iodine 123. A functioning adenoma can be separated from a nonfunctioning "cold" nodule. Several techniques, such as labeled white blood cells and gallium scanning, detect sites of active infection. More recently, positron-emission tomography (PET) and PET-CT, which uses glucose to assess metabolic function, have become useful in the diagnosis, management, and follow-up of many head and neck cancers.

■ Application Techniques in Specific Anatomical Regions

The character of the tissues and of the pathology determines the appropriate imaging strategy required to address a problem. Radiologists have varying opinions regarding the ideal imaging strategy in many clinical situations, and frequently the problem can be approached in more than one way. The following sections address various anatomical areas and approaches to clinical problems associated with pathology in those regions. The discussion includes the capabilities, strengths, and weaknesses of various imaging modalities in each region.

Temporal Bone

The temporal bone presents a system of fine bony structures with very little soft tissue. CT is the modality chosen for evaluation of many ear problems, particularly in the external and middle ears. CT visualizes the bone of the external auditory canal (EAC). Tumors erode that bone, so CT can demonstrate extension of tumor into the mastoid or into the bone of the wall of the EAC. Fat is seen on the outer margin of many of the walls of the EAC, so CT is quite effective in showing extension beyond the limit of the canal. CT can define the ossicles and detect subtle erosions of the tegmen, semicircular canals, and facial nerve canal. The plates separating the jugular vein and carotid arteries show as well-defined white lines. An aberrant carotid artery moves the lateral plate of the carotid canal into the middle ear or causes a defect in this thin plate of bone. A glomus jugulare gives a "smudgy" demineralization of the bone around the lateral jugular plate.

CT easily detects the contrast between the fluid of the inner ear and the surrounding otic capsule. Congenital anomalies, including dilation or undersegmentation of the cochlear lumen and dilation of the semicircular canals or vestibular aqueduct, are obvious on CT. Given its lower cost and shorter procedure time, CT is generally a better initial choice over MRI in the workup of pediatric patients with sensorineural or mixed hearing loss.

In the petrous apex, CT can show the septation of air cells. Therefore, it can demonstrate expansion, such as in a cholesterol granuloma or an epidermoid.

CT does not discriminate among various soft tissues or fluids as well as MRI, and so the usefulness of MRI increases in the deeper temporal bone.

CT demonstrates most tumors of the internal auditory canal (IAC) if IV contrast is used. Expansion of the bony canal is present in most tumors; however, MRI is more sensitive for small vestibular schwannomas. A gadolinium-enhanced MRI is extremely sensitive in this clinical situation and can detect tumors > 2 mm. Using high-resolution T2-weighted images, MRI can now resolve the individual nerves within the IAC. This approach is becoming competitive with gadolinium-enhanced MRI in evaluation of suspected acoustic neuroma.

The MRI appearance of a petrous apex cholesterol granuloma (hyperintense on both T1- and T2-weighted sequences) is very different from that of an epidermoid cyst or cholesteatoma (bright on T2-weighted images only). Thus MRI can be more specific in defining the identity of an apex lesion. However, CT will not "miss" the pathology.

When temporal bone pathology spreads intracranially, the effectiveness of MRI increases. Enhancement of the dura reflects the central spread of infection, and MRI is more sensitive for involvement of the brain. Though a glomus tumor (paraganglioma) is easily defined with CT, MRI is more accurate in defining the central extension into the posterior fossa. Flow-sensitive techniques of MRI can define the relationship of a tumor to any residual flow in the jugular vein.

MRI can be used to "prove" that there is flow in a venous structure, such as the jugular vein. Thrombosis is more difficult because there are many flow artifacts that can mimic thrombosis or absence of flow. Some radiologists prefer CT with a bolus of intravenous contrast to prove a vessel is thrombosed.

As stated, MRI does not show cortical bone detail as well as CT. Thus, for instance, the ossicles and mastoid septation are not well seen. Indeed, neither air nor cortical bone gives significant signal; both look black (signal void) on MRI so they cannot be separated. However, pathology, such as cholesteatoma, tumor, or infection in the middle ear and mastoid, is seldom completely missed. This is particularly true with diffusion-weighted MRI when one is looking for cholesteatoma recurrence. Nonetheless, CT still remains the gold standard.

Facial nerve pathology may be defined by CT or MRI. MRI shows enhancement in Bell palsy (idiopathic facial nerve paralysis) or in tumors. Verification of tumor requires demonstration of nerve enlargement. The canal is expanded at CT, and the resolution of MRI is reaching the point where more subtle enlargement can be defined. Many radiologists begin with MRI because it provides an excellent method of screening the entire pathway from the central nervous system through the temporal bone into the parotid. In positive cases, CT can be considered for assessing the bone architecture, helping narrow the differential diagnosis. Alternatively, CT can be performed if clinically the abnormality is localized to the temporal bone.

Sinus and Facial Bones

Plain films

Plain films provide a good survey of the facial bones, and most fractures can be detected. Frequently, the clinical examination combined with information from plain films is all that is required to rule out or to detect a fracture. However, CT provides much more information and is more sensitive for many fractures. Fracture lines can be followed through the ethmoid, orbital floor or roof, or skull base. The relationship of a fracture to key structures, such as the optic canal, can easily be defined using CT. The contiguous tissues, almost invisible on plain films, are well demonstrated on CT. For instance, CT defines the relationship of the inferior rectus to a blowout fracture of the floor. Subtle hemorrhage into the orbital fat can be appreciated as well. Newer techniques using solid and transparent volume-rendering and maximum intensity projection have been combined with high-resolution multiplanar reformation of CT images to improve detection of skull base fractures.

Computed Tomography

CT differentiates cortical bone and air from fluid or mucosal thickening extremely well. CT can always separate an obstructed sinus from a well-aerated one. The thin cortical bone in the ostiomeatal complex is an ideal subject for CT investigation. The uncinate process, ethmoid septations, and turbinates are all well seen. Therefore, CT is used for evaluation of inflammatory problems and for mapping the ostiomeatal complex prior to functional endoscopic sinus surgery. CT defines defects in the roof of the ethmoid, in the lamina papyracea, or in the bony plates of the sphenoid sinus covering the optic nerve and carotid artery. All of these structures are thin cortical plates of bone, ideally suited to CT investigation.

Fat-containing regions, such as the orbit and infratemporal fossa, border much of the sinus complex. CT detects tumor or inflammation extending from the sinus into these regions because pathology can always be differentiated from fat. The superior margins of the sinus are also cortical bone. CT defines erosion of these structures, but MRI is more sensitive in detecting tumor above the bone impinging on dura, CSF, olfactory bulbs, or brain.

Magnetic Resonance Imaging

MRI is better than CT in discriminating among various fluids and soft tissues. Thus MRI can almost always define the margin between tumor and obstructed sinus secretions and is more likely to differentiate tumor from inflammatory mucosal swelling. MRI demonstrates tumor on the other side of cortical bone, such as along the dura or in the orbit, infratemporal fossa, or pterygopalatine fossa. Chordomas, the most common primary malignant tumor of the skull base, are usually best seen on MRI as hyperintense masses on T2-weighted images with high-contrast enhancement at the clivus.

Secretions can have varying appearances on MRI. One problem with MRI is that desiccated secretions or fungal disease, such as aspergillosis, in an obstructed sinus can actually look black on MRI. This is the same as the signal void of air, so an obstructed sinus can be missed on MRI scans. For this reason, and because of poorer visibility of the important thin cortical bone structures, MRI is less effective than CT in evaluation of inflammatory disease of the sinus. Similarly, CT best discerns bony tumors and lesions of the paranasal sinuses, to include osteomas and fibrous dysplasia.

Recent Advances

Flash CT is a technique that is available at some centers. It can scan the neck or sinuses very rapidly with times measured in seconds. This technique offers a shortened exam time and lower radiation dose to patients. Thus patient motion is not problematic making it an appropriate study for pediatric and trauma patients.

In-office CT scanners are now available and afford the otolaryngologist with rapid CT scanning of the sinuses, which can be very helpful in distinguishing sinusitis from other entities with similar symptoms.

Oral Cavity, Pharynx, and Soft Tissues of the Head and Neck

CT and MRI are used to evaluate the deeper soft tissues of the head and neck. Although most sizable mucosal lesions can be detected, imaging is not as sensitive as direct visualization and is never considered a substitute for a complete head and neck examination that includes fiberoptic endoscopy. Again, an understanding of the basic capabilities of CT, MRI, and ultrasonography must be considered as one defines an imaging strategy for a head and neck problem.

Ultrasound is excellent for defining superficial soft tissues. Sound is reflected by air and bone, so there are limitations to the abilities of ultrasound. However, in the neck, ultrasound provides significant information. Ultrasound is very good at differentiating cysts from solids and is now able (with Doppler detection) to detect and quantify flow, such as in the carotid artery. The ability to analyze relatively superficial tissues makes ultrasound very useful in evaluating lesions, particularly in the upper neck, submandibular region, and thyroid. Ultrasonography can quickly and easily be performed in the office, and it has the benefit of improving diagnostic accuracy and expediting care when used to guide fine-needle aspiration biopsies of head and neck soft tissue lesions. The portability and affordability of newer ultrasound machines make ultrasonography a convenient and safe imaging modality in the office setting. It does have limitations in obese patients, for deeper structures in the neck, and in the presence of scar tissue from surgery or radiation.

CT and MRI can define both the deep anatomy and the location and extent of tumors. The diagnosis of many lesions is very dependent on anatomy, so either modality is effective. CT is considered better at defining cortical bone, whereas MRI has an advantage in separating soft tissues, particularly tumor and muscle. Both CT and MRI give a characteristic appearance to fat. Fat looks like nothing else on either exam, and because it is so important in organizing the anatomy of the head and neck, either modality is effective for defining it. When tumor is intimately associated with muscle, however, MRI has an advantage.

For instance, either CT or MRI can define the fat in the sublingual space or between the genioglossus/geniohyoid muscles, so either can localize lesions in the floor of the mouth, so long as a lesion, such as a ranula or an epidermoid/dermoid, does not invade the muscle. However, if a tumor, such as carcinoma, invades the muscles, MRI provides a slight advantage. MRI is also preferred when imaging the tongue in a patient with dental fillings secondary to dental artifact that occurs on CT scan. The tongue base, which comprises muscle, is well imaged using MRI, and, although bolus-injected contrast CT gives excellent soft tissue differentiation, MRI is still preferred in the tongue base.

The ability of CT to define calcification is important in certain clinical situations in the oral cavity region. Salivary calculi are easily seen, as are the subtle erosions of the inner cortex of the mandible or palate.

In the larynx, either CT or MRI results in good visualization, although, especially in the larynx, interpretation of MRI can be limited by motion artifact. The wall of the supraglottic larynx contains fat, whereas the wall of the glottic larynx contains only muscle (thyroarytenoid). CT or MRI can localize pathology. Tumors in the supraglottic larynx abut the paraglottic and pre-epiglottic fat. CT or MRI visualizes this interface easily. Tumor growing around the ventricle following the paraglottic space insinuates between the thyroid cartilage and the thyroarytenoid muscle. Imagers believe that MRI can better demonstrate this tumor–muscle interface and, therefore, can detect early extension across the ventricle. Subglottic extension from a glottic tumor is easily detected because the subglottic airway is distorted. Most radiologists would agree that MRI is more sensitive but less specific than CT for the diagnosis of early cartilage invasion. However, advances in high-resolution multichannel helical CT have resulted in CT being the primary imaging modality for tumors of the larynx at most institutions.

With regard to recurrent squamous cell carcinomas of the head and neck, 18F-fluoro-2-deoxy-D-glucose PET and PET-CT have a high sensitivity for detection. The higher metabolism of glucose by malignant cells allows early detection of persistent or recurrent disease. Inflammatory tissue, which is usually present following radiotherapy or surgery, also has a high metabolism of glucose on PET. As a result, interpretation of these scans can be difficult in the immediate postradiation or postsurgical timeframe. Therefore, PET scans should be obtained no sooner than 3 months following treatment.

Trauma evaluation requires visualization of the laryngeal cartilages. CT is excellent in performing this task. Even when incompletely ossified, the integrity of the cartilages can be assessed. Hematomas of the supraglottic larynx or distortion of the airway is also well defined with CT. If vascular injury is suspected and the patient is hemodynamically stable, CT angiography (CTA) should be performed.

In the lateral neck and in the parapharyngeal/masticator space regions, fat planes again are crucial in defining the anatomy and thus in defining the identity of a lesion. Either CT or MRI can show the relationship to the carotid artery, jugular vein, sternocleidomastoid and scalene muscles, brachial plexus, and other soft tissue structures. In the level of the oro- and nasopharynx, CT and MRI both show the fat planes of the parapharyngeal and masticator spaces, pterygoid muscles, carotid artery, and styloid process. The relationship of a tumor to these structures can help separate salivary gland lesions from more posterior neural lesions or paragangliomas, and more anterolateral lesions of the masticator space.

Because most lesions of any size will distort fat planes and will therefore be detected, CT and MRI are both used. MRI is more precise at differentiating a tumor from normal parotid tissue, so is considered slightly more sensitive. MRI can also show flow voids in a paraganglioma. Either CT or MRI can differentiate an avascular or cystic lesion from a soft tissue tumor that has a significant blood supply.

Because CT and MRI give comparable information, there is controversy regarding the most appropriate test in many clinical situations. Some radiologists prefer MRI for cancer evaluation or for differentiation of masses. CT is quicker and easier but uses ionizing radiation. MRI is slightly better in defining soft tissue interfaces; however, when fat is present, CT does an excellent job. For instance, lymph nodes in the neck are very well assessed using CT or MRI, but many radiologists prefer CT for a nodal screen. Some radiologists feel that an appropriate strategy for evaluation of head and neck cancer is to begin with CT and use limited MRI only when a question remains. Others prefer to use MRI. Close interaction between the otolaryngologist and the radiologist helps define the information most needed by the clinician and thereby helps define the most appropriate strategy.

Thyroid and Parathyroid

Ultrasonography, MRI, and CT have all been used in the thyroid area. However, because of its availability, low cost, and lack of radiation, ultrasound is the gold standard imaging modality of the thyroid. Biopsies or aspirations are also easily done in the office under ultrasound guidance. I-123 scans are sometimes obtained to characterize thyroid lesions. "Cold" lesions, however, may be benign or malignant, so the specificity is relatively low. If a lesion of concern is present, fine-needle aspiration biopsy under ultrasound guidance will usually provide a more reliable diagnosis. Tc-99m sestamibi scans are often used in the workup of suspected parathyroid adenomas and are very useful in postoperative patients with recurrent disease. Single-photon emission CT scans are often useful in locating ectopic parathyroid adenomas.

Blood Vessels

Dynamic CTA and MRA are commonly used to image the arterial and venous systems in the head and neck. MRA has become a popular noninvasive alternative to the traditional catheter-directed selective angiography and provides a roadmap to the vascularization of many head and neck vascular lesions and tumors, allowing development of a plan for embolization, if necessary preoperatively. Dual-energy CTA (DE-CTA) is a promising upcoming innovation that produces a three-dimensional vascular model by suppressing the bones, and is an attractive alternative to MRA.

■ Summary

Imaging provides information regarding deep tissues. The imaging strategy depends on the character of the tissues in question. Understanding basic imaging principles and consulting with a radiologist can result in optimal approaches. Several innovations in radiology, including DE-CTA and flash CT, may have useful applications in the head and neck.

■ Suggested Reading

Grossman RI, Zimmerman RD, Yousem DM. Neuroradiology: The Requisites. 3rd ed. St. Louis, MO: Mosby-Year Book; 2010

Harnsberger HR, Glastonbury CM, Michel MA, Koch BL. Diagnostic Imaging: Head and Neck. 2nd ed. Salt Lake City, UT: Amirsys, Inc.; 2010

Isles MG, McConkey C, Mehanna HM. A systematic review and meta-analysis of the role of positron emission tomography in the follow up of head and neck squamous cell carcinoma following radiotherapy or chemoradiotherapy. Clin Otolaryngol 2008; 33(3):210–222

Licameli G, Kenna MA. Is computed tomography (CT) or magnetic resonance imaging (MRI) more useful in the evaluation of pediatric sensorineural hearing loss? Laryngoscope 2010;120(12): 2358–2359

Schwartz JD, Loevner LA. Imaging of the Temporal Bone. 4th ed. New York, NY: Thieme; 2009

Sniezek JC. Head and neck ultrasound: why now? Otolaryngol Clin North Am 2010;43(6):1143–1147, v

Sofferman RA. Interpretation of ultrasound. Otolaryngol Clin North Am 2010;43(6):1171–1202, v–vi

Som PM, Curtin HD. Head and Neck Imaging. 4th ed. St. Louis: Mosby-Year Book; 2002

Valvassori GE, Mafee MF, Carter BL. Imaging of the Head and Neck. 2nd ed. New York, NY: Thieme; 2004

Vogl TJ, Harth M, Siebenhandl P. Different imaging techniques in the head and neck: assets and drawbacks. World J Radiol 2010; 2(6):224–229

22 Interventional Neuroradiology in Head and Neck Disorders

■ Introduction

Over the last 25 to 30 years, embolization of lesions in the head and neck has developed into a useful adjunct to surgery. An improved understanding of the vascular anatomy of the head and neck and refinements in angiographic technique, microcatheters, and embolic agents have all played important roles in increasing the number, safety, and effectiveness of head and neck embolization.

The primary goal of embolization is to precisely obliterate the blood supply to a tumor or vascular malformation, while preserving the supply to normal surrounding tissues. A detailed angiographic map of the lesion is visualized by selectively injecting contrast into each arterial trunk that can supply collaterals. Once this map has been evaluated, embolization is performed via the safest and most direct route to the lesion. After embolization, the adequacy of the results is evaluated by injecting all arteries that can anastomose with the occluded branch.

As embolization of head and neck lesions became more common and more successful, so too have other methods of radiographically assisted intervention become feasible. These include other vascular applications (e.g., intra-arterial chemotherapy, sclerotherapy, transvascular radiofrequency ablation, and venous sampling); and nonvascular applications (e.g., percutaneous biopsy, feeding tube placement, tracheobronchial balloon dilation, and abscess drainage). The unique experience gained by the use of computed tomography (CT) and magnetic resonance imaging has aided in the more complete understanding of the macroscopic and microscopic nature of various head and neck conditions, which has driven the desire to look for newer methods of achieving acceptable treatment results with reduced patient morbidity. **Table 22.1** provides an up-to-date listing of the types of head and neck procedures an interventional radiologist can perform. The remainder of this review considers only neuroradiological intervention, which is defined here as procedures involving access to the cerebrovascular circulation.

Vascular Anatomy

Advances in neuroembolization have almost completely eliminated the need for surgical ligation of the external carotid artery. In addition, surgical ligation of the external carotid artery is now contraindicated in most cases because it prevents vascular access for endovascular embolization. Moreover, as many senior surgeons can attest, ligation of the external carotid artery was often not effective due to the rich collateral network that exists between the external carotid, vertebral, and internal carotid arteries. The richness of these anastomoses explains not only the ineffectiveness of external carotid ligation but also the poor embolization results of individuals who incompletely understand the pertinent vascular anatomy.

A complete understanding of this complex vascular anatomy of the head and neck is critical to safe and effective embolization of lesions in these areas. Normal anatomy, variants, and important anastomoses must be mastered to avoid potentially devastating complications. As external carotid branches anastomose with branches to the brain and orbit, the prevention of cerebrovascular stroke and blindness is based on a clear understanding of these connections. Moreover, the cranial nerves have a complex blood supply arising from both the external and the internal carotid arteries that must be understood to prevent debilitating cranial nerve deficits. It is generally accepted that the risk of complications is higher for interventional procedures than for angiography alone, which can sometimes be completed without the use of catheters, as in the case of magnetic resonance angiography.

The head and neck receive their blood supply through a rich vascular network. The anterior por-

Table 22.1   Head and neck procedures performed by an interventional radiologist

Vascular Procedures
Tumor embolization
Treatment of epistaxis
Treatment of arteriovenous malformations
Intra-arterial chemotherapy
Percutaneous sclerotherapy
Radiofrequency ablation
Venous sampling
Nonvascular Procedures
Feeding tube placement
Foreign body removal
Balloon dilation of the tracheobronchial tree
Percutaneous needle biopsy
Needle aspiration of abscess

tion of the neck is supplied by the ascending cervical artery of the thyrocervical trunk. The posterior half of the neck is supplied by the deep cervical artery of the costocervical trunk. The vertebral artery supplies the posterior fossa, spinal cord, and vertebral bodies. The face and skull base are supplied primarily by the external carotid artery. The internal carotid artery (ICA) supplies the orbit and cerebrum.

There are many collaterals between these different vascular territories in the head and neck. These multiple points of connection may not be angiographically visible, but they are present in everyone. The ascending cervical, vertebral, deep cervical, and external carotid arteries all anastomose together at multiple points. For example, the occipital, deep cervical, and vertebral arteries all connect a few centimeters posterior to the ear. As another example, the ascending pharyngeal artery anastomoses with the vertebral artery and the distal internal maxillary artery to supply a large portion of the skull base. Virtually every location in the head and neck is supplied by two or more major arteries. Obviously, each one of these must be embolized to successfully devascularize complex head and neck lesions.

Blood Supply to the Skull Base, Pharynx, and Posterior Fossa

The *ascending pharyngeal artery* is a complex important artery supplying the base of the skull, the pharynx, and the posterior fossa. This artery anastomoses directly with the vertebral and internal carotid arter-

ies. These dangerous anastomoses are present in everyone, but they are often invisible on angiography. Frequently, they will begin to appear during the later stages of embolization when distal runoff decreases.

The ascending pharyngeal artery also supplies cranial nerves IX, X, XI, and XII. Improper embolization technique can result in paralysis of any or all of these cranial nerves. To safely and effectively devascularize a skull base lesion, one must be aware of all of the normal connections that exist between the ascending pharyngeal artery and the carotid and vertebral systems (**Tables 22.2** and **22.3**).

The *middle meningeal artery* is another important artery supplying the skull base and dura. Similar to the ascending pharyngeal artery, the middle meningeal artery has critical anastomoses and supplies cranial nerves. The middle meningeal artery normally anastomoses with the ophthalmic artery around the orbit and with the ICA via anastomotic branches coursing through the cavernous sinus. In addition, the middle meningeal artery supplies the seventh cranial nerve as it passes through the middle ear cavity. Proper placement of the microcatheter and judicious choice of embolic agents are essential for the safe and effective devascularization of lesions supplied by this artery.

Blood Supply to the Eye

In addition to receiving blood supply from the middle meningeal artery, the eye can be supplied by the anterior deep temporal, infraorbital, and sphenopalatine arteries that arise from the distal *internal maxillary artery*. The *facial artery* also has a rich vascular network; it can reconstitute the distal internal maxillary artery branches as well as provide collaterals to the eye. Knowledge of this facial artery reconstitution of the distal internal maxillary artery and potential supply to the eye becomes critical during embolization of intractable epistaxis.

Table 22.2   Ascending pharyngeal artery anastomoses

1. Vertebral, ascending cervical, deep cervical, and occipital arteries via odontoid arch, spinomuscular branch, and C1, C2, C3, and C4 collaterals
2. Internal carotid artery via carotid and mandibular branches of superior pharyngeal, clival branches of neuromeningeal trunk, and inferior tympanic artery
3. Internal maxillary, middle meningeal, posterior auricular, occipital arteries via anastomoses with the inferior tympanic artery
4. Distal internal maxillary artery branches with pharyngeal branches

Table 22.3 Vertebral artery anastomoses

1. Ascending pharyngeal artery
2. Occipital artery
3. Ascending cervical artery
4. Deep cervical artery
5. Internal carotid via trigeminal, otic, hypoglossal, or proatlantal arteries

Table 22.4 Blood supply to the middle ear

1. Superior tympanic artery from the middle meningeal artery
2. Anterior tympanic artery from the internal maxillary artery
3. Inferior tympanic artery from the ascending pharyngeal artery
4. Caroticotympanic artery from the internal carotid artery
5. Stylomastoid artery from the occipital or posterior auricular artery

Blood Supply to the Middle Ear

The middle ear cavity receives blood supply from five different arteries (**Table 22.4**). These five arteries to the middle ear all anastomose. If a middle ear lesion, such as a glomus tumor, is supplied by one of these five arteries, the other four also supply it. Therefore, all five arteries must be studied during the workup of tumors or vascular malformations that involve the ear and petrous bone.

Table 22.5 Sources of blood supply to the cranial nerves

Artery	Cranial nerve
ILT, MHT, trigeminal, middle meningeal, ascending pharyngeal, accessory meningeal, vertebrobasilar	III, IV, V, VI
Anterior inferior cerebellar, middle meningeal, stylomastoid	VII, VIII
Ascending pharyngeal	IX, X, XI, XII
Abbreviations: ILT, inferolateral trunk; MHT, meningohypophyseal trunk.	

Blood Supply to the Cranial Nerves

The cranial nerves are supplied by a variety of sources from both the external and the internal carotid arteries (**Table 22.5**). As the third, fourth, fifth, and sixth cranial nerves arise from the brainstem, they receive supply from both the internal carotid and the basilar arteries. Branches from the cavernous ICA supply the third and fourth nerves in the roof of the cavernous sinus. The ascending pharyngeal artery and the meningohypophyseal trunk (MHT) supply the sixth nerve near the dorsum sella.

In the cavernous sinus, cranial nerves III, IV, V, and VI are supplied by branches of the cavernous ICA. These cavernous ICA branches are referred to as the inferolateral trunk (ILT) and the MHT. The ILT is often referred to as the lateral mainstem artery. One common variation is for the accessory meningeal artery to replace all of the blood supply coming from the cavernous ICA ILT branches. This variation occurs in ~ 20% of the population.

The fifth cranial nerve is supplied by the trigeminal artery after it originates from the brainstem. More distally, the fifth cranial nerve receives supply from both the ascending pharyngeal and the middle meningeal arteries. Even more anteriorly, cranial nerve V receives supply from the artery of the foramen rotundum and the accessory meningeal artery.

The proximal portions of the seventh and eighth cranial nerves are supplied by the anterior inferior cerebellar artery, which arises from the basilar artery. More distally, the facial nerve is supplied by the middle meningeal artery via its superior tympanic branch (**Table 22.4**). The distal vertical portion of the facial artery is supplied by the stylomastoid artery, which originates from either the occipital or the posterior auricular artery.

Cranial nerves IX, X, XI, and XII are supplied by the neuromeningeal trunk of the ascending pharyngeal artery. The neuromeningeal trunk has hypoglossal and jugular branches. The eleventh cranial nerve also receives blood supply from the spinomuscular branch of the ascending pharyngeal artery.

Obviously, the blood supply to the skull base and cranial nerves is quite complex. Fortunately, with understanding of the vascular anatomy and knowledge of the properties of the different embolic agents, skull base and head and neck lesions can be safely devascularized prior to surgery.

■ Management

Methods and Materials of Embolization

Anesthesia, Anticoagulation, and Provocative Testing

Anesthesia

Anesthesia is essential for the safe and effective embolization of head and neck lesions. Nitrous oxide should be avoided because it can expand small air bubbles that might inadvertently be introduced into the arteries. These expanding air bubbles in small blood vessels can result in cerebrovascular compromise. General anesthesia is often required in the pediatric population. In particular, for embolizing juvenile angiofibromas, endotracheal intubation is usually necessary because of nasal obstruction and airway compromise caused by the tumor. General anesthesia is also commonly used during epistaxis embolization to provide better airway control and to limit the passage of blood into the airways and lungs. General anesthesia is advised for performing ethanol embolization because injection of this agent is often quite painful for the patient.

Neuroleptic Analgesia

The majority of interventional procedures are performed using neuroleptic analgesia. Neuroleptic agents allow for careful monitoring throughout the procedure, while inducing both sedation and analgesia in the patient. Propofol is the most commonly used neuroleptic analgesic and has the advantage of rapid onset and short half-life. If the patient needs to be awakened for neurological testing (e.g., provocative testing to avoid damage to cranial nerves), propofol is an excellent agent. However, an anesthesiologist should have considerable experience to titrate the propofol for patients undergoing neuroembolization procedures. Once anesthesiologists have gained experience in these procedures, they are quite comfortable using high enough levels of propofol to limit patient motion while maintaining good airway control.

Another very effective regimen is the combination of midazolam and nalbuphine hydrochloride. These two drugs can often provide adequate sedation for less lengthy and more straightforward neuroembolization procedures. One added benefit from nalbuphine is that it is an agonist-antagonist, which makes it difficult to overdose a patient with this narcotic. Midazolam has the added benefit of providing amnesia during the procedure.

Full Heparinization

Full heparinization is performed during most embolization procedures. This is particularly important during carotid test occlusions and balloon embolization procedures. Obviously, during the carotid test occlusion, the patient should be fully anticoagulated to prevent thrombus proximal to the balloon during inflation.

Coagulation Times

Coagulation times are obtained following heparinization to determine adequate anticoagulation. Following the completion of the procedure, protamine sulfate can be used to reverse the effects of heparin. This reversal of heparin can be confirmed with a second coagulation time. A normal coagulation time is required prior to femoral catheter removal.

The safety of embolization of arteries that supply the cranial nerves can be ascertained with intra-arterial lidocaine provocative testing. The judicious use of intra-arterial lidocaine is essential prior to arterial embolization with liquid embolic agents, such as alcohol or cyanoacrylate. With particulate embolization (e.g., polyvinyl alcohol [PVA]), it is virtually impossible to devascularize a cranial nerve. Therefore, lidocaine testing is not required prior to particulate embolization of the external carotid system.

Catheters and Embolic Agents

Catheters

Head and neck embolizations are now performed primarily via the transfemoral approach. The direct carotid artery approach is rarely used today. Routinely, a catheter up to 150 cm in length is used, which allows access to the vessels supplying the skull base. Often a 6F or 7F sheath is placed in the femoral artery, and then, through a stepwise set of coaxial catheters, access is gained to the common carotid artery. Microcatheters that have tips as small as 500 μm are then advanced coaxially to the target lesion. Guidewires as small as 0.010 in are placed through these microcatheters and steered to the target vessel. Using high-resolution digital fluoroscopy, live digital subtraction angiography, and digital road mapping, the catheter is then slowly advanced over the microguidewire to achieve the proper location for embolization. Placing the tip of the catheter immediately adjacent to the tumor or vascular malformation greatly increases the safety of embolization. The precise placement next to the lesion avoids inadvertent embolization of anastomoses to the brain and arteries supplying cranial nerves.

As a result of the different lumen sizes of modern microcatheters, surgeons are now able to embolize using a variety of embolic agents.

Particulate Agents

Particulate embolization refers to the mechanical blockage of a vessel with individual particles of uniform size and shape. The occlusive properties are directly related to particle size. PVA is a nonabsorbable biocompatible sponge material that is the most commonly used particulate agent with the longest track record. These dry particles come in sizes ranging from 150 to 1,000 μm. Although PVA particles are permanent, the vascular occlusion that results is not; recanalization occurs around the particles over time. For this reason, PVA particles are used primarily for embolization of epistaxis and preoperative embolization of tumors. Embospheres are a newer, more recently adopted synthetic bead-type material that is also being used for particulate embolization. They also range in size from 40 to 1,200 μm, with most head and neck applications being performed with the 100 to 300 μm or 300 to 500 μm beads.

Tumor embolization is routinely performed with 150 to 250 μm particles because this size allows deep penetration and increases the likelihood of tumor necrosis. Particles smaller than 150 μm are avoided because they are more likely to pass through dangerous anastomoses that exist between the external carotid artery and the ICA or eye. If a dangerous anastomosis is suspected, for instance between the distal internal maxillary artery and the eye, then larger particles, such as 700 to 1,000 μm, are chosen. The larger particles are less likely to pass through these anastomoses, but the tradeoff is that the overall embolization may not be as effective.

Other particulate agents include Gelfoam and silk suture. Gelfoam powder is a good temporary embolic agent, but because of the small particle size (40–60 μm), it can be quite dangerous, potentially passing through anastomoses to the internal carotid or vertebral arteries. Because of this high risk, it is now rarely used in head and neck embolization. Gelfoam sponge can be cut into fragments of various sizes (e.g., 3 × 2 × 5 mm), then rolled into a compact cylinder, compressed to an appropriate diameter, and used to temporarily block and protect arteries from undesired distal embolization with other particulate or liquid embolic agents. Gelfoam sponge in combination with PVA is quite effective in the embolization of recurrent epistaxis.

Surgical silk suture can also be used in head and neck embolization when cut into 1 to 2 cm lengths. These can be used in conjunction with PVA particles to devascularize lesions. Silk has the disadvantage of not being radiopaque, whereas PVA can be mixed with contrast media. One advantage of silk suture is that it is inexpensive.

Liquid Embolic Agents

Cyanoacrylate is a low-viscosity liquid with tissue adhesive properties that polymerizes quickly in ionic solution. It is the most effective and permanent liquid embolic agent in use today. In many cases of embolization of the head and neck and brain, there is no substitute for cyanoacrylate, because it is able to reach deep into vascular malformations and tumors. Because cyanoacrylates are the most permanent embolic agents available, they are often used in cases where surgery is not possible and embolization is the primary treatment. These situations are usually reserved for cases where surgery may be too disfiguring or dangerous.

Because of the complexities and hazards of cyanoacrylate embolization, considerable training and experience are necessary to safely use this embolic agent. More than for any other embolic agent, care must be taken to avoid cyanoacrylate passing through dangerous anastomoses into the intracranial circulation. Also, there is the risk of gluing the catheter in place. Cyanoacrylate polymerizes on contact with ionic solutions, such as saline or blood, but will not polymerize in solution with 5% dextrose and water. The polymerization of cyanoacrylate can be adjusted with oil-based compounds or acetic acid. The low viscosity of cyanoacrylates allows them to be easily injected through microcatheters. These microcatheters must be placed quite distally in blood vessels and deep in vascular lesions.

A newer alternative injectable liquid that will form a complete embolic plug involves the use of ethylvinyl copolymer (ethylene vinyl alcohol [EVOH]), or a mixture of EVOH, dimethylsulfoxide, and tantalum (Onyx, ev3 Neurovascular, Ervine, CA). Onyx is sometimes preferred to cyanoacrylate because it polymerizes and holds its shape well, while not being as adherent.

Ethanol is another effective and quite aggressive embolic agent. When injected intra-arterially, it produces cytotoxic damage and ischemic necrosis. These toxic effects occur only when ethanol is injected in high concentration. Ethanol is a suitable agent when necrosis and not just devascularization is desired, such as in cases of malignant tumor embolization. Such embolization is usually reserved for cases where surgical resection is not possible. Ethanol can also be used for direct embolization of venous malformations involving the head and neck.

Balloons

The development of the detachable balloon in 1974 was instrumental in the advancement of the field of interventional neuroradiology. The balloon is an outstanding embolic agent for several reasons. It can be placed precisely in a vessel or a fistula, and it can be easily removed or replaced if its size, shape, or position is not optimal. The balloon can be inflated to a large diameter once it is in the body, but entry into the femoral artery requires only a small percutaneous arteriotomy. As technology has improved, balloons smaller than a grain of rice can be placed through a catheter deep into the body and then inflated to diameters of 2 to 3 cm and lengths of over 4 cm.

Detachable balloons are made of either latex or silicone; the choice depends on the operator's personal preference. Both types come with self-sealing valves, both are detached by simple traction, and both come in a large variety of sizes and shapes that can be preselected for an individual lesion. Detachable balloons are used primarily to occlude arterial fistulas and major vessels, such as the internal carotid or vertebral artery.

Nondetachable balloons are also available. They are used for carotid test occlusions prior to either permanent surgical ligation or detachable balloon occlusion. These temporary occlusion balloon catheters come in a variety of shapes and sizes. The nondetachable balloons can also be made from either silicone or latex.

Coils

Over the past 20 years, coil technology has markedly improved. In the past, coils were known for imprecise placement and being impossible to retrieve. Detachable coils are now available that allow more precise coil placement. These coils can be removed prior to detachment if coil configuration or position is unsatisfactory. In addition, coils now come in a variety of shapes and sizes. Coils can contain thrombogenic Dacron fibers, which improve vessel occlusion.

Although coils are excellent embolic agents in selected situations, when improperly used, they can be as ineffective as external carotid ligation. Coils do not enter the nidus or interstices of the tumor; therefore, inadequate tumor necrosis and devascularization result. Moreover, if a coil is deposited in the vessel too proximally, distal collaterals will resupply the tumor or fistula, and correct embolization at a later date is prevented because the main feeding artery has been embolized with the coil.

Relying extensively on coils can be a warning sign that inadequate embolization is being performed. In particular, to occlude a carotid artery with coils is quite hazardous. As shown with transcranial Doppler, when a network of coils is deposited in the ICA, blood continues to flow through them, but as the coils start to thrombose, fragments of clot break off and embolize into the distal ICA. Because of the risk of embolic stroke, coil occlusion of major vessels is contraindicated, unless proximal vessel occlu-

sion can be first achieved using a temporary balloon occlusion catheter system.

Indications for Embolization

Embolization has proven to be of benefit in the treatment of various head and neck lesions. Indications for embolization include presurgical devascularization of tumors (e.g., juvenile angiofibromas, paragangliomas, meningiomas, neuromas); total cure or stabilization of vascular lesions (e.g., arteriovenous malformations and fistulas); intractable hemorrhage (e.g., epistaxis, trauma, tumor); and reduction of tumor volume, mass effect, or pain (e.g., metastases, primary tumors). Preoperative embolization provides a useful adjunct to surgery by decreasing blood loss; providing almost bloodless tumor exposure, thereby allowing identification of important structures, such as cranial nerves; decreasing operation time; increasing the rate of radical tumor removal; reducing surgical complication rates; and possibly lowering tumor recurrence rates.

Juvenile Angiofibromas

Juvenile angiofibromas are most commonly supplied by the distal internal maxillary, accessory meningeal, and ascending pharyngeal arteries. Quite often the supply is bilateral. All three of these vessels can have anastomoses to the internal carotid, and the distal internal maxillary artery can supply the eye. Because of these dangerous anastomoses, larger particles of PVA or Embosphere Microspheres (300 to 500 μm) (Merit Medical Systems, Inc., South Jordan, UT) are often used. All three of these vessels are embolized by placing the microcatheter as close to the tumor as possible. Again, particulate embolization allows for penetration deep into the tumor, which results in better devascularization and necrosis. Proximal occlusion of the feeding artery with an embolic agent, such as a coil, should be avoided because it does not thoroughly devascularize the tumor and allows collaterals to reconstitute the blood supply.

On occasion, these tumors are supplied by the ascending palatine artery (usually a branch of the facial artery), which may arise directly off the external carotid artery or the medial pharyngeal branch of the ascending pharyngeal artery. Larger tumors that grow into the sphenoid sinus often recruit supply from the ICA, which usually cannot be embolized. However, the supply from the ICA often is not substantial and can be easily managed at surgery.

Following embolization, the blood loss at surgery is markedly reduced. Before embolization came into widespread use, the primary risk from juvenile angiofibroma resection was exsanguination.

Paragangliomas

These hypervascular tumors occur most commonly in the middle ear cavity, jugular bulb, carotid bulb, and along the vagal chain. Ten percent of patients have multiple tumors, and vagal and carotid paragangliomas may be malignant in 15% of cases. Paragangliomas are all supplied by the ascending pharyngeal artery, but as these tumors enlarge they will parasitize supply from adjacent external carotid artery branches. These tumors are hypervascular and demonstrate arteriovenous shunting angiographically.

Embolization of these tumors begins with ascending pharyngeal artery catheterization. Usually the artery is markedly enlarged and easy to directly catheterize. The goal of embolization of these lesions is intratumoral devascularization. The agent of choice is PVA or Embospheres. Larger particles are used because they are less likely to pass through anastomoses between the ascending pharyngeal and the vertebral and carotid arteries and because these tumors demonstrate arteriovenous shunting. Once the ascending pharyngeal artery has been embolized, the surrounding external carotid branches can be devascularized as needed.

Hypertensive crisis due to catecholamine release can occur during the selective angiography and embolization of paragangliomas. Because of this potential complication, anesthesia backup should be readily available. However, the use of nonionic contrast over the last 10 to 15 years has significantly decreased the risk of hypertensive crisis in these patients. In the embolization of carotid body tumors, another possible complication that can occur is bradycardia and hypotension from carotid sinus stimulation. At times, atropine and dopamine are needed for 24 hours after embolization to control the bradycardia and hypotension. Medications used for pain control following embolization should be vagolytic or at least have little effect on heart rate and blood pressure, rather than narcotics, which typically accentuate bradycardia.

Skull Base Tumors

Meningiomas, neuromas, and other primary and metastatic lesions often involve the skull base. Over the last 5 to 10 years, transnasal approaches to the skull base have proven to be a useful method to treat patients with these tumors, improving upon a surgeon's ability to access them while also reducing patient morbidity. Embolization of skull base tumors is particularly useful because the blood supply of this region is difficult to reach surgically. Embolization of skull base lesions is usually performed with particles. Particle size is chosen to allow deep penetration into the tumor to maximize devascularization and

tumor necrosis. Embolization of these lesions is usually performed at the same time as the angiographic examination.

The typical branches that supply skull base tumors are the ascending pharyngeal and middle meningeal arteries. The distal internal maxillary branches supply the more anterior skull base lesions as well. It is important to remember that tumors involving the foramen magnum and clivus are supplied by the ascending pharyngeal and not the vertebral artery. Often the surgeon is told that a clival or foramen magnum tumor is avascular based on a vertebral artery injection, whereas in reality the tumor is quite vascular due to ascending pharyngeal supply.

Again, when embolizing internal maxillary, middle meningeal, and ascending pharyngeal arteries, care must be taken to prevent particles entering anastomotic branches to the eye, internal carotid, or vertebral arteries. Potential anastomoses are monitored throughout the embolization procedure using high-resolution fluoroscopy. Often larger particles are used to exceed the size of an anastomotic channel.

The timing of surgery following tumor embolization is variable. The effects of devascularization are immediate, and surgery can be performed the same day. Surgery is typically scheduled within 1 or 2 days. With PVA particles, embolization surgery can be performed 7 to 10 days later without significant recanalization.

Carotid Artery Occlusion

Head and neck tumors may involve the wall of the ICA. This invasion of the ICA represents a major limiting factor for radical tumor removal. Prior to balloon occlusion of the ICA, attempts of pericarotid tumor resection frequently resulted in laceration of the ICA with uncontrollable hemorrhage that led to significant morbidity and mortality. If the patient tolerates the carotid or vertebral test occlusion prior to surgery, then the surgeon has the option of sacrificing the carotid or vertebral artery with the tumor. Obviously, if the patient does not tolerate test occlusion prior to surgery, the surgeon is less likely to sacrifice the involved vessel.

Despite 25 years of experience and clinical research, occluding the ICA remains one of the most dangerous interventional procedures. Carotid artery occlusion consists of placing a series of detachable balloons in the ICA. Typically, three balloons are used to avoid problems if one balloon deflates.

The principal advantage of balloon occlusion of the internal carotid or vertebral artery over surgical ligation is that test occlusion can be performed on an awake patient before the vessel is permanently occluded. Another advantage of balloon occlusion is that the patient can be heparinized before and after the procedure, which may delay the formation of thrombus in the distal vessel, which can later embolize into the cerebral circulation.

With carotid and vertebral artery test occlusion, the patient is awake and fully heparinized. A balloon catheter is guided into the vessel of choice, and the patient is examined neurologically. The blood pressure is carefully monitored. At this point, the balloon is inflated. Once blood flow is completely arrested, the patient is closely monitored for 20 minutes. If the patient develops a neurological deficit during the test occlusion, the balloon is immediately deflated and normal flow is reestablished to the brain. It is also important to monitor the blood pressure during test occlusion, because the hemodynamics of the circle of Willis can change with reductions of blood pressure. If a patient tolerates carotid test occlusion at a given blood pressure, there is no guarantee that the patient will tolerate occlusion at a lower blood pressure.

Results from blind surgical occlusion of the ICA have shown a stroke rate of 20%. Balloon occlusion of the carotid artery with awake testing of the patient prior to carotid occlusion has reduced the stroke rate to ~ 10%. However, this 10% stroke rate is still unacceptably high. Transcranial Doppler monitoring, electroencephalographic monitoring, single-photon emission CT, positron-emission tomography, and xenon CT have been used to bolster the predictive value of the carotid test occlusion. Unfortunately, no randomized prospective trials have been conducted to prove the effectiveness of any of these techniques.

Stroke after carotid occlusion can be due to low flow through the compensating anterior and posterior communicating arteries or from emboli that developed in the more distal internal carotid artery and were washed into the middle cerebral circulation. Therefore, to reduce the risk of stroke from emboli, all patients should be heparinized for a few days following carotid occlusion. Despite this measure, there is still no statistical evidence that this significantly reduces the stroke rate.

Occasionally, the carotid artery must be occluded in emergency situations (e.g., gunshot wounds or carotid blowouts following tumor invasion). Unfortunately, in these situations performing test occlusions is usually not warranted. Transcranial Doppler monitoring can sometimes help, but the situation is often desperate, and there is no choice but to occlude the vessel.

Recurrent Epistaxis

Epistaxis can be due to hypertension, coagulopathy, atherosclerotic vascular disease, trauma, or vascular malformations secondary to such syndromes as Osler-Weber-Rendu disease. In cases where epistaxis does not respond to packing and standard surgical therapy, embolization can be quite beneficial.

Often the initial angiogram does not show active bleeding. The distal internal maxillary artery can anastomose with the orbital braches of the ICA, so one must be vigilant while identifying these dangerous anastomoses during embolization. In most cases, epistaxis can be effectively treated with bilateral embolization of the distal internal maxillary arteries using small (150–250 μm) PVA or Embosphere particles. Distal penetration with small particles is used to devascularize the nasal mucosa. Once the distal internal maxillary arteries have been embolized with particles, both facial arteries are embolized with Gelfoam pledgets. Usually five to seven pledgets are injected into each facial artery to block the distal facial supply that can reconstitute the distal internal maxillary artery and lead to recurrent bleeding. This technique of bilateral internal maxillary and bilateral facial artery embolization suffices in the vast majority of cases. Although it is not universally necessary to address all four arteries, an oft-cited Vitek report on endovascular therapy for idiopathic intractable epistaxis in 30 patients found an 87% success rate after embolization of the internal maxillary artery and a 97% success rate (with a 3% complication rate) after embolization of the internal maxillary and facial arteries.

The ICA should always be checked either before or after the embolization to determine the supply to the nasal mucosa from the ethmoidal arteries arising from the ophthalmic artery. In addition, rare cases of cavernous carotid false aneurysms can result in epistaxis.

Once embolization is complete, the catheter is placed on the side thought to be the source of bleeding. The surgical packs are then removed. If bleeding has stopped, then the procedure is terminated. If bleeding persists with the packs out, repeat angiography is immediately performed to ascertain the source of bleeding. If the blood supply is from ethmoidal branches from the ophthalmic artery, surgery is required to clip these vessels. There are rare occasions where arteries, such as the transverse facial artery, can resupply the nasal mucosa distally, and these vessels may have to be selectively catheterized and embolized.

Facial Venous Malformations and Arteriovenous Malformation

Vascular malformations of the face are rare. If surgical resection of an arteriovenous malformation (AVM) is planned, then preoperative embolization with particles is sufficient. If the lesion is too large or is in an unfavorable location, surgery may not be indicated, leaving embolization as the only treatment option. In these cases, cyanoacrylate or another polymerizing injectable liquid is the best embolic agent to use. It provides the most permanent occlusion of vessels, reduces recurrent bleeding from the AVM, and helps with controlling pain, which is sometimes a feature of the malformation.

Again, the basic technique is to place a microcatheter deep into the nidus of the vascular malformation. The nidus is then filled with cyanoacrylate or a similar liquid, which polymerizes shortly after contact with blood. Again, considerable skill is needed to safely perform this procedure. One must avoid injecting permanent, totally occlusive material into the dangerous branches that connect to the eye and ICA.

Venous malformations of the face can be embolized via direct puncture and alcohol injection, which scleroses and scars the lesion, resulting in bulk and mass effect reduction. During direct alcohol embolization of these venous malformations, the two main risks are skin necrosis and facial venous drainage into the cavernous sinus. Obviously, ethanol injection into a facial vein that drains into the brain can be catastrophic. Careful fluoroscopic monitoring and opacification of the alcohol with metrizamide powder are essential for safe performance of this procedure.

Trauma

Trauma to the face from gunshot wounds and motor vehicle accidents is often treated with the embolization techniques used for epistaxis. If the degree of extravasation is too great, however, coils are chosen instead of PVA. Gelfoam pledgets can be effective in cases of massive bleeding around the face and mouth. Traumatic injury to the carotid or vertebral arteries is treated with emergent permanent balloon occlusion. During vertebral artery occlusion, the anterior spinal artery should not be occluded because this can result in spinal cord infarction and paralysis.

Arteriovenous Fistulas

Fistulas of the face, head, and neck can be congenital or acquired secondary to trauma. Most fistulas are treated with balloon embolization. Smaller fistulas may not be amenable to balloon embolization and can be treated with cyanoacrylate, Onyx, or coil embolization. The goal is to place a balloon directly at the origin of the fistula. Proximal occlusion is to be avoided, due to the rich anastomotic network of the face and neck. Proximal balloon occlusion or external carotid ligation will result in rapid regrowth of the fistula, and this proximal blockage will prevent future proper embolization. In the unfortunate circumstance where the feeding artery has been ligated, direct puncture of the artery and direct embolization are sometimes effective.

The site of the fistula is where the artery enters the vein. Angiographically, the fistula location is determined by finding a change in the caliber of an enlarged artery when it suddenly dilates into a massive vein. Understanding the vascular anatomy, determining the exact location of the fistula, and precisely placing balloons are essential steps in the successful treatment of these lesions.

Complication Rate

When performed by highly trained and experienced individuals, the complication rate from head and neck embolization, such as epistaxis, tumor embolization, and fistulas, should be less than 1 to 2%. The complication rate will be substantially higher whenever carotid occlusion is performed, where the stroke rate is estimated to be 10 to 20%, depending on whether test occlusion can be performed prior to permanent parent vessel occlusion.

■ Controversial Issues

Controversial issues regarding interventional neuroradiology include the following:

- Definitive risk and benefit analysis of surgical intervention versus angiography with embolization for treatment of patients with refractory epistaxis
- Success being related to the level of a radiologist's experience with the technique; lack of consensus as to what constitutes adequate experience and level of safety
- Interventional radiologists and head and neck surgeons should be aware of and should fully understand the abundant and complex anastomoses between the branches of the external carotid artery, the intracranial branches of the ICA, and the vertobrobasilar system.

■ Conclusion

Embolization can be of great benefit to the otolaryngologist and head and neck surgeon. Close collaboration between the interventionalist and the surgeon is essential for managing these complex vascular lesions of the head and neck. Thorough understanding of the vascular anatomy, indications for embolization, and endovascular methods and materials and proper training are necessary prerequisites. When proper embolization technique is employed, the safety and effectiveness of head and neck surgery can be improved, and thus will lead to a better outcome for the patient.

■ Practice Guidelines, Consensus Statements, and Measures

To date, randomized, controlled trials evaluating safety and efficacy are lacking, in large part due to the rarity of hypervascular tumors. Standard definitions and uniformity across reports will aid in establishing best practice measures.

■ Suggested Reading

Becker SS, Chiu AG. Prevention and management of complications in sinus and skull base surgery. Otolaryngol Clin North Am 2010;43(4):xvii–xviii

Berenstein A, Lasjaunias P, ter Brugge KG. Clinical and Endovascular Treatment Aspects in Adults. Berlin, Germany: Springer-Verlag; 2004. Surgical Neuroangiography. Vol 2. 2nd ed

Broomfield S, Bruce I, Birzgalis A, Herwadkar A. The expanding role of interventional radiology in head and neck surgery. J R Soc Med 2009;102(6):228–234

Gandhi D, Gemmete JJ, Ansari SA, Gujar SK, Mukherji SK. Interventional neuroradiology of the head and neck. AJNR Am J Neuroradiol 2008;29(10):1806–1815

Lasjaunias P, Berenstein A, ter Brugge KG. Clinical Vascular Anatomy and Variations. Berlin, Germany: Springer-Verlag; 2001. Surgical Neuroangiography. Vol 1. 2nd ed

Lasjaunias P, ter Brugge KG, Berenstein A. Clinical and Interventional Aspects in Children. Berlin, Germany: Springer-Verlag; 2006. Surgical Neuroangiography. Vol 3. 2nd ed

Quadros RS, Gallas S, Delcourt C, Dehoux E, Scherperel B, Pierot L. Preoperative embolization of a cervicodorsal paraganglioma by direct percutaneous injection of onyx and endovascular delivery of particles. AJNR Am J Neuroradiol 2006;27(9):1907–1909

Snyderman CH, Harvey RJ. Skull base: meeting place for multidisciplinary collaboration. Otolaryngol Clin North Am 2011;44(5): xi–xii

Valavanis A, ed. Interventional Neuroradiology. New York, NY: Springer-Verlag; 2012

IV

Head and Neck Surgery

23 Cutaneous Melanoma of the Head and Neck

■ Introduction

Cutaneous melanoma is a malignant neoplasm that may have widely variable clinical features and survival. Very early lesions are highly curable if recognized and treated promptly. At the other end of the spectrum, some lesions behave in a highly malignant fashion and rapidly lead to a patient's demise. Recognition of suspicious lesions is important for the head and neck surgeon, because cutaneous melanoma may involve the head and neck region in 20 to 30% of cases. In addition, numerous studies have demonstrated that survival is directly related to early detection.

Etiology/Risk Factors

It is widely accepted that major risk factors for melanoma include ultraviolet (UV) light exposure, genetic influences, and immunologic deficits. Some studies have shown that there is a direct correlation with the total cumulative lifetime dose of UV light, whereas other investigators have noted a correlation with the number and severity of sunburns. Skin type (light complexion, freckling, sun sensitivity, inability to tan) and other phenotypical characteristics (light-colored eyes, blonde or red hair) are associated with increased risk of melanoma as well.

Those with a family history of melanoma and multiple and/or increased numbers of melanocytic nevi are at higher risk for developing melanoma. Hereditary dysplastic nevus syndrome (formerly known as familial atypical multiple mole-melanoma syndrome) is an inherited autosomal-dominant disorder that is characterized by large numbers of moles (melanocytic nevi), some of which are atypical. These atypical lesions carry a clear predisposition to cutaneous melanoma. In these patients, the estimated lifetime risk of developing melanoma has been estimated to be as high as 100%.

Lesions Associated with Increased Risk of Melanoma

Some melanomas arise in "precursor" pigmented lesions, whereas others appear de novo in normal-appearing skin. Pigmented lesions that are associated with increased risk of developing malignant melanoma are called markers. Congenital melanocytic nevi and dysplastic nevi are considered precursor lesions as well as markers, indicative of an increased risk of melanoma development.

Congenital Melanocytic Nevi

Congenital melanocytic nevi are categorized by size into small, medium, and large.

- Small—less than 1.5 cm in diameter
- Medium—1.5 to 19.9 cm in diameter
- Large—20 cm or more in diameter

Congenital melanocytic nevi occur in 1% of newborns. Most of these are of small or medium size. The lifetime risk of malignant melanoma in patients with large congenital melanocytic nevi has been estimated to be ~ 6%. There appears to be an increased risk for small- or medium-sized lesions as well, but the level of increased risk is controversial. When feasible, it is recommended that large congenital melanocytic nevi be treated with complete surgical excision. If the lesion is too large for excision, close clinical follow-up is necessary. Due to the controversy relating to small- and medium-sized melanocytic nevi, decisions relating to the necessity of surgical removal must be individualized according to the patient and the particular clinical setting.

Dysplastic Nevus

The dysplastic nevus is an *acquired* pigmented lesion of the skin. The cardinal features that separate dysplastic nevi from the more ubiquitous melanocytic nevi (moles) include the following: asymmetry, border irregularity, color variegation, a diameter greater than 6 mm, and evolution. Dysplastic nevi may occur in both familial and nonfamilial settings. The familial type has been studied and labeled dysplastic nevus syndrome. Patients with this syndrome generally have a triad that includes (1) more than 100 moles, (2) at least one mole 8 mm or larger in diameter, and (3) at least one mole with "atypical" features (as already described). The risks among individuals with dysplastic nevi vary with the total number of lesions present, as well as the specific family history of melanoma and dysplastic nevi.

Epidemiology

The incidence of melanoma in the United States is increasing at a rate greater than any other cancer. As of 2009, lifetime risk of melanoma is 1 in 39 for men and 1 in 58 for women. It is estimated that in 2012, 76,250 men and women will be diagnosed with melanoma, and 9,180 people died from this disease. This rise in incidence has partly been attributed to better screening and earlier detection. Along with increasing incidence has come increasing survival, with 5-year survival for localized, early-stage melanoma being ~ 98.2%.

Classification/Pathology of Cutaneous Melanoma

Cutaneous melanoma has been classified into morphological types that seem to share similar clinical, histological, and epidemiological characteristics. These include melanoma in situ (also known as lentigo maligna), lentigo maligna melanoma, superficial spreading melanoma, nodular melanoma, acral lentiginous melanoma (which is not seen in the head and neck), and desmoplastic melanoma. Clark was the first to observe that malignant melanomas tend to progress sequentially in two directions. Generally, in the early phase of growth, the *radial growth phase,* there is spread in a plane parallel to the skin surface. After a period of time, the direction of growth changes to a direction perpendicular to the surface of the skin and tumor growth takes on a *vertical growth phase.*

Melanoma in Situ

Melanoma in situ, which has been formerly labeled as lentigo maligna or Hutchinson freckle, represents the preinvasive stage of melanoma. Lesions are usually large and flat with asymmetric borders and heterogeneous pigmentation. They occur in sun-damaged areas of the skin, often affecting the face, ears, neck, and upper extremities. These lesions are usually greater than 10 mm in size and look histologically like malignant melanoma but are confined to the epidermis and adnexal epithelium. The risk of untreated lesions progressing to invasive melanoma has been estimated at 5 to 33%.

Lentigo Maligna Melanoma

Lentigo maligna melanoma has a predilection for the face, neck, and extremities. It is usually seen in older individuals and rarely seen in those younger than 50 years of age. Lentigo maligna melanoma has generally been regarded as the least invasive form of melanoma and makes up ~ 15% of melanomas of the head and neck region. It often arises from precursor melanoma in situ lesions, many of which have been present for years. As the progression to lentigo maligna melanoma takes place, a thickening or a nodule develops within the flat, pigmented patch of skin.

Superficial Spreading Melanoma

Superficial spreading melanoma is the most common type of cutaneous melanoma. It accounts for 30 to 50% of cases seen in the head and neck region. Lesions typically are flat to slightly raised. Superficial spreading melanoma is the type most often seen in individuals at risk for developing melanoma, such as those with a family history or those with prior dysplastic nevi.

Nodular Melanoma

Nodular melanoma exhibits a pure vertical growth phase. Tumor expansion occurs in a vertical direction, and there is very little horizontal spread. Nodular melanoma is considered the most aggressive and lethal type of melanoma. It presents as a tumor nodule and accounts for up to 30% of melanomas. Nodular melanoma is most often diagnosed in patients who are middle-aged. The lesions are usually 1 to 2 cm, are symmetric and smooth-surfaced, and typically have little color variegation, with pigmentation varying from dark brown to blue to gray.

Desmoplastic Melanoma

Desmoplastic melanomas often lack pigment and may be more difficult to recognize as suspicious for melanoma. Lesions may resemble fibromas or hypertrophic scars. It is a rare subtype of melanoma, but the majority of desmoplastic melanomas are seen in the head and neck. It has a high tendency for perineural invasion.

■ Evaluation

Clinical Features of Cutaneous Melanoma

The single most important factor in curing patients with melanoma is early detection. It is well established that the cure rate is inversely proportional to the depth of invasion of these lesions into the dermis and subcutaneous tissue. Thus it is extremely important for lesions to be detected at the earliest possible time. Early diagnosis coupled with prompt surgical removal can cut the death rate of melanoma to nearly zero. Thus it is essential that physicians be able to recognize the cardinal features of melanoma.

The characteristic clinical features of early melanoma lesions are the same as dysplastic nevi, and can be remembered by the ABCDE mnemonic:

A—asymmetry
B—border irregularity
C—color variegation
D—diameter greater than 6 mm
E—evolving lesion

It is estimated that cutaneous melanoma arises from a preexisting lesion 50% of the time. Clearly, any change in a preexisting pigmented lesion is one of the most suggestive features of early melanoma. Symptoms associated with lesions including bleeding, itching, pain, or ulceration are worrisome.

Diagnosis and Biopsy

All lesions presenting with signs suspicious for malignant melanoma should be biopsied to make a definitive diagnosis. Excisional biopsy (elliptical, punch, or saucerization) is the preferred method of obtaining tissue, while curettage, cryotherapy, and shave biopsies are contraindicated in this setting. The entire lesion should be removed with a narrow margin of normal skin, including subcutaneous fat with the specimen. Recommended excisional biopsy margins are 1 to 3 mm. If the lesion is so large or is located in an anatomical area for which excisional biopsy is not reasonable, punch biopsy should be performed in the most suspicious portion of the lesion.

Biopsies should ideally be read by a pathologist with experience in pigmented lesions, and reports should include the following minimal elements essential to staging melanoma:

1. Breslow thickness in mm
2. Histological ulceration present or absent
3. Dermal mitotic rate per mm squared (mm^2)
4. Peripheral and deep margin status
5. Clark level (encouraged for lesions < 1 mm, option for > 1 mm)

Additional encouraged elements in a pathology report as recommended by the American Academy of Dermatology include location, regression, tumor infiltrating lymphocytes, vertical growth phase, angiolymphatic invasion, neurotropism, histological subtype, and presence of pure versus mixed desmoplasia.

Patient History and Physical Examination

Further evaluation of the patient with a suspicious lesion includes a complete history and physical examination and assessment of risk factors as described earlier. Once diagnosis is confirmed, further evaluation for signs and symptoms of metastatic disease may be necessary. Any symptoms that cannot be readily accounted for should be evaluated with appropriate studies. Careful palpation should be performed to search for involved regional lymph nodes, and a careful skin survey should be made for any satellite lesions around the original lesion.

Imaging and Laboratory Tests

Routine imaging and laboratory tests are not recommended for patients with melanoma in whom no palpable lymphadenopathy has been identified. Specifically, the role of computed tomography (CT) and magnetic resonance imaging (MRI) in evaluating the neck for occult disease is not well established. Imaging is currently only recommended to evaluate specific signs or symptoms that cannot otherwise be explained, not to search for occult disease. However, in patients with clinically apparent lymphadenopathy or positive sentinel lymph node biopsy (discussed later in this chapter), baseline imaging such as CT, positron-emission tomography (PET)/CT, and/or MRI for staging and to evaluate for distant disease is recommended by the National Comprehensive Cancer Network (NCCN).

Laboratory tests that are useful in evaluating high-risk melanoma patients include liver function tests/lactate dehydrogenase, urinalysis, and stool guaiac. These tests are useful adjunct screening tests for distant metastatic disease.

Staging Systems

Multiple systems of staging melanoma have been used over the years. The system of the American Joint Council on Cancer was updated in 2009 and clinically implemented in the seventh edition of the *AJCC Cancer Staging Manual* in 2010. It includes tumor, nodes, and metastasis (TNM) staging categories, with expanded pathological staging regarding microstaging of the primary tumor and regional lymph nodes. Staging is shown in **Tables 23.1** and **23.2**. The current staging reflects that tumor thickness, mitotic rate, and ulceration are dominant prognostic variables in patients with localized melanoma.

Microstaging

Histological findings correlate directly with prognosis, and thus have a significant impact on recommendations for treatment. Therefore, it is crucial that the biopsy specimen be properly obtained and appropriately oriented for the pathologist. Historically, two microstaging systems have gained wide-

spread acceptance because of their correlation with prognosis: Clark levels and Breslow thickness. Clark levels are described here but are no longer used to a significant degree in the staging system. Breslow thickness, however, remains the most critical factor in staging/prognosis.

Clark Levels

The system devised by Clark classifies lesions based on the deepest level of skin invaded by melanoma cells:

- Level I—confined to the epidermis
- Level II—extension into the papillary dermis without completely filling this area

Table 23.1 Staging system for melanoma atomic stage and prognostic groups

Anatomic Stage—Prognostic Groups							
Clinical*				**Pathologic⁺**			
Group	**T**	**N**	**M**	**Group**	**T**	**N**	**M**
☐ 0	Tis	N0	M0	☐ 0	Tis	N0	M0
☐ IA	T1a	N0	M0	☐ IA	T1a	N0	M0
☐ IB	T1b	N0	M0	☐ IB	T1b	N0	M0
	T2a	N0	M0		T2a	N0	M0
☐ IIA	T2b	N0	M0	☐ IIA	T2b	N0	M0
	T3a	N0	M0		T3a	N0	M0
☐ IIB	T3b	N0	M0	☐ IIB	T3b	N0	M0
	T4a	N0	M0		T4a	N0	M0
☐ IIC	T4b	N0	M0	☐ IIC	T4b	N0	M0
☐ III	Any T	Any N > N0	M0	☐ IIIA	T1–4a	N1a	M0
☐ IV	Any T	Any N	M1		T1–4a	N2a	M0
				☐ IIIB	T1–4b	N1a	M0
					T1–4b	N2a	M0
					T1–4a	N1b	M0
					T1–4a	N2b	M0
					T1–4a	N2c	M0
				☐ IIIC	T1–4b	N1b	M0
					T1–4b	N2b	M0
					T1–4b	N2c	M0
					Any T	N3	M0
				☐ IV	Any T	Any N	M1

* Clinical staging includes microstaging of the primary melanoma and clinical/radiologic evaluation for metastases. By convention, it should be used after complete excision of the primary melanoma with clinical assessment for regional and distant metastases.

⁺ Pathologic staging includes microstaging of the primary melanoma and pathologic information about the regional lymph nodes after partial or complete lymphadenectomy. Pathologic Stage 0 or Stage IA patients are the exception; they do not require pathologic evaluation of their lymph nodes.

☐ Stage unknown   ☐ Stage unknown

Used with the permission of the American Joint Committee on Cancer (AJCC), Chicago, Illinois. The original source for this material is the AJCC Cancer Staging Manual, Seventh Edition (2010) published by Springer Science and Business Media LLC, www.springer.com.

Table 23.2 Staging system for melanoma of the skin   **151**

Melanoma of the Skin Staging Form

Clinical *Extent of disease before any treatment*	Stage Category Definitions		Pathologic *Extent of disease through completion of definitive surgery*
☐ clinical—staging completed after neoadjuvant therapy but before subsequent surgery	**Tumor Size:** _____	**Laterality:** ☐ midline ☐ left ☐ right ☐ bilateral	☐ pathologic—staging completed after neoadjuvant therapy AND subsequent surgery
Primary Tumor (T)			
☐ TX	Primary tumor cannot be assessed		☐ TX
☐ T0	No evidence of primary tumor		☐ T0
☐ Tis	Melanoma *in situ*		☐ Tis
☐ T1	Melanomas ≤ 1.0 mm in thickness		☐ T1
☐ T1a	without ulceration and mitosis < 1/mm²		☐ T1a
☐ T1b	with ulceration or mitoses ≥ 1/mm²		☐ T1b
☐ T2	Melanomas 1.01–2.0 mm		☐ T2
☐ T2a	without ulceration		☐ T2a
☐ T2b	with ulceration		☐ T2b
☐ T3	Melanomas 2.01–4.0 mm		☐ T3
☐ T3a	without ulceration		☐ T3a
☐ T3b	with ulceration		☐ T3b
☐ T4	Melanomas > 4.0 mm		☐ T4
☐ T4a	without ulceration		☐ T4a
☐ T4b	with ulceration		☐ T4b
Regional Lymph Nodes (N)			
☐ NX	Regional lymph nodes cannot be assessed		☐ NX
☐ N0	No regional lymph node metastasis		☐ N0
☐ N1	1 node		☐ N1
	micrometastasis*		☐ N1a
	macrometastasis**		☐ N1b
	2–3 nodes		☐ N2
	micrometastasis*		☐ N2a
	macrometastasis**		☐ N2b
☐ N2c	in transit met(s)/satellite(s) *without* metastatic nodes		☐ N2c
☐ N3	Clinical: ≥ 1 node with in transit met(s)/satellite(s); pathologic: 4 or more metastatic nodes, or matted notes, or in transit met(s)/satellite(s) *with* metastatic node(s)		☐ N3
	* Micrometastases are diagnosed after sentinel lymph node biopsy and completion lymphadenectomy (if performed).		
	** Macrometastases are defined as clinically detectable nodal metastases confirmed by therapeutic lymphadenectomy or when nodal metastasis exhibits gross extracapsular extension.		
Distant Metastasis (M)			
☐ M0	No distant metastasis (no pathologic M0; use clinical M to complete stage group)		
☐ M1a	Metastases to skin, subcutaneous tissues, or distant lymph nodes		☐ M1a
☐ M1b	Metastases to lung		☐ M1b
☐ M1c	Metastases to all other visceral sites or distant metastases to any site combined with an elevated serum LDH		☐ M1c

- Level III—melanoma fills and expands papillary dermis but without invasion of reticular dermis
- Level IV—infiltration into reticular dermis
- Level V—extension to subcutaneous fat

Even though Clark level is not used in official staging of all melanomas, it is still desirable to include this information in pathological reports, especially for lesions ≤ 1 mm thick and/or for lesions that are nonulcerated and for which mitotic rate is not determined.

Breslow Thickness

Breslow thickness classifies melanoma according to cross-sectional thickness as measured with a micrometer. The thickness is measured to the nearest tenth of a millimeter. Measurements are taken from the granular cell layer of the overlying epidermis to the deepest contiguous invasive malignant cell. In lesions that are ulcerated, the measurement begins at the base of the ulcer.

Table 23.3 Surgical margins for wide excision of primary melanoma

Tumor thickness	Recommended clinical margins[b]
In situ[a]	0.5–1 cm
< 1 mm	1 cm (category 1)
1.01–2 mm	1–2 cm (category 1)
2.01–4 mm	2 cm (category 1)
> 4 mm	2 cm (category 1)

[a] For large melanoma in situ (MIS), lentigo maligna type, surgical margins > 0.5 cm may be necessary to achieve histologically negative margins; techniques for more exhaustive histological assessment of margins should be considered. For selected patients with positive margins after optimal surgery, consider topical imiquimod (for patients with MIS0 or RT [category 2B]).

[b] Excision recommendations are based on clinical margins taken at the time of surgery and not gross or histological margins, as measured by the pathologist (category 1).

Data from NCCN Guidelines Version 1.2014 Melanoma. National Comprehensive Cancer Network, Inc.

◼ Management

Surgical Management of Primary Tumor

Surgical excision remains the treatment of choice for melanoma. Breslow thickness dictates excision margin. Previously, margins > 2 cm were used for melanomas that were > 2 mm thick. However, no survival or disease control benefit has been seen with margins > 2 cm. **Table 23.3** displays NCCN-recommended clinical margins based on tumor thickness. These are clinical margins measured by the surgeon at the time of excision, not gross or histological margins measured by the pathologist. Margins should be measured from the peripheral edge of the tumor or from the edge of the scar from the previous excisional biopsy. Within the head and neck, margin modification may be necessary due to anatomical constraints.

Frozen section is difficult to interpret in melanoma and thus frozen section margin analysis is not generally used in melanoma excisions. This brings up the issue of reconstruction in a setting of unconfirmed margin status. Delaying reconstruction until margin status is finalized via permanent histopathological examination ensures that further excision of any positive margins is not hindered by the reconstruction. Some surgeons will employ a split-thickness skin graft, or cover the wound with specialized dressing materials such as acellular dermis as temporary reconstruction until margins are finalized. When possible, delaying reconstruction that would compromise reexcision seems ideal. However, due to functional constraints in the head and neck, delayed

reconstruction of some defects, such as through and through cheek or lip defects, is undesirable. Ultimately, the decision regarding delayed versus immediate reconstruction is often surgeon-specific and based on the specific clinical scenario.

Mohs micrographic surgery is an area of controversy regarding surgical treatment of melanoma and has not been widely accepted at this time. Studies evaluating its efficacy are ongoing. Concerns regarding its usage include ability to evaluate 100% of the margin, the sometimes noncontiguous margins associated with melanoma lesions, and the ability to distinguish melanoma on frozen section.

Lymph Node Dissection

Without question, the most frequent site of metastasis from cutaneous melanoma of the head and neck is the regional lymph nodes. The nodes at risk vary with the specific site of the primary tumor and tend to follow known patterns of lymphatic drainage. Nodal involvement for lesions of the anterior face is predicted to first appear in the parotid or upper cervical nodes (levels I–III). Posterior scalp lesions may be associated with suboccipital and level V nodal disease. Lesions of the coronal and parietal scalp may be predicted to involve the parotid nodes and either anterior or posterior cervical nodes. However, lymphatic drainage of head and neck skin does not always follow known patterns, and location of potentially involved nodes may be outside of predictions. This has been observed in lymphoscintigraphic studies for sentinel lymph node biopsies.

Metastasis to regional lymph nodes has been shown to be the most important prognostic factor in patients with early-stage melanoma and is reported to occur in ~ 20% of patients with intermediate-thickness lesions. In patients with clinical evidence of nodal disease, neck dissection is performed to clear cervical and/or parotid nodal basins. However, if there is no palpable evidence of adenopathy, a decision must be made regarding evaluation and management of regional lymph nodes.

Historically, in the study of cutaneous melanoma, the role of elective lymph node dissection for occult disease was highly controversial. Over the past decade, studies have allowed more definitive data and recommendations regarding management of possible occult lymph node metastasis to emerge. Sentinel lymph node biopsy has now become part of the standard of care in evaluation and management of regional lymph nodes in melanoma, replacing observation and elective nodal dissection in patients with intermediate-thickness melanomas who lack clinical evidence of nodal disease.

The American Society of Clinical Oncology (ASCO) and Society of Surgical Oncology (SSO) recently performed a systematic review of literature on sentinel lymph node (SLN) biopsy and convened an expert panel to review the evidence and develop guideline recommendations. SLN biopsy is recommended for patients with intermediate-thickness melanomas (Breslow thickness 1–4 mm) of any anatomical site, including the head and neck. This provides accurate staging information to better predict prognosis. Completion lymph node dissection is recommended for all patients with a positive SLN biopsy and achieves regional disease control, even though this practice has not yet shown definitive improvement in overall disease survival.

For thin melanomas < 1 mm, risk of lymph node metastasis is considered low (~ 5.1%). For melanomas < 0.75 mm, SLN biopsy is generally not recommended. For melanomas 0.76 to 1 mm, a strong recommendation for SNL biopsy has not been made. However, with higher-risk tumor features, such as ulceration and mitotic rate > 1/mm, SNL biopsy can be discussed with the patient and offered as a reasonable option.

Controversy regarding thick melanomas and the use of SLN biopsy has also been present for years. In patients with T4 melanoma, it is estimated that the chance of lymph node involvement is 30% or more. This risk could argue in favor of immediate complete lymphadenectomy for a better chance of locoregional control. However, the chance of distant disease with T4 melanoma is higher than with intermediate thickness, and whether locoregional control actually conveys survival benefit is questionable. Morbidity rates of complete lymphadenectomy are inarguably higher than for SLN biopsy. According to the ASCO and SSO 2012 clinical practice guideline, SLN biopsy provides important staging and prognostic information and should be used for patients with thick melanomas as well.

Much of the information regarding SLN biopsy has been gleaned from all anatomical sites and is not specific to the head and neck. The test performance of SNL biopsy within the head and neck has been questioned, because lymphatic dissemination in head and neck melanoma is unpredictable, and the proximity of the primary lesion to nodal drainage basins can make identification of sentinel nodes more challenging. Several studies, including a large systematic review, have evaluated SLN biopsy in the head and neck and concluded that identification and excision of sentinel nodes is successful and safe but the false-negative rate (nodal recurrence in patients with negative SLN biopsy) may be higher in the head and neck compared with other locations. Recent advances in nuclear imaging using single-photon emission computed tomography (SPECT) fused with conventional CT allows for better localization of sentinel nodes compared with traditional lymphoscintigraphy. This is particularly useful in the head and neck. Regardless of the challenges encountered with head and neck SNL biopsy, recommendations for head and neck melanomas do not differ from those for other anatomical sites.

Other Treatment Modalities

Radiation Therapy

Melanoma has traditionally been considered a relatively radioresistant tumor. However, with variation in fractionation regimens, improved sensitivity of melanoma both in vitro and in vivo has been seen. Radiation therapy is generally not considered first-line treatment of cutaneous melanoma and is used as primary therapy only in selected cases for nonoperative candidates. Radiation is used more commonly as adjuvant therapy to facilitate locoregional control in surgically treated patients or as palliative therapy for metastatic disease. Current NCCN guidelines recommend that radiation be considered as adjuvant therapy for primary disease in selected patients with desmoplastic melanoma with narrow margins, recurrent disease, or extensive neurotropism. Additionally, radiation as adjuvant therapy is recommend for (1) nodal disease with gross nodal extracapsular extension, cervical lymph node basins with ≥ 2 clinically involved nodes, and/or if an involved node contains ≥ 2 cm of tumor; and (2) following resection of recurrent nodal disease. Improved locoregional control has been demonstrated with adjuvant radiation, though overall survival benefit has not definitively been shown.

For metastatic disease, radiation is used for brain metastasis, either stereotactic radiosurgery or whole-brain irradiation, as well as palliation for symptomatic soft tissue and/or bone metastasis.

Chemotherapy/Biological Response Modifiers/Immunotherapy

Chemotherapy has shown little success in treating melanoma. Several chemotherapeutic agents and combinations thereof have been studied and have generally been found to be only partly effective, with response rates of 6 to 15% and median progression-free survival of 2 to 3 months. High-dose interferon a-2b given for 1 year for high-risk patients has shown some survival benefit, but the side effects are often difficult for patients to tolerate. Dacarbazine is also approved by the U.S. Food and Drug Administration (FDA) as adjuvant chemotherapy but has not shown significant benefit. Since March 2011, two additional agents approved by the FDA are part of the preferred regimen for advanced metastatic disease. Ipilimumab is an immunotherapy anticytotoxic T-lymphocyte antigen 4 mono-

clonal antibody that has shown some improvement in overall survival for metastatic melanoma. However, response is highly unpredictable, and potentially severe immune toxicities can occur. Molecular pathway targeting is also an area of active research and has brought about approval of a second agent, vemurafenib, an inhibitor of BRAF in the oncogenic mitogen-activated protein kinase pathway. Tumor vaccines are similarly an area of active research but have yet to show definitive survival benefit. Research regarding medical therapy for melanoma continues with some promising findings, though the proper setting and patient population for each drug have yet to be determined.

■ Conclusion

Head and neck melanoma continues to be a problematic disease. Early recognition and evaluation of suspicious lesions has the greatest impact on survival. Knowledge of the risk factors, signs suggestive of melanoma, and appropriate therapy is critical to management of patients with this disease.

■ Practice Guidelines, Consensus Statements, and Measures

National Comprehensive Cancer Network. NCCN Clinical Practice Guidelines in Oncology for Melanoma version 1.2013. http://www.nccn.org/index.asp

Wong SL, Balch CM, Hurley P, et al. Sentinel lymph node biopsy for melanoma: American Society of Clnical Oncology and Society of Surgical Oncology joint clinical practice guideline. J Clin Oncol 2012;30(23):2912–2918

■ Suggested Reading

Balch CM, Gershenwald JE, Soong SJ, et al. Final version of 2009 AJCC melanoma staging and classification. J Clin Oncol 2009;27(36):6199–6206

Balch CM, Morton DL, Gershenwald JE, et al. Sentinel node biopsy and standard of care for melanoma. J Am Acad Dermatol 2009;60(5):872–875

Barker CA, Lee NY. Radiation therapy for cutaneous melanoma. Dermatol Clin 2012;30(3):525–533

Chandra S, Pavlick AC. Targeted therapies for metastatic melanoma. Dermatol Clin 2012;30(3):517–524

de Rosa N, Lyman GH, Silbermins D, et al. Sentinel node biopsy for head and neck melanoma: a systematic review. Otolaryngol Head Neck Surg 2011;145(3):375–382

Khan N, Khan MK, Almasan A, Singh AD, Macklis R. The evolving role of radiation therapy in the management of malignant melanoma. Int J Radiat Oncol Biol Phys 2011;80(3):645–654

Leong SPL. Role of selective sentinel lymph node dissection in head and neck melanoma. J Surg Oncol 2011;104(4):361–368

Morton DL, Thompson JF, Cochran AJ, et al; MSLT Group. Sentinel-node biopsy or nodal observation in melanoma. N Engl J Med 2006;355(13):1307–1317

Yao K, Balch G, Winchester DJ. Multidisciplinary treatment of primary melanoma. Surg Clin North Am 2009;89(1):267–281, xi

24 Nonmelanotic Skin Cancer

◼ Introduction

Nonmelanotic skin cancer (NMSC) is the most common cancer worldwide, with more than 1 million new cases diagnosed each year in the United States alone. NMSC has been increasing since the 1960s at a rate of ~ 5% per year; approximately one in six Americans will develop a skin cancer at some point in their lifetime. Cutaneous squamous cell carcinoma (cSCC) and basal cell carcinoma (BCC) constitute the vast majority of NMSCs, but more than 80 other types of NMSC exist. Although the vast majority of NMSCs are not life threatening, advanced cases can present treatment challenges and cause significant morbidity and mortality, taking the lives of ~ 2,500 people per year in the United States (**Tables 24.1** and **24.2**).

Epidemiology and Etiology

Ultraviolet (UV) light exposure plays a large role in the development of NMSC. The risk of cSCC rises in proportion to cumulative UV light exposure, whereas intermittent sun exposure, and exposure during childhood, is thought to be more important in the development of BCC. The relationship between sun exposure and the development of NMSC is highlighted by the increasing incidence of NMSC in the United States as latitude decreases, and by the fact that people with outdoor occupations are at a 10-fold risk of developing NMSC compared with those with indoor occupations. The relationship between sun exposure and cSCC, combined with the high rate of sun exposure in the head and neck, leads to more than 75% of cSCC arising in the head and neck.

The incidence of NMSC increases with age, with ~ 80% of cases occurring in people age 60 or older. The incidence of cSCC is more than 30 times higher in patients 70 years or older than in patients 50 to 55 years old, and almost 1/200 patients older than 85 develop cSCC yearly. Personal characteristics also play a role in the development of NMSC. People with fair skin, light eyes, and blond or red hair are at an increased risk of developing NMSC, as are people who tend to freckle or sunburn instead of tan when exposed to the sun. Routine application of sunscreen has been shown to potentially aid in the prevention of cSCC, but it has an unproven benefit in BCC. Many cSCCs arise from preexisting actinic keratoses, and up to 10% of actinic keratoses will develop into cSCC. Patients with 10 or more actinic keratoses are at over 100 times the risk of developing cSCC.

cSCC is also much more common in immunosuppressed patients than in the rest of the population. Patients with solid organ transplants have over a 50-fold increase in the risk of developing cSCC compared with the general population, and the risk increases with the length of immunosuppression; starting at ~ 7% at year 1 to ~ 70% at 20 years. In addition, a clear correlation has been established between the degree of immunosuppression and the incidence of NMSC, and reduction of immunosuppression is associated with better outcomes. Finally, an increased incidence of cSCC has been noted in patients with chronic wounds or chronic scarring, often associated with burns.

◼ Evaluation and Diagnosis

History and Physical

A complete history and physical is the initial step in the evaluation of any cancer patient and is the first step in the evaluation of a patient with suspected NMSC. The history should include information on the treatment of any previous skin cancers, the degree of lifetime sun exposure, and any history of immunosuppression. The presence of pain, paresthesia, or any signs of cranial nerve involvement should be noted, especially along the distribution of the

Table 24.1 Staging system for cutaneous squamous cell carcinoma

Primary Tumor (T)	
TX	Primary tumor cannot be assessed
T0	No evidence of primary tumor
Tis	Carcinoma *in situ*
T1	Tumor 2 cm or less in greatest dimension with less than two high risk features**
T2	Tumor greater than 2 cm in greatest dimension or Tumor any size with two or more high risk features*
T3	Tumor with invasion of maxilla, orbit, or temporal bone
T4	Tumor with invasion of skeleton (axial or appendicular) or perineural invasion of skull base
	* Excludes cSCC of the eyelid—See Chapter 48.

	** High Risk Features for the Primary Tumor (T) Staging:
	    Depth/Invasion: > 2 mm thickness, Clark level ≥ IV, Perineural invasion
	    Anatomic Location: Primary site ear, Primary site hair-bearing lip
	    Differentiation: Poorly differentiated or undifferentiated

Regional Lymph Nodes (N)	
NX	Regional lymph nodes cannot be assessed
N0	No regional lymph node metastasis
N1	Metastasis in a single ipsilateral lymph node, 3 cm or less in greatest dimension
N2	Metastasis in a single ipsilateral lymph node, more than 3 cm but not more than 6 cm in greatest dimension; or in multiple ipsilateral lymph nodes, none more than 6 cm in greatest dimension; or in bilateral or contralateral lymph nodes, none more than 6 cm in greatest dimension
N2a	Metastasis in a single ipsilateral lymph node, more than 3 cm but not more than 6 cm in greatest dimension
N2b	Metastasis in multiple ipsilateral lymph nodes, none more than 6 cm in greatest dimension
N2c	Metastasis in bilateral or contralateral lymph nodes, none more than 6 cm in greatest dimension
N3	Metastasis in a lymph node, more than 6 cm in greatest dimension
Distant Metastasis (M)	
M0	No distant metastasis (no pathologic M0; use clinical M to complete stage group)
M1	Distant metastasis

Pathologic

Group	T	N	M
☐ 0	Tis	N0	M0
☐ I	T1	N0	M0
☐ II	T2	N0	M0
☐ III	T3	N0	M0
	T1	N1	M0
	T2	N1	M0
	T3	N1	M0
☐ IV	T1	N2	M0
	T2	N2	M0
	T3	N2	M0
	T Any	N3	M0
	T4	N Any	M0
	T Any	N Any	M1
☐ Stage unknown			

Used with the permission of the American Joint Committee on Cancer (AJCC), Chicago, Illinois. The original source for this material is the AJCC Cancer Staging Manual, Seventh Edition (2010) published by Springer Science and Business Media LLC, www.springer.com.

Table 24.2 Staging system for Merkel cell carcinoma

Primary Tumor (T)	
TX	Primary tumor cannot be assessed
T0	No evidence of primary tumor
Tis	*In situ* primary tumor
T1	Less than or equal to 2 cm maximum tumor dimension
T2	Greater than 2 cm but not more than 5 cm maximum tumor dimension
T3	Over 5 cm maximum tumor dimension
T4	Primary tumor invades bone, muscle, fascia, or cartilage
Regional Lymph Nodes (N)	
NX	Regional lymph nodes cannot be assessed
N0	No regional lymph node metastasis Nodes negative by clinical exam* (no pathologic node exam performed) Nodes negative by pathologic exam
N1	Metastasis in regional lymph node(s) Micrometastasis** Macrometastasis***
N2	In transit metastasis****
	* Clinical detection of nodal disease may be via inspection, palpation, and/or imaging
	** Micrometastases are diagnosed after sentinel or elective lymphadenectomy
	*** Macrometastases are defined as clinically detectable nodal metastases confirmed by therapeutic lymphadenectomy or needle biopsy
	**** In transit metastasis: a tumor distinct from the primary lesion and located either 1) between the primary lesion and the draining regional lymph nodes or 2) distal to the primary lesion
Distant Metastasis (M)	
M0	No distant metastasis (no pathologic M0; use clinical M to complete stage group)
M1	Metastasis beyond regional lymph nodes
M1a	Metastasis to skin, subcutaneous tissues, or distant lymph nodes
M1b	Metastasis to lung
M1c	Metastasis to all other visceral sites

Pathologic			
Group	**T**	**N**	**M**
☐ 0	Tis	N0	M0
☐ IA	T1	pN0	M0
☐ IB	T1	cN0	M0
☐ IIA	T2/T3	pN0	M0
☐ IIB	T2/T3	cN0	M0
☐ IIC	T4	N0	M0
☐ IIIA	Any T	N1a	M0
☐ IIIB	Any T	N1b/N2	M0
☐ IV	Any T	Any N	M1
☐ Stage unknown			

Used with the permission of the American Joint Committee on Cancer (AJCC), Chicago, Illinois. The original source for this material is the AJCC Cancer Staging Manual, Seventh Edition (2010) published by Springer Science and Business Media LLC, www.springer.com.

trigeminal and facial nerves. Perineural invasion (PNI) has a large impact on prognosis but can often present with subtle symptoms, so care must be taken to look for signs of PNI in the patient history as well as the physical exam.

The physical exam should include a complete examination of the head and neck, including assessing for any other skin malignancies and cervical metastasis, as well as evidence of PNI. A whole-body exam by a dermatologist may be needed in high-risk patients.

Imaging

In patients with large or potentially deeply invasive lesions, computed tomography (CT) or magnetic resonance imaging (MRI) can be ordered to evaluate for invasion into adjacent structures and to look for cervical metastasis. If bone invasion is suspected, then a CT scan should be ordered, and if PNI is suspected an MRI scan is needed. If larger nerves are involved, PNI can be detected on MRI, but it is rare to find radiological evidence of PNI in asymptomatic patients. The role of positron-emission tomography (PET)-CT in patients with NMSC is unclear at this time.

Diagnosis

Early BCCs are usually small, translucent, or pearly with raised telangiectatic edges. Indurated edges and an ulcerative center are common features. Several distinct growth patterns of BCCs are noted. Nodular lesions, which constitute ~ 75% of BCC, often present as raised, pearly, well-circumscribed lesions with overlying telangiectasias. Superficial BCC accounts for 10% of BCC, is less common on the head and neck, and usually presents as a red, scaly plaque. Morphea-form or sclerosing-type BCC often shows a fibrotic yellowish plaque with indistinct borders, and is often the most aggressive form of BCC.

Cutaneous SCC is most common on actinically damaged skin, and can present as papules, nodules, or plaques. It can be hyperkeratotic or ulcerative, and may bleed or be painful. The most common presentation of cSCC is of an exophytic growth, with overlying hyperkeratosis and ulceration on a background of sun-damaged atrophic skin.

Diagnosis is made clinically but is confirmed with biopsy. The preferred method of biopsy depends on the size of the lesion and the judgment of the physician. For smaller lesions, an excisional biopsy is appropriate; for larger tumors, an incisional or punch biopsy is often sufficient for diagnosis. The pathology should mention grade, depth, size, and presence of perineural invasion.

■ Management and Treatment

Surgical excision is the preferred treatment for most NMSC and can involve conventional resection or Mohs micrographic surgery. Surgical excision allows for histological examination of excised tissues and ensures complete removal of all tumor. Other modalities, such as electrodessication and cryotherapy, radiation, photodynamic therapy, and such topical medicines imiquimod and fluorouracil, are occasionally used in the treatment of small cSCC or BCC of the head and neck; however, these modalities should be avoided in the management of high-risk cSCC.

Mohs Microsurgery

Mohs microsurgery is commonly used in the treatment of NMSC. In Mohs surgery the excised tissue is frozen and sectioned horizontally, and the margin is examined intraoperatively. Further excision is done only at the site of residual tumor, allowing for greater certainty of tumor excision and increased tissue conservation. Mohs surgery is commonly used in areas that demand maximal preservation of normal tissues. Very high cure rates between 95 to 98% have been reported in the high-risk subsites of ears and lips. In patients with large or aggressive NMSC, wide local excision with the patient under general anesthesia is often preferable to Mohs surgery, due to the possibility of invasion of deeper tissue or peripheral nerves.

Surgical Treatment of Primary Lesion

Excision of the primary site with appropriate margins is the first step in treating patients with NMSC. Studies have shown that excision of low-risk cSCC with 4 mm margins provides a cure rate of 95%, whereas a 6 mm margin is required for a 95% cure rate in high-risk lesions. The margin required for small BCCs is similar to that for cSCC. Larger or recurrent BCCs often require increased margins, with the literature supporting margins ranging from 5 to 15 mm.

Risk Stratification

The key to successfully treating cSCC while minimizing morbidity and maximizing survival is to identify the subgroup of patients who are at risk for local recurrence and for regional metastatic spread of disease. The vast majority of patients with cSCC and BCC of the head and neck are not at significant risk of developing nodal metastasis and can be classified as low risk. In this group of patients surgical excision alone is usually sufficient treatment. Regional lymph node metastases are rare in cSCC of the head and neck, with reported incidence generally being < 5%. However, patients with high-risk clinical and pathological features may present with up to a 20% risk of regional lymph node metastasis. This high-risk patient group may require treatment of the lymph nodes via either lymph node dissection or radiation.

One issue facing surgeons treating cSCC is that the definition of a high-risk patient is not consistently reported in the literature. The new American Joint Committee on Cancer (AJCC) Staging System recognizes the potential for metastasis and the risk of mortality in this high-risk subgroup by separating cSCC from other nonmelanotic skin cancers, and incorporating tumor-specific staging features that should help identify patients at risk.

Risk factors for cervical metastasis include size of the primary tumor greater than 2 cm, Breslow tumor thickness greater than 2 mm, Clark level IV or greater invasion, PNI, poor differentiation, high-risk anatomical sites, immunocompromised state, and local recurrent disease.

Tumor Size

Increased tumor size has been shown to correlate with local recurrence and metastasis. Several studies support 2 cm as the threshold above which tumors are more likely to metastasize to regional lymph nodes, and the AJCC has adopted 2 cm as a key delineating feature between T1 and T2 tumors. However, tumors less than 2 cm still pose a risk for regional metastasis in the presence of other high-risk features, with some studies showing up to 70% of skin cancers presenting with regional metastasis having a primary lesion less than 2 cm in diameter.

Tumor Thickness/Depth of Invasion

Both tumor thickness and depth of invasion have been recognized as important features in the prognosis of patients with cSCC, and studies have shown that both tumor thickness and depth of invasion correlate with an increased risk of metastasis. Studies have shown almost no patients with metastasis if the primary tumor was < 2 mm thick, approximately a 4% rate of metastasis in patients with tumors 2 to 6 mm, and approximately a 15% rate of metastasis if the depth of invasion is greater than 6 mm. Studies have also demonstrated increasing metastatic rates if the tumor invaded muscle or bone compared with subcutaneous tissue. In general, lesions greater than 2 mm in depth or Clark level IV or higher (invasion into subcutaneous tissue) are considered high risk.

Anatomical Site

The nonglabrous lip and ear have increased local and metastatic potential, and both are considered high-risk subsites.

Perineural Invasion

Tumors with PNI have a higher incidence of local recurrence as well as regional and distant metastasis, have the potential to extend into the skull base via cranial nerves, and demonstrate significantly reduced survival compared with those without PNI. Between 0.18 and 10% of patients with BCC and 2.5 to 14% of patients with cSCC demonstrate PNI on histopathology. Studies have shown a significant increase in local recurrence, nodal metastasis, and distant metastasis for patients with PNI compared with those without.

Patients with PNI are classified into two groups: those with PNI detected on microscopic evaluation and those who have clinical or radiographic findings. Patients with clinical features of PNI have a worse prognosis than those where PNI is just an incidental finding on histology, and patients with clinical PNI had worse 5-year local control rates than those with incidental PNI.

PNI can occur in primary tumors or in recurrent tumors. Studies have shown that, compared with primary tumors with PNI, recurrent tumors with PNI have a significantly higher rate of local and regional failures.

Recurrent Lesions

Recurrent cSCC is associated with approximately a 25% rate of local recurrence and a 30% risk of metastasis, significantly higher rates compared with nonrecurrent cSCC. Recurrent cSCC has a worse prognosis, partly because of its significantly increased rate of PNI compared with primary tumors. These factors lead to decreased survival in patients with recurrent lesions, with studies demonstrating that the 5-year survival in patients with recurrent cancer is only ~ 30% compared with almost 90% in patients at initial presentation.

Immunosuppression

Immunosuppressed patients with cSCC often present with more advanced tumors and have been shown to have worse outcome in advanced disease than immunocompetent patients. A staggering 5.2% of organ transplant patients die from skin malignancies, the majority of which are cSCC.

Grade

Poorly differentiated tumors have been found to have a significantly worse prognosis than well-differentiated tumors, with some studies showing almost 100% cure rate in well-differentiated tumors compared with only ~ 40% in poorly differentiated tumors.

Areas of Previous Scar

Patients with cSCC developing in scars from burns or trauma or in areas subject to chronic inflammation are at higher risk for aggressive behavior and metastasis. Cutaneous SCCs developing in scars have a metastatic rate of up to 40% and cSCCs arising in chronic ulcers have a regional metastatic rate of 36 to 54% and a 5-year survival of 52 to 75%.

Elective Nodal Treatment

Treatment—either surgery or radiotherapy—of clinically negative parotid and cervical lymph nodes in patients with high-risk features of the primary sites should be considered, but no consensus exists regarding when treatment of clinically negative nodal basins is needed. If radiation is being given to the primary site due to high-risk features, radiation may be considered as a potential treatment option for at-risk nodal basins. Elective treatment of at-risk nodal basins is more commonly used when multiple high-risk features are present in the primary site, such as recurrent cSCC with PNI. However, no data yet exist supporting or advocating against the use of radiation in the clinically negative neck in patients with high-risk primary cSCC, and treatment regimens can vary greatly among physicians.

Sentinel Lymph Node Biopsy

Sentinel lymph node biopsy (SLNB) is widely used in the treatment of melanoma and Merkel cell carcinoma, but is less commonly used in the treatment of cSCC. SLNB is a potentially useful means of assessing whether metastasis has occurred in patients with high-risk primary lesions. The ability of SLNB to identify specific patterns of drainage is particularly useful in cSCC, due to the variable drainage pattern of head and neck skin cancers, and the potential involvement of parotid and/or cervical lymph nodes. As of now all studies regarding the use of SNLB in cSCC are small case reports, but many show encouraging results. Although SLNB may prove useful in the treatment of cSCC, its role is currently unproven, and more studies need to be performed before specific recommendations can be made.

■ Treatment of Cervical Lymph Node Metastasis

Pattern of Spread

The nodal basins at risk from cSCC depend on both the location of the primary lesion and the unique drainage pattern of the individual. Parotid area nodes and levels I to V of the neck are the most frequent nodal basins involved; however, care must be taken to include the external jugular lymph nodes superficial to the SCM adjacent to the external jugular vein when performing neck dissections because they are also at risk in most cSCC.

Patients with anterior disease involving the nose, cheek, or lip are more likely to benefit from level I dissection, whereas posterior lesions rarely involve level I. Level V is rarely involved in isolation and is usually only dissected in posterior primary lesions involving the pinna, posterior neck, or posterior scalp of cSCC patients with nodal metastasis. Seventy to 80% develop nodal metastasis after treatment of the primary site (as opposed to presenting with both local and regional disease). The average time to presentation for regional metastatic disease is ~ 12 months after treatment of the primary site, and almost all metastases present within the first 2 to 3 years.

Extent of Surgery

All clinically positive lymphadenopathy, either by physical exam or by radiology, should be treated surgically if possible. This usually entails some combination of a superficial parotidectomy, in the case of facial and anterior scalp primaries, and neck dissection. An approximately equal distribution exists between patients with parotid metastasis alone, cervical metastasis alone, and combined parotid and cervical metastases. Studies show that when parotid area lymph nodes are involved, synchronous spread to level II to V nodes occurs in 15 to 30% of cases. As such, it is common practice to perform a selective neck dissection for the N0 neck in a patient with parotid metastasis.

Patients with parotid metastasis but a clinically N0 neck show approximately a 20% rate of metastasis to the neck, with level II being the most likely level involved. Although there is no consensus on the extent of neck dissection needed in cases with parotid metastasis, these data suggest that some form of neck dissection involving level II/III and the external jugular nodes should be performed. In cases with anterior primary sites a level I dissection may be added, and in cases with posterior primary sites a level IV/V dissection may be added.

If cervical metastases are present but the parotid is not clinically involved, there is no consensus on whether a parotidectomy should be performed. In general, it is more common to electively treat the neck in patients with parotid-only disease than it is to treat the parotid surgically in cases with cervical-only disease. Some centers advocate performing a parotidectomy in patients with cervical nodal disease only if the primary tumor arises from sites that commonly drain to the parotid, such as the root of the nose, eyelids, frontolateral scalp, pinnae, external auditory canal, and cheek. Other centers choose to radiate the parotid along with the postdissection neck in cases with clinical neck disease and no parotid disease because some studies have shown a high rate of occult parotid metastasis in patients with cN0 parotid but N+ neck.

Adjuvant Therapy

While earlier studies often recommended surgery alone for the treatment of cSCC, more recent studies support combined treatment with surgery and adjuvant radiation in operable patients with regional metastatic disease. With combined treatment of surgery and radiation, most studies demonstrate a 5-year disease-free survival rate of 60 to 70%, and many studies document the addition of adjuvant radiotherapy as a significant independent factor for increased survival.

In patients with both parotid and cervical metastatic disease, most centers would recommend a modified radical neck dissection with a superficial parotidectomy and adjuvant therapy to both nodal basins. The treatment of patients with disease in only cervical nodes or parotid nodes is more variable. Some centers forgo the dissection of the uninvolved nodal basins and instead treat with postoperative radiation, whereas others choose to operate on both uninvolved and involved basins. Although regional control for uninvolved basins is similar for both radiation and surgery, dissection of the clinically uninvolved neck or parotid may spare radiotherapy

to part of the neck or decrease the dose of radiation needed. Studies have shown that patients with a single node < 3 cm without extracapsular spread treated with surgery alone have a very low recurrence rate, suggesting that radiation may be spared in patients with small nodal disease without worrisome features.

Currently there is no proven role of chemotherapy in patients with cSCC, but because of its demonstrated benefit in advanced head and neck mucosal SCC, many centers treat advanced cases of cSCC with chemoradiation, despite the lack of evidence supporting its use in cSCC.

Merkel Cell Carcinoma

Merkel cell carcinoma is a rare but aggressive form of NMSC that occurs in ~ 1,000 patients a year. It arises from cutaneous mechanoreceptor cells (Merkel cells) located in the basal layer of the epidermis. Like cSCC, this lesion is more common in Caucasians with a history of significant sun exposure, as well as the immunocompromised. Typically, this neoplasm presents as a rapidly growing, dome-shaped, red or bluish nodule. In addition, the tumor may sometimes have a plaque-like appearance with small satellite lesions.

Merkel cell carcinoma is usually treated with wide local excision, followed by adjuvant radiation. Historically, Merkel cell carcinoma has been treated with 2 to 3 cm margins, but some studies suggest that 1 cm margins are adequate for small lesions. Regional lymphatics are often addressed with some combination of surgery and radiation, although there is no consensus as to ideal treatment, and some people suggest that lymphatic treatment is not needed for small lesions. In the N0 neck, SLNB is commonly used.

Merkel cell carcinoma is an aggressive cancer. The 5-year survival rate of these patients is 75%, 5%, and 25% for primary tumors, lymph node metastases, and distant metastases, respectively. More than one-third of patients diagnosed with Merkel cell carcinoma will die of the disease.

◼ Practice Guidelines, Consensus Statements, and Measures

National Comprehensive Cancer Network NCNN Guidelines. http://www.nccn.org/professionals/physician_gls/f_guidelines.asp

■ Suggested Reading

Bichakjian CK, Lowe L, Lao CD, et al. Merkel cell carcinoma: critical review with guidelines for multidisciplinary management. Cancer 2007;110(1):1–12

Brantsch KD, Meisner C, Schönfisch B, et al. Analysis of risk factors determining prognosis of cutaneous squamous-cell carcinoma: a prospective study. Lancet Oncol 2008;9(8):713–720

Ch'ng S, Maitra A, Allison RS, et al. Parotid and cervical nodal status predict prognosis for patients with head and neck metastatic cutaneous squamous cell carcinoma. J Surg Oncol 2008;98(2): 101–105

Ebrahimi A, Moncrieff MD, Clark JR, et al. Predicting the pattern of regional metastases from cutaneous squamous cell carcinoma of the head and neck based on location of the primary. Head Neck 2010;32(10):1288–1294

Farasat S, Yu SS, Neel VA, et al. A new American Joint Committee on Cancer staging system for cutaneous squamous cell carcinoma: creation and rationale for inclusion of tumor (T) characteristics. J Am Acad Dermatol 2011;64(6):1051–1059

Madan V, Lear JT, Szeimies RM. Non-melanoma skin cancer. Lancet 2010;375(9715):673–685

Veness MJ. High-risk cutaneous squamous cell carcinoma of the head and neck. J Biomed Biotechnol 2007;2007(3):80572

25 Oral Cavity Cancer

■ Introduction

Squamous cell tumors represent 90% of all oral malignancies. Survival following treatment for oral cavity carcinoma has not changed appreciably in the last half century. However, there have been significant new insights into the understanding of the behavior of this disease over the past 10 years.

Classification

The oral cavity consists of the alveolar ridge, buccal area, floor of mouth, tongue, retromolar trigone, and hard palate. These systems make an allowance for G-stage cancer, which is a histopathological grade, and for R-stage cancer, which is the presence or absence of residual tumor after treatment (**Table 25.1**).

Epidemiology

Six percent of all malignancies are head and neck carcinomas. Of these, 30% are oral cavity carcinoma. The National Cancer Institute reported an estimated 40,250 new cases of oral cancer in 2012 with 7,850 deaths. The peak incidence of oral cavity squamous cell carcinoma (SCC) is in the fourth and fifth decades of life, and the male-to-female ratio ranges from 2:1 to 4:1. Although smoking and alcohol have strong association with oral cancer, there has also been an increased awareness of the role of smokeless tobacco in the induction of oral cavity carcinoma. Chewing tobacco seems to be a distinct causal substance in the carcinogenesis of verrucous carcinoma of the oral cavity. Betel nut chewing continues to be a culprit in the etiology of carcinoma of the oral cavity in India, where the incidence is as high as 50% of all cancers.

A link between viruses and oral cavity cancer relating specifically to verrucous carcinoma and human papilloma virus has been described, but occurrence is more common in the pharynx than in the oral cavity. The use of advanced molecular biological techniques has helped to substantiate this association and identify additional potential biomarkers, although none are validated.

Biological Behavior

Basic Science

Much work has been performed in the past 10 years in the fields of immunology, cell biology, immunohistochemistry, and molecular biology. The specialty of head and neck oncology has made immense strides, with emphasis in many large centers on the basic science of oral SCC. Certainly, the improvement of existing immunohistochemical procedures and the discovery of major molecular biological techniques, such as polymerase chain reaction, have presented numerous opportunities to delve into previously uncharted territories regarding cellular behavior at its most fundamental level.

Investigators have studied many potential biomarkers for oral cancer. The use of the cell surface monoclonal antibody A9 antigen expression, combined with loss of expression of the normal blood group antigens, has been suggested as a good prognostic marker. It has also been shown that the cell surface molecule, integrin, which serves as a tumor suppressor, may be part of a multimolecular signal cascade that is disrupted in the process of carcinogenesis. The finding of overexpression of certain oncogenes, such as mutant p53, has also been implicated in the carcinogenesis of SCC. This conclusion has been reproducible in many centers. Furthermore, point mutations of p53 have been reported in 45% of head and neck SCCs. With respect to lymphocyte activity, there are reports that CD4+ T cells respond to autotumor by cytokinin production and proliferation and by inducing expansion of CD8+ effector T cells, which may be important in tumor immunosurveillance and destruction. Others have shown that

Table 25.1 Staging system for the oral cavity

TX	Primary tumor cannot be assessed
T0	No evidence of primary tumor
Tis	Carcinoma in situ
T1	Tumor ≤ 2 cm in greatest dimension
T2	Tumor > 2 cm but ≤ 4 cm in greatest dimension
T3	Tumor > 4 cm in greatest dimension
T4a	Moderately advanced local disease[a]
	(Lip) Tumor invades through cortical bone, inferior alveolar nerve, floor of mouth, or skin of face, that is, chin or nose
	(Oral cavity) Tumor invades adjacent structures only (e.g., through cortical bone [mandible or maxilla] into deep [extrinsic] muscle of tongue [genioglossus, hyoglossus, palatoglossus, and styloglossus], maxillary sinus, or skin of face)
T4b	Very advanced local disease
	Tumor invades masticator space, pterygoid plates, or skull base and/or encases internal carotid artery

Used with the permission of the American Joint Committee on Cancer (AJCC), Chicago, Illinois. The original source for this material is the AJCC Cancer Staging Manual, Seventh Edition (2010) published by Springer Science and Business Media LLC, www.springer.com.

[a] Superficial erosion alone of bone/tooth socket by gingival primary is not sufficient to classify a tumor as T4.

the T4 to T8 ratio of lymphocytes, when perturbed in SCC, portends a poor prognosis. These and other findings in cellular biology beg for further work to elucidate the complex interactions of cancer cells to lymphocytes.

Clinical Considerations

The local, regional, and distant biological activities of oral cavity SCC have been well described. The primary tumor tends to invade locally but may grow exophytically or invasively, the latter of which is associated with a poorer prognosis. With respect to the invasive pattern, the incidence of metastatic spread and survivorship is directly related to tumor thickness. These findings may play an important role in the evolution of future classification systems.

A major observation has been the substantiation of the metastatic patterns of spread of oral cavity carcinoma. These patterns have been noted in large cohorts of patients, with the important finding that a considerable frequency of patients has early occult

metastatic disease. This has led to the liberal performance of neck dissection for T1 and T2 lesions. Elective neck treatment is indicated for tongue tumors with thickness of ≥ 4 mm. For floor of mouth tumors, occult neck metastases occur in 33% of cases with thickness of 1.6 to 3.5 mm, and in 60% of cases with thickness > 3.6 mm. Depth of invasion is critical information to be obtained on diagnostic biopsy because this allows for preoperative determination of whether an elective neck dissection is to be performed. Pathological findings of perineural invasion (PNI) and perivascular invasion (PVI) independently serve as indications for adjuvant radiation. The N0 neck can also be treated electively with radiation therapy, and knowledge of PNI or PVI may influence the surgeon's management of the neck.

Histopathology

The histopathological reporting of SCC and all its precursors is well documented. Attempts have been made to grade histopathological patterns according to tumor factors (keratin production, grade, nuclear appearance, and mitoses), together with tumor host factors (inflammation, desmoplastic reaction, patterns of invasion, and vascular invasion). The incorporation of these parameters in tumor classification may assist in prognosticating and reporting results and aid in intercenter comparisons.

■ Evaluation

Diagnostic Imaging

In the 1980s and 1990s the application of existing technologies continued, and several new modalities showed promise in imaging of primary cancer and detection of metastases. The use of computed tomography (CT) and magnetic resonance imaging (MRI) is now standard in the mapping of the primary tumor in the oral cavity. The modalities complement each other in providing information on the extent of a soft tissue lesion (MRI) and the soft tissue and bone involvement. These applications removed the guesswork from determining the extent of lesions and have helped in decision-making as to the extent of resection, target localization for radiotherapy, proximity of vital structures, and extent of bone (mandible and maxilla) involvement. However, plain and panoramic dental radiographs are still very useful in assessing bone invasion.

CT and MRI have had limited application in staging the neck. Most series report sensitivities and specificities of 70 to 85%. Although accurate these statistics are not exact enough to make management decisions; in fact, in some studies, clinical examination is just as accurate as imaging. Therefore, clinicians must make recommendations regarding neck management (e.g., to perform an elective neck dissection) based on the T status and histological characteristics of the primary and historical evidence on the incidence of neck metastases in the particular situation. Many major studies have demonstrated that CT and MRI can upstage the clinically negative neck disease in a significant proportion of cases (~ 20%); this point is of obvious significant consequence in managing the neck.

There is also a role for ultrasonography in the assessment of cervical metastases from oral cavity SCC. It has been well described as a reliable determination of lymph node metastases in the neck using ultrasound-guided fine needle aspiration biopsy. Reports have noted sensitivities and specificities of up to 95% in accurately registering the status of the neck. To be successful, this methodology is dependent on experienced ultrasonographers, technicians, and cytopathologists. Notwithstanding these conditions, the results are very encouraging and may be, if reproducible, a significant breakthrough in neck management.

Positron-emission tomography (PET) and PET-CT fusion are commonly used in initial staging as well as surveillance imaging in head and neck cancers. Although there is some controversy with their use, these technologies have important utility in imaging distant metastasis and cervical node involvement. PET scans use focal fluorodeoxyglucose uptake to identify cells that are highly metabolic by their glucose uptake. They are full body scans and when fused with CT can be used to identify metastatic lesions as well as other primary tumors. PET-CT is an excellent modality for posttreatment evaluation where the anatomy is altered and recurrent disease may be difficult to detect on physical exam. Posttreatment PET-CT has good accuracy for identifying patients who can avoid neck dissection after definitive chemoradiotherapy for head and neck cancer. Physical exam and imaging remain important diagnostic modalities for primary oral cavity cancers.

◼ Treatment

The treatment of oral cavity SCC traditionally has involved surgery, radiation, or a combination of both. In the past 10 years, however, efforts have been made to introduce variations of these or newer means to treat oral cavity cancer. Generally, the treatment of early primary stages (T1 and T2) involves surgery, whereas the treatment of advanced disease (T3 and T4) involves surgery, combined surgery and radiation, radiation alone, or chemotherapy and radiation.

Photodynamic Therapy

This promising modality is undergoing further investigation. Its exact role has yet to be defined. Theoretically, photodynamic therapy (PDT) allows for the directed targeting of cancer cells with sparing of surrounding tissue. The complicated three-dimensional anatomy of the head and neck can make PDT challenging. Additionally, studies show upregulation of factors that confer resistance of cancer cells to PDT.

Chemotherapy

Chemotherapy plays an adjuvant and palliative role in oral cancer. Extracapsular spread of cervical nodes and positive resection margins of the primary tumor are indications for the addition of chemotherapy to radiation as adjuvant therapy. Chemotherapy as monotherapy is not used in oral cavity cancer. There is also an expanding use of concurrent chemotherapy and radiation therapy in stage III and IV cancer, particularly if a total glossectomy would be required for surgical management.

Radiation Therapy

As mentioned, radiation has been used as primary treatment, especially in advanced disease, or in combination with surgery. Indications of postoperative radiation therapy include more than one positive lymph node, extracapsular spread of cervical nodes, positive resection margins of the primary tumor, perineural or perivascular invasion, and advanced stage. Positive margins and extracapsular spread are indications for adjuvant chemoradiotherapy. The indications of primary radiotherapy for oral cavity cancer include T1-T2 disease in a patient who is a poor surgical candidate, early disease with poor expected cosmetic outcome (lip), and unresectable disease.

Important research has been conducted in attempting to improve radiation administration to oral cavity cancer. Trials in hyperfractionation (administration of more than one dose per day) have begun to show improved response rates in advanced disease. Intensity-modulated radiotherapy is being used as adjuvant therapy in the hope of reducing oral complications, such as osteoradionecrosis of the mandible. Interstitial radiotherapy (brachytherapy) delivers radioactive sources in direct proximity to the target tumor area and allows for rapid "fall off" of surrounding normal tissue. This can be used as a substitute for external beam radiation, but it has a high rate of osteoradionecrosis. Its use in the primary setting is mostly limited to superficial lesions that are more than 5 mm from the mandible.

Surgery

Surgery is the main treatment modality for oral cavity carcinoma. The issues that have to be addressed before undertaking a surgical intervention are the accurate staging of the disease, the precise assessment of the general condition of the patient, and the correct determination of the presence or absence of another primary tumor. Physical examination, appropriate laboratory investigations, and diagnostic imaging can deal with the first two concerns. Finally, before the surgical procedure, panendoscopy is necessary to evaluate the tumor as well as rule out synchronous primary tumors.

With regard to the surgical procedure, specific consideration must be given to dealing with the primary disease, the neck, the mandible, and, finally, the reconstruction.

Management of the Primary and Mandible

The surgical approach is dependent on the size and location of the primary tumor. Generally, T1 and T2 tumors can be adequately and appropriately removed by a transoral resection. Several surgeons report on lower morbidity if the laser is used instead of the scalpel or electrocautery. The resulting defect may be left open to heal by secondary intention, covered with split-thickness skin graft, or closed primarily. In some instances, a local mucosal flap can be employed with little impairment of speech and swallowing.

The "mandibular swing" approach to posterior oral cavity lesions has gained popularity for lesions that present difficult accessibility. This technique can also be safely performed in the postradiation patient. Recently, transoral laser surgery and transoral robotic surgery (TORS) have gained popularity in addressing these posterior lesions because this allows resection without mandibulotomy. TORS allows for unprecedented visualization and access to the posterior oral cavity and oropharynx and resection of tumors with decreased morbidity and improved cosmesis and function.

Larger lesions (T3 and T4), of course, necessitate the removal of more tissue, which has a greater impact on speech and swallowing function as well as potential cosmetic compromise. With respect to the mandible, over the past decade there has been an intense effort to spare the mandible or at least a rim, if at all possible, and thereby avoid the cosmetic disability rendered by a segmental resection. If a tumor presents with an area of normal tissue between it and the mandible, resection of the latter is usually not necessary. If the tumor is attached to the periosteum of the mandible without evidence of bone invasion, a rim resection can be performed. If direct invasion of bone is suspected or proven radiographically, segmental resection is mandatory. For additional bony defects, such as the hard palate, a prefabricated dental obturator can be inserted and secured at the time of surgery, or the defect can be closed by a free-flap reconstruction as an alternate method of closure.

Perioperative antibiotic coverage has played a major role in avoiding infectious complications. It is generally accepted that the choice of antibiotic should be targeted to the potential infecting organisms of the upper aerodigestive tract. These antibiotics usually include a third-generation cephalosporin combined with an antianaerobic drug. With respect to timing, the medication is commonly administered immediately preoperatively and for 24 to 48 hours postoperatively.

Management of the Neck

The purpose of a neck operation in oral cavity tumors is to remove clinical and/or occult disease. For oral cavity carcinoma, there is a menu of neck dissections that are less than radical but that still afford a comprehensive removal of metastatic neck disease. The options include the radical neck dissection (RND) or modified neck dissection (MND) (sparing the spinal accessory nerve while removing nodal levels I–V); selective neck dissections, such as a supraomohyoid neck dissection (sparing the accessory nerve, internal jugular vein, and sternomastoid muscle while removing nodal levels I–III); and an anterolateral neck dissection (sparing the accessory nerve, internal jugular vein, and sternomastoid muscle while removing nodal levels II–IV).

For oral cavity SCC, the type of neck dissection is determined by the extent of nodal disease. For the clinically negative neck (N_0) there is a high rate of occult metastases from oral cavity carcinoma, and the location of these potential metastases is predictable. Therefore, an "elective" neck dissection should be undertaken to encompass all potential metastatic nodes in the areas most likely to be involved (most often levels I–III, including level IV for anterior lesions). The supraomohyoid neck dissection is appropriate for this purpose. Should positive nodes be identified intraoperatively, the extent of dissection can be increased. More data are needed to ascertain with certainty whether this type of neck dissection is diagnostic (allowing for postoperative radiation) or therapeutic. If a lesion crosses the midline and the opposite neck is N_0, a contralateral selective neck dissection may be done because of the high incidence of occult contralateral nodal disease. The RND or MND is performed for the N+ neck—both with comparable control results with regard to disease. However, it is highly desirable to spare the spinal accessory nerve if there is no evidence of gross invasion. If a bilateral neck dissection is required for disease on both sides of the neck, every effort should be made to spare at least one internal jugular vein to avoid potential complications of increased intracranial pressure. Several indicators of poor prognosis in the neck have been identified: size of nodes > 3 cm; multiple nodes; very high or low nodes; extracapsular spread; tumor emboli; and extension to other structures, such as skin, nerve, bone, major vessel, and aerodigestive tract. When feasible, the neck dissection should be extended to encompass removal of such disease (extracapsular) extension.

Reconstruction

Small defects of the oral cavity can be managed with leaving the defects open, primary closure, or skin grafting. In the 1970s and early 1980s, major soft tissue reconstruction of the oral cavity was performed with regional flaps with the pectoralis major myocutaneous flap providing large, reliable bulky skin in one stage. This flap is still useful for lateral oral cavity defects.

The free vascularized flap for oral cavity reconstruction provides greater versatility of reconstruction and improved cosmetic results. Surgical success rates of flap viability are in excess of 90%. Furthermore, this technology, which requires highly specialized expertise, is now widely available. With regard to suitable donor sites for tissue transfer, the radial forearm skin or anterolateral thigh flap is optimal for defects requiring soft tissue only. For mandibular reconstruction only or with small skin requirements, the fibula free flap is best. These flaps allow for dental rehabilitation with implants. Reconstruction of the anterior mandible helps prevent the dreaded Andy Gump facial deformity. Reconstruction of the lateral mandible is less important in edentulous patients. There are also applications for the iliac, scapula, and lateral arm that can be tailored to specific defects. Some defects have been successfully rehabilitated with two simultaneous free flaps. The details regarding reconstruction of the oral cavity and the mandible can be found in Chapters 26 and 27.

Rehabilitation

Attention has been focused on rehabilitation of patients after surgery, and the impact of surgery on outcome measurements. Objective assessments of functional and cosmetic outcomes have helped surgeons, as well as radiation and medical oncologists, carefully evaluate patients prior to treatment, with the addition of quality-of-life and comorbidity scales to help all health care professionals assess head and neck cancer patients within a wider context. The evolution of the Brånemark titanium osseointegration peg has been a giant step forward in reconstruction because it has allowed fitting of dental prostheses in reconstructed oral cavities. This process has enhanced cosmesis, deglutition, and self-esteem for cancer patients.

Palliative Care

Unfortunately, many patients with oral cavity carcinoma fare poorly. Special palliative services have been developed to deal with a dying patient's needs, which may be substantial. The palliative team is trained and attuned to those myriad needs, which include pain relief, nutrition, feeding methods, and airway management. The liberal use of percutaneous gastrostomy has been very helpful. In addition, social, psychological, financial, and religious needs must be addressed. Although many of these services may be provided on an outpatient basis, at times, dying patients require more intensive care that, depending on availability, can be furnished in a hospice environment designed to serve complex needs.

■ Suggested Reading

Byers RM, El-Naggar AK, Lee YY, et al. Can we detect or predict the presence of occult nodal metastases in patients with squamous carcinoma of the oral tongue? Head Neck 1998;20(2):138–144

Edge SB, Byrd DR, Compton CC, et al., eds. American Joint Committee On Cancer Staging Manual. 7th ed. Springer, New York, NY: Springer; 2010

Ganly I, Patel S, Shah J. Early stage squamous cell cancer of the oral tongue—clinicopathologic features affecting outcome. Cancer 2012;118(1):101–111

Liao CT, Chang JT, Wang HM, et al. Analysis of risk factors of predictive local tumor control in oral cavity cancer. Ann Surg Oncol 2008;15(3):915–922

Rusthoven K, Ballonoff A, Raben D, Chen C. Poor prognosis in patients with stage I and II oral tongue squamous cell carcinoma. Cancer 2008;112(2):345–351

26 Soft Tissue Reconstruction of the Oral Cavity

■ Introduction

Advances in reconstruction of the oral cavity over the past 30 years have had a dramatic effect on the rehabilitative potential of patients who have had significant oncological ablative procedures or trauma involving this area. Prior to the mid-1980s, the major reconstructive options for oral cavity defects were the split-thickness skin graft, the deltopectoral flap, the platysma myocutaneous flap, and the pectoralis myocutaneous or myogenous flap. Since then, free tissue transfer for reconstruction of head and neck defects has been introduced and popularized, and has been adeptly applied in the oral cavity.

Anatomy and Goals of Reconstruction

When determining the appropriate option for reconstruction in the oral cavity, it is important to first gain an appreciation of what is needed to repair the defect. The oral cavity is made up of the following subsites: lips, buccal mucosa, mandible and maxillary alveolar ridges, retromolar trigones, hard palate, floor of the mouth, and oral tongue. Goals of the repair include achieving a watertight seal to avoid infection and fistula formation, reconstituting any lost bony support, and maximizing the function of the remaining tongue by restoring volume and, in some cases, sensation, while minimizing any restrictions in mobility. Therefore, the purpose of reconstruction is to optimize the patients' ability to speak, swallow, and breathe in a manner close to their premorbid state. This section focuses on defects of the oral cavity solely involving the soft tissue. Composite defects where adjacent bone of the mandible and/or maxilla are involved are discussed elsewhere.

■ Oral Cavity Reconstructive Techniques

As with any defect, surgeons should always refer to their reconstructive algorithm, starting from the simplest option to the most complex.

Primary Closure or Healing by Secondary Intention

Many defects in areas where there is adequate tissue laxity and little concern for tethering adjacent structures can be left to heal by secondary intention or closed by reapproximating the adjacent mucosal edges with absorbable sutures. Such situations include small to medium buccal mucosa and lateral tongue defects. For glossectomy closures, care must be taken to maintain adequate bulk of the tongue and to minimize tethering to the floor of the mouth, especially in dentate patients.

Skin Grafting

For defects where the defect is primarily one of mucosa, but there is significant concern for contracture with primary closure, split-thickness skin grafts can be considered. One example would be a small floor of mouth defect. The graft would be placed with the intent of decreasing the degree of restriction of tongue mobility. One disadvantage is the need for a bolster to remain in place for up to a week to optimize healing onto the underlying tissue. In situations where large bolsters are used, a tracheostomy should be considered.

Local and Regional Flaps

Despite the advances in microvascular reconstructive surgery over the past 30 years, many surgeons continue to rely on local or regional flaps for oral cavity reconstruction. Many oral cavity defects can be adequately reconstructed with these flaps, thus avoiding the potential morbidity of flap harvest, the increased operative time, and the potential vascular complications associated with the use of microvascular free tissue transfer. These local and regional flaps are very familiar to the head and neck surgeon, but several valuable modifications to these flaps have been described in the last decade.

Temporoparietal Fascial Flap

The temporoparietal fascial flap (TPFF) is the only pedicled thin fascia flap in the head and neck region. The fascia is the continuation of the superficial musculoaponeurotic system of the face and receives its blood supply from the superficial temporal artery and vein. The flap superiorly becomes the galea aponeurosis, and as such, can be difficult to harvest without prior experience. Once freed from the scalp and the underlying temporalis fascia, however, the fascia can be pedicled on its vessels inferior to the zygomatic arch. Therefore the fascia can be used for oral cavity reconstruction, as well as orbital, skull base, and auricular reconstruction.

The flap is harvested through a hemicoronal or a y-type incision placed behind the anterior and temporal hair line, incising only skin and dermis. Flaps are raised in a subdermal plane just deep to the level of the hair follicles, and care is taken to avoid the area of the frontal branch of the facial nerve. The posterior branches of the superficial temporal artery and vein are identified and kept intact and are followed proximally until the facial nerve branches are reached. Further proximal dissection puts the facial nerve at risk and should be avoided. Once adequate length and width of the flap are ensured, the flap margins are incised down to the temporal fascia and the flap is raised off the fascia in an avascular plane. The pedicle is then skeletonized if further flap length is necessary. The fascia is tunneled under the zygomatic arch and delivered into the oral cavity wound. The flap is sutured into the defect, and a split-thickness skin graft is applied.

The TPFF is best used for closing hemipalatal defects and re-creating buccal epithelial lining in cases where soft tissue injury or resection has involved the hard palate or cheek. Its advantages are its thin, pliable nature and reliable blood supply, which promotes healing and encourages skin graft survival. Its disadvantages include the risk to the frontal branch of the facial nerve during flap harvest, and temporary—and occasionally permanent—alopecia at the donor site.

Melolabial Flaps (Nasolabial Flaps)

The melolabial flap is well known to the otolaryngologist because of its use in facial reconstruction after trauma or tumor surgery. In almost all cases, it is harvested as a fasciocutaneous flap, with a random blood supply based superiorly or inferiorly, although its harvest as a myocutaneous flap has been described. In the case of oral cavity reconstruction, the flap is usually pedicled inferiorly and used to fill defects in the anterior and lateral floor of the mouth and to cover the mandibular alveolus. The process therefore requires a two-stage procedure, with flap division ~ 3 weeks after the definitive tumor removal, and first-stage flap insetting. Additionally, due to the risk of dental trauma to the pedicle during this time, the use of these flaps is not advisable in patients with associated dentition. Bilateral melolabial flaps may be needed for larger defects.

Complications associated with the melolabial flap include partial flap loss, facial scar, and intraoral hair growth. The main advantage of this flap is its thin, pliable nature and ease of harvest. However, it is nonsensate tissue and has a limited size, depending on facial skin laxity.

Submental Flap

The submental flap is a musculocutaneous flap pedicled on the submental branch of the facial artery and vein. Its design is an elliptical paddle extending from the ipsilateral mandibular angle to the contralateral submental area. The upper limb of the graft runs ~ 1 cm below the jawline, so care must be taken to avoid injury to the marginal mandibular branch of the facial nerve during elevation of this portion of the graft. The main limitation for width of the flap is what can be closed primarily.

The submental flap is usually harvested from distally to proximally (medial to lateral). Often the ipsilateral anterior belly of the digastric muscle is included with the flap, along with some of the associated submandibular space fat and lymph node contents. As a result, for patients being managed for malignancies of the oral cavity, use of the flap is contraindicated, especially if adjuvant radiation is not planned.

Pectoralis Major Myocutaneous Flap

Prior to the institution of free tissue transfer, the pectoralis rotational flap was the primary workhorse for repair of large soft tissue defects of the oral cavity. Based on the pectoral branch of the thoracoacromial artery, which pierces the claviopectoral fascia just medial to the superomedial portion of the pectoralis minor muscle, this robust flap provides a large amount of reliable soft tissue bulk and epithelial lining. Once harvested from distally to proximally, the humeral and sternal attachments are divided with the main pedicle in view to allow for adequate rotation into the neck. It is tunneled in a subplatysmal plain and is ultimately introduced into the oral cavity medial to the mandible. Upon completion of the elevation, the associated medial and lateral pectoral nerve branches can be divided to allow for muscle atrophy and to minimize the risk of banding across the pedicle that could create venous compromise. The resulting chest wall defect must then be widely undermined to allow for a tension-free closure over closed suction drains.

Free Flap Reconstruction of the Oral Cavity

In situations where the defect is sufficiently complex to demand a more detailed reconstruction than what can be offered by local or regional tissue, free flap reconstruction should be considered. Obviously, the use of these flaps, rather than local or regional pedicled flaps, demands the expertise of a trained microvascular surgeon and prolonged surgery, but the improved functional results have convinced many surgeons that the inconvenience is worth the effort. The great utility of revascularized flaps is based on several factors: (1) large surface areas can be reconstructed without introducing great bulk into the wound, thereby avoiding interference with normal tongue movement and preventing flap compression by an intact mandible; (2) the procedure avoids inferiorly based muscle pedicles, like those of pectoralis flaps, thus avoiding interference with tongue movement and potential tension on a suture line; and (3) the procedure has potential for sensation, which adds to quality of life and potentially improves function in deglutition and swallowing.

When selecting the appropriate flap, it is important to determine what needs to be replaced to optimize function. Specifically, is the defect one mainly in need of a pliable lining, or is additional bulk required? In addition, where multiple surfaces need to be relined, appropriate flap selection and surgical planning are critical to optimize the ultimate result.

Radial Forearm Free Flap

The radial forearm fasciocutaneous free flap (RFFF) was described in the late 1970s but did not gain widespread use in oral cavity reconstruction until the late 1980s. It is now considered by many authors to be the workhorse flap in modern oral cavity reconstruction because of its vascular reliability and its thin, pliable paddle.

The radial forearm flap is a fasciocutaneous flap based on the radial artery and two venae comitantes. Additional outflow from the flap occurs through the cephalic vein, which can be designed to be included in the flap. The fasciocutaneous paddle can be quite large and can encompass the entire forearm if necessary, although flaps 50 to 75 cm^2 are usually used for oral cavity reconstruction. A portion of the radius (up to 10 cm long and 40% in diameter) can also be harvested with the flap to create an osteofasciocutaneous flap; however, because of the risk of catastrophic pathological fractures of the radius, the vast majority of flaps are harvested with soft tissue only. The lateral antebrachial cutaneous nerve supplies the skin in its native site and can be harvested with the flap to allow this flap to become sensate when anastomosed to a sensory nerve in the head and neck region, usually the lingual or glossopharyngeal nerve. The median antebrachial cutaneous nerve can also be harvested with the flap when larger flaps are taken, and can be used similarly.

The RFFF is used primarily for reconstruction of moderate-to-large oral cavity defects without significant bone loss. These defects can be at any site in the oral cavity or oropharynx, but typically are composite defects involving both the tongue and the floor of the mouth. The thin flap provides for adequate mobility of the residual tongue, and its lack of bulk allows for free movement of food during oral deglutition. Also, the creation of a glossomandibular sulcus with the flap makes dental rehabilitation convenient, as compared with a bulky myocutaneous flap. Other sites for RFFF use in the oral cavity are the hard and soft palate and large, partial-thickness buccal defects.

The advantages of the radial forearm flap are numerous. The flap has a dependable blood supply with large vessels (2–4 mm) and a long vascular pedicle (up to 25 cm). Most large series report a flap success rate of > 90%. The skin paddle is thin and hairless, with sufficient size to cover even large defects. The distant location from the head and neck allows a two-team approach, so that the flap harvest can be performed simultaneously with the extirpative procedure, therefore reducing the time of the procedure and lessening potential perioperative morbidity.

There are a few major disadvantages to the use of the RFFF. The radial artery is the blood supply to the flap, and so must be sacrificed during the flap's harvest. An Allen test must be performed preoperatively to assess the patency of the deep palmar arch, which will allow adequate perfusion of the entire hand from the ulnar artery only. The absence of this circulation, or the congenital absence of the ulnar artery, is an absolute contraindication to the use of this flap.

The donor site must be closed with a skin graft. Since the paratenon is the only blood supply to this graft, loss of the skin graft and subsequent exposure of the underlying tendons have been reported in up to 30% of patients. This can usually be dealt with conservatively, but restriction of hand movement must be discussed with patients preoperatively. Bilobed local flap reconstruction of the donor defect has been evolving as well and avoids some of the donor site complications. As mentioned, pathological fracture can occur when bone is harvested and can be a devastating complication.

Anterolateral Thigh Free Flap

The anterolateral thigh free flap was initially described in the early 1980s, but its application in the head and neck was not outlined until the 1990s. The anterolateral thigh free flap's role in oral cavity reconstruction has blossomed in recent years due to its ease of harvest and relatively minimal donor site morbidity.

The procedure is based on the descending branch of the lateral femoral circumflex artery and the associated venae comitantes. The pedicle vessels are of excellent length (6–10 cm) and caliber (artery 1–3.5 mm, venae comitantes 1.8–4.5 mm) for use in the oral cavity. The main pedicle runs in the fascial interspace between the rectus femoris and the vastus lateralis muscle, giving off lateral-going perforating vessels to the overlying skin. Understanding the course of these perforators is essential for the successful harvest of the flap because up to 80% will course to a variable extent through the vastus lateralis. As a result, the graft must be taken with a cuff of associated muscle, or a meticulous perforator dissection must be employed.

The anterolateral thigh free flap was initially popularized in head and neck reconstruction in eastern Asia, where it was primarily employed as an alternative to the radial forearm free flap. Due to this population's relatively thin body habitus, a thin pliable flap can be harvested to assist in oral cavity repair. In the United States and many other areas of the world, where a considerably larger amount of subcutaneous fat is often encountered, the anterolateral thigh free flap is used to also replace bulk, as in patients who have undergone a subtotal glossectomy.

Lateral Arm Free Flap

Although the lateral arm fasciocutaneous free flap (LAFF) was described in the early 1980s, it has not gained the popularity of the RFFF in head and neck reconstruction. The LAFF is harvested from the lateral arm, starting just below the elbow and extending up to 12 cm proximal to the lateral epicondyle. It is centered on the lateral intermuscular septum, and it can be 6 to 8 cm wide and still allow for primary closure of the donor site. The flap is based on the posterior radial collateral artery, which is a terminal branch of the nonessential profunda brachii artery and the venae comitantes. The sensory supply of the flap skin is the posterior cutaneous nerve of the arm, a branch of the radial nerve that enters the flap posteriorly from the triceps muscle. The posterior cutaneous nerve of the forearm, which supplies the lateral forearm, accompanies the vascular pedicle, potentially causing some confusion during flap harvest and certain minor forearm numbness as a result of flap harvest.

The LAFF can be used as a substitute for the RFFF when the Allen test reveals poor ulnar flow to the hand. The flap has a dual thickness because the skin proximal to the elbow has a moderately thick subcutaneous component, whereas the skin distal to the elbow approximates the skin of the RFFF. It is thus especially useful for composite defects of the tongue base and adjacent structures, such as the anterior tongue, lateral pharynx, or floor of the mouth, where both thick and thin tissue are needed to reconstruct within a small overall area.

The greatest advantage of the LAFF is the thin, sensate, pliable skin paddle. Like the RFFF, it allows a two-team approach. It also has a long pedicle with moderate-sized vessels for anastomosis, leading to success rates comparable to those of the RFFF. The most common morbidities at the donor site include unsightly scar, elbow pain, and lateral forearm numbness. Hair growth at the recipient site can occasionally be a drawback.

Sensate Free Flaps

A major innovation in oral cavity reconstruction has been the introduction of flaps for soft tissue reconstruction that have the ability to restore sensation after loss of the lingual and/or glossopharyngeal nerves to tumor extirpation or trauma. Sensate flaps have the ability to distinguish two-point discrimination, pressure, pain, and hot and cold differences in their recipient site equally as well as native tissue, and better than in their original location. The success of restoring sensation has been borne out in the literature, but the functional benefits have yet to be established. Many outcomes studies investigating this topic are under way. The two flaps used in the oral cavity with this capability are the RFFF and the LAFF.

Reinnervation

For both the RFFF and the LAFF, success of reinnervation varies between 50 and 70%, with return of sensation occurring within 4 to 9 months. The success obviously differs, depending on surgical technique and the recipient nerve chosen for anastomosis. Generally, flaps with nerves anastomosed regain two-point discrimination, pressure, pain, and temperature sensation. The benefit of sensate flaps needs further study, but many authors' results suggest that the quality of life and swallowing are improved with the use of these flaps in large oral cavity defects, compared with previously available options.

Functional Tongue Reconstruction

The flaps already described can be used to reconstruct any part of the oral cavity. When they are used to reconstruct the tongue, function is provided by restoration of form while allowing unimpeded movement of the residual tongue remnant. In the case of near-total or total glossectomy, several surgeons have attempted to restore function by supplying both lining and muscle to the oral cavity. In these situations, the rectus myocutaneous free flap and the latissimus myocutaneous free flap have been the most common selections to attempt to restore the form and function of the tongue.

Latissimus Myocutaneous Free Flap

The latissimus myocutaneous free flap is based on the thoracodorsal artery and vein, which supply a broad, flat muscle with innervation from only the thoracodorsal nerve. This anatomy makes the flap an ideal candidate for total glossectomy reconstruction.

In this situation, the muscle is used as a sling on which to support the skin paddle above the body of the mandible bilaterally. The skin paddle is then closed to surrounding mucosa and the vallecula, and the thoracodorsal nerve is anastomosed to one hypoglossal nerve in an end-to-end fashion. The vessels are anastomosed to appropriate recipient vessels as in other microvascular cases. This eventually results in a muscular platform that maintains the overall bulk of the reconstruction, but that is really not actively involved in the coordinated process of swallowing. Still, this method has had success reported in protection of the larynx from aspiration during oral alimentation, thus allowing the maintenance of the larynx after total glossectomy.

Rectus Myocutaneous Free Flap

In a similar fashion to the latissimus flap just described, the rectus myocutaneous free flap can be used to reconstruct total glossectomy defects. The rectus muscle is a relatively broad, flat muscle with a moderately thick skin component (except in obese individuals) supplied by the deep inferior epigastric artery and vein. In contradistinction to the latissimus muscle, however, the rectus muscle has segmental innervation along its length via several distinct motor nerves, which makes reinnervation somewhat more difficult than in the previously discussed scenario. Still, the muscle and its fascia can be used to create a platform on which to suspend the skin component over the mandibular bodies and then closure and microvascular and microneural anastomoses are performed with routine technique. Success in reestablishing oral alimentation after total glossectomy has been reported by some authors using this technique.

■ Summary

Oral reconstruction has advanced to allow functional rehabilitation of a variety of ablative defects. A scaled approach, selecting increasingly complex techniques, is appropriate and will minimize complications from a given procedure. Free tissue transfer is the standard for sizeable defects and has resulted in significant improvements in the outcomes for these patients.

■ Suggested Reading

Burkey BB. The evolving use of sensate flaps in head and neck reconstruction. Curr Opin Otolaryngol Head Neck Surg 1996;4(4):259–261

Cheney ML, Varvares MA, Nadol JB Jr. The temporoparietal fascial flap in head and neck reconstruction. Arch Otolaryngol Head Neck Surg 1993;119(6):618–623

Evans GRD, Schusterman MA, Kroll SS, et al. The radial forearm free flap for head and neck reconstruction: a review. Am J Surg 1994;168(5):446–450

Kimata Y, Uchiyama K, Ebihara S, et al. Versatility of the free anterolateral thigh flap for reconstruction of head and neck defects. Arch Otolaryngol Head Neck Surg 1997;123(12):1325–1331

Sullivan MJ, Carroll WR, Kuriloff DB. Lateral arm free flap in head and neck reconstruction. Arch Otolaryngol Head Neck Surg 1992;118(10):1095–1101

Urken ML. Multidisciplinary Head and Neck Reconstruction: A Defect-Oriented Approach. New York, NY: Lippincott Williams & Wilkins; 2010

Urken ML, Cheney ML, Blackwell KE, Harris JR, Hadlock TA, Futran N. Atlas of Regional and Free Flaps for Head and Neck Reconstruction: Flap Harvest and Insetting. 2nd ed. New York, NY: Lippincott Williams & Wilkins; 2011

Urken ML, Moscoso JF, Lawson W, Biller HF. A systematic approach to functional reconstruction of the oral cavity following partial and total glossectomy. Arch Otolaryngol Head Neck Surg 1994;120(6):589–601

27 Advances in Mandibular Reconstruction

■ Introduction

Primary reconstruction of mandibular defects remains a formidable challenge to the head and neck surgeon. In general, reconstruction of composite defects involves tissue for lining, replacement of the mandibular bony segment, and, on occasion, external skin repair. The innumerable publications over the past 40 to 50 years attest to the surgeon's frustrations in achieving good cosmetic and functional results.

Ideal repair of mandibular defects includes, when necessary, thin pliable skin for lining, preferably with the potential for neurosensory reinnervation. In addition, the bone used for replacement should, if possible, be compatible with primary dental rehabilitation. It also should have minimal donor site morbidity. Finally, the technique should be compatible with either pre- or postoperative irradiation. The past 30 years have seen a renaissance in the techniques used to restore mandibular continuity. This chapter outlines a contemporary approach to mandibular reconstruction.

Anatomy and Principles of Reconstruction

The mandible is a continuous bony arch spanning from one temporomandibular joint (TMJ) to the other. It is made up of the following segments: condyle, subcondylar region, coronoid process, ramus, angle, body, parasymphysis, and symphysis. The most robust bone can be found at the symphysis and angle. The alveolar ridge in the adult houses 16 teeth, and an inferior alveolar neurovascular bundle enters the medial ramus at the mandibular foramen and exits as the mental nerve near the root of the second premolar. The mandible also provides for muscular attachments of the muscles of mastication (masseter, medial and lateral pterygoids, and temporalis), the digastric muscles, the mylohyoid muscle, and the intrinsic tongue muscles.

The length and location of the bony defect has a particular impact on what is necessary to allow for successful reconstruction. Lateral defects, especially those short in length (< 3 cm), can often be successfully rehabilitated with either a load-bearing plate or a free bone graft, provided there is adequate soft tissue coverage both internally and externally. For anterior defects, however, the posterior pull of the genial muscle attachments significantly increase the risk of plate extrusion, unless backed by vascularized bone. As a result, defects involving the parasymphysis and symphysis are best repaired with osseous or osseocutaneous free flaps.

■ Evaluation

Mandible Preoperative Assessment

Whether from trauma or involvement by an underlying benign or malignant neoplasm, the ability of the reconstructive surgeon to predict the extent of the bony defect has dramatically improved with the development of more robust imaging techniques. Although plain radiographs, such as mandibular series and panoramic X-rays can have a role, computed tomography (CT) is now the standard of care in assessing the extent of mandibular pathology. Magnetic resonance imaging (MRI) can also be used to assess for marrow extension or perineural invasion.

For cases where there is significant distortion of the mandible by trauma or tumor extension, a preformed mandible reconstructive plate can be considered to more accurately re-create the mandibular form. This can be accomplished by making a scale model (based on a high-resolution CT scan of the patient), where the plate can be bent by the surgeon. Alternatively, the plate itself can be prefabricated with the appropriate contour. In even more complex cases, a model or prebent plate can be designed based on the mirror image of the contralateral (normal) side of the mandible to best estimate the patient's anatomy.

■ Management

Reconstruction Plates without Bone Grafts

The advent of three-dimensional bendable mandibular reconstruction plates (MRPs), the adaptive optics (AO) reconstruction system, and the titanium-coated hollow screw reconstruction plate (THORP) system has provided not only a sufficiently adjustable system but also a system that gives the functional stability necessary for primary mandibular bridging.

The MRP technique is readily available to the head and neck surgeon, and its application is usually straightforward. Prior to resection of the bone segment, the mandible is exposed, and the proposed osteotomy sites are identified and marked. The plate is then contoured along the outer cortical plate, and the holes are drilled and tapped proximal and distal to the proposed segmental resection. Once the ablation is completed, the plate is affixed with screws, thus reestablishing mandibular contour and maintaining the segments in their proper alignment. The advantages of MRP compared with free composite tissue transfer include a lack of donor site morbidity, expediency in the operating room, excellent contour, and the ability to reconstruct the condyle.

The success of the soft tissue lining used concurrently with the reconstructive plates determines the percentage of early plate failure. However, late plate failure seems to be largely determined by the hardware resiliency. Five main factors must be taken into consideration with respect to "soft tissue" reconstruction: the amount of mucosa resected, the amount of bulk required, the location of the mucosal defect (anterior vs. lateral), the donor site availability and morbidity, and finally, the potential for flap reinnervation.

Patients with extensive mucosal resections that require replacement of extensive soft tissue loss, or patients with large-volume resections that require bulk replacement, may be best reconstructed with a myocutaneous flap or a free tissue transfer, such as the anterolateral thigh free flap. Patients with lateral or posterior defects likewise may be reconstructed with a pedicled flap or free tissue transfer because tongue mobility and oral function are largely inhibited by lateral bulk. Success of the bridging bar, therefore, is dependent on the soft tissue replacement; if this technique is employed in anterior defects, then a bone-containing free flap should be employed to minimize the risk of plate extrusion. When employed anteriorly to cover the plate, the pedicled myocutaneous flap will, in several patients, dehisce and result in delayed plate exposure and failure, especially in individuals with pre- or postoperative radiation.

Additional disadvantages of the flap-plate option include the deficiency of vertical height of the plate and the inability to employ dental implants. Potential complications include infection, fistula, flap loss, loosening of the plate, plate exposure, extrusion, or fracture.

Nonvascularized Bone Grafts

Nonvascularized free cortical bone grafts were used during World Wars I and II in the repair of traumatic mandibular defects. These free autologous bone grafts included the iliac crest, rib, tibia, and calvarium. The survival rates of these grafts, particularly in the irradiated wound, were dismal. Extrusion, resorption, and infection occurred in the majority of patients. Most authors therefore agree that, if used, free nonvascularized bone grafts should be limited to secondary reconstruction where the oral mucosa is intact.

Pedicled Osseous Flaps

Because of the poor results with free bone grafts in primary mandibular reconstruction, other techniques for providing improved outcome have been sought. Pedicled grafts were thought to be the solution. Pedicled flaps using the trapezius/scapula, sternocleidomastoid/clavicle, and temporalis/cortical bone have been described with marginal success. The poor reliability of these nonvascularized flaps, in addition to donor site defects and complications, made the pedicled flaps an unacceptable form of primary mandibular reconstruction, except in a very limited number of cases with benign bony tumors where resection had not violated the oral mucosa.

Osseous Free Flaps

The advent of microsurgical techniques raised the curtain on the second phase of mandibular repair. Initial reports demonstrated significant improvements over pedicled or nonvascularized bone grafts, but success rates were still less than 70% in most initial series. The failures were due mainly to a lack of experience and the use of complex free rib transfers. In addition, the more sophisticated fixation plates available today to stabilize the graft had not been employed. Subsequently, with the use of the "top four" osseocutaneous free flap options (fibular, iliac crest, scapula, and radius), combined with increased experience, the success rate of primary reconstruction, even in the irradiated patient, has increased to better than 96%. Mandibular reconstruction by free tissue transfer has rapidly become the gold standard against which all other techniques are now compared.

When determining the appropriate choice for mandibular reconstructive technique, it is important to assess the following factors: the location of the mandibular defect (anterior vs. lateral), involvement of the temporomandibular joint (TMJ), length of the bony defect, extent of mucosal and/or skin defect, bulk of soft tissue required in the repair, patient factors (comorbidities, prior or planned irradiation, prognosis, etc.), and likelihood of obtaining dental implantation. The final choice of tissue graft is influenced by the donor site availability and morbidity, the ease of flap dissection, the status of the recipient vessels, and the patient's overall medical condition. Although rib, metatarsus, humerus, and clavicle have all been used in mandibular repair, the most acceptable donor sites today include the fibula, iliac crest, scapula, and radius. The many advantages and limitations of each tissue type are summarized in **Table 27.1**.

Also, as previously mentioned, along with the emergence of microvascular free tissue transfer, there were significant advances and technical refinements in craniomaxillofacial surgery, resulting in more reliable implant devices. The development of durable mandibular reconstruction plates gave surgeons the option of reconstituting the mandibular arch without autogenous bone and its attendant donor site morbidity. In general, the plate–soft tissue flap option is indicated in edentulous patients with advanced disease, patients with poor prognosis, patients in poor physical shape, or patients unable to tolerate a more lengthy procedure (**Fig. 27.1**). This is ideally performed for short (< 3 cm) lateral mandibular defects.

Bone-Containing Free Flaps

The remaining portion of this chapter focuses on the bone-containing free flaps most commonly used in mandible reconstruction.

Fibular Flap

The fibular flap was initially used to reconstruct long bone defects of the extremities. However, over the last 3 decades, head and neck surgeons have suc-cessfully adapted this flap to the repair of segmental mandibular defects.

The fibular free osseous, osseocutaneous, or osseomyocutaneous flap is currently the most popular form of tissue used in complex mandibular repair. In general, the flap combines relatively good skin features of thinness, pliability, and potential sensory reinnervation with excellent osseous characteristics of bone length, depth, thickness, cortical content, and perfusion to allow full dental rehabilitation and a pedicle that is large, reliable, and expendable. The fibula can be harvested in situ around the prefabricated reconstruction plate concomitant with the extirpative procedure, thus minimizing operative time and the interval for flap ischemia. The fibular flap, therefore, represents the single composite free tissue transfer that best addresses the cosmetic and functional needs of a complex mandibular defect—that is, it includes a reliably perfused, reasonably thin, pliable skin paddle with potential for sensate skin innervation, and a long bicortical bone graft that is suitable for osseointegrated implants. The fibular osseous flap is currently the tissue of choice in mandibular repair.

Anatomy

The fibula is a long, thin, nonweight-bearing bone of the lower extremity. It has a tubular shape, with thick cortical bone around the entire circumference, rendering it one of the strongest bones available for transfer. Approximately 22 to 26 cm of bone can be harvested, while preserving 6 to 7 cm of bone both distally and proximally to maintain the integrity of the knee and ankle joints.

The peroneal artery and vein provide the primary blood supply to the fibular osseocutaneous flap. The popliteal artery is classically described as bifurcating into the anterior and posterior tibial arteries, with the latter vessel subsequently giving rise to the peroneal artery. This artery and its two venae comitantes descend in the lower leg between the flexor hallucis longus and the tibialis posterior muscles. In addition to supplying the nutrient artery of the fibula and musculoperiosteal vessels, the peroneal artery and

Table 27.1 Comparison of osteocutaneous donor sites[a]

| Flap | Tissue characteristics | | | Donor site characteristics | |
	Bone	Skin	Vessels	Position	Morbidity
Iliac	+++	+	++	+++	++
Fibula	++++	++	+++	++++	++++
Radius	+	++++	++++	++	+
Scapula	++	+++	+++	+	+++

[a] Plus signs show relative value of donor site from worst (+) to best (++++).

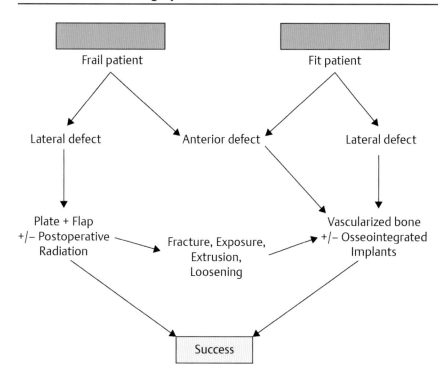

Fig. 27.1 Reconstructive algorithm.

its veins give rise to the fasciocutaneous perforators that run in the posterior crural septum to supply the overlying skin paddle. The vascular pedicle of the fibular flap, although consistent in location and caliber (6 cm long, 2–3 mm in diameter), is often limited in length by the bifurcation of the posterior tibial artery. Additional length can be obtained on the vascular leash by harvesting a more distal segment of bone and skin, while discarding the more proximal fibula.

A greater length of vascularized bone can be harvested from the fibula than from any other donor site. It can tolerate multiple osteotomies because of its profuse periosteal blood supply. Although the bone stock is adequate to support osseointegrated implants, the height of the neomandible is limited relative to that of the native dentate mandible. The overlying cutaneous skin paddle, although initially thought to be unreliable, is successful in 95% of cases with placement of the island of skin at the distal end of the fibula.

The ability to innervate and provide sensate tissue to this composite transfer is thought to enhance its functional outcome in oromandibular reconstruction. Based on preoperative nerve block patterns, one must select the donor nerve—either the lateral sural cutaneous nerve or the recurrent superficial peroneal nerve—that best subserves the skin paddle upon which the osseocutaneous flap will be transferred. If both nerves appear to supply the paddle, then both may be dissected, and the nerve with the best fascicles matched to the recipient nerve can be selected. The skin paddle is determined by the location of the peroneal artery perforators. Therefore, this flap has the potential for innervation, but the quality of the soft tissue is intermediate in thickness and pliability and thus ranks behind that of the radial forearm for soft tissue replacement. The fibular flap can also include the flexor hallucis longus muscle to provide soft tissue bulk where needed. Donor site morbidity with or without skin grafting following fibula free flap harvesting is minimal.

Preoperative Workup

As previously mentioned, when considering a fibula free flap, a detailed history should be taken regarding lower-extremity claudication or poor healing. This is especially critical to assess in individuals with significant peripheral vascular disease and/or diabetes mellitus. Moreover, any prior lower-leg trauma or surgery should be noted.

If the patient appears to be an acceptable candidate, the lower leg vascularity needs to be assessed with a magnetic resonance angiogram, CT angiogram, or lower-leg Doppler to ensure adequate three-vessel runoff to the foot. If adequate vascular flow is not present, an alternative donor site should be used.

Iliac Crest

The iliac crest flap is based on the deep circumflex iliac artery. Although the fibula is usually the osseous flap of choice, the iliac crest still has a significant role in primary mandibular reconstruction. Specific indications for the use of this flap include patients with significant peripheral vascular disease, a history of vein stripping or varicosity, prior leg trauma, or signs of venous or arterial insufficiency on physical examination.

The iliac crest is also the technique of choice in c-segment defects, which require intraoral lining, as well as cover. In this design, the skin paddle is draped over the bony reconstruction, providing intraoral lining, while the central deepithelialized segment provides a well-vascularized platform on which the lateral lip elements can sit. Restoration of this major central through-and-through defect is best repaired with free iliac osseocutaneous flap or the free scapula flap (to be described).

Anatomy

The iliac crest has a natural curvature not unlike that of the mandible. About 14 to 16 cm of bone can be harvested by extending the resection posteriorly to the sacroiliac joint. The bone graft can be contoured and tailored to reconstruct the anterior mandibular arch with osteotomies through the outer cortex, leaving its inner periosteum and blood supply intact. The height of the neomandible can be varied by positioning the transverse bone cut, making it well suited for placement of osseointegrated implants. Limitations associated with the flap include excess bulk of its cutaneous component, with an inability to freely move the soft tissue component independently of the bone. However, the internal oblique muscle has been shown to be an additional option for reliable intraoral lining when placed and allowed to epithelialize spontaneously.

The deep circumflex iliac vessels arise from the lateral surface of the external iliac artery and vein just cephalad to the inguinal ligament. The pedicle length averages 6 to 8 cm in the adult, and the vessel diameter is adequate, averaging 1 to 2.5 mm. The blood supply to the overlying skin paddle of the osseocutaneous flap comes from an array of perforators that are located in a zone along the medial aspect of the iliac crest. It is important when insetting the skin paddle to maintain the relationship of the skin to bone so as not to torque the perforators.

One of the disadvantages of the iliac crest is the morbidity at the donor site from abdominal wall weakness and potential herniation. Additionally, excessive traction or division of the lateral femoral cutaneous nerve may result in debilitating, persistent, postoperative pain. However, donor site morbidity may be diminished by splitting the ileum and taking the inner table with its overlying skin paddle. In this manner, the crest itself is left and the abdominal repair is much more secure. Holes are drilled in the remaining crest, to which the three layers of abdominal musculature are attached. Furthermore,

the muscles on the lateral side of the crest are undisturbed, minimizing the tendency for weakness of the abdominal wall. Finally, the cosmetic defect of this modification is significantly less compared with the original technique.

Preoperative Workup

Although no preoperative studies are required to determine candidacy for iliac crest harvest, it is essential to take a thorough history of prior abdominal surgery or hernia repairs or recent femoral arterial or central venous lines. More important, it is also necessary to scale the impact that gate disturbance would have on the patient, and to counsel the patient on the risk of abdominal hernia formation.

Free Scapular Flap

The use of the scapular free flap for mandibular reconstruction was popularized in the late 1980s. Its primary indication in the head and neck is for moderate composite mandibular defects, where the defect has a significant soft tissue component. Due to the ability to design two distinct skin paddles that are freely mobile from one another as well as the adjacent bone, it has proven to be of particular use for through-and-through mandible defects, where both the mucosa and the overlying skin need to be repaired. Although the bone of the lateral scapula is moderate in its thickness, its density is less robust than the fibula and iliac crest, making it less reliable for dental implantation.

Anatomy

The free scapular flap has a vascular supply consisting of a large interconnecting network of vessels originating from the circumflex scapular artery. The circumflex scapular artery is a branch of the subscapular artery. It courses to the back from the axilla by means of the triangular space, bordered by the teres major, the teres minor, and the long head of the triceps muscles, where it provides a vascular pedicle 6 to 8 cm long and 3.3 to 4 mm in diameter. The artery arborizes into several major branches, including the transverse cutaneous, descending cutaneous, and periosteal branches.

The periscapular and scapular skin flaps encompass large areas of the back skin and can be raised relatively independently of each other and of the bone graft itself. This provides greater flexibility in the positioning and tailoring of the graft for the reconstruction of the complex three-dimensional composite defects. The skin paddles of this flap vary in thickness with the amount of the patient's adipose tissue, but they tend to be much thicker than the radial forearm paddle and somewhat bulkier than that of the fibula. However, they are much less bulky than the soft tissue component of the iliac crest and can safely be used for intraoral lining.

The main limitation to the routine use of the scapular osseocutaneous flap is the inability to facilitate a two-team approach due to the need to reposition the patient during the harvest procedure. Additionally, only 10 to 12 cm of bone is reliably available with this transfer and may be too thin to support dental implantation. Finally, if this flap is used as an osseocutaneous flap, there is no distinct sensory cutaneous nerve available for primary neural reinnervation. The flap retains its popularity in soft tissue replacement about the head and neck area, particularly in the soft tissue defects of the face, but it is rarely used as an osseous flap, except in cases where fibular tissue transfer is not possible.

Preoperative Workup

The patient's history should include inquiry as to whether any prior shoulder or axillary surgery has been performed. In addition, if possible, the patient's nondominant hand should be used to minimize postoperative impairment. No preoperative imaging studies are necessary.

Radial Forearm Osseocutaneous Free Flap

Although initial descriptions of the radial forearm fasciocutaneous free flap occurred in the late 1970s, it wasn't until ~ 5 years later that the incorporation of a split thickness of the distal radius bone was described. This allowed this flap to be considered for use in segmental mandibular reconstruction.

Anatomy

The radial forearm flap is based on the radial vessels that course through the anterior lateral intermuscular septum (between the brachioradialis and flexor carpi radialis), with drainage from the venae comitantes or a superficial vein, such as the cephalic vein. The blood supply to the radius is preserved through periosteal attachments from the flexor pollicis longus and the pronator quadratus muscles.

The main advantage of this osseocutaneous flap rests with the skin paddle, which is abundant, thin, pliable, sensate, and thus ideal for the replacement of oral lining. About 10 to 12 cm and up to 40% of the circumference of the radius, which is supplied by septal perforators, can be harvested as an osseous flap.

The major disadvantage of this osseous flap is its quality of bone, having limited dimensions to satisfy the demands of functional mastication. In addition, forearm structural support is weakened, resulting in pathological fractures of the remaining radius in close to a quarter of reported flaps. Repair of this fracture will frequently necessitate a further bone graft. The occurrence of a pathological fracture, despite its subsequent successful repair, results in decreased range of motion, grip, and pinch compared with the hand on the unoperated side. Furthermore, a patient with an osseocutaneous radial forearm flap needs to be placed in a long arm cast postoperatively, which in itself causes significant functional morbidity, especially in the older patient. Although reinforcing titanium plates can be used to minimize the risk of fracture, this osseous flap is employed in a limited number of patients where other alternatives are not possible.

Preoperative Workup

Usually the patient's nondominant hand is considered the first choice for harvest. Any prior surgery or injury to the wrist should be documented. In addition, an Allen's test should be performed to ensure adequate circulation exists in the ulnar and palmar arch vessels.

■ Conclusion

The past 15 years have witnessed a growing popularity and enthusiasm for free osseous tissue transfer in mandibular reconstruction. Nonvascularized bone grafts, either free or pedicled, are used only in select cases where the mandibular defect segment is short, the oral cavity mucosa itself is intact, and the recipient bed is healthy and well vascularized.

The fibular osseous vascularized flap is the technique of choice in the majority of mandibular reconstructions because of its anatomical features and short- and long-term results, as well as its relatively insignificant morbidity at the donor site. The iliac crest, when harvested using the inner table alone, is a very acceptable alternative to the fibular graft. The scapular flap, although versatile and ideally suited for through-and-through defects with both a mucosal and a cutaneous component, is less popular because of the need to reposition the patient, therefore preventing a two-team approach. Finally, a combination of a myocutaneous pedicled flap or a free cutaneous tissue transfer in combination with a three-dimensional bendable reconstruction plate is an alternative form of reconstruction, especially in edentulous patients with poor prognosis, those with lateral defects, and those who would not otherwise tolerate a microvascular free tissue transfer.

■ Suggested Reading

Boyd JB, Mulholland RS, Davidson J, et al. The free flap and plate in oromandibular reconstruction: long-term review and indications. Plast Reconstr Surg 1995;95(6):1018–1028

Jewer DB, Boyd JD, Mankelow RT, et al. Orofacial and mandibular reconstruction with the iliac crest free flap: a review of 60 cases and a new method of classification. Plast Reconstr Surg 1989;84(3):391–403, discussion 404–405

Komisar A, ed. Mandibular Reconstruction. New York, NY: Thieme; 1997

Urken ML. Multidisciplinary Head and Neck Reconstruction: A Defect-Oriented Approach. New York, NY: Lippincott Williams & Wilkins; 2010

Urken ML, Cheney ML, Blackwell KE, Harris JR, Hadlock TA, Futran N. Atlas of Regional and Free Flaps for Head and Neck Reconstruction: Flap Harvest and Insetting. 2nd ed. New York, NY: Lippincott Williams & Wilkins; 2011

28 Oropharyngeal Cancer

■ Introduction

Each year 123,000 cases of pharyngeal cancer (both oropharyngeal and hypopharyngeal) are diagnosed worldwide; 79,000 patients die of their disease annually. Although classically associated with tobacco and alcohol abuse, oropharyngeal carcinoma (OPC) has recently been associated with chronic human papilloma virus (HPV) infection. With HPV infection rates approaching epidemic status, the incidence of HPV-associated OPC is on the rise, and new attention has been directed toward developing optimal treatment strategies.

Anatomy

The oropharynx is part of both the upper respiratory and the upper digestive tracts. It is an extremely dynamic segment that plays a crucial role in swallowing, speech, and breathing. Consequently, tumors of this region, as well as the treatment modalities used to eradicate them, can have serious effects on these critical functions.

The oropharynx is divided into several regions: the soft palate/faucial arch, the tonsillar fossa, the base of the tongue, and the posterior and lateral oropharyngeal walls. Tumors of each of these areas have certain peculiar clinical characteristics and may impact on therapeutic decisions. The oropharynx contains abundant lymphoid tissue, also known as the Waldeyer ring, and includes the palatine and lingual tonsils. Additionally, the oropharynx is characterized by a rich network of draining lymphatics that communicate freely across the midline. This explains the propensity of tumors of this region to metastasize to the regional lymph nodes, as well as the relatively high frequency of bilateral lymph node metastases. The lymphatic drainage of the oropharynx occurs predominantly toward the upper and midjugular lymph nodes (levels II and III). The retropharyngeal nodes are a less known but important echelon in the lymphatic drainage of the oropharynx. These nodes are found between the carotid bifurcation and the skull base. They are located within the loose fibrofatty tissue medial to the internal carotid artery and posterior and lateral to the pharyngeal constrictors.

■ Evaluation

Persistent throat pain is the most common presenting symptom of cancer of the oropharynx. Although this is common knowledge, the diagnosis of cancer is delayed in nearly one-third of the patients presenting with this complaint, and they are inappropriately treated with several courses of antibiotics. Cervical adenopathy is also a common presenting symptom and may also have been treated previously as a presumed infection. When evaluating a patient with a suspected oropharyngeal cancer, the physician must inquire about the presence and duration of other symptoms, such as otalgia, odynophagia, dysphagia, trismus, and hoarseness. A deep-seated parietal-retro-orbital unilateral headache may be indicative of retropharyngeal node metastases. The history should include documentation of risk factors, such as the use of tobacco and alcohol, and the occurrence and extent of weight loss and of all other medical conditions.

The physical examination includes inspection of all the areas of the oral cavity, pharynx, and larynx. If indirect laryngoscopy is not adequate, fiberoptic examination of the pharynx and larynx is necessary. The examination is not complete without palpating the floor of the mouth, tongue, base of the tongue, and/or tonsil to evaluate the depth of infiltration of the tumor and its proximity to the mandible. The examination also includes an assessment of the status of the mandible and the dentition, as well as an evaluation of the status of the airway. Finally, the clinical evaluation includes systematic palpation of both sides of the neck, recording the location, size, mobility, and relationship of nodes to adjacent structures.

Because oropharyngeal cancer often presents as a neck mass in an adult, fine-needle aspiration biopsy of the mass is among the first steps in diagnosis. Open surgical biopsy of such suspected lymph node metastasis is not advisable. Although it remains unclear that open biopsy would be detrimental in terms of local control or survival, it frequently affects the extent and possible morbidity of the definitive treatment with surgery, radiation, or both.

Examination under anesthesia via direct laryngoscopy is an important step in the evaluation of tumors of the oropharynx. Prior to it, however, the adequacy of the airway should be assessed. Fiberoptic intubation may be deemed safest due to tumor-altered anatomy or trismus, and patients with large tumors may require a tracheostomy under local anesthesia. Direct laryngoscopy and palpation of the base of the tongue and pharynx are essential to accurately assess the extent of the tumor, especially its inferior extent along the pharyngeal wall, and to rule out involvement of the larynx and hypopharynx. The routine use of esophagoscopy and bronchoscopy remains controversial. In the absence of abnormal clinical or radiographic findings, the yield of these procedures, particularly of bronchoscopy, does not seem to warrant performing them as a matter of course.

Imaging Studies

Computed tomography (CT) and magnetic resonance imaging of the primary tumor and neck are useful in assessing the extent of the primary tumor and its relationship to the mandible, the pterygoid muscles, the carotid arteries, and the prevertebral tissues. CT is useful in determining whether there is bony erosion of the mandible or the skull base. In the absence of palpable adenopathy in the neck, these imaging techniques may be useful in assessing the status of the cervical lymph nodes in patients who are obese or who have a thick, muscular neck. They are also useful in assessing the presence of parapharyngeal or retropharyngeal adenopathy. When a large node is palpable in the neck, these studies may help to clarify the relationship of the node to the carotid artery, the paraspinal muscles, or the cervical spine. Positron-emission tomography/CT scan is often used in treatment planning for radiation or chemoradiation, and to assess treatment response (performed at 3 months after treatment completion). Although it does provide information on possible distant metastasis, CT of the chest is an alternative option for metastatic workup.

Consultations

More often than not, comprehensive management of patients with oropharyngeal tumors is a multidisciplinary endeavor. Thus it is desirable to evaluate these patients in conjunction with both medical and radiation oncology. The patient may need postoperative radiation therapy (RT), or radiation may be used as the primary modality of treatment. Ideally, patients with OPC (and indeed all head and neck cancer patients) are presented at a multidisciplinary tumor board, where their case is discussed and an evidence-based treatment plan is formulated.

Dental evaluation is appropriate to assess the status of the teeth and the condition of the mandible prior to RT. The evaluating dentist should be versed in the effects of radiotherapy on dentition, and this evaluation should be done with knowledge of the treatment portals planned for RT. Preoperative counseling by a speech pathologist regarding possible postoperative speech and swallowing problems may facilitate rehabilitation.

Staging

The TNM (tumor-node-metastasis) staging system of the American Joint Committee on Cancer (AJCC) and Union for International Cancer Control (UICC) for OPC is provided in **Tables 28.1, 28.2, 28.3,** and **28.4.**

■ Treatment

Historically, the treatment of OPC has vacillated between primarily surgery-based treatment versus radiation-based therapy. For more advanced disease,

Table 28.1 Primary tumor (T)

TX	Primary tumor cannot be assessed
T0	No evidence of primary tumor
Tis	Carcinoma in situ
T1	Tumor ≤ 2 cm in greatest dimension
T2	Tumor > 2 cm but ≤ 4 cm in greatest dimension
T3	Tumor > 4 cm in greatest dimension or extension to lingual surface of epiglottis
T4a	Moderately advanced local disease. Tumor invades the larynx, extrinsic muscle of tongue, medial pterygoid, hard palate, or mandible[a]
T4b	Very advanced local disease. Tumor invades lateral pterygoid muscle, pterygoid plates, lateral nasopharynx, or skull base, or encases carotid artery

Used with the permission of the American Joint Committee on Cancer (AJCC), Chicago, Illinois. The original source for this material is the AJCC Cancer Staging Manual, Seventh Edition (2010) published by Springer Science and Business Media LLC, www.springer.com.

[a] Mucosal extension to lingual surface of epiglottis from primary tumors of the base of the tongue and vallecula does not constitute invasion of the larynx.

Table 28.2 Regional lymph nodes (N)[a]

NX	Regional lymph nodes cannot be assessed
N0	No regional lymph node metastasis
N1	Metastasis in a single ipsilateral lymph node, ≤ 3 cm in greatest dimension
N2	Metastasis in a single ipsilateral lymph node, > 3 cm but ≤ 6 cm in greatest dimension, or metastasis in multiple ipsilateral lymph nodes, ≤ 6 cm in greatest dimension, or in bilateral or contralateral lymph nodes, ≤ 6 cm in greatest dimension
N2a	Metastasis in a single ipsilateral lymph node > 3 cm but ≤ 6 cm in greatest dimension
N2b	Metastases in multiple ipsilateral lymph nodes, ≤ 6 cm in greatest dimension
N2c	Metastases in bilateral or contralateral lymph nodes, ≤ 6 cm in greatest dimension
N3	Metastasis in a lymph node > 6 cm in greatest dimension

Used with the permission of the American Joint Committee on Cancer (AJCC), Chicago, Illinois. The original source for this material is the AJCC Cancer Staging Manual, Seventh Edition (2010) published by Springer Science and Business Media LLC, www.springer.com.

[a] Metastases at level VII are considered regional lymph node metastases.

Table 28.3 Distant metastasis (M)

M0	No distant metastasis
M1	Distant metastasis

Used with the permission of the American Joint Committee on Cancer (AJCC), Chicago, Illinois. The original source for this material is the AJCC Cancer Staging Manual, Seventh Edition (2010) published by Springer Science and Business Media LLC, www.springer.com.

Table 28.4 Anatomical stage/prognostic groups

Stage	T	N	M
0	Tis	N0	M0
I	T1	N0	M0
II	T2	N0	M0
III	T3	N0	M0
	T1	N1	M0
	T2	N1	M0
	T3	N1	M0
IVA	T4a	N0	M0
	T4a	N1	M0
	T1	N2	M0
	T2	N2	M0
	T3	N2	M0
	T4a	N2	M0
IVB	T4b	Any N	M0
	Any T	N3	M0
IVC	Any T	Any N	M1

Used with the permission of the American Joint Committee on Cancer (AJCC), Chicago, Illinois. The original source for this material is the AJCC Cancer Staging Manual, Seventh Edition (2010) published by Springer Science and Business Media LLC, www.springer.com.

it is generally accepted that multimodality therapy is indicated, adding adjuvant RT for surgical patients and chemotherapy to primary RT regimens.

In general, early-stage tumors of the oropharynx (T1 or T2, N0) can be treated equally well with surgery or RT alone. The choice of treatment modality depends on the site of origin and the extent of the tumor, the patient's general condition, the anticipated functional consequences of the treatment, the patient's preference, and, in some instances, the philosophy and capabilities of the institution. In most patients with locoregionally advanced OPC (T3 or T4, and by definition, any N), combined therapy—that is, chemoradiation or surgery with postoperative radiation—appears to provide better locoregional control than surgery or RT alone. The oropharynx is noted to have a rich network of lymphatics draining all subsites, which creates a high risk of metastasis to the regional lymph nodes, even in the N0 neck. Thus, regardless of T stage, it is imperative to treat the cervical lymph nodes in all cases of OPC. In primary tonsil tumors that do not invade the base of the tongue or soft palate (i.e., are well lateralized), ipsilateral neck treatment is typically adequate; however, treatment of tumors of the base of the tongue, soft palate, and posterior pharyngeal wall must include bilateral neck treatment.

Early Oropharyngeal Cancer Treatment

Stage I and II OPC can typically be treated by surgery or radiation alone. When RT is selected, both the primary tumor and the neck are irradiated. If surgery is chosen, it should include resection of the primary tumor as well as selective neck dissection(s). Although no prospective trials comparing primary radiation with primary surgery exist for this patient group, retrospective studies indicate comparable locoregional control and survival rates. Indeed, most surgical studies tend to be small because less than 2 to 30% of OPC patients present with an N0 neck, and many studies include N1 disease in their analysis. That said, the most recent literature indicates over 80% 5-year disease-specific survival for surgically treated early-stage OPC. A prospective, multi-institutional study notes similar 2-year disease-free survivals of over 80% following primary intensity-modulated radiation therapy (IMRT) for early OPC (defined as T1–2, N0–1, M0). Direct comparisons of treatment modalities are hampered by the lack of randomized, controlled trials and variability both in patient selection (i.e., N0 only vs. inclusion of N1 disease) and in radiation and surgical techniques.

Radiation Treatment

Radiation treatment is an effective treatment for early OPC that spares the patient the morbidity of surgery, but it introduces its own spectrum of potential complications. At this time, it is generally accepted that IMRT is superior in the treatment of early OPC compared with conventional external beam RT and earlier iterations of conformal three-dimensional RT. IMRT allows for more accurate dosing of the primary tumor and draining lymphatics, as well as sparing of the vital functional anatomy of the oropharynx, salivary glands, and other uninvolved structures of the head and neck.

The RTOG 00–22 study included patients with clinical T1–2, N0–1, M0 OPC (some radiographic small-burden N2 patients were included as well); patients received 66 gray (Gy) at 2.2 Gy per fraction over 6 weeks. Mucositis, dysphagia, and overlying skin effects were the most common acute toxicities, as well as xerostomia, which was also the most common late toxicity. Two-year disease-free survival was over 80%, with estimated overall survival of over 95% and an estimated local-regional failure rate of less than 10%. Other contemporary prospective trials of primary RT for OPC that do not focus on single subsites or include advanced disease (and thus multimodality treatment) are lacking. However, when early-stage disease is examined within these studies, local control rates range from 84 to 88%, and 5-year cause-specific survival ranges from 86 to 100%.

Surgical Treatment

Early surgical approaches to the oropharynx involved extensive dissection, often including mandibulotomy and lip-splitting procedures that resulted in significant surgical morbidity, including swallowing and speech dysfunction. As RT techniques evolved and were noted to have comparatively less morbidity with similar efficacy, early OPC treatment became a primarily radiation-based approach at many institutions.

More recently, the development of minimally invasive transoral approaches to the oropharynx has resulted in the reintroduction of primary surgical treatment for early OPC. These techniques include transoral laser microsurgery (TLM) and transoral robotic surgery (TORS). Although retrospective in nature, small studies of TLM and TORS for OPC indicate that they are safe procedures with relatively low levels of morbidity. Permanent tracheostomy or feeding tube dependence is relatively low at 0 to 0.9% and 0 to 10%, respectively; most of these reports include both early- and advanced-stage disease. Two recent studies examined transoral surgery alone for OPC, both of which included patients with advanced OPC. These have demonstrated negative surgical margins in over 95% of cases and a local control rate of over 90%, with estimated 5-year locoregional control rates in the range of 90% for stage I, over 70% for stage II, and 70% for stage III OPC.

Although prospective clinical trials directly comparing transoral surgery to radiation for early OPC are lacking, retrospective studies argue that primary transoral surgery coupled with appropriate neck dissection allows for the most accurate staging of early OPC. At least one study noted that definitive surgical staging altered T stage in over 25% of patients, N stage in just under 25% of patients, and clinical stage in 40% of OPC patients treated with primary surgery. Tumors were upstaged in over 15% and downstaged in just under one quarter of patients. The argument follows that by performing primary surgery for early-stage OPC, there may be opportunity to identify patients in whom treatment may be safely deintensified, as well as those who may benefit from adjuvant treatment. Regardless, with only retrospective studies to guide us, there remains no evidence to suggest a superiority of either primary treatment for early OPC.

Locoregionally Advanced Oropharyngeal Cancer Treatment

Locoregionally advanced OPC consists of stage III and IVA/B disease; this includes T3 and T4 tumors, and all positive nodal disease, regardless of T stage. Indeed, by this definition, most OPC presents in advanced stages due to its propensity to metastasize to cervical lymph nodes; ~ 70% of OPC patients present with evidence of regional metastasis. Single-modality treatment of these tumors is considered insufficient; thus combined approaches have been developed.

The functional organ preservation approach typically consists of concurrent chemoradiation over radiation alone. Primary surgery for resectable stage III and IV disease should be followed by adjuvant radiation or chemoradiation, depending on the absence or presence of high-risk features on final pathology. These high-risk features include positive margins, perineural invasion, multiple and/or matted nodes, and extracapsular extension of tumor in lymph nodes. As with early OPC treatment, there are no large randomized trials comparing chemoradiation to surgery followed by adjuvant radiation or chemoradiation. Thus, while one approach has not yet demonstrated greater efficacy or lesser toxicity/morbidity over another, it is generally accepted that multidisciplinary treatment planning is needed to appropriately manage these patients.

Chemoradiation

A multitude of clinical trials have been undertaken using radiation in combination with chemotherapy. These include concurrent chemoradiation, neoadjuvant chemotherapy, and adjuvant chemotherapy. The Meta-Analysis of Chemotherapy on Head and Neck Cancer concluded that, for OPC, protocols that combined chemotherapy with radiation resulted in a significant reduction in the risk of death compared with radiation alone. Additionally, there was a 5% improvement in overall 5-year survival for patients treated with chemotherapy and radiation.

Contemporary chemoradiation schemes use three-dimensional conformal RT, typically IMRT and/or image-guided RT, usually in once-daily fractions of 1.8 to 2 Gy over 7 weeks, to a total dose of ~ 70 Gy (range 66–72 Gy). Hyperfractionation and accelerated RT have been investigated, but thus far results have been variable with respect to improvement of local control and overall survival. Generally speaking, platinum-based therapy is considered the standard of care for chemoradiation of OPC. Cisplatin, dosed at 100 mg per m^2 every 21 days for three doses, is the most commonly used concurrent chemotherapeutic, but other schedules and other drugs are in use. Carboplatin/5-fluorouracil combination therapy is also in common use. More recently, concurrent cetuximab with RT has been studied in comparison to RT alone; although the study population was only 60% OPC patients, combined cetuximab-RT resulted in improved overall survival and locoregional control. That said, there was some concern that this benefit was seen only in patients under 65 years of age and with higher performance scores. Finally, there are not yet data comparing cetuximab-RT with standard platinum-based chemoradiation, although a current RTOG trial (1016) is randomizing patients with locally advanced p16 positive OPC to IMRT with weekly cetuximab versus IMRT with cisplatin on days 1 and 22. Overall, a contemporary retrospective review of chemoradiation for locally advanced OPC at MD Anderson Cancer Center, which includes patients treated on protocols using all of the foregoing chemotherapeutics, shows 5-year actuarial overall survival, disease-free survival, and locoregional control rates of over 75%, just under 80%, and just under 90%, respectively.

The topic of induction chemotherapy is beyond the scope of this review, as is a full discussion of all the additional chemoradiation trials under way at this time. Induction chemotherapy has been shown in several trials to confer a survival benefit, but general opinion is that its use is best limited to within the context of a clinical trial.

Surgery with Adjuvant Radiation or Chemoradiation

As noted previously, the morbidity of traditional open approaches limited their widespread use as chemoradiation came into its own as an organ-preservation, function-focused approach. Surgery was reserved for T4b tumors invading the mandible (it is thought that chemoradiation is less effective in cases of bone invasion), or in cases of recurrent disease when surgical salvage was needed. With the advent of minimally invasive transoral approaches to oropharyngeal surgery, head and neck surgeons have begun to explore the utility of TLM and TORS for T3 and T4a disease. Additionally, T1 and T2 disease is often accompanied by advanced N stage disease. Although adjuvant RT is anticipated in this surgical group, early studies reveal that adjuvant chemoradiation is required in many, if not most, patients, due to advanced nodal burden. This fact raises the question if this group of patients would be better treated with primary chemoradiation, avoiding the additional modality of surgery. The role of primary surgery in locoregionally advanced OPC remains unclear, and it is under current investigation.

Role of HPV in OPC

In recent years, there has been an explosion of evidence linking HPV infection to the development of OPC. Although a comprehensive discussion of this association is beyond the scope of this brief review, the following is a summary of what is currently known about this new clinical entity.

- The majority of HPV-positive head and neck cancers arise in the palatine tonsils and base of the tongue. They demonstrate a poorly differentiated, basaloid histopathology. Immunohistochemistry for p16 is commonly used to identify HPV-related tumors because this protein is overexpressed in HPV-associated cancers. Tumors can also be tested for HPV deoxyribonucleic acid (DNA); concurrent HPV DNA positivity and high p16 expression portended a better prognosis over HPV DNA positive with low p16 expression in one study.

- HPV 16 is the most common viral serotype causing OPC, although HPV18, 31, and 33 have also been implicated.
- Patients with HPV-positive OPC tend to be young (often in their 30s and 40s), and tend to present with early T stage but advanced N stage disease. Large, bulky, cystic cervical adenopathy is the clinical hallmark of this disease.
- Current evidence suggests that HPV-positive OPC patients have a better prognosis compared with HPV-negative patients, and that their tumors are exquisitely

radiosensitive. The rate of second primary disease and distant metastasis also appears to be lower than in HPV-negative patients. That said, deintensification of treatment is not yet recommended for this patient group, pending the outcome of ongoing clinical trials.

Additional sources for more detailed information about HPV-positive OPC epidemiology, biology, clinical behavior, and treatment strategies are provided in this chapter's Suggested Reading list. In addition, evolving treatment guidelines can be found in the National Comprehensive Cancer Network (NCCN) Guidelines.

■ Suggested Reading

Ang KK, Harris J, Wheeler R, et al. Human papillomavirus and survival of patients with oropharyngeal cancer. N Engl J Med 2010;363(1):24–35

Blanchard P, Baujat B, Holostenco V, et al; MACH-CH Collaborative group. Meta-analysis of chemotherapy in head and neck cancer (MACH-NC): a comprehensive analysis by tumour site. Radiother Oncol 2011;100(1):33–40

Bonner JA, Harari PM, Giralt J, et al. Radiotherapy plus cetuximab for squamous-cell carcinoma of the head and neck. N Engl J Med 2006;354(6):567–578

Bourhis J, Sire C, Graff P, et al. Concomitant chemoradiotherapy versus acceleration of radiotherapy with or without concomitant chemotherapy in locally advanced head and neck carcinoma (GORTEC 99-02): an open-label phase 3 randomised trial. Lancet Oncol 2012;13(2):145–153

Eisbruch A, Harris J, Garden AS, et al. Multi-institutional trial of accelerated hypofractionated intensity-modulated radiation therapy for early-stage oropharyngeal cancer (RTOG 00-22). Int J Radiat Oncol Biol Phys 2010;76(5):1333–1338

Garden AS, Kies MS, Morrison WH, et al. Outcomes and patterns of care of patients with locally advanced oropharyngeal carcinoma treated in the early 21st century. Radiat Oncol 2013;8(1):21

Gillison ML, D'Souza G, Westra W, et al. Distinct risk factor profiles for human papillomavirus type 16-positive and human papillomavirus type 16-negative head and neck cancers. J Natl Cancer Inst 2008;100(6):407–420

Grant DG, Hinni ML, Salassa JR, Perry WC, Hayden RE, Casler JD. Oropharyngeal cancer: a case for single modality treatment with transoral laser microsurgery. Arch Otolaryngol Head Neck Surg 2009;135(12):1225–1230

Lim YC, Koo BS, Lee JS, Lim JY, Choi EC. Distributions of cervical lymph node metastases in oropharyngeal carcinoma: therapeutic implications for the N0 neck. Laryngoscope 2006;116(7):1148–1152

Moncrieff M, Sandilla J, Clark J, et al. Outcomes of primary surgical treatment of T1 and T2 carcinomas of the oropharynx. Laryngoscope 2009;119(2):307–311

Moore EJ, Olsen KD, Kasperbauer JL. Transoral robotic surgery for oropharyngeal squamous cell carcinoma: a prospective study of feasibility and functional outcomes. Laryngoscope 2009; 119(11):2156–2164

Moore EJ, Henstrom DK, Olsen KD, Kasperbauer JL, McGree ME. Transoral resection of tonsillar squamous cell carcinoma. Laryngoscope 2009;119(3):508–515

National Comprehensive Cancer Network. Guidelines. http://www.nccn.org/professionals/physician_gls/f_guidelines.asp. Accessed May 2, 2014

NIH Clinical trials database. http://www.clinicaltrials.gov/.

O'Hara J, MacKenzie K. Surgical versus non-surgical management of early stage oropharyngeal squamous cell carcinoma. Eur Arch Otorhinolaryngol 2011;268(3):437–442

Pignon JP, le Maître A, Maillard E, Bourhis J; MACH-NC Collaborative Group. Meta-analysis of chemotherapy in head and neck cancer (MACH-NC): an update on 93 randomised trials and 17,346 patients. Radiother Oncol 2009;92(1):4–14

Posner MR, Lorch JH, Goloubeva O, et al. Survival and human papillomavirus in oropharynx cancer in TAX 324: a subset analysis from an international phase III trial. Ann Oncol 2011;22(5):1071–1077

Sturgis EM, Ang KK. The epidemic of HPV-associated oropharyngeal cancer is here: is it time to change our treatment paradigms? J Natl Compr Canc Netw 2011;9(6):665–673

Walvekar RR, Li RJ, Gooding WE, et al. Role of surgery in limited (T1-2, N0-1) cancers of the oropharynx. Laryngoscope 2008;118(12):2129–2134

Weinstein GS, Quon H, Newman HJ, et al. Transoral robotic surgery alone for oropharyngeal cancer: an analysis of local control. Arch Otolaryngol Head Neck Surg 2012;138(7):628–634

29 Strategies for Nonsurgical Organ Preservation in Laryngeal Cancer

■ Introduction

The development of new strategies for organ preservation in laryngeal cancer is most pertinent to patients with advanced malignancy. Generally for small cancers (T1, T2), organ-preserving approaches using local excision, laser vaporization, partial laryngectomy, or definitive radiation are highly successful, and they preserve adequate-to-excellent laryngeal function and voice. In those 20 to 40% of patients where initial conservative treatment for an early cancer might fail, salvage conservation laryngeal surgical techniques often offer possible alternatives to total laryngectomy. This discussion emphasizes the emerging role and current status of the combination of chemotherapy and radiation as an alternative to total laryngectomy for patients with advanced (stages III and IV) cancers.

The frontiers of larynx preservation with partial laryngectomy for patients with moderately large lesions (selected T2, T3 transglottic or selected T3, T4 supraglottic) have been advanced with development of subtotal (75%) laryngectomy, supracricoid laryngectomy, and transoral laser techniques. The role of radiation therapy in the treatment of these more advanced lesions is controversial. Experiences from some radiation centers indicate excellent survival rates (~ 50%) and larynx preservation rates (~ 65%) with radiation alone for patients with either advanced glottic or supraglottic cancers; however, these results are achieved in patients without neck node metastases. Survival and larynx preservation rates in stage III or IV disease in patients with nodal metastases are considerably lower.

For the moderately advanced lesions one must consider the tradeoffs between definitive radiotherapy with laryngectomy held in reserve for salvage or an initial primarily surgical approach. The patient must be included in the decision-making process when the various treatment options are being formulated, because the patient may well decide to trade a few percentage points in terms of survival probability for a higher probability of voice preservation without a stoma.

■ Management

Alternative Strategies

In most cases, the traditional management of advanced glottic or supraglottic cancers has consisted of total laryngectomy with or without postoperative radiation. The past 15 years have seen the rapid proliferation of new treatment paradigms that incorporate initial or neoadjuvant chemotherapy for patients with advanced head and neck cancer. These approaches were predicated on the hypothesis that potent chemotherapy regimens capable of effecting major tumor regressions in previously untreated patients would reduce tumor burden, allow modifications in traditionally morbid local therapies, and have an impact on occult distant metastases.

Rationale for Neoadjuvant Chemotherapy for Organ Preservation

The Head and Neck Contracts Program and other trials that followed were consistent in demonstrating that patients achieving a complete clinical regression of cancer after neoadjuvant chemotherapy enjoyed a survival advantage. Also, response to chemotherapy tended to predict a favorable overall response after subsequent radiation therapy.

This led to the development of treatment paradigms that used chemotherapy to select patients for treatment that might avoid organ-sacrificing surgery. The first large, prospective, randomized trial combining neoadjuvant chemotherapy with radiation as an alternative treatment for patients who traditionally were felt to require surgical resection for optimal management was undertaken by a group of investigators from the U.S. Department of Veterans Affairs (VA). Advanced laryngeal cancer was selected because of the morbidity of total laryngectomy, the proven effectiveness of radiation on small laryngeal cancers, and the fact that some surgeons and patients would accept treatments with radiation alone as an alternative to laryngectomy, even if it meant risking lower survival rates.

Selection Criteria

Basic patient selection criteria for such an approach would include (1) patients with adequate hematologic, renal, audiological, and hepatic function to enable treatment with intensive chemotherapy; (2) previously untreated patients facing total laryngectomy as the optimal treatment alternative, rather than either radiation alone or conservation laryngeal procedure; and (3) patients with smaller tumors without extensive destruction of the laryngeal framework. In patients with extensive cartilage destruction, successful cancer eradication with chemoradiation often results in destruction of many of the structures in the larynx that were infiltrated by tumor and could result in chronic aspiration, poor voice, or chronic radiochondritis. Although these complications were rare in the VA trial, recent experience with more intensive regimens of accelerated fractionation radiation with concurrent chemotherapy have resulted in higher rates of radiation chondritis.

Survival and Larynx Preservation

Like its predecessor neoadjuvant trials, the VA trial failed to demonstrate that the addition of two to three cycles of chemotherapy (cisplatin and 5-fluorouracil) could improve survival or disease-free interval. In fact, disease-free interval was lower for chemotherapy-treated patients because of local recurrences in the larynx. Many of these patients with local failure underwent successful salvage laryngectomy, either as a planned procedure after a failure of chemotherapy to achieve major tumor regression or for persistent disease after completion of radiation. Overall survival was similar for both treatment groups, with an overall rate of preservation of the larynx among patients randomized to chemotherapy of over 60%. Likewise, an additional 5% of surviving patients retained a functioning larynx, although this group represented only one-third of the total number of patients initially randomized to chemotherapy. Long-term follow-up (median 98 months) of this well-studied cohort of patients continues to show similar survival curves with an overall survival rate of 35%. When analyzed by patterns of relapse, chemotherapy-treated patients had higher local recurrence rates and significantly lower distant relapse rates. This was based on an analysis of site of first relapse. Although these data suggested an impact of chemotherapy on distant disease, overall rates of distant metastases as a cause of death were similar in both treatment groups.

A large number of studies based on the carefully collected data from this trial have been published.

It has been shown that the addition of chemotherapy was not associated with increased radiation complications or surgical complications. The drugs were well tolerated, compliance was good, and few patients were lost to follow-up.

Analysis of neck disease documented that if a complete regression of clinical neck disease was achieved with neoadjuvant chemotherapy, radiation was quite effective in long-term control of disease. However, if any palpable neck nodes remained after chemotherapy in patients with advanced (N2, N3) neck disease, it was unlikely that radiation alone was curative in the neck. These findings have prompted either incorporation of earlier salvage neck dissections in nonresponders after chemotherapy or planned neck dissections after completion of radiation for patients with advanced, bulky neck disease.

The best clinical predictors of successful larynx preservation were achievement of a complete response after chemotherapy, smaller tumor size (T3 better than T4), and lack of the need for a pretreatment tracheostomy.

More recent approaches have looked at concurrent chemoradiotherapy for advanced laryngeal cancer. The 91–11 trial compared prospectively assigned patients to three groups: induction cisplatin plus fluorouracil followed by radiotherapy, concurrent cisplatin with radiotherapy, and radiotherapy alone. At 2 years, there was improved locoregional control with concurrent therapy compared with the other arms of the trial. Additionally, 88% of patients in the concurrent chemoradiation arm had an intact larynx at 2 years, compared with 75% in the induction chemotherapy arm and 70% in the radiotherapy-only arm. Interestingly, there was improvement in disease-free survival in the chemotherapy groups, but no difference in overall survival among the three arms.

The 2011 meta-analysis of chemotherapy in head and neck cancer (MACH-NC) update from the MACH-NC collaborative group found an overall benefit in the inclusion of chemotherapy to radiation. Concurrent chemoradiotherapy was superior to induction chemotherapy or adjuvant therapy. As long as patients have good performance status, chemoradiotherapy with cisplatinu is recommended for advanced-stage laryngeal cancers. Biologic therapies also have an evolving role in laryngeal cancer. In advanced cancers of the head and neck, cetuximab (anti-epidermal growth factor receptor [EGFR] antibody) given concurrently with radiation therapy improves local regional control and overall survival compared with radiotherapy alone.

Larynx Preservation in Hypopharyngeal Cancer

Another important randomized trial of combined chemotherapy and radiation for organ preservation was conducted by the European Organization for Research and Treatment of Cancer in patients with advanced hypopharyngeal cancer. Over 200 patients were randomly assigned to receive either surgery (total laryngectomy with partial pharyngectomy and neck dissection) with postoperative radiation (50–79 gray [Gy]) or induction chemotherapy (cisplatin and 5-fluorouracil). Complete responders to induction chemotherapy after either two or three cycles were treated with definitive radiation. Those not responding completely to chemotherapy underwent planned surgery and postoperative radiation. Salvage surgery for the primary tumor or neck metastases was performed for recurrences after chemotherapy and radiation.

With a median follow-up of 51 months, actuarial survival was similar for both treatment groups, with a longer median survival for the chemotherapy group (44 months vs. 25 months). Analysis of patterns of relapse showed similar recurrence rates for local, regional, or second primary tumor in the treatment groups, but a lower rate of distant relapse in the chemotherapy group was of borderline statistical significance. Unfortunately, the overall 3-year disease-free survival rates remained dismal for both groups of patients (31% of the surgery group, 43% of the chemotherapy group). At 3 years, 40% of patients randomized to chemotherapy were alive, disease-free, with an intact larynx, and without tracheostomy or feeding tubes.

Important Principles

The following important lessons learned in these two carefully performed and analyzed studies should guide current therapy and the further refinement of organ preservation approaches.

A Carefully Planned Program Can Be an Alternative to Immediate Laryngectomy

A carefully planned program using the response to neoadjuvant chemotherapy to select patients for definitive radiation can be an alternative to immediate laryngectomy for patients with advanced laryngeal or hypopharyngeal cancers. Although ~ 30 to 40% of patients can be expected to survive with a preserved larynx, the overall survival rates for these patients remain poor. Improved survival should continue to be the appropriate end point of future trials.

Surgeons Are Refocusing on Quality-of-Life Issues

In the absence of therapies that improve survival, organ preservation studies have refocused the attention of surgeons on quality-of-life issues. With this renewed interest, questions of cost, morbidity of

combining therapies, the inefficiencies of planned retreatment, and the prolonged length of treatment are being debated. This debate will continue to stimulate new studies that will lead to further therapy refinements. It remains axiomatic that treatment of potentially curable patients with newer combinations of chemoradiation should not and must not occur outside the setting of carefully designed clinical trials.

Neoadjuvant Chemotherapy Can Be Safely Combined with Surgery and Radiation

It has also been shown that neoadjuvant chemotherapy can be safely combined with surgery and radiation and that complete response rates of 40 to 50% can be expected with current drug regimens. An analysis of the success of organ preservation versus number of cycles of chemotherapy in the VA study has shown that a rapid tumor regression (after one or two cycles) predicts the likelihood of an eventual complete response. Achievement of a complete response, particularly a histologically confirmed response, is the best prognostication for successful organ preservation. The optimal number of cycles of neoadjuvant chemotherapy has not been defined, but it seems that the minimum number necessary to achieve a complete response is a reasonable guide.

Early Surgical Salvage Is an Integral Part of the Treatment Paradigm

Some investigators have questioned whether concomitant chemoradiation or simply more intensive (accelerated) radiation fractionation schemes might achieve similar organ preservation results. However, these approaches fail to appreciate the potentially important role that early surgical salvage plays in optimizing survival rates. In the successful organ preservation trials, most salvage surgical resections were performed as planned procedures after a failure of neoadjuvant chemotherapy. Thus surgery is an integral part of the treatment paradigm. If such patients were treated with radiation alone or combined chemoradiation, it is unlikely that they would have survival rates as high because immediate surgical salvage would be postponed for those 15 to 20% of patients who would have been selected for early salvage, thus leading to delays in the diagnosis of persistent or recurrent disease.

Careful Tumor Surveillance and Timely Detection of Recurrence Are Integral to Success

It is apparent that careful tumor surveillance and timely detection of recurrence after chemoradiation are integral to success and can often be difficult due to tissue fibrosis, edema, and tissue induration. An analysis of salvage neck dissections performed as part of the VA study demonstrated that patients with persistent neck disease after chemotherapy were rarely cured with subsequent full-course radiation, and that by the time persistent/recurrent neck disease was detected, it was often unresectable. Newer imaging studies using positron-emission tomography scanning may improve tumor surveillance abilities by reflecting physiological changes indicative of a tumor response to chemotherapy during and after treatment, and by detecting cancer recurrences in heavily treated tissues. It is clear that successful organ preservation approaches must incorporate careful tumor surveillance by experienced clinicians, especially head and neck surgeons who must be ready to intervene with appropriate biopsies as part of an aggressive approach to patient monitoring and timely surgical intervention.

Surgical Salvage after Combined Chemotherapy and Radiation Is Challenging

It has been shown that surgical salvage after combinations of chemotherapy and radiation is one of the most challenging oncological surgical endeavors. Major complication rates approach 60 to 70%. Complications may be reduced by meticulous surgical technique, free-tissue transfer reconstructions, and comprehensive nutritional and metabolic support. The extent of a salvage procedure must be aggressive and must completely encompass the original tumor volume and any areas of progressive disease. Pretreatment tattoos of the primary tumor resection margins are valuable adjuncts in this circumstance.

Primary recurrences after radiation are characterized by submucosal extensions that are often more extensive than the surface appearance of these cancers. Treatment of such cancers demands a thorough

knowledge of pathways of tumor spread in the larynx and hypopharynx, meticulous frozen section monitoring of deeper tissue planes, and an understanding of how radiation fibrosis may alter vascular and lymphatic drainage patterns. Naive management approaches that emphasize conservative resections for these recurrent cancers in a fashion similar to untreated cancers will lead to surgical misadventures and poor outcomes.

■ Future Approaches

The next frontier in neoadjuvant chemotherapy approaches for organ preservation will be improved patient selection and refinements in treatment paradigms. These approaches will allow the length of treatment to be shortened and the issues of disseminated disease and poor overall survival to be addressed. It is clear that not all patients benefit from the organ preservation approach, and some must be treated with three modalities, each with substantial morbidity without an expectation of improvement in survival. For those patients who achieve a complete tumor regression after chemotherapy, there is clearly a benefit. This benefit derives from selecting patients for curative radiation. Emerging laboratory data indicate that tumor kinetics and alterations in genes that regulate cell proliferation and apoptosis may be critical determinants of tumor response to chemotherapy and radiation and potentially useful aids in patient selection.

Through future approaches, improvements in survival are likely to be achieved. Until that time, existing trial results indicate that laryngeal preservation is an achievable goal in many patients with advanced laryngeal cancer if a carefully conducted program of patient selection using neoadjuvant chemotherapy and radiation is combined with appropriate tumor surveillance and timely surgical salvage.

■ Suggested Reading

Agrawal N, Goldenberg D. Primary and salvage total laryngectomy. Otolaryngol Clin North Am 2008;41(4):771–780, vii

Blanchard P, Baujat B, Holostenco V, et al; MACH-CH Collaborative group. Meta-analysis of chemotherapy in head and neck cancer (MACH-NC): a comprehensive analysis by tumour site. Radiother Oncol 2011;100(1):33–40

Bonner JA, Harari PM, Giralt J, et al. Radiotherapy plus cetuximab for squamous-cell carcinoma of the head and neck. N Engl J Med 2006;354(6):567–578

Forastiere AA, Goepfert H, Maor M, et al. Concurrent chemotherapy and radiotherapy for organ preservation in advanced laryngeal cancer. N Engl J Med 2003;349(22):2091–2098

Forastiere AA, Zhang Q, Weber RS, et al. Long-term results of RTOG 91-11: a comparison of three nonsurgical treatment strategies to preserve the larynx in patients with locally advanced larynx cancer. J Clin Oncol 2013;31(7):845–852

Posner MR, Hershock DM, Blajman CR, et al; TAX 324 Study Group. Cisplatin and fluorouracil alone or with docetaxel in head and neck cancer. N Engl J Med 2007;357(17):1705–1715

Vokes EE. Competing roads to larynx preservation. J Clin Oncol 2013;31(7):833–835

30 Contemporary Laryngeal Conservation Surgery

■ Introduction

Approaches in conservative laryngeal surgery can be divided into open procedures and endoscopic techniques. Technological advances have led to innovations in endoscopic techniques. Regardless of technique, goals remain the same and include achieving the local control rates similar to rates achieved with total laryngectomy while retaining the patient's ability to speak and swallow without permanent tracheostomy or gastrostomy tube. In the large majority of cases, the expected outcome is temporary dysphagia, temporary tracheostomy, and some degree of permanent hoarseness.

Although they share these mutual goals and drawbacks, there are some fundamental differences between open and endoscopic approaches. Transection of the tumor and piecemeal excision may be favored during endoscopic technique to determine the extent of tumor. In general, the tumor is totally excised with an endoscopic technique, with as much normal tissue preserved as possible; with an open technique, tumor margins are often defined by preset anatomical boundaries.

The Anatomical Basis of Conservation Laryngeal Surgery

The sine qua non for proper preoperative clinical evaluation of laryngeal cancers, prior to performing conservative laryngeal surgical techniques, is a three-dimensional understanding of how cancer invades the larynx. The key anatomical features of importance to the laryngeal surgeon are the (1) skeletal framework; (2) fibrous tissue barriers; (3) mucosal surfaces; (4) laryngeal spaces; and (5) soft tissue adnexae, including the blood vessels, nerves, lymphatics, musculature, and salivary glands.

Several reports have addressed the role of intralaryngeal barriers. Two studies have demonstrated that, although the conus elasticus plays a role as a temporary barrier for early cancers, it is not an effective barrier to invasion for larger lesions. Although opinions differ regarding cartilage invasion at the anterior commissure, Kirchner et al reported in 1987 that early carcinomas that extended to the anterior commissure rarely eroded the cartilage, whereas larger carcinomas spread along the anterior commissure tendon both inferiorly and superiorly. Cancer rarely extends through the hypoepiglottic ligament, which constitutes the superior fibrous barriers of the supraglottis. The traditionally held belief that a barrier prevents the spread of supraglottic carcinoma to the glottis has recently been disputed. Instead, the superior-inferior spread of supraglottic carcinoma appears to be impeded by the hourglass shape of the paraglottic space. This study also indicated that supraglottic carcinoma spreads to the glottis in 20 to 54% of cases.

In a whole-organ section study, Hirano et al noted that 50 to 65% of the entire adult airway is posterior to the anterior aspect of the vocal processes of the arytenoids. Therefore, they said the posterior glottis (interarytenoid area) should be regarded as the "respiratory larynx," and the anterior glottis (vocal cords) should be regarded as the "the phonatory larynx." Thus both cords can be resected with minimal impact on respiration and swallowing without a permanent tracheostomy.

■ Preoperative Evaluation

Extent of the Primary Laryngeal Tumor

The goal of the preoperative assessment is to provide a precise mapping of the superficial and deep extent of the lesion. The assessment of vocal cord and arytenoid mobilities through laryngoscopy provides an excellent indirect assessment of the depth of invasion of laryngeal carcinoma. An association has been noted between thyroarytenoid muscle invasion and impairment or fixation of the vocal cord. In 1991, Hirano et al reported that abnormalities of cord mobility are actually due to arytenoid invasion in the case of supraglottic carcinoma. In two-thirds of cases, arytenoid cartilage fixation is related to invasion of the cricoarytenoid musculature or joint, precluding performing conservative open laryngeal surgeries because of posterolateral cricoid involvement.

Radiological assessment is quite useful to corroborate the findings of the clinical exam. In many instances, computed tomography and magnetic resonance imaging are limited by their tendency to over- or underpredict tumor invasion. Nonetheless, they can be helpful in identifying submucosal invasion in the subglottis and the pre-epiglottic space. Involvement of the paraglottic space is difficult to assess, due to the inability to distinguish between deep invasion at the glottic level versus mass effect from pushing on the saccular and ventricular mucosa.

■ Surgical Treatment

Open Technique

The two standard types of open surgeries that have evolved are (1) vertical partial laryngectomies, primarily for glottic cancers, and (2) horizontal partial laryngectomies for supraglottic cancers. The role and the utility of the various conservation laryngeal surgeries have evolved over the past few decades in the United States, with large series of supraglottic laryngectomies being reported with great success in the appropriate situation. The role of vertical partial laryngectomy has become more limited since the advent of laser endoscopic surgical resection for early laryngeal carcinoma. The supracricoid laryngectomy has broadened the indications for conservation surgeries in the surgical treatment of selected laryngeal carcinomas.

Selected Surgical Techniques for Glottic Carcinoma

Laryngofissure and Cordectomy

This technique includes a midline thyrotomy approach for resection of vocal cord carcinoma. Its main utility is for the management of midcord lesions of the mobile true vocal cord. Outcomes for Tl glottic carcinoma revealed a 0 to 3.3% (2/61) recurrence rate. The advent of laser endoscopic approaches for similarly staged lesions has diminished the indications for laryngofissure and cordectomy. The expected functional swallowing outcome is excellent. Patients with false cord reconstruction

of the glottic level appear to have improved phonatory outcome.

Vertical Hemilaryngectomy

Vertical hemilaryngectomy can yield excellent local control of 93% for selected glottic carcinomas confined to the true vocal cord without anterior commissure involvement. However, involvement of the anterior commissure, reported in the same series, resulted in a 14 to 25% local failure rate. Other factors associated with local failure include impaired cord mobility and extension beyond the true cord into the ventricle. Two series have reported a local failure rate greater than 20% for T2 glottic carcinoma. The local failure rate following vertical hemilaryngectomy for T3 cancers has been greater than 36%.

In summary, vertical hemilaryngectomy can be expected to yield excellent oncological results for selected Tl glottic carcinoma limited to the true vocal cord, but it should be used with caution for Tl lesions with extensive invasion of the anterior commissure, or with early T2 glottic carcinomas with impaired mobility or extension beyond the glottis.

Extended Frontolateral Partial Laryngectomy with Epiglottic Laryngoplasty

This technique involves excision of both true vocal cords; both false cords, sparing a posterior strut of the thyroid cartilage bilaterally; and at least one arytenoid. Reconstruction is accomplished by advancing the epiglottis inferiorly and suturing it to the cricoid. Although Tucker et al reported no local failures in Tla, Tlb, or T2 lesions, they noted a 12.5% recurrence rate among T3 glottic carcinomas. Extension beyond 6 mm into the subglottis results in a local failure of 50%. Although this has been a useful procedure for selected glottic lesions, Nong et al have noted a breathy voice due to wide anteroposterior dimension of the reconstructed larynx.

Supracricoid Partial Laryngectomy with Cricohyoidepiglottopexy (SCPL c CHEP)

The SCPL c CHEP involves the resection of both true cords, both false cords, the entire thyroid cartilage, and the paraglottic spaces bilaterally, while sparing at least one arytenoid. Reconstruction is performed by direct closure between the cricoid, epiglottis, hyoid, and tongue base. The main indication is for advanced T2 glottic carcinomas, which are considered too extensive for vertical hemilaryngectomy, but this procedure has also been used for selected T1b, T3, and T4 glottic carcinomas. Laccourreye et al reported no local failures among nine patients with Tl glottic carcinoma. When this procedure was performed for selected T3 glottic carcinomas, with a fixed true cord but some residual mobility of the arytenoid, the local control was 90%. Similar control rates were reported by Piquet et al, who noted a 5% local failure rate with 104 patients (Tl = 12, T2 = 77, T3 = 15). Contraindications for the procedure include (1) subglottic extension greater than 10 mm anteriorly and 5 mm posteriorly, (2) arytenoid fixation, (3) invasion of the pre-epiglottic space, (4) extension to the pharynx or interarytenoid area, and (5) cricoid cartilage invasion. The expected functional outcome is temporary dysphagia and permanent hoarseness.

Surgical Techniques for Selected Supraglottic Carcinomas

Supraglottic Laryngectomy

The standard supraglottic laryngectomy results in resection of the epiglottis, pre-epiglottic space, false cords, and superior half of the thyroid cartilage. Reconstruction is accomplished by performing direct anastomosis between the remaining thyroid cartilage and the tongue base. Extended procedures can include resection of one arytenoid, the pyriform sinus, or a portion of the tongue base. Analysis of series of supraglottic laryngectomies performed in the United States revealed a 90% or higher local control rate in several large series. Although high local control has been reported for Tl and T2 lesions, the results for T3 and T4 lesions have been more variable in the literature. The expected functional outcome is temporary dysphagia with an excellent voice. From the swallowing perspective, Hirano et al reported that 84% of patients had removal of the feeding tube within 30 days; however, significant dysphagia has been associated with extended supraglottic laryngectomy.

Supracricoid Laryngectomy with Cricohyoidopexy (SCPL c CHP)

SCPL c CHP results in the resection of the epiglottis, pre-epiglottic space, true cords, false cords, and entire thyroid cartilage, sparing at least one arytenoid. The reconstruction is accomplished by suturing the cricoid to the hyoid and the tongue base. This procedure is most useful for selected T2 or T3 supraglottic carcinomas, which are not amenable to supraglottic laryngectomy.

The main indications for SCPL c CHP are supraglottic carcinomas with extension to the glottis. In whole-organ section series, these carcinomas have been noted to occur in 20 to 54% of cases and are a contraindication to standard supraglottic laryngectomy. Contraindications for the procedure include (1) subglottic extension greater than 10 mm anteriorly and 5 mm posteriorly, (2) arytenoid fixation, (3) massive invasion of the pre-epiglottic space or vallecula,

(4) extension to the pharynx or interarytenoid area, and (5) cricoid cartilage invasions. The expected functional outcome following SCPL c CHP is temporary dysphagia and permanent hoarseness. The world literature reveals variability in the duration of tube feeds from 13 days to 365 days. Resecting one arytenoid is associated with increased dysphagia. The factors important to optimizing functional outcome include patient selection, attention to intraoperative detail, and careful postoperative rehabilitation.

Endoscopic Technique

Endoscopic technique is also known as transoral laser microsurgery (TLM) resection. Advances in lasers, including fiber-based lasers and photoangiolytic lasers, as well as robotic access have allowed more extensive resections with less long-term swallow and voice dysfunction. Various studies have found local control rates for TLM resection for early glottic carcinomas to be similar to if not greater than rates for radiotherapy and a higher 5-year laryngeal preservation rate.

For early glottic carcinoma, less than 2% of patients require tracheostomy at the time of surgery. Many patients can be treated as ambulatory surgery or 23 hour observation. As a result, radiotherapy for an early glottis tumor was approximately four times more costly than TLM. A large meta-analysis found that the oncological and functional results of TLM for early glottis cancer appear to be comparable to radiotherapy, with a higher rate of laryngeal preservation and lower cost. Anterior commissure involvement in T2 and T3 glottic tumors can be successfully treated with local control. Voice outcomes with TLM may be equivalent to radiotherapy outcomes. In the event of early recurrence after laser resection, re-resection can be successfully accomplished while still preserving options for radiation or total laryngectomy.

T1 and T2 supraglottic tumors are frequently amenable to endoscopic excision, along with certain T3 and T4 lesions. Hinni et al reported an 86% laryngeal preservation and a 55% 5-year survival rate for T3 and T4 supraglottic tumors treated with TLM. Supraglottic tumors can be treated safely and effectively, with oncological results being similar between open and endoscopic techniques. Swallow is affected; the degree of injury is related to the extent of resection, but it generally improves.

Transoral Robotic Surgery (TORS)

TORS has shown to be a safe and feasible option for glottic and supraglottic carcinomas with low complication rates. Many appropriately selected patients preserve laryngeal function and do not need a long-term gastrostomy tube or tracheostomy tube. However, massive bleeding may require conversion to an open procedure. Excision is now enhanced with the use of fiber-based laser wave guides, which may be coupled to a robotic setup. TORS may be coupled to a thulium:yttrium-aluminum-garnet (Tm:YAG) laser, with equal hemostasis, less intraoperative pharyngotomies, and less pain.

There is a growing role for the use of photoangiolytic laser, such as the potassium-titanyl-phosphate or pulsed-dye laser wavelengths in the treatment of glottic cancers. Treatment is based on a tumor angiogenesis model and includes both excision and ablation of the mucosa in the surgical margins. Treatment is effective, and excisions can be repeated, while preserving excellent postoperative vocal function by preserving vibrations.

■ Summary

A wide spectrum of conservation laryngeal surgeries is available for the management of laryngeal carcinomas. The key to patient selection is an accurate assessment of the superficial and deep extent of the lesion. This assessment, coupled with an understanding of individual surgical techniques, permits a sound approach in choosing the appropriate surgical techniques for a particular lesion. The expected outcome in the majority of cases is permanent hoarseness, temporary dysphagia, and temporary tracheostomy, which would seem a reasonable price to pay if total laryngectomy can be avoided.

■ Suggested Reading

Blanch JL, Vilaseca I, Caballero M, Moragas M, Berenguer J, Bernal-Sprekelsen M. Outcome of transoral laser microsurgery for T2-T3 tumors growing in the laryngeal anterior commissure. Head Neck 2011;33(9):1252–1259

Brasnu D, Laccourreye O, Weinstein G, Fligny I, Chabardes E. False vocal cord reconstruction of the glottis following vertical partial laryngectomy: a preliminary analysis. Laryngoscope 1992;102(6):717–719

Chevalier D, Piquet JJ. Subtotal laryngectomy with cricohyoidopexy for supraglottic carcinoma: review of 61 cases. Am J Surg 1994;168(5):472–473

Grant DG, Repanos C, Malpas G, Salassa JR, Hinni ML. Transoral laser microsurgery for early laryngeal cancer. Expert Rev Anticancer Ther 2010;10(3):331–338

Hartl DM, Ferlito A, Brasnu DF, et al. Evidence-based review of treatment options for patients with glottic cancer. Head Neck 2011;33(11):1638–1648

Higgins KM. What treatment for early-stage glottic carcinoma among adult patients: CO_2 endolaryngeal laser excision versus standard fractionated external beam radiation is superior in terms of cost utility? Laryngoscope 2011;121(1):116–134

Higgins KM, Shah MD, Ogaick MJ, Enepekides D. Treatment of early-stage glottic cancer: meta-analysis comparison of laser excision versus radiotherapy. J Otolaryngol Head Neck Surg 2009; 38(6):603–612

Hinni ML, Salassa JR, Grant DG, et al. Transoral laser microsurgery for advanced laryngeal cancer. Arch Otolaryngol Head Neck Surg 2007;133(12):1198–1204

Hirano M, Kurita S, Kiyokawa K, Sato K. Posterior glottis: morphological study in excised human larynges. Ann Otol Rhinol Laryngol 1986;95(6 Pt 1):576–581

Hirano M, Kurita S, Matsuoka H. Vocal function following hemilaryngectomy. Ann Otol Rhinol Laryngol 1987;96(5):586–589

Hirano M, Kurita S, Matsuoka H, Tateishi M. Vocal fold fixation in laryngeal carcinomas. Acta Otolaryngol 1991;111(2):449–454

Holsinger FC, Nussenbaum B, Nakayama M, et al. Current concepts and new horizons in conservation laryngeal surgery: an important part of multidisciplinary care. Head Neck 2010;32(5):656–665

Kambic V, Radsel Z, Smid L. Laryngeal reconstruction with epiglottis after vertical hemilaryngectomy. J Laryngol Otol 1976; 90(5):467–473

Kirchner JA. Two hundred laryngeal cancers: patterns of growth and spread as seen in serial section. Laryngoscope 1977;87(4 Pt 1): 474–482

Kirchner JA, Carter D. Intralaryngeal barriers to the spread of cancer. Acta Otolaryngol 1987;103(5-6):503–513

Kirchner JA, Som ML. The anterior commissure technique of partial laryngectomy: clinical and laboratory observations. Laryngoscope 1975;85(8):1308–1317

Kujath M, Kerr P, Myers C, et al. Functional outcomes and laryngectomy-free survival after transoral CO_2 laser microsurgery for stage 1 and 2 glottic carcinoma. J Otolaryngol Head Neck Surg 2011;40(Suppl 1):S49–S58

Laccourreye H, Laccourreye O, Weinstein G, Menard M, Brasnu D. Supracricoid laryngectomy with cricohyoidoepiglottopexy: a partial laryngeal procedure for glottic carcinoma. Ann Otol Rhinol Laryngol 1990;99(6 Pt 1):421–426

Laccourreye H, Laccourreye O, Weinstein G, Menard M, Brasnu D. Supracricoid laryngectomy with cricohyoidopexy: a partial laryngeal procedure for selected supraglottic and transglottic carcinomas. Laryngoscope 1990;100(7):735–741

Laccourreye O, Weinstein G, Brasnu D, Trotoux J, Laccourreye H. Vertical partial laryngectomy: a critical analysis of local recurrence. Ann Otol Rhinol Laryngol 1991;100(1):68–71

Lee NK, Goepfert H, Wendt CD. Supraglottic laryngectomy for intermediate-stage cancer: U.T. M.D. Anderson Cancer Center experience with combined therapy. Laryngoscope 1990;100(8): 831–836

Lutz CK, Johnson JT, Wagner RL, Myers EN. Supraglottic carcinoma: patterns of recurrence. Ann Otol Rhinol Laryngol 1990;99(1): 12–17

Mohr RM, Quenelle DJ, Shumrick DA. Vertico-frontolateral laryngectomy (hemilaryngectomy). Indications, technique, and results. Arch Otolaryngol 1983;109(6):384–395

Murono S, Endo K, Kondo S, Wakisaka N, Yoshizaki T. Oncological and functional outcome after transoral 532-nm pulsed potassium-titanyl-phosphate laser surgery for T1a glottic carcinoma. Lasers Med Sci 2013;28(2):615–619

Nong HT, Mo W, Huang GW, Chen L. Epiglottic laryngoplasty after extended hemilaryngectomy for glottic cancer. Chin Med J (Engl) 1990;103(11):925–931

Olsen SM, Moore EJ, Koch CA, Price DL, Kasperbauer JL, Olsen KD. Transoral robotic surgery for supraglottic squamous cell carcinoma. Am J Otolaryngol 2012;33(4):379–384

Pérez Delgado L, El-Uali Abeida M, de Miguel García F, et al. CO_2 laser surgery of supraglottic carcinoma: our experience over 6 years. Acta Otorrinolaringol Esp 2010;61(1):12–18

Piquet JJ, Chevalier D. Subtotal laryngectomy with crico-hyoido-epiglotto-pexy for the treatment of extended glottic carcinomas. Am J Surg 1991;162(4):357–361

Remacle M, Matar N, Lawson G, Bachy V, Delos M, Nollevaux MC. Combining a new CO_2 laser wave guide with transoral robotic surgery: a feasibility study on four patients with malignant tumors. Eur Arch Otorhinolaryngol 2012;269(7):1833–1837

Remacle M, Van Haverbeke C, Eckel H, et al. Proposal for revision of the European Laryngological Society classification of endoscopic cordectomies. Eur Arch Otorhinolaryngol 2007;264(5):499–504

Roedel RM, Matthias C, Wolff HA, Christiansen H. Repeated transoral laser microsurgery for early and advanced recurrence of early glottic cancer after primary laser resection. Auris Nasus Larynx 2010;37(3):340–346

Thomas JV, Olsen KD, Neel HB III, DeSanto LW, Suman VJ. Early glottic carcinoma treated with open laryngeal procedures. Arch Otolaryngol Head Neck Surg 1994;120(3):264–268

Tucker HM, Benninger MS, Roberts JK, Wood BG, Levine HL. Near-total laryngectomy with epiglottic reconstruction. Long-term results. Arch Otolaryngol Head Neck Surg 1989;115(11):1341–1344

Van Abel KM, Moore EJ, Carlson ML, et al. Transoral robotic surgery using the thulium:YAG laser: a prospective study. Arch Otolaryngol Head Neck Surg 2012;138(2):158–166

Weinstein GS, Laccourreye O, Brasnu D, Tucker J, Montone K. Reconsidering a paradigm: the spread of supraglottic carcinoma to the glottis. Laryngoscope 1995;105(10):1129–1133

Weinstein GS, Laccourreye O, Brasnu D, Yousem DM. The role of computed tomography and magnetic resonance imaging in planning for conservation laryngeal surgery. Neuroimaging Clin N Am 1996;6(2):497–504

Weinstein GS, O'Malley BW Jr, Magnuson JS, et al. Transoral robotic surgery: a multicenter study to assess feasibility, safety, and surgical margins. Laryngoscope 2012;122(8):1701–1707

Zeitels SM, Burns JA, Lopez-Guerra G, Anderson RR, Hillman RE. Photoangiolytic laser treatment of early glottic cancer: a new management strategy. Ann Otol Rhinol Laryngol Suppl 2008;199:3–24

Zeitels SM, Kirchner JA. Hyoepiglottic ligament in supraglottic cancer. Ann Otol Rhinol Laryngol 1995;104(10 Pt 1, l0 Pt 1): 770–775

31 Nasopharyngeal Cancer

■ Introduction

Nasopharyngeal carcinoma (NPC), a type of squamous cell carcinoma arising in the nasopharynx, is a distinct entity among head and neck neoplasms, with a unique epidemiology and pathophysiology. Viral, genetic, and environmental factors can contribute to the etiology of NPC. NPC is endemic in Southeast Asia. The incidence of NPC in southern China is 30 to 80 cases per 100,000 people, whereas in North America the incidence is < 1 per 100,000 people. Therefore, it is incumbent upon physicians in North America to be familiar with the signs and symptoms of NPC.

World Health Organization Classification

The World Health Organization (WHO) has divided NPC into three distinct pathological subtypes: type 1, keratinizing squamous cell carcinoma (SCC); type 2, nonkeratinizing SCC; and type 3, undifferentiated carcinoma. Type 1, keratinizing SCC, accounts for less than 5% of the disease in endemic areas, but more than 50% of the cases in North America. Types 2 and 3 are similar in epidemiology and behavior, and are commonly grouped together as undifferentiated carcinoma of nasopharyngeal type. Type 2 cancers are sometimes referred to as transitional cell carcinomas. Type 3 cancers are also often referred to as lymphoepitheliomas because of the prominent nonneoplastic lymphoid component; they can be further subclassified into Regaud and Schmincke subtypes, depending on the pattern of invasion.

Large-cell non-Hodgkin lymphomas can also occur in the nasopharynx. In the past, they were sometimes confused with undifferentiated carcinomas. Modern immunohistochemical techniques allow for a reliable and accurate diagnosis of NPC because all three forms stain positively for cytokeratin and negatively for leukocyte common antigen.

Viral Causes

Epstein-Barr virus (EBV) deoxyribonucleic acid (DNA) is found by DNA hybridization techniques in all types of NPC in endemic areas. In North America, however, type 1 NPC has been variably associated with EBV, whereas type 3 disease remains an EBV-prevalent disease. Interestingly, the viral DNA found in these tumors is clonal, suggesting that the virus plays a role in the early stages of oncogenesis. Viral infection is thought to be seminal in the development of most NPC. Serological tests for the immunoglobulin A (IgA) antibody to viral capsid antigen (VCA) and early antigen (EA) have been used in endemic areas as a screening tool to determine populations at risk. Approximately 80% of patients with types 2 and 3 NPC will have IgA antibodies to EBV, whereas only 10 to 15% of those with type 1 tumors will test positive for these antibodies. In addition, some studies have shown that antibody levels will fall with successful treatment and rise with recurrence, even before the cancer is clinically evident.

Epidemiology

NPC is endemic in southern China, North Africa, the Philippines, the Caribbean, and among Aleut Indians. Evidence of a genetic risk factor for the development of this disease comes from studies showing that risk is associated with certain human lymphocyte antigen (HLA) histocompatibility loci. The relative risk of developing NPC is increased in people with HLA A2 and HLA B*Sin2*. It is also thought that nitrosamines in salted fish consumed during childhood are an important risk factor for the development of NPC in Hong Kong. When people from endemic areas of the world move to the West, their risk of developing NPC falls after several generations, but not to the risk level of the general population. Again, this is evidence for a genetic factor in the etiology of this disease. In North America, some clinicians believe that WHO type 1

NPC is related to the normal risk factors for upper aerodigestive tract SCC—namely, tobacco and alcohol exposure.

There appears to be a bimodal age distribution for the appearance of NPC, with peaks at 10 to 24 years and 40 to 60 years of age. Most of the disease in young people is of the type 3, undifferentiated form, which is more frequently observed in men.

■ Evaluation

History and Physical Exam

The presenting signs and symptoms of NPC are predictable, based on the anatomy of the region and the mode of spread of the tumor. The most common presentation is with a neck mass or fullness in the ear. Unilateral middle ear effusion in an adult without some obvious cause, such as an upper respiratory tract infection or barotrauma, warrants direct visualization of the nasopharynx and follow-up until the effusion clears. Because some NPCs are not visible on physical examination, a persistent unilateral serous otitis media may warrant imaging studies of the nasopharynx and/or biopsy of the fossa of Rosenmüller. Other presenting signs and symptoms include hearing loss, epistaxis, nasal obstruction, pain, weight loss, and double vision.

Tumors most commonly begin in the fossa of Rosenmüller or lateral nasopharyngeal recess, behind and superior to the torus tubarius or posterior lip of the eustachian tube cartilage. Here they may obstruct the eustachian tube, causing eustachian tube dysfunction and an effusion within the middle ear. From here they can spread upward through the soft tissue of the foramen lacerum to involve the cavernous sinus or superior orbital fissure with paralysis of cranial nerves III through VI. The abducens nerve is often the first cranial nerve to be involved for tumors with intracranial extension. The tumor may also spread posterolaterally along the skull base to the region of the jugular foramen to involve cranial nerves IX, X, and XI and even sometimes XII. Palsy of cranial nerves IX, X, and XI is known as Vernet syndrome. Palsy of cranial nerves IX, X, and XI plus nerve XII and Horner syndrome (paralysis of the cervical sympathetic chain) is known as Villaret syndrome.

The diagnosis of NPC has been greatly facilitated by the availability of flexible and rigid fiberoptic telescopes, which allow for easy visualization of the nasopharynx. For practical purposes, a biopsy of the nasopharynx is ultimately required to make a diagnosis of NPC. In selected patients, a biopsy can be done in the clinic with a biopsy forceps and fiberoptic telescope.

Special Investigation

Some clinicians have made the case that demonstration of EBV DNA in cervical lymph nodes from patients with an unknown primary SCC of the neck is also diagnostic of NPC, but such testing is not universally available or accepted.

In China, the detection of IgA antibodies to EBV VCA and EA has been successfully used to screen large populations for high-risk individuals who are then selected for examinations. In North America, however, where most of the tumors are WHO type I, such screening is not likely to be beneficial. In China, where most tumors are WHO types 2 and 3 and not related to tobacco and alcohol consumption, bronchoscopy, esophagoscopy, and direct laryngoscopy are not indicated. In North America, however, in a patient with WHO type 1 NPC, these diagnostic approaches are debatable because there may be a higher risk of a synchronous second primary cancer of the upper aerodigestive tract.

■ Management and Treatment

The current treatment standard for NPC includes both chemotherapy and radiation treatment. A clear survival advantage (hazard ratio 0.60; 95% confidence interval 0.48–0.76) has been associated with the use of concurrent chemoradiation over radiation therapy alone. The best evidence supports the use of radiation therapy (70 gray in 35 fractions) to the nasopharynx and both sides of the neck, with three cycles of concurrent cisplatin (100 mg/m²), followed by three cycles of adjuvant cisplatin and fluorouracil. Radiation is typically delivered using intensity-modulated radiation therapy (IMRT) techniques, which maximally exploit the spatial distances between the target tumor and other structures at risk. Thus the precision of IMRT techniques has made intracavitary brachytherapy and other approaches less common for the primary treatment of NPC.

Complications of irradiation for NPC include hypopituitarism, radionecrosis of the temporal bone, radiation myelitis, trismus from temporomandibular joint fibrosis, radionecrosis of the bone or soft tissues of the skull base, delayed palsy of cranial nerves (especially the hypoglossal), optic neuritis, cataracts, and retinopathy with loss of vision. In addition, there may be hypothyroidism from neck irradiation. The risk of complications increases with reirradiation for recurrence. Surgery is usually reserved for persistent neck disease when the primary tumor has been controlled with irradiation. Several authors have reported the results of surgical salvage of highly selected patients with localized recurrence in the nasopharynx through either a lateral skull base or a transpalatal approach.

Prognostic Factors

There are several staging systems for classification of NPC. In North America, the American Joint Committee on Cancer system is most commonly used (**Table 31.1**). Several studies have revealed poor prognostic indicators common to most staging systems. Cranial nerve involvement, intracranial extension, cervical lymph node metastases (especially to low in the neck), WHO type 1 histology, and older age have all been associated with poorer survival.

The overall 5-year survival rate for patients with NPC varies significantly across studies. In general, the survival rate for patients with WHO type 3 lymphoepithelioma is generally 20 to 30% higher than for those with SCC. For example, it has been reported that 5-year survival rates for WHO type 1, 2, and 3 tumors are 20%, 35%, and 56% respectively. Distant metastases occur in up to 20% of patients and have been correlated with advanced nodal disease.

Table 31.1 Staging system for nasopharyngeal cancer

Primary tumor (T)	
TX	Primary tumor cannot be assessed
T0	No evidence of primary tumor
Tis	Carcinoma in situ
Nasopharynx	
T1	Tumor confined to the nasopharynx, or tumor extends to oropharynx and/or nasal cavity without parapharyngeal extension[a]
T2	Tumor with parapharyngeal extension[a]
T3	Tumor involves bony structures of skull base and/or paranasal sinuses
T4	Tumor with intracranial extension and/or involvement of cranial nerves, hypopharynx, orbit, or with extension to infratemporal fossa/masticator space
Regional lymph nodes (N)	
Nasopharynx	
The distribution and the prognostic impact of regional lymph node spread from nasopharynx cancer, particularly of the undifferentiated type, are different from those of other head and neck mucosal cancers and justify the use of a different N classification scheme.	
NX	Regional lymph nodes cannot be assessed
N0	No regional lymph node metastasis
N1	Unilateral metastasis in cervical lymph node(s), 6 cm or less in greatest dimension, above the supraclavicular fossa, and/or unilateral or bilateral, retropharyngeal lymph nodes, 6 cm or less, in greatest dimension[b]
N2	Bilateral metastasis in cervical lymph node(s), 6 cm or less in greatest dimension, above the supraclavicular fossa[b]
N3	Metastasis in a lymph node(s)[b] > 6 cm and/or to supraclavicular fossa[b]
N3a	Greater than 6 cm in dimension
N3b	Extension to supraclavicular fossa[c]
Distant metastasis (M)	
M0	No distant metastasis
M1	Distant metastasis

[a] Parapharyngeal extension denotes posterolateral infiltration of tumor.

[b] Midline nodes are considered ipsilateral nodes.

[c] Supraclavicular zone or fossa is relevant to the staging of nasopharyngeal carcinoma and is the triangular region originally described by Ho. It is defined by three points: (1) the superior margin of the sternal end of the clavicle, (2) the superior margin of the lateral end of the clavicle, (3) the point where the neck meets the shoulder. Note that this would include caudal portions of levels IV and VB. All cases with lymph nodes (whole or part) in the fossa are considered N3b.

Used with the permission of the American Joint Committee on Cancer (AJCC), Chicago, Illinois. The original source for this material is the AJCC Cancer Staging Manual, Seventh Edition (2010) published by Springer Science and Business Media LLC, www.springer.com.

■ Practice Guidelines, Consensus Statements, and Measures

Practice guidelines for the management of NPC, as described in the chapter text, may be found at the National Comprehensive Cancer Network Web site.

National Comprehensive Cancer Network. Clinical Practice Guidelines in Oncology. Head and Neck Cancers (Version 2.2011). http://www.nccn.org/professionals/physician_gls/f_guidelines.asp#site. Accessed March 1, 2013

■ Suggested Reading

Al-Sarraf M, LeBlanc M, Giri PG, et al. Chemoradiotherapy versus radiotherapy in patients with advanced nasopharyngeal cancer: phase III randomized Intergroup study 0099. J Clin Oncol 1998;16(4):1310–1317

Baujat B, Audry H, Bourhis J, et al; MAC-NPC Collaborative Group. Chemotherapy in locally advanced nasopharyngeal carcinoma: an individual patient data meta-analysis of eight randomized trials and 1753 patients. Int J Radiat Oncol Biol Phys 2006;64(1):47–56

Hildesheim A, Wang CP. Genetic predisposition factors and nasopharyngeal carcinoma risk: a review of epidemiological association studies, 2000-2011: Rosetta Stone for NPC: genetics, viral infection, and other environmental factors. Semin Cancer Biol 2012;22(2):107–116

Ho FC, Tham IW, Earnest A, Lee KM, Lu JJ. Patterns of regional lymph node metastasis of nasopharyngeal carcinoma: a meta-analysis of clinical evidence. BMC Cancer 2012;12:98

Lee AW, Lin JC, Ng WT. Current management of nasopharyngeal cancer. Semin Radiat Oncol 2012;22(3):233–244

32 Management of Benign Salivary Tumors

■ Introduction

The major salivary glands include the parotid, submandibular, and sublingual glands. Hundreds of minor salivary glands are located throughout the upper aerodigestive tract (UADT), including the lip, palate, pharynx, nasopharynx, larynx, and parapharyngeal space. Tumors of the salivary gland are relatively uncommon and represent less than 5% of head and neck neoplasms. These lesions include tumorlike conditions, benign tumors, and malignant neoplasms. The majority of salivary gland tumors originate in the parotid gland (~ 70%), followed by the minor salivary glands (~ 20%) and the submandibular gland (~ 10%). Approximately 75 to 80% of parotid gland tumors and ~ 50% of submandibular gland tumors are benign. About 70% of minor salivary gland tumors are malignant. Pleomorphic adenomas are the most common benign salivary gland tumor, representing ~ 85% of all salivary gland neoplasms.

Relevant Anatomy and Surgical Landmarks

Parotid Gland

The parotid gland is located within a musculoskeletal recess formed by the mandible, temporal bone, atlas (C1), and their related musculature. The gland is surrounded by the deep cervical fascia that becomes the stylomandibular ligament in its anteroinferior extent. This ligament separates the parotid gland from the submandibular gland. The parotid gland has a superficial and deep lobe that is separated by the extratemporal portion of the facial nerve. The deep lobe abuts the parapharyngeal space.

The facial nerve exits the stylomastoid foramen just posterior to the base of the styloid and provides innervation to the postauricular and posterior belly of the digastric muscle. The main trunk turns anterolaterally and becomes embedded within the parotid tissue. At the pes anserinus, the nerve divides into temporofacial and cervicofacial branches. There is some degree of variation in the distribution of the facial nerve, which extends into five peripheral nerve branches: frontal, zygomatic, buccal, marginal mandibular, and cervical.

Surgical excision of a benign parotid mass requires identification and preservation of the facial nerve. Surgical landmarks for the main trunk of the facial nerve include the tragal pointer, sternocleidomastoid muscle, posterior belly of the digastric muscle, and tympanomastoid suture line. The posterior belly of the digastric muscle lies at the depth of the facial nerve.

Submandibular Gland

The submandibular gland fills most of the submandibular or digastric triangle. The gland is divided into superficial and deep lobes based on the relationship to the mylohyoid muscle. The lingual nerve and submandibular duct (Wharton duct) are located along the posterior border of the mylohyoid. The hypoglossal nerve courses deep to the tendon of the digastric triangle and lies medial to the deep cervical fascia.

The marginal mandibular branch of the facial nerve travels between the deep surface of the platysma and the superficial aspect of the fascia that overlies the submandibular gland. The facial artery and vein are located deep to the nerve, and ligation with gentle superior traction of these vessels during surgery may protect the nerve. However, the perivascular lymph nodes may not be appropriately removed with this maneuver. In excising the submandibular gland, the facial artery may be ligated distally at the lower border of the mandible and proximally at the border of the posterior belly of the digastric muscle.

Sublingual Gland

The sublingual gland is adjacent to the submandibular gland and lies between the mylohyoid and hyoglossus muscles. This gland is quite superficial and may be covered by only a thin layer of oral mucosa. The lingual nerve courses along the medial aspect of the gland.

Minor Salivary Gland

The minor salivary glands are widely dispersed along the UADT, including the palate, lip, pharynx, nasopharynx, larynx, and parapharyngeal space. The highest density of these glands is located in the hard and soft palates. Surgical landmarks are specific to the subsites of the UADT.

Etiology

Incidence/Epidemiology

Salivary gland tumors represent 2 to 3% of all head and neck neoplasms. These tumors are more common in women than in men, with a peak incidence in the third and fourth decades of life. Malignant tumors tend to present in older patients.

Approximately 85% of salivary gland tumors are pleomorphic adenomas, representing 70% of parotid gland tumors and 50% of submandibular gland tumors. Warthin tumors (papillary cystadenoma lymphomatosum) represent 5 to 15% of salivary gland tumors. They are the second most common tumors of the parotid gland. Warthin tumors are more common in men than in women, with a peak incidence in the fifth and sixth decades of life. An estimated 50% of neoplasms present in the minor salivary gland are malignant, with adenoid cystic carcinoma being the most common in that location.

Several environmental and genetic factors have been suggested for salivary gland tumors. Genetic alterations, including translocations, allelic loss, and amplification, may contribute to the development of salivary gland tumors. Radiation exposure has been linked to the development of the benign Warthin tumor and to malignant mucoepidermoid carcinoma. Epstein-Barr virus may be a factor in the development of lymphoepithelial tumors of the salivary glands.

Pathogenesis

The salivary gland unit is composed of an acinus located at the distal end. The acinus consists of pyramidal salivary-forming cells surrounding a central lumen, with myoepithelial cells present between the basal side of these cells and the basement membrane. The acinar cells may be serous, mucinous, or seromucinous. Serous acinar cells predominate in the parotid gland, whereas mucinous cells are present in greater proportion in the submandibular gland. The acinus leads into the intercalated duct, composed

of cuboidal cells also lined with myoepithelial cells. Intercalated ducts empty into striated ducts, which lead to excretory ducts. Stem cells (reserve cells) differentiate into the various cells along the salivary gland unit.

Two competing theories have been proposed regarding the origin of benign and malignant neoplasms of the salivary gland. The stem cell theory suggests that salivary gland neoplasms arise from the reserve of stem cells of the salivary duct unit. The type of neoplasm depends on the stage of differentiation of the stem cell at the time of transformation and the location of the stem cell within the salivary gland unit. The multicellular theory states that salivary neoplasms arise from differentiated cells along the salivary gland unit. Pleomorphic adenomas may originate from the intercalated duct cells and myoepithelial cells. Oncocytic tumors are derived from the striated duct cells. Acinic cell tumors arise from acinar cells. Mucoepidermoid and squamous cell tumors are derived from the excretory duct cells.

Pathology

Tumors of the salivary glands are classified based on cytological, architectural, and biological characteristics. The World Health Organization/International Agency for Research on Cancer classification divides benign and malignant tumors into epithelial and nonepithelial categories (**Table 32.1**).

Benign Epithelial Tumors

Benign epithelial tumors include pleomorphic adenoma, Warthin tumor, monomorphic adenoma, intraductal papilloma (IDP), oncocytoma, and sebaceous neoplasms.

Pleomorphic Adenomas

Pleomorphic adenomas (benign mixed tumors) are the most common tumors of the salivary glands. These tumors are composed of both epithelial and connective tissue components in varying amounts. They are classically described in the tail of the parotid gland. When identified in minor salivary glands, the hard palate is the most common site of involvement, followed by the upper lip. These lesions tend to be smooth, multiloculated, and surrounded by a thin, delicate, incomplete capsule. Transcapsular growth leads to pseudopod extensions that project into the surrounding parotid gland tissue. Thus a sufficient margin of normal glandular tissue needs to be excised with the tumor to ensure complete excision. Additionally, tumor spillage related to rupture of the capsule may lead to disease recurrence. These tumors do not contain focal calcification or necro-

Table 32.1 World Health Organization histological classification of salivary gland tumors

Malignant epithelial tumors			
Acinic cell carcinoma	8550/3	Oncocytic carcinoma	8290/3
Mucoepidermoid carcinoma	8430/3	Salivary duct carcinoma	8500/3
Adenoid cystic carcinoma	8200/3	Adenocarcinoma, not otherwise specified	8140/3
Polymorphous low-grade adenocarcinoma	8525/3	Myoepithelial carcinoma	8982/3
Epithelial-myoepithelial carcinoma	8562/3	Carcinoma ex pleomorphic adenoma	8941/3
Clear cell carcinoma, not otherwise specified	8310/3	Carcinosarcoma	8980/3
Basal cell adenocarcinoma	8147/3	Metastasizing pleomorphic adenoma	8940/1
Sebaceous carcinoma	8410/3	Squamous cell carcinoma	8070/3
Sebaceous lymphadenocarcinoma	8410/3	Small cell carcinoma	8041/3
Cystadenocarcinoma	8440/3	Large cell carcinoma	8012/3
Low-grade cribriform cystadenocarcinoma		Lymphoepithelial carcinoma	8082/3
Mucinous adenocarcinoma	8480/3	Sialoblastoma	8974/1
Benign epithelial tumors			
Pleomorphic adenoma	8940/0	Sebaceous	8410/0
Myoepithelioma	8982/0	Nonsebaceous	8410/0
Basal cell adenoma	8147/0	Ductal papillomas	
Warthin tumor	8561/0	Inverted ductal papilloma	8503/0
Oncocytoma	8290/0	Intraductal papilloma	8503/0
Canalicular adenoma	8149/0	Sialadenoma papilliferum	8406/0
Sebaceous adenoma	8410/0	Cystadenoma	8440/0
Lymphadenoma			
Soft tissue tumors			
Hemangioma	9120/0		
Hematolymphoid tumors			
Hodgkin lymphoma		Extranodal marginal zone B cell lymphoma	9699/3
Diffuse large B cell lymphoma	9680/3		

Note: Behavior is coded /0 for benign tumors, /3 for malignant tumors, and /1 for borderline or uncertain behavior.

Morphology code of the International Classification of Diseases for Oncology (ICD-0) [821] and the Systematized Nomenclature of Medicine (http://snomed.org).

Used with permission from Barnes L, Eveson J, Reichart P, et al. Chapter 5: Tumours of the Salivary Glands. In: Barnes L, Eveson J, Reichart P, et al., eds. World Health Organization Classification of Tumours--Pathology and Genetics: Head and Neck Tumours. France: IARCPress, 2005. http://www.iarc.fr/en/publications/pdfs-online/pat-gen/bb9/bb9-chap5.pdf. Accessed December 11, 2014.

sis. Microscopic features are quite diverse, including islands of spindle and stellate cells, commonly with a mixoid configuration.

Pleomorphic adenomas tend to grow very slowly, but they may still become quite significant in size. Tumor excision is recommended before the mass becomes physically disfiguring or the lesion undergoes malignant transformation (carcinoma ex pleomorphic adenoma). Complete excision requires removal of the entire affected gland. However, for the parotid gland, a superficial parotidectomy with facial nerve dissection and preservation is recommended. Enucleation may incompletely excise the tumor capsule or lead to tumor spillage, which may contribute to tumor recurrence. There is a growing experience with extracapsular dissection, a more limited excision than superficial parotidectomy and more extensive than enucleation. Early results suggest this technique has similar control rates to superficial parotidectomy with lower rates of gustatory sweating and facial nerve weakness. Long-term follow-up, however, is limited.

Warthin Tumor (Papillary Cystadenoma Lymphomatosum, Cystic Papillary Adenoma, Adenolymphoma)

This is a well-encapsulated benign lesion that contains multiple cysts and is typically found in the parotid gland. This lesion has a recurrence rate of ~ 5% following removal and tends to be bilateral in ~ 10% of patients. Malignant transformation has not been observed. Histological findings consist of a heavy lymphoid stroma and aciniform epithelial cells that line the cystic areas with papillary projections.

Monomorphic Adenomas

These slow-growing tumors represent less than 5% of all salivary gland tumors. They are composed of only one morphological cell type. They are subclassified by their epithelial or myoepithelial origin: basal cell adenoma, canalicular adenoma, oncocytoma, and myoepithelioma.

1. *Basal cell adenoma* This lesion accounts for ~ 2% of all epithelial salivary gland neoplasms. Histological subtypes include tubular, trabecular, cylindroma, and solid (most common). The parotid gland is the most commonly involved site.
2. *Canalicular adenoma* This lesion affects minor salivary glands. Although previously classified as a subtype of basal cell adenoma, this neoplasm is recognized as a distinct histological entity. Canalicular adenoma tends to be multifocal and may affect elderly patients along the upper lip mucosa. Although surgical excision is curative, recurrence or residual disease is possible if all disease foci are not addressed.
3. *Oncocytoma (oxyphil adenoma)* Oncocytomas of the salivary gland are quite uncommon. They occur twice as frequently in women and most commonly in the sixth decade of life. These lesions typically occur in the superficial lobe of the parotid gland, and they appear very rarely in the minor salivary glands. Oncocytomas are firm, slow-growing masses with a spherical shape. They have a distinct capsule, and histological findings include uniform cells arranged in solid sheets. As with other benign salivary gland tumors, oncocytomas will recur with incomplete excision.
4. *Myoepithelioma* This well-encapsulated lesion is composed almost exclusively of myoepithelial cells and commonly occurs in the parotid gland. Myoepitheliomas have no gender predilection and are commonly seen in the third to sixth decades of life.

Intraductal Papilloma

IDP presents as a small, tan, smooth lesion typically found in the submucosa. These lesions are commonly found in the major salivary glands; their presence in minor salivary glands has been described only in case reports. Histological findings include a cystically dilated duct partly lined with cuboidal epithelium with complex anastomosing papillary fronds of variable size filling the cystic area. Differentiation of this lesion from papillary cystadenoma can be challenging, but IDPs lack the intraductal hyperplasia and papillary folds and projections within the dilated duct.

Granular Cell Tumor

This lesion has malignant potential and is commonly found in minor salivary glands of the oral cavity. The mass is well circumscribed, mobile, and painless. Microscopic examination demonstrates polygonal cells with abundant eosinophilic granular cytoplasm and mildly pleomorphic nuclei that may be round to oval in shape.

Benign Nonepithelial Tumors

Benign nonepithelial tumors (mesenchymal derivatives) include hemangioma, angioma, lymphangioma (cystic hygroma), lipoma, and neural sheath tumors.

Hemangiomas

Hemangiomas are the most common salivary gland tumor in children. They frequently involve the parotid gland, although they may also occur in the submandibular gland. These vascular tumors are differentiated from vascular malformations because they tend to be present early in life, have a rapid growth phase in children (approximately age 1–6 months), and then involute over 1 to 12 years.

Capillary Hemangiomas

Capillary hemangiomas are the most common salivary gland tumor in children, representing more than 90% of parotid gland tumors in children less than 1 year of age. These lesions are usually asymptomatic, unilateral, and compressible. The mass tends to be lobulated, dark red, and unencapsulated. Microscopic examination reveals solid masses of cells and multiple anastomosing capillaries that replace the acinar structure of the gland. Some hemangiomas exhibit response to steroid treatment (2–4 mg/kg/d). Despite the tendency toward spontaneous involution, certain lesions may warrant surgical excision, especially if neighboring structures are infiltrated.

Lymphangioma (Cystic Hygroma)

These lesions are most likely related to lymphatic sequestration of primitive embryonic lymph ducts that undergo irregular growth and canalization. The gross mass is spongy and multiloculated and has a yellow-blue surface. These lesions are commonly found in infants and children. Approximately half are present at birth, and 80% manifest by 2 years of age. These endothelial-lined spaces are typically painless and rarely cause symptoms of airway obstruction. Surgical excision is the treatment of choice, typically due to cosmetic concerns.

Lipoma

This slow-growing lesion is relatively uncommon in major salivary glands. Lipomas are derived from fat cells and are smooth, well demarcated, and yellow in appearance. These masses are soft and mobile but may cause pain. They are 10 times more common in men than in women, and their peak incidence is in the fifth to sixth decade of life in men. Lipomas consist of mature adipose cells with uniform nuclei. Surgery is the treatment of choice.

Tumorlike Lesions

Necrotizing Sialometaplasia

Nontumor lesions are important in the differential diagnosis of parotid and other salivary gland masses. Necrotizing sialometaplasia may be mistaken for a malignant tumor. The lesion presents as a single, unilateral, and typically painless mass on the hard palate. However, this lesion is benign and self-resolving. The etiology is uncertain but may be a reparative response to ischemic necrosis of salivary gland tissue. The lesion is seen in adults over the age of 40 years and is two to three times more common in men than in women. A biopsy can differentiate the lesion from a malignancy, and no other treatment is indicated.

Lymphoepithelial Hyperplasia (Mikulicz Disease, Godwin Tumor, Sicca Complex, Chronic Punctate Sialadenitis)

The entire gland or a portion of the parotid gland may be diffusely enlarged. This disorder occurs more frequently in females than in males, with a peak incidence in the fourth and fifth decades of life. Bilateral parotid gland involvement may be seen. The growth is slowly progressive and may cause pain around the ear or in the retromandibular distribution. Histological findings include diffused, well-organized lymphoid tissue and lymphocytic interstitial infiltrate with obliteration of the normal acinar structure.

◼ Evaluation

Clinical Findings

The majority of salivary gland tumors present as painless, slow-growing masses on the face, neck, or floor of the mouth. Sudden change in size may be indicative of infection, cystic degeneration, or internal hemorrhage. Most worrisome is rapid size change of a long-standing mass, which may represent malignant transformation of a benign lesion. Benign salivary gland tumors are typically freely mobile. Depending on the location of the involved salivary gland, nerve compression symptoms may be present, especially with larger malignant masses.

History

The approach for a mass in the salivary glands begins with a thorough history and physical examination. Presentation of salivary gland tumors in the major salivary glands may be quite typical. Parotid masses present in the preauricular facial area or in the parotid tail posterior to the angle of the mandible. A submandibular gland mass lies inferior to the mandible and extends inferiorly into the neck. Given the widely varied locations for minor salivary glands, the presentation of these masses may be less typical. Salivary gland tumors of the nasal septum may present with epistaxis or nasal airway obstruction. Base of tongue salivary gland tumors may cause dysphagia or globus sensation. These presentations demonstrate that salivary gland tumors need to be part of the differential in patients with a suspected head and neck neoplasm. Parapharyngeal space masses may affect mouth closure, but the effect of a space-filling benign lesion needs to be distinguished from a malignant lesion that may invade the masseter and pterygoid musculature.

In distinguishing benign and malignant salivary gland tumors, metastatic disease to the major salivary glands must be considered. A remote history of skin cancer raises the possibility of a metastatic melanoma or squamous cell carcinoma to the parotid gland.

The patient should be assessed for a history of weight loss (anorexia nervosa); underlying infectious diseases (e.g., tuberculosis), which may be associated with cough; chest pain; lymphadenopathy; or lymphoma manifested in type B symptoms (e.g., fever and night sweats).

Nontumor lesions should be part of the differential in the consideration of parotid and other salivary gland tumors. These lesions include necrotizing sialometaplasia, benign lymphoepithelial lesions, cystic lymphoid hyperplasia (related to acquired immunodeficiency syndrome), and salivary gland cysts or mucoceles.

Physical Examination

Benign salivary gland tumors are typically painless and mobile. The consistency may vary, but the lesion is usually discrete. Involvement of the deep lobe of the parotid gland or a parapharyngeal space mass may cause either fullness in the retromandibular portion of the gland or asymmetric swelling of the soft palate. Bimanual palpation of a mass in the floor of the mouth can distinguish submandibular and sublingual lesions. Careful evaluation of the function of the facial nerve is critical for a parotid mass. Hypoglossal and lingual nerve function should be inspected for submandibular and sublingual gland lesions. Distinguishing a benign from a malignant lesion requires evaluation for new-onset pain, facial nerve weakness, rapid growth, paresthesias, hoarseness, skin involvement, fixed mass, and cervical lymphadenopathy.

Special Investigations

Fine-needle aspiration biopsy (FNAB) is extremely informative when properly performed and read by a pathologist with appropriate expertise and experience in evaluating salivary gland tumor cytology. Although not as sensitive or specific as for thyroid tumors, FNAB can be quite useful in differentiating between malignant and benign processes with an accuracy rate of ~ 85%. FNAB is being performed more frequently with ultrasound guidance to ensure accurate needle placement. In the case of cystic lesions, ultrasound guidance can improve the likelihood that the cyst wall is sampled, rather than adjacent salivary gland tissue or simply decompressing the cyst.

Clinical Laboratory Studies

Complete blood count may be useful to rule out an infectious process. Otherwise, typical laboratory testing facilitates the preoperative workup.

Imaging

Diagnostic imaging studies are not considered essential for the evaluation of small, mobile salivary gland lesions. Tumors that may be deep or fixed raise concern for invasion into adjacent structures. Additionally, a parotid gland lesion present in the preauricular region rather than the tail of the parotid gland may extend into the deep lobe of the gland. Imaging should be performed in that context to accurately delineate the location and extent of the tumor and to identify possible extraglandular extent.

The use of computed tomography (CT) versus magnetic resonance imaging (MRI) for salivary gland tumors tends to vary among institutions and is typically related to the individual preferences of surgeons and radiologists. CT scan is superior for delineating bony anatomy and potential invasion as well as lymph node metastasis. MRI provides excellent cranial nerve definition and soft tissue delineation, including potential deep lobe extension into the parapharyngeal space. In certain situations, both studies may complement each other well. Although the role of positron-emission tomography is evolving for malignant lesions it is not typically indicated for benign salivary gland tumors.

Differential Diagnosis

As described in the Pathology section, several benign processes and lesions may involve salivary glands. The possibility that a salivary gland tumor may be malignant must always be considered. The differential diagnosis should also include lymphoma and metastatic skin cancer.

■ Management

Surgery

There were initial attempts in the mid-19th century to perform parotid surgery with facial nerve preservation. By the late 19th century, total parotidectomy with facial nerve preservation was successfully performed. Facial nerve repair following resection was initially attempted in the early 1950s. The modern description of parotid gland surgery was published in the late 1950s and described the surgical landmarks for avoiding injury to the main trunk and branches of the facial nerve. It advocated complete removal of the superficial portion of the parotid gland for noninvasive lesions confined to that portion of the gland.

Surgery is the treatment of choice for benign tumors of the salivary gland. Masses of the face and neck can be bothersome and may cause cosmetic issues. More important, some benign masses may transform into malignant lesions (e.g., carcinoma ex pleomorphic). More concerning clinical signs for malignancy, including rapid growth of a long-standing mass, bleeding, airway compromise, and nerve dysfunction, are rare for benign lesions. The parotid gland can be approached through a modified Blair incision. A "facelift" incision may also be done for selected patients with benign lesions in the middle or lower portion of the parotid gland. The most widely accepted treatment for salivary gland tumors is a wide resection with a cuff of normal tissue when possible. Identification and preservation of critical nerves and structures should be possible with most benign lesions. In addition to facial nerve preservation, the greater auricular nerve can be preserved in many patients as well and may improve the postoperative quality of life.

Parapharyngeal space lesions can be typically removed through a transcervical approach with release of the stylomandibular ligament, although a transmandibular approach may be necessary for very large masses. Transoral robotic excision of some of these lesions has been reported, although long-term outcome data are still evolving.

Contraindications for surgical excision are generally related to comorbidities that may preclude the use of general anesthesia.

Recurrent Pleomorphic Adenoma

Surgical management of recurrent pleomorphic adenoma can be as challenging as aggressive parotid malignancies. Details regarding the initial lesion and previous surgical management need to be clearly understood. Certain variants of pleomorphic adenoma appear to increase the risk for recurrence, including large tumors, deep lobe tumors, tumors closely approximating the facial nerve, and previously recurrent lesions. Additionally, younger patients appear to be at increased risk for recurrent disease. Review of the previous pathology is critical to ensure proper initial diagnosis, and diagnosis of the present lesion(s) by FNAB is critical for confirmation and to rule out malignant transformation or a metachronous neoplasm. Diagnostic imaging is critical to ascertaining the extent of disease. Most recurrences may be multifocal, and quite often the extent of disease may still be underestimated.

The treatment for recurrent pleomorphic adenoma must be tailored to each patient. Factors that must be considered include the type of prior surgery, the extent and location of recurrence(s), facial nerve function, the patient's general health status, and the patient's needs. Given the multifocal nature of most recurrences, scar excision and total parotidectomy with facial nerve preservation to achieve complete resection of the remaining parotid gland should be performed whenever possible. If a total parotidectomy was previously performed, or the recurrence is unifocal, resection of the recurrent tumor mass alone by careful dissection may be appropriate. Management of recurrent pleomorphic adenoma that encases the facial nerve is controversial. Despite efforts to preserve the facial nerve, resection with immediate nerve grafting may be required for this difficult scenario. The patient must be carefully counseled regarding all risks of the treatment, and should be actively engaged in the treatment decision-making process. Observation alone of recurrent disease in elderly or infirm patients may be quite appropriate.

Significant scarring related to prior treatment can be expected in the surgical bed. Meticulous surgical technique is required with loupe/microscope magnification. The facial nerve may need to be identified within the mastoid or through retrograde dissection of a peripheral branch. Permanent facial paralysis, either partial or total, occurs in ~ 10 to 30% of patients. The marginal mandibular branch of the facial nerve is at most risk for injury and permanent paralysis. The use of electrophysiological monitoring of the facial nerve may assist in nerve identification and decrease facial nerve trauma.

Radiation Therapy

Radiation therapy may be used occasionally to control recurrent pleomorphic adenomas. Adjuvant postoperative therapy may also be useful to decrease further recurrences, especially when resection of gross residual tumor is possible. However, given frequent occurrence of recurrent pleomorphic adenoma in relatively young patients, radiation therapy must be carefully considered for these patients. Longer-term complications of sensorineural hearing loss and mandibular osteoradionecrosis are serious issues in this younger population. Preservation of the facial nerve with radiation therapy treatment of microscopic disease may offer improved quality of life for certain patients, rather than sacrifice of the nerve and facial function.

There are few, if any, indications for radiation therapy as the primary treatment for benign salivary gland tumors.

■ Controversial Issues

A mass in the region of the parotid gland is most likely a parotid neoplasm and should be considered as such until proven otherwise. Inappropriate open biopsy of parotid neoplasms continues to occur as a result of clinical confusion or a lack of understanding of this important concept. Inappropriate management carries not only the risk of facial nerve injury but also recurrent disease (e.g., recurrent pleomorphic adenoma).

There has been some recent increased advocacy for extracapsular dissection of benign parotid gland lesions. This was commonly performed prior to the 1950s, although often without facial nerve identification. At that time, this practice was complicated by unacceptably high tumor recurrence rates (20–45%) and facial nerve injury. Given the almost 10-year mean interval of time to first recurrence, most studies do not have adequate follow-up times on their patients to support such procedures. Currently, most surgeons advocate removal of any salivary gland mass with the entire gland (submandibular) or a sufficient cuff of normal salivary gland tissue (parotid). Complete excision ensures an excellent prognosis and may be appropriate treatment if the final pathology reveals a malignant lesion. Incomplete excision or tumor spillage raises the specter of disease recurrence. Repeated excision of recurrences is difficult, given the scarring and inflammation present in the surgical bed, and increases the risk of injury to the facial nerve.

Intraoperative monitoring of the facial nerve may be helpful in certain scenarios, including surgery for recurrent disease. At present, however, there are not sufficient data to advocate the routine use of intraoperative nerve monitoring for parotid gland surgery.

■ Practice Guidelines, Consensus Statements, and Measures

National Comprehensive Cancer Network guidelines are available for management of salivary gland tumors, but focus primarily on malignant lesions. Additionally, ENT-UK Head and Neck, the head and neck group of the British Association of Otolaryngologists–Head and Neck Surgeons, recently published a consensus statement regarding diagnosis and management of benign parotid gland disease.

■ Suggested Reading

Barnes L, Eveson JW, Reichart P, Sidransky D. Tumours of the salivary glands. In: Barnes L, Eveson JW, Reichart, P, Sidransky D, eds. Pathology & Genetics—Head and Neck Tumours. 3rd ed. Lyon, France: International Agency for Research on Cancer; 2005:209–281. World Health Organization Classification of Tumours, Vol 9

Bradley PT, Paleri V, Homer JJ. Consensus statement by otolaryngologists on the diagnosis and management of benign parotid gland disease. Clin Otolaryngol 2012;37(4):300–304

Donovan DT, Conley JJ. Capsular significance in parotid tumor surgery: reality and myths of lateral lobectomy. Laryngoscope 1984;94(3):324–329

Mehle ME, Kraus DH, Wood BG, et al. Facial nerve morbidity following parotid surgery for benign disease: the Cleveland Clinic Foundation experience. Laryngoscope 1993;103(4 Pt 1):386–388

National Comprehensive Cancer Network. NCCN Clinical Practice Guidelines in Oncology. Head and Neck Cancers. (Version 2.2013)

Phillips PP, Olsen KD. Recurrent pleomorphic adenoma of the parotid gland: report of 126 cases and a review of the literature. Ann Otol Rhinol Laryngol 1995;104(2):100–104

Scianna JM, Petruzzelli GJ. Contemporary management of tumors of the salivary glands. Curr Oncol Rep 2007;9(2):134–138

Seethala RR, LiVolsi VA, Baloch ZW. Relative accuracy of fine-needle aspiration and frozen section in the diagnosis of lesions of the parotid gland. Head Neck 2005;27(3):217–223

Spiro RH. Salivary neoplasms: overview of a 35-year experience with 2,807 patients. Head Neck Surg 1986;8(3):177–184

Thoeny HC. Imaging of salivary gland tumours. Cancer Imaging 2007;7:52–62

Witt RL. The significance of the margin in parotid surgery for pleomorphic adenoma. Laryngoscope 2002;112(12):2141–2154

33 Management of Salivary Gland Malignancies

◼ Introduction

Salivary malignancies encompass a diverse and fascinating array of histology and occur in major (parotid, submandibular, and sublingual) and minor salivary glands. Present treatment strategies are influenced by tumor size, cell type, anatomical location, nodal status, and a host of clinical factors that have been studied over the past half-century. Overall, the tumors are rare, accounting for 0.5% of all malignancies and 3 to 5% of head and neck cancers, occurring predominantly in the fifth and sixth decade. The relative paucity and numerous cell types of salivary malignancies have hindered their prospective study; thus present treatment strategies and understanding of clinical behavior rest largely on retrospective analyses.

Definitive surgical resection is the foundation of treatment, with radiotherapy having a role in large and high-grade tumors. The role of fast neutron radiotherapy continues to evolve in the management of recurrent and unresectable tumors. At present, chemotherapy is not routinely used in standard treatment strategies for salivary tumors. This section focuses on current management principles for salivary malignancies, highlighting the roles of preoperative diagnostics, surgical management, and radiotherapy.

◼ Evaluation

Clinical Findings

A comprehensive head and neck history and physical exam are critical because they may offer the initial clues to the malignant nature of a salivary gland tumor. Symptoms such as facial pain, facial numbness, and slow onset of facial weakness may be harbingers of malignancy. Similarly, findings of overlying skin involvement, fixation, cervical adenopathy, and facial weakness should raise suspicion for malignancy. Tumor staging initially arose from large retrospective studies that identified poor prognosti-

cators, including large tumor size, histology, anatomical location, extraparenchymal extension, neural involvement, and cervical metastasis. The American Joint Committee on Cancer primary tumor, regional nodes, metastasis (TNM) staging system for major salivary tumors is listed in **Table 33.1**. For minor salivary tumors, the TNM staging corresponds to the anatomical location of the tumor (e.g., soft palate, paranasal sinus).

Fine-Needle Aspiration

Fine-needle aspiration (FNA) with or without ultrasound guidance has become commonplace, given its wide availability, rapid acquisition, and low morbidity. Particularly if there is clinical suspicion for malignancy, FNA can be helpful in surgical planning and patient counseling. Because institutional cytopathological experience may influence accuracy, FNA results should not supersede the overall clinical picture. Much of the cytopathologist's challenge is that there are more than 40 salivary tumor histological cell types—more than any other tissue in the body. The World Health Organization risk classification of salivary histological cell types is shown in **Table 33.2**. The overall accuracy of FNA for parotid tumors approximates 90%, but for malignant tumors the results may be somewhat lower.

Imaging

The role of imaging in the management of salivary tumors continues to expand. For small tumors lacking ominous clinical features and limited to the lateral lobe or tail of the parotid, imaging is not routinely used. However, when malignancy is expected or there is concern for involvement of the deep lobe, parapharyngeal space, skull base, carotid artery, or extensive perineural involvement, computed tomography (CT) and/or magnetic resonance imaging (MRI) may prove invaluable for surgical plan-

Table 33.1 Staging system for the major salivary glands

TX	Primary tumor cannot be assessed
T0	No evidence of primary tumor
T1	Tumor ≤ 2 cm in greatest dimension without extraparenchymal extension
T2	Tumor > 2 cm but ≤ 4 cm in greatest dimension without extraparenchymal extension
T3	Tumor > 4 cm and/or tumor having extraparenchymal extension
T4a	Tumor invades skin, mandible, ear canal, and/or facial nerve
T4b	Tumor invades skull base and/or pterygoid plates and/or encases carotid artery

Used with the permission of the American Joint Committee on Cancer (AJCC), Chicago, Illinois. The original source for this material is the AJCC Cancer Staging Manual, Seventh Edition (2010) published by Springer Science and Business Media LLC, www.springer.com.

Table 33.2 World Health Organization risk classification of salivary malignancies

Low
Acinic cell carcinoma
Epithelial-myoepithelial carcinoma
Polymorphous low-grade adenocarcinoma
Clear cell carcinoma
Basal cell adenocarcinoma
Low-grade salivary duct carcinoma
Myoepithelial carcinoma
Oncocytic carcinoma
Sialoblastoma
Adenocarcinoma not otherwise specified (NOS), low grade
Cystadenocarcinoma, low grade
High
Sebaceous carcinoma and lymphadenocarcinoma
High-grade mucoepidermoid carcinoma
Adenoid cystic carcinoma
Mucinous adenocarcinoma
Salivary ductal carcinoma
Squamous cell carcinoma
Small cell carcinoma
Large cell carcinoma
Lymphoepithelial carcinoma
Metastasizing pleomorphic adenoma
Carcinoma ex pleomorphic adenoma
Carcinosarcoma
Adenocarcinoma and cystadenocarcinoma, NOS, high grade

Used with permission from Seethala RR. An update on grading salivary malignancy. Head Neck Pathol 2009;3(1):69–77.

ning and patient counseling. CT imaging provides excellent delineation of bony–soft tissue interfaces and can distinguish fat planes, tumor, and normal salivary tissue. Improvements in both MRI technology and protocols permit accurate identification of perineural spread and increasingly can effectively distinguish benign from malignant tumors. Additionally, both CT and MRI can identify clinically occult cervical nodal disease and are recommended for any tumors located in such sites as the floor of the mouth, oropharynx, and paranasal sinuses.

CT positron-emission tomography (PET) has an emerging but less established role in the management of salivary malignancy and is not routinely used. Because many benign salivary gland tumors have increased fluorodeoxyglucose (FDG) uptake, CT-PET should not be employed to distinguish benign from malignant disease. In selected patients with high-grade histology or advanced disease, CT-PET may provide clarity for lesions suspicious for regional or distant metastasis. Finally, further evaluation is needed to determine if this modality may be useful in restaging in the setting of known malignant disease.

■ Surgical Management and Principles

Facial Nerve Identification and Monitoring

There is no substitute for a thorough knowledge of the local anatomy and landmarks for the facial nerve when undertaking parotid surgery. For malignant

tumors, it is critical to anticipate and prepare for disease extension not fully appreciated during pretreatment evaluation. Although the classic landmarks (mastoid tip, posterior belly of the digastric muscle, tympanomastoid suture line, and cartilaginous pointer) for nerve identification are usually satisfactory, for large tumors epicentered over the stylomastoid foramen, the surgeon must be prepared to identify the marginal mandibular branch distally in the proximity of the angle of the mandible and perform a retrograde dissection. Occasionally, the surgeon may even need to consider a mastoidectomy to identify the vertical segment of the facial nerve prior to entry into the neck.

Increasingly, many surgeons now employ continuous neurophysiological monitoring of the facial nerve both to assist with identification and to enhance nerve integrity. Its use seems to be popular among surgeons who have completed their training more recently and those who perform infrequent parotid surgery. Although continuous neurophysiological facial nerve monitoring has become pervasive with parotid surgery, no study has yet demonstrated its superiority versus nonmonitoring in reducing complications.

Frozen Section

Intraoperative frozen section is still routinely performed for salivary malignancy. It may be of assistance when FNA is nondiagnostic. Although the sensitivity of intraoperative frozen section for determining exact histology may be modest, its accuracy for detecting malignant versus benign disease is very good, generally greater than 90%. Still, it is important to base intraoperative management on the sum of all of the clinical factors.

Management of Adjacent Nerves

The handling of nerves is always an important consideration for both parotid (facial) and submandibular (hypoglossal, lingual, marginal) malignancies, especially for tumors with a predilection for perineural involvement such as adenoid cystic carcinoma. Facial nerve involvement is a harbinger of poor prognosis. When a nerve is nonfunctional preoperatively, no attempts should be made to preserve it; rather, obtaining clear margins should be the focus. Similarly, even if a functioning nerve is grossly infiltrated or encased by tumor, it should be sacrificed, and margins should be cleared and the nerve repaired in the same setting. However, if a nerve is simply abutting tumor or can be dissected free of tumor, every effort should be made to preserve it. Although proximity to critical structures (nerves, skull base, carotid artery) frequently inhibits wide surgical margins, postoperative radiotherapy has improved local-regional control and survival in the setting of close margins.

Extent of Surgery: Primary Site and Neck

Again, the low incidence of salivary malignancies accounts for the lack of prospective clinical trials. Thus recommendations are based on retrospective data, and certain topics may lack complete consensus.

For parotid malignancies, the recommendation is for a total parotidectomy, with facial nerve preservation guided by the principles discussed previously. Occasionally, a superficial parotidectomy is performed where a definitive malignant histology is not known until the postoperative setting. For small,

low-grade tumors with wide margins (> 1 cm), an exception may be considered. For submandibular and minor salivary gland tumors, complete excision with wide margins as permitted by adjacent critical structures is the goal. For small (T1, T2) and low-grade tumors, these goals are generally straightforward to achieve.

For large (T3, T4) and high-grade tumors, close margins and involvement of surrounding structures are commonplace. A gross total resection should be achieved whenever possible. It is in this setting when surgical management of the neck must also be considered. Although not all of the indications for surgical treatment of the neck have universal agreement, a neck dissection is recommended when there is clinical nodal disease, presence of high-grade tumors with N_0 neck, advanced T stage (T3, T4), and histology with extensive infiltration. The incidence of the N_+ neck at presentation has a wide range, and there is no controversy regarding performing a neck dissection in this setting.

For the clinically N_0 neck, patient age, tumor size, histopathology, facial nerve involvement, extraparenchymal spread, and grade are believed to be significant predictors for nodal disease. Patients with N_+ disease have a considerably worse prognosis. Inevitably, a significant number of patients with clinically N_0 neck will harbor occult cervical metastasis. It is beneficial to consider the factors that predict occult metastasis, so that those who would best benefit from surgical management of the neck can be identified. Finally, the most consistent recommendations for elective neck dissection for major salivary malignancy include advanced T stage and high-grade histology.

■ Postoperative Radiation Therapy

Postoperative radiation therapy for resected salivary malignancies provides improved locoregional control and overall survival. The most common indications for postoperative radiation include close margins (< 2 mm), high-grade tumors, histology, advanced T stage, and perineural spread.

An important study by the Dutch Oncology Group evaluated 498 patients with malignant parotid tumors who were treated with surgery and postoperative radiation versus surgery alone. Their findings demonstrated that postoperative radiotherapy improved 10-year local control significantly compared with surgery alone in T3–4 tumors (84% vs. 18%), in patients with close margins (95% vs. 55%) and following incomplete resection (82% vs. 44%), in bone invasion (86% vs. 54%), and in perineural invasion (88% vs. 60%).

A confirmatory meta-analysis of 19 studies involving 4,638 patients treated from 1987 to 2005 supports the survival advantage afforded by postoperative radiation. Advanced T and N stage as well as high-grade tumors had a statistically significant worse survival: hazard ratio 1.8 (p = 0.041), 1.1 (p = 0.05), and high-grade 2.1 (p = 0.001), respectively. The effect of adjuvant radiation therapy improved overall survival, with a hazard ratio of 2.9 (p = 0.002). Thus postoperative radiation therapy has become a mainstay in the management of advanced salivary malignancy.

Neutron Beam Radiation

Availability and advances in fast neutron radiation therapy continue to hold promise for patients with salivary malignancies refractory to all other treatment options. Patients with skull base involvement, unresectable disease, and gross positive disease following surgery may potentially benefit from neutron radiotherapy.

For patients with locally advanced salivary malignancies treated with fast neutron therapy, the factors that were associated with more favorable local-regional control include tumors < 4 cm, lack of skull base involvement, no prior radiation, and prior surgical resection.

■ Summary

Salivary malignancies continue to present therapeutic challenges, given their diverse histology and clinical behavior, involvement of adjacent bony and neural structures, and difficulty in obtaining wide margins. Determination of histopathology and malignant status can be aided by FNA. Imaging with CT and MRI has become an important part of pretreatment evaluation, especially for advanced tumors. Complete surgical resection remains the mainstay for the treatment of salivary malignancy. For early and low-grade tumors lacking adverse histopathological features, observation postoperatively is usually adequate. For advanced tumors, complete resection is recommended with the addition of a neck dissection in the presence of cervical metastasis and for high-grade histology. Postoperative radiation is advocated for adenoid cystic tumors, advanced tumors, perineural spread, lymphovascular invasion, and close or positive margins. When unresectable disease is encountered, definitive radiation or reirradiation may be offered. Fast neutron beam radiation may provide an important role for the most recalcitrant, advanced tumors. Finally, clinical trials may be considered for metastatic disease.

■ Suggested Reading

Edge SB, Byrd DR, Compton CC, Fritz AG, Greene FL, Trotti A, eds. Major salivary glands (parotid, submandibular, and sublingual). In: AJCC Cancer Staging Manual. 7th ed. New York, NY: Springer; 2010

Jeannon JP, Calman F, Gleeson M, et al. Management of advanced parotid cancer: a systematic review. Eur J Surg Oncol 2009;35(9):908–915

Laramore GE. Role of particle radiotherapy in the management of head and neck cancer. Curr Opin Oncol 2009;21(3): 224–231

Mendenhall WM, Werning JW, Pfister DG. Treatment of head and neck cancer. In: DeVita VT, Jr, Lawrence TS, Rosenberg SA, eds. Cancer: Principles and Practice of Oncology. 9th ed. Philadelphia, PA: Lippincott Williams & Wilkins; 2011:729–780

Seethala RR. An update on grading of salivary gland carcinomas. Head Neck Pathol 2009;3(1):69–77

Terhaard CH, Lubsen H, Rasch CR, et al; Dutch Head and Neck Oncology Cooperative Group. The role of radiotherapy in the treatment of malignant salivary gland tumors. Int J Radiat Oncol Biol Phys 2005;61(1):103–111

34 Hypopharyngeal Cancer

■ Introduction

Incidence/Etiology

Cancer of the hypopharynx represents 5 to 10% of cancers of the upper aerodigestive system and ~ 0.5% of all malignancies. Patients with these cancers are difficult to treat because they present with advanced disease and severe nutritional problems.

Males are about eight times more susceptible than females, though a high incidence of cancer of the postcricoid region is found in females of Irish and Scandinavian descent who have Plummer–Vinson syndrome. This syndrome is characterized by glossitis, splenomegaly, esophageal stenosis, achlorhydria, and iron deficiency anemia, and is usually accompanied by severe gastroesophageal reflux. Gastroesophageal reflux may be part of the etiology of hypopharyngeal cancer in certain patients.

The prognosis for patients with advanced (stage III or IV) hypopharyngeal cancer is poor. Disease control and palliation have improved as a result of (1) modern imaging techniques that enable more precise staging of tumors, (2) increased knowledge of the nutritional deficiencies that must be corrected before treatment begins, (3) an expanding assortment of reconstructive procedures for the pharyngoesophageal region that allows aggressive resections and one-stage reconstitution of the gullet, and (4) improved sequencing of radiation therapy and chemotherapy in association with surgery (**Table 34.1**).

Relevant Anatomy

Certain aspects of the anatomy of the hypopharynx must be appreciated for successful treatment. The anatomical features include the following:

- The great vessels adjacent to the lateral walls of the hypopharynx may be invaded early in the natural course of the disease.

Table 34.1 Staging system for hypopharyngeal cancer

TX	Primary tumor cannot be assessed
T0	No evidence of primary tumor.
Tis	Carcinoma in situ
T1	Tumor limited to 1 subsite of hypopharynx and/or ≤ 2 cm in greatest dimension
T2	Tumor invades > 1 subsite of hypopharynx or an adjacent site, or measures > 2 cm but not > 4 cm in greatest dimension without fixation of hemilarynx
T3	Tumor > 4 cm in greatest dimension or with fixation of hemilarynx or extension to esophagus
T4a	Moderately advanced local disease
	Tumor invades thyroid/cricoid cartilage, hyoid bone, thyroid gland, or central compartment soft tissue
T4b	Very advanced local disease
	Tumor invades prevertebral fascia, encases carotid artery, or involves mediastinal structures

Used with the permission of the American Joint Committee on Cancer (AJCC), Chicago, Illinois. The original source for this material is the AJCC Cancer Staging Manual, Seventh Edition (2010) published by Springer Science and Business Media LLC, www.springer.com.

- The lymphatics of the hypopharynx are diffuse and drain superiorly to deep cervical and retropharyngeal nodes and inferiorly from the piriform apex and postcricoid regions to the lateral cervical (level II–IV), paratracheal, paraesophageal, and thyroid nodes.
- Extensive submucosal lymphatics are found in the hypopharynx, particularly in the inferior portions.
- Significant neural components of the swallowing mechanism are adjacent to the pharyngeal walls, including the glossopharyngeal, hypoglossal, superior laryngeal, and recurrent laryngeal nerves, and injury to any combination of these nerves may severely impair deglutition.

Pathology

The pathological concepts of hypopharyngeal cancer are as follows:

- Ninety-five percent of the malignancies are epidermoid carcinomas, and the remaining 5% are adenocarcinomas arising from glandular structures or from islands of ectopic gastric mucosa.
- Most hypopharyngeal cancers are located in the piriform fossae. The remainder are found, in decreasing incidence, in the posterior hypopharyngeal wall and postcricoid regions.
- The incidence of lymph node metastases is ~ 75% with bilateral disease present in 10% of patients.
- Submucosal spread of these cancers is common and is more prevalent as the location of the tumor approaches the cervical esophagus.
- Satellite tumors and/or "skip areas" are common.

The significance of submucosal spread and skip areas is that wide surgical margins and radiation therapy ports are essential. The superior margins are thought to be safe 2 to 3 cm (cm) from the grossly abnormal mucosa, but the inferior margin should be 4 to 6 cm from the gross tumor if there is involvement of the cervical esophagus.

■ Evaluation

Clinical Findings

Patients with hypopharyngeal cancer usually have social habits that include heavy tobacco exposure, moderate-to-severe alcohol ingestion, and poor dietary practices. Weight loss of up to 20 to 30% may be present with associated hypovitaminosis, dehydration, and anemia. Intra- and extravascular volumes are often depleted. A complete medical review and practical approach to chronic problems, such as pulmonary, liver, renal, and endocrine diseases, are essential in these patients, because most treatment protocols are rigorous and physiologically demanding.

Initial examination of the hypopharynx and larynx in the office begins the process of developing a three-dimensional concept of the tumor. In addition to evaluating the superior, medial, and lateral aspects of the tumor, the examiner looks for pooled secretions indicating obstruction, evidence of vocal cord paralysis, the state of the airway, and the presence of other cancers. The cranial nerves should be evaluated because preexisting neurological deficits

may signify tumor extension and other diseases or may affect rehabilitation efforts later on.

The neck examination includes a systematic evaluation of all major lymph node–bearing areas. The use of fine-needle aspiration for evaluation of neck masses in patients with gross evidence of hypopharyngeal cancer is rarely indicated because the presence of a neck mass in these patients requires its treatment as a metastatic lesion.

Flexible fiberoptic laryngoscopy, preferably with video documentation, is essential for determining the effects of the tumor on the laryngopharynx, such as vocal cord paralysis and fixation. After the physical examination and office endoscopy are completed, the remainder of the medical workup, imaging studies, and staging endoscopy are performed.

Imaging

The recommended radiological studies include the following:

- Chest X-rays are used to rule out metastases, determine whether there is a second primary tumor, and evaluate the parenchyma and mediastinal structures for other acute or chronic diseases.
- Computed tomography (CT) and magnetic resonance imaging provide excellent imaging of the primary tumor, involvement of the party wall between the trachea and the esophagus, and determination of mediastinal nodal metastases.
- Positron-emission tomography/CT can be useful for evaluating for nodal disease and the presence of distant metastasis, as well as extension of the primary tumor.
- Upper gastrointestinal series make it possible to evaluate the swallowing mechanism, the dynamic effects of the tumor, and the physiology of the esophagus, including both the upper and the lower esophageal sphincters, and to detect the presence of other tumors if warranted. The finding of gastroesophageal reflux disease merits treatment in the perioperative period to avoid adverse effects on both the healing and the rehabilitative processes. An assessment of the stomach and small intestine is helpful, given the potential for use of either of these structures for reconstruction.

Nutritional Evaluation

Evaluation of a patient's nutritional status is essential due to the compromise induced by the tumor. If appropriate, reversal of nutritional deficits requires several weeks in most patients. There should be immediate use of nasogastric feedings or intravenous hyperalimentation. In patients who will not require gastric pullup, a percutaneous esophagogastrostomy may be placed at the time of staging endoscopy.

Staging Endoscopy

Staging endoscopy should be performed under general anesthesia with complete muscle paralysis. The most important outcome of the endoscopy, other than obtaining a biopsy, is the determination of the inferior border of the tumor. Evaluation of the tumor inferiorly in relation to the piriform apex, cricopharyngeus muscle, cervical esophagus, and intrinsic larynx is essential. Invasion of the tracheal wall is uncommon and is usually apparent from imaging, but may require further evaluation with bronchoscopy.

Prognosis

The overall 5-year survival rate of patients with hypopharyngeal cancer is 35 to 40%, but the site, stage, and presence or absence of positive lymph nodes have a significant influence on these figures. In patients who have documented cervical metastases, the anticipated 5-year survival is less than 50% due primarily to the high incidence of local/regional recurrence and because there is a 20 to 25% incidence of distant metastases within 24 months of initial diagnosis and treatment.

Posterior hypopharyngeal wall cancers, often diagnosed in the early stages (I and II), do not have subclinical lymph node metastases, and thus have an excellent prognosis. Piriform fossa cancers, on the other hand, may have lymph node metastases, even when the primary lesions are small. Postcricoid cancer often presents as an advanced lesion associated with extensive paratracheal, paraesophageal, and mediastinal lymph node metastases and has a poor prognosis.

■ Management

The choice of treatment for hypopharyngeal cancer includes chemotherapy, radiation therapy, surgery, or a combination of these modalities. In general, most patients with advanced lesions (stage III or IV) require combination therapy. Concurrent chemoradiotherapy is commonly used to treat tumors in an advanced stage, whereas radiation therapy alone may be used for curative treatment of small (T1 and some T2) lesions, with surgery reserved for salvage therapy. The high incidence of lymph node metastases from hypopharyngeal cancer requires that treatment of the lymph nodes be considered even in patients with no palpable disease. Therefore, when surgery is chosen for control of the primary lesion, neck dissection or radiation therapy directed at the lymph nodes is necessary.

Surgery

The rules governing resection of hypopharyngeal cancers reflect the anatomy and pathology of the region. Neck dissection is performed in most patients because no relationship exists between the size of the primary lesion and the incidence of lymph node metastases. Most metastases are to level II or III cervical nodes, and lesions in the piriform fossa apex and arytenoid may metastasize to the paratracheal, paraesophageal, and level III nodes directly or may extend into the paralaryngeal compartments. Thyroid metastases may also occur.

Treatment of these cancers, therefore, requires special attention to lymph node groups that are not included in the standard neck dissections or radiotherapy ports. Superior mediastinal dissection is required when there are paratracheal, paraesophageal, or low cervical metastases. High retropharyngeal nodes should be removed along with the superior deep cervical nodes, because they may be involved through direct or retrograde metastases.

Tumors of the posterior hypopharyngeal wall often remain localized in their early stages and present an opportunity for wide excision with uncomplicated reconstruction. The most direct approach to this region is by suprahyoid pharyngotomy and the lateral pharyngotomy. This approach may be used for excision of more extensive posterior hypopharyngeal wall lesions as well. Most small posterior hypopharyngeal wall defects may be reconstructed with split-thickness or dermal skin grafts. In addition, there is a maturing experience with transoral resection, either transoral laser microsurgery (TLM) or transoral robotic surgery (TORS), for early primary tumors. The results are comparable to open surgery for these limited lesions and may not require reconstruction.

Posterolateral hypopharyngeal wall resections may be reconstructed with skin grafts sutured to bipedicled prevertebral or pectoralis myofascial muscle flaps. The ideal reconstruction for larger resections is a free flap, using either the thin pliable skin of the radial forearm or the jejunum as an open flap. Reconstruction of the posterior or posterolateral hypopharyngeal wall should not be carried below the level of the corniculate cartilages with the larynx in place, because of the potential for significant aspiration. In the case of significant extension below the corniculate cartilages total laryngectomy should be performed.

The amount and complexity of resection for cancers of the piriform fossa depend on the size and location of the tumor. A conservation surgery approach may be used, allowing for preservation of laryngeal function for lesions located in the superior aspect of the piriform fossa. These should be 2 cm or less, cause no impairment of vocal cord movement, and allow at least 1.5 cm of margin between the inferior aspect of the tumor and the piriform fossa apex. Resection of these small lesions, with preservation of the larynx, requires that the patient have good pulmonary function and excellent motivation. Postoperative swallowing rehabilitation is very difficult, and aspiration is common. This operation is an extension of the supraglottic laryngectomy—that is, "partial laryngopharyngectomy."

Transoral approaches have been used to treat early pyriform sinus and posterior hypopharyngeal primary cancers. However, in most patients, lesions are so significant that they will require total laryngectomy and partial pharyngectomy, with or without cervical esophagectomy, for adequate tumor resection. When partial pharyngectomy is performed, hypopharyngeal reconstruction may require a myocutaneous or free flap to avoid a tight primary closure. The adage "if there is enough mucosa to close over a no. 18 feeding tube, an adequate lumen will result" is incorrect and invariably will result in pharyngeal stenosis, which can be very challenging to reconstruct and will have many potential complications.

The most difficult surgical problems exist in patients who have primary tumors of the postcricoid region or the piriform apex. These lesions are associated with aggressive submucosal and lymphatic spread to the thyroid gland and to the paraesophageal, paratracheal, and level III and IV lymph nodes. The inferior line of resection must include the upper cervical esophagus, with the paraesophageal and paratracheal lymphatics and the ipsilateral lobe of the thyroid gland. If the inferior line of resection is below the mediastinal inlet, total esophagectomy is necessary because anastomoses within the mediastinum should be avoided. Gastric pull-up is then the reconstructive procedure of choice.

The use of regional or transplanted skin flaps for reconstruction of the hypopharynx with preservation of the larynx should be avoided in most patients who require more than 50% replacement of the hypopharynx. This amount of noncontractile or immobile pharyngeal wall interferes with the pharyngeal component of the swallowing process, and severe aspiration is inevitable.

The most common lesions of the hypopharynx are large and require extensive resection. When nontubular reconstruction is required, the choices for donor materials range from regional skin, myocutaneous, and myofascial flaps to transplanted skin or jejunal flaps. When a tubed reconstruction is required, because of partial or total esophagectomy, the choices range from regional skin flaps and myocutaneous flaps to transplanted skin or jejunal flaps and gastric interpositions. The major determinants in these choices should be simplicity, the overall condition of the patient, and the experience of the surgeon.

Radiation Therapy

Primary radiation may be used in selected patients with T1 or T2 lesions. Its use depends on the sophistication of the radiation oncologist in evaluating, planning, and delivering the treatment, on the patient's desires, and on the experience of the surgeon. Planned postoperative radiation therapy is the most common application of radiation therapy alone for treatment of hypopharyngeal cancer. Extensive lymph node metastases found low in the neck necessitate the addition of superior mediastinal ports to the postoperative radiotherapy regimen.

Concurrent chemoradiotherapy is commonly used for advanced stage hypopharyngeal cancer treatment. Initial trials also used induction chemotherapy prior to definitive radiotherapy; however, studies have shown that concurrent therapy reduces the incidence of distant metastasis. These organ-sparing modalities have largely replaced surgery (total laryngectomy) as the primary treatment for advanced hypopharyngeal cancer, with laryngopharyngectomy reserved for salvage treatment.

Choice of Treatment

Each site in the hypopharynx provides an opportunity for different approaches to treatment. In any one patient, decisions must be made between primary radiation therapy and surgical therapy, total laryngectomy and partial laryngectomy, partial esophagectomy and total esophagectomy, and neck dissection and radiation therapy for the "negative neck." As in all cancer treatment, the proper decision for each patient depends on information from accurate staging of the tumor, complete medical evaluation of the patient, the skills of the surgeon and radiation therapist, and, ultimately, the desires of the patient. Age is not as weighty a factor as is the physiological, mental, and social condition of the patient. An algorithm can aid with these decisions, but common sense and the integrity of the surgeon must prevail.

The National Comprehensive Cancer Network (NCCN) guidelines for early stage (I and II) cancers include either definitive radiotherapy with salvage surgery or upfront conservation surgery addressing the primary site and the neck.

Most patients with hypopharyngeal cancer present with advanced lesions that require aggressive combined therapy. The NCCN guidelines for advanced cancers recommend surgery with adjuvant therapy, induction chemotherapy, or concurrent chemoradiation therapy. Following surgery, the main question, after the decision to treat for cure has been made, relates to choosing the appropriate reconstructive procedure. When small cancers are treated surgically, usually the simplest approach, such as skin graft reconstruction, is the best. When large resections are performed, however, the enteral reconstructions (free jejunal autograft and gastric interposition), although more complicated, provide the most physiological rehabilitation compared with that provided by flaps and grafts.

■ Suggested Reading

Blanchard P, Baujat B, Holostenco V, et al; MACH-CH Collaborative group. Meta-analysis of chemotherapy in head and neck cancer (MACH-NC): a comprehensive analysis by tumour site. Radiother Oncol 2011;100(1):33–40

National Comprehensive Cancer Network. Clinical Practice Guidelines in Oncology. Head and Neck Cancers (Version 2.2013). http://www.jnccn.org/content/11/8/917.abstract

Pharynx. In: Edge SB, Byrd DR, Compton CC, et al., eds.: AJCC Cancer Staging Manual. 7th ed. New York, NY: Springer, 2010:41–56

Siegel R, Naishadham D, Jemal A. Cancer statistics, 2013. CA Cancer J Clin 2013;63(1):11–30

Steiner W, Ambrosch P, Hess CF, Kron M. Organ preservation by transoral laser microsurgery in piriform sinus carcinoma. Otolaryngol Head Neck Surg 2001;124(1):58–67

35 Evaluation of a Thyroid Nodule

■ Introduction

Thyroid nodules are a relatively common problem because of their high incidence. The Framingham Study reported an incidence of 3.9% of patients between the ages of 30 and 50 having nontoxic goiters, with an additional 0.3% having had nodules excised at some time in their past. The increasing use of ultrasonography as a screening study has identified thyroid nodules in 50% of a general population beyond the fifth decade of life. The overall incidence of malignancy in solitary thyroid nodules ranges between 10 and 30% and is in large part dependent on the patient population. Nodular thyroid pathology has been identified in nearly 40% of the patients reviewed in an autopsy series. Thus the number of patients presenting with thyroid pathology is considerable, and a cost-effective workup is necessary.

■ Clinical Evaluation

History and Physical Exam

In evaluating the patient with a solitary thyroid nodule, a thorough history and physical exam are indicated. Patients reporting a personal history of radiation exposure to the head and neck or a history of thyroid cancer in two or more immediate family members raises concern for malignancy. Many patients will present with an asymptomatic mass in the thyroid noted by either the patient or the primary care physician or identified incidentally by imaging studies. By the time a lesion becomes visible to the naked eye, it generally represents a large mass.

Symptoms, such as pain with rapid growth of the thyroid mass, are often indicative of either hemorrhage into a thyroid cyst or some form of thyroiditis.

The presence of hoarseness is suggestive of involvement of the recurrent laryngeal nerve. Shortness of breath or dyspnea on exertion suggests compression of the trachea, although many patients will unconsciously alter their lifestyle and decrease physical activity and may deny these symptoms. The presence of dysphagia suggests encroachment on the esophagus. Patients reporting dysphagia or pressure from small thyroid nodules should be evaluated for coexisting reflux. Hemoptysis may be a sign of invasion of the upper aerodigestive tract. Patients should be questioned for signs or symptoms of hypothyroidism or hyperthyroidism.

The physical examination should incorporate a complete head and neck evaluation. Attention should be directed toward the presence or absence of a normal voice. Similarly, stridor is a sign of advanced disease and when present is extremely worrisome. Asymmetrical vocal cord motion or paresis may be an early sign of recurrent laryngeal nerve invasion. Vocal cord paralysis coupled with an ipsilateral thyroid mass should be considered cancer until proven otherwise. Examination of the larynx, with either a mirror or a flexible laryngoscope, should focus on vocal cord mobility. In many instances, it is possible to examine the subglottic larynx with a flexible laryngoscope and evaluate the patient for evidence of subglottic compression.

In evaluating the thyroid mass, particular emphasis should be placed on the size and consistency of the mass and whether it is fixed to adjacent structures. The presence of bilateral or multiple thyroid masses is more indicative of benign disease. Hard, large masses, particularly in an elderly population, are consistent with thyroid cancer. A mass that replaces the central compartment and that presents over a short period of time is often consistent with anaplastic thyroid cancer or thyroid lymphoma. The lateral neck should be evaluated for lymphadenopathy. Again, the presence of enlarged lateral neck nodes with a thyroid mass is most consistent with metastatic thyroid cancer.

Risk Factors

In evaluating a patient with a solitary thyroid mass, consideration must be given to risk factors that may place patients in a high-risk group for thyroid cancer. Patients presenting with a thyroid mass during the first 2 decades of life have an increased incidence of thyroid cancer. However, it should be noted that such cases are associated with an excellent prognosis. In general, men older than 40 years and women older than 50 years are a high risk for thyroid cancer. Cancer tends to be more common in males and is associated with a worse prognosis. However, thyroid disease in general is more predominant in women. Patients who have received a low dose of radiation therapy for such conditions as tonsillitis, acne, or an enlarged thymus during childhood may be at increased risk for harboring a thyroid cancer and require lifelong follow-up. However, this point remains somewhat controversial.

Certainly, there has been increased reporting of thyroid cancer in patients directly exposed to the nuclear disaster at Chernobyl. The routine use of iodine in dietary salt in the United States has decreased the incidence of multinodular goiter. However, patients originating from endemic goiter regions in the Caribbean, Europe, the Himalayas, South America, and the Middle East are at increased risk for benign thyroid disease.

▪ Laboratory Studies

Laboratory studies should initially focus on obtaining thyroid function studies. T4, T3, free thyroid index, thyroid-stimulating hormone, and thyroglobulins should all be part of a standard laboratory evaluation. These tests will allow for the determination of the euthyroid state versus a hypothyroid or hyperthyroid condition. Although its use is controversial, thyroglobulin may be elevated in some patients with well-differentiated thyroid cancer and may serve as a serum marker reflecting disease status at presentation. The presence of hyperthyroidism in a unilateral thyroid mass will allow for the appropriate evaluation of such a patient to exclude a functioning thyroid nodule. Care must be taken interpreting these tests when patients are pregnant or on birth control medication.

In addition, thyroid peroxidase and thyroglobulin antibody studies allow for the determination of Hashimoto thyroiditis or other inflammatory diseases. The well-known propensity for lymphoma in association with Hashimoto thyroiditis must be considered in this clinical setting.

Endocrinology consultation should be considered in patients with a laboratory evaluation consistent with hypothyroidism or hyperthyroidism. A serum calcium should also be obtained in this patient population, due to the well-known propensity for parathyroid disease to arise at an increased rate in patients with thyroid disease.

One issue that remains unresolved is the routine use of calcitonin blood levels. To date, there have been no data to suggest the cost-effective use of calcitonin in screening the general population. Certainly, in patients with known familial multiple endocrine neoplasia syndromes, this is an effective test. In the past, provocative testing was used in an attempt to provide early identification of patients with this inherited disease. However, the routine use of RET (rearranged during transfection) proto-oncogene now allows for detection and intervention in this patient population at an early age before medullary thyroid cancer develops. Patients with medullary thyroid cancer will commonly have an elevated serum carcinoembryonic antigen level as well.

▪ Fine-Needle Aspiration Biopsy

The most commonly employed means of directly evaluating a thyroid nodule is the fine-needle aspiration (FNA) biopsy. Several technical issues must be considered. Patients with larger masses are more likely to have a higher yield. On the other hand, patients with a stocky neck or an ill-defined lesion may require the FNA biopsy to be performed under ultrasound guidance (USGFNA).

In performing FNA, the clinician must ensure that the patient is comfortably positioned so that the mass may be fixed between two fingers. Prior to attempting FNA, it is important to place 2 to 4 mL of air in the syringe. A 22-, 23-, or 25-gauge needle should be employed. In removing the syringe from the skin, the vacuum in the syringe must be decreased to prevent loss of cellular substance into the syringe.

The aspirate is fixed with 95% ethanol, and care is taken to immerse the specimen immediately to prevent drying artifact. When fluid is obtained, it is submitted for cell block preparation in a fixative. A minimum of two passes should be made for each suspicious thyroid mass. In patients where thyroid lymphoma is suspected, placement of the specimen into Roswell Park Memorial Institute (RPMI) solution will allow for proper pathological evaluation and flow cytometry studies.

Four broad categories have been used to classify FNA biopsies: (1) malignant, (2) suspicious, (3) benign, or (4) inconclusive. The fourth category requires additional attempts at needle biopsy. More recently, in an effort to standardize diagnostic terminology used in reporting thyroid cytopathology, many institutions have adopted a common reporting scheme known as The Bethesda System for Reporting Cytopathology (TBSRTC). This system uses six diagnostic categories for thyroid cytopathology as listed in **Table 35.1**.

This has resulted in improved consistency in reporting of thyroid cytopathology; however, management may differ among institutions regarding extent of surgery. Patients with repeat USGFNA that return as persistent category III may be offered diagnostic surgery.

Within the malignant category of thyroid cytology are papillary, medullary, thyroid lymphoma, and anaplastic thyroid cancers. Considerable difficulty is associated with the findings of follicular cells. The diagnosis of follicular thyroid cancer can be made only on complete evaluation of the thyroid neoplasm capsule, which would necessitate thyroidectomy for definitive diagnosis. Likewise, the finding of Hürthle cells may be difficult to interpret because they may represent neoplasm or inflammatory changes. Antithyroid antibody studies may differentiate between neoplasm and inflammation. Finally, the persistence of the thyroid mass after aspiration of a thyroid cyst should be viewed with some suspicion, even when the aspirant is benign on cytological evaluation, because persistence may represent a complex mass.

◼ Imaging

There are many radiographic studies for evaluating thyroid nodules. The routine use of all tests in any single patient would not be cost-effective and would be associated with an extremely expensive medical evaluation.

Thyroid Ultrasonography

Thyroid ultrasonography is relatively simple, noninvasive, and cost-effective. In some instances, surgeons and other physicians have ultrasound units in their offices, and they can perform the test on the day of evaluation. The ultrasound allows delineation of solid versus cystic masses. Some masses may have both cystic and solid components and are defined as complex masses. Thyroid ultrasonography has become a reliable method to allow more accurate sampling of thyroid nodules, whether cystic, solid, or complex. In addition, ultrasonography allows noninvasive surveillance of thyroid nodules followed over time, with or without thyroid suppression.

Radioactive Scans

Radioactive scans have been employed on a large scale in the past. The rationale for using this type of scan is that it allows determination of the functional status of a thyroid nodule. The preliminary scan is performed using pertechnetate, with radioactive iodine used with patients in whom there is a strong suspicion of malignancy. In patients in whom the nodule is isofunctioning (warm) or hyperfunctioning (hot), the risk of malignancy is relatively small—probably no greater than 3 to 5%. However, there is some evidence to suggest higher risk of malignancy in patients with toxic multinodular goiter. Thus patients with hyperthyroidism and multiple nodules may be considered for surgery rather than radioactive iodine (RAI), which addresses both the hyperthyroid state and possible malignancy. In suggested reading patients with hypofunctioning (cold)

Table 35.1 Bethesda system for reporting cytopathology

Category	Diagnosis	Risk of malignancy	Management
I	Nondiagnostic/unsatisfactory	1–4%	Repeat USGFNA
II	Benign	0–3%	Observation with ultrasound
III	AUS/FLUS	5–15%	Repeat USGFNA
IV	FN/SFN	15–30%	Lobectomy
V	Suspicious for malignancy	60–75%	Thyroidectomy
VI	Malignant	97–99%	Thyroidectomy

Abbreviations: AUS/FLUS, atypical ultrasound/follicular lesion unknown significance; FN/SFN, follicular neoplasm/suspicious for follicular neoplasm

Used with permission from Bongiovanni M, Spitale A, Faquin N, Mazzucchelli L, Baloch CW. The Bethesda System for Reporting Thyroid Cytopathology: a meta-analysis. Acta Cytol 2012;56(4):333–339.

nodules, the incidence of malignancy increases to 20 to 30%. However, this level of incidence leaves 70 to 80% of patients who do not have a malignancy, and this test does not distinguish between malignant and benign pathology. For this reason, with the exception of patients being evaluated for hyperthyroidism, radioactive scans have been largely abandoned.

Computed Tomography and Magnetic Resonance Imaging

The role of computed tomography (CT) and/or magnetic resonance imaging (MRI) has increased in the management of thyroid lesions. CT and MRI are most commonly used with patients with massive thyroid lesions, thyroid fixation, or large metastatic deposits in the lateral neck. More experience has been obtained with CT than MRI, but MRI has the advantage of improved soft tissue definition when compared with CT at other sites in the body. Both scans allow for the determination of the relationship of a thyroid mass to the trachea, esophagus, carotid sheath, mediastinum, and the great vessels within the mediastinum. For patients suspected of having lesions that encompass or invade any of the great vessels, MRI has the advantage of allowing simultaneous MR angiography (MRA). Depending on the findings with MRA, angiography with a test balloon occlusion may be necessary in a small proportion of patients. Determining the relationship of the mass to the great vessels within the mediastinum will allow the appropriate preoperative involvement of a thoracic or vascular surgeon to maximize the surgical results.

Chest X-Ray

In all patients undergoing thyroid surgery, a chest X-ray should be obtained. In many instances, a screening chest X-ray identifies previously undetected thyroid masses and necessitates an appropriate evaluation. Observations of thyroid calcifications, mediastinal widening, or lung nodules are suspicious for more substantial disease and should prompt additional evaluation, such as a chest CT scan.

Endoscopy, Laryngoscopy, Bronchoscopy, and Esophagoscopy

Finally, the presence of any of the worrisome symptoms, such as hoarseness, dyspnea on exertion, or hemoptysis, may result in the decision to use endoscopy at the time of the planned surgical resection.

Endoscopy can detect intraluminal tumors, which would necessitate a more extended resection. Direct laryngoscopy, bronchoscopy, and esophagoscopy should all be considered when evaluating patients with these ominous symptoms and should be routinely employed, with malignant invasion of the trachea noted on preoperative imaging.

■ Indications for Surgical Exploration

Surgery should be used as a diagnostic intervention under several circumstances:

- Patients with a unilateral thyroid mass who have undergone suppression with no response or progression of the size of the mass should be considered for thyroidectomy, even in the face of a previously benign needle biopsy.
- Patients with benign thyroid nodules that are enlarging on serial ultrasound should be given consideration for surgical intervention.
- Patients with symptoms of impingement on the central visceral structure (e.g., shortness of breath, dysphagia, or stridor) should be considered for surgery even in the face of presumed benign disease.
- Patients in whom a thyroid mass is associated with a unilateral vocal cord paralysis do not require needle aspiration cytology confirmation of malignancy and should undergo surgical intervention.

A common setting in which patients may present is open biopsy-proven metastatic papillary thyroid cancer with a previously undetected thyroid nodule. Thorough evaluation of the thyroid with ultrasound will often result in identification of the primary tumor in the thyroid. In addition, thyroglobulin stains of the metastatic nodule are helpful in confirming thyroid origin. In rare instances, a lateral neck mass may be the presenting finding of a patient with sporadic medullary thyroid cancer.

■ Summary

Thyroid nodules are commonly found among the general population and are usually benign. Some patients with a history of radiation or a family history of thyroid cancer may be at higher risk for malignancy. The standard physical examination should always include neck/thyroid palpation and visual laryngeal examination. With the use of ultrasound, thyroid nodules can be diagnosed, monitored, and biopsied with excellent clinical efficacy. Basic thyroid serology should affirm the presence or absence of the euthyroid state. Advanced imaging such as CT or MRI, as well as nuclear medicine studies, are not indicated in the vast majority of patients. Patients with a high historical risk, suspicious cytology or imaging, or increasing symptoms may be considered for thyroid surgery.

◼ Practice Guidelines, Consensus Statements, and Measures

Guidelines for the management of thyroid nodules can be found in the 2009 consensus guidelines of the American Thyroid Association, listed in the Suggested Reading section.

◼ Suggested Reading

Bongiovanni M, Spitale A, Faquin WC, Mazzucchelli L, Baloch ZW. The Bethesda System for Reporting Thyroid Cytopathology: a meta-analysis. Acta Cytol 2012;56(4):333–339

Cooper DS, Doherty GM, Haugen BR, et al. Revised American Thyroid Association Management Guidelines for Patients with Thyroid Nodules and Differentiated Thyroid Cancer. Falls Church, VA: American Thyroid Association; November 2009. http://thyroidguidelines.org/revised/taskforce

Crockett JC. The thyroid nodule: fine-needle aspiration biopsy technique. J Ultrasound Med 2011;30(5):685–694

Emerson CH. Can thyroid ultrasound and related procedures provide diagnostic information about thyroid nodules: a look at the guidelines. Thyroid 2011;21(3):211–213

Smith JJ, Chen X, Schneider DF, et al. Toxic nodular goiter and cancer: a compelling case for thyroidectomy. Ann Surg Oncol 2013;20(4):1336–1340

36 Management Options in Well-Differentiated Thyroid Cancer

■ Introduction

Thyroid cancer represents ~ 1% of all cancers in the United States. Histologically, thyroid cancers are divided into papillary, follicular, medullary, and anaplastic cancers. The papillary and follicular cancers are considered well differentiated and represent ~ 85% of all thyroid cancers. Pure follicular cancers represent 15 to 20% of well-differentiated cancers. The oxyphilic variant of follicular cancer, called Hürthle cell cancer, is included in this group (3–5%). The great majority (80–85%) of well-differentiated thyroid cancers are pure papillary tumors (15–20%) or mixed papillary-follicular tumors (65–70%); both are considered papillary cancers.

The prognosis of well-differentiated thyroid cancer is generally excellent: the cancer-specific survival is 80 to 95% at 20 years. The ideal treatment of differentiated thyroid cancer has been a source of controversy. The often indolent natural history of this cancer with a good prognosis in the majority of patients, regardless of treatment, contributes to the difficulty of analyzing available data. All the information and recommendations about this disease are based on retrospective studies of patients treated with many different approaches over a long period. The controversy is likely to persist because it is unlikely that any randomized study will ever be conducted.

No one disputes that surgery is the treatment of choice for differentiated thyroid carcinoma. However, the extent of necessary surgery, both to the thyroid and to the neck, the adjuvant use of radioactive iodine (RAI) and external irradiation, and the use and dosage of hormonal therapy are all controversial.

■ Prognostic Indicators

Retrospective analysis of large series of patients has identified pretreatment prognostic indicators for tumor recurrence and death from thyroid cancer. Depending on the study, all the following factors have been associated with a worse prognosis for tumor recurrence and death from thyroid cancer: older age, male sex, extrathyroidal extension, larger tumors, follicular lesions, higher tumor grade, nodal metastasis, distant metastasis, and delay in treatment. Different classification systems have evolved from these prognostic indicators.

The Age, Tumor Grade, Extent, and Size (AGES) Scoring System

A scoring system for papillary cancer is based on age, tumor grade, extent, and size (AGES). The prognostic score (PS) is computed as follows: PS = 0.05/ tumor size (ts)/age in years (if age 40 or older) or +0 (if younger than 40), +1 (if grade 2) or +3 (if grade 3 or 4), +1 (if extrathyroid) or +3 (if distant metastasis), + 0.2 /ts/ tumor size in centimeters (cm). This index was developed for 860 papillary cancer patients. Of those, over 85% had a prognostic score of less than 3.99 and a 25-year mortality of 2%. These patients were considered to be low risk. Patients with scores of 4 to 4.99, 5 to 5.99, and 6 and higher had mortality rates of nearly 25%, 50%, and over 90%, respectively. Collectively, for patients with scores above 4, the 25-year mortality rate was just under 50%. This group was considered high risk.

The Age, Distant Metastases, Extrathyroid Extension, and Size (AMES) Classification

The AMES classification is based on age, metastases, extent, and size (AMES). This resulted in a simplified definition of low risk and high risk for both papillary and follicular tumors, with low-risk patients being (1) all younger patients without distant metastases (men < 41 years and women < 51 years); and (2) all older patients with intrathyroidal papillary cancer or minor capsular involvement follicular carcinoma, of less than 5 cm in size, and with no distant metastasis. Using these criteria in over 300 patients treated from 1961 to 1980, almost 90% were classified in the low-risk group with a mortality of 2%, and the remainder in the high-risk group with a mortality of just under 50%.

Other Classification Systems

Other classifications have identified a difference in outcome based on patient and tumor factors at initial presentation. The American Joint Committee on Cancer (AJCC) also has a tumor, node, metastasis (TNM) classification, and others have recently modified the AGES scoring system by eliminating grade and adding completeness of resection (metastasis, patient age, completeness of resection, local invasion, and tumor size [MACIS]).

The question then becomes, does the initial therapy affect prognosis? Also, because surgery is the main treatment, does the extent of surgery alter the outcome? In addition, is the adjuvant use of RAI and thyroid suppression effective? The prognosis for nonaggressive tumors is so good that a large number of patients must be followed for a long period to detect any significant difference in survival among treatments.

■ Surgical Treatment

Thyroid Surgery

Surgery is the treatment of choice for well-differentiated thyroid cancer. In general, two management philosophies have been proposed for the treatment of the primary tumor in well-differentiated thyroid carcinoma: (1) the conservative approach, and (2) the aggressive approach (**Table 36.1**). Proponents of the conservative approach base the extent of thyroid surgery on prognostic indicators and recommend hemithyroidectomy for the low-risk group, which usually includes more than 80% of all patients. More extensive thyroid surgery is recommended for the high-risk group.

Because many scoring systems have been described, the definition of low risk varies from author to author, and recommendations for the same lesion may vary from institution to institution. Proponents of the aggressive approach recommend a total or near-total thyroidectomy in most cases; lobectomy is acceptable only for small, single lesions. Both philosophies describe the extent of surgery with a confusing array of terms. The minimal surgery recommended is a hemithyroidectomy and isthmectomy. At the other end of the spectrum is total thyroidectomy. From the conservative to the more radical, the following terminology is used: bilateral subtotal, unilateral total and contralateral subtotal, bilateral near-total, and unilateral total and contralateral near-total. The less-than-total techniques preserve a posterior portion of the gland in hopes of reducing the risk of injury to the recurrent laryngeal nerve and at least one parathyroid gland.

The theoretical advantages of total thyroidectomy are that (1) it addresses the problem of multicentricity, which has been reported to be as high as 80%; (2) it decreases the risk of local recurrence, not only in the thyroid bed but also in the regional nodes; (3) it decreases the risk of distant recurrence; (4) it reduces the risk of anaplastic transformation in the thyroid remnant; (5) it facilitates the diagnostic and therapeutic use of RAI; and (6) it allows the use of thyroglobulin as a tumor marker in the follow-up period. These advantages are appealing and would be accepted by the majority of surgeons if it were not for the proximity of the thyroid gland to the recurrent laryngeal nerves and parathyroid glands and the need for lifetime thyroid hormone replacement. Therefore, mainly because of a higher potential for complications in total thyroidectomy, but also because the majority of patients are considered to be low risk and are reported to do well regardless of the extent of surgery, a conservative thyroid resection in the low-risk group is favored by some surgeons.

There is ample support in the literature for a conservative approach in low-risk patients. In AGES low-risk patients with papillary cancers, mortality rates for lobectomy and total thyroidectomy patients are the same. In a series with nearly 250 patients with intrathyroidal papillary cancer, half of whom received hemithyroidectomy and half total thyroidectomy, the estimated recurrence rate at 20 years was less than 7%, and only two patients died of metastatic disease. No patient had recurrence in the thyroid bed or in the contralateral lobe. Interestingly, the 20-year recurrence rates were significantly lower in the unilateral group (~ 4%) than in the group with bilateral surgery (~ 13%). The complication rates were also lower in the unilateral group (1% vs. 8%), supporting the use of more conservative surgery for the treatment of intrathyroidal disease. Several investigators have shown similar survival in hemithyroidectomy patients with limited disease when compared with total thyroidectomy patients. This has led to controversy in the approach, with general consensus that patients with higher-risk disease, based on histology and extent of disease among others, should have total thyroidectomy in the hands of an experienced thyroid surgeon.

Despite some studies showing similar disease control, most thyroid surgeons acknowledge the higher incidence of tumor recurrence after conservative surgical treatment. An evaluation of the incidence of local recurrence in 963 patients with

Table 36.1   Extent of surgery for well-differentiated thyroid cancer

Study	Histology	Hemithyroidectomy	Total thyroidectomy	Comments/ conclusions
Hay and Klee (1993)[1]	AGES low-risk group, PTC	2% 25-year mortality	2% 25-year mortality	No difference in mortality between total and hemithyroidectomy
Vickery et al (1987)[3]	Intrathyroidal PTC	4.1% 20-year recurrence rate 1.1% complication rate	13.1% 20-year recurrence rate 8.2% complication rate	No recurrence in thyroid bed or contralateral lobe Recommend conservative surgery
Shah et al (1993)[4]	DTC, matched-pair analysis > 45 years of age	82% 20-year survival 7% local recurrence	79% 20-year survival 7% local recurrence	Recommend lobectomy for intrathyroidal tumors < 4 cm
Grant et al (1988)[5]	PTC	Low-risk AGES: 14% 30-year recurrence High-risk AGES: 59% 30-year recurrence	Low-risk AGES: 4% 30-year recurrence High-risk AGES: 20% 30-year recurrence	Difference in recurrence rate but no difference in survival
Mazzaferri and Jhiang (1994)[2]	DTC	40% 30-year recurrence 6% mortality	28% 30-year recurrence 9% mortality	Tumors < 1.5 cm may not require total thyroidectomy Larger tumors require total thyroidectomy, RAI remnant ablation/therapy
Segal et al (1995)[6]	PTC in setting of postoperative RAI ablation	28% local recurrence	8% local recurrence	Total or near-total thyroidectomy for PTC > 1 cm

Abbreviations: AGES, age, grade, extent, size; DTC, differentiated thyroid cancer; PTC, papillary thyroid cancer; RAI, radioactive iodine.
Data from:
1. Hay ID, Klee GG. Thyroid cancer diagnosis and management. Clin Laboratory Med 1993;13:725–734.
2. Mazzaferri EL, Jhiang SM. Long-term impact of initial surgical therapy and medical therapy on papillary and follicular thyroid cancer. Am J Med 1994;97:418–428.
3. Vickery AL, Wang C, Walker AM. Treatment of intrathyroidal papillary carcinoma of the thyroid. Cancer 1987;60:2587–2595.
4. Shah JP, Loree TR, Dharker D, Strong EW. Lobectomy versus total thyroidectomy for differentiated carcinoma of the thyroid: a matched-pair analysis. Am J Surg 1993;166:331–335.
5. Grant CS, Hay ID, Gough IR, Bergstrahl EJ, Goellner JR, McConahey WM. Local recurrence in papillary thyroid carcinoma: is the extent of surgical resection important? Surgery 1988;104:954–962.
6. Segal K, Fridental R, Lubin E, Shvero J, Sulkes J, Feinmesser R. Papillary carcinoma of the thyroid. Otolaryngol Head Neck Surg 1995;113:356–363.

papillary carcinoma showed that, in the low-risk AGES group, the 30-year recurrence rate was 14% after unilateral resection and 4% after bilateral resection; in the high-risk group, 30-year recurrence rates were nearly 60% for unilateral and 20% for bilateral surgery (both of which were statistically significant). The study also found that, 30 years after local recurrence, 50% of patients had died of cancer, but no deaths were related to recurrence limited to the thyroid remnant. Worse survival was reported in the low-risk group treated with unilateral resection, but this was not statistically significant. Survival curves for near-total thyroidectomy and total thyroidectomy were not statistically different, although the local recurrence rates for near-total resection, in both low-risk and high-risk patients, were definitely higher than for total thyroidectomy.

Many authors suggest that the ideal thyroid operation for differentiated cancer is a total thyroidectomy. Some authors found that a total thyroidectomy often revealed multicentric disease and could be performed with minimal morbidity, and others have reported a survival advantage to the more aggressive approach, even in the low-risk group.

In a large series of more than 1,300 patients, common risk factors were identified as important. Age at diagnosis, male sex, tumors larger than 1.5 cm, regional nodes, local invasion, and multiple thyroid tumors were all found to affect tumor recurrence and survival. When regional nodes were present, survival was decreased only in patients with follicular tumors. Treatment factors that influenced recurrence and survival were delayed therapy, extent of surgery, and medical therapy. The 30-year recurrence rates were just under 30% for total thyroidectomy and 40% for less than near-total resection ($P <$ 0.002); cancer mortality rates were just over 5% and just under 10%, respectively ($p = 0.02$). Recurrence rates were 40% without medical therapy, 30% with thyroid hormone alone, and 15% after RAI ($P < 0.001$). Death rates were similarly influenced. Despite more adverse risk factors in the RAI group, this group had a lower recurrence rate (16% vs. 38%, $P < 0.001$), and lower 30-year mortality rate (3% vs. 9%, $p = 0.03$). The authors suggested that tumors less than 1.5 cm may not require routine total thyroidectomy, whereas larger tumors require total thyroidectomy and RAI remnant ablation or RAI therapy for residual tumor.

Some authors have questioned the use of the conservative approach, even in single small lesions. A 1995 review of nearly 100 patients with primary tumors smaller than 1.5 cm showed that over a third of these patients had nodal disease, extrathyroidal extension, or metastatic disease. Multicentricity was found in 15 patients, and minimal residual disease after surgery was believed to be present in 6. The authors point out that small lesions should not be discounted as inconsequential because they can present with extrathyroidal extension and nodal and distant metastasis. The authors also believe that nodal disease increases the risk of tumor recurrence and possibly even death from cancer.

Central Nodal Surgery

Surgical therapy of the primary tumor is the critical step in controlling thyroid cancer. Treatment of the neck is secondary, but it is also controversial. The incidence of neck metastasis in well-differentiated thyroid carcinoma has been reported to be as high as 90%. The recommended treatment for clinical metastasis is the appropriate conservative neck dissection.

The many options mentioned for occult disease include expectant management or elective treatment with neck dissection, hormonal suppression, or RAI. One approach to minimize the morbidity and mortality associated with central compartment recurrence is to proceed to a routine prophylactic central nodal dissection for both diagnostic and therapeutic reasons. To rely strictly on RAI to detect and treat metastatic nodal disease could be risky, because only 75 to 80% of well-differentiated thyroid cancer lesions will concentrate RAI.

Another option is to perform a prophylactic central neck dissection in patients with high-risk features. It is a recent recommendation to perform a prophylactic central neck dissection on advanced primary tumors > 4 cm or those with extrathyroidal extension. Prophylactic central neck dissection can be avoided in patients with small tumors with no extrathyroidal invasion and most follicular cancers. A correlation analysis on central lymph node metastasis has found that tumors in the middle and lower poles, tumors > 0.5 cm in size, patients younger than 45 years, and capsular invasion were predictive of central lymph node metastasis.

It is the practice of some centers to avoid prophylactic neck dissection in the absence of clinically apparent nodes. Instead, careful intraoperative inspection of the central neck compartment and sampling of suspicious ipsilateral paratracheal nodes to detect disease can be performed. In the absence of metastasis, no further neck treatment is recommended. In the presence of microscopic nodal disease, a central neck dissection should be performed. These institutions believe that there is no convincing evidence of a benefit in survival or local recurrence (see **Table 36.2**). A central neck dissection should involve both level VI and level VII nodes.

The information gathered from a prophylactic neck dissection gives the best assessment of the nodal status, decreases the local recurrence rate, reduces the risks of a reoperation, and may guide the dosing of RAI. The clinical implications of nodal disease on presentation are controversial, with some

Table 36.2 Outcomes in prophylactic central neck dissection (CND) compared with controls

Study	Number of patients	Positive nodes (%)	Central recurrence after CND (%)	Central recurrence without CND (%)
Moreno et al[1]	252	71.4	1.8	2.4
Hughes et al[2]	143	62	2	2
Sywak et al[3]	447	38	0	1.7
Moo et al[4]	81	33	0	5.6

Data from:
1. Moreno MA, Edeiken-Monroe BS, Siegel ER, Sherman SI, Clayman GL. In papillary thyroid cancer, preoperative central neck ultrasound detects only macroscopic surgical disease, but negative findings predict excellent long-term regional control and survival. Thyroid 2012;22(4):347–355.
2. Hughes DT, White ML, Miller BS, Gauger PG, Burney RE, Doherty GM. Influence of prophylactic central lymph node dissection on postoperative thyroglobulin levels and radioiodine treatment in papillary thyroid cancer. Surgery 2010;148(6):1100-6.
3. Sywak M, Cornford L, Roach P, Stalberg P, Sidhu S, Delbridge L. Routine ipsilateral level VI lymphadenectomy reduced postoperative thyroglobulin levels in papillary thyroid cancer. Surgery 2006;140(6):1000–1005.
4. Moo TA, McGill J, Allendorf J, Lee J, Fahey T 3rd, Zarnegar R. Impact of prophylactic central neck lymph node dissection on early recurrence in papillary thyroid carcinoma. World J Surg 2010;34(6):1187–1191.

authors reporting an influence only on tumor recurrence, and others reporting a detrimental effect on survival. An accepted fact is that, of patients who die from well-differentiated thyroid cancer, 50% will die from central locally invasive disease. Some of these recurrences are local recurrences that should be minimized with a total thyroidectomy, but some are recurrences in the regional periglandular central neck nodes. A logical view that is gaining acceptance is that nodal metastasis on presentation denotes a more aggressive tumor, which increases the likelihood of distant metastasis and decreased survival.

Lateral Nodal Surgery

Given evidence of clinical lateral nodal disease, as diagnosed by fine-needle aspiration or intraoperative frozen analysis, a selective neck dissection is favored over isolated lymph node resection. There are data showing reduced recurrence rates and mortality of formal neck dissection. This should include levels II through IV and at least the inferior aspect of level V.

■ Special Considerations in Surgical Treatment

Extrathyroidal Extension

Extrathyroidal extension is a well-recognized sign of poor prognosis. A study of over 1,000 patients identified extrathyroidal extension in under 10%. The 30-year, disease-specific survival rate dropped from 87% in patients without extension to 29% in patients with extension. In general, total thyroidectomy followed by RAI, external irradiation, and hormonal suppression is recommended. The goal of surgery in patients with extrathyroidal extension is total tumor removal. However, extensive resection to establish wide margins is not appropriate, especially if it markedly increases morbidity. Multiple studies have examined the role of surgery when structures such as the recurrent laryngeal nerve, trachea, larynx, pharynx, and esophagus are involved. The recurrent laryngeal nerve has been identified as the most common important structure involved, and it is recommended that when the nerve is functional, every attempt should be made to dissect the tumor from the nerve and to preserve the nerve. If the nerve is paralyzed, it should be resected.

The extent of surgery recommended for the unfortunate 1% of patients with upper aerodigestive tract involvement has been controversial. The most recent publications recommend that no gross tumor be left behind. The shaving procedure seems to be acceptable when close margins are obtained or when only microscopic disease is left behind because survival is comparable to more aggressive procedures, and

morbidity is minimized. In the majority of patients where gross tumor excision requires removing part of the aerodigestive tract, a conservative procedure is often possible, and only occasionally are more extensive surgery and reconstruction necessary.

RAI should always be considered in patients with extrathyroidal disease. External radiation can also be considered, especially with microscopic or gross residual disease. The effectiveness of external radiation is greatly increased when only microscopic disease is left behind, although it remains useful in cases of incomplete resection as well.

Children and Adolescents

Approximately 3 to 10% of thyroid carcinomas are found in patients younger than 20 years of age. They usually present with more advanced disease: nodal metastasis, often bilateral, and distant metastasis. The prognosis, however, remains excellent. The recommended treatment is a total or near-total thyroidectomy for the primary tumor, followed by RAI and hormonal suppression.

Pathological Variants of Well-Differentiated Tumors

Within the well-differentiated thyroid carcinomas, there are special histological variants that carry a worse prognosis. These are the tall-cell variant of papillary carcinoma and insular carcinoma, which can be found in both the papillary and the follicular groups.

Tall-cell variants of papillary carcinomas are characterized by tall columnar cells with basal hyperchromatic nuclei and with a height of at least two to three times their width. They represent 4 to 10% of all papillary carcinomas and are often seen in older patients who typically present with a large tumor, extrathyroid extension, and nodal metastasis. Patients with this histological variant have a worse prognosis. An aggressive approach is recommended and commonly consists of total thyroidectomy with appropriate neck dissection, including paratracheal nodal dissection, followed by RAI ablation and therapy when necessary. External irradiation should also be considered for patients with tumors with extrathyroid extension.

Insular carcinoma is a poorly differentiated papillary or follicular tumor, situated histologically and biologically between the well-differentiated tumors and the anaplastic carcinomas. It represents ~ 3 to 6% of all thyroid carcinomas and also carries a worse prognosis. Patients with this tumor type tend to present at an older age. This variant is more aggressive than the tall-cell variant, with many patients dying of their thyroid cancer. Aggressive management is recommended for all patients with insular carcinomas.

Pregnancy and Thyroid Cancer

Thyroid cancer is more common in women of all ages, so the association of thyroid cancer and pregnancy can be encountered. The incidence of cancerous thyroid nodules found during pregnancy (~ 40%) seems to be higher than that among nonpregnant women. The hormonal effects of pregnancy on thyroid cancer are not well established; therefore, management is controversial.

In general, evaluation and treatment of thyroid cancer in pregnant women can be safely delayed until after delivery. When the diagnosis of malignancy is made during pregnancy, either with a fine-needle aspiration biopsy of a thyroid nodule or because of nodal metastasis, the patient should be placed on thyroid suppression. A tumor that grows rapidly despite suppression should be removed as soon as surgery will not endanger the fetus. The optimal time to perform surgery during pregnancy is during the second trimester. Earlier surgery carries the teratogenic risks of anesthetic agents, whereas surgery during the third trimester can induce premature labor. When the mother's survival may be at risk, a decision may have to be made to proceed surgically, regardless of the pregnancy stage.

Prior Exposure to Radiation

The incidence of thyroid cancer is higher in patients exposed to low-dose irradiation in childhood. The prognosis for these patients does not seem to be worse than for the rest of the population. Thyroid cancer occurring after irradiation is often multicentric and was considered high risk in a recent consensus conference. The Chernobyl nuclear disaster caused a rapid increase in the incidence of radiation-induced thyroid carcinoma, many of which are poorly differentiated tumors with nodal metastasis. Total or near-total thyroidectomy is recommended for the management of thyroid nodules and for carcinoma in patients previously exposed to radiation.

Hormonal Treatment

The effect of thyroid suppression on thyroid cancer has long been recognized. It is generally accepted that all patients with a history of thyroid cancer should be on sufficient doses of levothyroxine to suppress the thyroid-stimulating hormone (TSH) level. Surveys of clinical endocrinologists reveal that they all recommend hormonal therapy, and over 85% suggest a suppressive dosage. In cases of cancer requiring suppressive therapy, nearly all recommend that the TSH level be below the normal range.

■ Radiation Treatment

Radioactive Iodine

RAI can be used in the management of thyroid cancer, not only for thyroid ablation after thyroidectomy but also for the treatment of residual disease, nodal and distant metastases, and tumor recurrence. The initial scan obtained at the time of remnant ablation can also detect previously subclinical disease in the local bed or nodal compartments. Thyroid ablation is recommended after total or near-total thyroidectomy to eradicate residual normal and pathological thyroid tissue and to facilitate follow-up scanning to detect recurrent or metastatic disease. Thyroglobulin levels can then be used as reliable indicators of recurrent disease, because endogenous thyroid hormone is eliminated. A dose of ~ 150 mCi is usually recommended, both to ablate the gland and to treat micrometastases not seen on nuclear scanning.

RAI ablation after hemithyroidectomy is not very effective. Therefore, when residual thyroid is present, completion thyroidectomy is suggested if RAI is to be delivered. Recommendations are variable, but most recommend that patients receive RAI ablation. Thus far a benefit of RAI is not established in patients with a single lesion smaller than 1.5 cm. Therefore, in low-risk lesions of small size, the trend is not to treat with RAI, particularly given the possibility of secondary hematologic malignancies from the RAI.

Large retrospective studies have generally shown a decrease in disease recurrence and mortality with the use of RAI. The effect on mortality has not been shown on patients with a preablative low risk for mortality. Current guidelines recommend RAI for patients with (1) unresectable tumors, (2) persistent tumor after surgery, (3) primary tumor > 4 cm, (4) extrathyroid disease, (5) cervical and mediastinal nodal metastases, (6) recurrent disease, and (7) distant metastasis. RAI can also be considered for a combination of other high-risk features. Although quantitative dosimetric protocols have been described, the majority of patients are treated with standard fixed dosages that may vary according to the location and extent of the disease.

External Radiotherapy

External radiotherapy has been proposed for the treatment of thyroid carcinoma in a variety of situations. A review of over 1,000 T_3 and T_4 thyroid cancer patients found no advantage with external irradiation in patients younger than 40 years, and a slightly better survival ($p = 0.09$) in the irradiated patients older than 40 years. Other reports have shown benefit in patients over 40 with extrathyroidal papillary cancer and involved lymph nodes. This benefit was not seen in the absence of nodes and in patients with follicular cancer. In general, the use of external irradiation is limited to gross residual tumor after surgery and to unresectable tumors not given RAI in patients > 45 years of age.

Targeted Therapies

Recent progress in defining the molecular pathogenesis of thyroid cancer has led to the development of molecular markers and targeted therapies in recent years. Current applications of these targeted therapies include inoperable thyroid cancers that are refractory to RAI and cancers for which external beam radiation is not a good option. Limitation to this group is due to the significant cardiac, gastrointestinal, and skin-related side effects and overall toxicity of the drugs. Available agents are tyrosine kinase inhibitors and redifferentiation drugs, such as sorafenib, selumetinib, pazopanib, and sunitinib. Before therapy, a fluorodeoxyglucose positron-emission tomography scan is helpful to locate disease and determine the risk. The response rate range is under 50%. Phase 3 studies are ongoing and show some promising results. However, toxicities, side effects, and variable responses are limiting factors. Because many patients remain asymptomatic and disease may be indolent for some time, the commencement of targeted therapies must be carefully considered. It is also possible that the preoperative identification of genetic abnormalities such as BRAF, RB, and others may lead to the development of additional targeted therapies.

◼ Follow-Up

In addition to the regular clinical examination, whole-body RAI scans and thyroglobulin levels are standard follow-up tests for patients treated with total or near-total thyroidectomy. These two tests are complementary, and their optimal use requires the absence of residual normal thyroid tissue. These tests can be repeated annually for 2 years, and then every 5 years up to 20 years. After total thyroidectomy and ablation, the thyroglobulin level should be < 2 ng/mL on thyroid replacement and < 3 ng/mL off thyroid replacement. These tests are less reliable in patients with residual thyroid tissue and are not often used in this situation.

◼ Summary

The management of patients with well-differentiated thyroid cancer is controversial. Surgery is the mainstay of therapy. Prognostic factors, such as age, gender, extrathyroidal extension, and size, can be used to determine which patient will benefit from a more aggressive approach that combines total thyroidectomy, RAI ablation, and TSH hormonal suppression. The benefit of this aggressive approach is obvious for more advanced tumors, and disputable for early lesions. These benefits must be weighed against the risk of complications seen with total thyroidectomies performed by inexperienced surgeons.

◼ Suggested Reading

Cooper DS, Doherty GM, Haugen BR, et al; American Thyroid Association (ATA) Guidelines Taskforce on Thyroid Nodules and Differentiated Thyroid Cancer. Revised American Thyroid Association management guidelines for patients with thyroid nodules and differentiated thyroid cancer [published correction appears in Thyroid 2010;20(8):942. Hauger, Bryan R corrected to Haugen, Bryan R]. Thyroid 2009;19(11):1167–1214

Gyorki DE, Untch B, Tuttle RM, Shaha AR. Prophylactic central neck dissection in differentiated thyroid cancer: an assessment of the evidence. Ann Surg Oncol 2013;20(7):2285–2289

Kupferman ME, Patterson M, Mandel SJ, LiVolsi V, Weber RS. Patterns of lateral neck metastasis in papillary thyroid carcinoma. Arch Otolaryngol Head Neck Surg 2004;130(7):857–860

Lang BH, Law TT. The role of 18F-fluorodeoxyglucose positron emission tomography in thyroid neoplasms. Oncologist 2011; 16(4):458–466

Lundgren CI, Hall P, Dickman PW, Zedenius J. Influence of surgical and postoperative treatment on survival in differentiated thyroid cancer. Br J Surg 2007;94(5):571–577

Mazzaferri EL. Thyroid remnant 131I ablation for papillary and follicular thyroid carcinoma. Thyroid 1997;7:265–271

Mazzaferri EL, Jhiang SM. Long-term impact of initial surgical therapy and medical therapy on papillary and follicular thyroid cancer. Am J Med 1994;97(5):418–428

Mulla M, Schulte KM. Central cervical lymph node metastases in papillary thyroid cancer: a systematic review of imaging-guided and prophylactic removal of the central compartment. Clin Endocrinol (Oxf) 2012;76(1):131–136

Nixon IJ, Shaha AR, Tuttle MR. Targeted therapy in thyroid cancer. Curr Opin Otolaryngol Head Neck Surg 2013;21(2):130–134

Noguchi M, Kumaki T, Taniya T, et al. Impact of neck dissection on survival in well-differentiated thyroid cancer: a multivariate analysis of 218 cases. Int Surg 1990;75(4):220–224

Rosenbaum MA, McHenry CR. Contemporary management of papillary carcinoma of the thyroid gland. Expert Rev Anticancer Ther 2009;9(3):317–329

Sawka AM, Brierley JD, Tsang RW, et al. An updated systematic review and commentary examining the effectiveness of radioactive iodine remnant ablation in well-differentiated thyroid cancer. Endocrinol Metab Clin North Am 2008;37(2):457–480, x

Wang W, Gu J, Shang J, Wang K. Correlation analysis on central lymph node metastasis in 276 patients with cN0 papillary thyroid carcinoma. Int J Clin Exp Pathol 2013;6(3):510–515

Wong KP, Lang BH. New molecular targeted therapy and redifferentiation therapy for radioiodine-refractory advanced papillary thyroid carcinoma: literature review. J Thyroid Res 2012;2012:818204

Xing M. Molecular pathogenesis and mechanisms of thyroid cancer. Nat Rev Cancer 2013;13(3):184–199

37 Contemporary Screening Techniques for Medullary Carcinoma of the Thyroid

■ Introduction

Medullary carcinoma of the thyroid, or medullary thyroid cancer (MTC), is an uncommon malignancy that accounts for less than 1% of all thyroid masses and < 5% of all thyroid malignancies. MTC arises in the C cells, or the parafollicular cells, of the thyroid, and C-cell hyperplasia is usually found in conjunction with it. Up to 80% of MTC occurs sporadically, with no detectable family predisposition and with 20 to 25% being familial. Sporadic MTC tends to occur in a single lobe of the thyroid, whereas familial MTC is often bilateral and multicentric.

There are three inherited patterns of MTC: (1) familial MTC (FMTC); (2) multiple endocrine neoplasia type 2A (MEN2A); and (3) multiple endocrine neoplasia type 2B (MEN2B). MEN2A is characterized by MTC, pheochromocytoma, and parathyroid hyperplasia (in ~ 25% of cases). MEN2B is the most severe of the syndromes and is characterized by early onset of MTC and pheochromocytoma, aggressive and rapid progression of MTC, and rare parathyroid abnormalities, along with ophthalmological and skeletal abnormalities, mucosal neuromas, and intestinal ganglioneuromatosis. FMTC is characterized only by development of MTC, which usually develops later than in the MEN syndromes. It is important to identify whether the tumors develop in a sporadic or familial pattern, because subsequent evaluation, family screening, genetic counseling, and the prognosis of the disease are dependent on this distinction.

Hereditary MTC is inherited in an autosomal-dominant trait, with a high degree of penetrance but variable expression. Because penetrance is not complete, a negative family history is not sufficient in ruling out a familial disease in a patient with MTC. Germline mutations (mutations that are heritable in a germline) in the RET (rearranged during transfection) proto-oncogene have been identified in the familial MTC syndromes. The RET proto-oncogene has been located on chromosome 10 at 10q11.2 and consists of at least 20 exons. The codons involved vary among the three hereditary patterns. Although point mutations in the RET proto-oncogene have been seen in both sporadic and hereditary forms of MTC, they are more common in the hereditary forms. Of great clinical importance is the fact that the RET mutations can be identified in both family members with MTC and clinically normal family members.

■ Evaluation

The presentation of patients with MTC will depend on whether they have sporadic or familial MTC. Because a majority of patients with MTC present with the sporadic form, it is likely that their initial presentation will be with a thyroid mass. Therefore, customary evaluation of a thyroid mass would be indicated.

A careful patient history and clinical evaluation are critical to this assessment. The history and physical examination should focus not only on the thyroid mass or thyroid disease but also on identifying symptoms that might be consistent with MEN. These include diarrhea or flushing (hypercalcitonemia); hypertension, diaphoresis, tachycardia, palpitations, headache, or tremulousness (pheochromocytoma); and renal stones or bone abnormalities (hyperparathyroidism). A family history should be obtained regarding such symptoms or a history of MTC. Subsequent evaluation should be based on clinical judgment, but it is prudent to make a decision regarding subsequent diagnostic tests based on risk and discomfort to the patient, accuracy of testing, and cost.

The diagnosis of MTC can be challenging. Therefore, it is incumbent upon the thyroid surgeon to be aware of the potential diagnostic pitfalls in patients with MTC. The diagnosis of MTC is usually made in one of three clinical settings. MTC can be suspected after evaluation of a thyroid nodule, typically following fine-needle aspiration (FNA). It can also be identified at the time of surgery for excision of a thyroid nodule. Finally, MTC can be identified during screening of family members of a patient with known MTC, FMTC, or MEN2A or 2B.

FNA has become the workhorse of the initial presentation of thyroid masses. Because of the potential for insufficient cellular material for satisfactory cytologic interpretation, multiple biopsies may be required. Adequate material for evaluation would be expected in just under 100% of samples. FNA can identify a malignancy with high accuracy, although it often cannot determine the type of malignancy, particularly with follicular neoplasms. Since MTC is uncommon, the accuracy of FNA in patients with MTC is unknown. A high degree of clinical suspicion by the cytopathologist is usually the most important factor in making the diagnosis of MTC. Because MTC can show a variety of patterns, including papillary, follicular, and anaplastic patterns, immunohistochemical staining of calcitonin and carcinoembryonic antigen is needed to improve the reliability of FNA in MTC (**Fig. 37.1**).

Computed tomography (CT) or magnetic resonance imaging (MRI) can be used to evaluate possible extension of the tumor out of the thyroid into the larynx, mediastinum, or trachea. Iodinated contrast with CT is used in MTC for evaluation of cervical metastases and possible laryngotracheal invasion. Either CT or MRI scanning can be helpful in identifying occult neck metastases or clarifying the magnitude of palpable neck disease. MRI has been found to be useful in distinguishing postoperative cancer from scarring. Ultrasound, the workhorse of thyroid imaging, is critical for distinguishing benign from malignant thyroid nodules, although the reported number of patients evaluated with ultrasound who have MTC is small, making it difficult to determine the role of ultrasound in the screening of this disease.

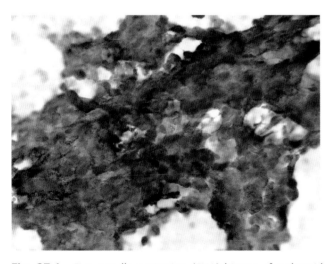

Fig. 37.1   Fine needle aspiration (FNA) biopsy of a thyroid nodule positive for calcitonin staining by immunohistochemistry and diagnostic of medullary thyroid carcinoma. (Image courtesy of David Sauer, MD.)

A chest X-ray can be performed to evaluate for metastatic disease. Patients with advanced-stage disease warrant CT evaluation of the chest to rule out distant metastases. Positron-emission tomography may also be useful in selected clinical settings.

■ Screening for Early Diagnosis of Medullary Thyroid Carcinoma

The parafollicular cells, or C cells, of the thyroid are members of a class of cells referred to as amine precursor uptake and decarboxylation (APUD) cells. C cells produce calcitonin, which has a somewhat imprecise role in calcium homeostasis. MTC has been shown to produce a variety of peptides and biologic amines, along with several other compounds, including prostaglandins, serotonin, substance P, somatostatin, histamine, gastrin-releasing protein, and several other products. Plasma calcitonin levels have been found to be elevated in the majority of MTC cases. This activity of MTC has led to the capability to screen for MTC by blood sampling.

Despite the fact that MTC accounts for well under 1% of thyroid masses, some clinicians have advocated for routine measurements of calcitonin in an effort to identify sporadic MTC. Some caution, however, should be exercised before routine screening of calcitonin is advocated because prevalence figures may not be similar in all areas of the world, and additional study is needed. Nonetheless, at this time, the threshold for performing calcitonin measurements in patients with nodular thyroid disease should decrease. These decisions should be guided by the individual patient and physician. Calcitonin testing should be considered for any patient with atypical malignant cytology noted on FNA.

One significant improvement in the ability to diagnose recurrent MTC has come from screening by provocative testing. Given that elevation of calcitonin levels strongly suggests MTC, measurement of stimulated plasma calcitonin is a sensitive and specific test for screening to detect recurrent or residual MTC following surgery. Pentagastrin, calcium, or a combination of pentagastrin and calcium infusion tests have all been used to detect elevation of calcitonin as detected by radioimmunoassay. The pentagastrin infusion test is performed by a bolus injection of pentagastrin with serum calcitonin measurements before, and 2 and 5 minutes after, injection. An alternative test is by calcium infusion with measurements of serum calcitonin 3 and 10 minutes after infusion of calcium. In general, calcitonin levels above 100 nanograms per liter (ng/L) are highly suggestive of MTC, and surgery is therefore advocated. Reproducibility on two separate tests may be recommended. When serum calcitonin levels of 30 to 100 ng/L are found, the significance is unclear, and further testing, such as repeat stimulation tests or deoxyribonucleic acid testing, may be indicated. Patients who have minimally elevated plasma calcitonin levels following provocative testing may also be candidates for selective venous catheterization, where basal and stimulated plasma calcitonin levels are taken from the inferior thyroid vein. However, routine calcitonin screening is not currently recommended for unselected patients with thyroid nodules given the limited availability of pentagastrin in North America.

Genetic Testing

The most important recent advance in screening and evaluating MTC has been due to the identification of the RET proto-oncogene. The RET gene was discovered in 1985. It has subsequently been shown that MEN2A, MEN2B, and FMTC are caused by germline RET mutations. Up to 25% of MTCs occur in familial patterns, with many of these occurring in the MEN syndromes. So, RET proto-oncogene testing is indicated in all patients with MTC and is ideally completed preoperatively with genetic counseling available. Once a germline RET mutation is identified, genetic testing should be offered to all first-degree relatives.

Without genetic testing, patients with known or suspected MTC should be evaluated for other possible endocrine disorders. In addition to serum calcitonin, serum calcium, albumin, and alkaline phosphatase tests are generally performed. Twenty-four-hour urine catecholamines are obtained to test for possible pheochromocytoma. If these are positive or if pheochromocytoma is suspected, an MRI scan of the adrenal glands would help to identify the tumor. Calcium, phosphate, chloride, and parathyroid hormone levels are measured in the fasting state to assess for parathyroid disease. Other tests can be performed based on the clinical evaluation and the level of suspicion of MEN, as well as specific tests based on the diagnosis of MEN2A or 2B.

■ Summary

MTC is an uncommon cancer of the thyroid gland. The diagnosis of MTC can usually be made by FNA. Most cases of MTC occur in a sporadic fashion, although 20 to 25% occur in the familial disorders FMTC, MEN2A, and MEN2B. Early identification and treatment affect outcome, so screening becomes an important part of evaluation of both sporadic and familial MTC. The discovery of the RET proto-oncogene and the ability to pinpoint mutations allow for a sensitive and specific way to assess risk of disease in families.

■ Practice Guidelines, Consensus Statements, and Measures

The current recommendations for the diagnosis and treatment of MTC are available at the National Comprehensive Cancer Network Web site: National Comprehensive Cancer Network. Thyroid Carcinoma (Version 2.2011). http://www.nccn.org/professionals/physician_gls/f_guidelines.asp#site. Accessed March 1, 2013

■ Suggested Reading

Daniels GH. Screening for medullary thyroid carcinoma with serum calcitonin measurements in patients with thyroid nodules in the United States and Canada. Thyroid 2011;21(11):1199–1207

Enewold L, Zhu K, Ron E, et al. Rising thyroid cancer incidence in the United States by demographic and tumor characteristics, 1980-2005. Cancer Epidemiol Biomarkers Prev 2009;18(3):784–791

Figlioli G, Landi S, Romei C, Elisei R, Gemignani F. Medullary thyroid carcinoma (MTC) and RET proto-oncogene: mutation spectrum in the familial cases and a meta-analysis of studies on the sporadic form. Mutat Res 2013;752(1):36–44

Kloos RT, Eng C, Evans DB, et al; American Thyroid Association Guidelines Task Force. Medullary thyroid cancer: management guidelines of the American Thyroid Association. Thyroid 2009; 19(6):565–612

Komminoth P, Kunz EK, Matias-Guiu X, et al. Analysis of RET proto-oncogene point mutations distinguishes heritable from nonheritable medullary thyroid carcinomas. Cancer 1995;76(3):479–489

Marsh DJ, Learoyd DL, Robinson BG. Medullary thyroid carcinoma: recent advances and management update. Thyroid 1995;5(5): 407–424

Rink T, Truong PN, Schroth HJ, Diener J, Zimny M, Grünwald F. Calculation and validation of a plasma calcitonin limit for early detection of medullary thyroid carcinoma in nodular thyroid disease. Thyroid 2009;19(4):327–332

38 Evaluation and Management of Hyperparathyroidism

■ Introduction

Primary hyperparathyroidism (HPT) results from hyperfunction of one or more parathyroid glands in the absence of an identifiable physiological stimulus. Elevated parathyroid hormone (PTH) secretion results in hypercalcemia. The prevalence is ~ 21 cases per 100,000 person-years and the mean age at diagnosis is between 52 and 56 years. There is a 3:1 female to male preponderance. Solitary parathyroid adenoma is the most common cause of primary HPT, occurring in ~ 85 to 90% of patients. Multiple gland disease accounts for ~ 9 to 14% of patients, which are mostly cases of four-gland hyperplasia but also include double adenomas. In cases of hyperplasia, the chief cell variety is more common than the clear cell. Parathyroid carcinoma is a rare cause of primary HPT, occurring in less than 1% of patients.

Secondary HPT is compensatory hyperfunction of parathyroid tissue due to prolonged hypocalcemia. It may occur in any disease setting in which hypocalcemia exists, including chronic renal failure, chronic vitamin D deficiency or rickets, malabsorption syndromes, and renal tubular acidosis. The parathyroid glands in secondary HPT from CRF demonstrate hyperplasia, pseudoadenomatous hyperplasia or nodular transformation. Renal transplantation may correct secondary hypercalcemia due to CRF. When this does not occur, the term *tertiary* or *pseudohyperparathyroidism* is used to describe a state of autonomous hypersecretion of PTH for which no pathophysiological stimulus can be identified. Patients with tertiary HPT often require parathyroidectomy to relieve symptoms of bone disease.

Pathology

Parathyroid adenomas typically demonstrate a monomorphic proliferation of chief cells within a morphologically enlarged parathyroid gland. A rim of normal parathyroid tissue may be found around the hypercellular portion of the gland. The concentration of stromal fat is useful in distinguishing between hyperfunctional and normal parathyroid tissue in that hypercellular tissue in adenoma or hyperplasia is noted to contain little or no stromal fat as compared with normal parathyroid tissue.

Chief cell hyperplasia may occur in parathyroid glands, often in all four glands and exhibiting nodular hyperplasia. Chief cell hyperplasia represents the pathological entity found in patients with multiple endocrinopathy syndromes (MEN I and II) and in familial (non-MEN) HPT. It is also the predominant lesion found in patients with secondary HPT produced by CRF.

The histological finding in secondary parathyroid hyperplasia is essentially the same as that found in primary disease, with the exception of increased fibrosis and nodularity noted in the former.

The true incidence of parathyroid carcinoma is difficult to accurately assess, primarily because of the difficulty in establishing a histological diagnosis. Grossly, lesions are noted to be hard and fibrous with a grayish-white color, demonstrating adherence to and invasion of surrounding structures (thyroid lobe). Carcinomatous glands demonstrate an inflammatory-like reaction that is characteristic and distinct from benign glandular enlargement. Histological features considered characteristic include a thick fibrous capsule, invasion of the fibrous capsule and vascular elements, with trabeculated regions of cells separated by thick fibrous septa. Mitotic figures, rarely seen in benign disease, are always present. Clinically, a firm palpable mass may be appreciated in the neck preoperatively, a rare finding in benign disease. Total serum calcium levels are usually elevated, in excess of 14 to 15 mg/dL, with markedly elevated levels of serum PTH characteristic (> 300 ng/dL). Malignant disease is more common in males than in females. Death from malignant disease is usually a result of persistent hypercalcemia and associated sequelae. Overall survival is noted to be poor regardless of treatment, with 5- and 10-year survival rates of ~ 50% and 10%, respectively.

■ Evaluation

Most patients with HPT are asymptomatic at presentation, having been diagnosed incidentally through routine blood chemistry testing. In general, however, ~ 50% of asymptomatic patients with primary hyperparathyroidism will become symptomatic within 5 years of its initiation. When present, clinical manifestations are described according to the organ system affected.

Kidney/Urinary Tract

Historically, over 50% of patients with HPT developed nephrolithiasis and/or nephrocalcinosis; this percentage decreased to ~ 4% following the widespread use of routine serum chemistries in the 1970s. Most stones are composed of calcium oxalate; however, calcium phosphate stones may also occur. The symptoms associated with urolithiasis include renal colic, hematuria, and pyuria. Metabolic acidosis may also be a part of the clinical syndrome, as is polyuria. Untreated HPT can result in kidney damage.

Skeletal System

Bone disease from HPT may present as bone and joint pain, pathological fracture, cystic bone changes, or focal areas of bone swelling; the latter can present in the head and neck as epulis of the jaw or "brown" tumors and represent accumulations of osteoclasts, osteoblasts, and fibrous matrix. Abnormalities of the skeletal system in the form of osteitis fibrosis cystica, once a common malady in patients with primary hyperparathyroidism, are now rarely encountered (less than 10% of patients). These changes include subperiosteal erosion of the distal phalanges, bone wasting and softening, chondrocalcinosis, and skull resorption noted as "salt and pepper skull" on imaging. Postmenopausal women with primary hyperparathyroidism exhibiting early signs of osteoporosis appear to be at significant risk for developing more severe bone disease and resultant sequelae (i.e., vertebral and hip fractures. The benefit of parathyroidectomy is most apparent in this population of patients.

Neuromuscular

Muscle weakness, particularly in the proximal extremity muscle groups, progressive fatigue, and malaise may occur. Subtle signs of muscle fatigue and weakness may be present in as many as 40% of patients with mild primary HPT; difficulty climbing the stairs or rising from a seated position are typical complaints.

Neurocognitive and Psychiatric

Primary HPT can result in neurological symptoms from anxiety and depression to frank psychosis. Depression, nervousness, and cognitive dysfunction may commonly occur to varying degrees in primary HPT.

Gastrointestinal

Gastrointestinal disorders that may occur in HPT include peptic ulcer disease and pancreatitis. Peptic ulcer disease occurs due to increased serum gastrin and gastric acid secretion stimulated by hypercalcemia. The colon may also be affected by HPT, with "sluggish bowels" or constipation that improves following surgery and achievement of normocalcemia.

Cardiovascular

Hypertension may occur in as many as 50% of patients with HPT. Definitive evidence of an underlying mechanism is lacking, and parathyroidectomy results in a reduction in blood pressure in only a few of these patients. Other cardiac manifestations include bradycardia, shortened QT interval, and left ventricular hypertrophy.

Hypercalcemic Abnormalities

Patients with calcium levels ≥ 15 mg/dL may present in "hypercalcemic crisis" with depressed mental status or coma. Acute renal failure and lethal dysrhythmias may ensue. Ectopic calcium deposits in various organs, including band keratopathy, skin changes, and pruritus can also occur.

Laboratory Testing

Given that most patients are asymptomatic at the time of diagnosis, laboratory testing remains the primary diagnostic tool in the workup of HPT. The definitive diagnosis of primary HPT depends on the concurrent demonstration of persistently elevated serum calcium together with elevation of circulating PTH. Remember that altered total protein levels will strongly influence measured serum calcium and may, under certain conditions, yield an underestimation of the hypercalcemia. In general, ~ 1 mg/dL of calcium may be added for each gram of total protein lost. It is, therefore, important to assess the status of serum calcium with concurrent measurement of serum albumin, especially where nutritional status is in question or in patients with an underlying metabolic disorder. The most accurate indication of hypercalcemia is measurement of the ionized calcium level. Determination of serum PTH represents the most efficient method of assessing parathyroid function. Because of the variance in both circulating serum calcium and PTH levels, both entities should be assessed concurrently.

In the absence of renal disease, it is important to assess the status of urinary calcium to eliminate the possibility of familial hypocalciuric hypercalcemia (FHH). FHH is an autosomal dominant disorder that represents a rare cause of hypercalcemia (< 1%). The disorder results from a defect yielding increased renal tubular absorption of calcium. Hypercalcemia with depressed 24 hour urinary calcium is the diagnostic hallmark of FHH. Serum PTH may be normal or mildly elevated. Urinary calcium levels in primary HPT are found to be normal or elevated, despite the direct action of PTH on the kidney to influence reabsorption. This is primarily due to the increased calcium burden in the circulation presented to the kidney.

Additional studies should be performed and may prove helpful in establishing the diagnosis and eliminating other causes of hypercalcemia. Albumin, creatinine, magnesium, 25-hydroxy vitamin D, and phosphorus levels should be assessed concurrently with serum calcium and PTH levels. Thyroid function studies should be obtained because of the effect of hyperthyroid conditions on serum calcium.

Imaging Studies

Localization studies are often used for surgical planning and are discussed in the surgical management section later in the chapter. They should not be used for diagnosis because that is done through biochemical studies as already described in the laboratory testing section.

Differential Diagnosis

In distinguishing the hypercalcemia of primary HPT from hypercalcemia due to other etiologies, the foremost cause to be eliminated is malignancy. HPT is the leading cause of hypercalcemia in the outpatient setting, whereas malignancy is the leading cause for inpatients. Primary HPT, together with malignancy, accounts for 90% of patients with hypercalcemia.

Generally, the hypercalcemia of malignancy is acute in onset and rapidly progressive, attaining serum calcium levels in excess of 13 mg/dL over a short period of time. There may be associated hypoproteinemia, anemia, and elevated erythrocyte sedimentation rates. The serum PTH level is usually low or undectable in these patients. PTH-related peptide may be elevated. Sarcoidosis and thiazide diuretic ingestion, as well as FHH, remain in the differential diagnosis of hypercalcemia.

In cases of sarcoidosis, hypercalcemia may be accompanied by hypercalciuria, but serum PTH is depressed because of increased calcium absorption by the gut and normally functioning parathyroids. Thiazide ingestion carries with it a history of medication usage but also demonstrates normal ionized calcium and a normal or depressed serum PTH. A 24-hour urinary calcium level below 100 to 150 mg may distinguish FHH. Other potential diagnoses include milk alkali syndrome, hypervitaminosis D, and hyperthyroidism.

In spite of the problems encountered in reconciling the differential diagnosis, the demonstration of a persistently elevated serum calcium level with a concurrent elevation in PTH level remains the most reliable indicator for the presence of HPT.

■ Management

Surgical therapy remains the mainstay of effective treatment for HPT. Excision of a solitary parathyroid adenoma is all that is required for cure in most cases. In patients with hyperplasia involving all four glands, subtotal parathyroidectomy or total parathyroidectomy with autotransplantation becomes necessary. It is generally accepted that surgery should be offered to patients with symptomatic primary HPT; there remains some debate over ideal management of the asymptomatic patient. Although age should not be an absolute determinant in patient selection, in general, younger patients with potentially longer exposure to hypercalcemia are at a substantially greater risk for developing complications. Surgery in postmenopausal women should be given special consideration; they are at greatest risk for development of long-term skeletal complications from generalized demineralization and osteopenia, such as hip and vertebral fractures.

The National Institutes of Health (NIH) 2nd Workshop on Asymptomatic Primary Hyperparathyroidism in 2002 provided the following guidelines for treatment and indications for surgery:

1. One mg/dL above the upper limit of the reference range for serum calcium
2. Twenty-four-hour urinary calcium > 400 mg/dL
3. A 30% decrease in creatinine clearance
4. Bone mineral density T-score less than − 2.5 at any site
5. Age < 50 years

Observation remains an option but must be vigilant, with serum calcium and creatinine levels checked every 6 months and yearly bone mineral density testing and monitoring for the development of symptoms.

Localization Studies

Localization studies may be separated into (a) those dealing with anatomical imaging of enlarged glands and (b) methods that exploit the physiological properties of hyperfunctional parathyroid tissue. Anatomical identification of parathyroid gland enlargement consists mainly of high resolution ultrasonographic imaging, magnetic resonance imaging (MRI), and computed tomography (CT). Ultrasound imaging has the advantage of being noninvasive, rapid, and reasonably inexpensive, with a sensitivity approaching 80 to 85%. Disadvantages of this technique include the image interference by hollow viscus (trachea, esophagus) and the inability to image the mediastinum. MRI, and to a certain extent CT, provides good to excellent resolution of enlarged tissue, especially in the mediastinum and, in the case of MRI, demonstrates a sensitivity of ~ 85%. Disadvantages include the necessity of contrast material, cost, and decreased resolution in the cervical region in the presence of thyroid nodular abnormalities. Some centers have shown four-dimensional CT to be an excellent localizing tool for parathyroid disease that localizes based on thin cuts and imaging timed for maximum contrast enhancement.

Studies that take advantage of the functional capacity of parathyroid tissue in an effort to identify hyperfunctional glands primarily use technetium 99m sestamibi, an isonitrile radiopharmaceutical of technetium 99m originally developed for nuclear studies of myocardial function. Sestamibi was noted, incidentally, to concentrate in thyroid and abnormally enlarged parathyroid tissue with a differential retention of the radiotracer between these tissues. This has allowed enlarged parathyroid tissue to be accurately imaged following intravenous administration of sestamibi with retention of the tracer in parathyroid adenoma and washout from normal thyroid gland. This method has demonstrated sensitivity for localizing parathyroid adenoma approximating 90 to 95%. It has a distinct advantage in that it images mediastinal parathyroid tissue readily. Further capabilities of sestamibi include application with single-positron emission computed tomography (SPECT) to produce a three-dimensional functional image and the ability to be detected by a handheld radio emission detector intraoperatively.

Embryology and Relevant Anatomy

Surgical exploration of the neck for HPT, regardless of the pathology suspected, requires meticulous dissection, maintenance of a bloodless field, attention to anatomical detail, and, most importantly, a thorough understanding of regional anatomy and embryology.

Parathyroid tissue originates from pharyngeal endoderm formed in the third and fourth pharyngeal pouches. The superior parathyroid glands originate from the fourth pharyngeal pouch and descend into the neck with the thyroid gland. The inferior glands derive from the third pharyngeal pouch and descend with thymic elements over a longer course to eventually rest lower in the neck. This embryological pattern has significant implications for the identification of both normal and ectopic glands during surgical exploration. Ectopic superior glands will often follow a path of descent posteriorly behind the esophagus or carotid sheath into the posterior superior mediastinum. Because of a shared common primordium in the fourth pharyngeal pouch with the thyroid, a missing superior gland may be located within the thyroid parenchyma. These intrathyroidal parathyroid lesions may appear as "cold" thyroid nodules on radioiodine scanning. If a parathyroid lesion is suspected, confirmation can be achieved by FNA and measurement of PTH in the needle washing. True intrathyroidal parathyroids are less than 1% in incidence. Inferior glands tend to follow the course of the thymus into the anterior superior mediastinum, and their ectopic locations are less predictable as a result of a longer pathway of descent during embryonic development.

Procedure

The operation begins with a low transverse incision ~ 2 fingerbreadths above the sternoclavicular notch and spanning the anterior borders of the sternocleidomastoid muscles. The incision can be as short as 2 cm in length. The anterior thyroid surface is accessed after separating the strap muscles. The lateral thyroid border is delineated bluntly, and, following division of the middle thyroid venous tributaries, medial mobilization allows blunt dissection of areolar tissue in the viscerovertebral angle. This permits visualization and/or palpation of enlarged parathyroid tissue with minimal dissection so as to prevent staining of tissues with blood. Depending on the surgical preference, the usual trend is to identify the inferior glands initially. They tend to be larger and more anterior; however, their location is also less constant. Typically, they are found adjacent to the inferior pole of the thyroid gland or within a tongue of thymic tissue inferior to the thyroid. Commonly, they may be located anterior and slightly medial to the juxtaposition of the inferior thyroid artery and recurrent laryngeal nerve.

The superior parathyroid glands are most commonly found along the posterior capsule of the thyroid gland at a point slightly lateral and posterior to the juxtaposition between the recurrent nerve and inferior thyroid artery. Blunt dissection along the posterior capsule will often reveal the superior gland to be suspended in a teardrop fashion within a centimeter of the entrance of the nerve under the cricothyroid muscle.

A thorough search is made to locate the second gland on the same side; if found, it can be biopsied if its identity is questioned. Some surgeons do not advocate proceeding to bilateral neck exploration if a histologically abnormal *and* a normal gland have been identified on the side explored first. It is prudent to eliminate the possibility of enlarged parathyroid tissue on the second side before terminating the procedure. An intraoperative PTH (IOPTH) assay can help with this matter. In general, unless equivocal findings are noted on the normal-appearing gland or should a normal gland not be identified on the first side, histological identification of additional glands is not necessary.

If the second gland is biopsied on the side explored first and is found to be abnormal, or if it appears enlarged, all four glands should be identified and histologically examined. In this instance, the presumptive diagnosis is hyperplasia that will require subtotal (three and a half glands) or total parathyroidectomy with auto transplantation. The distinction between adenoma and hyperplastic parathyroid tissue is difficult or impossible on frozen section analysis; therefore, the surgeon cannot rely on single-gland histological analysis for definitive therapy. Again, IOPTH assay may be helpful in these cases.

Failure to identify a missing gland suspected of being an adenoma or, in the case of hyperplasia, failure to locate all glands, mandates a thorough dissection in an effort to locate ectopic parathyroid tissue. A systematic approach is undertaken to examine all areas potentially harboring an ectopic gland. It is imperative that the surgeon knows which gland is missing with the understanding that a search is predicated on the likely ectopic sites. The surgical dissection should address all areas accessible through a cervical approach, including removal of thymic tissue within the superior mediastinum, examination of the retroesophageal space and carotid sheath to the hyoid bone, and rarely a thyroid lobectomy. Approximately 90% of all parathyroid adenomas are resectable through a transcervical approach, and thus a missing gland is usually harbored in an ectopic location accessible to the surgeon.

In a small percentage of patients, four glands are identified as being normal, indicating the presence of a supernumerary parathyroid gland(s). This is usually an inferior gland and may be located anywhere in the neck or in the mediastinum and frequently is associated with thymic tissue.

Approximately 2 to 5% of parathyroid glands are located in the mediastinum. Surgery for familial HPT (MEN 1 and 2) and tertiary HPT follows the same basic tenet as for routine exploration for primary disease.

Adjunctive Measures in Surgical Management

The introduction of several methods by which serum levels of PTH are rapidly determined intraoperatively has greatly enhanced the ability to assure satisfactory removal of all hyperfunctioning parathyroid tissues. These rapid assessments of serum PTH level may be obtained following removal of all abnormal parathyroid tissue, as judged by the surgeon, and compared with preoperative values while the patient remains on the operating table. Results demonstrating a greater than 50% drop in PTH from the preoperative baseline (and into the normal rage) at 10 minutes postexcision indicate a successful removal of hyperfunctioning tissue. Intraoperative PTH monitoring has allowed surgeons to perform "directed parathyroidectomy" in the appropriate patients; between preoperative localization studies and intraoperative PTH monitoring, a solitary adenoma may be located and removed and the physiological response confirmed without unnecessary additional dissection.

■ Medical Management of Hypercalcemia

Patients who may require medical stabilization of conditions unrelated to HPT prior to definitive surgery or those in whom HPT is secondary to chronic renal failure may need adequate management of symptomatic hypercalcemia. Those patients manifesting symptoms of mental derangement such as confusion, somnolence, or coma, and those in whom the risk of cardiac dysrhythmia is high, should receive aggressive intravenous hydration and diuresis with furosemide.

Patients with elevated serum calcium levels without overt symptoms may be medically followed while surgery is planned or contemplated. Adequate hydration should be encouraged with acceptable levels of exercise and avoidance of immobilization. Hypertension as a result of hypercalcemia should be treated. Administration of oral bisphosphonates is not recommended in that the shift in calcium will result in an increased stimulation of PTH production. PTH blockade (cinacalcet) can also be done and is approved for cases of secondary HPT.

■ Suggested Reading

AACE/AAES Task Force on Primary Hyperparathyroidism. The American Association of Clinical Endocrinologists and the American Association of Endocrine Surgeons position statement on the diagnosis and management of primary hyperparathyroidism. Endocr Pract 2005;11(1):49–54

Biskobing DM. Significance of elevated parathyroid hormone after parathyroidectomy. Endocr Pract 2010;16(1):112–117

Dudney WC, Bodenner D, Stack BC Jr. Parathyroid carcinoma. Otolaryngol Clin North Am 2010;43(2):441–453, xi

Fraker DL, Harsono H, Lewis R. Minimally invasive parathyroidectomy: benefits and requirements of localization, diagnosis, and intraoperative PTH monitoring. long-term results. World J Surg 2009;33(11):2256–2265

Lew JI, Irvin GL III. Focused parathyroidectomy guided by intraoperative parathormone monitoring does not miss multiglandular disease in patients with sporadic primary hyperparathyroidism: a 10-year outcome. Surgery 2009;146(6):1021–1027

NIH conference. Diagnosis and management of asymptomatic primary hyperparathyroidism: consensus development conference statement. Ann Intern Med 1991;114(7):593–597

Ruda JM, Hollenbeak CS, Stack BC Jr. A systematic review of the diagnosis and treatment of primary hyperparathyroidism from 1995 to 2003. Otolaryngol Head Neck Surg 2005;132(3):359–372

Siperstein A, Berber E, Barbosa GF, et al. Predicting the success of limited exploration for primary hyperparathyroidism using ultrasound, sestamibi, and intraoperative parathyroid hormone: analysis of 1158 cases. Ann Surg 2008;248(3):420–428

Stack BC Jr. Minimally Invasive Radioguided Parathyroidectomy (MIRP). Oper Tech Otolaryngol Head Neck Surg 2009;20(1):54–59

Stack BC Jr. Secondary Hyperparathyroidism. British Medical Journal (BMJ) Point of Care: www.pointofcare.bmj.com. https://online.epocrates.com/u/29111107/Secondary+hyperparathyroidism

Stack BC Jr, Moore ER, Belcher RH, Spencer HJ, Bodenner DL. Hormone relationships of parathyroid, gamma counts, and adenoma mass in minimally invasive parathyroidectomy. Otolaryngol Head Neck Surg 2012;147(6):1035–1040

Wermers RA, Khosla S, Atkinson EJ, et al. Incidence of primary hyperparathyroidism in Rochester, Minnesota, 1993-2001: an update on the changing epidemiology of the disease. J Bone Miner Res 2006;21(1):171–177

39 Complications of Endocrine Surgery

Introduction

Thyroidectomy and parathyroidectomy are common procedures performed by otolaryngologist–head and neck surgeons today. In experienced hands, these procedures are safe and reliable. However, despite using proper technique and taking appropriate precautions, complications can and do occur.

This chapter presents some of the more frequently encountered complications of head and neck endocrine surgery, their incidence, and the risk factors associated with them. Preventive strategies are discussed where applicable. In addition, recent years have seen the introduction of novel techniques such as minimally invasive video-assisted thyroidectomy (MIVAT) and robotically assisted thyroidectomy. These methods are also discussed in the context of their associated complication rates.

Influence of Surgeon Experience

It has been demonstrated repeatedly throughout the literature that higher-volume surgeons experience fewer complications during head and neck endocrine surgery. When compared with all other groups (and after controlling for case complexity and patient comorbidities), surgeons performing more than 100 endocrine cases per year have lower complication rates, shorter lengths of stay, and lower overall costs associated with thyroidectomy. Interestingly, however, a 2012 report by Duclos and colleagues found that performance during thyroidectomy also appears to be related to the number of years a given surgeon has been in practice. Though they did not control for the annual volume, they did find that the complication rates during thyroidectomy were highest among surgeons early and late in their careers. The highest-performing subgroup in their report was surgeons between the ages of 35 and 50.

Complications of Thyroid Surgery

Thyroidectomy has been practiced for hundreds of years. Thyroid surgery is considered to be safe and effective in the hands of modern-day surgeons. However, this has not always been the case. Early attempts at extirpation of the thyroid gland were fraught with danger, and mortality rates exceeded 40% as recently as the mid-19th century. Indeed, adverse outcomes became so commonplace during this period that the French Academy of Medicine actually banned thyroidectomy from being performed. However, refinements of surgical hemostasis, general anesthesia, and antiseptic technique led to dramatic improvements in surgical outcomes. These practices were adopted (and in many cases developed) by surgical pioneers such as Billroth and Kocher—leading to major reductions in thyroidectomy-associated mortality. However, it was the next generation of thyroid surgeons who eliminated much of the *morbidity* associated with these procedures. The modern techniques of thyroidectomy may be traced to the practices and teachings of individuals such as William Hallstead, who introduced the idea of parathyroid autotransplantation as a means of preventing postoperative tetany, and Frank Lahey, who first championed the idea of recurrent laryngeal nerve (RLN) preservation through meticulous dissection. Their contributions and those of their successors have further reduced the numbers of complications observed during thyroidectomy. And though the incidence of mortality is essentially negligible in the modern era of thyroid surgery, other adverse events, including hematoma/seroma, hypocalcemia, thyroid storm, superior laryngeal nerve injury, and RLN injury do continue to occur at varying rates. The rate at which these events occur may be related to the experience and expertise of the treating surgeon, the extent and nature of surgery performed, the patient's underlying condition, or any combination of these factors.

■ Hematoma and Seroma

Removal of the thyroid, either partial or complete, requires dissection deep to the strap musculature and the creation of a dead space. This space can be the eventual location of a seroma or hematoma. The rates of these complications are difficult to estimate, though a recent study that included over 3,600 thyroidectomies revealed the rate of hematoma requiring return to the operating room to be 2.1%. This was strongly correlated to advanced age and male gender. Moreover, a recent Cochrane review demonstrated that the use of a surgical drain does not reduce the risk of fluid collection and that it likely prolongs hospitalization after thyroidectomy. Factors that increase the risk of hematoma/seroma include surgery for mediastinal goiter (with or without sternotomy), elevation of subplatysmal flaps during thyroidectomy, elevated systolic blood pressure (> 150 mm Hg) in the recovery room, and cigarette smoking. Most hematomas do not develop until several hours after surgery. This has been a leading argument against same-day discharge after thyroidectomy because the consequences of delayed recognition and treatment can be serious. Though overnight observation will not prevent this complication, it does allow for more rapid detection and intervention, which may reduce the risk of life-threatening airway compromise.

■ Hypocalcemia

One of the most feared complications of thyroidectomy is hypocalcemia/hypoparathyroidism. As already mentioned, the risk of hypocalcemic tetany as a result of thyroidectomy has been recognized for nearly as long as the procedure has been performed. Given the variable definitions and criteria employed in the literature, accurate estimates of the true incidence of thyroidectomy-associated hypoparathyroidism are difficult to ascertain. However, in large current studies, transient hypocalcemia has been observed in ~ 8 to 25% of patients undergoing total thyroidectomy. The rates of permanent hypocalcemia range from 0 to 3% in these reports.

The underlying etiology of hypoparathyroidism after thyroid surgery is not entirely understood. Though inadvertent parathyroidectomy does occur in up to 12% of cases, clinical and biochemical hypoparathyroidism does not necessarily correlate to this occurrence. Inadvertent parathyroidectomy is more likely during extensive surgeries, such as those involving substernal goiter or central compartment lymph node dissection. A more likely cause, however, is devascularization of parathyroid glands left in situ during mobilization of the thyroid or during central neck dissection. Meticulous tissue technique with identification and preservation of the vascular supply of the parathyroid glands is thus advocated during all thyroidectomies and related procedures in the central compartment.

Despite excellent technique and attention to details, postoperative hypoparathyroidism does occur from time to time. It is imperative that this complication be identified early in the postoperative period so that appropriate interventions may be undertaken. Several different strategies have been employed for this purpose. The two most common are measurement of serial calcium levels and measurement of intact parathyroid hormone (iPTH) levels.

Serial calcium measurements are likely the most common means of assessing postoperative parathyroid hormone function. If this protocol is employed, it should be remembered that most serum calcium exists in a nonionized form and is bound to albumin. Consequently, hypoalbuminemia may artificially lower the total serum calcium level. In this circumstance, "corrected calcium" must be determined by the following formula:

$$\text{Corrected Ca} = (0.8 \times [\text{normal albumin} - \text{patient's albumin}]) + \text{serum Ca level}$$

The corrected calcium level is adequate for clinical decision making in most cases. However, ionized calcium may be a more accurate representation of calcium homeostasis—particularly in severe hypocalcemia. Thus, in patients with critically low total serum calcium levels (i.e., less than 7.0 mg/dL), where more rapid and precise correction is required, it may be more appropriate to trend the ionized calcium.

Hypocalcemia may manifest itself clinically in many different ways given the patient's calcium level and medical comorbidities. Most often, it provokes neuromuscular symptoms such as cramping, involuntary twitching, myalgias, and paresthesias. Early signs include a positive Chvostek sign (involuntary facial twitching during percussion over the facial nerve in the preauricular region) or Trousseau sign (elicitation of painful distal forearm spasm during sustained inflation of a sphygmomanometer cuff for 3 minutes). A Trousseau sign is thought to be more sensitive and specific for hypocalcemia than a Chvostek sign. In severe cases, there may be prolongation of the QTc interval, bronchospasm, laryngospasm, altered mental status, and/or tetany.

Given these potentially severe consequences, prompt intervention is vital. It is recommended that patients with serum calcium below 7 mg/dL or symptomatic patients with levels below 8 mg/dL receive intravenous replacement with calcium gluconate. These individuals should also be placed on telemetry for cardiac monitoring. Asymptomatic patients with serum levels above 8 mg/dL may receive oral supplementation with calcium and vitamin D. Several different calcium salts are available for oral replacement therapy. Each contains varying amounts of elemental calcium, and they all have inherent pros and cons associated with them. In general, patients should begin with 1,500 to 3,000 mg of elemental calcium (divided three times daily). They should then be titrated to symptoms and a low-normal serum calcium level.

Many centers are now using parathyroid hormone levels as a means of predicting hypocalcemia and the consequent need for inpatient admission and/or calcium replacement. It has been suggested that patients with iPTH levels ≥ 15 ng/L at 15 minutes post–total thyroidectomy may be safely discharged on the day of surgery without calcium supplementation. These same authors found that preoperative levels < 65 ng/L were also predictive of hypocalcemia. Other iPTH-derived criteria have been used to predict hypocalcemia and safety of same-day discharge after total thyroidectomy. Though the specific criteria, timing of iPTH sample collection, and normal ranges vary from study to study, a consistent theme throughout the literature is that severe hypocalcemia is highly unlikely in the context of a normal postoperative iPTH level.

One preventive measure that bears mentioning is parathyroid autotransplantation. As mentioned earlier, several cases of postoperative hypoparathyroidism are likely attributable to devascularization of parathyroid glands during dissection. For the most part, surgeons rely on their clinical judgment to determine whether a gland is viable. This principally entails a visual inspection of the glands to evaluate both their physical integrity and their color. Intraoperative change from the typical caramel brown/yellow to a more purple/gray hue is thought to indicate trauma to a gland and compromised vascularity. More often than not, this leads the surgeon to perform autotransplantation. Promberger and colleagues have called this practice into question in a recent study. The authors report that discoloration of at least three glands did correlate to a decrease in intraoperative PTH and temporary hypoparathyroidism. However, they also demonstrated that patients undergoing autotransplantation of one discolored gland developed more severe and prolonged hypoparathyroidism than patients in whom the discolored glands were left in situ. All patients in both groups did ultimately regain normal parathyroid function. Other large studies have demonstrated an increase in the frequency and severity of temporary hypoparathyroidism after autotransplantation. However, these have also revealed that autotransplantation is greater than 95% successful in preventing permanent hypoparathyroidism. Though some controversy does exist, it appears clear that any glands found to be inadvertently removed or separated from their dominant blood supply should be autotransplanted with

the expectation that long-term hypoparathyroidism may be avoided in a significant number of patients.

■ Complications Related to Central Compartment Dissection

The role and extent of central compartment dissection during surgery for thyroid carcinoma remains controversial. In the elective setting, this practice is thought to improve locoregional control and treat occult nodal metastases. In the N+ setting, it is aimed at improving locoregional control, biochemical cure rates, and the efficacy of radioiodine therapy. However, the procedure may carry with it an increased risk of complications. Specifically, it is thought that the RLNs and parathyroid glands may be at greater risk when central compartment dissection is added to thyroidectomy or performed as a staged procedure for recurrent disease. In response to these concerns, a meta-analysis was conducted to better evaluate the complications associated with the procedure. After analyzing over 1,100 patients across five studies, the authors reported no increased incidence of permanent hypocalcemia or RLN injury attributable to central compartment dissection. They did identify an increased risk of temporary hypoparathyroidism—with one episode per 7.7 dissections performed. This would suggest that patients undergoing this procedure should be appropriately counseled in the preoperative period and that they might benefit from prophylactic calcium and vitamin D supplementation after surgery.

■ Complications Related to Surgery for Hyperthyroidism

Though patients are more often referred for thyroidectomy in the context of nodular disease, goiter, or malignancy, surgery remains an option for the management of hyperthyroidism as well. Graves disease presents a particular problem in terms of surgical morbidity because hypervascularity is a hallmark—both clinically and sonographically. This could potentially translate to increased blood loss during surgery and increased difficulty in identifying and preserving critical structures such as the RLNs and parathyroid glands. Several strategies have been advocated as means of reducing thyroid vascularity in Graves disease over the years. Perhaps the two most commonly employed are antithyroid medication and Lugol solution. Though large-scale prospective and double-blinded studies are lacking, the available evidence does seem to suggest efficacy for both types of treatment. For Lugol solution, a 10 day preoperative course is recommended because it has been shown to reduce thyroid blood flow and microvessel density. In addition, it results in a ninefold reduction in intraoperative blood loss. Likewise, antithyroid medications such as methimazole and propylthiouracil have been shown to have a similar effect on thyroid gland vascularity and a more pronounced effect on intraoperative blood loss in patients with Graves disease. Moreover, patients who received antithyroid medications for more than 12 months leading up to surgery experienced significantly less blood loss during surgery than did patients with a shorter duration of antithyroid therapy.

More worrisome, perhaps, than intraoperative bleeding is the prospect of thyroid storm. This condition is an acute thyrotoxicosis characterized by severe autonomic dysfunction, hyperthermia, cardiovascular hyperactivity, hepatobiliary, gastrointestinal, and central nervous system disturbances. If a patient is not rendered euthyroid or if appropriate medical prophylaxis is not administered, surgery itself may precipitate thyroid storm. The American Thyroid Association currently recommends that all thyrotoxic patients be rendered euthyroid (via antithyroid medications) prior to surgical intervention for Graves disease. A combination of inorganic iodine solution (such as Lugol iodine) and antithyroid medication may be used to rapidly decrease systemic levels of T_4 and T_3. Corticosteroids may also be administered in situations where surgery needs to be done on an urgent basis. Likewise, perioperative b blockade should be performed in these situations to reduce the risk of cardiovascular complications.

Superior Laryngeal Nerve Injury

Though the RLN receives much attention from surgeons and patients alike with respect to thyroidectomy, injuries to the superior laryngeal nerve (SLN) may also occur during this procedure and can have significant functional consequences. The SLN arises from the vagus nerve at the level of the skull base and descends medial to the carotid sheath before splitting into an internal and external branch at the level of the thyrohyoid membrane. The internal branch enters the thyrohyoid membrane with the superior laryngeal artery and vein, where it provides sensory innervation to the supraglottic larynx. The external branch provides motor neurons to the cricothyroid muscle. Many surgeons do not routinely identify the SLN during thyroidectomy; consequently, the rates of SLN injury are higher than those observed for the RLN. Electromyographic evidence of SLN injury has been observed in up to 58% of patients postthyroid-

ectomy. Dysfunction of the SLN can be subtle both on clinical exam and on laryngoscopy. Adjunct studies such as stroboscopy and electromyography are required for confirmation. These tests are not routinely employed in the postoperative setting; thus the true incidence of thyroidectomy-related injury is largely unknown.

Due to its close proximity to the upper pole of the gland, the nerve is at greatest risk during the ligation and division of the superior thyroid vascular pedicle. In 70 to 80% of cases, the nerve crosses the superior thyroid vessels in a "high-risk" position (i.e., at the level of the upper pole or within 1 cm of it). Careless clamp placement or electrocautery in this region can result in injury to the nerve and may result in clinically relevant dysphonia, dysphagia, and even aspiration.

Recurrent Laryngeal Nerve Injury

RLN injury is perhaps the most dreaded complication of thyroid surgery. RLN injury has immediate and profound effects on both the patient's ability to communicate and the surgeon's self-confidence. It is also the most common reason for thyroidectomy-related malpractice litigation. Unfortunately, over two-thirds of these decisions have historically favored the plaintiff. As a consequence, it is important to understand this potentially devastating complication and the means by which it may be prevented.

Prior to the 1920s, it was dogmatic that if the RLN was seen during surgery, it was almost assuredly injured. This assertion was challenged and ultimately disproven by Frank Lahey, who pioneered the modern-day techniques of RLN identification, dissection, and preservation. Nearly 100 years after Lahey's last thyroidectomy, his RLN injury rate of 1% (covering over 10,000 procedures) remains the benchmark against which all other surgeons are compared. Though 1% is indeed an oft-quoted benchmark in the literature and during patient counseling, it is somewhat difficult to ascertain the true risk of RLN injury from modern-day series for several reasons. Principal among these is the fact that the definition of RLN injury varies between authors. Several authors define RLN injury by the presence of subjective or observed changes in voice. As most otolaryngologists are aware, subjective voice complaints and hoarseness do not necessarily correlate to objective findings on laryngoscopy. Given that a large number of thyroid surgeons do not routinely perform postoperative laryngoscopy, the true incidence of RLN injury may be underestimated. Despite this inherent limitation, the best available evidence suggests that the rate of temporary RLN paresis ranges from ~ 1 to 6%, whereas permanent RLN paralysis occurs in 0.05 to 2.5% of cases. Reoperative thyroid surgery appears to increase the risk of both temporary paresis and permanent paralysis, with incidence rates of up to 10.1% and 8.1%, respectively.

The most significant advance in thyroidectomy technique with respect to risk of iatrogenic RLN injury has been identification and dissection of the nerve. This technique sufficed for nearly 80 years, but recent years have seen the introduction of RLN monitoring devices to the operating room. These devices can provide the surgeon with real-time feedback regarding the identity and integrity of the RLN. The most commonly used commercially available device employs electrodes coupled to an endotracheal tube. These electrodes record surface potentials from the vocalis muscles on a continuous basis. Shifts in the baseline electromyographic activity may be indicative of nerve injury. Likewise, electrical stimulation of the nerve may be used to confirm integrity (provided that an evoked suprathreshold response is observed on the monitor). Statistically, it has been shown that the sensitivity and specificity of RLN monitoring for the detection of permanent paralysis are 85.7 and 97.3%, respectively. Positive and negative predictive values range from 23.7 to 40% and 99.8 to 100%, respectively.

Advocates of nerve monitoring argue that the technique facilitates nerve identification and thus preservation. It also allows for confirmation of electrical integrity and planning for second-side surgery during difficult dissections. Additionally, it may be a valuable teaching tool for resident trainees. Detractors cite the costs, the potential for nerve fatigue after use of the electrical stimulator, and the potential for disregarding anatomy in favor of a technology that has limitations of sensitivity and specificity. The available literature unfortunately does not provide any definitive conclusions regarding routine use of nerve monitoring during thyroid surgery. To date, only one large study comparing thyroidectomy with and without nerve monitoring has been able to demonstrate a statistically significant difference in the rates of RLN paresis. In this study of over 7,100 nerves at risk, the use of monitoring resulted in a 33% reduction in the rate of temporary paresis and a 50% reduction in the rate of permanent paresis. A subsequent meta-analysis published in 2011 considered nearly 65,000 nerves at risk and found no statistically significant differences in RLN paresis between cases in which nerve monitoring was or was not used. As a consequence, the use of nerve monitors during thyroidectomy continues to be controversial and at present cannot be considered "standard of care" for these procedures.

◼ Complications Related to Emerging Minimally Invasive Techniques

The last decade has seen a shift across nearly all disciplines toward minimally invasive surgery. Minimally invasive procedures use smaller and more cosmetically appealing incisions that are often placed at great distances from the ultimate surgical site. Advances in fiberoptic endoscopy, computer software, hemostatic devices, and miniaturization of surgical instruments have enabled this shift toward "incisionless" surgery. Despite these advances, much of the popularity of minimally invasive surgical approaches remains largely patient driven, and controversy exists regarding the potential risks, benefits, and costs of the associated techniques and technologies.

Minimally invasive video-assisted thyroidectomy (MIVAT) (and parathyroidectomy) has become a commonly employed alternative to traditional open thyroidectomy/parathyroidectomy. This procedure involves placement of a small (1.5 cm) incision in the central neck and removal of the thyroid using blunt dissection and harmonic scalpel technique under endoscopic visualization. Miccoli and colleagues, who developed MIVAT in Italy in the late 1990s, report complication rates that are consistent with those observed after traditional open thyroidectomy. In their 2008 series of over 1,300 patients, they reported a 0.15% rate of bilateral RLN paralysis; unilateral temporary and permanent RLN paralysis rates of 2.65 and 1.13%, respectively; a 2.72% rate of permanent hypoparathyroidism; and wound-related complications occurring in less than 0.005% of patients.

As a means of further reducing scar visibility, transaxillary approaches to the thyroid and parathyroid glands have also been employed. This technique has been successfully accomplished using gasless endoscopic and robotic technologies. A facelift-type robotic approach has also been described. Standard metrics such as RLN paralysis, hypoparathyroidism, and wound complications are similar to those experienced after traditional open thyroid/parathyroid surgery or the MIVAT approach. The transaxillary robotic approach has the disadvantage of potentially putting the brachial plexus at risk during positioning and dissection. It has been reported that brachial plexopathy may be observed in up to 0.3% of these cases. A patient with a short neck and elevated body mass index may be at increased risk for this complication. Though both the MIVAT and the robotic approaches to the thyroid and parathyroid glands are still relatively novel, they appear to be at least as safe as open thyroidectomy in experienced hands. Additional clinical experience and honest and accurate reporting of complications are required before definitive statements can be made regarding their widespread applicability, safety, and efficacy.

■ Complications of Parathyroidectomy

Much of this chapter has been devoted to a discussion of thyroidectomy and its potential complications. Owing to the fact that there is, to the author's knowledge, no body of literature specifically addressing issues such as bleeding, SLN and RLN injury, and risks associated with minimally invasive techniques during parathyroidectomy, the thyroidectomy data must unfortunately be extrapolated. The presumption that the rates of these complications are similar for these two procedures may be somewhat flawed due to the fact that most modern parathyroidectomy techniques entail significantly less dissection than do thyroidectomies. This is particularly true in an era where four-gland exploration is no longer commonplace and minimally invasive and directed parathyroidectomy has become the norm. However, a recent report by Untch et al indicates that right superior parathyroid adenomas are significantly closer to the RLN nerve and are more likely to physically abut the nerve than adenomas in other positions. In their study, the right upper pole adenomas were in contact with the RLN in nearly 50% of cases. The implications of this on parathyroidectomy technique are yet to be determined, though it does seem to suggest that increased vigilance may be required with respect to the RLN if preoperative imaging suggests a right superior adenoma.

■ Metabolic Complications and Sequelae of Parathyroidectomy

Perhaps more common than SLN/RLN injury and wound complications are issues related to postoperative calcium homeostasis. The two principal scenarios of concern are persistent hypercalcemia/hyperparathyroidism and postresection hypocalcemia.

The main potential risk associated with the minimally invasive approach to parathyroid disease is the risk of a negative neck exploration (i.e., a "missed" adenoma). The risk of "missing" a second (or third) adenoma also exists. Though the vast majority of cases of hyperparathyroidism are due to a single adenoma (over 90% in most series), double adenomas occur in ~ 2 to 4% of patients. Preoperative sestamibi scanning allows for unilateral/focused neck exploration and significantly reduces the risk of missed adenomas. This study has a sensitivity of 73

to 100% for single or multiple adenomas. The addition of preoperative surgeon-performed ultrasound has been shown to improve the detection and localization of adenomas as well.

Despite these methods, adenomas still may not be detected or localized preoperatively, and intraoperative adjuncts may be needed. Intraoperative iPTH assays, methylene blue injections, and radioguidance have all been used to localize parathyroid glands during surgery. iPTH has a half-life of ~ 5 minutes and is helpful in confirming successful adenoma removal. Intraoperative iPTH assays allow for the assessment of biochemical response to surgery in a rapid and relatively inexpensive fashion. However, with respect to complications, use of iPTH has been shown to reduce the number of reoperations, shorten the surgical time, and minimize the extent of dissection during minimally invasive parathyroidectomy.

Owing to its selective staining of parathyroid tissue, intravenous methylene blue has long been used for adjunct identification and localization of the glands. However, methylene blue may result in factitious lowering of pulse oximetry after injection, and the anesthesia team must be made aware of its use. Methylene blue has also recently been shown to inhibit monoamine oxidase (MAO). This places patients at risk of the serotonin syndrome if they are concurrently taking selective serotonin reuptake inhibitors (SSRIs), serotonin/norepinephrine reuptake inhibitors (SNRIs), or tricyclic antidepressants (TCAs). The serotonin syndrome is characterized by diffuse and often severe encephalopathy. To prevent this occurrence, it is recommended that methylene blue be avoided in patients taking SSRIs, SNRIs, TCAs, or other drugs that increase central serotonin levels. It is also recommended that there be a washout period of at least 5 weeks prior to the use of methylene blue in patients who have recently discontinued use of these medications.

Similar to methylene blue, intravenous sestamibi has an affinity for parathyroid tissue. As noted earlier, this property has improved preoperative localization and has likely reduced the morbidity and length of parathyroid surgery. Concentration of sestamibi within parathyroid tissue has also allowed for intraoperative identification of the glands using handheld gamma probes.

Although persistent hypercalcemia is of great concern to the parathyroid surgeon, there is also a risk of hypocalcemia after this procedure. In patients with primary hyperparathyroidism, postoperative hypocalcemia occurs in 47% of patients and is typically mild and of short duration. The risk and severity may be increased if the postoperative reduction in iPTH exceeds 85%. Patients undergoing subtotal parathyroidectomy for secondary hyperparathyroidism/hyperplasia experience postoperative hypocalcemia in 97% of cases. This is typically more severe (mean postoperative calcium levels less than 8 mg/dL) and long lasting (mean duration of nearly 5 days) than what is observed in patients with single or double adenomas.

Given the low risk of severe or symptomatic hypocalcemia after removal of single or double adenomas, same-day discharge after surgery is thought to be safe and cost-effective. Vasher and colleagues presented a series of 6,000 outpatient parathyroidectomies and found that hypocalcemia was rare and that symptoms almost never developed before postoperative day 2. The authors indicate that the risk of postoperative hypocalcemia increases concordantly with the preoperative calcium level. Patients with preoperative calcium levels below 11.5 mg/dL had less than a 5% risk of developing hypocalcemia, whereas those with preoperative levels of 13 mg/dL had a 33% risk. Based on the elevated risk associated with preoperative hypercalcemia, bone density T-score below − 3, morbid obesity, and removal of more than one gland, the authors suggest a sliding scale of calcium replacement that all but eliminates symptoms of hypocalcemia in the parathyroidectomy population and facilitates same-day discharge. They recommend that all patients undergoing parathyroidectomy be placed on calcium replacement beginning 3 hours after surgery.

Severe cases of postoperative hypocalcemia may be associated with the so-called hungry bone syndrome. This complication is seen in up to 12.6% of parathyroidectomies and is a metabolic response to rapid declines in serum PTH. The sudden drop in PTH levels leads to rapid bone remineralization and results in severe and prolonged hypocalcemia in some patients. Risk factors for hungry bone syndrome include severely elevated preoperative blood urea nitrogen (BUN), calcium and alkaline phosphatase levels, PTH levels > 96, and age > 61. Preoperative bisphosphonate therapy has been advocated as a potential strategy to prevent hungry bone syndrome, though controlled trials have not yet been performed.

One final complication of parathyroidectomy that pertains to calcium homeostasis is pseudogout. Rapid reductions in serum calcium levels—as may be seen after parathyroidectomy—may lead to shedding of calcium pyrophosphate crystals from the articular cartilage to the synovial fluid. These deposits lead to painful joint swelling—most commonly in the knee. This complication is typically observed in the first few days postoperatively and is recognized based on clinical and radiographic signs and symptoms. Definitive diagnosis requires needle aspiration of the affected joint. Treatment generally includes anti-inflammatory medications such as NSAIDs.

■ Summary

Thyroid and parathyroid surgery are safe and effective in the vast majority of patients. However, complications can and do occur, even in the most experienced of hands. Knowledge of these complications, their incidence, risk factors, preventive measures, and management strategies will undoubtedly help the head and neck endocrine surgeon to provide safer and more effective care to their patients.

■ Suggested Reading

Bahn Chair RS, Burch HB, Cooper DS, et al; American Thyroid Association; American Association of Clinical Endocrinologists. Hyperthyroidism and other causes of thyrotoxicosis: management guidelines of the American Thyroid Association and American Association of Clinical Endocrinologists. Thyroid 2011;21(6):593–646

Barczyński M, Konturek A, Stopa M, Honowska A, Nowak W. Randomized controlled trial of visualization versus neuromonitoring of the external branch of the superior laryngeal nerve during thyroidectomy. World J Surg 2012;36(6):1340–1347

Bergenfelz A, Jansson S, Kristoffersson A, et al. Complications to thyroid surgery: results as reported in a database from a multicenter audit comprising 3,660 patients. Langenbecks Arch Surg 2008;393(5):667–673

Byrnes MC, Huynh K, Helmer SD, Stevens C, Dort JM, Smith RS. A comparison of corrected serum calcium levels to ionized calcium levels among critically ill surgical patients. Am J Surg 2005;189(3):310–314

Cavicchi O, Piccin O, Caliceti U, De Cataldis A, Pasquali R, Ceroni AR. Transient hypoparathyroidism following thyroidectomy: a prospective study and multivariate analysis of 604 consecutive patients. Otolaryngol Head Neck Surg 2007;137(4):654–658

Cernea CR, Brandão LG, Hojaij FC, et al. Negative and positive predictive values of nerve monitoring in thyroidectomy. Head Neck 2012;34(2):175–179

Crea N, Pata G, Casella C, Cappelli C, Salerni B. Predictive factors for postoperative severe hypocalcaemia after parathyroidectomy for primary hyperparathyroidism. Am Surg 2012;78(3):352–358

Duclos A, Peix JL, Colin C, et al; CATHY Study Group. Influence of experience on performance of individual surgeons in thyroid surgery: prospective cross sectional multicentre study. BMJ 2012;344:d8041

Erbil Y, Barbaros U, Ozbey N, Aral F, Ozarmağan S. Risk factors of incidental parathyroidectomy after thyroidectomy for benign thyroid disorders. Int J Surg 2009;7(1):58–61

Erbil Y, Ozluk Y, Giriş M, et al. Effect of lugol solution on thyroid gland blood flow and microvessel density in the patients with Graves' disease. J Clin Endocrinol Metab 2007;92(6):2182–2189

Godballe C, Madsen AR, Pedersen HB, et al. Post-thyroidectomy hemorrhage: a national study of patients treated at the Danish departments of ENT Head and Neck Surgery. Eur Arch Otorhinolaryngol 2009;266(12):1945–1952

Grodski S, Serpell J. Evidence for the role of perioperative PTH measurement after total thyroidectomy as a predictor of hypocalcemia. World J Surg 2008;32(7):1367–1373

Gurevich Y, Poretsky L. Possible prevention of hungry bone syndrome following parathyroidectomy by preoperative use of pamidronate. Otolaryngol Head Neck Surg 2008;138(3):403–404

Higgins TS, Gupta R, Ketcham AS, Sataloff RT, Wadsworth JT, Sinacori JT. Recurrent laryngeal nerve monitoring versus identification alone on post-thyroidectomy true vocal fold palsy: a meta-analysis. Laryngoscope 2011;121(5):1009–1017

Huang SM. Do we overtreat post-thyroidectomy hypocalcemia? World J Surg 2012;36(7):1503–1508

Lee HS, Lee BJ, Kim SW, et al. Patterns of post-thyroidectomy hemorrhage. Clin Exp Otorhinolaryngol 2009;2(2):72–77

Luginbuhl A, Schwartz DM, Sestokas AK, Cognetti D, Pribitkin E. Detection of evolving injury to the brachial plexus during transaxillary robotic thyroidectomy. Laryngoscope 2012;122(1):110–115

Miccoli P, Berti P, Ambrosini CE. Perspectives and lessons learned after a decade of minimally invasive video-assisted thyroidectomy. ORL J Otorhinolaryngol Relat Spec 2008;70(5):282–286

Miller MC, Spiegel JR. Identification and monitoring of the recurrent laryngeal nerve during thyroidectomy. Surg Oncol Clin N Am 2008;17(1):121–144, viii–ix

Mitra I, Nichani JR, Yap B, Homer JJ. Effect of central compartment neck dissection on hypocalcaemia incidence after total thyroidectomy for carcinoma. J Laryngol Otol 2011;125(5):497–501

Morton RP, Mak V, Moss D, Ahmad Z, Sevao J. Risk of bleeding after thyroid surgery: matched pairs analysis. J Laryngol Otol 2012;126(3):285–288

Nagar S, Reid D, Czako P, Long G, Shanley C. Outcomes analysis of intraoperative adjuncts during minimally invasive parathyroidectomy for primary hyperparathyroidism. Am J Surg 2012;203(2):177–181

Pollack G, Pollack A, Delfiner J, Fernandez J. Parathyroid surgery and methylene blue: a review with guidelines for safe intraoperative use. Laryngoscope 2009;119(10):1941–1946

Promberger R, Ott J, Kober F, et al. Intra- and postoperative parathyroid hormone-kinetics do not advocate for autotransplantation of discolored parathyroid glands during thyroidectomy. Thyroid 2010;20(12):1371–1375

Randolph GW, Dralle H, Abdullah H, et al; International Intraoperative Monitoring Study Group. Electrophysiologic recurrent laryngeal nerve monitoring during thyroid and parathyroid surgery: international standards guideline statement. Laryngoscope 2011;121(Suppl 1):S1–S16

Rosato L, Avenia N, Bernante P, et al. Complications of thyroid surgery: analysis of a multicentric study on 14,934 patients operated on in Italy over 5 years. World J Surg 2004;28(3):271–276

Samraj K, Gurusamy KS. Wound drains following thyroid surgery. Cochrane Database Syst Rev 2007;4(4):CD006099

Sheahan P, O'Connor A, Murphy MS. Comparison of incidence of postoperative seroma between flapless and conventional techniques for thyroidectomy: a case-control study. Clin Otolaryngol 2012;37(2):130–135

Shindo M, Wu JC, Park EE, Tanzella F. The importance of central compartment elective lymph node excision in the staging and treatment of papillary thyroid cancer. Arch Otolaryngol Head Neck Surg 2006;132(6):650–654

So YK, Seo MY, Son YI. Prophylactic central lymph node dissection for clinically node-negative papillary thyroid microcarcinoma: influence on serum thyroglobulin level, recurrence rate, and postoperative complications. Surgery 2012;151(2):192–198

Stavrakis AI, Ituarte PH, Ko CY, Yeh MW. Surgeon volume as a predictor of outcomes in inpatient and outpatient endocrine surgery. Surgery 2007;142(6):887–899, discussion 887–899

Terris DJ, Singer MC. Qualitative and quantitative differences between 2 robotic thyroidectomy techniques. Otolaryngol Head Neck Surg 2012;147(1):20–25

Testini M, Gurrado A, Avenia N, et al. Does mediastinal extension of the goiter increase morbidity of total thyroidectomy? A multicenter study of 19,662 patients. Ann Surg Oncol 2011;18(8):2251–2259

Testini M, Rosato L, Avenia N, et al. The impact of single parathyroid gland autotransplantation during thyroid surgery on postoperative hypoparathyroidism: a multicenter study. Transplant Proc 2007;39(1):225–230

Tomoda C, Hirokawa Y, Uruno T, et al. Sensitivity and specificity of intraoperative recurrent laryngeal nerve stimulation test for predicting vocal cord palsy after thyroid surgery. World J Surg 2006;30(7):1230–1233

Untch BR, Adam MA, Danko ME, et al. Tumor proximity to the recurrent laryngeal nerve in patients with primary hyperparathyroidism undergoing parathyroidectomy. Ann Surg Oncol 2012;19(12):3823–3826

Vaiman M, Nagibin A, Hagag P, Kessler A, Gavriel H. Hypothyroidism following partial thyroidectomy. Otolaryngol Head Neck Surg 2008;138(1):98–100

Vasher M, Goodman A, Politz D, Norman J. Postoperative calcium requirements in 6,000 patients undergoing outpatient parathyroidectomy: easily avoiding symptomatic hypocalcemia. J Am Coll Surg 2010;211(1):49–54

Verloop H, Louwerens M, Schoones JW, Kievit J, Smit JW, Dekkers OM. Risk of hypothyroidism following hemithyroidectomy: systematic review and meta-analysis of prognostic studies. J Clin Endocrinol Metab 2012;97(7):2243–2255

Walker Harris V, Jan De Beur S. Postoperative hypoparathyroidism: medical and surgical therapeutic options. Thyroid 2009;19(9):967–973

40 General Concepts in Free Flap Reconstruction

■ Introduction

Since the mid-1980s, microvascular free tissue transfer has become a standard in the armamentarium for head and neck reconstructive surgery. It offers significant advantages over traditional methods of reconstruction, such as primary closure or pedicled rotational flaps. Although regional flaps are still useful in head and neck reconstruction, they may not be appropriate for every defect because of the limited quantity or type of tissue that is available and the limited arc of rotation of the pedicle.

Advantages of Microvascular Free Flaps

The main advantage offered by microvascular free flaps is that head and neck defects can be custom fitted with tissue of appropriate size and composition to achieve restoration of function and aesthetics in a single stage. When performed by experienced head and neck microvascular reconstructive surgeons, success rates > 95% can be expected. Free flaps also eliminate the problem of limited arc of rotation, which minimizes problems with wound dehiscence and plate exposure that frequently result from gravitational pull of a pedicled flap. Furthermore, the morbidity and deformities associated with local and regional flaps, such as shoulder dysfunction and breast distortion, can be avoided. Coverage of defects with well-perfused tissue from successfully revascularized free flaps (1) improves primary wound healing, especially when the vascularity in the recipient bed is compromised by previous irradiation or trauma, and (2) protects against radionecrosis and injury to vital underlying structures that can result from postoperative radiotherapy.

Disadvantages of Microvascular Free Flaps

Although free tissue transfer offers many advantages for reconstruction of large, complex head and neck defects, it has some disadvantages. The major disadvantages are the complexity of the technique, requiring the expertise of a head and neck microvascular reconstructive surgeon, and prolonged anesthetic time. Although the operative time for head and neck cancer ablation and primary reconstruction with free flaps is longer by an average of 4 hours compared with reconstruction with pectoralis myocutaneous flaps, the length of hospitalization and incidence of medical complications are similar. With many of the free flaps (i.e., fibula, iliac crest, radial forearm, lateral arm, anterolateral thigh, lateral thigh, rectus, and jejunum), the graft can be harvested at the same time of recipient-site surgery to reduce operative time. With this simultaneous two-team approach, the operative time is not significantly longer than when pedicled flaps that require repositioning are used, such as trapezius and latissimus dorsi flaps.

Recent Advancement in Head and Neck Reconstruction

A recent advancement in head and neck reconstruction since the introduction of free flaps is the capability to restore sensation to the skin lining of the defect. This is achieved by harvesting a neurofasciocutaneous flap (a cutaneous paddle with a sensory nerve that innervates that skin territory), and performing microneural anastomosis between that nerve and a recipient sensory nerve, such as lingual, superior laryngeal, or glossopharyngeal. The afferent sensory input from the reinnervated skin may not always have the same cortical representation as that from the site of the defect; however, this may be achieved over time with training. Although sensory reinnervation has added a new dimension to head and neck reconstruction, the question of whether it truly improves or expedites functional rehabilitation still needs to be answered.

■ Donor Sites

Fibula Flap

The fibula flap is the workhorse of osteocutaneous flaps and mandibular reconstruction, with the skin paddle centered over the lateral aspect of the leg. It is supplied by the peroneal artery and two accompanying veins. The vascular anatomy of the leg must be assessed preoperatively with dye injection angiography, magnetic resonance angiography, or computed tomographic angiography. The flap should not be used if any of the three vessels supplying the lower extremity is not patent to the ankle. Up to 22 cm of bone can be attained, along with large areas of thin, pliable skin if perforators exist to the skin. The advantages include easy harvest, large-caliber vessels, and ability to work with two teams. The main disadvantage of this flap is the tenuous blood supply to the skin paddle. A sensory nerve can be harvested with the skin for sensory reinnervation.

Iliac Crest Flap

The iliac crest flap was originally described as an osseous or osteocutaneous flap and was later modified to include the internal oblique muscle (osseomyocutaneous flap). As an osseomyocutaneous flap, the two soft tissue components—skin and muscle—can be independently used to resurface two different sites, such as the floor of the mouth and the lower cheek. The flap is supplied by the deep circumflex iliac artery and accompanying veins. It is very bulky, which can be an advantage or a disadvantage, depending on the type of defect. However, the skin is not very pliable. Disadvantages of the flap include the postoperative pain, loss of sensation to the lateral thigh, and a significant risk of hernia development.

Scapula Flap

The scapula flap is an osteocutaneous flap based on the circumflex scapula artery and vein. A unique feature of this flap is the ability to harvest two independent skin paddles with the bone based on a single

vascular pedicle. Another advantage is the flap's large-caliber vessels. Major disadvantages are inability to simultaneously harvest, the need to reposition the patient into a lateral decubitus position during the case, and postoperative shoulder dysfunction.

Radial Forearm Flap

The radial forearm flap can be harvested as an osteocutaneous free flap, providing up to 10 cm of radial bone for mandibular reconstruction. It is often used for lateral mandibular defects, but some have used it in anterior composite defects. It carries a risk of radial bone fracture so the remaining radial bone is typically plated to help prevent future fractures. Other major disadvantages are the inability to implant the radial bone and the limited bone stock available.

Myocutaneous Flaps

Rectus Flap

The rectus flap is historically one of the workhorse soft tissue flaps because it is easy to harvest and is reliable. However, it has largely been replaced by the popular anterolateral thigh flap. The rectus flap's dominant blood supply is the inferior epigastric artery. The skin paddle can be designed transversely, vertically, or obliquely, which makes it very versatile for three-dimensional complex reconstruction. The main disadvantage is that it can be quite bulky in some individuals. Previous abdominal and pelvic surgery, the presence of inguinal hernia, and obesity are contraindications to the use of this flap. Development of abdominal or inguinal hernia is a potential complication.

Latissimus Dorsi Flap

The latissimus flap is the flap of choice when a skin paddle with a large surface is required. The blood supply to this flap is the thoracodorsal artery. Disadvantages include the need for lateral decubitus positioning, the inability to simultaneously harvest, and postoperative shoulder dysfunction, which is generally limited to extreme flexion and extension, thus affecting such activities as swimming and cross-country skiing.

Gracilis Flap

The gracilis flap is primarily used for facial reanimation. It is based on a muscular perforator from the profunda femoris artery. The obturator nerve is harvested with the muscle for neural reinnervation.

Fasciocutaneous Flaps

Radial Forearm Flap

The radial forearm flap is one of the most common fasciocutaneous flaps in head and neck surgery. It is a thin, pliable, versatile, and robust flap that is easy to harvest. A large surface area of skin, up to 120 cm², can be harvested. A major advantage of this flap is the availability of a very long pedicle, which is ideal when the ipsilateral neck is void of recipient vessels resulting from previous radical neck dissection or extensive gunshot blast injury. Unique to this flap is its venous drainage, which occurs through two systems: (1) the superficial system via the cephalic vein, and (2) the deep system via the venae comitantes that accompany the radial artery. Either or both systems can be used, allowing flexibility of venous drainage and size matches for the recipient veins.

An Allen test must be performed to assess the contribution of the radial artery to the blood supply of the hand to ensure viability of the hand after harvesting the radial artery. In addition, the arm should be protected from any venipuncture prior to surgery. This flap can also be harvested as a neurofasciocutaneous flap for sensory reinnervation. The forearm defect is usually covered with a split- or full-thickness skin graft, although a bilobed rotational flap may also be used for primary closure of the donor site. Potential major complications associated with the radial forearm flap are hand ischemia and tendon exposure. The major disadvantage with this flap is the unappealing scar at the donor site.

Lateral Arm Flap

The lateral arm flap is a moderately thick flap that is useful for reconstruction of small- to medium-size defects. It is based on the posterior radial collateral artery. Advantages of this flap over the radial forearm flap are (1) the donor site is closed, primarily leaving only a linear scar along the posterolateral aspect of the upper arm, and (2) the flap has more subcutaneous fat than the radial forearm flap, which may be preferred in some situations. A vascularized nerve graft may be harvested along with the flap for facial nerve reconstruction. The disadvantages of this flap include small-caliber vessels and a limited quantity of available skin. The flap can also be made sensate.

Anterolateral Thigh Flap

The blood supply to the anterolateral thigh flap is based on the descending branch of the lateral circumflex femoral artery and can be harvested as a fasciocutaneous or myocutaneous flap depending on the location of the perforators. The flap has become one of the workhorses in soft tissue head and neck reconstruction and has supplanted the lateral thigh flap. It has more subcutaneous fat than the radial forearm flap, and it can be harvested with or without a large portion of the vastus lateralis muscle. Because a large area of skin can be harvested, the anterolateral thigh flap is an excellent choice for defects requiring a flap with a large surface area and some bulk. The donor site is closed primarily, leaving only a linear scar along the anterolateral aspect of the thigh.

Scapula Flap

The vascular anatomy of the scapula flap is similar to that of the osseous flap. Two skin paddles can be harvested based on a single pedicle. Additionally, the latissimus system can be included on this pedicle, allowing a significant amount of versatility and tissue if needed. The scapula flap is the only fasciocutaneous flap that does not have the potential for sensory reinnervation.

■ Specific Applications

The most common application of free tissue transfer in the head and neck region is oromandibular reconstruction. Other applications include reconstruction of pharyngoesophageal defects, large cranial and skull base defects, massive facial soft tissue defects, orbitomaxillary defects, facial soft tissue augmentation, and facial reanimation (**Table 40.1**).

Oromandibular Reconstruction

The absolute indication for using an osteocutaneous free flap in mandibular reconstruction is an anterior arch defect. Other indications are significant mandibular defects, associated extensive soft tissue defects, and the presence of osteoradionecrosis. Lateral defects can be reconstructed with bone if dentate or with a plate and soft tissue flap if edentulous. Appropriate flap selection is important to achieve optimal functional and aesthetic results. The requirements at the recipient site as well as donor site availability should dictate the selection.

Fibula Flap

The fibula flap is the most popular osseous flap because of ease of harvesting, large-caliber vessels, and large amount of bone stock. It can be used to reconstruct defects involving any portion of or

Table 40.1 Microvascular flaps

Flap	Bone	Advantages	Disadvantages	Applications
Fibula	Yes	– Large bone stock – Dental implants possible – Thin skin paddle – Long pedicle	– Prone to atherosclerosis – Skin paddle less reliable then other flaps – Not good for large-volume defects – Risk of foot ischemia	– Mandible – Midface
Iliac crest	Yes	– Large bone stock – Dental implants possible – Large amount soft tissue and skin	– Small vessels – Significant hernia risk – Skin/soft tissue bulky and not flexible	– Mandible – Midface – Orbit
Scapula	Yes	– Two skin paddles with or without bone – Lastissimus system can be employed on same vessels – Large amount of bone – Generally free of atherosclerosis	– Bone usually not implantable – Unable to harvest simultaneously with two teams – Shoulder dysfunction	– Oral cavity with internal and external paddles – Midface
Radial forearm	Yes	– Thin pliable skin with bone – Often a good alternative when patient not a good fibula candidate	– Short bone stock – Risk of radial fracture – Bone not implantable	– Tongue, floor of mouth, oropharynx, pharynx, esophagus – Mandible – Skull base/dural reconstruction
Latissimus	No	– Large amount of skin/muscle – Long pedicle – Can be harvested with scapula on one pedicle	– Requires lateral positioning – Two-team harvesting not possible – Shoulder dysfunction	– Large soft tissue defects (scalp, neck)
Rectus	No	– Large amount of skin, subcutaneous fat, and muscle – Easy to harvest	– Hernia risk	– Skull base defects – Total glossectomy
Gracilis	No	– Thin – Ideal for facial reanimation	– Not always successful – Requires multiple surgeries for reanimation	– Facial reanimation
Radial forearm	Yes	– Large amount of thin, pliable tissue – Long pedicle with versatile venous drainage options	– Unappealing scar on arm – Risk of tendon exposure and hand ischemia	– Tongue, floor of mouth, oropharynx, pharynx, esophagus – Mandible – Skull base/dural reconstruction
Lateral arm	No	– Favorable donor site with good cosmesis – More fat then many flaps – Good color match for facial defects	– Small-caliber vessels – Risk to radial nerve	– Parotid with or without facial nerve grafts – Tongue, base of tongue, pharynx
Anterolateral thigh	No	– Large amount of skin and fat – Muscle optional depending on location of perforators – Favorable donor site	– Variable vascular anatomy	– Large soft tissue defects – Total glossectomy – Laryngopharyngeal defects

near-total mandibular defects. Up to 22 cm can be harvested and osteotomized to achieve the desired contour. It is the preferred flap for composite defects with mild to moderate soft tissue loss, particularly losses resulting from floor-of-mouth and partial glossectomy resections. The thin cutaneous paddle is ideal for coverage of the bone and for re-creating the floor of the mouth and labial sulci. Similarly, with composite tonsillar defects, the skin paddle of the fibula flap can be used to reconstruct the pharyngeal and soft palate defects.

Iliac Crest or Scapula Flap

The iliac crest flap can also be used in this situation, though it may be too bulky if the soft tissue defect is small. If one chooses to use the iliac crest flap, the bulkiness can be minimized by using the thin, flat internal oblique muscle covered with a split-thickness skin graft to reconstruct the floor of the mouth or the tonsillar defect.

With composite defects that involve resection of more than half of the tongue, an iliac crest or scapula flap is preferred because of the need for soft tissue bulk. Through-and-through composite defects resulting from removal of external skin and intraoral soft tissue (i.e., floor of the mouth, tongue, buccal mucosa) are best reconstructed with a scapula flap with two cutaneous paddles—one for intraoral soft tissue reconstruction, and the other for external coverage. Alternatively, the iliac crest flap can also be used if the oral cavity soft tissue defect is small, using the cutaneous paddle for external coverage and the internal oblique muscle for intraoral lining.

Customized Soft Tissue Free Flaps

The most significant recent advancement in oral cavity and oropharyngeal soft tissue reconstruction is the capability for early restoration of speech and swallowing functions with the use of customized soft tissue free flaps. The radial forearm flap has been the workhorse flap for this application. For tongue, floor-of-mouth, pharynx, and soft palate defects, it can be divided into multiple lobes to reconstruct each subunit due to the extensive pliability of the radial forearm skin.

Pharyngoesophageal Reconstruction

The goal of reconstruction is to reestablish a pharyngeal conduit that will not stricture at the distal anastomosis and that will be optimal for alaryngeal speech. Although partial hypopharyngeal defects can be repaired by primary closure or regional myocutaneous flaps, reconstruction of circumferential hypopharyngeal defects and cervical esophageal defects requires reconstruction with visceral interposition procedures (gastric pull-up, colon interposition), or microvascular free flaps, either jejunum or a tubed fasciocutaneous flap. Selection of method should consider successful restoration of swallowing and speech functions, as well as morbidity from the procedure.

From a functional standpoint, free flaps have proven to be far superior to traditionally used pedicled myocutaneous flaps or colon interposition for circumferential defects. In a review of 145 cases of reconstruction of the total hypopharynx and cervical esophagus, the incidence of functional failure (inability to take oral feeds) with free jejunal transfer (20%) was similar to that with gastric pull-up (17%), but much lower compared with tubed myocutaneous flaps (40%) and colon interposition (42%). Though the swallowing function is reliably restored with gastric pull-up, the morbidity and mortality are much higher due to the need for a laparotomy. With regard to free flaps, the choice between a jejunum flap and a tubed fasciocutaneous free flap is a surgeon's preference, with each method having its advantages and disadvantages.

The most commonly used cutaneous flap is the radial forearm flap, though the anterolateral thigh flap is a good alternative. The specific anatomical and technical advantages of the radial forearm flap have previously been stated. The incidences of fistula and stricture formation at the pharyngoesophageal anastomosis are similar between the radial forearm flap and the jejunum flap. A major advantage of the radial forearm flap over the jejunum flap is the better outcome with speech rehabilitation. In a patient who does not receive postoperative radiotherapy, the mucous production in the jejunum causes difficulty with speech production, with a "wet" voice through the tracheoesophageal puncture. The tubed cutaneous flap, however, provides a stiffer tube without excessive mucous, which allows better apposition of the walls during speech production.

Orbitomaxillary Defects

Orbitomaxillary defects resulting from radical maxillectomy and/or orbital exenteration can be reconstructed with soft tissue flaps or osteocutaneous flaps. The most commonly used soft tissue flaps are anterolateral thigh, rectus, and latissimus myocutaneous flaps, which provide sufficient skin and bulk that are usually required to reconstruct these composite maxillectomy defects. One would need to use an osteocutaneous flap, most commonly the scapula, to restore the contour of the malar eminence or to reconstruct the alveolar ridge with bone for subsequent placement of osseointegrated dental implants.

Alternative methods include fibular, osteocutaneous forearm, and iliac crest flaps; the use of pericranial bone grafts to restore the bony contour; and coverage of the bone grafts with the radial forearm flap.

Cranial and Skull Base Defects

Most skull base defects do not require free tissue transfer. Free flaps should be considered for large skull base defects and those with a high potential for cerebrospinal fluid leaks, such as postradiation defects or a large dural defect.

Anterolateral thigh and rectus muscle flaps are ideal and routinely used for skull base reconstruction because of their reliability, long pedicle, versatility in the design of the skin paddle, and presence of tendinous insertions that allow the muscle to be firmly suspended with transosseous sutures in the deepest regions of the skull base. Furthermore, the vascularized tensor fascia lata or anterior rectus sheath can be used to reliably repair dural defects, and the vascularized fat that lies between the anterior rectus sheath and skin can be used to obliterate deep, irregular skull base defects.

The latissimus dorsi myocutaneous flap is suitable for complex craniofacial defects. It can be divided into vertical and transverse segments to reconstruct cranial and orbitomaxillary defects; free bone grafts can also be sandwiched between the two segments.

Dynamic Facial Reanimation

The ultimate goal of dynamic facial reanimation is to restore emotional facial expression. Various muscles—including gracilis, latissimus dorsi, pectoralis minor, and serratus anterior—have been described in the literature for facial reanimation. Of these, the gracilis has gained the most popularity because of the ease of flap harvest, thin muscle, and the least donor site morbidity. After the gracilis muscle is transferred and revascularized, it is anchored between the orbicularis oris muscle and the zygomatic arch to restore the mimetic function of the midface. Neural anastomosis is then performed between the obturator nerve and the recipient nerve. The proximal stump of the facial nerve, cross-facial sural nerve graft, hypoglossal nerve, ansa hypoglossi, or masseter nerve can be used as the recipient nerve to reinnervate the gracilis muscle. The proximal stump or a branch of the ipsilateral facial nerve is the optimal choice because it offers the best potential for restoring natural facial mimetic function.

When the proximal facial nerve stump is not available, the contralateral branch(es) of the facial nerve can be used; however, this procedure requires two-staged reconstruction. In the first stage, a sural nerve is harvested and anastomosed to the buccal and zygomatic branches of the intact contralateral facial nerve and tunneled subcutaneously across the upper lip to the paralyzed side. The nerve graft is then left there for ~ 9 to 12 months to allow axons to regenerate to the distal stump. This can be assessed clinically by an advancing Tinel sign, where the patient perceives a tingling sensation to percussion along the regenerating nerve. In the second stage, microvascular transfer of the gracilis muscle is performed, and the obturator nerve is anastomosed to the distal stump of the sural nerve graft. The presence of regenerated axons is confirmed histologically by biopsy prior to the neural anastomosis.

O'Brien et al reported excellent to good facial symmetry at rest in 66% of 69 patients, and symmetry with smiling in 56%. Restoration of facial symmetry at rest is usually evident by 4 months, and some motion can be expected by 6 months. The disadvantages of using cross-facial nerve graft include risk of facial weakness on the nonparalyzed side, potential failure of axonal regeneration across the sural nerve graft, and additional time required to achieve ultimate reanimation. Alternatives to the use of the cross-facial nerve graft would be to use other motor nerves, such as the branch of the fifth cranial nerve to the masseter muscle, the hypoglossal nerve, or the ansa hypoglossi. Reinnervation of the gracilis can be consistently achieved with any of these nerves; however, the facial mimetic function is less natural because the act of smiling must be coordinated with simultaneous tongue movement or swallowing. Extensive training of and practice by the patient postoperatively are required for the patient to learn how to initiate emotional facial expressions.

Preservation of Recipient Vessels in the Neck

The success rate of head and neck free tissue transfer is > 95% when performed by experienced head and neck microvascular reconstructive surgeons. Several factors contribute to the high success rate: achieving a perfect anastomosis, appropriate selection of recipient vessels, careful attention to geometry of the vascular pedicle, and diligent postoperative care.

The most important consideration in selection of a recipient vessel is that it must appear to be healthy and demonstrate good flow. Other considerations are size match between donor and recipient vessels and final orientation of the axis of the vascular pedicle. The following principles should be adhered to in the selection and preservation of the recipient vessels:

1. Recipient vessel diameter should be similar to that of the donor vessels.
2. Ligation and division of the vessels that are being preserved for anastomosis should be performed at least 1 cm away from their

origin (i.e., from the external carotid artery or internal jugular vein).

3. Vessels should be handled gently, atraumatically, and meticulously, and thermal injury should be avoided.
4. Appropriate geometry of the vascular pedicle should be ensured to avoid kinking or compression of the vessels.

It appears that for head and neck reconstruction, the facial, superior thyroid, and transverse cervical arteries are the most commonly used recipient arteries because of size, similarity, and good geometry. Therefore, these arteries should be handled atraumatically and be carefully preserved. If oncologically sound, the transverse cervical vessels should also be preserved. There are several advantages to using the transverse cervical artery: (1) the anastomosis can be performed with ease without the mandible being in the way; (2) the vessel is often not damaged by radiation; and (3) several veins in the supraclavicular fossa, including the transverse cervical vein, can be used, which will result in optimal vessel geometry for both the arterial and the venous systems.

Frequently used recipient veins are the external jugular, common facial, and anterior facial veins. The external jugular vein often serves as an excellent recipient vein because it can be preserved without violating oncological principles, and it is usually adequately long and a good size match for easy primary end-to-end anastomosis. If there is a possibility that the internal jugular vein may have to be resected, it is imperative that the external jugular vein(s) be meticulously preserved during the skin flap elevation and transected as far cephalad as possible toward the angle of the mandible to attain an adequate length for primary end-to-end anastomosis. The common facial vein also serves as an excellent recipient vein and should be carefully preserved when a modified neck dissection is performed.

■ Postoperative Care

In the early postoperative phase, attention must be paid to preventing external compression of the vascular pedicle. No compression neck dressings or tracheostomy ties should be used. The head should be placed in a neutral position to avoid kinking of the vascular pedicle.

Many microvascular surgeons administer antithrombogenic agents perioperatively, though none of them has been clearly proven to reduce the incidence of thrombosis. The most commonly used agents are salicylic acid and low-molecular-weight Dextran (40% at 20–30 mL/h). Subcutaneous injection of mini-dose (5,000 units) heparin is also used by some surgeons. Because of the risk of systemic bleeding, intravenous heparin is generally not used unless there is vessel thrombosis and the patient has a hypercoagulable state.

Flap Monitoring

Diligent, close monitoring of the flap and careful management of hemodynamics in the postoperative period are essential to the success of a microvascular free flap. Because long primary and secondary ischemic times significantly jeopardize ultimate flap viability, early detection of vascular compromise and immediate return to the operating room are crucial for salvage of a compromised flap. Primary ischemic time is the length of ischemia during transfer of the flap (from the time the pedicle is transected to the time that the flap is reperfused). Secondary ischemic time is the length of ischemia from the onset of vessel thrombosis to the time of successful reperfusion. Prolonged ischemia, particularly secondary ischemia, causes irreversible damage to the capillary bed and results in a "no reflow" phenomenon, where the tissue cannot be reperfused despite successful reanastomosis.

Thrombosis due to anastomotic failure generally occurs within 24 to 48 hours after reperfusion. However, thrombosis may also occur much later because of vessel kinking, extrinsic compression (due to tissue edema, hematoma, seroma), or inflammation resulting from infection or fistula formation. It is difficult to salvage a flap in the setting of failure due to infection.

A variety of methods can be used to assess flap perfusion. Clinical assessment includes color, temperature, capillary refill, and dermal bleeding from a needle prick. The choice of monitoring method should be individualized. In some patients, the natural skin color may be too light or too dark to appreciate adequate perfusion or to assess capillary refill. Many of the flaps are placed in the oral cavity or pharynx where the ambient warm temperature will affect the accuracy of the flap temperature. Therefore, if the color, capillary refill, and temperature are difficult to assess, the flap should be pricked with a needle to assess cutaneous bleeding. A healthy flap should appear pink, be warm to the touch, demonstrate good capillary refill, and readily bleed bright red to needle prick. A pale, cool flap with reduced capillary refill that does not bleed to a needle prick indicates arterial compromise. Duskiness of the cutaneous paddle indicates venous thrombosis. A previously healthy-appearing flap that suddenly becomes edematous, has a very brisk capillary refill, and demonstrates return of venous-color blood suggests early venous congestion.

The most commonly used objective test for monitoring head and neck free flaps is an ultrasonic Doppler to detect flow in the vascular pedicle. One pitfall with using the Doppler in head and neck free flaps is that a false-positive reading can be attained due to the blood flow signal from other neck vessels in proximity to the vascular pedicle. An implantable Doppler can be used to overcome this but necessitates delayed removal of the wires and can give false-positive results for vascular compromise. Other objective tests for monitoring flaps have been described, such as fluorescence dye injection, temperature probes, and measurement of tissue oxygenation with a laser pulse oximeter; however, none of these methods is practical in head and neck free flaps. The flaps should be diligently monitored hourly or every 1 to 2 hours during the first 48 hours for evidence of arterial insufficiency as well as venous congestion. If there is any evidence of vascular compromise or any doubt with regard to the patency of the vascular pedicle, the patient should be taken to the operating room immediately for exploration. In the event of venous congestion, medicinal leeches can be applied to the flap to somewhat decongest it while preparations are being made to return to the operating room.

Hemodynamics

The goals of hemodynamics are to (1) maintain a good perfusion pressure (generally at the level of the patient's baseline blood pressure), (2) maintain adequate intravascular volume, (3) avoid rapid large shifts in the patient's fluid status, and (4) reduce blood viscosity by maintaining the hematocrit between 25 and 30%. Blood pressure is best maintained by administration of fluids and/or blood. Alpha-adrenergic agents, such as epinephrine, should not be used to treat hypotension, except in a life-threatening situation, because they cause vasoconstriction in the flap. If adequate perfusion pressure cannot be maintained despite volume replacement, low-dose dopamine (1 to 2 g/kg/min), which has very little a-adrenergic effect at this dose, can be administered. Although maintenance of intravascular volume is essential, it is also important not to overload the patient with fluids. If the need arises to diurese the patient, diuretic agents should be used in a very low dose (i.e., furosemide 20 mg).

◼ Suggested Reading

Bak M, Jacobson AS, Buchbinder D, Urken ML. Contemporary reconstruction of the mandible. Oral Oncol 2010;46(2):71–76

Futran ND, Mendez E. Developments in reconstruction of midface and maxilla. Lancet Oncol 2006;7(3):249–258

O'Connell DA, Teng MS, Mendez E, Futran ND. Microvascular free tissue transfer in the reconstruction of scalp and lateral temporal bone defects. Craniomaxillofac Trauma Reconstr 2011;4(4): 179–188

Shnayder Y, Tsue TT, Toby EB, Werle AH, Girod DA. Safe osteocutaneous radial forearm flap harvest with prophylactic internal fixation. Craniomaxillofac Trauma Reconstr 2011;4(3):129–136

Wong CH, Wei FC. Microsurgical free flap in head and neck reconstruction. Head Neck 2010;32(9):1236–1245

41 Current Classification, Staging, and Management of Lymphomas

■ Introduction

Hodgkin lymphoma (HL) and non-Hodgkin lymphomas (NHLs) represent ~ 5% of new cancer cases and are the fifth leading cause of cancer death in the United States annually. Both types of lymphoma can occur in nodal and extranodal regions of the head and neck. Lymphomas are a diverse group of malignancies with differing clinical presentations, disease courses, and prognoses. Hence, diagnostic characterization, accurate staging, and individualized treatment are critical to therapeutic success.

■ Hodgkin Lymphoma

The incidence of HL in the United States is ~ 7,500 new cases annually. The etiology of HL remains poorly characterized, but there is an increased incidence in the Jewish population, suggesting a genetic predisposition. The two major subtypes of HL are classic Hodgkin lymphoma (CHL) and nodular lymphocyte predominant Hodgkin lymphoma (NLPHL). Both diseases are monoclonal lymphoid neoplasms that usually arise from B cells. More than 90% of HL cases are CHL, which is diagnosed most frequently between 15 and 30 years of age and less frequently after 55 years of age.

Lymph nodes involved by CHL harbor malignant mononuclear cells termed Hodgkin cells and multinucleated Reed–Sternberg cells. In contrast, NLPHL-affected lymph nodes contain lymphocyte-predominant cells that are known as popcorn cells because they microscopically resemble popped kernels of corn. The surface antigenicity of each group of cells is unique, which permits immunophenotypic characterization and impacts their response to treatment.

Classification

The World Health Organization classification scheme for CHLs categorizes them by morphological and clinical features into nodular sclerosis, mixed cellu-

larity, lymphocyte-rich, and lymphocyte-depleted subtypes. Nodular sclerosis CHL is the most common subtype, representing 60 to 80% of cases, followed by mixed cellularity CHL (15–30%), lymphocyte-rich CHL (5%), and lymphocyte-depleted CHL (< 1%). Mediastinal involvement is most frequently seen in nodular sclerosis CHL, whereas abdominal lymph node and splenic involvement are more common in mixed cellularity CHL. Lymphocyte-rich CHL has a slightly better prognosis than other subtypes of CHL.

Evaluation

Clinical Presentation and Natural History

An enlarged, nontender, freely movable lymph node in the upper cervical or supraclavicular region is the most common clinical presentation in 60 to 80% of cases of CHL. The next most frequent location is the axillary region, followed by the inguinal and femoral regions. Mediastinal involvement may be identified on a routine chest X-ray.

Abdominal symptomatology is usually associated with the location and size of the tumor mass. Symptoms associated with extranodal involvement may also occur. A significant number of HL patients present with systemic symptoms before the discovery of lymphadenopathy. Fever and drenching night sweats occur in up to 25% of patients at the time of presentation, and weight loss is also common. These constitute the "B" symptoms associated with HL. Other symptoms include fatigue, pruritus, and pain after drinking alcohol. Symptoms attributable to extranodal disease occur less frequently in HL than in NHL patients.

HL typically begins in a single group of lymph nodes and subsequently spreads to adjacent lymph nodes with eventual hematologic spread. Contiguous spread to other regional lymph nodes most frequently occurs with the nodular sclerosis and mixed cellularity subtypes: the neck and mediastinum are involved in more than 60% of these patients, which is at least four times more frequent than any other region above or below the diaphragm. Bilateral cervical nodal involvement is uncommon, unless mediastinal involvement is also present, raising the possibility that spread to the contralateral neck occurs via the mediastinum. Splenic involvement is suggestive of extranodal spread and is more common in patients with adenopathy below the diaphragm, systemic symptoms, and mixed cellularity subtype. Bone marrow involvement is usually local and is typically associated with extensive disease and systemic symptoms.

Diagnostic Evaluation

Diagnosis of HL usually requires excisional lymph node biopsy for immunophenotyping, immunohistochemistry, morphological assessment, and other special testing. Core needle biopsy may be sufficient, if diagnostic. Fine-needle aspiration (FNA) for cytological assessment is generally not adequate, despite the use of flow cytometry. Most of the treating oncologists will want additional information provided by an open biopsy and histological assessment.

History and physical evaluation should be directed toward systemic symptoms, such as weight loss, fevers, and night sweats (B symptoms). Fevers in HL patients characteristically occur intermittently and recur at varying intervals over the course of several days or weeks. Other systemic symptoms that may be present include fatigue, pruritus, and the development of pain at the site of nodal involvement shortly following alcohol intake. The following diagnostic tests should be performed: complete blood count (CBC) with differential; erythrocyte sedimentation rate (ESR); liver and renal function tests; plain film chest radiographs; computed tomography (CT) of the neck, chest, abdomen, and pelvis; positron-emission tomography (PET)-CT scan; bone marrow biopsy (stage IB, IIB, and III–IV); and human immunodeficiency virus (HIV) test for complete evaluation. This will often be performed by the medical oncologist after the open biopsy.

Staging

Staging for HL is based on the Ann Arbor staging system (**Table 41.1**). Each stage is subdivided into A and B categories. The absence of systemic symptoms is designated by *A*, whereas the presence of unexplained weight loss of > 10% of body weight, unexplained fevers, or drenching night sweats is designated by *B* (B symptoms). Addition of the letter *E* also denotes involvement of a single extranodal site that is contiguous or proximal to the known nodal site. The Cotswolds classification system, a modification of the Ann Arbor classification that was proposed in 1989, designates other prognostically

Table 41.1 Cotswolds modification of Ann Arbor staging system

Stage	Area of involvement
I	Single lymph node group
II	Multiple lymph node groups on same side of diaphragm
III	Multiple lymph node groups on both sides of diaphragm
IV	Multiple extranodal sites or lymph nodes and extranodal disease
Designations applicable to any disease stage	
A	No symptoms
B	Symptoms: weight loss > 10%, fever (temperature > 38°C), drenching night sweats
X	Bulky disease: nodal mass > 10 cm or widening of mediastinum by more than one-third
E	Extranodal extension or single isolated site of extranodal disease

Data from Lister TA, Crowther D, Sutcliffe SB, et al. Report of a committee convened to discuss the evaluation and staging of patients with Hodgkin's disease: Cotswolds meeting. J Clin Oncol 1989;7(11):1630–1636.

important information using letter suffixes, including *X* when bulky mediastinal disease is present.

Treatment and Outcomes

Patients with HL are usually classified into three groups: early-stage favorable disease (stage I–II with no unfavorable factors); early-stage unfavorable disease (stage I–II with any unfavorable factor, such as large mediastinal adenopathy, B symptoms, numerous sites of disease, or significantly elevated ESR); and advanced-stage disease (stage III–IV). Each of these groups is treated in accordance with the aggressiveness of the disease:

1. Early-stage favorable disease: two to three cycles of chemotherapy plus involved field radiation therapy (IF-RT), total dose of 20 to 30 gray (Gy)
2. Early-stage unfavorable disease: four cycles of chemotherapy plus IF-RT, 30 to 36 Gy
3. Advanced-stage disease: eight cycles of chemotherapy with or without consolidation RT (to residual tumors), 30 to 36 Gy
4. Bulky disease at any stage: RT dose of 30 to 36 Gy

IF-RT is limited to the site of the clinically involved lymph node group. The most common chemotherapy regimens for CHL include **a**driamycin, **b**leomycin, **v**inblastine, and **d**acarbazine (ABVD) and Stanford

V (Adriamycin [doxorubicin/hydroxydaunorubicin], vinblastine, mechlorethamine, etoposide [VP-16], vincristine, bleomycin, and prednisone).

Treatment with chemotherapy and RT for early-stage favorable disease results in 5-year event-free survival rates of > 90%. Combined modality therapy for early-stage unfavorable disease results in 5-year, event-free survival and overall 10-year survival of ~ 85%. Various chemotherapy regimens have been evaluated for the treatment of advanced-stage HL. In one important randomized multicenter clinical trial, ABVD treatment without RT resulted in a 61% 5-year, failure-free survival rate and a 73% overall 5-year survival rate, which was equally effective and less toxic than mechlorethamine, vincristine (**O**ncovin, Genus Pharmaceuticals, Huddersfield, England), **p**rocarbazine, and **p**rednisone (MOPP)/ABVD, supporting the use of ABVD alone as first-line therapy. In another large clinical trial that compared ABVD to Stanford V with or without consolidation RT, there was no difference in 5-year, progression-free (75%), and overall survival (90%) rates.

■ Non-Hodgkin Lymphomas

NHLs comprise a diverse group of lymphoproliferative disorders arising from B-lymphocytes, T-lymphocytes, or natural killer (NK) cells. In the United States, 80 to 85% of NHL cases are B-cell lymphomas, 15 to 20% are T-cell lymphomas, and < 1% are NK-cell lymphomas. Over the past 4 decades, the incidence of NHL has markedly increased. The reasons for this NHL epidemic are not completely clear, but acquired immune deficiency syndrome (AIDS)-related NHLs explain some of this increase.

Etiology

Although the etiology of most cases of NHL is unknown, infectious agents and other exposures have been associated with various types of NHLs. Epstein-Barr virus (EBV) deoxyribonucleic acid is associated with 95% of Burkitt lymphomas, as well as posttransplant lymphoproliferative disorders and some AIDS-associated lymphomas. Hepatitis C virus is also associated with NHL. The risk of NHL is increased in subjects with herbicide exposure and may also be elevated in individuals who have used recreational drugs or tobacco. Following treatment for HL, the risk of NHL may be increased more than 20-fold. In addition, ~ 5% of all patients afflicted by the autoimmune disease Primary Sjögren syndrome develop NHL. Sjögren syndrome increases the risk of developing NHL of the parotid gland and other body regions by at least 15-fold, and this risk continues to increase risk over time. The relationship between other autoimmune diseases such as immunoglobulin G4 (IgG)-associated sialadenitis and the development of NHL remains less clear. Multicentric head and neck Castleman disease, also termed angiofollicular lymph node hyperplasia, has been associated with an increased risk of developing NHL.

The Lymphoid Tissues and Non-Hodgkin Lymphomas

Lymphoid tissues are divided into the primary lymphoid tissues, which include the bone marrow and thymus, and secondary lymphoid tissues, which include the lymph nodes, spleen, and mucosa-associated lymphoid tissue (MALT). MALT is specialized lymphoid tissue that is found in the pharynx (Waldeyer ring), the gastrointestinal tract, and the lung. NHLs develop from B and T cells in these tissues at various stages of antigen-independent and antigen-dependent differentiation, resulting in the heterogeneous group of NHLs that have been characterized. In addition, NK cells represent a third line of lymphoid cells that are derived from a common progenitor with T cells and are able to kill cells that lack certain surface antigens, possibly resulting from viral infection or malignancy. NHLs rarely develop from NK cells.

Classification

The fourth edition of the World Health Organization (WHO) classification of lymphoid neoplasms includes 86 distinct entities divided into five major categories: precursor B- and T-cell neoplasms, mature B-cell neoplasms, mature T/NK cell neoplasms, HL, and immunodeficiency-associated lymphoproliferative disorders. This classification scheme lists the lymphoid neoplasms first by differentiation stage (precursor or mature), then by lineage (B or T/NK), and finally by specific disease entities in accordance with their distinct clinical presentation. Histological grade is applied within a disease entity, rather than across the whole range of lymphoid neoplasms.

Evaluation

Clinical Presentation and Natural History

The WHO classification separates the 86 recognized lymphoid neoplasms into three broad categories based on their clinical presentation:

1. Predominantly disseminated diseases, which frequently involve the bone marrow and may be leukemic
2. Primary extranodal lymphomas

3. Predominantly nodal disease entities, which are frequently disseminated and can also involve extranodal sites

Extranodal involvement has been reported to occur in 25 to 40% of all NHL cases. The head and neck region is the second most common extranodal site after the skin. Extranodal locations in the head and neck region include the Waldeyer ring, mucosa of the oral cavity, pharynx and larynx, nasal cavity, and parotid, submandibular, and thyroid glands. Lymphomas of the palatine tonsils represent more than 50% of the lymphomas that arise from the Waldeyer ring.

Diagnostic Evaluation

Diagnosis of NHL usually requires excisional lymph node biopsy for immunophenotyping, immunohistochemistry, morphological assessment, and other special testing. Core needle biopsy is usually discouraged unless it is the only safe method of obtaining a diagnostic tissue sample. FNA by itself is not a sufficient diagnostic tool for NHL because classification is based on both morphology and immunophenotyping. However, FNA in combination with flow cytometry and immunohistochemistry markedly improves diagnostic accuracy. In situations where NHL arising from an extranodal site is suspected, adequate tissue sampling, such as tonsillectomy or open parotid or thyroid biopsy, may be required for diagnosis.

Immunophenotyping of B and T lymphoid cells—by detecting the presence of surface or cytoplasmic antigens (cluster designations or CDs) with labeled monoclonal antibodies and detection of chromosomal translocations, additions, and deletions using polymerase chain reaction—is essential to accurately diagnose lymphoid neoplasms. Initial immunophenotyping permits characterization of a neoplasm as either B cell (e.g., CD19, CD20, CD79a) or T cell (e.g., CD2, CD3. CD5, CD7) antigen-positive. Initial morphological analysis subdivides B-cell positive lymphomas into small, medium, and large cells (two to three times the size of normal lymphocytes) and T-cell positive lymphomas into anaplastic versus nonanaplastic morphology. Clinical features, such as age and location (cutaneous, nodal, extranodal), are also considered. Additional immunophenotypic and genetic testing is then performed to accurately diagnose the lymphoid neoplasm. For example, morphological assessment of a biopsy specimen demonstrates *medium-sized cells*, which test *positive for B-cell antigens*. Four types of NHL fit this profile: Burkitt lymphoma, diffuse large B-cell lymphoma, mantle cell lymphoma–blastic variant, and B-cell lymphoma–unclassifiable. Additional immunophenotypic and genetic testing is performed to make the diagnosis.

History and physical examination should document night sweats, fever, and unexplained weight loss, as well as symptoms that could be associated with involvement of a specific organ system. A history of waxing and waning lymphadenopathy should also be documented because spontaneous regression can occur with follicular lymphomas. Examination of all lymph node–bearing areas and evaluation for splenomegaly and hepatomegaly are essential. Physical examination should also evaluate for pharyngeal involvement, thyroid or salivary gland masses, pleural effusions, and abdominal or testicular masses.

Laboratory evaluation should include complete blood count (CBC), studies of renal and hepatic function, lactate dehydrogenase (LDH), hepatitis B and C testing, and evaluation for HIV. Bone marrow aspirate and biopsy should be performed in most cases. Computed tomography (CT) of the neck, chest, abdomen, and pelvis should be performed. A growing body of literature suggests that positron-emission tomography (PET)-CT is more sensitive and specific than CT scan and can be used for initial staging, restaging, and follow-up of NHL patients.

Staging and Prognosis

Although the Ann Arbor staging system and the subsequent Cotswolds modification were developed for patients with HL, these staging systems are also employed for NHL and have demonstrated their value for effective prognostic stratification and treatment planning. However, the International Prognostic Index (IPI) has become the most valuable and widely used method of stratifying lymphoma patients according to prognosis. Five different disease-related factors have been shown to adversely impact survival: age > 60 years, Karnofsky performance status ≤ 70, Ann Arbor stage III or IV, extranodal involvement at two or more sites, and abnormal LDH level. IPI scores of 0 and 1 are classified as low, whereas scores of 4 and 5 are classified as high and are associated with worse survival.

Treatment and Outcomes of Specific Disease Entities

Diffuse Large B-Cell Lymphomas

Diffuse large B-cell lymphomas (DLBCLs) are the most common form of lymphoma, representing ~ 30% of the NHLs diagnosed in the United States. An enlarging mass is the most common clinical presentation, and one-third of the patients manifest B symptoms. Extranodal disease is present in 30 to 40% of patients. DLBCLs account for 50 to 70% of primary lymphomas of the thyroid gland and are the second most common type of lymphoma of the parotid gland in patients with Sjögren syndrome. Clinical trial outcomes have demonstrated that disseminated DLBCL is curable.

Most patients with DLBCL and other aggressive lymphomas receive CHOP-based CT (cyclophosphamide, hydroxydaunorubicin [adriamycin/doxoid rubicin], oncovin [vincristine], prednisone). Rituximab in combination with CHOP (R-CHOP) has demonstrated lower rates of treatment failure, relapse, and death, and thus has emerged as the standard initial therapy for DLBCL in the United States.

Follicular Lymphoma

Follicular lymphoma (FL) is a B-cell lymphoma. It is the second most common lymphoma in the United States, representing ~ 22% of all NHLs and 70% of low-grade lymphomas. FL affects largely older adults with a slight female predilection. Disease is usually widespread at the time of diagnosis and predominantly involves lymph nodes, but it may also involve extranodal sites. Although most patients are diagnosed at an advanced stage, median survival is > 10 years. RT is the recommended treatment for most patients with stage I and II FL. The role of chemotherapy in combination with RT for early-stage FL is unclear. When chemotherapy is used to treat FL, the monoclonal antibody rituximab is frequently combined with chemotherapy. Combination chemotherapy results in more rapid complete remission in patients with disseminated FL, but data suggesting improved long-term control results are lacking. Most patients with FL eventually relapse and undergo salvage therapy, requiring treatments, such as second-line chemotherapy and bone marrow transplantation.

Mucosa-Associated Lymphoid Tissue Lymphoma

Extranodal marginal zone MALT lymphoma is divided into gastric and nongastric MALT lymphoma. Sites of nongastric MALT lymphoma include small/large bowel, breast, lung, ocular adnexa, ovary, prostate, salivary gland, and Waldeyer ring. MALT lymphomas are small B-cell lymphomas that represent 50 to 75% of the parotid gland lymphomas associated with Sjögren syndrome and are the most common lymphomas involving the salivary glands. Moreover, 25 to 30% of primary thyroid lymphomas are MALT lymphomas. These lymphomas generally run an indolent disease course with > 85% 5-year survival.

Extranodal Natural Killer/T-Cell Lymphoma, Nasal Type

Extranodal NK/T cell lymphoma, nasal type, is an aggressive rare extranodal lymphoma that is designated as NK/T to denote that, although most cases have an NK lineage, some cases have a cytotoxic T-cell phenotype. This lymphoma, which is also known as lethal midline granuloma and polymorphic reticulosis, most frequently occurs in middle-aged males and presents in the midfacial region, nose, and palate. Patients present with midfacial swelling, nasal obstruction, epistaxis, and rhinorrhea. Multiple biopsies are frequently required because there are variable degrees of necrosis and an atypical polymorphic infiltrate. Lymphoid cells are medium-sized, manifest a characteristic immunophenotype, and demonstrate infection with EBV (EBV-encoded small nuclear ribonucleic acid). Curative treatment usually requires RT with or without chemotherapy. The usual RT dose is 40 to 55 Gy administered once a day at 1.8 to 2 Gy/fraction, but RT alone is associated with a high rate of treatment failure. Chemotherapy protocols used to treat other lymphomas are not effective treatments for NK/T-cell lymphoma. Regimens containing L-asparaginase have shown promise in the treatment of advanced disease. The prognosis of patients with disseminated disease is very poor.

■ Controversial Issues

The utility of FNA for the diagnosis of lymphoproliferative disorders remains controversial. There are several arguments against the use of FNA:

1. Nondiagnostic results require a second procedure, which increases cost and discomfort and delays diagnosis and treatment.
2. Limitations of FNA include loss of architecture, sampling error, difficulty distinguishing malignant cells from reactive cells, and lack of adequate material that may not allow for additional stains or flow cytometry.
3. Diagnosis of lymphoma with FNA in the community setting may by impacted by limited resources and training in diagnostic cytology.
4. Grading lymphomas is difficult.
5. Certain lymphomas are particularly difficult to diagnose with FNA, including the following:
   a. HL, especially lymphocyte-depleted, due to the paucity of Reed-Sternberg cells
   b. Differentiation between T-cell NHL, T-cell–rich B-cell lymphomas, and HL

In contrast, several academic centers have published favorable experiences with FNA for the diagnosis of lymphomas. As an example, The University of Texas MD Anderson Cancer Center has used FNA for more than 15 years to diagnose lymphomas, applying a multiparameter approach. Immediate evaluation of the adequacy of the cytological aspirate is essential. Microscope slides that have been air dried and alcohol fixed are stained with the Diff-Quik method to highlight cytoplasmic features and the Papanicolaou method to evaluate nuclear features. The rest of the aspirated material is rinsed in a cell preservative such as RPMI-1640. A minimum of three to four FNAs are required to aspirate at least 700,000 cells. However, collection of 10 million cells will provide the highest diagnostic yield so that ancillary studies can be performed. Common ancillary studies include immunophenotyping with flow cytometry or immunocytochemistry and proliferative markers such as Ki-67 or DNA ploidy analysis. Other studies are performed in certain cases, such as fluorescence in situ hybridization (FISH) to detect a translocation associated with mantle cell lymphoma, or polymerase chain reaction (PCR) when T-cell lymphoma is suspected. Although this multiparameter approach can be effectively employed to diagnose most lymphomas, open biopsy is still required for the diagnosis of HL, which is the most difficult lymphoma to diagnose by FNA for a variety of reasons.

■ Suggested Reading

Caraway NP. Strategies to diagnose lymphoproliferative disorders by fine-needle aspiration by using ancillary studies. Cancer 2005;105(6):432–442

Engert A, Eichenauer DA, Harris NL, Mauch PM, Diehl V. Hodgkin lymphoma. In: DeVita VT, Lawrence TS, Rosenberg SA, eds. DeVita, Hellman, and Rosenberg's Cancer Principles & Practice of Oncology. 9th ed. Philadelphia, PA: Lippincott Williams & Wilkins; 2011:1819–1854

Friedberg JW, Mauch PM, Rimsza L, Fisher RI. Non-Hodgkin lymphomas. In: DeVita VT, Lawrence TS, Rosenberg SA, eds. DeVita, Hellman, and Rosenberg's Cancer Principles & Practice of Oncology. 9th ed. Philadelphia, PA: Lippincott Williams & Wilkins; 2011:1855-1893

Hoskin PJ, Lowry L, Horwich A, et al. Randomized comparison of the stanford V regimen and ABVD in the treatment of advanced Hodgkin's Lymphoma: United Kingdom National Cancer Research Institute Lymphoma Group Study ISRCTN 64141244. J Clin Oncol 2009;27(32):5390–5396

International Agency for Research on Cancer. Swerdlow SH, Campo E, Harris NL, et al., eds. WHO Classification of Tumours of the Haematopoietic and Lymphoid Tissues. Lyon, France: IARC Press; 2008.

Jaccard A, Hermine O. Extranodal natural killer/T-cell lymphoma: advances in the management. Curr Opin Oncol 2011;23(5): 429–435

National Comprehensive Cancer Network. Hodgkin Lymphoma. NCCN Clinical Practice Guidelines in Oncology. (Version 2.2012). www.nccn.org

National Comprehensive Cancer Network. Non-Hodgkin's Lymphomas. NCCN Clinical Practice Guidelines in Oncology. (Version 3.2012). www.nccn.org

Pollard RP, Pijpe J, Bootsma H, et al. Treatment of mucosa-associated lymphoid tissue lymphoma in Sjogren's syndrome: a retrospective clinical study. J Rheumatol 2011;38(10):2198–2208

Solans-Laqué R, López-Hernandez A, Bosch-Gil JA, Palacios A, Campillo M, Vilardell-Tarres M. Risk, predictors, and clinical characteristics of lymphoma development in primary Sjögren's syndrome. Semin Arthritis Rheum 2011;41(3):415–423

42 Metastatic Cancer of Occult Origin to Cervical Lymph Nodes

■ Introduction

Metastatic disease to the neck may be a first sign of malignancy. The metastasis may originate from an occult primary tumor of the upper aerodigestive tract, thyroid, or skin, or it may represent a metastasis from an infraclavicular primary cancer. Although a primary care physician may be called upon to recognize an enlarged lymph node in the neck of an adult as being potentially malignant, it is incumbent upon an otolaryngologist not only to diagnose the cervical metastasis but also to appropriately direct cancer care.

Squamous cell carcinoma metastatic to cervical lymph nodes from an occult head and neck primary tumor accounts for up to 5% of head and neck cancers. The prognosis for these patients is relatively favorable. Metastatic carcinoma to cervical lymph nodes from an infraclavicular occult primary, however, carries a dismal prognosis, with a median survival of less than 6 months and a 10 to 15% treatment response. Therefore it is critical to determine whether the site of origin is above or below the clavicles and to direct appropriate cancer care.

For occult head and neck primary cancers, early diagnosis, attempted identification of the primary site of origin, and development of a comprehensive treatment plan are all important to achieving a favorable outcome. Unfortunately, untimely biopsies are sometimes still performed prior to a thorough and systematic search for a primary tumor. This may result in the mandatory need for irradiation due to tumor spillage, complicate definitive surgery, and increase operative morbidity. As with any head and neck malignancy, the workup begins with a thorough history and physical examination.

■ Relevant Anatomy

When evaluating a neck mass suspicious for metastatic carcinoma, identification of the lymph node group involved is important for determining the putative primary site of origin. A mass presenting in upper level II is most commonly associated with metastatic disease from the oral cavity, oropharynx, supraglottic larynx, hypopharynx, and nasopharynx. A mass arising more posteriorly may represent metastatic disease from the nasopharynx, posterior oropharynx, or maxillary sinus. In contrast, a metastatic lymph node in level I may result from a primary tumor of the oral cavity, including the anterior tongue, floor of the mouth, alveolar ridge, or retromolar trigone. With metastatic disease in level I, a skin primary should also be considered because the facial and parotid nodes are the most likely site of involvement for these malignancies. A submental mass may be due to metastasis from the lips, skin of the nose, or anterior floor of the mouth.

A single metastasis in level III or the midjugular chain often represents spread from a primary tumor of the larynx, hypopharynx, or thyroid. The presentation of a mass in level IV suggests the primary tumor site resides in the subglottic larynx, thyroid, cervical esophagus, or infraclavicular locations, such as the lungs, esophagus, or gastrointestinal tract. This is particularly true on the left side when metastatic disease involves the Virchow node. Supraclavicular masses (level V) usually represent an infraclavicular primary tumor, or metastatic disease from the nasopharynx, cervical esophagus, or thyroid. In addition to identifying the involved level of the neck, the examination should document the mass's size, mobility, and fixation to underlying structures.

■ Patient Evaluation

History

In the clinical setting of a patient with a neck mass of undetermined etiology, it is most critical to determine whether the neck mass represents a malignancy and, if so, whether the site is identifiable. A mass suspected of harboring malignancy should be approached in an organized fashion, beginning with a pertinent history. Factors associated with an increased probability of malignancy include (1) excessive use of tobacco and alcohol; (2) age over 40; (3) a mass that is nontender and enlarging; (4) symptoms of airway impairment, dysphagia, otalgia, or odynophagia; and (5) prior history of head and neck cancer or previous radiotherapy to the head and neck. Other important history includes symptoms of pulmonary or gastrointestinal disturbance, such as dyspepsia, hematemesis, hematochezia, or melena. History of prior treatment for a skin malignancy should also be elicited. The patient should be queried about symptoms of weight loss, fever, chills, or night sweats, which may be suggestive of a systemic etiology for the neck mass.

A complete examination of the entire head and neck is mandatory. Among patients with metastatic disease from a primary upper aerodigestive tract carcinoma, the primary tumor can be identified in 90% of patients through a careful examination. The location in the neck of metastatic squamous carcinoma may predict the primary site of origin and guide evaluation.

Physical Examination

Physical examination includes thorough inspection of the oral cavity after removal of any denture appliances. Complete inspection of the floor of the mouth, tongue, alveolar ridge, hard palate, and buccal areas should be documented. Primary squamous carcinoma of the oral cavity will almost always be identifiable on physical exam. The oropharynx, including the base of tongue, vallecula, tonsil regions, and soft palate are best evaluated by visual exam and palpation. This is especially important for the tonsil and base of tongue, where the surface component of a malignancy may be minimal. Palpable induration may identify the presence of the primary carcinoma. Examination of the nasopharynx, hypopharynx, and larynx may be performed by mirror examination, the flexible fiberoptic endoscopic visualization. Asymmetry of the nasopharynx, fullness in the fossa of Rosenmüller, or the presence of friable tissue that bleeds readily with minimal manipulation requires a biopsy. Systematic evaluation of the laryngopharyngeal structures is critical. Tongue protrusion will open the vallecula and expose the lingual surface of the epiglottis to closer inspection. The pyriform sinuses and postcricoid area are carefully examined with the patient breathing normally, and again following a cheek puff maneuver to insufflate the hypopharynx if using fiberoptic visualization. Pooling of secretions, asymmetry, or failure of the pyriform sinus to open may point to the presence of an occult tumor. The laryngeal structures are closely examined to assess any asymmetry, fullness of the false cords, or diminished mobility of the larynx, any of which may suggest the presence of a neoplasm.

Fine-Needle Aspiration

Initial biopsy of the neck mass should be by fine-needle aspiration (FNA). Open biopsy of head and neck masses is generally condemned. FNA biopsy avoids an open biopsy, which may result in tumor spillage, placement of an incision that cannot be easily incorporated into a definitive surgical procedure, and unnecessary expense to the patient. Also, often the treatment choice for metastatic lymphadenopathy relies on a fascial dissection, which is fundamentally disrupted by open biopsy. Information obtained by FNA will direct the remaining evaluation and focus the search for the primary tumor site.

With an experienced cytopathologist, FNA diagnosis is 98 to 99% accurate for diagnosing metastatic squamous cell carcinoma in a cervical lymph node, provided adequate material is obtained for examination. The aspiration can be performed rapidly with minimal patient discomfort, and the material can be examined immediately for verification of adequacy of sample.

Rapid cytological stains can provide an immediate diagnosis, especially with squamous cell carcinoma. When the aspirate reveals a poorly differentiated carcinoma or is predominantly lymphoid, special immunocytological staining is necessary to establish a diagnosis. Special stains can include cytokeratins, thyroglobulin for differentiated thyroid cancer, calcitonin for medullary carcinoma, S-100 and human melanoma black 45 (HMB-45) for melanoma, vimentin for sarcomas, and leucocyte common antigen for lymphoma. Numerous other immunocytochemical studies are available, depending on the cellular morphology. Finally, selective use of ultrasonographic or computed tomographic (CT) guidance may enhance the accuracy of FNA. When lesions are necrotic or located close to vascular structures, image guidance may provide a better means of obtaining tissue.

When a poorly differentiated carcinoma is obtained in the needle aspirate, nasopharyngeal or oropharyngeal carcinoma is a possibility. Clonal Epstein-Barr virus (EBV) genomes are present in the tumor cells of nasopharyngeal carcinoma and may be used to identify the source of the metastatic carcinoma. The cellular deoxyribonucleic acid (DNA) from the aspirate is expanded by polymerase chain reaction and analyzed for the presence of the EBV genomes. The detection of EBV DNA supports the probability of the primary site arising in the nasopharynx. In addition, expression of p16 or human papilloma virus (HPV) is suggestive of a tonsil or tongue base primary, and diagnostic attention should be directed to those areas.

At times an open biopsy is necessary, especially when FNA biopsy is suggestive of lymphoma or is nondiagnostic. Flow cytometry and special studies will permit immunotyping and precise characterization of the cell lineage of the lymphoma. When an open neck biopsy is performed, the patient should be prepared for the possibility of neck dissection, especially in the setting of epithelial malignancy (e.g., squamous cell carcinoma), for which treatment is primarily surgical.

Diagnostic Radiology

After FNA, the next step in the diagnostic pathway should be to obtain a radiographic evaluation of the head and neck region. This should be obtained before any incisions are made. The benefit of diagnostic imaging for a mass in the neck may be questioned from a cost-effectiveness standpoint; however, when a malignancy in the neck is suspected, these studies provide further information. They confirm the exact location of the neck mass and the relationship to the great vessels, and they may demonstrate characteristics suggestive of the histopathological process present. Also, imaging may identify a putative primary site by revealing areas of asymmetry in the nasopharynx, base of the tongue, tonsil, or pyriform sinus.

The principal imaging modalities for evaluation of a neck mass of undetermined etiology are CT with contrast or CT/positron-emission tomography (PET). CT is recognized as the primary imaging modality for evaluation of metastatic cervical lymphadenopathy. On CT, a discrete nonenhancing mass located in the lymph node–bearing region of the neck has a high probability of being malignant if it (1) is > 1.5 cm in diameter, (2) displays central hypolucency and peripheral enhancement, (3) has poorly defined or irregular borders, and (4) is associated with a loss of adjacent tissue planes. Peripheral enhancement is also indicative of malignancy. The size criteria for identifying a node as being metastatic is > 1.5 cm for level I nodes and > 1 cm for all other nodes. It has been reported that, when the size criteria were met, 80% of these nodes were pathologically infiltrated by tumor. The presence of one or more of these radiographic findings is strongly suggestive of metastatic disease in lymph nodes. The CT scan may also iden-

tify metastatic disease in other lymph node stations that cannot be directly examined, such as the retropharyngeal nodes. In patients with a large or muscular neck, involved lymph nodes that escape detection by physical examination may be imaged with CT. Extracapsular spread, if present, may also be well demonstrated by CT.

Magnetic resonance imaging (MRI) also has utility for the evaluation of a neck mass of undetermined etiology. Although this modality provides superior soft tissue detail and multiplanar imaging capabilities, data are lacking as to MRI's cost-effective benefit over CT. The resolution capabilities of MRI have been enhanced with the use of a neck surface coil. Recently, with administration of gadolinium and fat-suppression techniques, the utility of MRI for evaluation of metastatic disease has been reassessed. Most studies show CT to have a higher accuracy and sensitivity than MRI for nodal metastasis. At present, CT must be considered superior to and more cost-effective than MRI for determining the likelihood of a lymph node harboring metastatic disease. Therefore, CT is the modality of choice for evaluating a suspicious neck mass in an adult.

More recently, fluorine-18 fluorodeoxyglucose (18F-FDG) PET has been investigated for identifying occult primary tumors of the head and neck. This imaging modality uses the radionuclide glucose analogue FDG, which is incorporated by rapidly dividing cells. It holds promise for providing metabolic images of tumor tissues. The scientific basis is that the differential metabolic activity of the tumor will contrast with the surrounding normal tissue, thus allowing detection of an occult lesion. In general, PET has the capability of identifying squamous cell carcinoma with tumor volumes estimated at > 1 mL. The combination of PET and CT, which is common at this time, further enhances the utility of this imaging technique by providing both metabolic and anatomical information. Studies have demonstrated this modality to be superior to either alone in the situation of an unknown primary. Although the use of PET-CT is now commonplace in the workup of the unknown primary, false-positives and false-negatives continue to be present, so direct inspection is very important.

Other Considerations

Panendoscopy with directed biopsies of the nasopharynx, tonsil, tongue base, and pyriform sinuses has been advocated for detection of occult carcinomas since the 1940s. The tonsillar fossa may often harbor occult malignancy followed by the base of the tongue. Tonsillectomy will detect malignancy in ~ 25 to 40% of patients, and most authors advocate bilateral tonsillectomy to maximize the yield of primary identification. Recent reports have advocated a transoral resection of the tongue base as well, identifying the occult primary in the majority of those patients who did not have a primary site identified during tonsillectomy and guided biopsies. Despite imaging and endoscopic evaluation, identification of the primary site may remain elusive in some patients due to (1) spontaneous regression of the tumor; (2) low tumor volume, which may be hidden within the crypts of the Waldeyer ring; or (3) submucosal origin of the tumor. Finally, a chest radiograph should be obtained to exclude a lung primary site, especially in patients with lower cervical metastasis.

In summary, identification of an occult tumor through physical examination and imaging studies has an important therapeutic impact. If a head and neck primary site is identified, a patient is treated as if he or she presented with that primary. Knowledge of the primary site allows for administration of a higher total radiation dose to the tumor site and substantially reduces the volume of tissue irradiated to the maximum dose levels. Conversely, complete surgical excision may be the treatment of choice for some primary sites. Thus localization of the primary site may increase the likelihood of local control, reduce side effects and late complications, and have the potential benefit of increasing patient survival.

■ Management and Treatment

At this juncture, the patient should be prepared for an examination under anesthesia and endoscopic evaluation of the nasopharynx, oropharynx, hypopharynx, larynx, and oral cavity. When the FNA is inconclusive, an open neck biopsy is indicated to obtain tissue for pathological examination. If an open neck biopsy is necessary, an excisional biopsy is preferable to avoid tumor spillage, and the incision should be appropriately placed so that it will not compromise further surgery. Surgical management is deferred until the diagnosis is certain.

With the patient under general anesthesia, direct visualization of the likely primary sites should be performed, including palpation of the nasopharynx, base of the tongue, and tonsil regions. Rigid endoscopy of the oropharynx, hypopharynx, and larynx is also performed. The esophagus can be evaluated by rigid or flexible esophagoscopy.

Biopsies of all suspicious areas should be performed, and frozen sections should be requested; however, random biopsies have a low yield and are not indicated. Directed biopsies may be obtained in areas of high probability, based on the predictability of lymphatic drainage and abnormalities seen on endoscopy. These areas would include the naso-

pharynx, tonsils, pyriform sinus, and base of the tongue. If a primary site is not identified, bilateral tonsillectomy is warranted because a malignancy may develop in one of the deep tonsillar crypts. With the foregoing diagnostic procedures, the majority of occult primary tumors will be identified. As noted previously, there are some authors who advocate transoral tongue base resection as well, which has been very successful in identifying the primary site in those who have not had their primaries identified, despite all the other procedures.

Despite a careful and thorough search, the origin of the primary tumor may remain elusive. The clinician must address management of the metastatic disease in the neck, and in the case of squamous cell carcinoma, the likely primary site(s) of origin. The traditional surgical approach for metastatic squamous carcinoma to the neck has been a radical neck dissection. Many authors have demonstrated the utility of performing less than a radical neck dissection for limited cervical metastasis when the neck has not been violated. The concept of performing a selective neck dissection for metastatic squamous cell carcinoma is based on the efficacy of radiotherapy to control microscopic disease once all gross disease is removed. Studies have shown external beam radiotherapy to be 90% effective for controlling occult disease in the neck.

For an N1 metastatic node in level I or II, a selective neck dissection is appropriate. This may take the form of a supraomohyoid (levels I, II, and III) or anterolateral (levels II, III, and IV) neck dissection. Unless there is radiographic evidence of extracapsular spread or fixation, the spinal accessory nerve, sternocleidomastoid, and internal jugular vein may be preserved. This dissection removes the lymph nodes in the submental and submandibular triangles, and the upper and midjugular lymph nodes as well. The posterior limit of the dissection is the posterior border of the sternocleidomastoid and the cutaneous branches of the cervical plexus. The inferior limit is the omohyoid muscle where it crosses the internal jugular vein. Whenever more extensive disease is encountered at the time of surgery, the dissection can be modified to include resection of the sternocleidomastoid muscle, internal jugular vein, or spinal accessory nerve. In addition, lymph nodes in levels IV and V can be removed as indicated.

Patients having more advanced neck disease (N2 or N3) will require a more extensive neck dissection due to higher incidence of extracapsular spread and the implications of multimodal disease. In these patients it is frequently necessary to sacrifice the sternocleidomastoid muscle and internal jugular vein. Provided the tumor is not in the upper posterior aspect of level II or along the posterior strip of level V, the spinal accessory nerve can generally be preserved. When an open neck biopsy has been performed, prior to the definitive surgical procedure a more extensive dissection is usually warranted as well.

In some instances, the neck biopsy will reveal metastatic carcinoma of the thyroid, malignant melanoma, or adenocarcinoma. When differentiated thyroid cancer is encountered, an ultrasound of the gland is obtained to search for the primary site. Further management will include a total thyroidectomy and ipsilateral neck dissection of levels II to V and VI. Melanoma metastatic from an unknown primary site in the absence of distant metastases requires a comprehensive neck dissection. Adenocarcinoma in the lower neck is usually metastatic from an infraclavicular primary tumor, and biopsy alone is sufficient. With metastatic adenocarcinoma in the upper neck, a salivary gland primary site should be excluded prior to performing a complete neck dissection, so primary site surgery can be included in the treatment plan.

Adjuvant Radiotherapy for Squamous Cell Carcinoma

For patients with cervical adenopathy in whom a suspected primary head and neck tumor cannot be found, several treatment options are available. These include (1) neck dissection alone, (2) neck dissection combined with radiotherapy to the dissected neck, (3) elective irradiation of the mucosal sites at risk and the contralateral neck, and (4) the use of chemotherapy concurrent with the radiation.

Outcome data are available on the effectiveness of surgery as a single-modality treatment for isolated metastatic squamous cell carcinoma to levels I and II. When no extracapsular spread is identified and a single positive lymph node metastasis is present, careful observation without the addition of postoperative radiation is justified. Close follow-up is essential to diagnose the primary tumor, should it become apparent. However, subsequent failure in the dissected neck will decrease the ultimate control in the surgical area and survival.

Comprehensive adjuvant radiotherapy following neck dissection for patients with metastatic squamous cell carcinoma to the neck from an unknown primary is controversial. Nevertheless, well-established criteria exist for treatment to the neck based on important pathological findings. Key pathological data include the number of lymph nodes involved, the levels of involvement, and the presence or absence of extracapsular spread. Indications for postoperative radiation are (1) multiple positive nodes, (2) multiple levels of involvement, (3) extracapsular spread, and (4) prior open neck biopsy.

If elective radiation is to be administered, it should cover the likely mucosal sites of origin and

both sides of the neck with a boost to the operated neck. Therefore, patients receive external beam radiotherapy to the nasopharynx, oropharynx, hypopharynx, and larynx. Treatment morbidity is often significant and includes xerostomia, loss of taste, sore throat, and weight loss during the course of treatment. Xerostomia is generally permanent, and progressive neck fibrosis may also occur. If indications exist for treatment of the neck, then the likely primary sources should also receive comprehensive radiation. The benefits of radiotherapy are that it can improve local control in an operated high-risk neck, and it can reduce the risk for emergence of a mucosal primary site and contralateral neck disease. Mucosal emergence rates after comprehensive neck irradiation are in the ranges of 2 to 13% (median 9.5%) and 5 to 44% (median 8%) after unilateral neck irradiation. There are no compelling data that single-neck radiation and comprehensive-neck irradiation differ in outcome. Although radiotherapy has not clearly been shown to increase survival, it is important to improve control above the clavicles.

As has been the case with the larynx and pharynx, chemotherapy is also employed in the primary and adjuvant treatment of the unknown primary. Because spread to the neck places the patient in at least stage 3, and chemotherapy with irradiation has been shown to be beneficial in advanced-stage patients, many patients receive chemotherapy with their irradiation. This increases both the control rates and the toxicities, so it is important to balance the benefit and the morbidity for each patient. In general, however, a platinum-based drug or a taxane should be administered if radiation is delivered. Concurrent delivery has been shown more effective than neoadjuvant chemotherapy and is also recommended if the patient can tolerate it. The use of an epidermal growth factor receptor (EGFR) inhibitor with the radiation may also be considered if a patient is not a candidate for platinum or taxanes.

Outcome

Factors affecting regional control and survival following treatment for metastatic cancer to the neck from an unknown primary site depend on (1) the histological type of cancer; (2) the volume or stage of disease in the neck; (3) the presence of extracapsular spread, particularly for squamous carcinoma; and (4) the location of the metastasis.

The overall survival rate for patients with occult metastatic squamous cell carcinoma to the neck is in the range of 50 to 60% at 5 years. Although a decrease in survival has been reported with subsequent appearance of the primary tumor, the data are conflicting, with some demonstrating worse prognosis and others showing no difference. Metastatic adenocarcinoma to the supraclavicular area generally originates below the clavicles and has a poor prognosis, with few patients surviving beyond 6 to 12 months. For patients with squamous cell carcinoma to the supraclavicular area, long-term survival is ~ 15%. In contrast, metastatic differentiated thyroid cancer has an excellent prognosis.

Control in the neck is also dependent on stage. Regional control rates for combined surgery and radiation for metastatic N1 disease in the setting of the unknown primary is ~ 80%, but falls to 30% for patients with N3 disease. Extracapsular spread is associated with more advanced nodal stage, a higher regional recurrence rate, and poorer survival despite combined therapy. Data are conflicting on the potential adverse effect of incisional biopsy performed prior to the definitive procedure. Some studies have shown that pretreatment open neck biopsy increases the risk of regional complications and distant metastasis. Other studies have found no difference in survival or recurrence if the neck was biopsied prior to definitive treatment.

Long-term follow-up is needed to identify the emergence of a primary tumor site. Approximately 6 to 22% of patients with metastatic squamous cell carcinoma will develop an obvious primary tumor. Patients who receive comprehensive radiation to the likely mucosal sites of origin and the neck have a lower incidence of clinical appearance of the occult primary. Although neck control has improved in patients with metastatic squamous cell carcinoma who receive combined modality therapy, an improvement in overall survival is not evident. Multiple factors are contributory and include disseminated disease, relapse in the neck among patients with advanced regional disease, and the development of second primary tumors. Nevertheless, it is mandatory that these patients have frequent and close follow-up, so that should the primary become identifiable, it may be treated with surgery and/or radiation.

■ Summary

A systematic approach is necessary to evaluate the neck mass in an adult suspected of having metastatic disease. In the high-risk patient, FNA will determine the etiology of the mass and focus the search for the primary site. Imaging and staging endoscopy should follow. Open biopsy is seldom necessary as an initial procedure, unless FNA is inconclusive. For squamous carcinoma metastatic to the neck from an unknown primary site, a neck dissection is indicated to remove all gross disease. Neck dissection alone is adequate for patients with small N1 disease at levels I or II without extracapsular spread and in whom the primary tumor is not identified. For patients with more advanced neck disease, a comprehensive neck dissection with radiation to the neck and potential primary sites is indicated. Concurrent chemotherapy and radiotherapy also constitute a valid option for initial treatment as well. Current guidelines for therapy may be found at http://www.nccn.org/professionals/physician_gls/f_guidelines.asp.

■ Suggested Reading

Balaker AE, Abemayor E, Elashoff D, St John MA. Cancer of unknown primary: does treatment modality make a difference? Laryngoscope 2012;122(6):1279–1282

Cianchetti M, Mancuso AA, Amdur RJ, et al. Diagnostic evaluation of squamous cell carcinoma metastatic to cervical lymph nodes from an unknown head and neck primary site. Laryngoscope 2009;119(12):2348–2354

Iganej S, Kagan R, Anderson P, et al. Metastatic squamous cell carcinoma of the neck from an unknown primary: management options and patterns of relapse. Head Neck 2002;24(3):236–246

Mehta V, Johnson P, Tassler A, et al. A new paradigm for the diagnosis and management of unknown primary tumors of the head and neck: a role for transoral robotic surgery. Laryngoscope 2013;123(1):146–151

Miller FR, Karnad AB, Eng T, Hussey DH, Stan McGuff H, Otto RA. Management of the unknown primary carcinoma: long-term follow-up on a negative PET scan and negative panendoscopy. Head Neck 2008;30(1):28–34

National Comprehensive Cancer Network. www.nccn.org

Nieder C, Gregoire V, Ang KK. Cervical lymph node metastases from occult squamous cell carcinoma: cut down a tree to get an apple? Int J Radiat Oncol Biol Phys 2001;50(3):727–733

Wong WL, Sonoda LI, Gharpurhy A, et al. 18F-fluorodeoxyglucose positron emission tomography/computed tomography in the assessment of occult primary head and neck cancers—an audit and review of published studies. Clin Oncol (R Coll Radiol) 2012;24(3):190–195

43 The N0 Neck: Diagnostic Evaluation and Management of Upper Aerodigestive Tract Malignancies

◼ Introduction

The management of patients with an N0 neck with head and neck squamous cell carcinoma (HNSCC) remains controversial. Definitive data regarding the management of the neck in this situation are not currently available. The primary options have been elective neck dissection (END), radiation therapy, or observation. Recent investigations have evaluated the role of sentinel lymph node biopsy (SLNB), especially for early T stage tumors (e.g., T1–2 oral cavity SCC [OCSCC]), but the indications remain unclear.

Incidence/Epidemiology

Depending on the anatomical subsite, the likelihood of nodal metastasis is quite variable relative to primary tumor stage. The decision to potentially treat the N0 neck requires the determination of an appropriate treatment threshold that balances the potential benefits of treatment and possible treatment-related morbidity. This predefined threshold for action serves as a framework for the interpretation of the risk for nodal metastases. The often-quoted treatment threshold of 20% was derived by Weiss et al using a decision tree analysis. This analysis was based on the risk of nodal disease, the effectiveness of primary and salvage surgery, and a subjective assignment of the usefulness of treatment outcomes. More recent studies have recommended treatment thresholds between 17 and 40%. However, there is an overall lack of high-quality evidence surrounding any of these treatment thresholds. Rather than serving as absolute values that define when treatment is appropriate, they should serve as guidelines to support clinical judgment.

The incidence of nodal metastases for various sites and stages of the primary cancer of the head and neck has been reported by many authors (**Table 43.1**). Certain sites, such as the base of the tongue, tonsil, and supraglottis, have a richer lymphatic supply and are more likely to have nodal metastases. Generally, the larger the tumor, the greater the likelihood of lymph node metastases. The term *occult node* represents a clinically negative neck with a pathological positive lymph node. Numerous papers have shown certain sites have a higher incidence of occult nodal disease, and that the higher the T stage, the higher the incidence of occult nodes. In principle, the neck should not require treatment if no metastases exist. The problem is that occult nodes may be present due to the inaccuracies of evaluation, either palpation or diagnostic imaging.

Regional lymph node metastases are the most important prognostic factor for survival in patients with HNSCC. Neck staging should include both the clinical exam and various diagnostic tests. For many years, clinical palpation was the standard for staging a neck, and the inaccuracy was as high as 50%, even when the examiners were experienced. Current staging should take into account more objective tests, such as ultrasonography, magnetic resonance imaging (MRI), and computed tomography (CT). This chapter focuses specifically on HNSCC, although the general principles apply to other upper aerodigestive tract malignancies.

Relevant Anatomy

Classification of Cervical Nodes

Although superior mediastinal nodes were previously defined as level VII, efforts to create consensus on lymph node classification have recommended using an anatomical name to define a region outside the typical boundaries of the neck. Thus the superior mediastinal lymph nodes extend from the suprasternal notch to the innominate artery, including lymph nodes in the anterosuperior mediastinum and tracheoesophageal grooves.

Table 43.1 Incidence of cervical node metastases based on primary tumor site

Primary tumor	T stage	Nodal metastasis rate (%)
Oral tongue[1]	T1	18
Oral tongue[1]	T2	33
Oral tongue[1]	T3	60
Floor of mouth[2]	T1	38
Floor of mouth[2]	T2	65
Floor of mouth[2]	T3	71
Oropharynx[3]	Tx	72
Supraglottis[4]	Tx	33
Supraglottis[5]	T1–3	22
Supraglottis[5]	T4	44
Transglottic[6]	Tx	52
Subglottis[4]	Tx	19
Hypopharynx[6]	T2	63
Hypopharynx[6]	T3	68
Hypopharynx[6]	T4	100

Data from:
1. Mendelsohn BC, Woods JE, Beahrs OH. Neck dissection in the treatment of carcinoma of the anterior two-thirds of the tongue. Surg Gynecol Obstet 1976;143:75–80.
2. Krause CJ, Lee JG, McCabe BF. Carcinoma of the oral cavity. Arch Otolaryngol 1973;97:354–358.
3. Shah JP. Patterns of cervical lymph node metastasis from squamous carcinomas of the upper aerodigestive tract. Am J Surg 1990:160:405–409.
4. McGavran MH, Bauer WC, Ogura HL. The incidence of cervical lymph node metastases from epidermoid carcinoma of the larynx and their relationship to certain characteristics of the primary tumor: a study based on the clinical and pathological findings for 96 patients treated by primary en bloc laryngectomy and radical neck dissection. Cancer 1961;14:55–66.
5. Gavilan C, Gavilan J. Five-year results of functional neck dissection for cancer of the larynx. Arch Otolaryngol Head Neck Surg 1989;115:1193–1196.
6. Murakami Y, Ikari T, Haraguchi S, et al. A rationale for bilateral neck dissection in hypopharynx cancer surgery: a histological analysis of metastatic nodes in the neck. Keio J Med 1987;36:399–406.

■ Evaluation

Although a thorough history and physical examination are critical for every patient with an upper aerodigestive tract malignancy, there are no specific signs and symptoms that would suggest occult neck disease. The site of the primary lesion provides a basis for determining the risk of occult cervical lymph node metastasis. As previously mentioned, the staging of the neck for metastases includes palpation and clinical tests, such as ultrasonography, CT, or MRI.

Assessment of the N0 neck is typically done in the context of imaging of the primary tumor. The identification of an enlarged lymph node does not necessarily mean the lymph node contains cancer. Therefore, the workup should involve not only identifying enlarged lymph nodes but also determining whether they are positive or negative for cancer.

By definition, an N0 neck is one that has no clinical evidence of regional lymph node metastases. Because of the inaccuracy of palpation for cervical lymph nodes, some guidelines for obtaining additional tests can be established. Given the changing landscape of medical care, every conceivable imaging test available for evaluating the neck cannot and should not be ordered. The factors that need to be considered include (1) the patient's neck size, (2) the site of the primary tumor, (3) the stage of the primary tumor, and (4) previous treatment.

Examining a patient with a long and thin neck for nodes using palpation can be very accurate. On the other hand, a patient with a short or full neck can be very difficult to evaluate by palpation. If other factors, such as an advanced-stage primary cancer, are present, imaging tests should be considered.

The site of the primary cancer is important. Certain sites, such as the floor of the mouth, tongue, pharynx, and supraglottic larynx, have a richer lymphatic supply and are more likely to have nodal metastases. The stage of the primary is also important, with the incidence of node metastases increasing as the stage increases. Previous treatment can also be an important factor. Secondary primaries are not uncommon, and the patient may have had previous surgery or radiation therapy, which can make it difficult to assess the neck by palpation and thus increase the importance of imaging.

Imaging

Computed Tomography

CT became available in the 1970s, and over the years it has gained widespread popularity in the staging of head and neck cancer. Many studies demonstrate the advantages of CT over palpation. High-resolution CT scanning can give excellent anatomical information. An iodine-containing contrast agent given intravenously during a CT scan can enable the examiner to reliably discriminate between lymph nodes, vessels, muscles, and salivary glands. If a lymph node is identified with CT, the question is whether the node has metastatic cancer.

Several different radiological criteria can be used to assess the presence or absence of metastasis in the lymph nodes. These criteria include the maximal axial diameter, the irregular enhancement due to tumor necrosis, the shape of the nodes, and the grouping of nodes. Of these criteria, irregular contrast enhancement in nodes is the most reliable criterion. It can represent tumor necrosis, cystic tumor growth, or avascular keratinization. Adipose metaplasia in lymph nodes may stimulate tumor necrosis and can give a false-positive.

The cost of a CT scan is usually less than half the cost of MRI and has a similar predictive value. However, CT exposes patients to ionizing radiation.

Magnetic Resonance Imaging

MRI is based on the principle of nuclear magnetic resonance. Energy is absorbed and subsequently released by nuclei, following excitation by electromagnetic waves of a specific resonant frequency. The acquisition of these data and subsequent image generation are beyond the scope of this chapter. The use of paramagnetic contrast agents, such as gadolinium-diethylenetriamine pentaacetic acid (Gd-DTPA) has further increased the soft tissue discrimination potentials of MRI, by selective enhancement of mucosal linings, tumor tissue, and inflammatory lesions. MRI has the advantage of being able to discriminate soft tissues.

MRI has been compared with palpation to detect cervical lymph node metastases. The accuracy of gadolinium-enhanced MRI was found to be over 80%, compared with under 70% for palpation. The use of MRI reliably upstaged nearly two-thirds of the necks that were deemed negative by palpation. However, MRI should not be the only criterion for selecting patients for prophylactic neck treatment. On MRI, nodes are interpreted as malignant if (1) central necrosis is depicted, (2) the minimal axial diameter of nodes exceeds 11 mm in the subdigastric region or 10 mm in other lymph node regions, and (3) groups of three or more borderline nodes are seen in the first or second echelons of the primary tumor.

MRI is an expensive imaging technique and does not seem to have a clear advantage over other methods. There is no ionizing radiation exposure with MRI.

Ultrasonography and Ultrasound-Guided Fine-Needle Aspiration Cytology (FNAC)

Ultrasonography uses the reflected high-frequency sound waves that are intermittently generated and detected by piezoelectric crystals in a transducer as a signal. By electric transformation and computerized processing, the reflected sound waves are transformed into a two-dimensional image. For the neck, 7.5 to 10 megahertz transducers give the best resolution. Because bone and air interfaces reflect all sound waves, no signal from underlying structures can be visualized.

Most studies involving ultrasonography of the neck show that ultrasound (US) is superior to palpation for the detection and quantification of cervical lymph node metastasis. However, US alone does not enable differentiation between enlarged reactive nodes and enlarged metastatic nodes. This can be explained by the fact that US does not reliably depict tumor cells, necrotic tumor tissue, or tumor keratinization in lymph nodes.

In a prospective study on the value of US and US-guided FNAC for the assessment of the N0 neck authors in the Netherlands determined that US alone is an unreliable method for detecting occult lymph node metastases. They found that the accuracy never exceeded 70%, with a sensitivity of 60% and a specificity of 77%. In contrast, US-guided FNAC had an accuracy of 89%, a sensitivity of 76%, and a specificity of 100%. The authors concluded that the sensitivity and specificity of the US-guided FNAC were higher than those reported for CT or MRI in the literature and recommended that this technique play an important role in directing treatment of the palpably negative neck. Thus far, however, this modality has not gained widespread acceptance. There is no radiation exposure with US, and US-guided FNAC is usually less expensive than CT or MRI.

Positron-Emission Tomography (PET)

PET uses metabolic imaging agents that are positron emitters. This imaging modality evaluates metabolic activity and perhaps cell proliferation of any site in the body, such as cervical lymph nodes. Fusion of PET and CT images provides anatomical localization of areas of increased metabolic activity. Although these imaging characteristics suggest the potential for improved detection of occult nodal metastases, prospective data are still being acquired. Meta-analysis of studies comparing PET, US, CT, and MRI have not established a clear advantage for any of these modalities in the setting of an N0 neck.

PET imaging is relatively expensive compared with the other modalities, and the evolution of its role in assessment of the N0 neck and unknown primary disease continues.

Other Imaging Modalities

Lymphoscintigraphy involves the local injection of sulfur colloid labeled with technetium (Tc)-99m to depict the anatomy of the lymphatic drainage pathways. For melanoma this technique can be helpful to identify the first echelon or "sentinel" node(s) for biopsy purposes when deciding whether further surgery is indicated. Evidence has been accruing with regard to this imaging modality and lymph node mapping for early-stage oral cavity tumors.

Although palpation of the neck has been the most common method of evaluating the neck for metastases, it is important to consider performing imaging techniques to make the neck evaluation more accurate. At present, no single test will ensure that the clinical N0 neck will be a pathological staged N0 neck. Currently, it appears that the best test available to detect occult metastatic neck disease may be US-guided FNAC. However, this test is not 100% accurate and depends a great deal on the skill and motivation of the examiner and the cytopathologist.

Many patients require CT or MRI for staging of their primary tumor. If the CT or MRI leaves no doubt about the nodal status, then no US-guided FNAC is needed. However, if the nodal staging is unsure with CT or MRI or if no CT or MRI has been obtained and palpation is not clearly positive, then a US-guided FNAC of the neck is indicated. The most accurate assessment for an N0 neck would be an END and pathological evaluation of the nodes. However, even this assessment is not 100% accurate because of the possibility of missing micrometastases in lymph nodes histologically. In this situation, an END would serve as a staging procedure to determine prognosis and adjuvant treatment.

■ Management

If no cervical metastases are present, the neck should not require treatment. However, based on the previous discussion, it is difficult to be absolutely sure that occult metastases do not exist. For head and neck cancer patients, the status of the cervical lymph nodes is the single most important tumor-related prognostic factor. Prognosis can decrease by 50% if lymph node metastases are present at initial presentation or develop during follow-up; therefore, it is important to know the neck node status as accurately as possible to make a rational decision regarding treatment. The major dilemma is whether delayed treatment has an adverse effect on prognosis. The options for management of the N0 neck include (1) observation, (2) END, and (3) elective irradiation. A potential role for SLNB is developing with respect to OCSCC.

Observation

If diagnostic evaluation techniques were more accurate, the no-treatment option would be more popular. The most important disadvantage of elective treatment of the neck is that many patients are treated unnecessarily. These patients face the risk of postoperative complications and functional or aesthetic problems unnecessarily.

There is still no proof that prophylactic treatment versus delayed therapeutic treatment improves prognosis. Most studies on this subject found a benefit of END over therapeutic neck dissection on survival, but these were primarily retrospective analyses. Several reports from the MD Anderson Cancer Center show

that a combination of a "wait-and-see" policy for patients with an N0 neck and treating the neck when clinically positive nodes appear may be successful in controlling regional disease. However, because these patients are at an increased risk of developing distant metastasis, they have a poorer prognosis. Only four prospective studies have been reported, and none has demonstrated a significant difference in overall survival. Unfortunately, the most significant limitation of currently available studies is the lack of adequate statistical power to detect a meaningful difference in survival.

Critical factors in the strategy of observation include patient compliance for follow-up and the effectiveness of salvage surgery in patients who develop delayed node metastases. Retrospective studies have demonstrated a relatively high proportion of patients who return will do so with advanced cervical disease that is not operable. Most head and neck surgeons are predisposed to believe that a delay of treatment will have an adverse effect on survival; therefore, the wait-and-see policy is unpopular.

Patients who are profoundly ill, have significant comorbidities, or are elderly may be appropriate for observation of the neck.

Elective Neck Dissection

The incidence of occult nodal metastases per site and T stage has been widely reported. Generally, the larger the tumor, the greater the likelihood of lymph node metastases. Based on the information available from the literature, it is fairly easy to give a probability figure for occult metastases for a given site and stage of the primary tumor. Most head and neck surgeons and radiation therapists believe that a frequency of occult lymph node metastases approaching 15 to 20% is enough to justify the elective treatment of cervical nodes. Other indications include (1) if the neck must be entered for excision of the primary tumor, (2) if a patient is judged to be unreliable for follow-up visits, or (3) if the primary tumor is able to be managed solely with surgery.

For the N0 neck, there is little justification for a radical neck dissection. The primary type of neck dissection used for the N0 neck would be the selective neck dissection. This is based on the predictable pattern of lymphatic spread in previously untreated cancers. Of the selective neck dissections, the most commonly used would be the supraomohyoid, the lateral, and the posterolateral neck dissections. The supraomohyoid neck dissection includes nodes in levels I, II, and III; the lateral neck dissection includes levels II, III, and IV; and the posterolateral neck dissection includes nodes in levels II, III, IV, and V and the suboccipital and retroauricular nodes.

The supraomohyoid neck dissection is the appropriate treatment for T1–4, N0 SCC of the oral cavity, although consideration should be made to also remove level IV nodes. Node metastases from cancers in the oral cavity have been shown to be related to the thickness of the lesion versus the diameter. A thickness of more than 2 mm histologically has a significantly higher rate of node metastasis, and depth of invasion should be considered when considering an END. Some surgeons suggest that 4 mm depth of invasion may be a better predictor of occult nodal metastasis.

The lateral neck dissection is the appropriate treatment for T1–4, N0 of the oropharynx, hypopharynx, supraglottic larynx, and T3–4, N0 of the glottic larynx. Dissection of the posterior triangle (level V) should be considered for T3–4, N0 of the base of the tongue. In cases where a cancer approaches or crosses the midline, a bilateral neck dissection is indicated. These sites include the tip of the tongue, floor of the mouth, base of the tongue, and epiglottis.

Elective Radiation Therapy

Elective irradiation has been proposed as an alternative to END to control microscopic or occult cervical node metastases. Fletcher reported over 20 years ago that metastatic lymph nodes < 2 cm can be sterilized with 5,000 cGy or more of irradiation. It would be unusual for an N0 neck, assessed with palpation and one of the imaging techniques, to have nodes 2 cm or larger. Therefore, elective irradiation should be effective in controlling occult metastasis. Several reports showed a 13 to 19% recurrence in the neck after elective radiotherapy, which improved to 1 to 4% after excluding patients who had developed recurrence at the primary site.

The main advantages of radiotherapy as treatment in the clinically negative neck are the apparent decreased incidence of cervical recurrences in the ipsilateral and contralateral neck and the ease of administering radiotherapy to the neck when the primary lesion is being irradiated. The disadvantages of radiotherapy are that (1) many patients may undergo unnecessary treatment if radiotherapy is routinely administered; (2) morbidity and mortality are increased if subsequent surgical therapy is needed; (3) a large field of radiotherapy increases problems

during treatment, especially mucositis, pain, and weight loss; (4) long-term side effects, such as dryness of the mouth and pharynx, as well as fibrosis of the neck tissues, usually occur; and (5) radiation fibrosis increases the difficulty of diagnosing recurrent disease, especially in patients with a thick neck.

Sentinel Lymph Node Biopsy (SLNB)

There has been increasing interest in the use of SLNB for early-stage OCSCC. Evidence of potential effectiveness has come primarily from retrospective series from Europe. A multi-institutional American College of Surgeons Oncology Group trial in the United States also demonstrated the feasibility and safety of the procedure for T1–2, N0 OCSCC. Negative predictive value on routine analysis was 94% when comparing the pathology findings from the sentinel lymph node(s) and END nodes. The surgeon's experience with SLNB also improves the accuracy of the procedure. There is also some suggestion that SLNB may be less morbid than END.

The available evidence supports the need for continued examination of SLNB for staging the neck for early-stage OCSCC in clinical trials. Results from the multi-institutional prospective European trial are expected to be reported soon and should provide more information regarding the procedure.

◼ Controversial Issues

Several prospective trials are currently accruing patients to address the issue of observation versus END for OCSCC.

◼ Practice Guidelines, Consensus Statements, and Measures

The National Comprehensive Cancer Network guidelines provide recommendations with regard to neck dissection for specific disease stage (TNM [tumor-node-metastasis]) at each physical subsite.

■ Suggested Reading

Ferlito A, Robbins KT, Shah JP, et al. Proposal for a rational classification of neck dissections. Head Neck 2011;33(3):445–450

Liao LJ, Lo WC, Hsu WL, Wang CT, Lai MS. Detection of cervical lymph node metastasis in head and neck cancer patients with clinically N0 neck—a meta-analysis comparing different imaging modalities. BMC Cancer 2012;12:236

Robbins KT, Shaha AR, Medina JE, et al; Committee for Neck Dissection Classification, American Head and Neck Society. Consensus statement on the classification and terminology of neck dissection. Arch Otolaryngol Head Neck Surg 2008;134(5):536–538

van den Brekel MW, Catelijns JA, Stel HV, et al. Occut metastatic neck disease: detection with US and US-guided fine-needle aspiration cytology. Radiology 1991;180(2):457–461

van den Brekel MW, Stel HV, Castelijns JA, et al. Cervical lymph node metastasis: assessment of radiologic criteria. Radiology 1990;177(2):379–384

Weiss MH, Harrison LB, Isaacs RS. Use of decision analysis in planning a management strategy for the stage N0 neck. Arch Otolaryngol Head Neck Surg 1994;120(7):699–702

44 The N+ Neck: Diagnostic Evaluation and Management of Upper Aerodigestive Tract Malignancies

■ Introduction

Regional metastatic disease in patients with squamous carcinoma of the upper aerodigestive tract (UADT) adversely impacts disease-specific survival (DSS). Over the past decade, the role of radiation therapy and surgery in the management of node positive (N+) disease has become better defined, and the survival benefit of chemotherapy and other novel therapeutic modalities has been rigorously evaluated. This chapter reviews the evaluation and management of N+ patients diagnosed with cancer arising from a known primary site and who are being treated with curative intent.

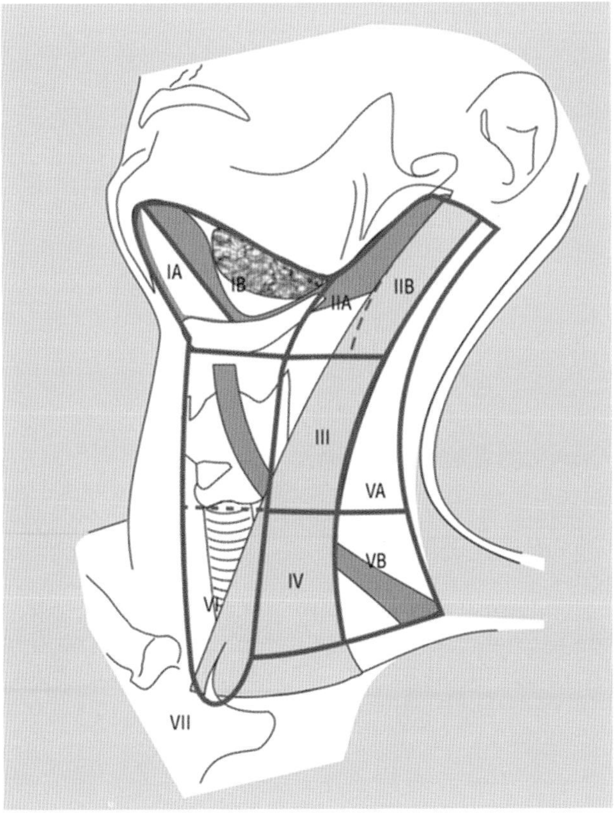

Classification of Cervical Lymph Nodes

Historically, the cervical lymph nodes were thought to be organized into "chains" that were named by their proximity to nearby anatomical structures or by their topographical distribution, such as the "spinal accessory chain," which was synonymous with the posterior cervical nodes, or the "transverse cervical chain," which was synonymous with the supraclavicular lymph nodes. This nomenclature has been supplanted by the "level"-based system, which uses anatomical boundaries to divide the lymph node groups on either side of the neck into six levels and six sublevels. These lymph node groups and their corresponding levels include the following: submental (IA) and submandibular (IB); upper jugular (IIA and IIB); middle jugular (III); lower jugular (IV); posterior triangle (VA and VB); and anterior compartment (VI). Although superior mediastinal nodes were previously defined as level VII, efforts to create consensus on lymph node classification have recommended using an anatomical name to define a region outside the typical boundaries of the neck. Thus the superior mediastinal lymph nodes extend from the suprasternal notch to the innominate artery, including lymph nodes in the anterosuperior mediastinum and tracheoesophageal grooves. Cancer of the UADT typically requires evaluation, and potentially management, of lymph node levels I through V on both sides of the neck (**Table 44.1; Fig. 44.1**).

Fig. 44.1 Anatomical structures defining the boundaries of the neck levels and sublevels.

Table 44.1   Anatomical structures defining the boundaries of the neck levels and sublevels

Level	Boundary			
	Superior	Inferior	Anterior (medial)	Posterior (lateral)
IA	Symphysis of mandible	Body of hyoid	Anterior belly of contralateral digastric muscle	Anterior belly of ipsilateral digastric muscle
IB	Body of mandible	Posterior belly of muscle	Anterior belly of digastric muscle	Stylohyoid muscle
IIA	Skull base	Horizontal plane defined by the inferior body of the hyoid bone	Stylohyoid muscle	Vertical plane defined by the spinal accessory nerve
IIB	Skull base	Horizontal plane defined by the inferior body of the hyoid bone	Vertical plane defined by the spinal accessory nerve	Lateral border of the sternocleidomastoid muscle
III	Horizontal plane defined by inferior body of hyoid	Horizontal plane defined by the inferior border of the cricoid cartilage	Lateral border of the sternohyoid muscle	Lateral border of the sternocleidomastoid or sensory branches of cervical plexus
IV	Horizontal plane defined by the inferior border of the cricoid cartilage	Clavicle	Lateral border of the sternohyoid muscle	Lateral border of the sternocleidomastoid or sensory branches of cervical plexus
VA	Apex of the convergence of the sternocleidomastoid and trapezius muscles	Horizontal plane defined by the lower border of the cricoid cartilage	Posterior border of the sternocleidomastoid muscle or sensory branches of cervical plexus	Anterior border of the trapezius muscle
VB	Horizontal plane defined by the lower border of the cricoid cartilage	Clavicle	Posterior border of the sternocleidomastoid muscle or sensory branches of cervical plexus	Anterior border of the trapezius muscle
VI	Hyoid bone	Suprasternal	Common carotid artery	Common carotid artery

Data from Deschler DG, ed. Quick Reference Guide to TNM Staging of head and Neck Cancer and Neck Dissection Classification, 4th ed. Alexandria, VA: American Academy of Otolaryngology–Head and Neck Surgery Foundation; 2014.

■ Initial Diagnostic Evaluation

Clinical Presentation

Head and neck cancer patients with clinically positive nodes typically report a history of a painless unilateral neck mass that has been slowly enlarging over the course of months. Metastatic spread to the lymph nodes generally follows a predictable pattern based on the primary tumor site. Large retrospective series that used histopathological assessment to evaluate the lymph nodes harvested from neck dissection specimens have characterized the typical patterns of regional metastatic spread (**Table 44.2**). Based on this knowledge of the patterns of nodal metastasis, the location of a metastatic node may help to identify the primary tumor site in a patient with an unknown primary site .

Physical Examination

Palpation of cervical lymph node metastases typically underestimates the size of clinically positive nodes, especially if the lymph node measures < 3 cm in diameter. The sensitivity and specificity of palpation of metastatic cervical lymph nodes are both in the range of 60 to 70%. Therefore, imaging should always be performed in the case of lymph node metastases.

Radiographic Evaluation

Contrast-enhanced computed tomography (CT) and contrast-enhanced magnetic resonance imaging (MRI) provide excellent anatomical imaging that permits systematic comprehensive evaluation of the

Table 44.2   Pattern of cervical lymphatic drainage by head and neck subsite

	Neck level								
	IA	IB	II	III	IV	V	VI	VII	RP
Oral cavity		X	X	X					
Lip	X								
Anterior mandibular alveolar ridge	X								
Floor of mouth	X								
Anterior nasal cavity		X							
Nasal cavity			X						
Nasopharynx			X	X		X			X
Soft tissues and structures of the midface		X	X						
Maxilla		X	X						X
Oropharynx			X	X	X				X
Hypopharynx			X	X	X				X
Pyriform sinus (apex)							X		X
Larynx			X	X	X		X		
Cervical esophagus					X		X		X
Thyroid					X		X	X	

Abbreviation: RP, retropharynx.

cervical lymph nodes. Contrast-enhanced imaging is essential to appreciate parenchymal changes within nodes that may be due to small metastatic deposits and to distinguish lymph nodes from vessels. Lymph node metastasis may be suggested by increased lymph node size, changes in morphology, and/or the presence of internal defects. Lymph node size is a relatively poor predictor of malignancy because small nodes may contain micrometastases and larger nodes may be inflamed or hyperplastic. In addition, normal lymph node size differs by location, with normal level II nodes measuring up to 15 mm. In cases where the risk of cervical metastasis is likely unilateral, comparison with the contralateral nodes at the same level may increase suspicion for metastasis. Comparison with lymph node morphology has also been associated with the presence of nodal metastases: normal or reactive lymph nodes are typically flat and ovoid, whereas malignant lymph nodes are more likely to be round. However, malignant nodes harboring micrometastases frequently maintain their ovoid shape and lymph nodes in the parotid and submandibular regions are frequently round, limiting the predictive value of shape as a criterion for malignancy. Central nodal necrosis is a late finding of nodal metastatic disease with a specificity of 95%. Early indicators of metastatic disease include the presence of focal parenchymal defects such as areas of low density or lucency, focal enhancement, and/or dystrophic calcification. These parenchymal abnormalities, which are frequently found in the periphery of the node, are particularly useful in identifying metastatic nodes measuring less < 1 cm. CT detects focal metastatic deposits with greater sensitivity and accuracy than MRI. However, MRI may be preferred over CT to evaluate for carotid artery invasion or encasement, tracheal or esophageal invasion, and prevertebral fascia invasion, and to evaluate patterns of submucosal tumor invasion in areas such as the nasopharynx and base of the tongue. Ultrasonography, which is less expensive than other diagnostic imaging modalities and can be performed in real time, permits fine-needle aspiration for cytological diagnosis of malignancy. Ultrasonographic features that increase the likelihood of malignancy include (1) increased size; (2) round shape, as defined by a short axis to long axis ratio of > 0.5; 3) irregular nodal borders, which suggest extracapsular spread (ECS); (4) the absence of an echogenic lymph node hilum, which suggests tumor infiltration of the hilum; (5) intranodal necrosis, changes in architecture or calcifications, and; (6) increased peripheral vasculature. It is also an accurate and useful means of reevaluating cervical lymphadenopathy for cancer surveillance after definitive therapy. The role of positron-emission tomography and computed tomography (PET-CT) for initial nodal staging of UADT malignancies has not been defined. A recent systematic review that was performed to evaluate the utility of PET for staging patients with head and neck cancer concluded that PET should be used when conventional imaging is equivocal or in situations where treatment recommendations could be significantly modified. Because PET-CT cannot detect small metastatic foci, it should be used to supplement anatomically based axial imaging such as CT or MRI that can detect subtle intranodal changes. PET-CT may also be used to aid in the localization of unknown primary tumors, evaluate for distant metastatic disease, and identify infraclavicular malignancy when an isolated metastatic level IV or supraclavicular lymph node is present.

Tissue Diagnosis

In most situations, biopsy of the primary tumor site is preferred as part of the initial diagnostic evaluation. However, cytological assessment using ultrasound- or CT-guided fine-needle aspiration (FNA) or core needle biopsy may be required if the primary tumor site has not been identified or if biopsy of the primary site is contraindicated (e.g., medical comorbidity). Open cervical lymph node biopsy should not be performed because histological diagnosis can usually be achieved via biopsy of the primary tumor or FNA, and this procedure has been associated with poorer treatment outcomes in at least one retrospective study. However, the association between open cervical lymph node biopsy and its impact on survival remains controversial given that subsequent research has not shown an adverse impact on survival if patients were treated with definitive radiation therapy (RT) following open biopsy.

Staging

Nodal staging using the universally adopted tumor, node, metastasis (TNM) staging system is identical for cancers arising from the oral cavity, oropharynx, hypopharynx, and larynx. The presence of a single ipsilateral cervical lymph node metastasis measuring 3 cm or less in greatest diameter is designated as N1. The nodal stage is designated as N2 if there is (1) a lymph node > 3 cm but not > 6 cm in greatest diameter; (2) multiple ipsilateral nodes ≤ 6 cm in diameter; or (3) bilateral or contralateral nodes. Metastasis in a lymph node measuring > 6 cm is designated as N3 (**Table 44.3**).

All possible TNM permutations are assigned to a stage grouping of I through IV based on progno-

Table 44.3 Staging of regional lymph nodes

	Oral cavity, oropharynx, hypopharynx, larynx	Nasopharynx
NX	Regional lymph nodes cannot be assessed	
N0	No regional lymph node metastasis	
N1	Metastasis in a single ipsilateral lymph node ≤ 3 cm	Unilateral metastasis in lymph node(s), ≤ 6 cm, above the supraclavicular fossa,[a] and/or unilateral or bilateral retropharyngeal lymph nodes ≤ 6 cm (midline nodes are considered ipsilateral nodes)
N2		Bilateral metastasis, ≤ 6 cm, above the supraclavicular fossa[a]
N2a	Metastasis in a single ipsilateral lymph node > 3 cm but ≤ 6 cm	
N2b	Metastasis in multiple ipsilateral lymph nodes, ≤ 6 cm	
N2c	Metastasis in bilateral or contralateral lymph nodes, ≤ 6 cm	
N3	Metastasis in a lymph node > 6 cm	
N3a		Metastasis in a lymph node > 6 cm
N3b		Metastasis to the supraclavicular fossa[a]

[a] The supraclavicular fossa is a triangular region that includes the caudal portions of levels IV and VB and is defined by three points: *Note:* 1, The superior margin of the sternal end of the clavicle; 2, The superior margin of the lateral end of the clavicle; 3, The point where the neck meets the shoulder.

Used with the permission of the American Joint Committee on Cancer (AJCC), Chicago, Illinois. The original source for this material is the AJCC Cancer Staging Manual, Seventh Edition (2010) published by Springer Science and Business Media LLC, www.springer.com.

sis. Patients with a nodal stage of N1 and a tumor stage of T1–3 are designated as stage III cancers. The stage IV grouping includes patients with T4 primary tumors (e.g., T4N1), patients with N2 or N3 disease, and patients with distant metastasis. Hence all patients with nodal metastatic disease are diagnosed with stage III or IV cancer. Most clinical trials are focused on the treatment outcomes of patients with local-regionally advanced stage III and IV head and neck cancer.

■ Principles of Management

The preferred management approach for the primary cancer frequently guides initial therapy for the N+ neck. As examples, neck dissections are typically performed if surgical management of the primary is chosen, whereas concurrent chemoradiotherapy (CRT) may be used to treat the neck if a nonsurgical approach is used for primary management. Single-modality therapy, such as surgery or RT alone, should be used if a cure rate of > 70% can be achieved to avoid increased morbidity. However, most patients with local-regionally advanced stage III or IV cancer realize a survival benefit from combined modality therapy.

Nonsurgical Therapy

Radiation Therapy

If external-beam RT is used, treatment may be administered to the primary site and positive nodal basin(s), either with conventional once-daily fractionation to 66 to 70 gray (Gy) at 2 Gy per fraction 5 days a week in a continuous course, or with an altered fractionation schedule. Higher rates of local-regional control have been shown with the concomitant boost technique and with hyperfractionation, which uses an increased number of fractions at a lower dose per fraction in the same overall treatment time and total dose. A recent meta-analysis calculated an 8% improvement in overall survival for patients treated with hyperfractionation versus those treated with standard fractionation.

Radiation Therapy and Concurrent Chemotherapy

The addition of chemotherapy to RT is equivalent to a radiation dose escalation of 12 Gy and improves disease-specific survival in local-regionally advanced head and neck cancer compared with treatment with RT alone. A meta-analysis of randomized clinical trials that evaluated the outcomes of treatment with

chemotherapy and RT for more than 17,000 patients demonstrated a 4% increase in overall 5-year survival and found that concurrent CRT resulted in an 8% increase in overall 5-year survival. Platinum-based therapy is associated with the greatest benefit.

However, the treatment outcomes described in this meta-analysis do not account for the unmeasured impact of human papillomavirus (HPV) infection, which is an independent prognostic factor for survival in patients with oropharyngeal cancer. Oropharyngeal cancer is the most frequently studied primary tumor site in head and neck cancer outcomes research. Patients with oropharyngeal cancer can be stratified into low-, intermediate-, and high-risk groups based on their HPV status and pack-years of tobacco use. The group of low-risk patients who are HPV negative with 10 or fewer pack-years of tobacco use demonstrate the best overall 5-year survival following concomitant CRT, whereas the group of high-risk patients who are HPV-positive with more than 10 pack-years have the lowest rate of survival.

Radiation Therapy Plus Cetuximab

Treatment with high-dose RT and cetuximab, a monoclonal antibody against the epidermal growth factor receptor, has been shown to improve local-regional control and overall survival compared with high-dose RT alone in patients with stage III to IV head and neck cancer. Cetuximab is an effective therapeutic target in the treatment of head and neck cancer that has also been shown to enhance the cytotoxic effects of chemotherapy. Although early investigations suggested that the potential toxicity associated with cetuximab therapy was relatively trivial, treatment with cetuximab is associated with severe skin reactions, sepsis, and hypomagnesemia.

Induction Chemotherapy Followed by Concomitant Chemoradiation

Although concomitant CRT has emerged as the preferred nonsurgical treatment modality for local-regionally advanced head and neck cancer, analysis of the outcomes following induction chemotherapy is impacted by methodological limitations of most published studies. In a recent prospective, randomized, multicenter trial that compared the treatment of stage III to IV head and neck cancer patients with docetaxel, cisplatin, and fluorouracil versus cisplatin and fluorouracil followed by CRT and surgery, improved overall survival and local-regional control were demonstrated with the three-agent induction regimen. There was no significant difference in the rates of gastrostomy tube and tracheotomy dependence between the studied cohorts. These promising results reopened the door to consider induction chemotherapy as a potential treatment option for appropriate candidates.

Although these results demonstrated the superiority of three-agent induction chemotherapy over two-agent therapy, the survival benefit of induction therapy has not been proven. The same multicenter research group conducted another randomized clinical trial that compared three-regimen induction chemotherapy followed by concurrent CRT with cisplatin-based concurrent CRT alone. There was no difference in overall survival between these two treatment groups. This head to head comparison of two different treatment paradigms failed to demonstrate a role for induction chemotherapy in locally advanced head and neck cancer. Hence the role for induction chemotherapy in the treatment of head and neck cancer remains unclear.

Evaluation and Management of the Neck following RT or CRT

Historically, most patients who were treated for N1 neck disease and achieved a complete response were observed, whereas patients with N2 or N3 neck disease were usually treated with a planned neck dissection due to concerns that there was persistent nodal disease. This treatment paradigm resulted from outcomes of treatment with RT alone, which demonstrated low response rates in patients with advanced nodal disease prior to the routine use of CRT. More recently, refinements in radiotherapy techniques and chemotherapy regimens, improved patient selection, and an increasing proportion of HPV-positive patients have led to improved rates of complete response to treatment. Despite these advances in treatment and outcomes, some patients will have persistent regional metastatic cancer, which, if undetected, will likely result in the need for more radical surgery or unresectability and a worse prognosis. This begs the question as to whether planned neck dissections are indicated following RT or CRT.

In the past, planned neck dissections were performed because the diagnostic accuracy of posttreatment evaluation for residual neck disease was poor. Over the past decade, however, several improvements in posttreatment surveillance have been realized that improve our ability to identify patients who have residual disease in the neck. Following CRT, PET-CT that is performed 12 or more weeks following completion of treatment has a negative predictive value of > 95% for persistent nodal metastatic disease. A PET-CT that is performed < 12 weeks after treatment will have a higher false-positive rate and should not be performed. Some clinicians are not comfortable with a 12 week waiting period because this permits the development of increased

treatment-related fibrosis and potential postsurgical morbidity, and it also delays definitive surgical management for several additional weeks. These clinicians advocate the performance of a contrast-enhanced CT 4 to 6 weeks after treatment: a radiographic complete response, defined as lymph node size < 1.5 cm and normal radiographic morphology with no filling defects or calcifications, has also been associated with a negative predictive value of at least 95%. If CT evaluation of residual nodal metastatic disease is equivocal, PET-CT may still be performed 12 weeks following treatment as a complementary imaging modality.

A growing body of literature has substantiated the value of PET-CT and CT for posttreatment surveillance. As an example, investigators from Memorial Sloan-Kettering Cancer Center recently published a 97.7% rate of regional control over 5 years in a large cohort of patients who were treated with CRT and were evaluated with posttreatment clinical examination, PET-CT, and in some cases CT or MRI. In addition, a literature review conducted by the International Head and Neck Scientific Group led them to conclude that a complete radiographic and clinical response to CRT is associated with a very low risk of neck recurrence, and the "strategy of systematic planned neck dissection is no longer justified." Adoption of this approach will markedly lower the rate of pathologically node-negative neck dissections and avoid the morbidity of surgery. However, it is critical that high-quality diagnostic imaging is obtained and radiological interpretation is rigorously performed to guide decision making so that comparable outcomes may be achieved.

Surgical Therapy

Neck Dissection

Since the original description of the radical neck dissection (RND) in 1906, various neck dissection procedures have evolved from our increased understanding of the patterns of lymph node metastasis and the need to decrease postoperative morbidity. The extent of cervical lymphadenectomy should be guided by the extent and pattern of lymph node metastases that are identified on radiographic imaging and that are expected based on the location of the primary tumor.

Seminal research by Jatin Shah at Memorial Sloan-Kettering Cancer Center and Robert Byers at MD Anderson Cancer Center provided the foundation for our present understanding of the patterns of lymph node metastasis and the rationale for modified radical neck dissections (MRNDs) and selective neck dissections (SNDs). In Shah's review of neck dissections performed for the N+ neck, oral cavity cancers most frequently metastasized to lymph node levels I through III, whereas cancers of the oropharynx, hypopharynx, and larynx usually metastasized to lymph node levels II through IV. The prevalence of lymph node metastasis to the posterior triangle (level V) in the N+ neck is 5%, and metastasis to the apex of level V is rare. More recently, variable rates of metastatic involvement in neck dissection specimens of sublevel IIB and level IV have been documented, giving rise to a wide range of SND options.

Our improved understanding of the patterns of lymph node metastasis coupled with the desire to decrease the morbidity resulting from surgery has led to the increased performance of spinal accessory nerve-sparing comprehensive (levels I–V) and selective neck dissections. In general, more conservative lymphadenectomy procedures result in lower mean numbers of harvested lymph nodes: RND, 40 lymph nodes; MRND, 30 lymph nodes; and SND, 20 lymph nodes. Although lower lymph node yields raise concerns that the risk of regional nodal recurrence could increase, the literature does not bear this out. A recent compilation of nine studies from the retrospective literature found that MRND was as effective as RND in the management of N1 and N2 disease. Furthermore, several investigators who evaluated the outcomes of SND for the pathologically positive neck independently concluded that SND with or without postoperative RT provides regional control rates that are comparable to those achieved with MRND or RND with or without postoperative RT.

In general, the choice of neck dissection procedure should balance the anticipated extent of cervical nodal metastatic disease with the potential for treatment-related morbidity. However, the risk of shoulder dysfunction and pain following nerve-sparing lymphadenectomy remains significant and must be routinely discussed during the preoperative counseling session.

Postoperative Radiation Therapy

No randomized trials have addressed the efficacy of postoperative adjuvant RT. Some of the best available data are from the Medical College of Virginia, where two groups of surgeons operated on patients with head and neck cancer. The two groups were general surgical oncologists who employed surgery alone and reserved RT for treatment of recurrent disease and otolaryngologists who routinely referred patients with locally advanced disease for postoperative RT. Disease-specific survival rates at 3 years were 41% for surgery alone and 72% for surgery and postoperative RT ($p = 0.0003$).

Postoperative RT should be considered if the risk of local-regional recurrence is > 20%. Postoperative RT is indicated for T4 status, positive or close margins at the site of primary tumor resection, perineural or vascular invasion, and multiple positive nodes or

ECS. Radiation therapy should be initiated within 6 to 8 weeks of surgery. The dose-fractionation schedule depends on the surgical margins: negative, 60 Gy in 30 fractions; close (< 5 mm), 66 Gy in 33 fractions: and positive, 74.4 Gy in 62 twice-daily fractions. Concurrent chemotherapy is also administered to high-risk patients with ECS or positive margins.

Adjuvant Chemotherapy

Two randomized clinical trials recently defined the indications for and the survival benefit of supplementing postoperative RT with concurrent chemotherapy. Both randomized trials compared RT alone to RT in combination with three cycles of high-dose cisplatin in treatment groups with similar rates of ECS and positive margins. Disease-free survival and progression-free survival were significantly greater in the groups of patients treated with CRT. Consequently, concurrent chemotherapy and RT are indicated in the presence of ECS or positive surgical margins.

Preoperative Radiation Therapy

Preoperative RT may be indicated if (1) there are fixed lymph nodes, (2) the initiation of postoperative RT would be delayed for more than 8 weeks, or (3) open biopsy of a positive neck node was performed. Patients are treated to 50 to 60 Gy at either 2 Gy/fraction once daily or 1.2 Gy/fraction twice daily, and fixed nodes are boosted to higher doses.

Salvage Neck Dissection

Approximately 10% of patients with an N+ neck who have been treated with definitive RT with or without chemotherapy and/or neck dissection eventually develop regional nodal failure within 18 months of the completion of initial treatment. Patients with isolated nodal metastases are the best candidates for surgical salvage, so early detection and prompt treatment are paramount.

If persistent nodal disease is identified in a single lymph node on posttreatment PET-CT or CT, a selective neck dissection is appropriate. A comprehensive neck dissection should be considered if multiple positive nodes are present. If regional failure subsequently occurs, salvage neck dissection should be considered. Patients with isolated nodal recurrences are acceptable candidates for salvage neck dissection. Regional failure in multiple nodes following RT or CRT has a very poor prognosis, and the likelihood of surgical salvage is very low. The patient should be counseled at length regarding the poor prognosis and morbidity associated with salvage neck dissection, and consultation with radiation oncology may also be considered to discuss the possibility of reirradiation following salvage surgery. Carotid artery invasion or encasement following RT or CRT is likely noncurative disease with a high risk of significant morbidity and death and should be considered only after extensive patient counseling and careful preoperative planning.

■ Miscellaneous

Classification of Neck Dissection

American Academy of Otolaryngology–Head and Neck Surgery standardized neck dissection terminology in 1991. More recent consensus statements have addressed classification and terminology for neck dissections.

- *Radical neck dissection (RND)* En bloc resection of lymph node containing tissue in levels I–V with removal of the sternocleidomastoid (SCM) muscle, internal jugular vein (IJV), and spinal accessory nerve (CN XI). Recent classification of neck dissection would denote ND (I–V, SCM, IJV, CN XI).
- *Modified radical neck dissection (MRND)* Resection of lymph node–bearing tissue from levels I–V, with preservation of one or more nonlymphatic structures. The current recommended nomenclature proposes clear statement of the neck levels removed and the nonlymphatic structures removed. For example, an MRND with preservation of CN XI would be described as ND (I–V, SCM, IJV).
- *Selective neck dissection (SND)* Lymphadenectomy of selected cervical lymph node–bearing levels. The following SNDs are most frequently performed:
- *Supraomohyoid* Levels I, II, and III, or ND (I–III)
- *Lateral* Levels II, III, and IV, or ND (II–IV)
- *Posterolateral* Levels II, III, IV, and V; suboccipital and retroauricular nodes; or ND (II–V)
- *Anterior* Level VI (pretracheal, paratracheal, and prelaryngeal nodes) or ND (VI)
- *Extended radical neck dissection* RND with resection of lymphatic and/or nonlymphatic structures not normally encompassed by RND. Examples of lymphatic structures are parotid, suboccipital, paratracheal, and mediastinal nodes. Nonlymphatic structures include muscle, nerve, skin, carotid artery, and viscera of the neck.

Specific Aspects of Neck Dissection

Elective and therapeutic neck dissection are valuable means of predicting prognosis and planning adjuvant therapy, particularly in the clinically N0 neck. Neck dissection alone is highly effective in patients with N1 and limited N2 disease without extracapsular spread (ECS). However, neck dissection has limited value in cervical metastasis with ECS, N3 necks, and patients with nodal metastasis fixed to structures, such as the carotid artery and brachial plexus. Such patients require adjuvant irradiation and/or chemotherapy.

Spinal Accessory Nerve (CN XI)

Resection of CN XI may cause "shoulder syndrome"—that is, weakness and wasting of the trapezius muscle and pain and adhesive capsulitis of the shoulder. CN XI may be preserved when cervical metastasis does not invade the nerve without adversely affecting regional control. However, this does not ensure normal shoulder function. CN XI dysfunction following dissection of only the proximal segment of the nerve, as in supraomohyoid and lateral SND, may be due to stretching of the nerve during dissection and delivery of the supraspinal accessory lymph node pad of level 2 or may result from devascularization of the nerve from ligation of the occipital artery. Even patients who have only had SND should have their shoulder function monitored because they may require physiotherapy to minimize morbidity related to CN XI dysfunction.

Internal Jugular Vein (IJV)

Simultaneous ligation of both IJVs may cause venous congestion and edema of the head and neck, raised intracranial pressure, and syndrome of inappropriate antidiuretic hormone secretion. A functioning IJV may also be required for venous anastomosis of a free flap. Preservation of the external jugular vein may theoretically avoid the sequelae of bilateral IJV ligation. Preservation of the IJV in modified neck dissections results in IJV patency rates ranging from 86 to 99% if patients with compression of the IJV by tumor recurrence or myocutaneous flaps are excluded.

Endothelial damage should be avoided by atraumatic handling of the IJV, by tying as opposed to cauterizing tributaries of the IJV, and by avoiding desiccation of the IJV during surgery. Compression of the preserved IJV should be minimized by avoiding tight dressings and by securing the tracheotomy tube with sutures, not ties.

Prior or subsequent irradiation does not appear to affect IJV patency. When carcinoma involves the second IJV, the therapeutic options are to stage the second neck dissection or to proceed with bilateral IJV resection with or without IJV reconstruction. The IJV may be reconstructed with various materials, including spiraled saphenous vein, a segment of contralateral IJV, or external jugular vein. Patients with a jugular stump pressure of > 30 mm Hg are more likely to maintain graft patency.

Carotid Artery

Carotid artery invasion is associated with a poor prognosis. Stripping tumor off the carotid artery does not provide adequate oncological margins. Therefore, the principal options are no treatment, debulking with adjuvant therapy, or, for carotid encasement, carotid artery resection with or without revascularization. Carotid artery resection is associated with 22% 2-year disease-free survival, and major and minor neurological sequelae occur in 17% and 11% of patients, respectively. Patients with invasion of the carotid artery should undergo cerebral blood flow studies prior to surgery. Patients who fail the study may benefit from revascularization.

Nerve Invasion

Perineural invasion (PNI) is associated with increased risk of local recurrence, and perineural propagation of tumor up to 12 cm has been reported. Therefore, PNI is equivalent to a positive margin, and adjuvant therapy should be considered. When invasion of the lower cranial nerves, or brachial or cervical plexus, is found at surgery, the decision to resect involved nerves as opposed to debulking and adjuvant therapy is dependent on the goals of treatment. Morbidity of nerve resection should be weighed against the prospect of cure or local control.

◾ Practice Guidelines, Consensus Statements, and Measures

National Comprehensive Cancer Network. Head and Neck Cancers. NCCN Clinical Practice Guidelines in Oncology. (Version 2.2013). www.nccn.org

◾ Suggested Reading

Adelstein DJ, Rodriguez CP. Current and emerging standards of concomitant chemoradiotherapy. Semin Oncol 2008;35(3):211–220

Ang KK, Harris J, Wheeler R, et al. Human papillomavirus and survival of patients with oropharyngeal cancer. N Engl J Med 2010;363(1):24–35

Bernier J, Domenge C, Ozsahin M, et al; European Organization for Research and Treatment of Cancer Trial 22931. Postoperative irradiation with or without concomitant chemotherapy for locally advanced head and neck cancer. N Engl J Med 2004;350(19):1945–1952

Bonner JA, Harari PM, Giralt J, et al. Radiotherapy plus cetuximab for squamous-cell carcinoma of the head and neck. N Engl J Med 2006;354(6):567–578

Bourhis J, Overgaard J, Audry H, et al; Meta-Analysis of Radiotherapy in Carcinomas of Head and neck (MARCH) Collaborative Group. Hyperfractionated or accelerated radiotherapy in head and neck cancer: a meta-analysis. Lancet 2006;368(9538):843–854

Cooper JS, Pajak TF, Forastiere AA, et al; Radiation Therapy Oncology Group 9501/Intergroup. Postoperative concurrent radiotherapy and chemotherapy for high-risk squamous-cell carcinoma of the head and neck. N Engl J Med 2004;350(19):1937–1944

Goenka A, Morris LG, Rao SS, et al. Long-term regional control in the observed neck following definitive chemoradiation for node-positive oropharyngeal squamous cell cancer. Int J Cancer 2013;133(5):1214–1221

Haddad R, O'Neill A, Rabinowits G, et al. Induction chemotherapy followed by concurrent chemoradiotherapy (sequential chemoradiotherapy) versus concurrent chemoradiotherapy alone in locally advanced head and neck cancer (PARADIGM): a randomised phase 3 trial. Lancet Oncol 2013;14(3):257–264

Hamoir M, Ferlito A, Schmitz S, et al. The role of neck dissection in the setting of chemoradiation therapy for head and neck squamous cell carcinoma with advanced neck disease. Oral Oncol 2012;48(3):203–210

Kasibhatla M, Kirkpatrick JP, Brizel DM. How much radiation is the chemotherapy worth in advanced head and neck cancer? Int J Radiat Oncol Biol Phys 2007;68(5):1491–1495

Lorch JH, Goloubeva O, Haddad RI, et al; TAX 324 Study Group. Induction chemotherapy with cisplatin and fluorouracil alone or in combination with docetaxel in locally advanced squamous-cell cancer of the head and neck: long-term results of the TAX 324 randomised phase 3 trial. Lancet Oncol 2011;12(2):153–159

Mendenhall WM, Riggs CE, Vaysberg M, Amdur RJ, Werning JW. Altered fractionation and adjuvant chemotherapy for head and neck squamous cell carcinoma. Head Neck 2010;32(7):939–945

Robbins KT, Clayman G, Levine PA, et al; American Head and Neck Society; American Academy of Otolaryngology–Head and Neck Surgery. Neck dissection classification update: revisions proposed by the American Head and Neck Society and the American Academy of Otolaryngology–Head and Neck Surgery. Arch Otolaryngol Head Neck Surg 2002;128(7):751–758

Yeung AR, Liauw SL, Amdur RJ, et al. Lymph node-positive head and neck cancer treated with definitive radiotherapy: can treatment response determine the extent of neck dissection? Cancer 2008;112(5):1076–1082

45 Paragangliomas of the Head and Neck

■ Introduction

Paragangliomas of the head and neck are unusual neoplasms that arise from extra-adrenal paraganglia. Variously termed glomus tumor, nonchromaffin paraganglioma, and chemodectoma, the paraganglioma is derived from chief cells that populate the paraganglia, and it is categorized based on the particular paraganglion of origin. These tumors have a slow growth rate and rarely metastasize, but they can be locally invasive and frequently occur in young people. Tumors can be multicentric and may occur in a familial inheritance pattern. Diagnosis of lesions has been greatly facilitated by the advent of magnetic resonance imaging (MRI), as well as newer nuclear medicine imaging modalities. Debate persists on the optimal management of paragangliomas of the head and neck; the three primary alternatives are surgical resection, radiation therapy, and observation.

This chapter delineates the nomenclature, physiology, and pathophysiology of the extra-adrenal paraganglia, outlines diagnostic techniques, and presents management options with particular regard to treatment-specific outcomes.

Nomenclature

Each paraganglion is composed of two cell types, a Schwann-like satellite cell, and the neural-crest-derived chief cell. The chief cells migrate with autonomic ganglion cells to a variety of locations closely associated with sympathetic ganglia, the aorta, and its main branches. The extra-adrenal paraganglia are distinguished from the adrenal paraganglion or the adrenal medulla and have been grouped according to their anatomical location and innervation as branchiomeric, intravagal, aorticosympathetic, and visceral autonomic paraganglia. This discussion focuses on tumors of the branchiomeric paraganglia as well as the intravagal paraganglia.

The branchiomeric paraganglia are related to the cranial nerves and arteries of the ontogenetic gill arches and include the jugulotympanic, intercarotid, subclavian, laryngeal, coronary, aorticopulmonary, and pulmonary paraganglia. Orbital and intravagal paraganglia are not closely associated with arteries and are therefore considered separate groups. The tumors arising from these paraganglia within the head and neck are classified according to their site of origin. These include the jugulotympanic paraganglioma, the intercarotid paraganglioma or carotid body tumor, and the intravagal paraganglioma. Less common tumors include orbital and laryngeal paragangliomas.

Many other names for these tumors exist throughout the literature, with the most frequently cited being glomus tumors, such as glomus jugulare, glomus tympanicum, and glomus vagale tumors. This designation was derived from the misconception that these tumors arose from pericytes that make up the normal glomus body, a specialized arteriovenous anastomosis that extends from a preterminal arteriole to an efferent vein and helps regulate blood pressure, temperature, and the interstitial cellular environment. The term *chemodectoma* has been applied to these tumors, primarily in reference to the chemoreceptor function of the carotid body or intercarotid paraganglia.

Anatomy and Physiology

The chief cells of the paraganglia are functionally and ultrastructurally linked with thyroid C cells, ultimobranchial cells, and adrenaline and noradrenaline cells of the adrenal medulla as members of the amine and amine precursor uptake and decarboxylase (APUD) series. This family of cells has been renamed as the diffuse neuroendocrine system (DNES) by the same author, because the products of APUD cells include both neuropeptides and catecholamines and may function as neurotransmitters, neurohormones, hormones, and parahormones. Paraganglia are richly vascular, providing a favorable environment for chief cells both to sample the chemical milieu and to influence homeostatic mechanisms through catecholamine and neuropeptide release. This may occur via a humoral mechanism or through the release of a neurotransmitter to influence afferent nerve activity. Although essentially all paragangliomas have the potential to secrete catecholamines, few extra-adrenal paragangliomas produce symptomatic levels of catecholamines.

The incidence of functional activity in jugular paragangliomas is 1%. Virtually all documented craniocervical catecholamine-secreting paragangliomas produced norepinephrine. This low incidence of documented secreting tumors may be due in part to the fact that a four- to fivefold increase in norepinephrine levels is necessary to produce symptoms. These symptoms include headache, excessive perspiration, palpitations, pallor, and nausea. The most common physical finding is episodic or sustained hypertension. Laboratory findings may confirm the presence of a catecholamine-secreting tumor. Metabolic breakdown products of dopamine, norepinephrine, and epinephrine include normetanephrine and metanephrine, which are further broken down into vanillylmandelic acid (VMA). Twenty-four-hour urine screening for metanephrine and VMA levels detects the expected breakdown products of epinephrine- and norepinephrine-secreting tumors. Serum catecholamine levels may be measured as well, and associated findings may include elevated blood glucose, low insulin levels, and an elevated hematocrit. If elevated serum epinephrine levels are detected, a coexisting pheochromocytoma must be ruled out.

Although all paraganglia and, likely, a variety of neuropeptides are capable of secreting catecholamines, no physiological function of the jugulotympanic paraganglia or the intravagal paraganglia has been established. However, a physiological role for the intercarotid paraganglia, or the carotid body, is clearly defined. The carotid body and carotid sinus function as complementary chemoreceptor and baroreceptor to effect homeostatic regulation of both ventilation and perfusion. An understanding of the functional role of both structures is critical in determining optimum treatment strategies for tumors of the carotid paraganglia. Feedback from these two structures passes through the carotid sinus nerve, also known as the nerve of Hering, which joins the glossopharyngeal nerve 1.5 cm distal to the jugular foramen.

The carotid sinus is a grossly imperceptible structure composed of stretch receptors. It lies in the adventitia of the carotid bulb. The active component of the stretch receptors is composed of spray-type nerve endings that are stimulated when stretched. They are concentrated on the lateral aspect of the carotid bulb, extending up to the carotid bifurcation.

The carotid body is consistently located along the medial aspect of the carotid bifurcation. The average size of the normal gland is ~ 5 × 3 × 1.5 mm. Normal variation in carotid body size occurs, and bilateral hyperplasia, slowly increasing with age, has been associated with high-altitude dwellers.

The carotid body–sinus complex functions as both a chemoreceptor and a baroreceptor. The chemoreceptor function, which is primarily mediated through the carotid body, has been shown to be sensitive to changes in partial pressure of oxygen (Po_2) and carbon dioxide (Pco_2) in the blood, acidity or alkalinity (pH), and blood flow. As the Po_2 decreases, there is an increase in the rate of firing within the carotid sinus nerve, increasing the rate of ventilation. An increase in ventilation is also seen as the Pco_2 increases. The effects of both hypoxia and hypercapnia together are more than just additive resulting in a marked increase in firing within the sinus nerve. Chronic hypoxia is regulated by central mechanisms with little input from the carotid body.

The physiological role of the carotid sinus baroreceptor is in regulation of blood pressure during changes in body posture or other stress. Pooling of blood in the lower extremities upon rising from a supine or sitting position robs the head and upper extremities of needed blood flow. An immediate response to this change is through the baroreceptors, with a decrease in neural discharge in the nerve to the carotid sinus and a resultant decrease in parasympathetic discharge affecting heart rate and peripheral vasomotor tone. A corresponding increase in sympathetic discharge is elicited, and blood pressure is maintained. The carotid body–carotid sinus complex, therefore, exerts control over the regulation of ventilation and perfusion through chemoreceptor and baroreceptor mechanisms. Input from both is mediated via a common neural pathway. Therefore, function of the entire system is affected with resection of tumors involving the intercarotid paraganglia.

Although no physiological role for the jugulotympanic or intravagal paragangliomas has been established, their anatomical locations are well characterized. Paraganglia of the temporal bone are smaller than the carotid body, measuring 0.1 to 1.5 mm in diameter, and are usually three in number. They are adjacent to the tympanic branch of the glossopharyngeal nerve (Jacobson nerve) or the auricular branch of the vagus nerve (Arnold nerve). About 50% of temporal bone paraganglia are located in the jugular fossa, 10% are found in the mucosa of the promontory, and 20% are found in the inferior tympanic canaliculus, transmitting Jacobson nerve from the jugular fossa to the tympanic cavity. The primary blood supply to these paraganglia is the ascending pharyngeal artery via its inferior tympanic branch. The intravagal paraganglia are described as dispersed cell groups within the perineurium of the vagus nerve. Their location can be in either the jugular ganglion or the ganglion nodosum, or just inferior to the latter. Exceedingly rare are tumors involving paraganglia in the larynx and orbit. Paraganglia exist in the larynx deep to the epithelium superior to the anterior aspect of the vocal fold in relation to the internal branch of the superior laryngeal nerve, and between the cricoid and thyroid cartilages in relation to the recurrent laryngeal nerve.

Clinical Features

Tumors of the branchiomeric and intravagal paraganglia share many common features. Paragangliomas are typically solitary but may present with multicentricity, particularly in familial syndromes, such as Carney syndrome (Carney triad) and multiple endocrine neoplasia (MEN) syndromes, types 2A and 2B. Carney syndrome consists of the triad of gastric epithelioid leiomyosarcomas, pulmonary chondromas, and extra-adrenal paragangliomas. Neurofibromatosis and von Hippel–Lindau are also associated with paragangliomas. Familial paragangliomas constitute ~ 28% of paraganglioma cases. Approximately 8 to 25% of sporadic paraganglioma cases have germline succinate dehydrogenase (SDH) mutations, leading to a probable underestimation of the hereditary factor. Thus the familial paraganglioma prevalence is likely much higher because genetic testing of every patient is not common. The presentation is typically at younger ages and often involves multiple sites. Multicentricity is present 10% of the time in sporadic paragangliomas versus 30 to 40% in the familial version.

The primary gene (PGL1) responsible for hereditary paragangliomas of the head and neck has been identified at the 11q23 locus, and other less common genes have been found. The PGL genes code for the SDH complexes subunit D (SDHD, 11q23), B (SDHB, 1p36), and C (SDHC, 1q21), which are part of mitochondrial complex II. Mutations of these genes are hypothesized to lead to defective oxygen sensing and cellular proliferation, similar to conditions produced by chronic hypoxia. This may explain the higher incidence of paragangliomas at higher altitudes. Of the familial cases, mutated SDHD, SDHB, and SDHC are found at rates of 51%, 34%, and 14.2%, respectively. The PGL1 (SDHD) gene is inherited in an autosomal-dominant fashion with genomic imprinting, leading to "skipping" of generations. Males with the gene can produce children with a 50% chance of developing paragangliomas. Females can inherit the gene and pass it along, but they will not have affected children. Interestingly, the genes encoding for SHDB and SDHC are inherited in the standard autosomal-dominant fashion. Multicentricity is found in about two-thirds of SDHD mutation patients. Malignant paragangliomas are more prevalent in SDHB patients (37.5%) than in SDHD (3.2%) and SDHC patients (0%).

Paragangliomas of each type generally exhibit a very slow growth rate. Although growth rates of individual tumors can be determined only by serial radiological imaging studies, reports of patients who have been followed in this manner suggest tumors may remain stable in size over several years, or may increase in size at rates < 0.5 cm per year. To date there is no reliable indicator that predicts the growth rate or aggressiveness of these usually slowly enlarging tumors.

Another feature common to all paragangliomas is a low potential for malignancy. Malignant paragangliomas, as defined by the presence of metastatic lesions in sites other than known locations of other paraganglia, likely occur in < 5% of tumors, with reported incidences of malignant lesions varying from < 1% in a series of 108 craniocervical paragangliomas, to as high as 19% among vagal paragangliomas. The most common sites of metastases are to regional lymph nodes, with rare distant spread to lungs, liver, bone, and spleen.

■ Evaluation

Workup of the patient with suspected paraganglioma begins with a careful history and physical examination. Pertinent findings within the history include other family members with neck masses or previous head and neck surgery for tumors of unknown types. A known family history of paragangliomas is helpful, and counseling with regard to inheritance patterns is initiated to ensure that appropriate family members are screened. Symptoms of secreting tumors are elicited. Pertinent physical findings include the presence of a cervical mass, oropharyngeal findings of a parapharyngeal space lesion, and neurotologic findings characteristic of a temporal bone tumor. Cranial nerve deficits are searched for and documented. Screening laboratory evaluation includes 24-hour urine and serum analysis for the presence of excess catecholamines.

Screening MRI scans, which are virtually diagnostic for these tumors, are obtained, including the head and cranial base, neck, and upper mediastinum. MRI is preferred both for its sensitivity and because of the characteristic appearance these tumors have based on their vascularity, for its diagnostic capability. Lesions can be followed with either computed tomography (CT) or MRI once their size and location have been documented. CT scans of the temporal bone are obtained on all patients with evidence of temporal bone involvement or intracranial extension if surgical resection is entertained. This modality provides unparalleled bony detail of the cranial base structures in a format familiar to the surgeon. Octreotide scintigraphy is a useful modality to assess total body involvement by paragangliomas. Although not yet routinely obtained, octreotide scintigraphy will be of most utility in the patient with a strong family history or in whom multicentric or metastatic disease is suspected.

If surgery is planned, bilateral carotid arteriography is considered. Arteriography was once necessary to make the diagnosis, but it has been supplanted for this purpose by MRI. Similarly, the finding of multiple lesions on arteriography is just as well documented by MRI. This practically limits the usefulness of arteriography to those patients with moderate to large paragangliomas in whom surgery is planned. Arteriography is performed for two primary reasons: tumor embolization and diagnostic studies relative to the patency of collateral cerebral circulation. Preoperative embolization is gaining a wider acceptance for all larger lesions and should be performed within 24 to 48 hours of resection to prevent formation of collateral circulation.

■ Management and Treatment

Treatment options for craniocervical paragangliomas must be measured against the natural history of these tumors, with particular regard to their slow rate of growth, tendency toward multicentricity, presentation in relatively young patients, and tendency toward locally aggressive behavior with rare malignant potential. Treatment can consist of observation alone, particularly in the context of multiple tumors or tumors presenting in the elderly or infirm patient. Observation is an optional initial management strategy in any patient with a craniocervical paraganglioma to document the rate of growth of a particular lesion. There is rarely any need to pursue therapy urgently for these tumors in the absence of functionally significant catecholamine secretion.

Surgical Resection and Radiotherapy

If a therapeutic intervention is desired, the two primary options are surgical resection or radiotherapy. Comparison between treatment modalities is difficult based on a literature review. The surgical literature judges successful treatment by complete tumor resection without evidence of recurrence. The radiation therapy literature judges successful treatment by the absence of radiographic progression of disease. Very few large series exist carefully comparing the two treatment modalities. Patients treated with primary radiotherapy are often selected based on large tumor size and relative "unresectability." Treatment arms are rarely equivalent and are evaluated retrospectively.

Perhaps the most significant confounding factor, however, is the slow growth rate of these tumors and thus the need for careful follow-up over many years,

preferably 10 to 30 years. Few studies achieve this goal, and even those that do are further confounded by the significant advances that have occurred during the past 30 years in both surgical and radiotherapeutic treatment modalities.

Radiation doses, like surgical techniques, have varied widely over the past 30 years. However, more recent studies have evaluated optimal treatment regimens by retrospective case review. Past studies of patients treated with primary radiation therapy for jugulotympanic paragangliomas found a historical failure rate of just over 20% for doses < 40 gray (Gy) over 4 weeks, compared with 2% for doses > 40 Gy/4 wk, leading to a recommendation of radiation doses of 40 to 45 Gy. A similar review found equal local control with radiation doses of 35 Gy/3 wk for paragangliomas of the temporal bone. Such treatment has led to local control rates of ~ 90% at a median follow-up of 10 years. Most current radiation therapy regimens favor doses of 40 to 45 Gy/4 wk, with the primary stated advantage of this dose being its low morbidity. Although this is frequently reported, there is a paucity of carefully analyzed data on treatment-related morbidity in the radiation therapy literature.

Surgical therapy for paragangliomas of all types has also advanced tremendously in the past 20 years. The following sections review specific features and treatment modalities for the three common craniocervical paragangliomas.

Carotid Body Tumors

Although the carotid body tumor (CBT) is the most common of head and neck paragangliomas, the incidence is still quite low. CBTs are commonly treated outside major medical centers, with no record of these tumors in the literature. The average age at the time of treatment is 42 to 44 years, with ages at presentation varying widely from as young as 6 months to 80 years. Essentially equal sex distributions exist for familial tumors, whereas reports vary for sporadic tumors.

The most common presenting symptom and physical finding associated with CBTs is a painless neck mass. Although this is classically described as a mass that can be moved horizontally but not vertically by the examiner, our experience suggests this finding has little clinical utility. A carotid bruit is infrequent but may be present if the tumor causes sufficient compression of the carotid artery. Up to 10% of CBTs may extend into the parapharyngeal space to produce a noticeable medial bulging of the oropharyngeal wall. Differential diagnosis includes any of the many etiologies of level II neck masses in general, and parapharyngeal space masses in particular. Of particular interest are the carotid artery aneurysm and neurolemmomas of the vagal nerve or sympathetic trunk. Cranial nerve deficits may occur at presentation (11% with vagal paralysis, and 4% with hypoglossal paralysis). Horner syndrome from involvement of the cervical sympathetic nerves has also been reported. To date there has been no widely used staging system for CBTs.

Traditional therapy for unilateral CBTs has been surgical resection. In experienced hands, resection of CBT is a very safe procedure, with complete resection in 96 to 98% of cases. The two major risks of surgical resection are cranial nerve injury and carotid artery injury with excessive bleeding. The carotid artery is at risk for injury during the dissection in direct proportion to tumor size. In tumors < 5 cm, only 15%, or less, of patients may require resection and reconstruction of the carotid during tumor removal, whereas up to 50% of patients with tumors > 5 cm might require resection and reconstruction. There is a low perioperative stroke rate. The Shamblin classification groups carotid body tumors into three classes to predict those tumors that are more or less likely to require vascular resection and reconstruction. Group I tumors are easily dissected away from the vessels and minimally attached to the vessels. Group II tumors are more adherent and partially surround the vessels. Group III tumors surround the vessels and are intimately associated with the vessels, making carotid dissection impossible without sacrifice and reconstruction.

Cranial nerve deficits remain the most troubling morbidity following surgical resection of unilateral CBTs, with a rate of 5 to 40% in reported series. This reference has provided a detailed outline of a surgical technique designed to minimize cranial nerve dysfunction, the crux of which is to achieve high cervical exposure with careful identification of all cranial nerves prior to dissection of the tumor.

Although resection of unilateral CBTs is generally well accepted, treatment of bilateral CBTs, or a unilateral CBT with a contralateral vagal paraganglioma, is more problematic. The first issue involves the vagus nerve, and the potential for bilateral vagal paralysis as a consequence of bilateral resections. Certainly if bilateral resections are planned, they should be performed in a staged fashion to verify that vocal fold function is intact on the operated side following the first resection. If vagal paralysis occurs with the initial resection, then it is prudent to consider observation or radiation therapy for the contralateral lesion. The side with the smaller tumor and higher success rate of vagal preservation is typically approached first. If vagal preservation is confirmed postoperatively, then the contralateral side with the bigger tumor is resected.

A less obvious but equally troubling potential clinical sequela of bilateral CBT resections is baroreceptor dysfunction as a consequence of bilateral denervation of the carotid sinus. The postoperative course is characterized by severe labile hypertension and hypotension, headache, diaphoresis, and emotional instability. Loss of the baroreceptor negative feedback on blood pressure control can result in minor stimuli causing rapid changes in blood pressure. Stress may result in a hypertensive crisis, with antianxiety drugs playing a vital role in the management of these patients. The unopposed sympathetic system is responsible for most of the cardiovascular morbidity seen after bilateral resection because the parasympathetic regulatory system is lost.

The efficacy of radiation therapy for CBTs is similar to its efficacy for other paragangliomas. Local control rates for stereotactic or traditional fractioned radiation may reach 95%. This is a viable option to consider in medically inoperable patients, elderly patients, and bilateral vagal or carotid body tumors. Typical radiation doses range from 45 to 60 Gy.

Jugulotympanic Paragangliomas

Jugulotympanic paragangliomas are the second most common of the craniocervical paragangliomas. They represent the most common tumor of the middle ear and the second most common tumor of the temporal bone. Nevertheless, like CBTs, they are rare lesions. Age at presentation is usually in the fourth to fifth decades, and unlike CBTs, there seems to be a clear female sex predilection as high as four to six times that of males for sporadic tumors. Recalling the inheritance pattern for familial tumors, there is an equal male and female distribution for all types of paragangliomas among kindreds.

Presenting symptoms vary depending on tumor location. Tumors limited to the middle ear more commonly present with aural symptoms relating to the mass effect of tumor impinging on the ossicular chain, or less commonly as a vascular polyp extending into the external auditory canal. Tumors originating in the jugular bulb region more commonly present with clinical involvement of cranial nerves IX through XII. Mastoid growth can result in facial paralysis. Intracranial extension can lead to signs of intracranial pressure or cerebellar dysfunction.

Physical findings correlate with symptomatology. Predominantly aural symptoms commonly yield the finding of a vascular mass visible in the middle ear or external auditory canal. This mass may be pulsatile and may blanch with positive pneumatoscopic pressure (Brown sign). Cranial nerve deficits and central signs can be discovered on physical examination. Initial cranial nerve deficit is more common for jugulotympanic paragangliomas as compared with CBTs. Cranial nerve deficits among jugulotympanic tumors are as high as 18% for the facial and cochlear nerves, 10% for the glossopharyngeal nerve, 14% for the vagal nerve, 4% for the spinal accessory nerve, and

8% for the hypoglossal nerve. Differential diagnosis includes meningioma; neural lesions; carcinoma (primary, metastatic, and nasopharyngeal); primary cholesteatoma; and more unusual lesions, including rhabdomyosarcoma, plasmacytoma, melanoma, giant cell tumor, osteoblastoma, lipoma, chondrosarcoma, petrositis, and histiocytosis.

The natural history of jugulotympanic paragangliomas is one of slow growth along pathways of least resistance. This includes along air cell tracts within the temporal bone, the eustachian tube, the vascular lumens, and the neurovascular foramina of the cranial base. Intracranial extension to the posterior fossa occurs along the hypoglossal canal or via the sigmoid sinus. Unlike CBTs, jugulotympanic paragangliomas have two meaningful staging systems based on anatomical location; however, neither system is uniformly used.

Fisch categorized tumors as A through D, based on location within the temporal bone relative to the labyrinth and on degree of intracranial extension (**Table 45.1**). Jackson et al divided tumors into glomus tympanicum and glomus jugulare based on presumed site of origin and intracranial extension (**Table 45.2**).

When craniocervical paragangliomas are under discussion, perhaps the greatest debate arises between radiotherapists and surgeons concerning the optimum treatment of jugulotympanic paragangliomas. Traditionally, surgical therapy for these lesions has been associated with high morbidity, particularly with regard to multiple cranial nerve deficits. For this reason, the literature is replete with reports of radiation therapy used in small series with variable follow-up in the treatment of jugulotympanic paragangliomas. As already noted, local control rates of 80% have been reported. Higher control rates of 94% have been reported in 15 of 16 tumors followed for more than 10 years when only megavoltage radiation is considered. At the recommended radiation dose of 40 to 45 Gy, complications are expected to be minimal, although this is poorly documented. However, as also noted, local control is generally reported as no progression of disease. Biological response to radiotherapy among these lesions is unpredictable. Given the highly variable follow-up among reported series, it remains unclear what will be the long-term outcome in young patients treated with primary radiotherapy.

Although radiotherapy for jugulotympanic paragangliomas deserves strong consideration, surgical resection remains the only definitively curative therapy for these tumors. The infratemporal fossa approach of Fisch and the surgical modifications of

Table 45.1 Jugulotympanic paraganglioma: Fisch classification

Type	Physical findings
A	Tumors limited to the middle ear cleft
B	Tumors limited to the tympanomastoid area with no infralabyrinthine compartment involvement
C1	Tumors destroying the jugular foramen and jugular bulb, with limited involvement of the vertical portion of the carotid canal
C2	Tumors destroying the infralabyrinthine compartment of the temporal bone and invading the vertical portion of the carotid canal
C3	Tumors involving the infralabyrinthine and apical compartments of the temporal bone, with invasion of the horizontal portion of the carotid canal
D1	Tumors with intracranial extension < 2 cm in diameter; removal in one stage through infratemporal fossa approach possible
D2	Tumors with intracranial extension > 2 cm in diameter that require a combined two-staged otologic and neurosurgical removal
D3	Tumors with inoperable intracranial invasion

Used with permission from Fisch U. Infratemporal fossa approach for glomus tumors of the temporal bone. Ann Otol Rhinol Laryngol 1982;91:474–479.

Table 45.2 Jugulotympanic paraganglioma: Glasscock-Jackson glomus tumor classification

Type	Physical finding
Glomus tympanicum	
I	Small mass limited to promontory
II	Tumor completely filling middle ear space
III	Tumor filling middle ear and extending into mastoid
IV	Tumor filling middle ear, extending into mastoid or through tympanic membrane to fill external auditory canal; may also extend anteriorly to internal carotid artery
Glomus jugulare	
I	Small tumor involving jugular bulb, middle ear, and mastoid
II	Tumor extending under internal auditory canal; may have intracranial extension
III	Tumor extending into petrous apex; may have intracranial extension
IV	Tumor extending beyond petrous apex into clivus or infratemporal fossa; may have intracranial extension

Used with permission from Jackson CG, Glasscock ME, Harris PF. Glomus tumors: diagnosis, classification and management of large lesions. Arch Otolaryngol 1982;108:401–406.

this approach as proposed by Jackson have helped to decrease the morbidities of cranial nerve loss and cerebral fluid leakage.

Large series in the surgical treatment of jugulotympanic paragangliomas yielded significant cranial nerve deficits with a twofold increase in vagal and facial paralysis with resection, and a three- and fourfold increase in hypoglossal and glossopharyngeal paralysis, respectively, following resection. This review of jugulotympanic paragangliomas cannot settle the debate between radiotherapists and surgeons over optimal treatment. In general, radiotherapy yields lower morbidity with regard to cranial nerve dysfunction, although the long-term complications of radiation in doses of 40 to 50 Gy to the temporal bone are unknown. For smaller tumors of the middle ear and mastoid, resection appears to be the treatment of choice. For large tumors with intracranial extension in the elderly or infirm patient, radiation therapy provides clear advantages over surgical resection. No definitive answer yet exists for the preferred treatment of large jugular paragangliomas in the young or middle-aged healthy patient.

Vagal Paragangliomas

Vagal paragangliomas are the least common of the three primary craniocervical paragangliomas, representing < 5% of head and neck paragangliomas. Age at presentation is similar to other craniocervical paragangliomas, and like jugulotympanic tumors there appears to be a female sex predilection for sporadic lesions. The most common presenting complaint is a painless neck mass, with other symptoms including hoarseness and dysphagia. Physical findings include a palpable neck mass, medial oropharyngeal wall bulging indicative of a parapharyngeal space mass, and evidence of cranial nerve involvement. Cranial nerve dysfunction at the time of presentation occurs at a rate intermediate between CBTs and jugulotympanic tumors. Horner syndrome may result from involvement of the cervical sympathetic nerves. Intracranial extension occurs via the pars nervosa of the jugular foramen. Differential diagnosis is similar to that for CBTs. No staging system exists for vagal paragangliomas.

Treatment recommendations for vagal paragangliomas involve the same dilemmas as already noted. Vagal paragangliomas arising in the high cervical region present similar considerations as do CBTs. Vagal paragangliomas arising at the skull base, with or without intracranial extension, warrant a combined cervicotemporal approach. Radiation therapy

for vagal paragangliomas has been reported primarily in the context of isolated cases within larger series of jugulotympanic paragangliomas, with similar long-term control rates as described earlier for jugulotympanic tumors. Surgical resection of high cervical vagal tumors is the most common treatment. The incidence of vagal paralysis following resection is virtually 100%; however, 15 to 30% of the patients present with preoperative vagal palsy. With excellent rehabilitation of unilateral vocal cord paralysis, this argues in favor of resection of unilateral high cervical lesions.

Vagal tumors presenting at the skull base may mimic jugular paragangliomas. Clinical suspicion of a vagal tumor rather than a jugular paraganglioma is heightened by the presence of vocal cord paralysis or hoarseness early in the patient's course. Resection of such tumors can be accomplished by a variety of surgical approaches, which vary on surgeon preference and location of tumors.

Rare Craniocervical Paraganglioma

Other paragangliomas of the head and neck are exceedingly rare. Laryngeal paragangliomas have been reported and commonly present with symptoms of hoarseness and dysphagia due to mass effect, rather than cranial nerve involvement. The clinical behavior of laryngeal paragangliomas is thought to be more aggressive, with a higher malignant potential than other paragangliomas. Paragangliomas of the thyroid have been reported, but given the fact that no known location of normal paraganglia exists within the thyroid, it is likely that these tumors represent inferior laryngeal paraganglionic tissue presenting in continuity with the thyroid gland. Orbital paragangliomas are the least common of all craniocervical paragangliomas and must be distinguished from alveolar sarcoma. Presenting symptoms relate to the effects of a retrobulbar mass, and intracranial extension may occur.

Metastatic Paragangliomas

Rare cases of metastatic paragangliomas provide unique treatment dilemmas. This situation is very difficult to treat, and the results have been poor in the past. Chemotherapeutic regimens have not been successful. Radiation therapy provides complete relief of pain in many patients with bone metastases. There appears to be a limited role for surgical resection of metastatic lesions.

■ Suggested Reading

Fishbein L, Nathanson KL. Pheochromocytoma and paraganglioma: understanding the complexities of the genetic background. Cancer Genet 2012;205(1–2):1–11

Gulya AJ. The glomus tumor and its biology. Laryngoscope 1993; 103(11 Pt 2, Suppl 60):7–15

Langerman A, Athavale SM, Rangarajan SV, Sinard RJ, Netterville JL. Natural history of cervical paragangliomas: outcomes of observation of 43 patients. Arch Otolaryngol Head Neck Surg 2012;138(4):341–345

McCaffrey TV, Meyer FB, Michels VV, Piepgras DG, Marion MS. Familial paragangliomas of the head and neck. Arch Otolaryngol Head Neck Surg 1994;120(11):1211–1216

Netterville JL, Reilly KM, Robertson D, Reiber ME, Armstrong WB, Childs P. Carotid body tumors: a review of 30 patients with 46 tumors. Laryngoscope 1995;105(2):115–126

Robertson D, Hollister AS, Biaggioni I, Netterville JL, Mosqueda-Garcia R, Robertson RM. The diagnosis and treatment of baroreflex failure. N Engl J Med 1993;329(20):1449–1455

Schiavi F, Boedeker CC, Bausch B, et al; European-American Paraganglioma Study Group. Predictors and prevalence of paraganglioma syndrome associated with mutations of the SDHC gene. JAMA 2005;294(16):2057–2063

van der Mey AGL, Frijns JHM, Cornelisse CJ, et al. Does intervention improve the natural course of glomus tumors? A series of 108 patients seen in a 32-year period. Ann Otol Rhinol Laryngol 1992;101(8):635–642

Woods CI, Strasnick B, Jackson CG. Surgery for glomus tumors: the Otology Group experience. Laryngoscope 1993;103(11 Pt 2, Suppl 60):65–70

46 Tumors of the Parapharyngeal Space

■ Introduction

Parapharyngeal space (PPS) tumors are uncommon, representing only 0.5% of all neoplasms of the head and neck region. Consequently, the evidence pertaining to the diagnostic evaluation and management of these tumors is largely derived from retrospective case series, case reports, and expert opinion papers. Nonetheless, refinements in assessment and treatment have been realized over the past decade, providing clinicians with an increasingly evidence-based approach to the management of these neoplasms. A thorough understanding of the anatomy of the PPS and an individualized approach to each PPS neoplasm are critical to achieving optimal patient outcomes.

Anatomy

The PPS is an inverted pyramid- or cone-shaped potential space that is situated medial to the mandibular ramus and lateral to the pharynx and extends from the skull base to the hyoid bone. The PPS is defined by six anatomical boundaries, which define the superior base of the pyramid, its inferior apex, and each of its four "sides":

1. *Superior* Temporal bone lateral to the attachment of the pharyngobasilar fascia and medial to the foramen ovale and foramen spinosum
2. *Inferior* Greater cornu of the hyoid bone and the posterior belly of the digastric muscle
3. *Medial* Fascia covering the tensor and levator palatini muscles and the superior constrictor muscle
4. *Lateral* Fascia overlying the deep lobe of the parotid gland, the medial pterygoid muscle, and the mandibular ramus

5. *Anterior* The pterygomandibular raphe, which extends from the hamulus of the medial pterygoid plate to the posterior aspect of the mylohyoid line on the lingual surface of the mandible.
6. *Posterior* Fascia overlying the spine and paraspinal muscles

The parapharyngeal space is divided into anterolateral prestyloid and posteromedial poststyloid compartments by the tensor-vascular-styloid fascia, which overlies the tensor veli palatini muscle and extends medially from the styloid process toward the pharynx. The prestyloid space is the *true PPS*, whereas the poststyloid PPS may be referred to as the *carotid space*. The prestyloid or true PPS contains fat, a variable portion of the retromandibular deep lobe of the parotid gland, minor or ectopic salivary glands, the maxillary and ascending pharyngeal arteries, and the auriculotemporal nerve. The poststyloid or carotid space contains lymph nodes; the internal carotid artery and internal jugular vein; cranial nerves IX, X, XI, and XII; the cervical sympathetic chain; and glomus bodies (**Table 46.1**).

Pathology

Tumors of the PPS can arise de novo from tissues within the PPS or from neoplasms that extend into the PPS from adjacent regions, such as the nasopharynx or the masticator space. The majority of malignant tumors that directly invade the PPS are squamous cell carcinomas that arise from the oropharynx or nasopharynx. Pharyngeal squamous cell carcinomas can also metastasize to the parapharyngeal lymph nodes. Rarely, the PPS is a site of distant metastases arising from other malignancies, such as lung cancer.

Table 46.1   Components of the parapharyngeal space

Prestyloid parapharyngeal space (true parapharyngeal space)
Fat
Retromandibular deep lobe of the parotid gland
Minor or ectopic salivary glands
Maxillary and ascending pharyngeal arteries
Auriculotemporal nerve
Poststyloid parapharyngeal space (carotid space)
Lymph nodes
Internal carotid artery
Internal jugular vein
Cranial nerves IX, X, XI, and XII
Cervical sympathetic chain
Glomus bodies

Salivary Gland Neoplasms

Approximately 50% of the neoplasms arising within the PPS are of salivary gland origin, 20% are neurogenic tumors, and various benign and malignant neoplastic processes make up the remaining 30%. Most salivary gland tumors arise from the deep lobe of the parotid gland and are usually pleomorphic adenomas that may become considerably large without any external deformity. Spread into the PPS via a "dumbbell" extension through the stylomandibular tunnel can occur, but more commonly, tumors arising from the tail and retromandibular portions of the parotid extend below the ligament and displace the pharyngeal wall more diffusely. Neoplasms of ectopic salivary gland tissue within the PPS can also occur. It is important to preoperatively differentiate minor salivary gland tumors that arise from the pharyngeal mucosa from those that arise from ectopic salivary gland tissue within the PPS, because pharyngeal wall tumors will require partial pharyngectomy to achieve complete resection.

Schwannoma

Schwannoma (neurilemmoma) is the most common neurogenic tumor arising within the PPS. The vagus is the nerve of origin in 50% of cases, followed by the cervical sympathetic chain. These tumors rarely present with symptoms referable to their nerve of origin and grow slowly. They may extend intracranially, but malignant transformation rarely occurs. Treatment consists of enucleation with preservation of the involved nerve, and intraoperative nerve monitoring may facilitate such a resection. Removal

of larger tumors inherently increases the risk of temporary or permanent nerve damage.

Neurofibromas, Vagal Paragangliomas, and Other Benign and Malignant Disorders

Neurofibromas are uncommon and occur as multiple lesions that can undergo malignant degeneration. Vagal paragangliomas are the most common paragangliomas arising in the PPS. They may be associated with other multicentric lesions and can secrete catecholamines, but these tumors rarely undergo malignant change. Thirty percent may present with vagal deficits or jugular foramen syndrome, characterized by neuropathy of cranial nerves IX, X, and XI. Various other benign and malignant disorders have been reported in the PPS, including vascular malformations, lipomas, lymphoma, and various sarcomas.

■ Diagnostic Evaluation

Clinical Presentation and Natural History

PPS tumors are frequently asymptomatic. They are often detected incidentally on a radiographic imaging study that was performed for an unrelated medical problem. Signs and symptoms of PPS are more likely to be present in malignant and larger tumors. A neck mass is the most common initial sign, and parotid fullness or a submucosal bulge or fullness in the soft palate or pharyngeal wall may be present. Vague symptoms, such as dysphagia, aural fullness or decreased hearing, hoarseness, or unilateral anhydrosis, may occur. Pain and cranial nerve palsies are highly suggestive of malignancy. Otalgia, facial pain, and patients diagnosed with temporomandibular joint disorder who do not respond to treatment may also have a malignant PPS neoplasm. First-bite syndrome has also been reported in association with malignant lesions, and other unusual symptoms, such as bradycardia and syncopal episodes, may be reported in tumors affecting the carotid sinus and glossopharyngeal nerve. A history of neurofibromatosis or a family history of paragangliomas should also be noted.

Physical Examination

A comprehensive physical examination of the head and neck region should be performed, including careful evaluation for mucosal lesions of the upper aerodigestive tract, suggestive of squamous carcinoma. Evaluation of all head and neck mucosal surfaces, through fiberoptic endoscopy or mirror inspection, should be routinely performed to evaluate the nasopharynx, oropharynx, hypopharynx, and larynx, including vocal cord mobility. The soft palate, tonsillar fossa, and lateral pharyngeal wall should be evaluated for evidence of submucosal fullness or bulging. Thorough assessment for cranial neuropathies of cranial nerves VII and IX through XII should be completed. Ptosis of the upper eyelid and miosis are suggestive of Horner syndrome. Otoscopic examination may demonstrate unilateral middle ear effusion or tympanic membrane retraction. Palpation of the parotid gland and neck region is also performed to evaluate for masses.

Radiographic Evaluation

Computed tomography (CT) and magnetic resonance imaging (MRI) are most commonly employed to evaluate PPS tumors. MRI is superior to CT for the evaluation of retrograde perineural spread and recurrent pleomorphic adenoma. CT angiography (CTA) or magnetic resonance angiography (MRA) should be used for poststyloid lesions, so that paragangliomas can be differentiated from nerve sheath tumors. Flow voids are diagnostic of paragangliomas, but they may not be appreciated with MRA until the tumor measures 2 cm in diameter. Nerve sheath tumors occasionally enhance on CTA and MRA, but paragangliomas typically enhance much more intensely, particularly on contrast-enhanced CT.

MRA is valuable in determining the degree of vascularity of the mass and its relationship to the great vessels, as well as in identifying larger feeder vessels. However, MRA is not yet able to detect subtle carotid involvement and has not yet replaced angiography, particularly if preoperative embolization is being considered.

The fat of the PPS has a distinct appearance on CT and MRI; it is often displaced in a characteristic manner by tumors of the PPS or adjacent areas. Tumors of the *pharyngeal mucosal space*, which is defined medially by the squamous mucosa of the nasopharynx and oropharynx and laterally by the pharyngeal constrictor muscles, displace the PPS fat *posterolaterally*. On the other hand, tumors of the *masticator space*, which extends from the inferior border of the mandible to the skull base and contains the posterior body and ascending ramus of the mandible, the muscles of mastication, and the mandibular branch of the trigeminal nerve, displace the PPS fat *posteromedially*. Deep lobe parotid gland tumors displace the PPS fat *anteromedially*, and tumors of the poststyloid compartment or carotid space displace the PPS fat *anterolaterally*. Obvious tumor infiltration of the PPS fat is a reliable indicator of malignancy.

Cytological Assessment

Applying transoral or transcervical fine-needle aspiration (FNA) for cytological evaluation provides complementary information to radiographic imaging, which can be used to differentiate between benign and malignant lesions. Cytological evaluation can detect or exclude malignancy with 90% diagnostic accuracy when the cytological aspirate is satisfactory for evaluation. However, FNA provides a correct specific diagnosis in only one-third of cases when compared with final histopathology. Moreover, approximately one-third of FNA specimens are nondiagnostic, which may result from technical challenges associated with CT-guided FNA or hypocellular aspirates.

However, FNA or core needle biopsy may be valuable if lymphoma or distant metastases are suspected, if the tumor is unresectable, or if observation would be a treatment option for a benign process. Furthermore, cytological diagnosis can be used in combination with radiographic evaluation to reaffirm the indications for surgery and to determine the most appropriate surgical approach. Transoral open biopsy is not recommended because it may result in tumor spillage and adherence of the pharyngeal wall to the tumor, and injury to adjacent neurovascular structures.

Other Diagnostic Tests

Urinary catecholamines should be obtained if a paraganglioma is suspected, so that optimal perioperative management for a secreting tumor is performed. Direct laryngoscopy with endoscopic evaluation of the upper aerodigestive tract is indicated if nodal metastases are identified. Additional tests, such as chest radiography and positron-emission tomography, are performed when they are clinically indicated.

◼ Management

The available treatment options for a particular PPS neoplasm are based on the clinical, radiographic, and cytological findings. Observation may be appropriate for asymptomatic benign tumors, especially in elderly or debilitated patients. The surgeon must carefully weigh the indications for surgery against the risks of surgical resection, particularly if cranial nerve injury is likely. Because the exact procedure that will be required to safely resect the tumor is frequently unclear preoperatively, care must be taken to provide the patient with a detailed informed consent that includes all possible approaches, including mandibulotomy and the potential sequelae and complications associated with cranial nerve palsies and vascular injury.

Selection of a surgical approach for PPS tumor resection should be based on the size and location of the tumor, its relationship to the internal carotid artery and internal jugular vein, the expected vascularity of the tumor, and the likelihood of malignancy. Surgical approaches to gain access to and resect PPS tumors include transoral, transcervical, transparotid-transcervical, transparotid-transcervical-transmandibular, infratemporal fossa, and skull base surgery. The infratemporal fossa and skull base surgery approaches are indicated for carefully selected tumors located near the skull base or those that invade the skull base and are not discussed in this chapter.

Transoral Approach

The transoral approach is usually not recommended for treating PPS tumors because it increases the risk of tumor rupture and neurovascular injury. However, relatively small benign tumors that are located in the medial prestyloid space may be amenable to a transoral approach. These are often pleomorphic adenomas originating in the minor salivary glands. This approach is contraindicated in the management of malignant tumors. Dissection posterior to the stylopharyngeus and styloglossus muscles and lateral to the superior constrictor muscle increases the risk of injury to the internal carotid artery, internal jugular vein, and cranial nerves. Transoral robotic surgery, which has been successfully employed at some centers to remove benign PPS tumors, may enhance the safety of transoral PPS surgery.

Transcervical and Transparotid-Transcervical Approaches

Benign tumors in the prestyloid compartment, such as extraparotid tumors, may be removed via a transcervical approach if adequate exposure can be achieved. Video-assisted dissection supplemented by intraoperative image guidance has been used to improve visualization and ease of dissection, so that more extensive surgery is not required.

The transparotid-transcervical approach, also known as the cervical-parotid approach, is the most commonly employed technique to resect deep lobe parotid tumors, extraparotid salivary gland tumors, and many poststyloid nerve sheath tumors. This approach uses a preauricular parotidectomy incision that is extended into a neck incision. A superficial parotidectomy is completed, the spinal accessory and hypoglossal nerves are exposed, and the internal jugular vein and carotid artery are visualized. The

stylohyoid muscle and posterior belly of the digastric muscle are divided at their origin on the styloid process. If exposure is still insufficient, the stylomandibular ligament is divided along the posterior aspect of the mandible, which allows the surgeon to displace the mandible slightly forward. This frequently increases the portal of dissection sufficiently to permit safe dissection around the tumor. Care is taken to establish a plane of dissection between the internal carotid artery and the tumor. Ligation of branches of the external carotid artery is frequently required to improve access to the PPS.

Mandibulotomy

A transmandibular approach is typically used in concert with a transparotid-transcervical approach when the transparotid-transcervical approach will not provide sufficient exposure for safe tumor removal. A mandibulotomy should be considered for large benign tumors, infiltrating malignant tumors that cannot be readily dissected away from the surrounding soft tissues, and highly vascular tumors. Tracheotomy may also be necessary if significant postoperative pharyngeal edema is expected.

◼ Complications of Treatment

Complications can be minimized by careful preoperative planning, evaluation of the anatomical relationships between the tumor and the adjacent structures within the PPS, and an appreciation for the infiltrative behavior of the tumor based on radiological imaging. Adequate surgical exposure is paramount to minimize morbidity during PPS surgery.

The most frequent serious complication is injury to one or more cranial nerves (VII and IX–XII). An injury of the vagus nerve is associated with the greatest morbidity, particularly if it is severed above the nodose ganglion, because of the impact on the pharyngeal branches and the superior laryngeal nerve. Dysphagia and dysphonia are the sequelae of such an injury. Younger patients who have an isolated vagal injury may be able to compensate over time, but elderly patients are more likely to require a gastrostomy tube and early vocal cord medialization. Injury to the internal carotid artery can occur, so careful preoperative radiographic assessment, choice of surgical approach, and attainment of adequate exposure are critical.

Potential complications resulting from mandibulotomy include malocclusion, malunion, and lingual nerve injury. First-bite syndrome, a disorder that is characterized by severe spasms or cramping in the parotid region with the first bite of each meal that diminishes over the next several bites, develops in ~

20% of patients who undergo PPS surgery. Partial or total symptomatic resolution is eventually achieved in 80% of these patients. These patients may have severe, debilitating symptoms, and gabapentin (Neurontin, Pfizer, New York, NY) has been used successfully in some patients. As stated, resolution is expected over time and reassurance should be part of the treatment plan.

■ Suggested Reading

Arnason T, Hart RD, Taylor SM, Trites JR, Nasser JG, Bullock MJ. Diagnostic accuracy and safety of fine-needle aspiration biopsy of the parapharyngeal space. Diagn Cytopathol 2012;40(2):118–123

Beswick DM, Vaezi A, Caicedo-Granados E, Duvvuri U. Minimally invasive surgery for parapharyngeal space tumors. Laryngoscope 2012;122(5):1072–1078

Dallan I, Seccia V, Muscatello L, et al. Transoral endoscopic anatomy of the parapharyngeal space: a step-by-step logical approach with surgical considerations. Head Neck 2011;33(4):557–561

Kanzaki S, Nameki H. Standardised method of selecting surgical approaches to benign parapharyngeal space tumours, based on preoperative images. J Laryngol Otol 2008;122(6):628–634

Lieberman SM, Har-El G. First bite syndrome as a presenting symptom of a parapharyngeal space malignancy. Head Neck 2011; 33(10):1539–1541

Linkov G, Morris LG, Shah JP, Kraus DH. First bite syndrome: incidence, risk factors, treatment, and outcomes. Laryngoscope 2012;122(8):1773–1778

Olsen KD. Tumors and surgery of the parapharyngeal space. Laryngoscope 1994;104(5 Pt 2, Suppl 63):1–28

Stambuk HE, Patel SG. Imaging of the parapharyngeal space. Otolaryngol Clin North Am 2008;41(1):77–101, vi

47 Contemporary Adjunctive Cancer Therapy

■ Introduction

Adjunctive local and systemic therapies have been integrated into the overall management of cancer of the head and neck because of the continued poor response of patients to the standard mainstays of treatment: surgery and radiation. Although improvements in survival and functional outcomes have been seen using standard therapies for early-stage disease, similar success has not been achieved for advanced-stage disease, with the problems of local-regional recurrence, distant metastasis, and poor overall survival still significant.

Adjunctive therapies administered to patients with head and neck cancer include variations in radiation dosing and scheduling, use of cytotoxic chemotherapeutic drugs, and/or targeted molecular therapies with or without radiation. The goals of these treatment strategies have been to improve local-regional control rates, increase disease-free survival intervals, improve overall survival outcomes, and decrease the rates of distant metastases and development of second primary malignancies. In general, the regularly updated National Comprehensive Cancer Network clinical practice guidelines are an excellent resource for up-to-date consensus recommendations for the application of adjunctive therapies for head and neck cancer (see this chapter's Suggested Reading section). At present, advances in therapy have made headway into achieving these goals, but more research is needed to fully define the rationale for application of adjuvant therapies to head and neck cancer. This chapter focuses on the most common malignancy of the head and neck: head and neck squamous cell carcinoma (HNSCC).

■ Management and Treatment

Adjunctive Chemotherapy Treatment Schemes

Historically, chemotherapy has been used mainly as a palliative treatment for patients with locally recurrent, unresectable, or metastatic disease. Several agents have been used with this intent, with clinical response rates averaging < 30%. Although complete responses have been reported, the overall survival for most patients following chemotherapy in this setting is typically 6 to 12 months. Because clinical responses (i.e., reduction in tumor burden) can be seen with chemotherapy alone, investigators have been encouraged to combine chemotherapy with surgery and radiation in the hope of improving outcomes. Given this history, chemotherapy for HNSCC has been administered in three general treatment schemes: adjuvant, neoadjuvant, and concurrent chemotherapies.

Adjuvant Chemotherapy

In adjuvant chemotherapy the agents are administered in a well-defined number of cycles after the primary treatment, whether surgery and/or radiation therapy. In this treatment approach, gross clinical disease is not measurable; thus it is not possible to monitor an individual patient for a response to the chemotherapy. Adjuvant chemotherapy is rarely applied.

Neoadjuvant Chemotherapy

In this approach, also known as induction or sequential chemotherapy, drugs are administered in a predetermined number of chemotherapy cycles prior to the definitive therapy, such as surgery, radiation, or chemotherapy and radiation. The theoretical advantages of this scheme are that the systemic therapy is provided before disruption of the tumor microvasculature by surgery and radiation. Additionally, it is theoretically possible that a reduction in tumor bulk might permit a less aggressive surgical resection and improved functional outcomes. The downside to neoadjuvant chemotherapy is that it adds to the overall length and toxicity of treatment. It is also possible for disease to progress during neoadjuvant chemotherapy, such that a patient never receives definitive treatment.

Neoadjuvant chemotherapy can be applied solely for research purposes as part of a "window" study. In this setting, chemotherapy is given in a nontherapeutic manner after an initial biopsy and before surgery or other therapy to test the biology of the tumor.

Concurrent Chemotherapy

In this approach, chemotherapy and radiation therapy are administered simultaneously. The major theoretical advantage is that the chemotherapy can increase the local-regional activity of radiation therapy, thereby enhancing the tumor response to this treatment. The radiosensitizing effect of chemotherapy is counterbalanced by the increase in acute and long-term toxicity seen with this treatment approach.

Chemotherapeutic Agents

Although several different agents have been used in the treatment of HNSCC, the most studied agents are cisplatin and 5-fluorouracil (5-FU). These agents have direct cytotoxic effects as well as radiation-sensitizing effects. Taxanes, and carboplatin have also been shown to be effective in treating HNSCC, alone or in combination with other drugs. More recently, targeted molecular therapies have been used in the treatment of HNSCC. Biologic agents that target the epidermal growth factor receptor (EGFR) are the best characterized. Cetuximab, a prototypic anti-EGFR monoclonal antibody, is currently available for clinical use.

It is important to note that use of specific chemotherapeutic agents can vary depending on the site of disease, patient performance status and comorbidities, treatment strategies and goals, and physician and patient preference. For example, if induction chemotherapy is planned, then there is level 1 evidence to support the use of combined docetaxel, cisplatin, and 5-FU. Alternatively, if palliative chemotherapy is planned, then there is level 1 evidence to support the use of combined cisplatin or carboplatin, 5-FU, and cetuximab. Cisplatin alone or cisplatin and 5-FU have been the traditional standard for patients treated with concurrent chemotherapy. However, there are also strong data supporting the use of cetuximab concurrent with radiation therapy, particularly in patients whose tumors test positive for the human papillomavirus (HPV). A phase 3 randomized, controlled trial comparing radiation and cisplatin versus radiation and cetuximab is under way for patients with HPV-associated HNSCC treated with concurrent chemoradiation. At this point, however, the data regarding treatment alterations for HPV-related tumors are preliminary.

Advances in Radiotherapy for Head and Neck Cancer

Radiation therapy for HNSCC has traditionally been used as either a primary therapeutic modality or a postoperative adjuvant therapy. Postoperative adjuvant radiation therapy has been a cornerstone of treatment for advanced-stage HNSCC, particularly oral cavity cancers. Adjuvant use of radiation therapy has been shown to improve local-regional control. Adjuvant radiation therapy does not alter the rate of distant metastasis or prevent the development of second primary malignancies.

Altered Fractionation Schemes for Radiation Therapy

In an effort to improve local-regional control and reduce late complications due to damage of normal tissue, altered fractionation schemes for radiation therapy have been used. Altered fractionation schemes attempt to address the issues of tumor cell repopulation during treatment, tumor cell hypoxia, and intrinsic radioresistance of tumor cells, all of which have been implicated as causes of failure after primary radiation therapy. Conventional fractionated radiation therapy for HNSCC usually consists of 1.8 to 2 gray (Gy) daily to maximum doses of 60 to 75 Gy. In this conventional scheme, treatment breaks are avoided because of the associated risk of increased local-regional recurrence.

Altered fractionation schedules that have been used fall under two general categories:

- *Hyperfractionation* uses a treatment scheme of more than one dose a day (usually two) with smaller-than-conventional radiation dose fractions, yielding an overall treatment total dose in excess of conventional radiation total dosage.
- *Accelerated fractionation* uses multiple daily treatments (two to three) administered to total doses equal to or less than conventional radiation doses. In this manner, treatment is delivered in a more intense but shorter time frame.

Retrospective studies of accelerated fractionated radiotherapy and hyperfractionated radiotherapy have demonstrated an approximate 20% improvement in local-regional disease control when compared with historical control rates of conventional radiation therapy. A prospective randomized trial of the European Organization for the Research and Treatment of Cancer (EORTC) demonstrated a 20% increase in 5-year local-regional control, and a 14% improvement in survival for patients with oropharyngeal carcinoma treated with hyperfractionated radiation therapy compared with once-daily treatment. Although this improvement in 5-year local-regional control was statistically significant ($p = 0.007$), the improvement in survival was not significant ($p = 0.08$). The incorporation of altered fractionation radiation schemes into current treatment algorithms continues to evolve and remains an area of active clinical research.

Combination Chemotherapy and Radiation Therapy for Head and Neck Cancer

In an effort to improve the treatment outcome for patients with locally advanced HNSCC, several treatment strategies that incorporate both chemotherapy and radiation therapy have been developed and investigated. These therapies aim to improve survival, lower the rate of distant metastases, and decrease the functional morbidity associated with primary surgery.

Traditionally, radiation and chemotherapy are given concurrently. However, there are also data to support the use of an induction strategy. Several phase 1 and 2 studies using induction chemotherapy followed by radiation therapy for treatment of primary disease demonstrated high overall partial and complete response rates frequently exceeding 50%. A randomized phase 3 clinical trial has confirmed the use of docetaxel, cisplatin, and 5-FU if an induction strategy is planned. These studies suggest that chemotherapy used for primary disease might have greater benefit than when used for recurrent or metastatic head and neck carcinoma. However, no randomized trial using induction chemotherapy has demonstrated a significant survival benefit from the addition of chemotherapy over conventional treatment approaches.

Organ Preservation Treatment

The use of induction chemotherapy has received the greatest attention as a result of two randomized trials using cisplatin and 5-FU prior to definitive radiation for laryngeal and hypopharyngeal cancer, respectively. These studies have sought to determine whether use of chemotherapy in combination with conventional radiotherapy could provide local-regional control and overall survival rates equivalent to total laryngectomy and pharyngolaryngectomy.

The Veterans Affairs Laryngeal Cancer Study Group trial evaluated induction chemotherapy with three cycles of cisplatin and 5-FU followed by radiation therapy in stage III or IV SCC of the larynx. In this study, the estimated 2-year survival rate was found to be 68% for both the chemotherapy and radiation therapy and the surgery and postoperative radiotherapy groups, with larynx preservation in approximately two-thirds of the patients receiving the chemotherapy and radiotherapy. A similar study performed by EORTC evaluating larynx preservation in advanced-stage hypopharyngeal carcinoma demonstrated similar data, suggesting that neoadjuvant chemotherapy plus radiation therapy is equivalent to surgery and postoperative radiation with respect to survival, with a resultant higher degree of organ preservation. However, both of these studies failed to provide a radiation therapy alone treatment group for comparison. Thus there are no data to support neoadjuvant chemotherapy as being more effective than radiation therapy alone in these malignancies.

In two large retrospective reviews of radiotherapy and chemotherapy combinations for treatment of HNSCC, the data suggest that a small but clinically significant benefit in overall survival is present with the use of combination chemotherapy and radiation therapy. In one of these studies, a meta-analysis of 54 randomized, controlled trials of chemotherapy was performed. Concurrent chemotherapy and radiation therapy offered a higher survival benefit than neoadjuvant chemotherapy (increased overall survival by 12% vs. 3%, respectively). This suggests that further use of concurrent radiation and chemotherapy may prove to offer the greatest benefit to patients with advanced-stage disease.

A phase 3 randomized prospective trial directed as an intergroup study by the Southwest Oncology Group, the Radiation Therapy Oncology Group, and the Eastern Cooperative Oncology Group has recently been completed. The trial investigated the effectiveness of chemotherapy and radiation therapy administered concurrently versus radiation therapy alone in patients with stages III and IV nasopharyngeal carcinoma. This study demonstrated a statistically significant difference in progression-free and overall survival for the combination therapy group, with 2-year survival of 55% in the radiation therapy alone group, versus 80% in the chemotherapy and radiation therapy treatment group. At present, this study supports the standard use of concurrent chemotherapy and radiation therapy using cisplatin and 5-FU in patients with advanced-stage nasopharyngeal carcinoma.

The use of chemotherapy in the adjuvant setting is well defined. Two randomized phase 3 clinical trials explored the role of radiation versus chemoradiation after surgery for HNSCC. These studies established the role for the addition of chemotherapy to radiation after surgery for patients with either positive surgical margins or evidence of extracapsular spread. Of course, these studies predated our current understanding of the impact of HPV on prognosis for patients with HNSCC. In the future, it is likely that the recommendations will differ, depending on HPV status, particularly with respect to extracapsular spread. Further, the optimal choice and dosing schedule of chemotherapy have yet to be defined in the adjuvant setting.

Chemoprevention of Head and Neck Cancer

Prevention of head and neck cancer by chemotherapeutic means can be defined as pharmacological intervention using specific nutritional agents or other chemical derivatives to suppress or reverse carcinogenesis and prevent the development of invasive malignancy. The concept of chemoprevention for HNSCC is highly relevant for the following reasons:

- Many patients have significant tobacco and alcohol exposure, which delineates a population at risk for HNSCC.
- Premalignant lesions, such as leukoplakia and erythroplakia, are relatively common.
- The risk of developing a second primary malignancy of the head and neck after treatment for HNSCC approximates 1 to 2% per year.

For these reasons, a safe and effective chemopreventive agent would be a major advance for patients with risk factors for developing new or secondary HNSCC. Chemopreventive strategies should be recognized as "secondary" prevention measures, as opposed to "primary" prevention measures, which in the population at risk for HNSCC would be avoidance of environmental carcinogens, such as tobacco and alcohol. The ideal chemopreventive agent has not been developed. However, the characteristics desired of such a therapeutic modality include that it be nontoxic, easily administered, inexpensive, readily available, and effective against the promotion stage of carcinogenesis.

Several different agents have been evaluated as chemopreventive, including retinoids, antioxidants, arachidonic acid cascade inhibitors, and prostaglandin inhibitors. Retinoids have been the most studied chemopreventive agents for HNSCC.

Retinoids

The retinoids, synthetic analogues of vitamin A, have been extensively studied and demonstrate promise as inhibitors of carcinogenesis. Clinically, their use has been limited by the onset of significant toxicity in patients treated with higher doses as well as by the cost associated with their use. Several retinoids have been tested for efficacy in head and neck cancer, including retinol, 13-cis retinoic acid (13-cRA), etretinate, N-4-(hydroxyphenyl)retinamide (4HPR), and N-4-(hydroxycarbophenyl)retinamide (4HCR).

Retinoids for Oral Premalignancy

Retinoids have been studied extensively as chemopreventive agents useful in reversing oral premalignant lesions and preventing progression to invasive cancers. This treatment has focused on reversal of the clinical finding of leukoplakia and the histological finding of dysplasia. One early randomized study demonstrated that two-thirds of the patients treated daily with high-dose 13-cRA had partial or complete resolution of leukoplakia, as compared with only 10% of the patients in the placebo group. Unfortunately, at the doses used (2 mg/kg/d), 13-cRA was found to be unacceptably toxic. In addition, once treatment was discontinued, new or original lesions rapidly recurred. Studies evaluating other retinoids, including 4HPR, 4HCR, and retinol, have demonstrated similar effects. At present, treatment of oral premalignant lesions by retinoids appears to be effective at reversing both the leukoplakia and the histological dysplasia. However, the effect is short lived, with prompt recurrence once the drug is discontinued. Therefore, use of retinoids for treatment of oral premalignancy and prevention of invasive oral cancer should be considered experimental for the time being.

Beta Carotene

Beta carotene is another agent that has undergone extensive clinical testing as a chemopreventive agent for HNSCC. It is nontoxic and inexpensive and is readily available. Unfortunately, the majority of studies evaluating β-carotene as a chemopreventive for HNSCC have been nonrandomized trials. Although initial clinical results were promising for treatment of oral premalignant lesions, subsequent prospective studies failed to support β-carotene's routine use for this purpose. In addition, the potential use of β-carotene for head and neck cancer prevention has been compromised by findings that suggested that such use may increase the risk of lung cancer in heavy smokers.

Inconclusive Results

The conflicting findings regarding the use of the most common chemopreventive agents, retinoids and b-carotene, suggest that the value of these agents as chemopreventives in HNSCC remains unknown. For this reason, these agents should be viewed as experimental in any setting of chemoprevention for HNSCC at present.

■ Practice Guidelines, Consensus Statements, and Measures

National Comprehensive Cancer Network. Clinical Practice Guidelines in Oncology. Head and Neck Cancers (Version 2.2011). http://www.nccn.org/professionals/physician_gls/f_guidelines.asp#site. Accessed March 1, 2013

■ Summary

This chapter covers many applications of adjunctive therapy. In the neoadjuvant setting, most agents are used for primary therapy, not as a tumor "debulking" prior to therapy. However, there are some studies supportive of neoadjuvant chemotherapy as a means to predict biologic behavior and stratify treatment according to response. In these applications, a good response would prompt continuation on to concurrent chemotherapy and radiotherapy, and a lack of response would prompt surgical intervention. In the postoperative, adjuvant setting radiation therapy or chemotherapy and radiation may be used in circumstances such as positive margins, extracapsular extension of nodal disease, multiple lymph node metastasis, and tumor features such as perineural invasion, lymphovascular invasion, the infiltrative pattern of the tumor, and other factors.

■ Suggested Reading

Bernier J, Cooper JS, Pajak TF, et al. Defining risk levels in locally advanced head and neck cancers: a comparative analysis of concurrent postoperative radiation plus chemotherapy trials of the EORTC (#22931) and RTOG (# 9501). Head Neck 2005;27(10): 843–850

Bernier J, Domenge C, Ozsahin M, et al; European Organization for Research and Treatment of Cancer Trial 22931. Postoperative irradiation with or without concomitant chemotherapy for locally advanced head and neck cancer. N Engl J Med 2004;350(19): 1945–1952

Bonner JA, Harari PM, Giralt J, et al. Radiotherapy plus cetuximab for squamous-cell carcinoma of the head and neck. N Engl J Med 2006;354(6):567–578

Cooper JS, Pajak TF, Forastiere AA, et al; Radiation Therapy Oncology Group 9501/Intergroup. Postoperative concurrent radiotherapy and chemotherapy for high-risk squamous-cell carcinoma of the head and neck. N Engl J Med 2004;350(19):1937–1944

The Department of Veterans Affairs Laryngeal Cancer Study Group. Induction chemotherapy plus radiation compared with surgery plus radiation in patients with advanced laryngeal cancer. N Engl J Med 1991;324(24):1685–1690

Forastiere AA, Zhang Q, Weber RS, et al. Long-term results of RTOG 91-11: a comparison of three nonsurgical treatment strategies to preserve the larynx in patients with locally advanced larynx cancer. J Clin Oncol 2013;31(7):845–852

Hong WK, Lippman SM, Itri LM, et al. Prevention of second primary tumors with isotretinoin in squamous-cell carcinoma of the head and neck. N Engl J Med 1990;323(12):795–801

Kalinsky K, Hershman DL. Cracking open window of opportunity trials. J Clin Oncol 2012;30(21):2573–2575

Lefebvre JL, Chevalier D, Luboinski B, Kirkpatrick A, Collette L, Sahmoud T; EORTC Head and Neck Cancer Cooperative Group. Larynx preservation in pyriform sinus cancer: preliminary results of a European Organization for Research and Treatment of Cancer phase III trial. J Natl Cancer Inst 1996;88(13):890–899

Omenn GS, Goodman GE, Thornquist MD, et al. Risk factors for lung cancer and for intervention effects in CARET, the Beta-Carotene and Retinol Efficacy Trial. J Natl Cancer Inst 1996;88(21):1550–1559

Pignon JP, Bourhis J, Domenge C, Designé L. Chemotherapy added to locoregional treatment for head and neck squamous-cell carcinoma: three meta-analyses of updated individual data. MACH-NC Collaborative Group. Meta-Analysis of Chemotherapy on Head and Neck Cancer. Lancet 2000;355(9208):949–955

Posner MR, Hershock DM, Blajman CR, et al; TAX 324 Study Group. Cisplatin and fluorouracil alone or with docetaxel in head and neck cancer. N Engl J Med 2007;357(17):1705–1715

Thomas F, Rochaix P, Benlyazid A, et al. Pilot study of neoadjuvant treatment with erlotinib in nonmetastatic head and neck squamous cell carcinoma. Clin Cancer Res 2007;13(23):7086–7092

Vermorken JB, Mesia R, Rivera F, et al. Platinum-based chemotherapy plus cetuximab in head and neck cancer. N Engl J Med 2008;359(11):1116–1127

48 Function and Quality of Life after Therapy for Squamous Cell Cancer of the Head and Neck

■ Introduction

Health-related quality of life (QOL) is a concept that has garnered increasing attention over the past 2 decades and in many instances is considered as important as other treatment outcomes, such as survival and recurrence. QOL is a complex concept that is a measure of the patient's own perspective of mental, physical, and social well-being. Treatment is no longer considered successful simply if there is the absence of disease. QOL may vary significantly among individuals and across culture, gender, age, and disease states. Thus QOL can be a challenge to measure and requires disease-specific tools for accurate assessment. QOL surveys are designed following a rigorous process that includes focus group feedback, relevant literature review, understanding of disease natural history, and statistical and psychometric analyses that culminate in a process termed validation. The validation process ensures that the concepts to be measured are actually measured. Moreover, validated QOL instruments have the property of maintaining integrity and precision over time and with retesting.

For patients with squamous cell cancer of the head and neck (SCCHN), QOL encompasses the factors that are most relevant to patients impacted by their disease and its treatment. This population includes patients with primary tumors arising in the larynx, pharynx, oral cavity, paranasal sinuses, and salivary glands. Global general health QOL instruments that measure a wide range of medical conditions (heart disease, diabetes mellitus, etc.) frequently do not have adequate sensitivity and specificity to capture important issues for patients with SCCHN. Thus disease-specific head and neck QOL instruments have been designed that measure a patient's perspective on the mental, social, and physical aspects relating to speech, eating, xerostomia, swallowing, breathing, head and neck pain, sleeping, work, recreation, and appearance. Certainly, it is important for both physicians and patients to understand both the overall and the specific health impacts of disease and its treatment effects on patients with SCCHN. Often, when treatment outcomes are comparable, patients will desire the option that best preserves QOL.

Physicians, including surgeons, radiation oncologists, and medical oncologists, who care for patients with SCCHN continue to work diligently to provide treatment options that preserve QOL. Even before health-related QOL was fully conceptualized or capable of being measured, practitioners aspired to provide treatment paradigms that would improve survival outcomes, while minimizing deficits to patients' physical and emotional well-being, QOL, socialization, and aesthetics. Examples of such efforts include external beam radiation to avoid ablative surgery; chemoradiation protocols (organ preservation) to avoid laryngectomy, pharyngectomy, or base-of-tongue resection; intensity-modulated radiotherapy; microvascular free-tissue reconstruction; transoral laser microsurgery; and transoral robotic surgery. Each of the aforementioned treatment advances recognizes the commitment and emphasis that both patients and physicians hold on the importance of QOL as a critical clinical outcome. With the advent of tools to measure QOL, researchers have attempted to better understand the important components that constitute QOL, as well as the clinical factors that impact and predict QOL.

■ Evaluation

At present, the routine use of QOL instruments in evaluating individual patients with SCCHN is not in practice. QOL questionnaires are still largely used to study specific populations or subpopulations of patients. For the head and neck cancer patient, QOL instruments are now available to evaluate every important aspect of the disease and treatment. **Table 48.1** presents a list of QOL instruments that have commonly been used and by no means is intended to be inclusive of every tool available. Some instruments

Table 48.1 Head and neck health-related QOL instruments

European Organization for Research and Treatment of Cancer—Quality of Life Questionnaire (EORTC QLQ-C30 and -HN 35)
Functional Assessment of Cancer Therapy (FACT)
University of Washington Quality of Life (UW QOL)
University of Michigan Head and Neck Quality of Life (HN QOL)
Quality of Life Radiation Therapy Instrument (QOL-RTI)
Performance Status Scale for Head and Neck Cancer (PSS-HN)
Voice Handicap Index (VHI)
Liverpool Oral Rehabilitation Questionnaire (LORQ)
Neck Dissection Impairment Index (NDII)
Swallowing Quality of Life Questionnaire (SWAL-QOL)

have been designed to focus on specific parameters (such as swallowing, xerostomia, and shoulder function), whereas others attempt to capture and measure broad aspects expected to be affected by the disease and treatment. In each QOL instrument, the questions are generally organized in "domains," which are questions that cluster to a common theme—for example, communication, eating, pain, mood, cognition. Typically, a higher score indicates a better QOL. The QOL instruments currently in use assume that patients have the requisite language, reading, and cognitive skills to complete the questionnaire themselves, and thus are self-report questionnaires that use simplified language and request a response to a specific question with several options to choose from. Ultimately, a patient's responses can be scored and tabulated for both domain and overall scores.

Many of the head and neck QOL researchers and instrument developers have also used global health-related QOL instruments in parallel while evaluating QOL in head and neck cancer populations. The most widely employed global health-related QOL instrument is the Medical Outcomes Study (MOS) Short-Form Health Survey (SF-36). The SF-36 has two components—a Physical Component Scale and a Mental Component Scale—both with attendant domains that evaluate a broad range of health-related factors. Large amounts of QOL data across all disease states have been accumulated using the SF-36; thus any disease can be viewed in the context of both normative respondents (healthy individuals) as well as sick patients with a broad range of illnesses. Although global instruments like the SF-36 can demonstrate changes in health-related QOL over time or in response to interventions across a host of

diseases, they may fail to query or measure important specific aspects of head and neck cancer health-related QOL, such as eating and speech. Numerous studies of SCCHN patients using both the SF-36 and a head and neck cancer–specific QOL instrument have demonstrated the utility of the SF-36 to track global health-related QOL but have also confirmed that head and neck cancer-specific tools are essential to detect important nuances related to the disease or treatment of head and neck cancer.

■ Management

Although there has been tremendous growth in the field of QOL research, as well as universal acceptance of the importance of health-related QOL, complex treatment decisions for individual patients is not influenced by QOL questionnaire results. Treatment decisions for any individual patient should still best be driven by present standard-of-care protocols, careful consultation with patients and their families, and clinical trials under the purview of national and institutional governing bodies.

Over the past couple of decades, numerous prospective and retrospective studies have been completed using head and neck QOL instruments. A wide variety of topics among head and neck cancer populations have been studied, including comprehensive issues encompassing head and neck cancer health as well as specific topics such as swallowing, xerostomia, speech, pain, shoulder mobility, sleep, and mood. Rather than tailoring treatment decisions for any individual patient, a more constructive manner in which to view and interpret head and neck QOL data is to understand broad themes that can be derived from the numerous studies. These themes may have the benefit of strategically targeting concerns and risks during pretreatment consultation. Practitioners may decide to preemptively address important issues, including nutrition or depression concerns that have been demonstrated to significantly impact long-term QOL.

For patients with SCCHN, myriad clinical issues must be managed that relate to their disease and treatment. A great deal of research has been performed with the intent to understand how and to what extent these factors impact head and neck QOL. Some of these issues include alterations in diet and feeding, communication disorders, pain, depression, loss of work and income, and deterioration of social and family relationships. This can create the sentiment of an overall lack of usefulness and self-value. For any individual patient, each clinical issue may have varying degrees of impact, but practitioners can take away an understanding as to which clinical factors routinely predict worse QOL.

As a general rule, SCCHN patients' long-term physical QOL is negatively impacted following treatment, whereas their mental QOL will frequently recover, regardless of treatment modality. Prospective analysis has been completed to evaluate head and neck specific indices over time, with one study of over 300 patients evaluating the University of Michigan's Head and Neck (HN) QOL questionnaire and the SF-36 prior to treatment and 1 year following treatment. Although physical components of QOL were significantly diminished from baseline, mental components of QOL continued to increase and approach baseline at 1 year. Clinical factors, including prolonged gastrostomy tube, smoking, and depressive symptoms, were major predictors of worse QOL. Other studies have consistently established that clinical factors predictive of poorer QOL include the presence of a gastrostomy tube, prolonged tracheostomy, radiation therapy, chemotherapy, neck dissection, and advanced-stage disease.

Additionally, multiple studies have demonstrated that patients who begin with higher baseline QOL have better long-term QOL. Analysis of nearly 175 patients using the University of Washington QOL instrument concluded that baseline QOL and comorbidity were both the strongest predictors for QOL at 1 year following treatment. Other clinical factors that were significant and predicted worse QOL included gastrostomy tube and T (tumor) and N (node) stages; treatment modality was not significantly predictive. Clinical factors that have consistently predicted favorable QOL in addition to baseline QOL include prevention of unintentional weight loss and earlier-stage disease. Some practitioners advocate early gastrostomy placement to prevent weight loss and preserve QOL, with the goal of early removal as soon as oral intake can sustain weight.

Not surprisingly, patients with depressive symptoms will also have reduced long-term QOL. A prospective assessment of over 300 patients prior to initiation of treatment for SCCHN evaluated depressive symptoms. While controlling for age, gender, marital status, site and stage of disease, tobacco and alcohol intake, comorbidity, and pretreatment QOL score, patients with depressive symptoms present prior to treatment had significantly lower QOL scores at 3 and 12 months in the areas of speech, eating, aesthetics, and social disruption. QOL researchers have suggested that

patients known to have depressive symptoms prior to treatment should be more aggressively and proactively treated for their depression to potentially minimize long-term QOL deficits.

Finally, numerous studies assert QOL may predict survival. For example, in a prospective study that evaluated nearly 500 SCCHN patients, while controlling for age, marital status, education, time since diagnosis, and tumor site and stage, both the HN QOL and the SF-36 physical correlates of QOL significantly predicted survival, whereas emotional QOL correlates did not. Similarly, another assessment of over 500 patients being treated for SCCHN to evaluate the relationship between QOL and survival used the European Organization for Research and Treatment of Cancer—Quality of Life Questionnaire Core 30. Patients' physical functioning QOL independently and significantly predicted overall survival. Using multivariable analysis, change in physical function QOL was the strongest predictor of overall survival.

◼ Controversial Issues

Although QOL has emerged as an important clinical outcome measure, many practitioners still do not know precisely how to implement it in their routine management. The assessment of QOL in SCCHN is now a routine part of prospective, randomized clinical trials, and the findings from these high-quality studies will continue to provide themes that are significant and practical for the management of head and neck cancer patients.

◼ Summary

Health-related QOL is a complex concept that is a measure of the patient's own perspective of mental, physical, and social well-being. It is a clinical outcome that has become established conceptually by both health care workers and patients as having relevance similar to recurrence, survival, and treatment risks. Individuals who care for patients with SCCHN should be aware of the factors that portend better or worse QOL, even though management decisions for an individual will not be based singularly on QOL questionnaires.

■ Suggested Reading

Curran D, Giralt J, Harari PM, et al. Quality of life in head and neck cancer patients after treatment with high-dose radiotherapy alone or in combination with cetuximab. J Clin Oncol 2007;25(16):2191–2197

El-Deiry MW, Futran ND, McDowell JA, Weymuller EA Jr, Yueh B. Influences and predictors of long-term quality of life in head and neck cancer survivors. Arch Otolaryngol Head Neck Surg 2009;135(4):380–384

Karvonen-Gutierrez CA, Ronis DL, Fowler KE, Terrell JE, Gruber SB, Duffy SA. Quality of life scores predict survival among patients with head and neck cancer. J Clin Oncol 2008;26(16):2754–2760

Meyer F, Fortin A, Gélinas M, et al. Health-related quality of life as a survival predictor for patients with localized head and neck cancer treated with radiation therapy. J Clin Oncol 2009;27(18): 2970–2976

Ronis DL, Duffy SA, Fowler KE, Khan MJ, Terrell JE. Changes in quality of life over 1 year in patients with head and neck cancer. Arch Otolaryngol Head Neck Surg 2008;134(3):241–248

49 Advances in Head and Neck Diagnostic Pathology

■ Introduction

The field of head and neck pathology is evolving. It is imperative that the head and neck surgeon stay abreast of changes and how they affect the day-to-day practice of otolaryngology. Specifically, advances in biopsy techniques, histological interpretation, and molecular diagnostics have had dramatic impacts on the profession in recent years. This chapter discusses these developments in the context of otolaryngology because they have undoubtedly resulted in improved diagnosis, prognostication, and, in many cases, treatment of surgical head and neck disease. The chapter is organized into four principal sections that reflect changes in percutaneous biopsy practices, cytology analysis, interpretation of histopathology, and molecular diagnostics. Consensus guidelines for reporting standards are also discussed, where applicable.

■ Advances in Percutaneous Biopsy Techniques

Fine-Needle Aspiration (FNA) Cytology

Fine-needle aspiration (FNA) has long been used in the evaluation and management of thyroid nodules. It has now attained a prominent role in the evaluation of other neck masses. The sensitivity, specificity, positive, and negative predictive values of head and neck FNA are reported to be 90%, 97%, 96%, and 90%, respectively. On average, 90% of head and neck FNA specimens are deemed adequate for cytological diagnosis, though this clearly depends on the experience and training of the person performing the procedure.

Standard FNA techniques are straightforward, but proper handling and fixation of the specimen are crucial for accurate cytological evaluation. It is important for the otolaryngologist to discuss sample preparation techniques with the cytopathologist.

Because cytological diagnosis is a specialized pathology skill, it is also important for the otolaryngologist to know the experience level of the cytopathologist.

FNA techniques have been extensively described. The use of 22- to 25-gauge needles has been clearly shown to be adequate for sample procurement, while virtually eliminating the risk of tumor cell seeding. Cytological preparations fall into three categories: (1) alcohol-fixed (e.g., ethanol/Papanicolaou method), (2) air-dried, and (3) placed in specialized media for preparation as cytospins. If a lymphoproliferative process is suspected, the pathologist should be informed so that the specimen may be appropriately collected and prepared for flow cytometry.

One potential advantage of air-dried slides is that they may be evaluated on site using Diff-Quik staining. This process allows for immediate examination by the cytopathologist and determination of specimen adequacy. Whenever feasible, a cytotechnologist or cytopathologist should be present during performance of an FNA to perform this task; it has been clearly demonstrated that both the rates of specimen adequacy and the ability to obtain a definitive diagnosis by FNA are improved with immediate analysis.

If sufficient material is available, a cell block may be prepared from an FNA specimen as well. Cell blocks are derived from small tissue fragments, blood clots, and mucus within the FNA needle. This material is then compressed into a "block" and processed as if it were a solid biopsy sample (i.e., it is embedded in paraffin, sectioned, and subsequently stained with hematoxylin and eosin). Additionally, special stains (including immunohistochemistry) can be performed on cell blocks.

Core Needle Biopsy

When compared with FNA cytology, core biopsies provide a more substantial and intact piece of tissue for analysis. This procedure is generally performed using a large-bore needle (18 or 20 gauge). There are several commercially available devices for core needle biopsy.

Despite the potential diagnostic benefits, core needle biopsy has yet to gain widespread popularity for head and neck applications. This may be due to concern regarding bleeding and trauma to cranial nerves, complications that have indeed been reported. However, larger studies specifically addressing head and neck biopsies have demonstrated complication rates similar to those reported for FNA. Another concern regarding head and neck core biopsy is that it may have the potential to seed tumor cells along the needle track, though this has not been shown to be the case in controlled studies. Further experience with this technique is required before definitive recommendations can be made regarding its applicability in the head and neck.

Image Guidance

Although not an advance in pathology per se, the addition of image guidance has had a significant effect on the practice and ultimate success of FNA. Computed tomography (CT) and ultrasound-guided biopsy have been shown to improve the diagnostic yield of needle biopsy. Ultrasonography has the advantages of reduced cost, improved sensitivity, avoidance of radiation, and portability. It has consequently become the imaging modality of choice for this purpose. Ultrasound-guided FNA has effectively reduced the number of false-negative biopsies, and has substantially improved FNA's diagnostic accuracy and adequacy rates. Now that office-based ultrasonography has become common in otolaryngology practices, the numbers of inadequate FNA specimens are likely to continue to decrease, with reports of a 30% improvement in adequacy rates when ultrasound was used to perform FNA in the otolaryngology clinic.

■ Advances in Cytology Analysis

Reporting Standards

One of the principal difficulties in interpreting thyroid cytopathology reports has been the inconsistent application of diagnostic criteria and terminology from laboratory to laboratory over the past several decades. This has created confusion on the part of clinicians and has likely resulted in unnecessary surgery for many patients with indeterminate cytology. In response to this problem, the National Cancer Institute convened an expert panel in 2009 and charged the panelists with clarifying both ter-

Table 49.1 Bethesda System diagnostic categories and risk of malignancy

Bethesda System category	Risk of malignancy (%)
Nondiagnostic/unsatisfactory	1–4
Benign	0–3
Atypia of undetermined significance or follicular lesion of undetermined significance	5–15
Follicular neoplasm or suspicious for follicular neoplasm	15–30
Suspicious for malignancy	60–75
Malignant	97–99

Used with permission from Ali, SZ, Cibas, ES. The Bethseda System for Reporting Thyroid Cytopathology. New York: NY: Springer; 2010.

minology and morphological criteria with respect to thyroid cytology. Ultimately, this group developed the Bethesda System for Reporting Thyroid Cytopathology, which is a set of guidelines that have now been widely adopted.

The Bethesda System aims to simplify cytopathology reports, allowing for only six general diagnostic categories: nondiagnostic/unsatisfactory, benign, atypia of undetermined significance, follicular neoplasm, suspicious for malignancy, and malignant. Each of these categories may have several possible subcategorizations. If the criteria for each category are strictly adhered to, a corresponding risk of malignancy is implicit in the diagnosis, and the appropriate intervention may be chosen (**Table 49.1**). The widespread adoption of this system has reduced both the number of specimens designated as "indeterminate" and the number of thyroidectomies performed. It is recommended that otolaryngologists treating thyroid diseases consult with their local cytopathologists and urge them to adopt this system if they have not already done so.

Molecular Diagnostic Adjuncts to Cytopathology

Using the aforementioned Bethesda System, less than 30% of thyroid FNAs will fall into an indeterminate category. Among these nodules, it is thought that ~ 5 to 30% will ultimately prove to be malignant. Molecular diagnostic techniques now allow the surgeon to further risk-stratify patients with indeterminate cytopathology. This is accomplished by exploiting the knowledge that up to 50% of papillary thyroid cancers will possess a mutation in the gene $BRAF^{V600E}$. In the context of thyroid neoplasia, BRAF mutation is highly specific for the presence of malignancy. Using the polymerase chain reaction (PCR), cytology specimens may be analyzed for the presence of BRAF mutation. Given the sensitivity of PCR, even scant samples may be tested using this technique. Consequently, BRAF analysis has been advocated as a useful refinement to FNA cytology in the context of indeterminate thyroid nodules.

After a patient has received definitive therapy for a thyroid malignancy, detection of recurrence may be difficult in certain contexts. Circulating antibodies may confound the interpretation of serum thyroglobulin levels, and imaging modalities may not be able to readily distinguish between benign and malignant masses—particularly lymph nodes. Cytology may be less sensitive when cystic masses are encountered. Consequently, many clinicians have advocated for the use of molecular diagnostics as a means to identify recurrent neck disease after treatment of thyroid malignancy. Specifically, immunoassays for thyroglobulin have been employed for this purpose.

Thyroglobulin is a glycoprotein that is produced exclusively by benign and neoplastic thyroid follicular cells. Its presence in cervical lymph nodes or within the soft tissues of the thyroid bed is thus indicative of persistent or recurrent disease. Levels > 29 ng/mL have been found to be 100% sensitive, over 95% specific, and nearly 100% accurate in this context. Thus, in circumstances where the clinical picture is not entirely clear or if cytology is inconclusive, thyroglobulin staining of FNA specimens may be quite illuminating. Neither thyroglobulin testing nor BRAF testing is routine in most laboratories. It is thus critical that the surgeon communicate the specific clinical concerns to the pathologist. This will ensure that the assays are used appropriately and cost-effectively.

Similar to the use of thyroglobulin and BRAF to confirm the presence of thyroid malignancy, identification of human papillomavirus (HPV) within the cervical lymph nodes can both confirm malignancy and suggest the site of origin in unknown primary head and neck cancers. HPV has emerged as a leading cause of oropharyngeal carcinoma in the United States, with growing numbers of these tumors now being attributed to the virus. In addition to the primary tumor site, HPV type 16 (HPV-16) deoxyribonucleic acid (DNA) has been identified within the cervical lymph nodes of patients with oropharyngeal carcinoma. It has also been found in the lymph nodes of nearly 30% of patients with unknown primary head and neck cancers. Given the high specificity of HPV to oropharyngeal carcinomas, it has been postulated that the presence of HPV in the lymph nodes of unknown primary head and neck cancers all but confirms the tonsils/tongue base as the site of origin.

◼ Interpretation of Histopathology

Squamous cell carcinoma remains the predominant cell type and continues to account for > 90% of all nonthyroidal head and neck cancers. Although the appearance of the disease under the light microscope has not changed significantly, the clinical implications of certain pathological features are now being characterized throughout the literature. Likely underrecognized and underreported in years past, these "adverse pathological features" are now being used routinely to prognosticate and to guide therapy. Both the histological variant of squamous carcinoma and the nature of its relationships to the surrounding tissues are important in this context.

Histological Variants of Squamous Cell Carcinoma

Invasive head and neck carcinoma may be present as either conventional type squamous cell carcinoma (SCC) or as one of a variety of subtypes, including basaloid, spindle cell, and verrucous carcinoma, among others. Conventional SCC may be well, moderately, or poorly differentiated, depending on the degree of keratinization and cytological/nuclear atypia.

Basaloid squamous (basosquamous) carcinoma is a high-grade variant of SCC that is characterized by basaloid and squamous components. Basaloid squamous carcinoma is most commonly seen in the oropharynx and was classically thought to be more aggressive than conventional squamous cell carcinoma. Many of these tumors are now believed to be related to HPV and are actually thought to be less aggressive than their non-HPV-related counterparts.

Spindle cell carcinoma derives its name from the fact that the predominant cells in this poorly differentiated tumor possess a spindle or sarcomatoid appearance. This renders histological diagnosis somewhat difficult, and immunostaining is typically required for confirmation. These tumors are thought to carry a worse prognosis than conventional SCC and warrant aggressive treatment.

In contrast to the basaloid and spindle cell variants, verrucous carcinomas are low-grade malignancies. These tumors are named for the fact that they resemble verrucous warts on both gross and histological inspections. They typically behave in an indolent but locally destructive fashion. Verrucous carcinomas became of interest after reports surfaced that radiation therapy resulted in poor rates of local control and, in some cases, transformation to a highly malignant form known as anaplastic carcinoma. Although the tumors have subsequently been shown to be less radiosensitive than conventional SCCs, large controlled studies have failed to demonstrate any increased risk of anaplastic transformation.

Adverse Features in Squamous Cell Carcinoma

Given the potential therapeutic implications, reporting of SCC should include not only a description of tumor grade and subtype but also a description of histological features of known prognostic significance. Primary tumors should be evaluated for perineural and lymphovascular invasion. It has been repeatedly demonstrated that perineural spread is an independent risk factor for locoregional recurrence and mortality. Lymphovascular invasion also has deleterious effects on locoregional control and survival. The depth of tumor invasion also appears to bear prognostic significance, particularly for oral cavity cancers. Depth of invasion corresponds to an increased risk for occult nodal disease in early-stage tongue and floor-of-mouth cancer. A 2009 meta-analysis confirmed this and concluded that early-stage tumors > 4 mm thick require elective treatment of the neck.

Lymph nodes should also be carefully scrutinized under the light microscope for the presence or absence of extracapsular extension. In previous studies, the presence of extracapsular nodal extension indicated a worse overall survival. These patients subsequently also experienced a survival benefit from the addition of chemotherapy to adjuvant radiotherapy in the postoperative setting. Subsequent analysis found that this was significant only among patients with extracapsular nodal extension and/or positive margins. In advanced-stage disease, it is therefore critical that the pathologist comment on the presence or absence of these features, so that appropriate counseling and adjuvant therapy may be pursued. This has been called into question in patients with HPV-related tumors and will require further evaluation.

Reporting Standards in Head and Neck Histopathology

Appropriate and meaningful pathology reports are critical to providing comprehensive cancer care. Site-specific guidelines and standards for reporting in the context of cancer diagnoses have been established by the College of American Pathologists. These guidelines and standards are updated regularly to reflect the current literature. The most current iteration recommends that perineural invasion, lymphovascular invasion, extracapsular extension, margin status, and tumor thickness all be specifically addressed in the reporting of head and neck cancers.

■ Advances in Molecular Diagnostics

Refinements in molecular diagnostics over the past decade have enhanced the ability to diagnose and treat several diseases encountered by otolaryngologist–head and neck surgeons. Specifically, the ability to identify specific gene mutations, such as BRAF^{V600E}, and overexpressed receptors, such as the epidermal growth factor receptor (EGFR) and vascular endothelial growth factor receptor (VEGFR), has led to the burgeoning field of targeted therapy. Moreover, the presence or absence of these mutations and overexpressed proteins may have significant prognostic implications. As already noted, it is now also understood that HPV-16 is responsible for a growing number of oropharyngeal carcinomas, and that these tumors are distinct from their HPV-negative counterparts from clinical, pathological, and prognostic standpoints. This has led to considerable advances in the detection and characterization of HPV.

Molecular Diagnosis: Implications for Prognosis and Treatment

Several subcellular structures identified in recent years have been shown to carry significant prognostic value in head and neck tumors. As mentioned earlier, a subset of papillary thyroid carcinomas possesses a mutated BRAF^{V600E} gene. The presence of this mutation is a marker for extrathyroidal extension, more aggressive histology, and a more advanced clinical stage of disease. Consequently, BRAF testing on thyroidectomy specimens is now routine in many laboratories. Its judicious use can be helpful in planning therapy and follow-up in a subset of patients with papillary carcinoma. Interestingly, BRAF mutations are also seen in malignant melanoma, where they have been correlated with an increased risk of death and a significant reduction in survival time.

Numerous molecular markers of prognosis also exist for SCCs. Tests for many of these markers are commercially available. Well-characterized examples in routine clinical use include in situ hybridization testing for HPV-16 and immunohistochemical (IHC) staining for p16 and EGFR. As previously mentioned, HPV-related cancers are clinicopathologically distinct from conventional SCCs. Patients with HPV-related oropharyngeal cancers are typically younger, and their prognosis is improved when compared with cohorts with HPV-negative tumors. Knowledge of the HPV status in the context of oropharyngeal carcinoma carries with it tremendous prognostic and counseling implications. Because HPV-related tumors share overlapping histological features with non-HPV-related disease, special tests are required to confirm the presence of the virus.

The gold standard for diagnosis of HPV is polymerase chain reaction (PCR). Although this test is highly sensitive and specific for the detection of viral DNA, it has the disadvantages of high cost and the lack of widespread availability. Alternative methods include in situ hybridization (ISH) for HPV DNA and IHC staining for p16, a protein that is upregulated in virally induced oropharyngeal cancers. It is recommended that all oropharyngeal cancers now be tested for HPV, using either HPV ISH or p16 IHC. Given its improved sensitivity as compared with HPV ISH, p16 IHC is considered to be the preferred assay. Additional prognostic information can be gleaned from the expression of EGFR in oropharyngeal carcinomas. Some investigators have found incremental improvements in responsiveness to induction chemotherapy, disease-specific survival, and overall survival that were directly related to p16 expression and inversely related to EGFR staining. This information is useful for both prognosis and treatment planning. Consequently, EGFR staining should be considered in addition to HPV assays for oropharyngeal cancers.

Numerous other molecular markers have been shown to carry prognostic value for head and neck tumors and may be available in clinical laboratories. Although a comprehensive review of these is beyond the scope of this chapter, a sampling is included in **Table 49.2**. Many of these markers are now also used to guide the selection of therapy. For instance, numerous monoclonal antibodies have been developed as targeted therapies for squamous and nonsquamous malignancies of the head and neck. Perhaps the best known and most widely used is cetuximab, which targets EGFR and is used in combination with radiation therapy for the treatment of SCCs. Other targeted therapies currently in use for head and neck tumors include BRAF inhibitors, such as vemurafenib (melanoma), and VEGFR inhibitors, such as sorafenib (melanoma and thyroid cancers). Numerous other therapies are currently being investigated in phase 2 and phase 3 clinical trials as well. In the future, it is likely that panels of these molecular targets will be generated for individualized tumors. In conjunction with the histopathology report, this panel will allow for more thorough characterization of the tumor and highly targeted therapy.

Table 49.2 Sample molecular markers

Markers of improved prognosis	Markers of worsened prognosis
p16 overexpression in oropharyngeal carcinoma	Increased EGFR expression in oropharyngeal carcinoma
Low p53/Bcl-xL expression in oropharyngeal carcinoma	BRAF mutations in PTC and malignant melanoma
	ret/PTC rearrangement in PTC
	Loss of heterozygosity in p53, p16, E-cadherin, and pRB in hypopharyngeal cancers
	p53 overexpression in laryngeal carcinoma
	p21, p53, and pRB alterations in HPV-negative tonsil cancers

Abbreviations: EGFR, epidermal growth factor receptor; HPV, human papilloma virus; PTC, papillary thyroid carcinoma; RET, RET proto-oncogene.

■ Suggested Reading

Allen CT, Lewis JS Jr, El-Mofty SK, Haughey BH, Nussenbaum B. Human papillomavirus and oropharynx cancer: biology, detection and clinical implications. Laryngoscope 2010;120(9):1756–1772

Ang KK, Harris J, Wheeler R, et al. Human papillomavirus and survival of patients with oropharyngeal cancer. N Engl J Med 2010; 363(1):24–35

Chirilă M, Bolboacă SD, Cosgarea M, Tomescu E, Mureşan M. Perineural invasion of the major and minor nerves in laryngeal and hypopharyngeal cancer. Otolaryngol Head Neck Surg 2009; 140(1):65–69

Chung YL, Lee MY, Horng CF, et al. Use of combined molecular biomarkers for prediction of clinical outcomes in locally advanced tonsillar cancers treated with chemoradiotherapy alone. Head Neck 2009;31(1):9–20

Cibas ES, Ali SZ; NCI Thyroid FNA State of the Science Conference. The Bethesda system for reporting thyroid cytopathology. Am J Clin Pathol 2009;132(5):658–665

Compton AM, Moore-Medlin T, Herman-Ferdinandez L, et al. Human papillomavirus in metastatic lymph nodes from unknown primary head and neck squamous cell carcinoma. Otolaryngol Head Neck Surg 2011;145(1):51–57

Gillison ML, D'Souza G, Westra W, et al. Distinct risk factor profiles for human papillomavirus type 16-positive and human papillomavirus type 16-negative head and neck cancers. J Natl Cancer Inst 2008;100(6):407–420

Huang SH, Hwang D, Lockwood G, Goldstein DP, O'Sullivan B. Predictive value of tumor thickness for cervical lymph-node involvement in squamous cell carcinoma of the oral cavity: a meta-analysis of reported studies. Cancer 2009;115(7):1489–1497

Kumar B, Cordell KG, Lee JS, et al. EGFR, p16, HPV Titer, Bcl-xL and p53, sex, and smoking as indicators of response to therapy and survival in oropharyngeal cancer. J Clin Oncol 2008;26(19): 3128–3137

Lee JH, Lee ES, Kim YS. Clinicopathologic significance of BRAF V600E mutation in papillary carcinomas of the thyroid: a meta-analysis. Cancer 2007;110(1):38–46

Mendelsohn AH, Lai CK, Shintaku IP, et al. Histopathologic findings of HPV and p16 positive HNSCC. Laryngoscope 2010;120(9): 1788–1794

Moberly AC, Vural E, Nahas B, Bergeson TR, Kokoska MS. Ultrasound-guided needle aspiration: impact of immediate cytologic review. Laryngoscope 2010;120(10):1979–1984

Pitman MB, Abele J, Ali SZ, et al. Techniques for thyroid FNA: a synopsis of the National Cancer Institute thyroid fine-needle aspiration state of the science conference. Diagn Cytopathol 2008; 36(6):407–424

Robitschek J, Straub M, Wirtz E, Klem C, Sniezek J. Diagnostic efficacy of surgeon-performed ultrasound-guided fine needle aspiration: a randomized controlled trial. Otolaryngol Head Neck Surg 2010;142(3):306–309

Ryerson AB, Peters ES, Coughlin SS, et al. Burden of potentially human papillomavirus-associated cancers of the oropharynx and oral cavity in the US, 1998-2003. Cancer 2008;113(10, Suppl): 2901–2909

Sang-Hyuk Lee SH, Lee NH, Jin SM, Rho YS, Jo SJ. Loss of heterozygosity of tumor suppressor genes (p16, Rb, E-cadherin, p53) in hypopharynx squamous cell carcinoma. Otolaryngol Head Neck Surg 2011;145(1):64–70

Tandon S, Shahab R, Benton JI, Ghosh SK, Sheard J, Jones TM. Fine-needle aspiration cytology in a regional head and neck cancer center: comparison with a systematic review and meta-analysis. Head Neck 2008;30(9):1246–1252

V

Laryngology and Bronchoesophagology

50 Esophageal Dysmotility and Dysphagia

■ Introduction

The main function of the esophagus is to transport food from the pharynx to the stomach and prevent its return. Coordinated timing and strength of muscle contraction are necessary to generate effective peristalsis. Broadly stated, a failure of the esophagus to carry out this function can be attributed to either (1) a motility disorder, characterized as a failure of peristalsis, sphincter function, or both; or (2) a structural obstruction.

Esophageal Motility

The primary symptoms associated with *esophageal motility* disorders include dysphagia, chest pain, and symptoms of gastroesophageal reflux disease (GERD). The dysphagia tends to be intermittent, and it progresses very slowly if at all. Difficulty is noted with liquids and solids right from the outset. On the other hand, *structural obstructions* tend to produce constant and progressive dysphagia, beginning with solids then progressing to liquids. The dysphagia of esophageal dysfunction tends to be nonspecific and nonlocalizing. Patients often indicate the sternal notch and above, even when afflicted with pathological conditions of the lower esophagus. Problems with esophageal dysmotility tend to increase with age; older individuals have a higher incidence of nonperistaltic contractions, as well as occasional swallows that produce incomplete peristalsis.

Esophageal disease is a frequent cause of noncardiac chest pain, due to either GERD or a motility disorder. High-pressure nonperistaltic contractions may produce episodic chest pain that may be severe enough to simulate the pain of myocardial infarction. Symptoms that may distinguish an esophageal etiology from cardiogenic pain include symptoms of GERD, dysphagia, and chest pain that is associated with the ingestion of hot or cold foods or relieved with antacids.

Before discussing the diagnostic evaluation of dysphagia, a word about *globus pharyngis* is necessary. The etiology of this sensation of a lump in the throat remains controversial and is probably multifactorial. Esophageal dysmotility needs to be carefully considered in the differential diagnosis of patients presenting with globus symptoms.

■ Diagnostic Evaluation

Methods for testing esophageal function may be categorized as imaging techniques, direct visualization, and functional studies. Often, these studies complement each other.

Imaging Techniques

Barium Esophagram

A barium study is generally the best initial test to identify an esophageal disorder. It is reported that careful fluoroscopy and maximal esophageal distention constitute the most sensitive single test for a fixed structural lesion of the esophagus. In contrast, endoscopy alone may miss up to 42% of lower esophageal rings. In addition, fluoroscopic observation of multiple single swallows of barium may provide some assessment of esophageal motility and has a high correlation with manometry. Recent studies suggest that radiological evaluation has better than 90% sensitivity for detecting abnormal motility.

Regardless of a patient's symptoms, the entire swallowing sequence should be evaluated. A routine barium swallow focuses on the pharynx, upper esophageal sphincter (UES), body of the esophagus, and lower esophageal sphincter (LES). To identify a specific problem, it may be helpful to have the input of a speech pathologist, particularly if there is difficulty with the oral or pharyngeal phases of swallowing, or cricopharyngeal dysfunction (also known as UES achalasia) is suspected, with or without a hypopharyngeal (Zenker) diverticulum. A modified barium swallow uses varying consistencies and quantities of barium and can be particularly useful in delineating the function of all phases of swallowing, as well as an anatomical survey. Provocative maneuvers include various test feeding techniques, bolus modification, and altering patient position in an attempt to simulate the patient's problem with dysphagia. If aspiration is a concern, it is best to use a thin suspension of barium, which is less irritating to the tracheobronchial tree. Water-soluble materials, such as meglumine diatrizoate (Gastrografin, Bracco Diagnostics, Inc., Monroe Township, NJ), are appropriate only if an esophageal perforation is suspected. A barium study is not a sensitive test for GERD.

Computed Tomography (CT) and Magnetic Resonance Imaging (MRI)

Computed tomography (CT) and magnetic resonance imaging (MRI) are used for evaluating esophageal disease and are particularly effective for pretreatment staging of esophageal carcinoma. These imaging techniques are rarely indicated in the initial workup of dysphagia of esophageal origin or esophageal dysmotility.

Direct Visualization

Endoscopy

Motility disorders lend themselves poorly to endoscopic assessment because some factors, such as peristaltic contractions and sphincter competence, are not easily visualized. On the other hand, complications, such as reflux esophagitis and esophageal stricture, or the presence of a hypopharyngeal diverticulum, are readily detected.

Esophagoscopy is the best method for assessing mucosal integrity, inflammation, and malignancy of the esophagus, as well as providing the opportunity for direct tissue examination. Patients with persistent symptoms, such as dysphagia, whose cause has not been determined by history and other preliminary testing, are considered for endoscopic examination. Disorders that have been associated with malignant degeneration, such as Barrett epithelium, lye stricture, achalasia, or Plummer–Vinson syndrome, need to be considered for regular endoscopic follow-up.

Gastroenterologists generally prefer flexible instruments that allow air insufflation for distention and better access to the lower esophagus and stomach. Otolaryngologists are usually trained with rigid esophagoscopes with telescopes that have superior optics and provide a better view of the esophageal inlet and postcricoid area. Recently, use of transnasal esophagoscopy (TNE) has become widely adopted in otolaryngology. TNE offers the clinician the opportunity to perform unsedated direct visualization (with insufflation) under topical anesthesia at initial presentation in the clinic. The role of TNE in motility disorders includes an anatomical survey, evaluation for GERD and Barrett esophagitis, ability to perform LES Botox injection (Allergan, Irvine, CA), and placement of a pH probe.

Functional Studies

Manometry

Esophageal manometry is used to assess (1) peristaltic activity within the body of the esophagus, and (2) LES pressure and relaxation. The laryngeal cartilages cause an asymmetry within the UES, making pressure readings in this location difficult to interpret. Intraluminal pressures may be measured by either external water-perfused transducers or small solid-state transducers placed directly on the manometric catheter, the latter being standard today. The former system is low cost and flexible, whereas the latter is somewhat more accurate.

In the clinical setting, esophageal manometry is used to determine whether primary peristalsis is weak, absent, or disordered, and whether LES relaxation is impaired. Such findings are very sensitive for detecting motility disorders but are sometimes nonspecific. The American Gastroenterological Association advocates the use of manometry to establish the diagnoses of achalasia, ineffective esophageal motility disorder, and diffuse esophageal spasm or to detect esophageal motor abnormalities associated with systemic diseases. More common disorders should first be excluded with barium study or endoscopy. Manometry may now be combined with impedance testing for patients whose dysmotility is suspected as being related to GERD refractory to standard medical therapy, such as instances where bile reflux or nonacidic reflux is suspected.

Recent technical advances have led to the widespread use of high-definition manometry combined with pressure topographic plots. This differs from conventional manometry in recording pressures by solid-state microtransducers at 12 points around the circumference at every centimeter of esophageal length and displaying the data in pseudo-three-dimensional format using a topographic plot, representing esophageal pressures by different colors. These technical advances have improved the sensitivity in detecting certain motility disorders.

Intraluminal pH Studies

Esophageal pH monitoring is considered the most sensitive method for detecting clinically significant GERD and is not indicated for the initial evaluation of esophageal dysmotility. Reflux and esophagitis can be associated with abnormal motility. This may occur as esophageal contractility decreases with increasing mucosal injury. Although barium studies and manometry may not be the most sensitive single screening tools for detecting GERD, they may provide complementary information, such as degree of tissue sequelae of chromic irritation or presence of concomitant dysmotility. The pH monitoring is generally performed over a 24-hour period to provide the most comprehensive and reproducible information. This can be accomplished with a single or dual-sensor pH channel or, more recently, monitoring may occur over 48 hours with a wireless Bravo capsule (Given Imaging, Ltd., Mattawan, MI). Patients are encouraged to continue normal activity while avoiding particularly acidic foods.

The parameter most consistent with a diagnosis of esophagitis is the percentage of time that esophageal pH is below 4, which usually does not exceed 7% over a 24-hour period in normal subjects. Six components are used to determine a composite pH score (DeMeester score), including the percentage of total, upright, and supine time with a pH < 4; the number of recorded reflux episodes; the number of recorded reflux episodes > 5 minutes; and the length of time of the longest recorded reflux event. A composite score of > 14.72 indicates the presence of GERD.

Multichannel intraluminal impedance is now frequently combined with pH monitoring and employed in patients with suspected bile reflux, nonacidic reflux, or GERD nonresponsive to standard medical therapy.

Radionuclide Scintigraphy

Esophageal scintigraphy was developed as a noninvasive and quantitative measurement of esophageal transit. It is a functional study and does not provide direct anatomical information. The patient is given water mixed with technicium-99m-sulfur colloid in a single swallow and then swallows the mixture at 15-second intervals for 10 minutes. Counts are recorded by a gamma camera and processed by computer. If indicated, the radioisotope can be bound to specific foods. When esophageal contractions are nonperistaltic, such as in distal esophageal spasm (DES), repetitive retrograde-antegrade movement of the bolus is apparent. Other motility disorders, such as achalasia and secondary motility disorders (e.g., scleroderma) may also cause bolus retention.

Scintigraphy is not an ideal screening test for esophageal dysmotility. As long as contractions are peristaltic and the LES does relax, transit time may be normal. For example, the relatively common diagnosis of nonspecific esophageal motility disorder (NEMD) is frequently missed by esophageal scintigraphy alone.

Esophageal scintigraphy provides no anatomical information. This disadvantage, along with its relative insensitivity, precludes it from being a first-line test in the evaluation of dysphagia or suspected dysmotility. Esophageal scintigraphy's primary advantage is in providing quantitative information that may be used to gauge response to therapeutic intervention. It may also be useful when manometry is unavailable or its results are equivocal. GERD scintigraphy (and gastric emptying scan) is used widely with infants and children to investigate reflux in relation to pulmonary disorders, vomiting, and failure to thrive.

■ Evaluation and Management of Motility Disorders

Dysphagia is a nonspecific symptom and not a diagnosis unto itself. Although a thorough history is essential for elucidating the cause of dysphagia, it is best to approach any patient with esophageal symptoms as though an obstructing lesion is the cause until proven otherwise. This requires diagnostic tests as already described, including TNE at the initial evaluation, if available.

Normal individuals swallow more than 1,000 times a day. This complicated process requires the coordination of at least 26 muscles and five cranial nerves. Not only must effective peristalsis be generated but the airway must be protected. With recent advances in computerization and solid-state electronics, esophageal dysmotility has been more precisely defined.

Esophageal motility disorders are classified as either primary, affecting just the esophagus, or secondary, in which esophageal dysfunction is part of a systemic illness or specific injury (**Table 50.1**).

Primary Motility Disorders

Classification and Diagnostic Criteria

Numerous manuscripts have been published dealing with esophageal motility disorders. Spechler and Castell published a widely accepted classification scheme and diagnostic criteria for esophageal motility disorders in 2001. They classified disorders

Table 50.1 Esophageal motility disorders

Primary
Achalasia
Distal esophageal spasm
Nutcracker esophagus
Ineffective esophageal motility (nonspecific esophageal motility disorder)
Secondary
Collagen vascular diseases
– Scleroderma (CREST syndrome)
– Polymyositis
– Dermatomyositis
Diabetes mellitus
Alcoholism
Chagas disease
Neuromuscular disorders (Parkinson disease)
Multiple endocrine neoplasia (type IIb)
Eosinophilic esophagitis
Neurofibromatosis (type 1)
Paraneoplastic syndrome

tosis and regurgitation may occur because of retained material within the esophagus. Chronic aspiration with chronic bronchitis or recurrent pneumonia may infrequently occur. Odynophagia is unusual and may suggest underlying malignancy.

In advanced cases, a plain chest radiograph may reveal an air–fluid level in a dilated esophagus. The barium study shows marked esophageal dilation, tapering to a "bird's beak" deformity at the LES (**Fig. 50.1**). Manometry demonstrates high resting pressure of the LES, usually > 35 mm Hg above gastric pressure, with failure of relaxation during swallowing (**Fig. 50.2**). Secondary causes of achalasia need to be excluded, such as a malignant lesion at the LES.

Therapy for achalasia has centered on decreasing LES pressure. Historically, temporizing improvement could be achieved by balloon or rigid dilation, or by intrasphincteric injection of botulinum toxin (Botox). Definitive treatment may be in the form of a surgical myotomy (Heller procedure) or Toupet fundoplication, both of which are now being reported via a laparoscopic approach. Pneumatic dilation is considered by many clinicians as the current treatment of choice for achalasia, although response rates for pneumatic dilation and laparoscopic Heller myotomy are similar

as inadequate LES relaxation (achalasia and atypical disorder of LES relaxation), uncoordinated contraction (diffuse esophageal spasm), hypercontraction (nutcracker esophagus and isolated hypertensive LES), and hypocontraction (ineffective esophageal motility). The major entities are delineated next.

Achalasia

Achalasia is perhaps one of the most common and best understood of the primary motor disorders. It is characterized by incomplete relaxation of the LES, with elevated resting tone and absent esophageal peristalsis, which leads to stasis with esophageal dilatation. Although the etiology remains unknown, histological evidence demonstrates degenerative changes within the dorsal vagal nucleus, vagal trunks, and myenteric ganglia of the esophagus. In addition to the neurodegenerative hypotheses, recent research has considered viral causes, an autoimmune connection, and the role of eosinophilic infiltrate.

Achalasia occurs at a frequency of ~ 1 per 100,000 people, without a gender bias. Dysphagia is the most prevalent symptom, usually slowly progressing over several years, with the majority of patients being diagnosed in the third and fourth decades of life. Patients often point to the xiphoid as the point of obstruction. Chest pain is a common symptom. Hali-

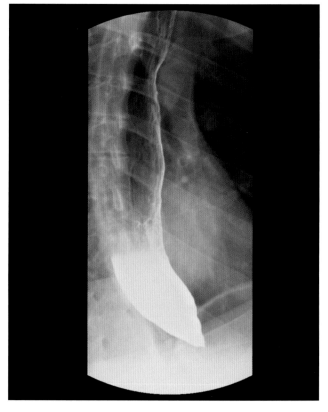

Fig. 50.1 Barium esophagram demonstrating marked esophageal dilation tapering to a "bird's beak" deformity at the lower esophageal sphincter, characteristic of achalasia.

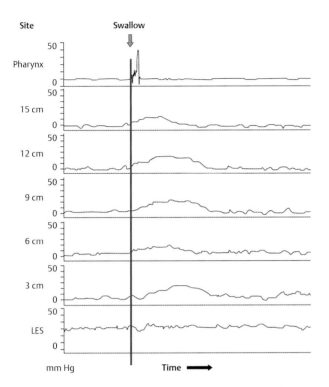

Fig. 50.2 Schematic representation of manometry demonstrating high resting pressure of the lower esophageal sphincter, usually > 35 mm Hg above gastric pressure, with failure of relaxation during swallowing, characteristic of achalasia.

in some published reviews. The choice of pneumatic dilation versus laparoscopic myotomy seems to be an issue of controversy. Response rates vary widely from report to report, and relapses requiring "touchups" are not uncommon.

Distal Esophageal Spasm

DES is characterized by repetitive, nonperistaltic, high-amplitude contractions of the smooth muscle portion of the esophagus. These contractions occur intermittently and vary in severity but are associated with more than 20% of swallows. The upper striated portion of the esophagus and LES generally function normally. DES is a relatively rare condition compared with achalasia.

The etiology of DES is unknown, although there appear to be degenerative changes in esophageal branches of the vagus nerve as well as muscular hypertrophy. DES and achalasia may be part of the same spectrum of abnormal esophageal motility related to varying degrees of neurogenic damage to the esophagus.

The prevailing symptoms of DES are chest pain and dysphagia. The pain is substernal, and may radi-ate to the arms and back. Because DES pain may occur with or without swallowing, it is difficult to distinguish from cardiogenic pain. The absence of exertional pain and the occasional association with swallowing and dysphagia are helpful clues. The typical patient tends to be anxious. In fact, symptoms can be triggered by emotional stress. Other precipitating factors include the ingestion of hot or cold liquids and GERD.

The barium esophagram is quite characteristic (**Fig. 50.3**). The nonperistaltic, simultaneous contractions produce segmentation of the barium column in the lower two-thirds of the esophagus, a so-called corkscrew or rosary bead appearance. The barium study may also be entirely normal in the setting of DES. Manometry findings of prolonged, high-amplitude nonperistaltic or tertiary contractions on more than 20% of swallows are considered diagnostic (**Fig. 50.4**). Simultaneous contractions can occur in up to 10% of swallows in normal individuals. Radionuclide scintigraphy may be useful in demonstrating a prolonged transit time of more than 20 seconds, along with fragmentation of the radioactive bolus.

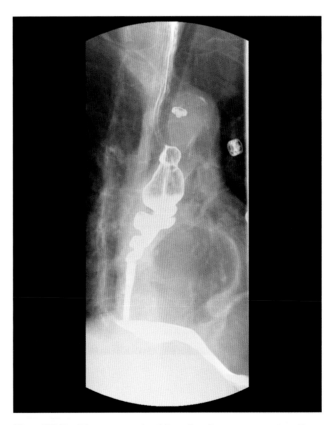

Fig. 50.3 The nonperistaltic, simultaneous contractions produce segmentation of the barium column in the lower two-thirds of the esophagus, a "corkscrew" or "rosary bead" appearance, characteristic of diffuse esophageal spasm. Note the incidental finding of a large hiatal hernia.

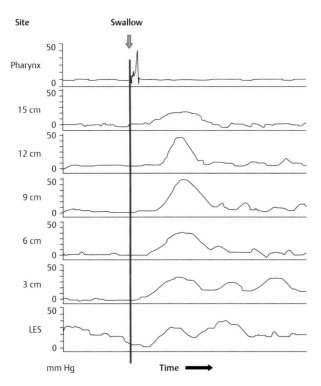

Fig. 50.4 Schematic representation of manometry demonstrating prolonged, high-amplitude nonperistaltic or tertiary contractions, characteristic of diffuse esophageal spasm.

Treatment begins by reassuring the patient that the pain is not cardiac after diagnostic workup confirms that it is not. Avoiding factors that trigger symptoms is helpful; for the patient to do so may require treatment of any associated GERD. Clinical improvement has been reported with sublingual nitroglycerin for acute attacks and longer-acting nitrates for prophylaxis. Calcium channel blockers, tricyclic antidepressants, and anticholinergic agents have met with limited success. Balloon dilation may help if there is associated LES dysfunction, but it does little to alleviate the chest pain. Intraluminal Botox injections appear to be the best available current treatment option. When patients are incapacitated and have not responded to conservative therapy, surgical myotomy may be helpful in some patients. The surgery is quite extensive given that the myotomy needs to include the entire smooth muscle portion of the esophagus.

Nutcracker Esophagus

Similar to DES, nutcracker esophagus is characterized by high-amplitude esophageal contractions that produce chest pain and dysphagia. The contractions remain peristaltic, however, and there is in fact some debate as to whether this represents a true motility disorder or whether it is simply within the range of normal esophageal function.

Unlike achalasia and DES, nutcracker esophagus cannot be diagnosed radiographically. A barium esophagram is usually normal or may demonstrate nonspecific tertiary contractions. Esophageal transit is also usually normal. On the other hand, manometry (**Fig. 50.5**) will indicate normal peristalsis but with distal peristaltic pressure amplitudes > 180 mm Hg (normal mean distal esophageal amplitude is 100 mm Hg).

Treatment is aimed at reducing the amplitude of distal peristaltic contractions. Smooth muscle relaxants such as nitrates and calcium channel blockers have been tried with variable results. Interestingly, there is a poor correlation between reduction of contraction amplitude and improvement of chest pain. A recent study suggests a high incidence of GERD in patients with nutcracker esophagus, and demonstrated that acid suppression therapy was effective in alleviating the pain.

Ineffective Esophageal Motility (IEM) Disorder

IEM is a relatively new, *manometrically defined*, esophageal motility disorder, associated with severe GERD, GERD-associated respiratory symptoms, delayed acid clearance, and mucosal injury. A barium esophagram appears to be relatively insensitive in the workup of

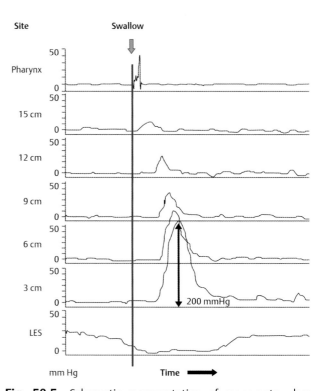

Fig. 50.5 Schematic representation of manometry demonstrating normal peristalsis, but with distal peristaltic pressure amplitudes > 180 mm Hg, characteristic of nutcracker esophagus.

suspected IEM. The condition is defined by at least 50% ineffective contractions out of 10 wet swallows on manometry. Symptoms of dysphagia as well as the typical and atypical symptoms of GERD predominate. Treatment is individualized to the patient's symptoms, and frequently involves an antireflux regimen and aggressive acid-suppression therapy.

NEMD is a vague category used to include patients with poorly defined esophageal contraction abnormalities. The criteria include "ineffective" contraction waves (i.e., peristaltic waves that either are of low amplitude or are not transmitted). Most patients previously classified as having NEMD would now meet the criteria as having IEM to describe abnormalities characterized by hypocontraction. The term *NEMD* has been dropped from many current classification schemes for esophageal motility disorders.

Presbyesophagus and *presbyphagia* are terms originally used to describe esophageal dysmotility that occurs with aging. Many of these patients now meet the manometric criteria for IEM, or they are found to have some other primary or secondary motility disorder. Clinically significant esophageal dysfunction as a consequence of age alone is rare, and the terms *presbyesophagus* and *presbyphagia* are misnomers.

Secondary Motility Disorders

Collagen Vascular Diseases

This group of diseases includes several inflammatory disorders that tend to have multisystem involvement. Although esophageal dysphagia is not commonly the presenting symptom, significant functional impairment may develop during later stages of disease. Esophageal involvement is seen most often with scleroderma, polymyositis, and dermatomyositis.

Eighty percent of patients with scleroderma may have head and neck manifestations; 52% report some type of dysphagia as a primary symptom. Esophageal involvement has been found in 75 to 90% of patients. The presence of Raynaud phenomenon is closely correlated with esophageal involvement. Scleroderma is characterized by a generalized small vessel arteritis with excessive collagen deposition. In the esophagus, smooth muscle atrophy and collagen deposition have been found within the submucosa. The striated upper portion of the esophagus remains normal; aperistalsis occurs within the lower esophagus. Nevertheless, the esophagus empties with gravity, and patients may be relatively asymptomatic. A decrease in LES pressure allows reflux to occur, while the lower aperistalsis prevents the esophagus from readily clearing the acid. This leads to esophagitis with potential complications, including stricture, which has been found in as many as 48% of patients with scleroderma. Dysphagia, particularly in response to solid food, generally occurs and may be due to abnormal motility, reflux esophagitis, or stricture.

Evaluation begins with a barium esophagram that typically shows a patulous LES and diminished peristalsis or tertiary contractions of the lower two-thirds of the esophagus. In more advanced cases, a long stricture with upper esophageal distention may occur (**Fig. 50.6**). Endoscopy is indicated to assess the severity of esophagitis and to rule out malignancy. All patients with scleroderma should be evaluated to detect esophageal involvement. Therapy is directed toward preventing GERD and its complications.

Other Secondary Motility Disorders

Several metabolic and endocrine disorders may alter esophageal function. Both diabetes and alcoholism can produce a peripheral neuropathy that may result in disordered peristalsis. Various neuromuscular diseases may affect the pharynx and striated portion of the esophagus and may also disrupt motility within the distal smooth muscle portion.

Chagas disease is a systemic infection caused by the parasite *Trypanosoma cruzi*. It is endemic to South America and may involve multiple organ systems. When the esophagus is involved, patients may present with such symptoms as achalasia, which is primarily dysphagia without associated pain. Chagas

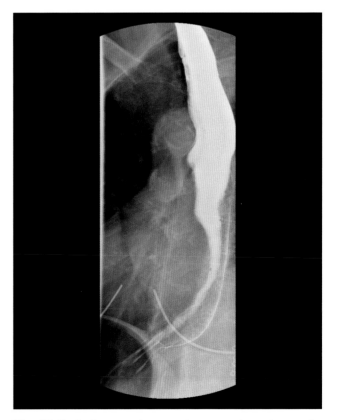

Fig. 50.6 Barium esophagram demonstrating a long stricture with upper esophageal distention, characteristic of scleroderma.

disease is diagnosed by a history of endemic exposure, detection of antibody (serology), and evidence of other organ involvement.

One large study reports that the recent widespread use of bariatric surgery to treat obesity has led to the development of secondary motility disorders by radiographic criteria in 68% of patients having undergone laparoscopic adjustable gastric banding. The long-term effects of an occlusive gastric band could produce dilation of the esophagus, as is seen in achalasia, in some cases necessitating emptying of the device or outright surgical removal. As experience grows with these relatively new devices, the clinical picture should become clearer.

Eosinophilic esophagitis (EoE) is another relatively newly described entity clinically relevant in the etiology and workup of dysphagia. First described in the early 1990s, EoE has rapidly evolved as a distinctive chronic inflammatory esophageal disease with increasing incidence and prevalence in developed countries. This disease is more prevalent in males and is frequently associated with allergies. Its diagnosis is established based on the presence of esophageal symptoms and dense eosinophilic esophageal infiltration, once other conditions associated with esophageal eosinophilia are excluded. Topical corticosteroids lead to a rapid improvement of active disease. At least one study has demonstrated manometric motility abnormalities. Although the long-term effects of EoE on esophageal motility have yet to be elucidated, it already appears to play a significant role in esophageal phase dysphagia.

The number of secondary causes of dysmotility continues to grow at a significant pace. The interested reader is directed to the work of Hirano.

■ Suggested Reading

Aly YA. Digital radiography in the evaluation of oesophageal motility disorders. Clin Radiol 2000;55(7):561–568

Amin MR, Postma GN, Setzen M, Koufman JA. Transnasal esophagoscopy: a position statement from the American Bronchoesophagological Association (ABEA) [Erratum appears in Otolaryngol Head Neck Surg 2009;140(2):280]. Otolaryngol Head Neck Surg 2008;138(4):411–414

Aviv JE. Transnasal esophagoscopy: state of the art. Otolaryngol Head Neck Surg 2006;135(4):616–619

Bashashati M, Andrews C, Ghosh S, Storr M. Botulinum toxin in the treatment of diffuse esophageal spasm. Dis Esophagus 2010;23(7):554–560

Belafsky PC, Postma GN, Daniel E, Koufman JA. Transnasal esophagoscopy. Otolaryngol Head Neck Surg 2001;125(6):588–589

Boeckxstaens GE, Annese V, des Varannes SB, et al.; European Achalasia Trial Investigators. Pneumatic dilation versus laparoscopic Heller's myotomy for idiopathic achalasia. N Engl J Med 2011;364(19):1807–1816

Castagliuolo I, Brun P, Costantini M, et al. Esophageal achalasia: is the herpes simplex virus really innocent? J Gastrointest Surg 2004;8(1):24–30, discussion 30

DeMeester TR, Peters JH, Bremner CG, Chandrasoma P. Biology of gastroesophageal reflux disease: pathophysiology relating to medical and surgical treatment. Annu Rev Med 1999;50:469–506

Dent J, Holloway RH. Esophageal motility and reflux testing. State-of-the-art and clinical role in the twenty-first century. Gastroenterol Clin North Am 1996;25(1):51–73

Färkkilä MA, Ertama L, Katila H, Kuusi K, Paavolainen M, Varis K. Globus pharyngis, commonly associated with esophageal motility disorders. Am J Gastroenterol 1994;89(4):503–508

Hirano I. Pathophysiology of achalasia and diffuse esophageal spasm. GI Motility online. (2006) doi:10.1038/gimo22. Published 16 May 2006

Hoppo T, Jobe BA. Is laparoscopic Heller myotomy superior to pneumatic dilation to treat achalasia? Semin Thorac Cardiovasc Surg 2011;23(3):178–180

Kahrilas PJ. Esophageal motor disorders in terms of high-resolution esophageal pressure topography: what has changed? Am J Gastroenterol 2010;105(5):981–987

Katzka DA, Castell DO. Review article: an analysis of the efficacy, perforation rates and methods used in pneumatic dilation for achalasia. Aliment Pharmacol Ther 2011;34(8):832–839

Martín Martín L, Santander C, Lopez Martín MC, et al. Esophageal motor abnormalities in eosinophilic esophagitis identified by high-resolution manometry. J Gastroenterol Hepatol 2011;26(9):1447–1450

Mayberry JF. Epidemiology and demographics of achalasia. Gastrointest Endosc Clin N Am 2001;11(2):235–248, v

Naef M, Mouton WG, Naef U, van der Weg B, Maddern GJ, Wagner HE. Esophageal dysmotility disorders after laparoscopic gastric banding—an underestimated complication. Ann Surg 2011;253(2):285–290

Pandolfino JE, Richter JE, Ours T, Guardino JM, Chapman J, Kahrilas PJ. Ambulatory esophageal pH monitoring using a wireless system. Am J Gastroenterol 2003;98(4):740–749

Boeckxstaens GE, Annese V, des Varannes SB, et al; European Achalasia Trial Investigators. Pneumatic dilation versus laparoscopic Heller's myotomy for idiopathic achalasia. N Engl J Med 2011; 364(19):1807–1816

Popoff AM, Myers JA, Zelhart M, et al. Long-term symptom relief and patient satisfaction after Heller myotomy and Toupet fundoplication for achalasia. Am J Surg 2012;203(3):339–342, discussion 342

Postma GN. Transnasal esophagoscopy. Curr Opin Otolaryngol Head Neck Surg 2006;14(3):156–158

Rees CJ. In-office transnasal esophagoscope-guided botulinum toxin injection of the lower esophageal sphincter. Curr Opin Otolaryngol Head Neck Surg 2007;15(6):409–411

Richter JE, Boeckxstaens GE. Management of achalasia: surgery or pneumatic dilation. Gut 2011;60(6):869–876

Shakespear JS, Blom D, Huprich JE, Peters JH. Correlation of radiographic and manometric findings in patients with ineffective esophageal motility. Surg Endosc 2004;18(3):459–462

Spechler SJ, Castell DO. Classification of oesophageal motility abnormalities. Gut 2001;49(1):145–151

Tutuian R, Vela MF, Shay SS, Castell DO. Multichannel intraluminal impedance in esophageal function testing and gastroesophageal reflux monitoring. J Clin Gastroenterol 2003;37(3):206–215

51 Evaluation and Management of Gastroesophageal Reflux

■ Introduction

Revolutionary changes in the diagnosis and management of gastroesophageal reflux disease (GERD) have occurred within the past 40 years. Yet many aspects of the "prevalent cult of 'reflux disease'" remain unanswered.

Many manifestations of GERD are of particular interest to the otolaryngologist. Acid reflux may cause or exacerbate a variety of otorhinolaryngological symptoms, such as chronic cough, wheezing, hoarseness, throat pain, and dysphagia. Disorders, including chronic laryngitis, laryngeal edema, subglottic stenosis, and laryngeal cancer, have been implicated in patients with GERD as their only risk factor. This review evaluates the current literature, with particular attention to the extraesophageal manifestations of GERD. Unfortunately, the definitive diagnosis, elucidation of the pathophysiology, and effective treatment of suspected extraesophageal reflux remain controversial and are limited by the paucity of evidence from randomized, placebo-controlled, large-scale population studies.

Numerous terms have been applied to the manifestations of reflux disease that are extraesophageal, including extraesophageal reflux disease (EERD), laryngopharyngeal reflux (LPR), atypical GERD, and reflux laryngitis. Many of these terms are used interchangeably. *LPR* seems to be the most frequently used of these labels in the otolaryngology literature and is common enough to appear as its own search term. In the past 10 years, more than 200 publications have been matched to the term *laryngopharyngeal reflux*. However, significant controversy still exists regarding whether LPR or EERD represents a distinct disease process unto its own or is solely an extraesophageal sibling of GERD.

The true incidence of "reflux disease" is difficult to define because GERD is not just one disease. Heartburn is believed to affect 40% of the U.S. adult population. Symptomatic gastroesophageal reflux affects 11% of Americans daily, 12% weekly, and 15%

monthly. Extraesophageal manifestations of GERD, such as asthma, hoarseness, chronic cough, and globus, are more difficult to define. Extraesophageal GERD may affect at least 5 million Americans. It has been estimated that extraesophageal GERD symptoms represent 30% of patients presenting for GERD evaluation and management.

■ Pathophysiology

Key physiological factors contributing to the development of GERD include the following:

1. Lower esophageal sphincter (LES) competence
2. Upper esophageal sphincter (UES) function
3. Esophageal motility
4. Gastric contents
5. Gastric motility

The degree to which each of these factors contributes to LPR specifically has been studied as well. These factors appear to be much less predictive of the presence of LPR symptoms or response to therapy.

Lower Esophageal Sphincter Competence

The LES is the major sphincteric barrier between gastric contents and the esophagus. Basal LES pressures have a resting value that transiently decreases during swallow, then is restored after the bolus passes. LES resting pressures have been measured with manometry and are expressed relative to gastric pressure. Although LES hypotonia has been believed to be the major determinant of gastroesophageal reflux and esophagitis, this concept has been questioned because most patients with GERD have normal basal LES pressures. More recent studies have clarified the pathophysiology of GERD by identifying transient LES relaxation in patients with otherwise normal LES tone.

Despite controversy as to when and why reflux occurs, LES incompetence with reflux of stomach contents into the esophagus is the basic pathophysiological process of GERD. With 24 hour pH monitoring and simultaneous recordings of LES pressures, transient acid reflux has been documented as a normal phenomenon. A study by Dent et al demonstrated that LES pressure varied significantly, and that episodes of reflux were primarily related to transient complete episodes of inappropriate relaxation, rather than decreased basal resting LES pressures. This may indicate that a proportion of reflux events is random, rather than something persisting.

The degree of acid exposure and host mucosal defenses have been implicated as additional factors in the pathophysiology of GERD. Further study will elucidate the role of the LES and stomach in the pathogenesis of GERD. Surgical management of GERD primarily involves enhancement of LES function as a keystone of therapy.

Upper Esophageal Sphincter Function

The role of the UES as a barrier to gastroesophageal reflux and its extraesophageal manifestations has not been studied systematically. This is due in part to the asymmetric and complex dynamics of the UES at rest and during swallow. The UES has a slitlike configuration, with radial asymmetric zones. Higher pressures are recorded anteriorly and posteriorly than laterally and medially. In Koufman's study of normal volunteers using multichannel, 24-hour pH-metry, pharyngeal acid reflux was not detected. With pH probes above and below the UES, Shaker et al showed a higher incidence of acid events in the pharynges of laryngitis patients (compared with normal healthy people and patients with classic symptoms of GERD), implying the role of pharyngeal acid penetration in laryngeal manifestations of GERD. However, the normal group also exhibited episodes of pharyngeal acid reflux, and in other studies the rate of false-positives ranged from 7 to 17%. Vaezi reviewed 12 previous studies and found that only 54% of 1,217 patients clinically suspicious for having reflux laryngitis had evidence of pharyngeal acid exposure. Clinically, Ulualp et al found that even LPR-suspected patients who tested positive for pharyngeal acid exposure by pH-metry were no more likely to respond to acid suppression therapy than those who tested negative on a pH test.

Esophageal Motility

Esophageal clearance of acid in the pathogenesis of GERD appears to be an important cofactor. A comparison of normal healthy volunteers and GERD patients showed that, in healthy people, most episodes of gastroesophageal reflux occurred spontaneously and were cleared from the lower esophagus by peristaltic contractions. During episodes of gastroesophageal reflux in GERD patients, esophageal motility was less, with fewer peristaltic contractions than in controls.

Belafsky et al believe that a subset of proton pump inhibitor (PPI)-refractory LPR patients have esophageal-pharyngeal reflux, which they characterized as regurgitation of proximal esophageal contents into the laryngopharynx, caused by a disorder of volume clearance and esophageal dysmotility instead of acidic or peptic injury. Knight et al found a significant association between esophageal dysmotility and extraesophageal manifestations; however, they demonstrated no statistically significant association between esophageal motility disorders and abnormal acid reflux in this same population. The authors suggested that these problems exist as an accompanying condition or pathogenic cofactor in some patients with atypical GERD.

Gastric Factors: Pepsin and Acid

Acid concentration and duration of esophageal exposure are significant in causing esophageal injury, but the composition of the refluxate is the major factor that determines how damaging the refluxed material will be. The damage caused by acid is enhanced by pepsin. Dent showed that abnormally prolonged or frequent exposure of the lower esophagus to a pH < 4 is the major factor. Pepsin activity is a major determinant of the aggressiveness of refluxate; full activity of gastric pepsin requires a pH < 3. Thus acid suppression may protect the mucosa from injury indirectly by preventing the activation of pepsin. Peptic activity, and hence the aggressiveness of refluxate, are reduced markedly when pH rises from 3 to 4.

Gastric Motility

The role of gastric emptying in the pathogenesis of GERD is unclear. Prolonged gastric emptying has not been found in patients with GERD. Although prokinetic agents had been frequently used for management of GERD, abnormalities of gastric emptying have not been established as significantly contributing to GERD, and these medications by and large are no longer used as first-line therapy for GERD or LPR.

Other Factors

Recently, genetic factors and molecular pathways in laryngopharyngeal disease have been evaluated. Although this line of study is still in its infancy, differentiating the "sibling diseases" of GERD and LPR may offer better insight into the pathogenesis of LPR, opening new, disease-specific therapeutic trends.

Pathology of GERD and Extraesophageal GERD

EERD versus GERD

Shaker et al studied the pathophysiology of EERD to compare the pharyngoesophageal distribution of gastric refluxate between patients with laryngitis attributed to gastroesophageal reflux and three control groups. Between-group comparison showed no significant difference in the reflux parameters in the lower esophagus, whereas a significantly higher percentage of reflux episodes reached the upper esophagus in the laryngitis group. The number of pharyngeal reflux episodes and time of acid exposure were significantly higher in the laryngitis group. Thus exposure of the pharynx to reflux may be the most important parameter in the evaluation of EERD. The use of a three-channel pH probe for the detection of extraesophageal reflux in these patients is important in the definition of pharyngolaryngeal manifestations of GERD.

There is some evidence in dog studies that gastric juices (acid and pepsin) are more damaging than duodenal substances (bile acids and trypsin). Barry and Vaezi hint that the larynx may be more sensitive to injury than the esophagus. A study of pig larynges indicates that laryngeal tissues are essentially resistant to isolated acidic damage at pH of 4, unless pepsin is present, with the clinically relevant exception of the subglottic mucosa, found to be the most sensitive laryngeal site to isolated acid injury at pH of 4. The posterior glottis was noted to be the least sensitive. Clinically, this would correlate with the common finding of posterior laryngitis in the setting of suspected LPR, expected to be the first anatomical site of exposure in the larynx, and the relatively uncommon finding of subglottic tissue injury or stenosis in (nonintubated) individuals. Intuitively, this accounts for the relatively proadaptive resistance of the posterior glottis and maladaptive susceptibility of the subglottis. Pepsin itself has been considered an important target for therapy and a marker of LPR. There is good evidence of pepsin endocytosis by hypopharyngeal epithelial cells causing mitochondrial damage and changes in the expression of several genes implicated in stress, even under conditions of nonacidic reflux, providing a rationale for targeting pepsin in the treatment of reflux disease and a promising topic for future research.

GERD: The Histopathology of Esophagitis

Morphological changes in patients with esophagitis are associated with inflammatory cells and are therefore important criteria in the diagnosis of esophagitis. Neutrophilic infiltration of the squamous epithelium is characteristic of reflux esophagitis. However, it occurs in only a minority of such patients. Intraepithelial eosinophilia is also a sensitive histological marker for GERD.

Riddell reviewed the role of biopsy in GERD and concluded that the location most likely to show inflammatory changes of the squamous mucosa, such as neutrophils or eosinophils, is close to the Z line, whereas traditional reactive changes in the squamous mucosa are found only in biopsies taken at least 3 cm above the Z line. Endoscopic criteria for GERD have a morphological counterpart in capillary congestion and hemorrhage into the papillae. Other findings of esophagitis in biopsies from the gastroesophageal junction include basal zone thickening and increased papillary height. The need for multiple biopsies and the interpretive aspects of biopsy and tissue orientation make the histopathological alterations of GERD not completely reliable, but useful in understanding the pathology of esophagitis.

GERD: Risk Factors

Physiological changes may promote LES dysfunction and GERD. Heartburn occurs in approximately two-thirds of all pregnancies. The origin is multifactorial, but the predominant factor is a decrease in LES pressure. Smokers have chronically diminished LES pressure, and periods of smoking are associated with an increased number of reflux events. Smoking also causes chronically diminished salivary function that causes prolonged acid clearance time. Drugs, such as alcohol, theophylline, and caffeine, decrease LES tone. Large meals, chocolate, carbonated beverages, and diets high in fat have also been implicated. Pathological conditions that affect peristalsis and LES function may increase reflux. There is a strong correlation with the presence and size of a hiatal hernia, LES function, and GERD. Common drugs and conditions associated with GERD are shown in **Table 51.1**. The stress-induced increase in gastric pressure that occurs with exercise, singing, bending, and restrictive clothing may promote GERD in patients with a mild decrease in LES pressure.

GERD Symptoms

Heartburn and regurgitation are typical GERD symptoms. Symptoms alone, however, cannot predict the presence or absence of esophageal inflammation or tissue injury, because GERD includes the person with recurrent symptoms but without objective disease, as well as the person with objective disease but without symptoms. GERD may be differentiated as having the following:

1. Typical symptoms
2. Atypical symptoms
3. Symptoms with complications

Table 51.1   Causes of decreased lower esophageal sphincter (LES) pressure

Dietary
High-fat diet
Peppermint and spearmint
Caffeine
Alcohol
Chocolate
Tobacco
Drugs
Theophylline
Calcium channel blockers
Barbiturates
Diazepam
Anticholinergic drugs
Hormones
Estrogen
Progesterone
Glucagon

Typical GERD symptoms include postprandial substernal burning, often associated with bitter or sour taste. Symptoms are worse reclining and with cough or exercise. Typical GERD events occur more often after meals and at night. Nocturnal reflux events, such as cough, choking, or epigastric distress, may awaken the patient from sleep. Chest pain of uncertain origin may also be caused by GERD.

GERD: Complications

Esophageal complications of GERD include Barrett metaplasia, esophageal ulceration, and esophageal stricture. Esophageal stricture follows esophageal ulceration and fibrosis. Progressive dysphagia for solids is the typical symptom of a stricture. Esophageal ulceration due to chronic acid exposure cannot be distinguished radiographically from other causes of esophageal ulceration and should be investigated by endoscopy and biopsy.

Barrett metaplasia is the presence of specialized columnar epithelium replacing the normal stratified squamous epithelium of the lower esophagus. It is an acquired condition secondary to GERD. Barrett metaplasia represents response to acid injury and requires both injury to esophageal squamous epithelium and an acidic esophageal environment during the period of repair. Barrett metaplasia may be diagnosed by biopsy of the abnormal-appearing mucosa. Barrett metaplasia has a strong association with ade-

nocarcinoma, the prevalence of which is rising in the United States. Every other year, endoscopic examination for dysplasia is recommended for patients with Barrett metaplasia. If mild dysplasia is found on biopsy, intensive antireflux therapy is indicated with follow-up biopsy; high-grade dysplasia is managed surgically.

GERD: Extraesophageal Manifestations

The many head and neck manifestations of gastroesophageal reflux include hoarseness, frequent throat clearing, dysphagia, globus pharyngeus, laryngeal granulomas, and subglottic stenosis. Postnasal drip, exacerbation of sleep disorders, laryngospasm, and chronic sinonasal disease have recently been added to the growing list as well. GERD causes various symptoms; some are merely nuisances, and some are life threatening.

The original report of association of gastroesophageal reflux and vocal fold contact ulcer was made by Cherry and Margulies in 1968. Since then, other authors have further delineated the role of acid in the pharynx in the pathogenesis of chronic posterior laryngitis and studied the response of chronic laryngitis attributed to acid reflux; with endoscopic documentation and questionnaires, improvement with treatment for GERD have been documented. The laryngoscopic findings of reflux laryngitis may be characteristic or subtle, spanning a spectrum from a normal appearance to severe laryngitis with stenosis.

Endoscopic biopsy and acid output studies in patients with posterior chronic acid laryngitis have identified histological changes typical of the hyperregenerative or atrophic phases of reflux esophagitis. Posterior laryngitis can be attributed to a combination of gastroesophageal reflux, friction of the vocal processes during phonation, and vocal abuse.

Other benign lesions in which gastroesophageal reflux is suspected to play an important role include contact ulcers and vocal process granulomas. Suspected LPR, whether symptomatic or not (also known as "silent reflux") is anecdotally considered an exacerbating factor in recurrence rates of laryngeal papillomatosis and laryngeal dysplasia. As such, most experts place these patients of long-standing acid suppression under therapy unless contraindicated.

There are conflicting reports on the role of GERD in causing symptoms of globus and dysphagia. The appropriate workup and differential diagnosis of isolated globus pharyngeus are extensive, a subject of great controversy, and beyond the scope of this text. Also, the literature is incomplete. Globus is a very frequent complaint in LPR, isolated as well as part of an extraesophageal symptom complex, with or without typical GERD complaints. In a study of patients with globus symptoms, pH-metry abnormalities did not correlate directly with laryngeal findings. In all likelihood, globus pharyngeus is multifactorial. The response rates of isolated complaints of globus to an antireflux regimen of dietary and lifestyle modifications and empirical acid-suppression PPI therapy have been underwhelming.

In Ossakow et al's study of cervical dysphagia and the role of GERD, patients with cervical symptoms but no heartburn were found to have a high incidence of reflux, dysmotility, and reduced acid clearance. These patients appear to have diminished esophageal sensitivity, despite frequent and long acid exposure.

Increased risk of laryngeal cancer associated with reflux in lifetime nonsmokers has been reported. Patients were documented as being at low risk for developing carcinoma from smoking or environmental exposure; chronic laryngitis due to acid reflux was the only risk factor identified. **Fig. 51.1** demonstrates an example of multifocal laryngeal carcinomatosis in a lifetime nonsmoker with severe, chronic, untreated GERD as the patient's only risk factor.

The role of acid reflux in the development of subglottic stenosis after intubation trauma has been reported with abnormal reflux in patients intubated in the intensive care setting and undergoing surgery. Most clinical pathways recommend the routine use of acid suppression therapy in all patients during prolonged intubation.

There is conflicting evidence on the prevalence of GERD in the genesis of cough and hoarseness in the general population. It is possible that patients with cough and hoarseness present to the otolaryngolo-

gist because of (1) low esophageal reflux exposure but abnormal pharyngeal exposure; (2) insensitivity of the esophageal mucosa to acid exposure; or (3) pharyngeal and laryngeal sensitivity to episodic pharyngeal reflux. Although it is recognized that GERD is an important consideration in patients with chronic cough and hoarseness, controversy remains as to its prevalence.

In the pediatric population, acid reflux is increasingly recognized as an important comorbid factor in acquired subglottic stenosis, recurrent idiopathic croup, sudden infant death syndrome, and feeding disorders of infancy. The role of reflux has also been implicated in otitis media and sinusitis in the pediatric population, both areas of ongoing research. Unlike in adults, physiological gastroesophageal reflux is common in infants and children. It is distinguished from the disorder in the adult population by the large number of thriving infants with functional reflux and by the large proportion of older infants and children with secondary pathological reflux.

■ Evaluation

Diagnosis of GERD

A careful history and physical examination with a high index of suspicion are the first steps in the assessment of a patient suspected of GERD or EERD. Attention should be paid to both typical and atypical symptoms, dietary and patient factors, and predisposing factors (medications, certain systemic illnesses, etc.). The role of a patient-reported reflux symptom index has been established. The range of diagnostic testing in the workup for reflux is summarized in **Table 51.2**.

Endoscopy

Endoscopic evaluation of the laryngopharynx and esophagus has a role in the diagnosis of reflux disease. Esophageal endoscopy can be performed transnasally in an awake, unsedated patient in the clinic; in a sedated patient in an endoscopy suite with a flexible scope; or in the operating room, usually with a rigid instrument. Flexible fiberoptic laryngoscopy, with or without stroboscopy, is frequently the first diagnostic test performed by otolaryngologists on patients presenting to otolaryngology with laryngeal complaints.

Esophagoscopy is used to establish a diagnosis and stage reflux esophagitis, to exclude other esophageal disease, and to permit directed biopsy if columnar metaplasia, dysplasia, or carcinoma is suspected. The lesions of reflux esophagitis (erosions,

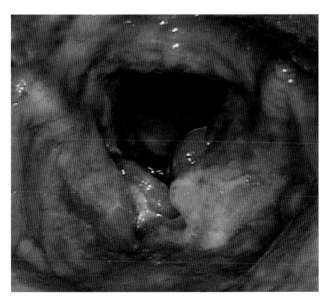

Fig. 51.1 Multifocal laryngeal carcinomatosis in a lifetime nonsmoker with severe, untreated gastroesophageal reflux disease as the patient's only risk factor.

Table 51.2   The range of diagnostic testing in the workup for reflux

Endoscopy
Transnasal esophagoscopy in clinic
Sedated flexible esophagoscopy in endoscopy suite
Rigid esophagoscopy in operating room
Flexible fiberoptic laryngoscopy in clinic
pH-metry
Catheter-based single or dual sensor
24-, 48-, 72-plus-hour wireless monitoring
Radiography
Barium esophagram
Impedance
Multichannel intraluminal impedence (MII)
MII/manometry
MII/pH-metry
Hypopharyngeal MII (investigational)
Others
Pepsin assay (investigational)
Bilirubin assay (investigational)

ulceration, stricture, and metaplasia) are identified and graded independently. Absence of abnormal findings on endoscopy does not exclude GERD. Gastroenterologists generally prefer flexible instruments that allow air insufflation for distention and better access to the lower esophagus and stomach. Otolaryngologists are usually trained with rigid esophagoscopes with telescopes that have superior optics and provide a better view of the esophageal inlet and postcricoid area. Recently, use of transnasal esophagoscopy (TNE) has become widely adopted in otolaryngology. TNE offers the clinician the opportunity to perform unsedated direct visualization (with insufflations and biopsy) under topical anesthesia at initial presentation in the clinic.

The role of laryngoscopy in the diagnosis of LPR remains an area of intense controversy. Many of the symptoms of LPR, including hoarseness, are nonspecific and could suggest the presence of malignancy, indicating the need for laryngoscopy. Once cancer has been excluded, there is a tendency to attribute the symptoms to reflux and assign a diagnosis of LPR. The most common findings on laryngoscopy attributable to reflux are erythema, edema, ventricular obliteration, postcricoid hyperplasia, and pseudosulcus, with edema being the most frequent finding used to diagnose LPR. Unfortunately, these findings on laryngoscopy are nonspecific, and are subject to significant interrater variability. In one study, at least

one of these LPR-associated signs was found in 80 to 90% of asymptomatic patients tested who had no clinical or diagnostic history of GERD or LPR. Belafsky et al created a scoring system for the presence and severity of laryngoscopic findings—the reflux finding score (RFS)—in an attempt to improve interrater reliability and standardize a grading system. However, criticisms that a large-scale randomized trial validating the RFS has not been done limit its widespread incorporation in clinical otolaryngology practices.

pH-Metry

Esophageal pH monitoring is considered the most sensitive method for detecting clinically significant GERD. The pH monitoring is generally performed over a 24-hour period to provide the most comprehensive and reproducible information. This can be accomplished with a single- or dual-sensor pH channel, or more recently, monitoring may occur over 48 or more hours with a wireless Bravo capsule (Given Imaging, Ltd., Mattawan, MI). Patients are encouraged to continue normal activity while avoiding particularly acidic foods. The parameter most consistent with a diagnosis of esophagitis is the percentage of time that esophageal pH is below 4. Generally, this does not exceed 7% over a 24 hour period in normal subjects. Six components are used to determine a composite pH score (DeMeester score), including the percentage of total, upright, and supine time with a pH of < 4 the number of recorded reflux episodes, and episodes > 5 minutes, and the length of time of the longest recorded reflux event. A composite score of > 14.72 indicates the presence of GERD.

Considered the gold standard in reflux diagnosis, ambulatory pH probes have been shown to be unreliable in patients with laryngeal symptoms, even when pharyngeal pH monitoring is employed. This has prompted the search for an LPR-specific diagnostic test with better sensitivity and specificity.

Radiography

Radiographic evaluation of patients with otorhinolaryngological manifestations of GERD primarily consists of the barium esophagram, which detects gross morphological changes of reflux esophagitis and may demonstrate free regurgitation of refluxate during the examination. A baseline barium esophagram is indicated in all patients with esophageal complaints and dysphagia, providing complementary information to that of endoscopy alone. A midesophageal stricture, not a rare complication of chronic reflux disease or finding on barium esophagram, is considered pathopneumonic for GERD (**Fig. 51.2**). However, the presence of a malignant process should also be excluded with esophagoscopy. Although there appear to be

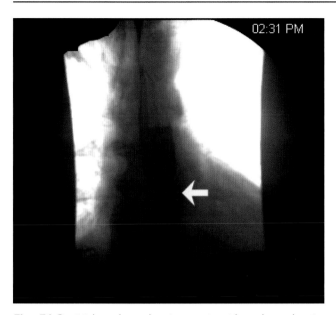

Fig. 51.2 Midesophageal stricture. A midesophageal stricture (*white arrow*) is considered a pathognomonic radiological finding in gastroesophageal reflux disease. A malignant process must be excluded.

radiographic signs of severe esophagitis on barium esophagram, none of these are considered specific for Barrett metaplasia.

A hiatal hernia, generally easy to find on barium esophagram, is considered a risk factor for GERD. However, its presence radiographically is neither specific nor sensitive in predicting the degree or presence of esophagitis per se.

Impedance Testing

Esophageal impedance testing is a newer technology that measures electrical resistance (impedance) along different points of the esophagus to detect the reflux of acid and nonacidic materials. Multichannel intraluminal impedance (MII) can be combined with pH monitoring (MII-pH) as well as manometry. The role of impedance testing is evolving as the test becomes a standard part of the diagnostic armamentarium. Initially, the test was used in refractory cases of GERD to establish a diagnosis of "nonacidic" or bile reflux in patients nonresponsive to standard medical therapy. An initial complaint was the lack of specificity and sensitivity for LPR. Recently, studies have begun to establish normative data for the hypopharynx, using hypopharyngeal MII-pH monitoring. Recently, the success of acid suppression in the setting of chronic reflux laryngitis could be better predicted using reflux parameters detected using the combination 24 hour MII-pH monitoring, which appeared strongest among patients having increased laryngopharyngeal bolus exposure time.

Other Testing

The role of manometry in patients with isolated extraesophageal symptoms has not been established. GERD, which certainly has a role in dysmotility, can be evaluated with combined MII/manometry. However, this combined test most likely would not be useful in the absence of dysphagia or a suspected motility disorder. Newer assays have been developed to detect pepsin and bilirubin. Pepsin has been posited to be a reliable biological marker of the upper airway manifestations of extraesophageal reflux, as when found in the lung, bronchi, or paranasal sinuses. A pepsin assay has been used to identify refluxate in the trachea, lung, sinus, middle ear, and breath. One review of the literature determined that an immunological pepsin assay was 100% sensitive and 89% specific for detection of extraesophageal reflux based on pH-metry. Bilirubin assays are also available, with a good correlation of gastric bile acid concentrations; however, their utility in LPR is less certain.

■ Management of GERD

The goals of management of GERD are (1) relief of symptoms, (2) healing of esophagitis/ laryngitis, (3) prevention of complications, and (4) maintenance of remission. Lifestyle changes may control GERD in up to 20% of patients. The best results of promotility therapy achieved only 50 to 60% control using cisapride. Cisapride was removed from the U.S. market because of cardiac arrhythmias. Effective use of older agents (metoclopramide and bethanechol) is limited by side effects; therefore, these have largely been abandoned as standard first-line treatments. Acid suppression using histamine receptor antagonists controls GERD in 50 to 60% of patients, whereas PPIs offer the most effective control (80–100%). A surgical approach (especially using newer laparoscopic techniques) provides effective therapy of GERD in many patients, but comparisons are needed to define the long-term efficacy and related costs of surgical and chronic medical therapy.

Simple lifestyle changes, diet modification, and reflux precautions effectively manage reflux in many patients. Nonmedical management is used first or in conjunction with medical therapy. Absolute smoking cessation is mandatory. Dietary restriction of fat, alcohol, peppermint, citrus juices, and caffeine is recommended. For laryngopharyngeal symptoms, patients are frequently asked to avoid the five "Cs":

1. Carbonated beverages
2. Caffeine
3. Cigarettes
4. Cocktails
5. Chocolate

The maintenance of a height gradient between the UES and LES by head-of-bed elevation and upright posture after meals are simple yet often effective measures, as is avoidance of meals or snacking 2 hours before bedtime. Noncompliance with an antireflux diet and lifestyle significantly limits the effectiveness of medical management and frequently results in an overreliance on pharmacotherapy.

Medical Management

GERD is frequently a chronic, often lifelong illness with periodic exacerbations. Some gastroenterologists suggest maintenance therapy for most patients. In some patients, GERD may not be invariably a chronic, unremitting condition, and acceptable long-term management may require only intermittent symptomatic therapy or no medication at all. Clinical trials and management algorithms that presume the abolition of symptoms and complete resolution of esophagitis to be the desirable therapeutic goals may not be necessary for all patients. Individual therapy based on symptoms and severity may be appropriate for a large percentage of patients. The essence of effective medical treatment of esophagitis is to reduce the acidity of the refluxate to a level above the optimum proteolytic pH range of pepsin (> pH 3.5).

The keystone of medical management of GERD is acid suppression. Two classes of drugs that have shown effectiveness in acid suppression are the histamine-2 receptor antagonists (H2 blockers: cimetidine, ranitidine, famotidine, nizatidine) and the proton pump inhibitors (omeprazole, lansoprazole, and others). Newer versions of omeprazole are available as combination therapy with time-released sodium bicarbonate. PPIs are more effective than H2 blockers in total acid suppression.

Given the wide variety of effective agents available, a stepwise approach to therapy using several drug classes is reasonable. Comparisons of treatment strategies for biopsy-proven esophagitis have shown complete endoscopic normalization of the esophageal mucosa in 90% of patients with grade I esophagitis within 4 weeks of treatment with omeprazole, 40 mg once daily, compared with 55% of those treated with ranitidine. In comparisons based on the results of clinical healing trials, omeprazole has been found to be the most cost-effective drug for treatment of reflux esophagitis. The addition of prokinetic drugs to H2 blockers has shown little, if any, benefit over H2 blockers alone.

Use of drugs in long-term maintenance therapy needs to be tailored to the severity of the disease. Comparative trials have shown that 82% of patients with esophagitis can be maintained in endoscopic and symptomatic remission for 12 months when treated with omeprazole, 20 mg once daily, compared with only 36% of patients in remission when given "full-dose" H2 blocker therapy (ranitidine,

300 mg daily). The addition of H2 blocker therapy (typically at bedtime) to PPIs has not been shown to improve LPR symptom relief or decrease objective reflux events. Additionally, very few PPI-nonresponsive patients receive benefit from H2 blocker therapy, relegating this class of medication to a category of poor second-line therapy.

Most clinicians in otolaryngology and gastroenterology recommend a minimum of a 2-month trial of empirical twice-daily acid suppression therapy using PPIs for suspected LPR. In responders, tapering the pharmacotherapy to once daily would be prudent, and ultimately to minimal acid suppression to control symptoms, while stressing the dietary and lifestyle components. It is important to note that in patients with both GERD and LPR symptoms, the extraesophageal symptoms typically take much longer to respond to PPI therapy than the esophageal ones, necessitating 3 to 6 or more months of therapy. In PPI nonresponders, additional testing may be indicated, as well as careful consideration of other causes of the patient's symptoms. The duration of an empirical trial varies widely in the literature and points to the lack of an accepted clinical decision pathway. Finally, some authors have found empirical PPI therapy disappointing, given a study by Vaezi et al, which found that, in patients with isolated LPR symptoms, twice-daily acid PPI therapy was no better than placebo, with each group reporting a statistically insignificant proportion of resolution of symptoms at 4 months.

Although empirical PPI therapy appears to be safe in the short term, PPIs as a class have been linked with an increased risk of osteoporosis in at-risk individuals. Finding the least amount of drug necessary to control symptoms and maintain integrity of esophageal mucosa minimizes cost and potential long-term risk.

Surgery

Several antireflux procedures yield good to excellent results when performed by skilled and experienced surgeons. Surgery is designed to correct a mechanically defective LES. Laparoscopic fundoplication can result in long-term success in more than 90% of patients. However, complications and poor results need to be compared with the alternative of long-term medical acid suppression. With recent surgical and medical advances, it is difficult to compare results. Surgery is a reasonable alternative in the following cases:

1. Failed medical therapy
2. Healthy patients with personal preference for surgery
3. Refractory extraesophageal manifestations of GERD, such as reflux laryngitis and asthma
4. Bleeding from refractory esophagitis

Multiple studies have evaluated the role of surgical fundoplication for isolated LPR symptoms nonresponsive to standard medical therapy. By and large, authors conclude that surgery is *not* recommended for patients whose symptoms do not respond to PPI therapy, and that the only useful preoperative predictor of postfundoplication relief of extraesophageal symptoms is preoperative response to aggressive acid suppression therapy.

Recently, there has been an explosion in the field of bariatric surgery. Body mass index has long been associated with increased risk for GERD. Interestingly, this has not been established in patients with isolated LPR. Early reports seem to indicate an improvement in self-reported reflux symptoms following bariatric gastric banding and other bariatric procedures. The degrees of improvement in extraesophageal symptoms and objective measures of reflux are areas of active research. There now appear to be indications for bariatric surgery as the primary surgical option over fundoplication for surgical candidates with GERD in the morbidly obese population.

■ Conclusion

GERD has been recognized as an important contributor to otorhinolaryngological disorders affecting the pharynx, larynx, sinuses, ears, and trachea. Although GERD is usually mild and can be treated by lifestyle modifications, an antireflux diet, and medication, the clinical head and neck spectrum of GERD includes life-threatening complications, such as pulmonary fibrosis, asthma, laryngeal cancer, and subglottic stenosis. Evaluation of suspected GERD or EERD includes history, physical examination, and endoscopy of the larynx and esophagus. Further testing may be indicated in nonresponders. An antireflux regimen, including dietary and lifestyle modifications, and medical therapy with total acid suppression are the treatments of choice for initial treatment and long-term management of severe complications. Step-down therapy is appropriate for long-term symptom management. Surgery is considered only for a small subset of well-selected patients. Although LPR seems to be part of a reflux epidemic, the golden test and a critical pathway are still lacking. There are major differences between existing protocols for reflux disease in the literature, reflecting many clinical controversies resulting in more questions than answers.

The interested reader is referred to Pearson et al for an excellent review of recent research, diagnostic testing, and clinical progress in GERD and LPR.

■ Suggested Reading

Adhami T, Goldblum JR, Richter JE, Vaezi MF. The role of gastric and duodenal agents in laryngeal injury: an experimental canine model. Am J Gastroenterol 2004;99(11):2098–2106

Amin MR, Postma GN, Setzen M, Koufman JA. Transnasal esophagoscopy: a position statement from the American Bronchoesophagological Association (ABEA) [Erratum appears in Otolaryngol Head Neck Surg 2009;140(2):280]. Otolaryngol Head Neck Surg 2008;138(4):411–414

Aviv JE. Transnasal esophagoscopy: state of the art. Otolaryngol Head Neck Surg 2006;135(4):616–619

Barry DW, Vaezi MF. Laryngopharyngeal reflux: More questions than answers. Cleve Clin J Med 2010;77(5):327–334

Belafsky PC, Postma GN, Koufman JA. The validity and reliability of the reflux finding score (RFS). Laryngoscope 2001;111(8):1313–1317

Belafsky PC, Postma GN, Koufman JA. Validity and reliability of the reflux symptom index (RSI). J Voice 2002;16(2):274–277

Belafsky PC, Rees CJ, Rodriguez K, Pryor JS, Katz PO. Esophagopharyngeal reflux. Otolaryngol Head Neck Surg 2008;138(1):57–61

Bulmer DM, Ali MS, Brownlee IA, Dettmar PW, Pearson JP. Laryngeal mucosa: its susceptibility to damage by acid and pepsin. Laryngoscope 2010;120(4):777–782

Chen YM, Gelfand DW, Ott DJ, Wu WC. Barrett esophagus as an extension of severe esophagitis: analysis of radiologic signs in 29 cases. AJR Am J Roentgenol 1985;145(2):275–281

Cherry J, Margulies SI. Head and neck manifestations of gastroesophageal reflux. Laryngoscope 1968;78:1937–1940

DeMeester TR, Peters JH, Bremner CG, Chandrasoma P. Biology of gastroesophageal reflux disease: pathophysiology relating to medical and surgical treatment. Annu Rev Med 1999;50:469–506

Eubanks TR, Omelanczuk PE, Maronian N, Hillel A, Pope CE II, Pellegrini CA. Pharyngeal pH monitoring in 222 patients with suspected laryngeal reflux. J Gastrointest Surg 2001;5(2):183–190, discussion 190–191

Hoppo T, Sanz AF, Nason KS, et al. How much pharyngeal exposure is "normal"? Normative data for laryngopharyngeal reflux events using hypopharyngeal multichannel intraluminal impedance (HMII). J Gastrointest Surg 2012;16(1):16–24, discussion 24–25

Jacob P, Kahrilas PJ, Herzon G. Proximal esophageal pH-metry in patients with 'reflux laryngitis'. Gastroenterology 1991;100(2):305–310

Johnston N, Wells CW, Samuels TL, Blumin JH. Rationale for targeting pepsin in the treatment of reflux disease. Ann Otol Rhinol Laryngol 2010;119(8):547–558

Knight RE, Wells JR, Parrish RS. Esophageal dysmotility as an important co-factor in extraesophageal manifestations of gastroesophageal reflux. Laryngoscope 2000;110(9):1462–1466

Koch OO, Kaindlstorfer A, Antoniou SA, Asche KU, Granderath FA, Pointner R. Influence of the esophageal hiatus size on the lower esophageal sphincter, on reflux activity and on symptomatology. Dis Esophagus 2012;25(3):201–208

Kotby MN, Hassan O, El-Makhzangy AM, Farahat M, Milad P. Gastroesophageal reflux/laryngopharyngeal reflux disease: a critical analysis of the literature. Eur Arch Otorhinolaryngol 2010;267(2):171–179

Koufman JA. The otolaryngologic manifestations of gastroesophageal reflux disease (GERD): a clinical investigation of 225 patients using ambulatory 24-hour pH monitoring and an experimental investigation of the role of acid and pepsin in the development of laryngeal injury. Laryngoscope 1991;101(4 Pt 2, Suppl 53):1–78

Milstein CF, Charbel S, Hicks DM, Abelson TI, Richter JE, Vaezi MF. Prevalence of laryngeal irritation signs associated with reflux in asymptomatic volunteers: impact of endoscopic technique (rigid vs. flexible laryngoscope). Laryngoscope 2005;115(12):2256–2261

Miura MS, Mascaro M, Rosenfeld RM. Association between otitis media and gastroesophageal reflux: a systematic review. Otolaryngol Head Neck Surg 2012;146(3):345–352

Oridate N, Takeda H, Asaka M, et al. Acid-suppression therapy offers varied laryngopharyngeal and esophageal symptom relief in laryngopharyngeal reflux patients. Dig Dis Sci 2008;53(8):2033–2038

Ossakow SJ, Elta G, Colturi T, Bogdasarian R, Nostrant TT. Esophageal reflux and dysmotility as the basis for persistent cervical symptoms. Ann Otol Rhinol Laryngol 1987;96(4):387–392

Pandolfino JE, Richter JE, Ours T, Guardino JM, Chapman J, Kahrilas PJ. Ambulatory esophageal pH monitoring using a wireless system. Am J Gastroenterol 2003;98(4):740–749

Pearson JP, Parikh S, Orlando RC, et al. Review article: reflux and its consequences—the laryngeal, pulmonary and oesophageal manifestations. Conference held in conjunction with the 9th International Symposium on Human Pepsin (ISHP) Kingston-upon-Hull, UK, 21–23 April 2010. Aliment Pharmacol Ther 2011;33(Suppl 1):1–71

Postma GN. Transnasal esophagoscopy. Curr Opin Otolaryngol Head Neck Surg 2006;14(3):156–158

Prachand VN, Alverdy JC. Gastroesophageal reflux disease and severe obesity: Fundoplication or bariatric surgery? World J Gastroenterol 2010;16(30):3757–3761

Samuels TL, Johnston N. Pepsin as a marker of extraesophageal reflux. Ann Otol Rhinol Laryngol 2010;119(3):203–208

Shaker R, Milbrath M, Ren J, et al. Esophagopharyngeal distribution of refluxed gastric acid in patients with reflux laryngitis. Gastroenterology 1995;109(5):1575–1582

So JB, Zeitels SM, Rattner DW. Outcomes of atypical symptoms attributed to gastroesophageal reflux treated by laparoscopic fundoplication. Surgery 1998;124(1):28–32

Ulualp SO, Toohill RJ, Shaker R. Outcomes of acid suppressive therapy in patients with posterior laryngitis. Otolaryngol Head Neck Surg 2001;124(1):16–22

Vaezi MF. Gastroesophageal reflux disease and the larynx. J Clin Gastroenterol 2003;36(3):198–203

Vaezi MF, Hicks DM, Abelson TI, Richter JE. Laryngeal signs and symptoms and gastroesophageal reflux disease (GERD): a critical assessment of cause and effect association. Clin Gastroenterol Hepatol 2003;1(5):333–344

Vaezi MF, Richter JE, Stasney CR, et al. Treatment of chronic posterior laryngitis with esomeprazole. Laryngoscope 2006;116(2):254–260

Vardouniotis AS, Karatzanis AD, Tzortzaki E, et al. Molecular pathways and genetic factors in the pathogenesis of laryngopharyngeal reflux. Eur Arch Otorhinolaryngol 2009;266(6):795–801

Wang AJ, Liang MJ, Jiang AY, et al. Predictors of acid suppression success in patients with chronic laryngitis. Neurogastroenterol Motil 2012;24(5):432–437, e210

Wood JM, Hussey DJ, Woods CM, Watson DI, Carney AS. Biomarkers and laryngopharyngeal reflux. J Laryngol Otol 2011;125(12):1218–1224

Yang YX. Proton pump inhibitor therapy and osteoporosis. Curr Drug Saf 2008;3(3):204–209

52 Caustic Ingestion

■ Introduction

Esophageal, pharyngeal, and laryngeal injury can occur from ingestion of bases (alkalines or caustics), acids, and, rarely, bleaches. Denture cleaners contain various combinations of these chemicals. Ingestion of substances containing bases produces the most significant injury in the esophagus. These substances include lye, which is found in drain cleaners such as Drano, ammonia, and electric dishwasher soaps.

Epidemiology

It is estimated that more than 1.3 million nonpharmaceutical toxic exposures occur annually in the United States. Of these, ~ 77% occur by caustic ingestion. Available data show that most accidental ingestions occur in children aged 12 to 48 months. Typically, the offending caustic substance in these cases is an alkali agent in the form of household bleach, laundry detergent, and a variety of other household agents, such as oven, toilet, tile, and drain cleaners. In this young age group, most ingestions do not result in fatality, given their accidental nature. In adolescents, however, the fatality rate is higher because ingestion is deliberate, with higher amounts of volume and concentration of the caustic agent. In series with a high rate of intentional ingestions, acid ingestions represent a higher fraction of the total ingestions, whereas in series of accidental ingestions, alkali agents typically predominate.

Mechanism of Injury

The principal mechanisms of injury are alkalis and acids (**Table 52.1**). Alkalis are usually odorless and tasteless, and depending on their pH level will result in varying degrees of liquefactive necrosis, with rapid penetration of the esophageal wall. Alkalis with a pH between 9 and 11, including many household deter-

Table 52.1 Mechanism of caustic injury

Alkali ingestions	Acid ingestions
Esophageal injury	Gastric injury
Liquefactive necrosis	Coagulation necrosis
Accidental ingestion	Deliberate ingestion

gents such as bleaches, rarely cause serious injury following ingestion. Ingestion of even small quantities of an alkali with a pH above 11 on the other hand may cause severe burns. Ingestion of a product with a pH more than 12.5 will cause injury regardless of the concentration. As mentioned, specific examples of strong alkali are sodium hydroxides (lye products, drain cleaner, oven cleaner, and dishwashing detergents) and sodium phosphates (dishwashing and laundry detergents).

Acids are usually foul tasting and smelling. As such, their volume of ingestion will usually be small during accidental injuries. They produce coagulation necrosis, with more limited esophageal wall penetration. Gastric injury is more common than esophageal injury, especially in the prepyloric area. Specific strong acids include sulfuric acid (drain cleaner), hydrochloric acid (toilet bowl cleaner), sodium bisulfate (toilet bowl cleaner), hydrofluoric acid (metal cleaner, photography products), and phosphoric acid.

Clinical Presentation

The most common symptoms following a caustic ingestion are dysphagia, drooling, feeding refusal, retrosternal pain, abdominal pain, and vomiting. Symptoms involving the airway are less common, although if present, dyspnea is associated with a high risk of significant gastrointestinal injury. But most important is that studies have demonstrated that the presence or absence of symptoms does not necessarily predict the severity of ingestion injury to the gastrointestinal tract. In a landmark review of 378 pediatric ingestions by Gaudreault et al, 12% of asymptomatic children had severe esophageal burns, whereas 82% of symptomatic children had no esophageal burns. The presence or absence of oral lesions is also a poor indicator of esophageal injury. In a recent series of 473 pediatric caustic ingestions, primarily of alkaline agents, 61% of patients without oral cavity burns had esophageal lesions found at endoscopy.

■ Evaluation

Because rational therapy is based on a precise diagnosis, the essence of the evaluation is to determine the extent of injury. This begins with a careful history, including the type, amount, and brand name of the ingested product. A parent may be sent home to retrieve the container. Any previous home or hospital treatment is documented. Physical examination of the face, extremities, and chest should not be overlooked in the examiner's enthusiasm to focus on the oral cavity, pharynx, and upper digestive tract. The precise location and the extent of any burn or edema is noted. If possible, the larynx is examined with a flexible laryngoscope, depending on the age and degree of cooperation of the patient and whether the patient has significant symptoms of airway obstruction. In the presence of serious airway obstruction, this part of the examination may be deferred until the airway has been stabilized, so as not to precipitate an acute severe obstructive episode.

Radiological examination may include chest radiograph and airway films, particularly if any symptoms of airway obstruction are present. Barium esophagram is of little value under acute conditions because it delays the endoscopic evaluation, and it will not show first- or second-degree injury. If an esophagram is obtained, an atonic, dilated esophagus is an indication of a severe (full-thickness) injury.

Indications for Esophagoscopy

Patients with a history of ingesting household bleach rarely require therapy, and observation is usually the only treatment required unless they become symptomatic. However, with other caustic substances, because signs and symptoms do not accurately predict the presence or severity of injury, esophagoscopy is performed in virtually every patient who is suspected of having ingested a caustic substance. Esophagoscopy is more accurate than any other means to evaluate involvement of the esophagus following a caustic ingestion.

Esophagoscopy should be performed with extreme caution, or should be deferred in the pres-

ence of a severe burn with evidence of laryngeal edema and in patients who have been on high doses of steroids. Typically, esophagoscopy is performed under general anesthesia within 24 to 48 hours of ingestion to the upper limit of any full-thickness burn encountered. The type of injury and the depth are noted; circumferential burns are more likely to cause strictures than linear injuries. Endoscopy is required in all cases of intentional ingestion, even if the patient is asymptomatic, because there is a higher likelihood of oropharyngeal sparing due to rapid swallowing of the caustic, and the presence or absence of oral burns or symptoms in this setting is a poor indicator of the extent of oral or gastric injury.

Esophageal injury is graded at the time of endoscopy (**Table 52.2**). The likelihood of complications correlates with the degree of injury. Grade 1 injury, seen in 60 to 80% of patients who have injury, consists of edema and erythema. In these instances, patients can be fed normally and can be managed as outpatients. Grade 2 esophageal injury consists of linear ulcerations and necrotic tissue with whitish plaques. Grade 2a lesions are superficial and noncircumferential and rarely progress to esophageal stenosis. Grade 2b lesions are deeper and more circumferential and are thus associated with an increased risk of stricture formation. Grade 3 esophageal injury is characterized by circumferential injury, which may be transmural with mucosal sloughing. Patients require intravenous nutrition, and strictures will often develop in a majority of cases.

■ Management

Gastric lavage and induced vomiting with emetics is contraindicated following a caustic ingestion because of potential reexposure of the esophageal mucosa to the caustic agent. Oral dilution or neutralizing agents are also contraindicated because they may also result in vomiting, with further esophageal injury. Nasogastric tubes should not be placed blindly because of the risk for esophageal perforation if there is severe esophageal ulceration. Corticosteroid administration is controversial and is usually confined to patients with symptoms involving the airway. The concomi-

Table 52.2 Grade of esophageal injury

Grade 1	Erythema, edema
Grade 2	Linear ulcerations, whitish plaques
2a	Superficial, noncircumferential
2b	Deeper, more circumferential
Grade 3	Transmural, circumferential, muscle exposed, tissue sloughing

tant administration of broad-spectrum antibiotics is required if corticosteroids are initiated, given the theoretical risk of aggravating or masking infection during full-thickness burns with potential visceral perforation. Separate meta-analyses have not shown a benefit to steroid administration in terms of long-term complications, such as stricture formation.

If no burns are present in the hypopharynx or esophagus, the patient is discharged and scheduled for an esophagram and reevaluation in 3 weeks. Should there be evidence of stricture at that time, dilation is begun. If first- or second-degree burns are discovered at esophagoscopy, the patient is hospitalized and treated with antibiotics. Pain and agitation may require analgesics and sedation. Clindamycin, 25 mg/kg/d in four doses every 6 hours is administered for 14 days. Antibiotics work by decreasing infection, pyogenic granulation tissue, and scar formation. Gastroesophageal reflux disease may exacerbate any esophageal injury. Aggressive antireflux therapy is initiated. When third-degree burns are present, the patient is hospitalized, and supportive therapy is initiated. Nasogastric tubes are sometimes placed as a stent during endoscopy (and never a priori) in patients with severe circumferential burns, to keep the esophagus open when the development of strictures is anticipated.

Long-Term Management

Barium esophagrams are performed to follow the progress of the developing stricture. Strictures may develop as early as 3 weeks following ingestion.

Esophageal perforation may also occur as a result of initial or subsequent dilations performed to alleviate esophageal strictures. Therefore, initial dilations should be performed as gently as possible using esophageal bougie dilators or balloons. Initially, this may be done on an outpatient basis under general anesthesia. Severe strictures and those resistant to dilation require gastrostomy and placement of a string for prograde dilation with Tucker retrograde esophageal dilators.

Dilations are most effective when performed early, before a hard, fibrous, mature cicatricial stenosis has formed. Two or three dilations may be undertaken the first week, one or two the second week, and one the third week. An attempt is made to double the length of time between subsequent dilations, once an adequate lumen has been attained. When attempts at dilation are repeatedly unsuccessful, esophageal replacement surgery, either by colonic interposition or gastric pull-up, is considered.

Esophageal carcinoma (both adenocarcinoma and squamous cell carcinoma) is a late but serious complication of severe caustic injury. The incidence following caustic ingestion ranges from 2 to 30%, depending on the series, with the carcinoma developing 1 to 3 decades after the ingestion. The incidence is 1,000 times the expected occurrence rate in patients of a similar age. This long-term risk of cancer increases in patients with caustic ingestion who require years of dilations. It should not be assumed that increasing dysphagia is necessarily due to recurrence of the stricture; cancer of the esophagus needs to be ruled out.

■ Suggested Reading

Betalli P, Falchetti D, Giuliani S, et al; Caustic Ingestion Italian Study Group. Caustic ingestion in children: is endoscopy always indicated? The results of an Italian multicenter observational study. Gastrointest Endosc 2008;68(3):434–439

Doğan Y, Erkan T, Cokuğraş FC, Kutlu T. Caustic gastroesophageal lesions in childhood: an analysis of 473 cases. Clin Pediatr (Phila) 2006;45(5):435–438

Eliçevik M, Alim A, Tekant GT, et al. Management of esophageal perforation secondary to caustic esophageal injury in children. Surg Today 2008;38(4):311–315

Fulton JA, Hoffman RS. Steroids in second degree caustic burns of the esophagus: a systematic pooled analysis of fifty years of human data: 1956-2006. Clin Toxicol (Phila) 2007;45(4):402–408

Gaudreault P, Parent M, McGuigan MA, Chicoine L, Lovejoy FH Jr. Predictability of esophageal injury from signs and symptoms: a study of caustic ingestion in 378 children. Pediatrics 1983; 71(5):767–770

Havanond C, Havanond P. Initial signs and symptoms as prognostic indicators of severe gastrointestinal tract injury due to corrosive ingestion. J Emerg Med 2007;33(4):349–353

Kay M, Wyllie R. Caustic ingestions in children. Curr Opin Pediatr 2009;21(5):651–654

Riffat F, Cheng A. Pediatric caustic ingestion: 50 consecutive cases and a review of the literature. Dis Esophagus 2009;22(1):89–94

Watson WA, Litovitz TL, Belson MG, et al. The Toxic Exposure Surveillance System (TESS): risk assessment and real-time toxicovigilance across United States poison centers. Toxicol Appl Pharmacol 2005;207(2, Suppl):604–610

53 The Contemporary Clinical Voice Laboratory: Its Role in the Diagnosis of Laryngeal Disorders

Introduction

Programs specializing in voice disorders frequently use a clinical voice laboratory. The contemporary clinical voice laboratory provides measures of vocal function that can assist in the diagnosis and management of voice disorders. Such a facility has measurement capabilities that are aimed at assessing the fundamental processes involved in the production of voice. Thus, to understand the design of the contemporary clinical voice laboratory, it is helpful to first briefly review the primary steps that are involved in the initiation of normal voice production.

Normal voice is produced by (1) vocal fold adduction and appropriate adjustment of vocal fold tension via laryngeal muscle activity; (2) exhalation to build up positive subglottal air pressure to blow the vocal folds into air flow–induced vibration; and (3) the release of air pulses from the glottis (volume velocity waveform) as the vocal folds vibrate, which generates the acoustic energy that is heard as the voice. The contemporary clinical voice laboratory is designed to assess all of these aspects of the voice production process, including laryngeal muscle activity, aerodynamic forces, vocal fold vibration, and the acoustic signal.

The Voice Team

The value of the contemporary clinical voice laboratory is enhanced if it is used as part of a team-based approach to the diagnosis and management of voice disorders. Laryngeal production of voice involves a variety of both physical (muscle activity, aerodynamics, etc.) and behavioral (cognition, emotional state, etc.) processes that can be additionally affected by environmental influences. Thus a multitude of factors, both individually and in combination, can cause or contribute to a voice disorder.

This acknowledgment of the complex, multidimensional nature of many voice disorders and their treatment has led increasingly to the realization that such disorders are most effectively managed by a multidisciplinary team. The primary members of the team are the otolaryngologist/laryngologist and the speech-language pathologist, who often takes the lead in performing and interpreting much of the vocal function testing. Team membership is sometimes supplemented by neurologists, radiologists, psychiatrists, internists, gastroenterologists, allergists, rheumatologists, pulmonologists, laryngeal physiologists, and speech and voice scientists, as needed. Team review of cases is enhanced by the presentation of clinical objective test results.

Objective Measures

The types of tests performed in the contemporary clinical voice laboratory are often referred to as objective voice measures. This terminology stems from a long-standing desire in the field to develop measures that would be less subjective and provide more reliable insights into vocal function than judgments that rely heavily on auditory perception—that is, the clinician's impression that the voice "sounds" better or worse following treatment. Although methods currently available in the contemporary voice laboratory can clearly enhance the clinician's ability to diagnose and manage voice disorders, limitations in each of the various approaches to vocal function testing necessitate caution in their use and interpretation. These limiting factors are discussed in the review of measurement approaches later in the chapter.

The types of vocal function test procedures that are commonly available in the contemporary clinical voice laboratory include electromyography (EMG), videostroboscopy, aerodynamic assessment, electroglottography (EGG), and acoustic assessment.

Primary Diagnostic Measures

Laryngeal Electromyography

EMG of the laryngeal muscles has been increasingly used to assist in the differential diagnosis of laryngeal neuromotor disorders, particularly in cases involving restriction of vocal fold adduction and abduction. (e.g., differentiating arytenoid fixation from neuromotor pathology). EMG is conducted in special cases and is not generally included in the battery of vocal function tests performed routinely on most patients in a clinical voice laboratory. Diagnostic laryngeal EMG usually involves the insertion of a needle or hooked-wire electrodes into intrinsic laryngeal muscles. Surface EMG has had limited application in attempts to evaluate overall levels of muscle activity and tension (e.g., vocal hyperfunction) in the laryngeal region of the neck, and as biofeedback to reduce vocal hyperfunction.

Videostroboscopy

The most useful voice laboratory tool from a diagnostic point of view is endoscopy with videostroboscopy. Modern videostroboscopic units use an automatically obtained estimate of the basic rate of vocal fold vibration (i.e., an estimate of fundamental frequency from a microphone or EGG signal) to set the flash rate of a xenon strobe light at a frequency that creates the optical illusion of slow-motion vocal fold vibration. The strobed images are recorded on videotape with a camera attached to the endoscope. In reality, each slow-motion vibratory cycle is an averaging across many cycles, so that true cycle-to-cycle details of vocal fold vibration are not captured.

It is not possible to obtain reliable stroboscopy for voices that are too severely disordered (aperiodic) to allow sufficiently consistent estimates of fundamental frequency for triggering the strobe. However, in such cases, the source of the dysphonia is usually obvious, and stroboscopy is not required for diagnosis.

Videostroboscopy may be performed using a rigid transoral or flexible transnasal endoscope. Video recording of endoscopic/stroboscopic images has the advantages of allowing for (1) repeated review of an examination, which is particularly valuable in cases where only a very brief view can be obtained (e.g., gagging, negative reaction of the patient to the procedure); and (2) direct comparison of multiple exams (e.g., pre- vs. posttreatment). Videostroboscopy provides the opportunity to evaluate critical parameters of vocal fold vibration during phonation that are not possible to assess with the constant halogen light sources that are typically used to perform laryngeal endoscopy. The evaluation of the videostroboscopic recording currently relies on subjective visual assessment by the examiner, so that in a strict sense, this test does not produce objective measures. Parameters that can be subjectively evaluated with the strobe light include glottal closure, amplitude of vocal fold vibration, mucosal wave activity, and symmetry of vocal fold vibratory phases (right vs. left). A disruption in any of these parameters is often further specified in terms of severity (e.g., mild, moderate, severe). Following is a brief description of the primary clinical diagnostic implications of each of these parameters.

Glottal Closure

A posterior opening (chink) of the cartilaginous glottis during phonation is a normal phenomenon. Clear extension of the posterior chink into the membranous portion of the glottis (i.e., anterior to the vocal processes of the arytenoids) is typically associated with vocal dysfunction (e.g., vocal hyperfunction). Any pathological/functional process that interferes with complete closure of the membranous glottis is likely to result in the generation of excess unmodulated (turbulent) glottal air flow and the perception of increased breathiness. During normal (chest register) phonation, the glottis is closed an average of 40 to 60% of each vibratory cycle. A significant increase or decrease in this glottal closed phase (sometimes referred to as open quotient or duty cycle) can be an indication of vocal dysfunction. Additional terms that are commonly used to describe abnormal patterns of glottal closure include the following:

1. *Anterior glottal chink* Lack of vocal fold contact in the anterior glottis with posterior closure
2. *Hourglass* Vocal fold contact in the midmembranous glottis with a lack of anterior and posterior closure, often seen with bilateral lesions, such as vocal nodules
3. *Irregular* Some ragged areas of vocal fold contact along the membranous glottis but a lack of complete closure
4. *Bowed* Lack of vocal fold contact in the midmembranous glottis, with anterior and posterior closure, usually associated with vocal fold atrophy
5. *Incomplete* Lack of glottal closure

Amplitude of Vocal Fold Vibration

Amplitude of vibration is judged separately for each vocal fold. It essentially refers to the maximum lateral excursion (relative to the midline of the glottis) displayed by each vocal fold during vibration. Some evaluation systems further specify the integrity of vibratory activity for subsegments of each vocal fold (e.g., division of vocal folds into anterior, middle, and posterior thirds).

Mucosal Wave Activity

The presence of a smooth, uninterrupted wavelike motion on the surface of a vocal fold during vibration is a sign that the upper layers of the vocal fold (i.e., the structures of the vocal fold cover, including the epithelium and the three layers of the lamina propria) are healthy. Like amplitude of vibration, mucosal wave activity is judged separately for each vocal fold, and often for subsegments (e.g., thirds) of each fold. Mucosal wave activity is highly correlated with amplitude of vocal fold vibration during normal phonation in the chest (modal) register (i.e., the larger the amplitude of vibration the larger the mucosal wave).

In the presence of vocal fold pathology, the normal covariance between vibration amplitude and mucosal wave activity may be maintained (i.e., both can display similar magnitudes of reductions/disruptions), or it can be disrupted, necessitating the option of evaluating each of these parameters separately. For example, postsurgical scarring of the vocal fold (i.e., fixation of the vocal fold cover to the underlying vocalis muscle) can significantly disrupt mucosal wave activity (e.g., the appearance of an adynamic segment of the vocal fold cover), while overall vibratory amplitude may continue to appear normal.

Symmetry of Vocal Fold Vibratory Phases

Under normal conditions, the right and left vocal folds display symmetry of vibratory motion (i.e., lateral and medial movements are in synchrony along the entire membranous glottis). A lack of symmetry in vibratory phase between the vocal folds is often associated with some degree of dysphonia or vocal dysfunction. Such asymmetry can be present with or without obvious accompanying vocal fold pathology. For example, asymmetry of vocal fold vibration in the absence of vocal fold lesions can be a confirmatory sign of functional dysphonia (secondary to vocal hyperfunction), sometimes referred to as musculoskeletal tension dysphonia.

Other Vocal Function

The remaining vocal function measures that are typically available in the contemporary clinical voice laboratory (i.e., acoustic, aerodynamic, EGG) are not currently at a stage of development that merits their being viewed as primary diagnostic tools. In a strict sense, these approaches are often referred to as objective voice measures because they produce data in hard numbers. They are implemented when possible as supplemental measures that are integrated into the clinical evaluation process. Such integration of measures enhances the quality of diagnosis and treatment by providing further insights into underlying vocal mechanisms. As such, objective measurement data are used to support and validate clinical impressions, diagnoses, and treatment recommendations, not in place of them.

The data provided by objective vocal function measures are useful for determining (1) the extent to which a patient's typical vocal function is within normal limits; (2) the potential for voice therapy to improve vocal function by measuring the effects of "trial therapy" on function; and (3) the extent to which vocal function has been altered by treatment, which, in addition to helping evaluate treatment efficacy and outcomes (i.e., there is increasing pressure to demonstrate efficacy in the growing managed care environment), can help inform decisions about whether additional treatment is required, when to dismiss patients from voice therapy, and which patients are "at risk" for recurrence of functionally related vocal pathology (e.g., vocal hyperfunction). The availability of pre- and postoperative objective measurement data can also enhance ongoing efforts to design and improve surgical procedures. In addition, because of their noninvasive nature, some objective vocal function measures can readily be used as biofeedback during voice therapy treatment.

The primary clinical impact of technical advances in objective vocal function measures over the past 10 years has been the increased availability of user-friendly, computer-based measurement systems for clinical use. The three most common objective measurement approaches are aerodynamic assessment, EGG, and acoustic assessment.

Aerodynamic Assessment

Clinically based aerodynamic assessment of vocal function primarily involves obtaining estimates of average glottal air flow rates (liters per second) and average subglottal air pressures (centimeters of water) via noninvasive oral measurements during a well-controlled utterance (i.e., strings of /pi/ syllables). Both measures are easy to obtain, even in young children. It has been shown that average glottal air flow rates can display a relatively high degree of variation across repeated recordings of normal speakers, which cannot be easily corrected for. There is circumstantial evidence that a likely source of this normal variation is a change in the extent to which the posterior glottis closes across repeated phonations (i.e., variation in posterior glottal chink size). Thus average air flow rate is most useful and reliable as an indicator of relatively large changes in vocal function (e.g., comparing vocal function before and after medialization for vocal fold paralysis).

Subglottal air pressure is highly correlated with the sound pressure level (SPL) of the voice. Thus the sensitivity and usefulness of subglottal pressure estimates can be greatly increased if simultaneous measures of vocal SPL are obtained. This is accomplished by using age- and gender-specific normative data as a basis for predicting what the appropriate subglottal pressure should be for a patient phonating at a particular SPL. In this way, it is possible to determine whether a patient is using excessive subglottal driving pressure to produce a given SPL output, even if the absolute pressure value is within normal limits. Such a scenario is often interpreted as evidence of vocal hyperfunction.

The commonly used method of estimating subglottal air pressure from the intraoral air pressure during bilabial stop consonant production (i.e., during /pi/ syllable strings) assumes that laryngeal conditions (e.g., muscle tension) do not vary significantly across the test utterance. Although this approach has been validated via tracheal puncture in healthy volunteers there is concern that absolute pressure value estimates need to be viewed cautiously when obtained from patients in whom laryngeal conditions can vary significantly across the test utterance (e.g., spasmodic dysphonia). However, in such cases, the finding of abnormally high pressures and the monitoring of the relative change in pressure with treatment are still useful and valid.

Electroglottography

EGG is a noninvasive method for evaluating aspects of vocal fold contact during phonation. This is accomplished through the use of surface electrodes to monitor changes in the electrical impedance of the neck. Of the objective measures, EGG is the least robust and useful. It can be difficult to obtain a clear, interpretable EGG signal for certain types of neck morphologies (e.g., excessive fatty tissue) and in cases where the voice disorder causes too much disruption in the pattern of vocal fold contact during phonation. It is possible to obtain an adduction quotient (duty cycle) measure from the EGG signal that is most useful as an indicator of the extent to which the voice is abnormally "pressed" (overadduction/hyperfunction) or "breathy" (underadduction) during attempts to stimulate a better voice (i.e., trial voice therapy). The EGG signal is immune to airborne noise, and thus it can be used in noisy environments to obtain estimates of fundamental frequency (it is used in some videostroboscopy systems as a triggering signal).

EGG results are most reliably interpreted if they can be related to videostroboscopic assessment. This is primarily because other structures, in addition to the vocal folds, can make contact at the glottal level. For example, mucous stranding across the glottis

can influence the EGG signal, and severe ventricular compression can mask glottal incompetence.

Acoustic Assessment

Current clinical methods for acoustic analysis are designed primarily to evaluate physical parameters that are related to the salient perceptual characteristics of the voice—namely, vocal pitch, loudness, and quality. The general goal of acoustic analysis has high face validity because listeners hear the acoustic signal, and it is the basis for perceptual judgments. Several user-friendly acoustic analysis systems currently on the market can provide clinical estimates of (1) average fundamental frequency (hertz [Hz]) and sound pressure level (decibel [dB]) during running speech (standard reading passage) to reflect habitual pitch and loudness; (2) perturbation (percentage of jitter and shimmer) and harmonics-to-noise ratio (dB) from sustained vowels to characterize voice quality; and (3) maximum phonation time (seconds), maximum frequency range (Hz), and maximum intensity range (dB) to evaluate maximum vocal capabilities.

Most of the methods available for clinical evaluation of vocal pitch and quality rely on accurate pitch period detection (i.e., tracking of fundamental frequency), which can be unreliable when voices become too dysphonic. The danger is that some automated clinical systems still provide measures, even when the underlying pitch period detection is faulty. It has recently been recommended that these types of commonly used time-based analyses be applied only to signals that meet certain criteria, thus reducing the potential for obtaining erroneous results.

Accurate SPL measures can provide a highly reliable means of tracking vocal function. Accurate measurement of SPL requires simply that the microphone be kept a constant distance from the patient's lips and that it be calibrated.

There is growing evidence that spectrally based measures may be able to overcome some of the difficulties that negatively influence more traditional time-based measures of voice quality. For example, it is more likely that spectral measures can be acquired from running speech, whereas time-based measures are essentially restricted to sustained vowels, which are not always representative of a patient's typical speaking voice. In addition, some spectral measures appear to have better potential for providing insights into underlying vocal mechanisms (e.g., degree of glottal closure or vocal fold adduction) than more traditional time-based measures.

■ Suggested Reading

Bacon RJ, Orlikoff RF. Clinical Measurement of Speech and Voice. Boston, MA: Little, Brown and Company; 1987:53–144

Baken RJ. Electroglottography. J Voice 1992;6:98–110

Carding PN, Wilson JA, MacKenzie K, Deary IJ. Measuring voice outcomes: state of the science review. J Laryngol Otol 2009; 123(8):823–829

Chang JI, Bevans SE, Schwartz SR. Otolaryngology clinic of North America: evidence-based practice: management of hoarseness/dysphonia. Otolaryngol Clin North Am 2012;45(5):1109–1126

Hillman RE, Holmberg EB, Perkell JS, Walsh M, Vaughan C. Objective assessment of vocal hyperfunction: an experimental framework and initial results. J Speech Hear Res 1989;32(2):373–392

Hillman RE, Holmberg EB, Perkell JS, Walsh M, Vaughan C. Phonatory function associated with hyperfunctionally related vocal fold lesions. J Voice 1990;4(1):52–63

Hillman RE, Montgomery WW, Zeitels SM. Appropriate use of objective measures of vocal function in the multidisciplinary management of voice disorders. Curr Opin Otolaryngol Head Neck Surg 1997;5:172–175

Hirano M, Bless D. Videostroboscopic Examination of the Larynx. San Diego, CA: Singular Publishing Group; 1993

Holmberg EB, Hillman RE, Perkell JS, Gress C. Relationships between intra-speaker variation in aerodynamic measures of voice production and variation in SPL across repeated recordings. J Speech Hear Res 1994;37(3):484–495

Löfqvist A, Carlborg B, Kitzing P. Initial validation of an indirect measure of subglottal pressure during vowels. J Acoust Soc Am 1982;72(2):633–635

Mehta DD, Hillman RE. Current role of stroboscopy in laryngeal imaging. Curr Opin Otolaryngol Head Neck Surg 2012;20(6): 429–436

Qi Y, Hillman RE. Temporal and spectral estimations of harmonics-to-noise ratio in human voice signals. J Acoust Soc Am 1997; 102(1):537–543

Redenbaugh MA, Reich AR. Surface EMG and related measures in normal and vocally hyperfunctional speakers. J Speech Hear Disord 1989;54(1):68–73

Rickert SM, Childs LF, Carey BT, Murry T, Sulica L. Laryngeal electromyography for prognosis of vocal fold palsy: a meta-analysis. Laryngoscope 2012;122(1):158–161

Smitheran JR, Hixon TJ. A clinical method for estimating laryngeal airway resistance during vowel production. J Speech Hear Disord 1981;46(2):138–146

Titze I. Workshop on Acoustic Voice Analysis. Denver, CO: National Center for Voice and Speech; 1995

54 Laryngeal Neurological Dysfunction

Introduction

Neurological dysfunction manifests itself in the larynx as either hyperfunction (overactivity, spasm, tremor, or tics) or hypofunction (weakness, paralysis, bradykinesia). The evaluation of neurological disorders of the larynx begins with a good history of the onset of the disorder; the vocal characteristics (harshness, pitch breaks, decreased loudness, tremor); the presence of dyspnea or stridor; and the presence of dysphagia (liquids, solids). Also extremely important in assessing neurological disorders of the larynx are other areas of bodily dysfunction, weakness, tremor, and sensory deficit; predisposing factors; a review of gastrointestinal, pulmonary, and endocrine systems; and a medication history.

Diagnostic Techniques

Flexible Fiberoptic Laryngoscopy and Stroboscopy

The flexible endoscope is an essential part of the evaluation of neurological disorders of the larynx. A mirror examination will not allow for evaluation of normal speaking tasks, which are often impaired. Allowing the patient to speak with a flexible laryngoscope in place will display tremor, spasms, myoclonic jerks, weakness, or paralysis. The use of the video stroboscope will allow for examination and video documentation. The video can then be played at a slow speed to assess detail of the motion. The stroboscope allows for very accurate evaluation of the mucosal wave along the vocal fold. The stroboscope also allows for evaluation of vocal fold motion, tremor, subtle weakness, or loss of coordination.

Vocal Dynamics Laboratory

Acoustic signal analysis, airflow, duration of phonation, and pitch control can all be tested and yield important diagnostic information.

Laryngeal Electromyography

The electrical activity of the laryngeal muscles may be studied with needle or hooked-wire electrodes to help diagnose neurological abnormalities of the larynx. The most common use in the larynx is to study the immobile vocal cord. The presence of fibrillation potentials or positive waves suggests a denervating process, whereas normal electrical activity suggests mechanical fixation. Synkinesis (a mixed abductor and adductor signal) may produce an immobile vocal fold. Tremors can more easily be defined with analysis of electromyography (EMG). Distinctions between neuropathy, anterior horn cell disease, brainstem lesions, myopathy, and neuromuscular transmission disorders are more easily made with EMG.

Evaluation and Treatment

Site of Neurological Lesion and Laryngeal Deficit

Neurological lesions occur in several sites. The type of impairment or disorder varies with the site.

Cortical Lesions

Cortical lesions may result from strokes, tumors, or trauma. They typically impair memory and the planning and execution of motor activity. Because of diffuse representation, cortical damage usually does not produce flaccid or spastic paralysis. The patients usually present with aphonia or apraxia of speech, and may cause inappropriate vocal fold adduction with inspiration, causing stridor.

Extrapyramidal System Lesions

Extrapyramidal system lesions from tumors, trauma, Parkinson disease, essential tremor, or dystonia produce motor control abnormalities (excessive muscle tension, tremor, and involuntary spasmodic muscle contractions) causing vocal stridor, voice arrests, pitch breaks, and pitch instability.

Cerebellar Lesions

Cerebellar lesions impair the coordination of motor activity and may produce vocal strain and dysarthria. The patients may also have intention tremors, disdiadochokinesia, ataxia, and nystagmus.

Brainstem Lesions

Brainstem lesions cause flaccid paralysis of muscles. Because of the close proximity of motor nuclei in the brainstem, tumors or injury cause severe dysfunction, with weakness or paralysis of the larynx, pharynx, and/or tongue, with associated sensory deficits.

Peripheral Nerve Lesions

Peripheral nerve lesions may result in paralysis or paresis of the vocal folds. The glottic configuration and vocal fold position (intermediate, paramedian, cadaveric) are not reliable indicators of the site of the lesion. The cricothyroid muscle does not appreciably influence the position of the vocal fold.

Neuromuscular Junction Disorders

Neuromuscular junction disorders (myasthenia gravis, botulism, and Eaton-Lambert syndrome) cause depletion of acetylcholine, leading to easy fatigability and weakness of the oropharyngeal and laryngeal musculature.

Diffuse Central Nervous System (CNS) Lesions

Diffuse CNS lesions may produce a variable spectrum of signs and symptoms, depending on the location and extent of the lesions. Multiple sclerosis (MS) and amyotrophic lateral sclerosis (ALS) are examples of diffuse disorders.

Hypofunctional Disorders

Myopathic Disorders

Primary muscle diseases may result in weakness of the oral cavity, pharynx, and larynx, which puts the patient at risk for aspiration and dyspnea with stridor. Polymyositis is an acquired myopathy characterized by acute and subacute weakness evolving in weeks or months. There is usually histological evidence of muscle inflammation. Dermatomyositis is characterized by a rash in addition to proximal limb weakness. Many patients with dermatomyositis have oropharyngeal weakness with severe dysphagia, leading to aspiration and respiratory complications. The muscular dystrophies are characterized by inherited, progressive weakness with variable age of onset, distribution, and disability. In the adult-onset cases, there is evidence of myotonia with facial, oropharyngeal, and limb weakness. Severe oropharyngeal and laryngeal weakness occurs late in the disease, when aspiration is common.

Neuromuscular Junction Disease

Myasthenia gravis is perhaps the most common disease of the neuromuscular junction. It occurs in fewer than 10 per 100,000 of the population. It causes a depletion of acetylcholine, leading to easy fatigability. Ocular involvement is most common, causing ptosis and diplopia. About 30% of myasthenia gravis patients have dysphagia, dysarthria, hypernasality, and dysphonia. Some of the patients develop progressive weakness of the posterior cricoarytenoid muscle, causing increasing dyspnea and stridor. Severe oropharyngeal and laryngeal weakness as well as ineffective cough predispose the patient to aspiration and possible myasthenic crisis, requiring mechanical ventilation.

Examination with the flexible laryngoscope may show velopharyngeal insufficiency and incomplete adduction or abduction of the vocal cords. With continued activity, the patient's muscle will fatigue and the symptoms will exacerbate. This diminution of activity can be documented with EMG and can be reversed with edrophonium (Tensilon). Eighty percent of myasthenia patients have circulating antibody to acetylcholine, which confirms the diagnosis. Treatment is generally with the administration of anticholinesterase drugs, such as pyridostigmine (Mestinon, Valeant Pharmaceuticals International, Aliso Viejo, CA). Some patients have an associated thymoma and require thymectomy as part of their overall management.

Parkinson Disease

This extrapyramidal syndrome is caused by cell death in the substantia nigra. It may be idiopathic or secondary (due to drugs, strokes, or encephalitis). Patients usually present with a resting tremor, muscle rigidity, bradykinesia, and/or loss of postural reflexes. They characteristically have a flat facial expression and abnormal posture, as well as a "pill-rolling" tremor of the hands. Speech is frequently impaired from the generalized bradykinesia, resulting in sluggish articulation, decreased loudness, and a monotone voice. There is also an associated vocal tremor. A less common variant of Parkinson disease produces rigidity of the larynx, causing a strained voice with breaks similar to those of spasmodic dysphonia. Some patients may present with intermittent stridor, due to a lack of coordination between the laryngeal and respiratory muscles. Swallowing is usually not markedly impaired, but patients often drool because voluntary swallowing does not occur.

There are several Parkinson plus syndromes, including multisystem atrophy (MSA or Shy-Drager syndrome) and progressive supranuclear palsy (PSP). In patients with MSA there is an idiopathic failure of the autonomic nervous system characterized by orthostatic hypotension, impotence, sphincter dysfunction, and anhydrosis. Many of these patients have failure of vocal cord abduction on inspiration, causing stridor. These patients often need tracheostomy. There is often a decreased sensation in the larynx, making aspiration more probable. In PSP patients, characteristically there is progressive Parkinsonism and ocular motility disturbance. The speech difficulties include a spastic, hypernasal, monotonous, low-pitch dysarthria.

Current treatment for Parkinson disease voice disorders consists of a combination of neuropharmacological dopamine agonist therapy and behavioral speech therapy. Although neurosurgical procedures such as deep brain stimulation, ablative surgeries, and fetal cell implantation have improved limb motor function, the voice results have been inconsistent.

Nuclear Damage

Lower motor neuron damage of the tenth nerve nucleus will produce a flaccid paralysis and hypoadduction. This damage can occur from brainstem infarction secondary to vascular occlusion of the posterior inferior cerebellar artery. Patients usually present with dysphagia, dysphonia, and, often, dysarthria. In addition, they may have an ipsilateral Horner syndrome, ipsilateral face, and contralateral body pain and temperature impairment (Wallenberg lateral postmedullary syndrome). Other causes of nuclear lesions include Arnold-Chiari malformations, syringobulbia, tumors, and trauma.

Mixed Disorders

Mixed disorders have a variety of cerebellar, upper (spastic), and lower (flaccid) motor neuron signs and symptoms. ALS is a progressive degenerative disorder, displaying upper and lower motor neuron signs. Currently, ALS is thought to be an autoimmune disorder. The incidence is 0.4 to 1.8 per 100,000, with an average age of onset of 58 years. The median survival is 17 months from the time of onset of symptoms. The initial symptoms are muscle weakness, cramps, and fasciculations. The majority of ALS patients have slurred speech patterns, with ~ 15% with hoarseness and dysphagia. The dysphonia of ALS is a mixed flaccid-spastic dysarthria with a harsh, strained voice with episodes of breathiness and reduced loudness and a "wet hoarseness" due to pooled secretions. Some patients exhibit a rapid tremor or "flutter" in their voice. Many begin to have poor vocal cord motion and develop stridor, requiring tracheostomy.

Multiple Sclerosis (MS)

MS is a disease of demyelination of the brainstem, brain, and spinal cord. The symptoms vary and wax and wane. Many MS patients have "scanning speech," in which each syllable is produced hesitantly with a pause after each syllable. There is also a paroxysmal dysarthria, at times making speech unintelligible. The voice may be harsh, with poor loudness control. These symptoms vary considerably. Speech therapy may help several MS patients.

Hyperfunctional Disorders

Essential Tremor

Essential tremor is a common neurological disorder of middle to late adulthood. It produces shaking of the hands, head titubation, and a tremulous voice (in up to 20% of cases). The vocal tremulousness is related to shaking of the larynx, pharynx, soft palate, and cervical strap muscles. Tremors are described according to frequency, regularity, amplitude, body distribution, and exacerbating factors. Essential tremor has a prevalence of 4 to 60 per 1,000 people. A hereditary family history is reported in ~ 50% of affected patients. Although the etiology is unknown, recent positron-emission tomography shows abnormalities in the olivocerebellar tracts.

The laryngeal examination in these patients shows abnormal movements at rest and on phonation. Vertical oscillations of the larynx and strap muscles may also be seen. EMG studies of the thyroarytenoid and strap muscles usually show a regular tremor at 4 to 8 Hz. The treatment has been with systemic pharmacotherapy with propranolol, pyrimidone, acetazolamide, alprazolam, and phenobarbital. Systemic therapy is usually more efficacious for head and hand tremor and less effective for vocal tremor. Recently, injections of botulinum toxin have proven effective in limiting the amount of tremor in these patients.

Myoclonus

This condition has sudden, brief, shocklike involuntary movements caused by muscular contractions (positive myoclonus) or inhibition of motion (negative myoclonus or asterixis), which is due to a central nervous system (CNS) abnormality. Brachial myoclonus consists of myoclonic symptoms affecting cranial structures. The most focal forms of myoclonus involve the palate only. These forms are usually bilateral and symmetric, from 1.5 to 3 Hz, causing clicking of the ears. More extensive forms involve the pharynx and larynx as well. The jerky motion in these patients produces a broken speech pattern simulating a slow tremor. Examination of the larynx shows a rhythmical adduction and abduction of the vocal cords at the same frequency as the palate and pharynx. The myoclonic jerks may also be seen in the eyes, face, neck, shoulders, and/or diaphragm.

Spasmodic Dysphonia (Laryngeal Dystonia)

Spasmodic dysphonia is a neurological disorder of central motor processing, characterized by action-induced spasms of the vocal cords. The spasms are poorly controlled by the patient, and the symptoms are exacerbated by stress. Patients with this disorder are usually middle-aged at disease onset.

The vocal characteristics of patients with the adductor form of spasmodic dysphonia have been described as having a staccato, jerky, squeezed, labored, hoarse, or groaning voice, with voice arrests (from hyperadduction of the true and false cords), intermittent phonation, segmented vowels, difficulty with loudness control, deviated pitch, vocal tension, intermittent aphonia, strangled voice, breathiness, glottal fry, glottal spasms, syllable repetitions, vowel prolongations, whispered speech, choked vocal attacks, and hard glottal initiation. Some of these parameters are easily documented with a sound spectrogram of the speech pattern. Telephone calls and stress exacerbate the disorder and make the speech pattern more unintelligible. Tremor activity in patients with spasmodic dysphonia has been described by several authors.

A less common variety of spasmodic dysphonia produces abductor spasms of the vocal folds. Patients exhibit a breathy, effortful voice quality with abrupt termination of voicing, resulting in aphonic whispered segments of speech. The voice is reduced in loudness, and vocal tremor is frequently observed. The dysphonia may begin as nonspecific hoarseness or breathiness, and over a period of days to weeks begins to show signs of intermittent breathy breaks.

Other patients may have a mixed abductor-adductor dysphonia with an admixture of breathy breaks and tight, harsh sounds. Some authors have proposed that both conditions exist in all patients, and the symptoms depend on whether there is more adductor or abductor activity. There is also a small group of patients who have adductor spasms on inspiration, causing paradoxical vocal fold motion and stridor. These patients are not hypoxic, but they produce moderate to severe inspiratory stridor. This symptom disappears as soon as patients go to sleep, and reappears a short while after they awaken. These patients may also have discoordination of the respiratory muscles on breathing, with paradoxical diaphragmatic movements, as well as chest wall abnormalities.

During the evaluation, patients should undergo vocal tasks to observe for tremor and hyperadduction. This is often completely missed on indirect mirror laryngoscopy. The motion disorder is better studied with fiberoptic laryngoscopy. The hyperadduction may just produce a slightly open posterior commissure (laryngeal isometric), cause closure of the false vocal cords, cause a narrowing of the anteroposterior dimension of the glottis due to the tipping of the arytenoids anteriorly, or cause complete apposition of the arytenoids against the petiole of the epiglottis. The laryngostroboscope may be useful in defining tremor and in better demonstrating the hyperadduction.

In abductor patients, the laryngostroboscopic examination reveals a synchronous and untimely abduction of the true vocal folds, exposing an extremely wide glottic chink. These spasms are triggered by consonant sounds, particularly when they are in the initial position in words. Patients are usually worse under stress or on the telephone. They often have a normal laugh, normal yawn, normal humming, and, occasionally, normal singing.

Laryngeal dystonia may present focally or in association with other dystonic movements. Examples of other focal dystonia that may occur in these patients include blepharospasm (forced, involuntary eye closure); oromandibular dystonia (face, jaw, or tongue); torticollis (neck); and writer's cramp (action-induced dystonic contraction of hand muscles). Family history is significant, with nearly 20% of the primary laryngeal dystonias having a family history of dystonia. Intensive molecular genetic studies have established linkage of the same region of chromosome 9 (9q32–34) to idiopathic torsion dystonia in a large non-Jewish family with high penetrance (0.75) and in 12 Ashkenazi Jewish families with low penetrance (0.3).

In the past, therapy for spasmodic dysphonia has consisted of psychotherapy, speech therapy, and biofeedback. These approaches have been generally unsuccessful in alleviating the symptoms. Recurrent laryngeal nerve section had been the best treatment. However, it does not have universal long-term success, and patients have continued vocal cord paralysis. This failure rate may be related to hyperfunction of the opposing hyperfunctional dystonic muscle, which usually exaggerates the dystonic symptoms, or there may be some evidence for tonic reinnervation of the recurrent laryngeal nerve stump by local fibers of surrounding muscles. Systemic pharmacotherapy provides little relief of symptoms.

Improvement in symptoms of spasmodic dysphonia with local injections of Botox (Allergan, Irvine, CA) has been dramatic. Botulinum toxin is produced by the bacteria *Clostridium botulinum,* which produces seven immunologically distinct toxins that are potent neuroparalytic agents. Botulinum toxin exerts its effect at the neuromuscular junction by inhibiting the release of acetylcholine, causing a flaccid paralysis. The degree of clinical improvement correlates with weakness produced by the blockade of neuromuscular transmission. Clinically, there is typically a delay of 24 to 72 hours between administration of toxin and onset of clinical effect. It is possible that this delay is secondary to the time necessary for botulinum toxin's enzymatic disruption of the synaptosomic release process.

Toxin is injected through a monopolar hollow Teflon-coated injection EMG needle connected to an EMG recorder. The purpose of the EMG is to identify actively contracting muscle sites. The adductor injections are given percutaneously, through the cricothyroid membrane into the thyroarytenoid muscle. Either unilateral or bilateral injections are given. Some authors have used an indirect laryngoscopic approach to inject the vocal folds with toxin. The abductor spasmodic dysphonia patients may be treated with botulinum toxin injections of the posterior cricoarytenoid muscles.

Botox injections have several advantages over surgical therapy in the management of intractable disease. The patient is awake, and there is no risk of anesthesia. Graded degrees of weakening can be achieved by varying the dose injected. Most adverse effects are transient and are due to an extension of the pharmacology of the toxin. If the patient has a strong response to therapy and too much weakness occurs, strength gradually returns. Follow-up therapy is carefully individualized for each patient.

The disadvantages of Botox injections for the treatment of spasmodic dysphonia include the need for repeat injections, the unpredictable relationship between dose and response, and potential short-term dysphagia and breathiness. Selective adductor denervation-reinnervation (SLAD-R) is a surgical strategy first described by Berke et al in 1999. This technique involves selectively denervating the adductor branches of the recurrent laryngeal nerve and reinnervating the distal stump with a branch of the ansa cervicalis. In a recent comparative study, SLAD-R outcomes were found to be greater than or equal to standard results for Botox injections as measured by patients' Vocal Handicap Index-10 scores. This same study reported that objective voice ratings indicated similar levels of breathiness and overall voice quality among the surgical and Botox injection cohorts.

■ Suggested Reading

Armin BB, Head C, Berke GS, Chhetri DK. Useful landmarks in arytenoid adduction and laryngeal reinnervation surgery. Laryngoscope 2006;116(10):1755–1759

Benninger MS, Gardner G, Grywalski C. Outcomes of botulinum toxin treatment for patients with spasmodic dysphonia. Arch Otolaryngol Head Neck Surg 2001;127(9):1083–1085

Birkent H, Maronian N, Waugh P, Merati AL, Perkel D, Hillel AD. Dosage changes in patients with long-term botulinum toxin use for laryngeal dystonia. Otolaryngol Head Neck Surg 2009;140(1): 43–47

Blair RL, Berry H, Briant TD. Laryngeal electromyography: techniques and application. Otolaryngol Clin North Am 1978; 11(2):325–346

Blitzer A. Spasmodic dysphonia and botulinum toxin: experience from the largest treatment series. Eur J Neurol 2010;17(Suppl 1): 28–30

Blitzer A, Crumley RL, Dailey SH, et al. Recommendations of the Neurolaryngology Study Group on laryngeal electromyography. Otolaryngol Head Neck Surg 2009;140(6):782–793

Chhetri DK, Berke GS. Treatment of adductor spasmodic dysphonia with selective laryngeal adductor denervation and reinnervation surgery. Otolaryngol Clin North Am 2006;39(1):101–109 Review

Chhetri DK, Mendelsohn AH, Blumin JH, Berke GS. Long-term follow-up results of selective laryngeal adductor denervation-reinnervation surgery for adductor spasmodic dysphonia. Laryngoscope 2006;116(4):635–642

Colosimo C, Suppa A, Fabbrini G, Bologna M, Berardelli A. Craniocervical dystonia: clinical and pathophysiological features. Eur J Neurol 2010;17(Suppl 1):15–21

Colosimo C, Tiple D, Berardelli A. Efficacy and safety of long-term botulinum toxin treatment in craniocervical dystonia: a systematic review. Neurotox Res 2012;22(4):265–273

Eskander A, Fung K, McBride S, Hogikyan N. Current practices in the management of adductor spasmodic dysphonia. J Otolaryngol Head Neck Surg 2010;39(5):622–630

Hallett M, Albanese A, Dressler D, et al. Evidence-based review and assessment of botulinum neurotoxin for the treatment of movement disorders. Toxicon 2013;67:94–114

Hillel AD. The study of laryngeal muscle activity in normal human subjects and in patients with laryngeal dystonia using multiple fine-wire electromyography. Laryngoscope 2001;111(4 Pt 2, Suppl 97):1–47

Hillel AD, Maronian NC, Waugh PF, Robinson L, Klotz DA. Treatment of the interarytenoid muscle with botulinum toxin for laryngeal dystonia. Ann Otol Rhinol Laryngol 2004;113(5):341–348

Klotz DA, Maronian NC, Waugh PF, Shahinfar A, Robinson L, Hillel AD. Findings of multiple muscle involvement in a study of 214 patients with laryngeal dystonia using fine-wire electromyography. Ann Otol Rhinol Laryngol 2004;113(8):602–612

Ludlow CL. Spasmodic dysphonia: a laryngeal control disorder specific to speech. J Neurosci 2011;31(3):793–797

Ludlow CL, Adler CH, Berke GS, et al. Research priorities in spasmodic dysphonia. Otolaryngol Head Neck Surg 2008;139(4):495–505

Mao VH, Abaza M, Spiegel JR, et al. Laryngeal myasthenia gravis: report of 40 cases. J Voice 2001;15(1):122–130

Maronian NC, Waugh PF, Robinson L, Hillel AD. Tremor laryngeal dystonia: treatment of the lateral cricoarytenoid muscle. Ann Otol Rhinol Laryngol 2004;113(5):349–355

Mehta DD, Hillman RE. Current role of stroboscopy in laryngeal imaging. Curr Opin Otolaryngol Head Neck Surg 2012;20(6):429–436

Mendelsohn AH, Berke GS. Surgery or botulinum toxin for adductor spasmodic dysphonia: a comparative study. Ann Otol Rhinol Laryngol 2012;121(4):231–238

Simpson DM, Blitzer A, Brashear A, et al; Therapeutics and Technology Assessment Subcommittee of the American Academy of Neurology. Assessment: Botulinum neurotoxin for the treatment of movement disorders (an evidence-based review): report of the Therapeutics and Technology Assessment Subcommittee of the American Academy of Neurology. Neurology 2008;70(19):1699–1706

Sulica L, Louis ED. Clinical characteristics of essential voice tremor: a study of 34 cases. Laryngoscope 2010;120(3):516–528

Woodson G. Management of neurologic disorders of the larynx. Ann Otol Rhinol Laryngol 2008;117(5):317–326 Review

55 Evaluation and Management of Unilateral Vocal Fold Paralysis

■ Introduction

Phonation is dependent on highly coordinated activity of the laryngeal muscles, which requires both anatomical and neurophysiological integrity. An immobile vocal fold may be a manifestation of several different disease entities. As such, neurological disorders of central and peripheral etiology, muscular disorders, and anatomical abnormalities, such as ankylosis, must all be considered and systematically evaluated. It is important to accurately identify the etiology and the residual pathophysiology so that treatment can be planned rationally. An understanding of neurolaryngology and a systematic, logical approach to evaluation and treatment of vocal fold paresis will improve treatment outcome. This section reviews the following:

1. The relevant neuroanatomy and neurophysiology of the larynx
2. The causes and pathophysiology of vocal cord paralysis
3. A variety of state-of-the-art diagnostic modalities that are currently used to aid in diagnosis and treatment planning
4. The surgical treatment modalities for unilateral paralysis, their relative advantages and disadvantages, and treatment selection

■ Anatomy

The evaluation and management of laryngeal paralysis require a thorough knowledge of the laryngeal biomechanics, laryngeal neuroanatomy, and physiology of vocal fold movement. Vocal fold movement is controlled by groups of laryngeal musculature that exert different vectors of forces on the arytenoid cartilage. These muscles consist of a group of adductors—the thyroarytenoid, lateral cricoarytenoid, and interarytenoid, and the sole abductor—the posterior cricoarytenoid. The cricothyroid muscle increases the tension of the vocal cords, though it may function as an abductor during stressed respiration. All of the muscles are paired and receive innervation separately from each side, except the interarytenoid muscle, which is a single muscle that receives bilateral innervation.

The vagal nervous system controls the functions of the larynx by providing motor innervation to the laryngeal musculature and carrying sensory fibers from the larynx. Laryngeal motor fibers arising from the cerebral cortex and midbrain pass caudally to the lower pontine levels as part of the pyramidal tracts, enter the medulla, and terminate in various motor nuclei within the nucleus ambiguus. Before entering the medulla, some of these fibers decussate, giving bilateral innervation to the nucleus ambiguus.

As its name implies, the nucleus ambiguus is a motor nucleus without clearly defined boundaries. It contains motor neurons to the larynx, upper cervical esophagus, and pharynx. Nerve fibers arising from the nucleus ambiguus form the peripheral vagus trunk and exit the skull through the jugular foramen. In addition to containing motor fibers to the laryngeal, pharyngeal, and upper esophageal musculature, the vagus nerve carries sensory (visceral afferent) fibers from these sites. These sensory fibers terminate in the nucleus solitarius in the brainstem. Immediately below the jugular foramen, the vagus nerve swells to form the nodose ganglion. The superior laryngeal nerve arises just inferior to the nodose ganglion. It divides into an external branch, which innervates the cricothyroid muscle, and an internal branch that carries sensory fibers from the supraglottic larynx. The cell bodies for these sensory fibers are located in the nodose ganglion. The vagus nerve continues its course in the neck along the carotid arteries and terminates in the chest as recurrent laryngeal nerves (RLNs). On the right, the RLN courses anterior to the subclavian artery, loops around it, and courses cephalad in the tracheoesophageal groove to enter the larynx. On the left, the RLN courses anterior to the aorta, loops around it, and courses cephalad in the tracheoesophageal groove to enter the larynx. The RLN divides into abductor and adductor branches to innervate these respective groups of muscles.

■ Etiology

Because laryngeal paralysis is a symptom, not a disease, a diligent search for the etiology of the paralysis is essential. The causes of laryngeal paralysis are listed in **Table 55.1**. Unilateral vocal fold paralysis typically results from injury to the vagus nerve, its branches, or its lower motor neurons. However, upper motor neuron lesions may also manifest as vocal fold paresis or paralysis and should be considered in the differential diagnosis. Paralysis of the peripheral tenth cranial nerve may result from a variety of etiologies. Iatrogenic injury to the tenth nerve and its branches remains one of the most common causes of vocal cord paralysis. Neoplasms along the long course of the tenth nerve may affect its function by compression or direct invasion.

Cancers of the thyroid, esophagus, and lung, and metastatic carcinomas to the neck and base of the skull are common neoplasms that cause vocal cord paralysis. Therefore, they should be ruled out prior to considering symptomatic treatment. Rarely, primary tumors affecting the tenth nerve, such as vagal schwannomas and glomus vagale tumors, may cause flaccid paralysis. Peripheral neuropathy due to chemotherapeutic agents (vincristine), diabetes, renal failure, and dialysis may affect tenth nerve function. Viral inflammation (e.g., postpolio syndrome, Guillain-Barré syndrome) can also affect tenth nerve function. Cardiovascular diseases may cause paralysis of the left vocal cord by compression or stretch injury. Cardiomegaly, aortic aneurysm, mitral stenosis, and cardiac surgery are some specific causes.

Inflammatory etiologies include rheumatoid arthritis, endotracheal intubation, chronic nasogastric tube, and gastroesophageal reflux. Cricoarytenoid arthritis due to rheumatoid arthritis manifests during the inflammatory period as an erythematous, immobile joint. Later, the presence of an affected immobile joint can best be confirmed by diagnostic laryngoscopy and palpation of the joint. Posterior glottic stenosis or web should be suspected in patients with a recent history of prolonged intubation and head injury. In patients with prolonged nasogastric tube use, erosion of the posterior cricoid lamina by the nasogastric tube has been described, resulting in injury to the posterior cricoarytenoid muscle along the posterior cricoid plate.

Laryngeal trauma may result in fracture of the thyroid lamina or cricoid ring, dislocation of the arytenoid cartilage, or blunt injury to the RLN, all of which can result in paralysis of the vocal folds. Ary-

Table 55.1 Causes of vocal cord paralysis

| Surgery |
| Neoplastic processes |
| Bronchogenic/lung cancer |
| Thyroid cancer |
| Laryngeal cancer |
| Cancer of the upper esophagus |
| Mediastinal lymphoma |
| Paragangliomas |
| Iatrogenic |
| Thyroidectomy |
| Cardiothoracic surgery |
| Skull base surgery |
| Neck and pharyngoesophageal surgery |
| Cervical spine surgery |
| Laryngeal and penetrating neck trauma |
| Neurological diseases |
| Parkinson disease |
| Multiple sclerosis |
| Myasthenia gravis |
| Cerebrovascular accident |
| Inflammatory |
| Intubation |
| Rheumatoid arthritis |
| Gastroesophageal reflux |
| Chronic nasogastric tube |
| Idiopathic |

tenoid dislocation can also result from endotracheal intubation. The diagnosis of arytenoid dislocation is made by a combination of careful indirect endoscopic examination, computed tomographic (CT) scan of the larynx, and direct laryngoscopy with palpation.

Various central nervous system disorders may affect vocal fold movement. These disorders include amyotrophic lateral sclerosis, syringobulbia, poliomyelitis, multiple sclerosis, Shy-Drager syndrome, Parkinson disease, bulbar palsy, and pseudobulbar palsy. Neuromuscular junction disorder and diseases of muscle may also result in flaccid dysphonia. Myasthenia gravis is a neuromuscular junction disorder resulting from immunological damage and loss of acetylcholine receptors from the postsynaptic membrane, causing generalized progressive muscle weakness. It may affect the laryngeal muscles, causing bilateral vocal fold weakness, incomplete adduction, abduction, bowing, and loss of rapid diadochokinesis. The diagnosis is made by enzyme testing and the Tensilon test. Other muscular disorders, such as muscular dystrophy, myositis, and dermatomyositis, may affect muscles of the larynx and pharynx preferentially.

Idiopathic vocal cord, a diagnosis of exclusion, is considered a mononeuropathy, possibly related to viral inflammation. The majority of such cases recover spontaneously. If the vocal cord function does not return after a reasonable period of time, usually 4 to 6 months, a diligent search for the etiology should continue.

■ Clinical Evaluation

A systematic approach should be taken in the evaluation of a patient with an immobile vocal fold. A thorough patient history; physical, endoscopic, and flexible examination of the vocal fold movement; and stroboscopic examination of the vibratory pattern of vocal folds are essential. Radiographic evaluation of the neck and chest, including the skull base region, should be undertaken if the etiology is not obvious. Operative endoscopy, laryngeal electromyography, and objective testing of vocal function should be performed as indicated to assess nerve integrity, determine prognosis for return of function, and assess treatment results.

Patient History

The patient history should include a review of the onset, duration, character, and severity of the dysphonia. A general medical history should include questions regarding prior intubation, heart disease, medications, and systemic medical illnesses, such as rheumatoid arthritis, diabetes mellitus, renal failure, and neurological disorders. Associated viral illness may precede sudden idiopathic vocal fold paralysis.

Patients with vocal cord paralysis typically complain of a weak, soft voice that is difficult to project beyond a whisper. They describe difficulty in being heard in a crowded environment, such as a party or restaurant. They also frequently complain of dyspnea, vocal fatigue, and effortful speaking. These complaints correspond directly with the physiological findings of high air leakage during phonation, shortened phonation time, and loss of high-frequency acoustic energy associated with the breathy voice. The voice characteristic of vocal cord paralysis is one of stable breathy dysphonia with little fluctuation. Fluctuations in voice quality suggest paresis. Some patients with paresis do not complain of voice difficulties until the end of the day after heavy usage.

Complaints of swallowing difficulties are common. Although many patients with vocal cord paralysis do not have overt aspiration, some notice that extra care is necessary to prevent aspiration of liquids. Patients with high vagal injury have pharyngeal paralysis and are much more debilitated by their aspiration than those with unilateral vocal cord paralysis. Aspiration of liquids may occur early in the course of RLN injury; however, adequate compensation and improvement are seen in most patients over time. Patients with advanced age, cancer, weight loss, and prior prolonged intubation are at greater risk for aspiration than young, neurologically intact patients with ability to compensate. Cough and dyspnea are also frequent complaints. The cough is ineffective and sometimes leaves the patient with residual excess phlegm and a sensation of the need to continually cough.

When possible, the level of the injury or lesion should be localized because it has prognostic and therapeutic implications. When the lesion is high in the jugular foramen or at the exit of the tenth nerve from the skull base, branches to the pharynx, superior laryngeal nerve, and RLN will be affected. Such patients often have severe aspiration, breathy dysphonia, and levator palatine weakness. Isolated superior laryngeal nerve palsy limits a patient's ability to raise the pitch, but aspiration and dysarthria are rare. With RLN paralysis, the voice will be breathy and hoarse. Vocal fold position helps in the differential diagnosis but is by no means diagnostic. In differentiating a flaccid lower motor neuron lesion from an upper motor neuron injury, it is important to assess the quality of the voice and to look for evidence of other multisystem involvement. Patients with supranuclear lesions, such as Parkinson disease, often present with hypophonia and difficulty in producing voicing after voiceless consonants. Similarly, dysarthria and poor breath support are overt comorbid processes in the voice production of patients with bulbar and pseudobulbar lesions. Swallowing function is often affected more than voice in patients with bulbar lesions. This is in contrast to the peripheral nerve palsies, which affect voice but in general spare articulation and swallowing. **Table 55.2** lists some common central nervous system disorders and their findings.

Physical Examination

A thorough head and neck examination should include specific neurological examination of cranial nerves II through XII, examination of the neck and thyroid landmarks, and maneuvers designed to assess laryngeal function. The neck and larynx should be carefully palpated to evaluate cricothyroid contraction with phonation, assess laryngeal elevation with each swallow, assess voice improvement with various head positions and neck turning, and deter-

Table 55.2 Central and neuromuscular system diseases affecting vocal fold movement

Disorder	Features	Voice Characteristic
Parkinson disease	Fading with tremor Onset of voice difficult Rapid glottal stops difficult	Reduced intensity and range
Shy-Drager syndrome	Slow dysarthric speech Hypotension, apnea, autonomic symptoms, bilateral abductor paralysis	Slow speech, reduced intensity, unintelligible
Amyotrophic lateral sclerosis	Spastic and flaccid picture, asymmetric movement of vocal folds, velopharyngeal insufficiency	Hoarseness or harsh wet voice, hypernasal, poor articulation
Multiple sclerosis	Fluctuation in symptoms Intermittent spasticity or flaccidity, other sensory or motor involvement	Variation on rate of speech; disrupted, tremulous, spastic voice
Upper motor neuron atrophy	Swallow affected, muscle wasting, aspiration, stridor	Voice weak, dysarthric, breathy
Myasthenia gravis	Fatigue of voice with use of small muscle affected, e.g., eye	Hypophonia, breathy, voice fluctuations

mine the degree of voice improvement with medial compression testing. Medial compression testing has been advocated as a predictor of whether medialization laryngoplasty will result in a better voice. Voice improvement with neck turning and position may indicate that such patients will improve with speech therapy. Assessment of vocal function with the help of a speech pathologist may reveal a particular pitch range that gives the patient an optional voice. The "better" voice may then be used by the patient with appropriate training by the speech pathologist.

Physical examination by endoscopy is a well-recognized method for visual documentation of vocal fold movement. Mirror examination, though simple and easy to perform, often fails to detect fine details, which are better revealed by telescopic examination or telescopic examination with video. Rigid indirect telescopic examination affords an excellent view of the vocal folds but has poor capability to assess motion of the vocal cord apparatus in the natural state. Therefore, paresis and compensatory changes of the vocal tract mechanism are often not appreciated by rigid endoscopic examination of the vocal folds.

The preferred method is to use the rigid telescope to assess lesion and anatomy, whereas flexible endoscopy is used to assess motion and vocal function. Rigid endoscopic examination should assess the normal capability of the vocal folds to change length with increasing pitch and assess the vocal folds for ulcerations and structural abnormalities that are easily missed by the flexible fiberoptic examination. Flexible examination of the larynx is done with a standard set of vocal maneuvers that test voice and other vegetative functions of the larynx. Specifically, the larynx is examined during sustained vowels and during running speech, readings of "The Rainbow Passage," whistle,

cough, and swallow. Flexible laryngoscopy is also used to assess palatal function and the nasopharyngeal port, if such documentation is necessary or desirable.

The pathological changes of vocal fold movement with unilateral vocal cord paralysis typically show the pyriform sinus to be open with pooling. The arytenoid is often rolled forward and the vocal process is in the paramedian-to-abducted position. With phonation, the contralateral innervated vocal cords may overcompensate and cross the midline. Vocal fold length comparisons show the denervated vocal cord during inspiration to be shorter than the innervated side. During phonation, the innervated side actually shortens to match the length of the innervated vocal cord. If there is excessive contraction by the innervated side, the paralyzed side will appear longer than the innervated side during phonation and shorter during inspiration. Compensatory gestures of the larynx and pharynx are common in patients as they try to produce better phonation. These findings on fiberoptic laryngoscopy may show anteroposterior (AP) supraglottic squeezing, ventricular phonation, and pharyngeal constriction with laryngeal elevation. Abnormal pitch elevation into falsetto and habitual phonation in falsetto are common findings in many patients with vocal cord paralysis.

Flexible video laryngoscopy is used to assess (1) the closure of the glottis; (2) the extent of pharyngeal compensation; (3) compensatory supraglottic hyperadduction; and (4) the extent of spontaneous movements. During the flexible video examination, estimates of the phonation time, maximum phonation decibel output, and fundamental frequency may be made. With modern endoscopy equipment, estimates of statistics, such as decibel and frequency output, may be directly displayed on screen.

Objective Testing

A variety of objective tests can be used to assess the breathy voice quality, glottic configuration, vibratory characteristics of the vocal folds, and degree of muscle denervation. These objective tests are important for both assessment and documentation.

Laryngeal Function Studies

Breathy voice quality in vocal cord paralysis is associated with reduced phonation time, need for frequent inhalations during conversational speech, and increased mean airflow rates. Airflow measures show an increase in the mean flow rates and an increase in glottal leakage flows. Measures of the efficiency of airflow conversion show reduction in the alternating current/direct current flow ratio. Analyses of the frequency component of airflow signal show an increase in the turbulent energy and a decrease in the harmonic energy. With surgical rehabilitation, phonation time, mean flow rates, and other aerodynamic factors revert toward more normal values.

Acoustic Measures

Studies of acoustic voice measures show several common features. Besides reduction in phonation time, there is reduction in the dynamic range, in both loudness and frequency range. Spectrogram analysis shows loss of high-frequency energy and higher format peaks on the spectrogram. Increase in the signal-to-noise ratio, and increase in the aperiodicity, jitter, and shimmer are other common features in patients with vocal cord paralysis.

Glottography

At this time, electroglottography has only limited clinical application in the diagnosis of vocal fold paralysis, although it has research applications in understanding vibratory functions of the vocal fold. In general, there is a short contact period, a prolonged open period, and a reduced rate of vocal fold opening and closing velocity. Photoglottography complements the electroglottography finding by providing some information on the pattern of vocal fold function during the opening period.

Videostroboscopy

Glottal configuration during phonation is best assessed with videostroboscopy. Typical patterns of vocal fold closure include midcord gap, posterior gap, and height differences between the vocal folds.

This information is important in selection of the medialization procedures. Denervation pattern and early reinnervation can be differentiated by direct inspection of vibratory behavior of the vocal folds using videostroboscopy. The stroboscopic examination often shows incomplete closure, prolonged open phase, amplitude reduction, asymmetry, and loss of mucosal wave. Phase differences between vibration of the vocal folds will show the innervated vocal fold to open earlier than the denervated vocal fold. The denervated vocal fold often shows a floppy "flag in the breeze" appearance. With early reinnervation, there is reversal of many of these findings before gross movement restoration. This is correlated with improvement of the voice.

Electromyography

Assessment of the innervation status of the intrinsic laryngeal muscles with electromyography (EMG) is important for both diagnostic and prognostic purposes. Neuropathic and myopathic disorders are differentiated by monopolar needle examination of the intrinsic laryngeal muscles as well as the limb muscles. Diagnosis of vocal cord paralysis versus ankylosis is easily differentiated using EMG. Vagal paralysis, superior laryngeal paralysis, and recurrent nerve paralysis can be differentiated by testing the cricothyroid muscle and the thyroarytenoid muscle sequentially. Indications for laryngeal EMG in the management of vocal cord paralysis include its use as a tool for prognostication of return of function. Electrical patterns are analyzed for spontaneous and evoked activity. The presence of polyphasic and/or giant motor unit potentials indicates reinnervation. Electrical silence and spontaneous discharge of low-voltage and fibrillation potentials are evidence of denervation with poor reinnervation. Presence of evoked giant polyphasic potentials mixed with fibrillation potentials indicates partial denervation and reinnervation. Recruitment patterns during voluntary activity, such as phonation and cough, give an estimate of the degree of voluntary activity in the particular muscle of interest. In general a three- to fivefold difference between maximal recruitment pattern and minimal voluntary recruitment activity can be expected in normal muscles.

Diagnostic Imaging

With advanced imaging modalities, both a chest X-ray and a CT scan of the course of the vagus nerve are the state of the art in investigation of unexplained vocal cord paralysis. CT scan from the base of the skull to the chest, including the jugular foramen, thyroid gland, root of the neck, and carina, should be done to investigate the cause of unexplained vocal fold paralysis. When endoscopic evaluation is not possible and it is necessary to assess the level differences between the vocal folds, a fluoroscopic examination in the AP plane or CT of the larynx in the AP plane during phonation can offer additional information. Magnetic resonance imaging of the brain and neck structures is indicated in selected patients, depending on their history and physical examination. In cases of laryngeal trauma, including intubation injury, thin-cut CT scan of the larynx (2 mm cuts) should be obtained to look for evidence of arytenoid dislocation and/or laryngeal fracture.

Operative Laryngoscopy

Occasionally the etiology of vocal fold immobility is not clear even after office examination and radiographic investigation. In such patients, operative laryngoscopy may be warranted. Operative laryngoscopy is performed to rule out laryngeal pathology, assess joint mobility, and evaluate esophageal pathology, which may mimic vocal cord paralysis. Examination of the posterior cricoid plate, palpation of arytenoid motion, and examination of the integrity of the cricoarytenoid joint are best done under operative conditions.

■ Management

The management options for unilateral vocal fold paralysis include observation, speech therapy, and surgical intervention. The choice of therapy is determined by the degree of functional deficit, etiology, and prognosis for recovery. It is important in the management of vocal cord paralysis to have an appreciation of the wide variety of functional deficits with which patients present. A functional rating should be noted on their initial presentation and followed.

The voices of many patients with unilateral vocal cord paralysis will improve over time as the contralateral vocal cord compensates; therefore, these patients do not require surgical intervention. Most of the improvement is noted over the first 3 to 6 months. Typically, the voice stabilizes but remains weak. Occasionally, the voice will become more diplophonic and hoarse. This has been attributed to vocal fold atrophy and the effect of asymmetric mass. The voice fluctuates with use and is typically better early in the day before heavy use.

Speech Therapy

Speech therapy is important to educate the patient regarding vocal mechanisms that improve voice quality as well as prevent the development of potentially harmful vocal habits from compensatory efforts. It is also essential to help reduce hyperkinetic and hyperadductive compensatory gestures before and after surgery to attain optimal surgical results. By working with breath control and exploring areas of the voice that can be produced with the greatest ease, functional improvement can be obtained in many patients without the need for surgery. However, speech therapy cannot be used to rehabilitate the aphonic patient nor significantly improve a severely breathy voice. It also cannot be expected to correct differences due to vocal fold atrophy. A variety of speech therapy techniques, such as vocal range exercises, hum, aspirate voice, trill, Valsalva, and other voice awareness programs can be used, depending on the voice problem. Speech therapy can be used in tandem with surgical treatment.

Surgical Intervention

In considering treatment options for the patient with vocal cord paralysis, it is important to consider the needs of the patient, the natural course of the disease, and the expected result from each type of therapy. The indications for surgical intervention are aspiration, disabling breathy hypophonia, and inability to produce an effective cough.

The options for surgical intervention are medialization and reinnervation. Medialization can be accomplished through vocal cord injection, medialization laryngoplasty (thyroplasty), or arytenoid adduction. Substances currently used for vocal cord injection are collagen, autologous fat, micronized dermis, and various synthetic injectables, such as calcium hydroxylapatite and dermal fillers. The injection is accomplished through direct laryngoscopy or in the unsedated setting through the mouth or cervical skin. In the past, Teflon injections were a popular choice for unilateral vocal fold paralysis. Potential complications of Teflon vocal cord injection include failure to achieve the desired voice result, airway obstruction, and Teflon granuloma. Failure to achieve a good voice may be due to overinjection, underinjection, decreased vibration of the vocal cord due to mass effect, or failure to close the posterior glottic chink. Airway obstruction is rare and usually results from injection into the subglottic space.

Medialization laryngoplasty (ML) and arytenoid adduction (AA) are external approaches to medialization of vocal cords. ML is accomplished by excising a rectangular window of cartilage from the thyroid lamina at the level of the true vocal cords and placing an alloplastic implant to push the vocal fold medially. The size of the window is 3 to 6 mm × 10 to 13 mm. The superior border of the window is determined by a horizontal line drawn from the midway point of the thyroid notch to the inferior border and paralleling the inferior border. The anterior border is placed ~ 6 to 8 mm from the midline to avoid injury to the anterior commissure. The best results with ML are obtained when the glottic gap is along the midportion of the cord. It is difficult to correct a large posterior gap or a vocal cord that lies at a lower level with ML. Complications of ML include implant extrusion, airway obstruction, wound infection, and fistula formation. Implant extrusion usually occurs intralaryngeally through the ventricle.

To perform AA, the posterior border of the thyroid lamina is exposed, and the cricothyroid joint is separated. The muscular process of the arytenoid cartilage is identified and a 3–0 nylon suture is placed through it. Using a straight needle, the suture is then passed through the thyroid lamina near its anterior inferior border and then tied. This rotates the vocal process medially toward the midline to medialize the vocal cord. Because the procedure is performed under local anesthesia with intravenous sedation, when the suture is tied the patient can be asked to phonate to confirm good medialization. AA is ideal for correction of a glottic gap involving the posterior and midcord. ML may need to be performed in conjunction with AA to correct very large gaps. Complications of AA include slipped suture, airway obstruction, wound infection, and fistula formation. One case of carotid artery injury has been reported with this procedure when it was performed in an irradiated patient.

Various reinnervation procedures have been advocated for rehabilitation of the paralyzed larynx. The ultimate goal of reinnervation is to restore purposeful movement—that is, adduction during phonation or swallowing, and abduction with inspiration. However, purposeful movement does not always occur, even if the laryngeal muscles are successfully reinnervated. The most likely reason for failure to restore purposeful movement is nonselective reinnervation of the adductor and abductor muscles, resulting in cancellation of the vectors of pull of the arytenoid cartilage, a phenomenon known as "laryngeal synkinesis." Nevertheless, even if purposeful movement is not restored, muscle bulk and normal joint position can be maintained with reinnervation. For unilateral paralysis, reanastomosis of the RLN, selective reanastomosis of the abductor and adductor branches of the RLN, ansa-omohyoid neuromus-

cular pedicle implantation onto the thyroarytenoid muscle, and ansa cervicalis–RLN anastomosis have been performed in human subjects with variable success.

The decision regarding when to surgically intervene depends on the degree of functional deficit, etiology of the paralysis, and prognosis for recovery. It is important to remember that the resting position of a paralyzed vocal cord can change with time, depending on the degree of muscle atrophy and the ultimate resultant vector of muscle pull on the arytenoid cartilage. Atrophy of the thyroarytenoid muscle may result in progressive bowing of the vocal cord. On the other hand, should spontaneous reinnervation occur, the vocal fold may shift back toward the midline, even if movement is not restored. Early surgical intervention is indicated when severe functional disability exists, such as aspiration; ineffective cough; or disabling breathy hypophonia, as evidenced by phonation time of < 5 seconds, high mean flow rates > 250 mL/s, or reduced maximal decibel output (< 75 dB). Disability from breathy hypophonia varies among individuals. For example, vocal fatigue and mild breathiness in a professional voice user can be quite disabling. Surgical therapy at 6 to 9 months after injury is indicated in patients who demonstrate evidence of denervation or little activity on EMG and who have had a poor response to a reasonable trial of speech therapy.

Though these static medialization procedures offer a significant improvement in the intensity of the voice, patients should be warned that their voice probably will not be normal. Static procedures may not always restore symmetrical mucosal wave. Early postoperative voice quality is usually diplophonic, harsh, high pitched, and gravelly. It is frequently strained, especially in patients who have had long-standing paralysis. It is likely that most of these patients have developed mechanisms to compensate for the breathy hypophonia. It is well recognized that the paralyzed vocal fold is often shortened, probably due to the scar contracture, and the normal vocal fold will shorten and hyperadduct to attain approximation with the paralyzed vocal fold. Such compensatory mechanisms persist following medialization. For these reasons, speech therapy is an essential component in the management of vocal cord paralysis, both preoperatively and postoperatively.

■ Suggested Reading

Aynehchi BB, McCoul ED, Sundaram K. Systematic review of laryngeal reinnervation techniques. Otolaryngol Head Neck Surg 2010; 143(6):749–759

Fang TJ, Li HY, Gliklich RE, Chen YH, Wang PC, Chuang HF. Outcomes of fat injection laryngoplasty in unilateral vocal cord paralysis. Arch Otolaryngol Head Neck Surg 2010;136(5):457–462

Friedman AD, Burns JA, Heaton JT, Zeitels SM. Early versus late injection medialization for unilateral vocal cord paralysis. Laryngoscope 2010;120(10):2042–2046

Li AJ, Johns MM, Jackson-Menaldi C, et al. Glottic closure patterns: type I thyroplasty versus type I thyroplasty with arytenoid adduction. J Voice 2011;25(3):259–264

Misono S, Merati AL. Evidence-based practice: evaluation and management of unilateral vocal fold paralysis. Otolaryngol Clin North Am 2012;45(5):1083–1108

Paniello RC, Edgar JD, Kallogjeri D, Piccirillo JF. Medialization versus reinnervation for unilateral vocal fold paralysis: a multicenter randomized clinical trial. Laryngoscope 2011;121(10):2172–2179

Paquette CM, Manos DC, Psooy BJ. Unilateral vocal cord paralysis: a review of CT findings, mediastinal causes, and the course of the recurrent laryngeal nerves. Radiographics 2012;32(3):721–740

Rickert SM, Childs LF, Carey BT, Murry T, Sulica L. Laryngeal electromyography for prognosis of vocal fold palsy: a meta-analysis. Laryngoscope 2012;122(1):158–161

Sulica L, Rosen CA, Postma GN, et al. Current practice in injection augmentation of the vocal folds: indications, treatment principles, techniques, and complications. Laryngoscope 2010;120(2): 319–325

Tan M, Woo P. Injection laryngoplasty with micronized dermis: a 10-year experience with 381 injections in 344 patients. Laryngoscope 2010;120(12):2460–2466

56 Surgical Therapy of Voice Disorders

Introduction

In the last decade, the substantive innovations in endoscopic surgery have been in the design of the procedures, a result of improved understanding of the layered microstructure of the vocal fold, the physiological principles of laryngeal sound, and the use of stroboscopy to analyze vocal fold oscillation. This approach, called phonomicrosurgery, is based on maximally preserving the vocal fold's layered microstructure, epithelium, and lamina propria.

Instrument Selection

The glottiscope that provides the widest aperture for visualizing the glottal surgical field should be selected. Placing the largest tubed laryngoscope that can be admitted from the lips to the vocal folds can be hard work and may be the lengthiest portion of the surgical case. If not achieved, the precision of the procedure may be compromised because of both limited exposure of the lesion and limited ability to angulate hand instrumentation for tangential tissue dissection in the lamina propria.

The use of a smaller-lumened glottiscope is slightly less important when the laser is used because only one hand instrument requires angulation. However, many otolaryngologists believe that for most benign glottal pathology, precise microdissection is optimally performed by exclusive use of cold instruments. This requires a glottiscope that can accommodate angulation of two hand instruments. The subepithelial infusion of saline and epinephrine into the superficial lamina propria (SLP) has further enhanced precision in microlaryngoscopic vocal fold surgery with the use of both the laser and cold instruments.

In recent years, a variety of improvements in hand instruments relate primarily to finer size and greater selection of the angles of previously designed mechanics. The greatest attributes of cold instru-mentation are that the surgeon can palpate the tissues and can perform delicate tangential dissection in the SLP (**Fig. 56.1**) with minimal trauma to the lamina propria and epithelium. The thermal trauma of the CO_2 laser can be detrimental to the delicate loosely arranged elastic tissue of the SLP. The use of the microspot CO_2 laser may be less precise than carefully selected cold instruments during delicate tangential dissection of microflaps. The laser is optimally used in more vascular lesions, because bleeding otherwise obscures the operative site, and for larger lesions that cannot be effectively retracted within the lumen of the laryngoscope.

General Endoscopic Technique and Principles

Suspension microlaryngoscopy is performed with general anesthesia and paralysis, most commonly using a small endotracheal tube. A true suspension gallows is preferable; however, a fulcrum laryngoscope holder is usually adequate. *External counterpressure* and *internal distension* can be very helpful in visualization. An appropriately selected endotracheal tube provides a stable point from which the largest lumened laryngoscope is intercalated between the endotracheal tube and the infrapetiole region of the supraglottis (for glottal surgery) to internally distend the surgical field. Jet ventilation may not be practical for many lesions and precludes adequate internal distension of the laryngeal introitus.

The patient is placed in the classic Boyce-Jackson position, with the neck flexed and the head extended at the atloid-occipital joint. The authors feel this position is optimally maintained with a modified Killian gallows (Pilling Surgical, Inc., Durham, NC). External laryngeal counterpressure is first applied manually to determine its value for improving exposure and then is applied with silk tape that is stretched from the lower laryngeal framework to the operating table. The magnitude of the pressure and vector

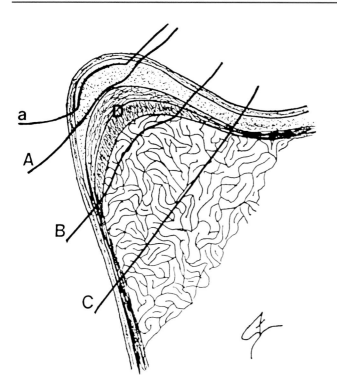

Fig. 56.1 A drawing of the layered microstructure of the vocal fold demonstrating the variety of procedures that vary in depth. a: dissection just below the basement membrane. (**a**) Dissection in the superficial lamina propria with preservation of the vocal ligament D. (**b**) Dissection between the vocal ligament and the thyroarytenoid muscle. The vocal ligament is used as the deep margin. (**c**) Dissection within the thyroarytenoid muscle. Used with permission from Zeitels, S. Phonomicrosurgical treatment of early glottic cancer and carcinoma in situ. The American Journal of Surgery, 1996; 172(6): 704-709.

of the force are adjusted to optimize the exposure of the lesion and the anterior glottis. If a CO_2 laser or other laser is to be used primarily or in conjunction with sharp microlaryngeal instrumentation, both the patient and the endotracheal tube should be protected appropriately.

An operating microscope fitted with a 400 mm front lens is used to examine the glottal surgical field at ×15, ×25, and ×40. In addition to the magnified visual examination, the lesion is palpated with a blunt probe to help assess its texture and the depth of deep tissue involvement. Subepithelial infusion of saline and 1:10,000 epinephrine into the SLP may be used to aid dissection of glottal lesions. If the epithelial lesion has not invaded nor obliterated the SLP, the infusion will hydrodissect under the lesion and lift it from the vocal ligament. Preoperative stroboscopy is helpful but is not always reliable for determining the depth of invasion of epithelial lesions, such as keratosis. Pre-excisional knowledge about the depth of penetration of the lesion is critical for selecting instrumentation (cold vs. laser), as well as for adjusting the deep margin precisely. Both of these factors are crucial to the patient's postoperative vocal outcome.

During superficial glottal procedures, hemostasis is achieved by topical application of epinephrine-soaked cotton. For deeper glottal lesions, a CO_2 laser may be employed with a defocused spot, or, when available, a vascular laser, such as the potassium-titanyl-phosphate (KTP) or pulsed-dye laser (PDL). In certain circumstances, electrocoagulation is useful. When the surgery is completed, any residual blood or secretions that are in the laryngeal introitus or hypopharynx are suctioned, and the larynx is sprayed with plain lidocaine to avoid laryngospasm during extubation. Postoperatively, the patient is placed on humidified room air and is managed for laryngopharyngeal reflux as necessary. Antibiotics, steroids, and/or analgesics are prescribed selectively based on surgeon preference and the extent of the surgery.

After vocal fold surgery, complete voice rest is advised, usually for 1 week, and modified voice use for 2 weeks. The patient has preoperative and postoperative appointments with a speech pathologist for objective voice assessment and vocal hygiene discussion. Formal voice therapy is administered as is necessary.

■ Assessment and Rehabilitation of Patients Undergoing Phonomicrosurgery

The majority of endoscopic surgery in the glottis is performed to treat benign processes. The most frequent presenting symptom for glottal disease is hoarseness. Benign lesions typically occur in vocal overdoers and seldom occur in individuals who are reticent and shy. Many individuals with benign lessons require preoperative and postoperative vocal therapy to eliminate habits that predispose to the original lesion and/or to remove compensatory strategies that have developed as a result of the lesions. Because the timing and decision about surgery are frequently linked to the response to vocal therapy, the surgeon must know the speech language pathologist well to accurately assess the adequacy of therapy.

The preoperative evaluation ideally should include flexible and rigid laryngeal stroboscopy as well as acoustic and aerodynamic assessment. At a minimum, a presurgical workup should include a preoperative and postoperative voice recording. Stroboscopy has become an invaluable tool for understanding the oscillatory characteristics of pathological vocal folds and for assessing the postsurgical voice. Telescopic stroboscopy provides superior optics for analyzing the anatomy of the vocal folds, the details of the lesion, and the characteristics of the mucosal wave oscillation. Flexible stroboscopy is superior for analyzing generalized laryngeal configuration during sound production, which is necessary for assessing the magnitude of muscle tension that accompanies the lesion.

The aforementioned visual information, along with acoustic and aerodynamic data, provide the surgeon with objective information about laryngeal sound production. The acoustic and aerodynamic information should be obtained for normal and loud voice tasks. The aerodynamic (pressure, flow, and resistance) efficiency is an excellent indicator of a patient's work and effort to phonate.

Ideally, the complete assessment should be repeated ~ 1 month postoperatively to analyze the result. This provides valuable information to the surgeon for postoperative discussions with patients about what to expect from their voice. It also provides information to the speech language pathologist, who may be instituting vocal therapy. Finally, the postoperative assessment documents the result in the event of future voice disturbances.

■ Phonomicrosurgery for Benign Lesions

Lesions along the glottal introitus impair entrained oscillation by creating stiffness in the diseased vocal fold and by preventing smooth vocal-edge closure. These factors result in an aerodynamically inefficient glottal valve. Phonomicrosurgical procedures are designed to improve aerodynamic efficiency and vocal quality by creating a smooth vocal fold edge that is not excavated with overlying epithelium that is flexible.

Optimal phonomicrosurgical management of benign glottal lesions requires maximal preservation of normal lamina propria and epithelium. Therefore, it is valuable to assess the microlayers of involvement of any lesion. This should involve both high-magnification visual inspection as well as gentle retraction and palpation. Given the choice of sacrificing or disturbing normal SLP or normal epithelium, it is wiser to preserve normal SLP.

There is little difficulty in the growth and regeneration of normal epithelium, as is seen after a cordectomy that is left to heal secondarily. Normal SLP does not regenerate if it has been removed. Postoperative stroboscopic findings further reveal that if extensive dissection in normal SLP is performed to raise a wide microflap, stiffness will be noted in the field of dissection. Regenerated epithelium essentially reflects the viscoelastic properties and the oscillation characteristics of the tissue that it overlies.

Vocal Polyps

Vocal polyps present in a variety of sizes and are typically the result of trauma to the microvasculature of the SLP. They are most commonly found in the mid-

musculomembranous region, because the aerodynamically induced shearing forces on the microvasculature of the SLP are greatest in this region. The lesions may present as sessile or pedunculated. The classic appearance of a vocal fold polyp is a unilateral, translucent polypoid lesion at the midmembranous position of the vocal fold at the point of maximal collision force during phonation, as seen in **Fig. 56.2**. Subepithelial infusion of saline and epinephrine can be used to enhance the precision of the resection of these lesions.

The sessile lesions can often be removed by means of a microflap and a subepithelial resection of the polyp contents. Pedunculated lesions are optimally resected by retraction and amputation. Care should be taken to palpate the component of the polyp that is in the SLP so that it is adequately excised. The small lesions (0–3 mm) and medium-sized (3–6 mm) lesions can usually be removed with greater precision by cold instruments. When removing these lesions, the surgeon may encounter a small feeding vessel. Application of cotton soaked in saline/epinephrine (1:10,000 concentration) will usually stop the bleeding. Occasionally, the judicious use of a vascular laser is necessary to microcauterize the vessel. Larger sessile lesions (> 6 mm) are best managed with the microspot CO_2 laser. The bleeding that occurs after incising these lesions with cold instruments will usually obscure the magnified operative field.

Vocal Nodules

Vocal nodules may present visually in a varied manner. There are divergent opinions as to the value of phonomicrosurgical intervention, which may very

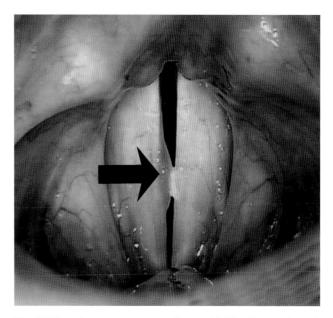

Fig. 56.2 Classic appearance of a vocal fold polyp. Unilateral, translucent, and found at the midmembraneous portion.

likely be due to confusion in the literature about what constitutes vocal nodules. There is little disagreement that these lesions are the result of vocal abuse or phonotrauma. Therefore, irrespective of the decision regarding whether to excise vocal nodules, all of these patients will require vocal therapy. A common laryngoscopic appearance of nodules is bilateral subepithelial fibrovascular changes involving the midmembranous portions at the point of maximal collision force during phonation, as seen in **Fig. 56.3**.

In most cases, it is advantageous to employ surgery as secondary management. An initial trial of vocal therapy should reduce the hyperfunctional behavior and the generalized edema of the SLP that typically accompany these lesions. Even if the nodules do not resolve and disappear visually, the patient may be satisfied with the quality and stamina of the voice, so that surgical intervention is not necessary. If the patient desires further improvement and clear nodules are seen, phonomicrosurgical excision may further enhance vocal quality. The prior vocal therapy will benefit the patient during the postoperative rehabilitative process to prevent injury and recurrence.

Patients who are not typically candidates for surgery will present with "nodular swelling." Anatomically, these vocal folds have fusiform swelling of the SLP, which is usually bilateral and symmetric and in the midmusculomembranous region. A discrete mass is not seen on telescopic laryngostroboscopy. Prioritization of vocal activities and vocal therapy should adequately treat these individuals.

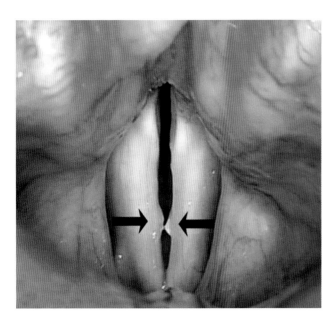

Fig. 56.3   A common appearance of vocal fold nodules. Bilateral and found at the midmembraneous portion.

Similar to the aforementioned techniques for excising vocal polyps, phonomicrosurgical resection of vocal nodules can be performed by means of a microflap or by amputation. Cold instruments provide improved precision, considering the small size of these lesions and the need for palpation during the procedure. The subepithelial infusion technique should be used selectively. Nodules that are less well defined visually and by palpation may become obscured by the infusion-induced distension of the SLP.

Subepithelial Cysts

Subepithelial cysts arise in the SLP and present in a variety of sizes. They may be attached to the vocal ligament and/or the epithelial basement membrane. Small cysts may also be freely suspended within the SLP. Subepithelial cysts may be confused with nodules if visual examination is performed without stroboscopy. Stroboscopic examination typically reveals a characteristic asymmetric, disordered oscillation of the mucosa because of the well-circumscribed stiffness in the area of the cyst. If the cyst protrudes from the medial surface of the glottal edge, reactive nodularity may be observed at the striking zone of the contralateral vocal fold.

Subepithelial cysts probably arise from obstructed ducts within the SLP. They may contain mucus or may be composed of an epithelial rest (similar to a cholesteatoma). On occasion, small ovoid subepithelial masses that are thought preoperatively to be a cyst within the SLP are found at microlaryngoscopy to be fibrous masses. These masses are usually firmer to palpation and may be the result of an old microvascular injury or a rheumatoid lesion. The submucosal infusion technique is extremely helpful in well-defined cysts. The infusion can obscure the boundaries of small cysts and lead to unnecessary dissection and trauma of normal SLP.

Masses within the SLP should be resected with cold instruments with few exceptions. The need for extremely delicate tangential dissection precludes effective use of the CO_2 laser. Great care should be taken to minimally disturb any normal SLP and epithelium. This approach will optimize postoperative mucosal-wave oscillation and vocal quality.

Most phonosurgeons would agree that, of all the common benign subepithelial pathologies encountered, cysts can be the most challenging in terms of technique. The technique to excise a cyst illustrates several technical points that may be broadly applied to most phonomicrosurgery. First and foremost are adequate preoperative assessment, planning, and availability of sufficient instrumentation. The surgical plan is confirmed after achieving wide exposure, magnified visual inspection, and blunt palpation of the lesion (**Fig. 56.4a**). A subepithelial infusion of the epinephrine/lidocaine mixture will expand the SLP prior to the cordotomy incision and development of the microflap (**Fig. 56.4b**). The interface between the lesion and the SLP is critical and should be well identified so as not to unnecessarily resect uninvolved SLP. Frequently, cysts and other benign lesions can be dissected free from the uninvolved overlying epithelium (**Fig. 56.4c**). The pathology should be excised in its entirety without disturbing adjacent SLP or overlying epithelium or leaving attachments in the case of a cyst (**Fig. 56.4d**). This technique maximally preserves the layered microstructure (**Fig. 56.4e**) and postoperative outcomes.

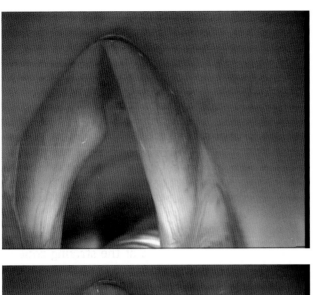

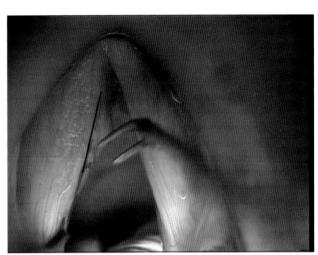

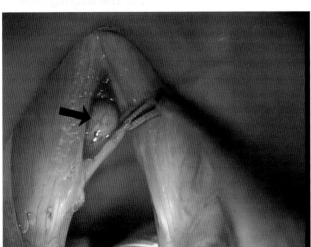

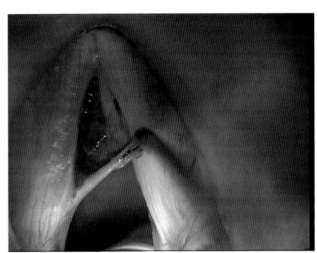

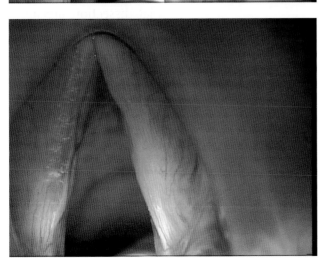

Fig. 56.4 (**a**) Intraoperative view through a Universal Modular Glottiscope, operating microscope, 400 mm lens, maximum magnification. A large subepithelial lesion is noted within the left vocal fold, with severe deformation of the left vibratory edge. (**b**) After subepithelial infusion of lidocaine with epinephrine (note the subepithelial bubbles visible through the epithelium on the superior surface), an epithelial cordotomy incision is fashioned just lateral to the lesion (*black line*). (**c**) After careful dissection, an epidermoid cyst is clearly visible (*black arrow*). (**d**) The epidermoid cyst is dissected free from the overlying epithelium and underlying superficial lamina propria (SLP) and excised intact. (**e**) Postexcision examination. The cyst was excised without violation of the SLP or resection of the overlying epithelium. When the operated vocal fold is reinfused with the epinephrine/lidocaine mixture, expansion of the SLP indicates integrity, and visual inspection reveals no significant vibratory edge defect.

Granulomas

Although the majority of granulomas are found in the arytenoid region, they may occur in other areas where there has been traumatic disruption of mucosa. These lesions typically arise in patients with laryngopharyngeal reflux. Reflux creates an environment of generalized mucositis, and the traumatic disruption of glottal epithelium predisposes patients to a hypertrophic inflammatory reaction. The frequent throat clearing noted in patients with vocal process granulomas is thought to fuel a chronic chrondritis of the cartilaginous posterior glottis that many clinicians consider to be a critical component of the hypertrophic inflammatory reaction in reflux laryngitis–related pathology. These lesions may be bilateral or unilateral, as seen in **Fig. 56.5**.

Classical descriptions of posterior glottal granulomas have occurred after an endotracheal intubation. In this instance, the posteriorly situated endotracheal tube has disrupted the periarytenoid epithelium. These patients will frequently have simultaneous endotracheal and nasogastric tubes, with the latter predisposing to extraesophageal reflux.

The typical outpatient posterior glottal granuloma is the result of vocally induced trauma in a reflux environment. These patients demonstrate vocal hyperfunction that causes high-impact collision forces of the arytenoids during phonation. Videolaryngoscopy reveals hyperfunction of the lateral cricoarytenoid musculature that results in hyperrotation of the arytenoids and abnormal concussion. This in turn leads to epithelial trauma. It is common to find granulomas that show a bilobed configuration, which reflects the conformation of the contralateral arytenoid from the closure pattern of the

arytenoids during phonation. These patients require vocal therapy as an adjunct to their treatment, which includes antireflux management and possible microlaryngeal resection.

Granulomas are frequently exophytic with a surprisingly narrow base. When they are small or medium in size, they may not impair glottal closure. However, large granulomas will result in a substantial glottal chink in the musculomembranous region that leads to further glottal insufficiency during laryngeal sound production and increased vocal hyperfunction.

Phonomicrosurgical resection should be performed when behavior modification and medication have not led to a resolution or there is concern about a neoplastic process. On rare occasions, granulomas will require excision due to airway compromise, especially in older patients. The use of the laser or cold instruments alone is individualized, based on surgeon preference and the anatomical characteristics of the lesion. The critical surgical principle is to remove the mass without disturbing the arytenoid perichondrium. Injecting the base of the granuloma with a small amount of an aqueous-based steroid, such as Depo-Medrol (Pfizer, New York, NY), may help to prevent recurrence.

The necessity of treating vocal hyperfunction, a predisposing traumatic behavior, cannot be overstated. Abusive vocal behavior is usually the culprit with recurrent, recalcitrant arytenoid granulomas. If the hyperfunctional activity of the lateral cricoarytenoid muscles is still observed, low-dose botulinum toxin can be used to chemically unload this closure pattern. Administration of 1.5 international units of botulinum toxin is a good initial dose. Based on the severity of the hyperfunction, one or both vocal cords can be injected. The injection can be placed at the time of the endoscopic excision of the granuloma. The botulinum toxin should be directed toward the lateral cricoarytenoid muscle, rather than the thyroarytenoid muscle. This will help minimize the vocal insufficiency, for which the patient must be prepared.

Polypoid Corditis (Reinke Edema)

Polypoid corditis presents as extensive swelling of the Reinke space. The swelling is usually situated on the superior surface of the musculomembranous vocal fold, as presented in **Fig. 56.6**. This entity is another manifestation of vocal fold pathology that is of multifactorial genesis. These patients typically smoke extensively, have laryngopharyngeal reflux, and demonstrate vocal hyperfunction. The swelling probably occurs from the increased aerodynamic pressures that drive vocal fold mucosal oscillation in a general environment of glottal mucositis, which is secondary to smoking and reflux.

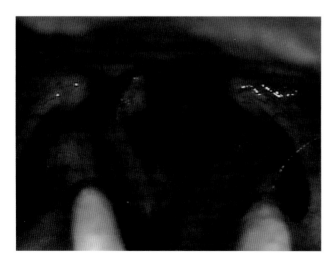

Fig. 56.5   A right-sided vocal process granuloma is marked and can be appreciated against a background of chronic laryngitis.

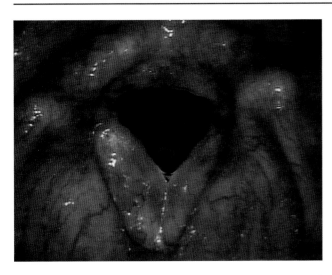

Fig. 56.6 An example of Reinke edema, also known as polypoid corditis.

Individuals with polypoid corditis have abnormally low-pitched voices because the mass-loaded folds oscillate at an inordinately low frequency. Females present more frequently than males, and they undergo phonomicrosurgical management more frequently because of the greater discrepancy from their normal fundamental voice frequency.

Before undergoing surgery, individuals with polypoid corditis should discontinue smoking, have their reflux controlled, and have preoperative vocal therapy. The technique for the surgical procedure is based on raising a thin epithelial microflap after incising the mucosa near the vestibular fold. A microscissor is used for the initial incision, unless there is prominent subepithelial vascular injection. The gelatinous hypertrophied SLP should then be carefully contoured and reduced to a more normal volume. This can be done by suctioning or by direct removal. The vocal ligament should never be visualized directly.

Great care must be taken not to overreduce the SLP, which results in an inordinately stiff vocal system. Overreduction of the SLP can result in a severely strained, harsh voice, given that these individuals generally employ high subglottal pressures to drive their floppy, mass-loaded folds. Vocally, it is preferable to leave a larger fold than to create a visually pleasing smaller fold.

Once the SLP has been reduced, the epithelium is redraped and trimmed appropriately. If there is keratotic or dysplastic epithelium, it should be excised and sent to pathology for histopathological analysis. After an initial period of vocal rest (10 days), patients should receive vocal therapy and should be monitored closely. Preventing recurrence is dependent on modification of the predisposing factors, especially smoking.

Respiratory Papillomatosis

Patients who have respiratory papillomatosis of the glottis most frequently present with hoarseness. Most commonly, the glottal disease is confined to the musculomembranous region, although it is not unusual to find extension into the ventricle and subglottis, as can be seen in **Fig. 56.7**. Adult glottal papillomatosis tends to be more plaquelike than the juvenile variety.

Because the disease is confined to the epithelium, great care should be taken to maximally preserve the underlying SLP. An en bloc resection by means of a microflap can frequently be accomplished for very limited disease. However, a motorized microlaryngeal debrider is commonly employed for debulking and may be safely used, even on diseased vibratory epithelium, in experienced hands. The learning curve for motorized microlaryngeal debrider can be steep, with severe inadvertent resection of normal epithelium, SLP, or even anterior commissural ligament possible if the instrument is not carefully employed.

The use of vascular lasers in the treatment of papillomatosis is beyond the scope of this chapter. Readers are encouraged to familiarize themselves with the multitude of emerging technologies and minimally invasive techniques now employed routinely. Use of the CO_2 laser to vaporize papillomas has been largely abandoned in favor of safer, less invasive techniques.

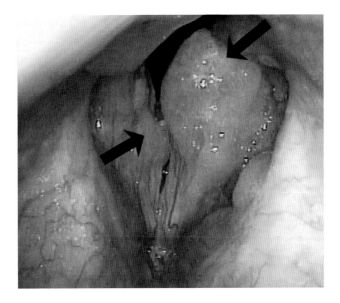

Fig. 56.7 Respiratory papillomatosis involving both musculomembranous vocal folds (marked). There is also extension into the left laryngeal ventricle (not marked). Note the numerous capillary ectasias leading into the metabolically active abnormal vocal fold epithelium.

Premalignant Vocal Fold Epithelium

Disease Presentation

Premalignant vocal fold epithelium is essentially a smoking-induced disease. Lesions will frequently be confined geographically to the superior surface of the vocal fold. This allows for complete preservation of layered microstructure on the medial valving surface of the glottis. Keratotic (white) lesions of the vocal fold represent most of the dysplastic lesions of the glottis (**Fig. 56.8**). Unfortunately, the magnitude and appearance of the keratosis may belie the severity of the cellular atypia or the presence of microinvasive carcinoma. Erythroplasia (red lesions) typically contains carcinoma in situ and is an infrequent finding. Isolated ulceration of the vocal fold in an immunocompetent smoking host who does not have an infectious process typically reflects carcinoma.

Philosophy of Management

Recently, otolaryngologists have incorporated physiological principles of laryngeal sound production into the design of the oncological procedures. By definition, premalignant epithelium is confined to the nonkeratinizing, stratified squamous epithelium and does not affect the layered microstructure of the SLP.

Endoscopic excision is associated with a very low complication rate, which consists mainly of minor

postoperative bleeding and granuloma formation. An en bloc excisional biopsy provides an accurate diagnosis, as well as an effective treatment, and does so with minimal morbidity. Whole-mount-section histological examination of resected specimens prevents overtreatment or undertreatment of small glottic lesions.

Endoscopic Technique

The goal of endoscopic treatment of dysplastic epithelium of the musculomembranous vocal fold is eradication of the disease with maximal preservation of the normal layered microstructure. This approach results in the optimal postoperative voice without compromising complete extirpation of the abnormal epithelium.

The technique for phonomicrosurgical excision of dysplastic laryngeal epithelium is similar in principle to that previously delineated for benign pathology: wide exposure, adequate preexcisional assessment, sufficient preoperative and perioperative planning, knowledge of the delicate layered vocal fold microanatomy, and experience with sharp microlaryngeal instrumentation to be able to perform a complete en bloc resection of only the involved epithelium and a 1 mm rim of normal-appearing margin. In the example presented in **Fig. 56.8**, involvement of the anterior commissure requires two additional technical considerations: (1) a vocal fold spreader should be used for work at the anterior commissure, and (2) the two sides should be staged at 2 to 3 months to avoid webbing.

In addition to improving preexcisional assessment of lesion depth, part of the preexcision planning—the subepithelial saline–epinephrine infusion into the Reinke space—assists with the technical execution of the surgery in several ways:

1. The infusion facilitates mucosal incisions by improving visualization of the lateral border of the lesion and by distending the SLP so that the overlying epithelium is under tension.
2. The infusion also increases the depth of the SLP, which facilitates less traumatic dissection in this layer and leads to regenerated epithelium that is more flexible.
3. The epinephrine and hydrostatic pressure of the infusion vasoconstricts microvasculature in the SLP, which improves visualization and precise dissection.
4. If the CO_2 laser is used, the saline acts as a heat sink, which decreases thermal trauma to the normal vocal fold tissue.

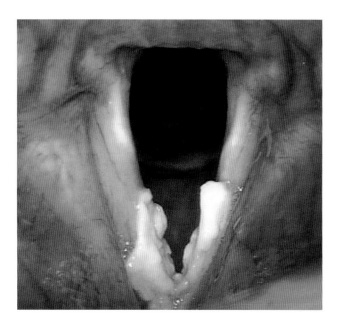

Fig. 56.8 An example of a bilateral laryngeal keratosis involving the anterior commissure. Work on these lesions should be staged to avoid webbing.

Summary

Every substantive innovation in endoscopic surgery of the larynx enhanced precision and, in turn, improved postoperative laryngeal function (airway, swallowing, and voice). Endoscopic voice surgery for both benign and malignant disease is a physiologically based phonomicrosurgical approach. It has developed from the convergence of microlaryngoscopic surgical technique theory with mucosal-wave theory of laryngeal sound production. Furthermore, phonomicrosurgery will continue to evolve as a result of the collaboration of surgeons with voice scientists, speech pathologists, and other voice professionals.

Suggested Reading

Eckel HE, Thumfart WF. Laser surgery for the treatment of larynx carcinomas: indications, techniques, and preliminary results. Ann Otol Rhinol Laryngol 1992;101(2 Pt 1):113–118

Ford C, Bless D, eds. Phonosurgery: Assessment and Surgical Management of Voice Disorders. New York, NY: Raven; 1991

Haben MC. Adult Laryngotracheal Papillomatosis. February 2009. http://www.entnet.org/academyu

Hirano GM. Phonosurgical anatomy of the larynx. In: Ford C, Bless D, eds. Phonosurgery. New York, NY: Raven; 1991:25–41

Hirano GM. Structure of the vocal fold in normal and diseased states: anatomical and physical studies. In: Ludlow CK, O'Connell-Hart M, eds. Proceedings of the Conference on the Assessment of Vocal Pathology. ASHA Report 11. Rockville, MD: American Speech-Language-Hearing Association; 1981:11–27

Hirano M, Hirade Y, Kawasaki H. Vocal function following carbon dioxide laser surgery for glottic carcinoma. Ann Otol Rhinol Laryngol 1985;94(3):232–235

Isshiki N. Phonosurgery: Theory and Practice. New York, NY: Springer-Verlag; 1989

Isshiki N. Vibration of the vocal folds. In: Isshiki N. Phonosurgery: Theory and Practice. Tokyo, Japan: Springer-Verlag; 1989:7–11

Kass ES, Hillman RE, Zeitels SM. Vocal fold submucosal infusion technique in phonomicrosurgery. Ann Otol Rhinol Laryngol 1996;105(5):341–347

Koufman JA. The endoscopic management of early squamous carcinoma of the vocal cord with the carbon dioxide surgical laser: clinical experience and a proposed subclassification. Otolaryngol Head Neck Surg 1986;95(5):531–537

McGuirt WF, Blalock D, Koufman JA, Feehs RS. Voice analysis of patients with endoscopically treated early laryngeal carcinoma. Ann Otol Rhinol Laryngol 1992;101(2 Pt 1):142–146

Shapshay SM, Rebeiz EE, Bohigian RK, Hybels RL. Benign lesions of the larynx: should the laser be used? Laryngoscope 1990; 100(9):953–957

Zeitels SM. Laser versus cold instruments for microlaryngoscopic surgery. Laryngoscope 1996;106(5 Pt 1):545–552

Zeitels SM. Phonomicrosurgical treatment of early glottic cancer and carcinoma in situ. Am J Surg 1996;172(6):704–709

Zeitels SM. Premalignant epithelium and microinvasive cancer of the vocal fold: the evolution of phonomicrosurgical management. Laryngoscope 1995;105(3 Pt 2):1–51

Zeitels SM, Hillman RE, Bunting GW, Vaughn T. Reinke's edema: phonatory mechanisms and management strategies. Ann Otol Rhinol Laryngol 1997;106(7 Pt 1):533–543

Zeitels SM, Vaughan CW. "External counterpressure" and "internal distention" for optimal laryngoscopic exposure of the anterior glottal commissure. Ann Otol Rhinol Laryngol 1994;103(9): 669–675

57 Management of Chronic Aspiration

■ Introduction

Aspiration is defined as misdirection of pharyngeal contents below the vocal cords. It can result from oropharyngeal dysphagia or laryngopharyngeal reflux. This chapter discusses chronic aspiration secondary to oropharyngeal dysphagia. The reader should understand that there is debate in the literature regarding the evaluation and treatment of aspiration.

Consequences of Aspiration

Nocturnal aspiration is known to occur in a large percentage of normal adults without known clinical consequences. What, then, determines whether a patient with oropharyngeal aspiration will develop pneumonia or other pulmonary sequelae, such as diffuse aspiration bronchiolitis or chronic obstructive pulmonary disease? Although the answer to this question is not yet clear, such factors as the quantity and frequency of aspiration, the pH of the aspirated material, and underlying host defenses are all important.

Causes of Aspiration

The causes of chronic aspiration are myriad, and a detailed discussion is beyond the scope of this review. However, causes can be briefly outlined as follows:

1. *Neurologic* Cerebrovascular accident, head trauma, cerebral palsy, myasthenia gravis, multiple sclerosis, amyotrophic lateral sclerosis, and Parkinson disease
2. *Muscular* Oculopharyngeal muscular dystrophy, inclusion body myositis,

inflammatory myopathy, dermatomyositis/polymyositis, muscular dystonias, and Zenker diverticulum
3. *Structural* Strictures, webs, neoplasia, and postsurgical and postradiation fibrosis
4. *Other* Tracheotomy tube, salivary gland dysfunction, and medications (e.g., phenothiazines, benzodiazepines)

Of these, tracheotomy bears some elaboration. There are several reasons a tracheotomy tube predisposes patients to aspiration. This includes tethering of the larynx, which prevents full upward motion on swallowing; loss of laryngeal adductor reflexes, leaving the glottis open during swallowing; esophageal compression by the inflated balloon; and interference with the rise of subglottic pressure during swallowing.

■ Evaluation

Patients can be evaluated for dysphagia and aspiration by bedside evaluation, head and neck examination with flexible laryngoscopy, and modified barium swallow (MBS).

Bedside Evaluation

Bedside evaluation, usually performed by a speech-language pathologist (SLP), may include observing a patient swallow a 50 or 90 mL bolus of water from a cup. The ability to complete the bolus swallow and the presence or absence of coughing are noted. A few clinicians believe this examination is well correlated with the presence of aspiration detected on videofluoroscopy, whereas others disagree. Nevertheless, most clinicians agree that the bedside evaluation provides only limited information.

Flexible Fiberoptic Laryngoscopy

A full head and neck examination, including flexible fiberoptic laryngoscopy, is most helpful in determining whether there are any structural abnormalities in the head and neck (e.g., tumor) that are causing dysphagia with aspiration. Laryngoscopy is also useful in documenting pooling of secretions in the pharyngeal recesses or postcricoid area, the mobility of the vocal cords, and gross aspiration of oropharyngeal secretions. Also, the presence or absence of coughing in reaction to aspiration can identify silent aspiration. With laryngoscopy, a functional endoscopic evaluation of swallowing (FEES) may be performed, which may also include sensory testing (FEESST).

Modified Barium Swallow

An MBS consists of giving the patient small measured volumes of barium in liquid, paste, and solid forms. The presence of aspiration is easily visualized but cannot be quantified on this examination. If aspiration is present, it can occur before, during, or after the pharyngeal phase of the swallow. Aspiration before the swallow is due to either a loss of bolus control in the oral phase or a delay in initiation of the pharyngeal phase. Aspiration during the swallow results from inadequate protection of the larynx during the pharyngeal phase. Contributing factors include decreased laryngeal elevation, incomplete epiglottic deflection, and incomplete vocal cord adduction. Aspiration after the pharyngeal phase occurs when incompletely cleared residue in the vallecula, piriform sinuses, or pharyngeal diverticulum spills over into the pharynx and then into the unprotected larynx. Identifying which of these dynamics is contributing to aspiration is crucial in determining which textures, positions, and maneuvers are effective in decreasing aspiration in an individual patient.

The MBS and the FEES examinations may be complementary, with each having relative advantages. Advantages of the MBS include being able to evaluate the entire swallow, including the esophageal phase, and better assess upper esophageal sphincter opening and posterior tongue movement. However, the MBS requires transporting the patient to a fluoroscopy suite where radiation is used. FEES examination allows for better examination of the mucosal surfaces, as well as the ability to distinguish "native" secretions from ingested oral challenges. A FEES examination can be performed bedside without the need for radiation equipment. A prospective, randomized study found no difference in pneumonia incidence whether MBS or FEESST was used to guide oral intake.

■ Treatment of Chronic Aspiration

Nonoral Feeding

In treating chronic aspiration, the first decision that needs to be made is whether the patient can tolerate oral feedings. This decision is usually based on the presence or absence of clinical sequelae, such as recurrent pneumonia, rather than solely on the results of the MBS. For example, if a patient is tolerating oral feedings even in the presence of mild-to-moderate (but not severe) aspiration on the MBS, then oral feedings can often be continued. These feedings can be modified with regard to texture and positioning based on the MBS findings, to decrease the chance of untoward sequelae of aspiration. If it is determined that continued oropharyngeal feeding poses too great a risk for aspiration, then the patient should not be fed orally, and alternative nonoral feeding is instituted.

Tracheotomy Tube Manipulation

Although sometimes a tracheotomy tube is useful as a stopgap measure in patients who are aspirating their secretions, it is often a contributing cause of aspiration. Therefore, if a tracheotomy tube is present, every effort should be made to decannulate the patient. If airway constraints preclude this, plugging the tube as often as possible or using a Passy-Muir Tracheostomy and Ventilator Swallowing and Speaking Valve (Passy-Muir, Inc., Irvine, CA) has been shown to decrease aspiration.

Medialization

Patients with laryngeal incompetence secondary to abnormal laryngeal closure might have improved swallowing function from medialization for two reasons. One is that the closure of the glottis can decrease aspiration during the swallow, and the other is that the restored increase in subglottis pressure can improve swallowing efficiency and therefore decrease aspiration from pharyngeal residue. Techniques of medialization include vocal cord injection and thyroplasty type I.

Laryngeal Suspension

Any interference with laryngeal elevation during swallowing can predispose patients to aspiration because the larynx is no longer adequately positioned in the more protected position under the tongue base, and because there will also be decreased epiglottic deflection. Laryngeal suspension is sometimes performed during the primary operation for head and neck tumors. The procedure may be performed in conjunction with the cricopharyngeal myotomy or epiglottopexy.

Cricopharyngeal Myotomy

The cricopharyngeus muscle forms the main portion of the pharyngoesophageal sphincter (PES). In some patients with diffuse pharyngeal muscle weakness, the PES fails to open because the suprahyoid muscles are too weak to effect the anterior-superior laryngeal motion that is largely responsible for PES opening. The bolus then is retained not only in the pharyngeal recesses but also above the functionally narrowed PES. A cricopharyngeal myotomy (CPM) can at least remove a relative outflow obstruction to bolus flow, although it does not address the other issues of pharyngeal dysfunction. A CPM has also been described in conjunction with translaryngeal resection of the cricoid lamina. Botulinum toxin can be injected into the cricopharyngeus to assess effect.

Surgery for Intractable Chronic Aspiration

If the measures already discussed are either not applicable or ineffective in preventing the sequelae of recurrent chronic aspiration, then more definitive measures need to be contemplated. Such measures include laryngeal closure or stenting, laryngotracheal separation, and laryngectomy, all of which have been well documented. In selecting which of these procedures to perform, many factors should be considered, including efficacy in preventing aspiration; risk of complications, including breakdown of the laryngeal closure; voice preservation; reversibility of the procedure; and level of technical difficulty in performing the procedure. Most papers describe these procedures with various modifications, and a few discuss results. There are no studies comparing the efficacy of each of these procedures, probably because there are too few patients in any given study.

In summary, the management of chronic aspiration depends on various factors, including the underlying condition of the patient, the dynamics and etiology of the chronic aspiration, and the severity of aspiration. The literature to date is replete with many possible options, without any large studies to assess the efficacy of one approach compared with another.

■ Suggested Reading

Aviv JE. Prospective, randomized outcome study of endoscopy versus modified barium swallow in patients with dysphagia. Laryngoscope 2000;110(4):563–574

Aviv JE, Kim T, Sacco RL, et al. FEESST: a new bedside endoscopic test of the motor and sensory components of swallowing. Ann Otol Rhinol Laryngol 1998;107(5 Pt 1):378–387

Blitzer A, Krespi YP, Oppenheimer RW, Levine TM. Surgical management of aspiration. Otolaryngol Clin North Am 1988; 21(4):743–750

DePippo KL, Holas MA, Reding MJ. Validation of the 3-oz water swallow test for aspiration following stroke. Arch Neurol 1992; 49(12):1259–1261

Dettelbach MA, Gross RD, Mahlmann J, Eibling DE. Effect of the Passy-Muir Valve on aspiration in patients with tracheostomy. Head Neck 1995;17(4):297–302

Eibling DE, Gross RD. Subglottic air pressure: a key component of swallowing efficiency. Ann Otol Rhinol Laryngol 1996;105(4): 253–258

Eibling DE, Snyderman CH, Eibling C. Laryngotracheal separation for intractable aspiration: a retrospective review of 34 patients. Laryngoscope 1995;105(1):83–85

Eisele DW. Surgical approaches to aspiration. Dysphagia 1991; 6(2):71–78

Feinberg MJ, Ekberg O. Videofluoroscopy in elderly patients with aspiration: importance of evaluating both oral and pharyngeal stages of deglutition. AJR Am J Roentgenol 1991;156(2):293–296

Finucane TE, Bynum JP. Use of tube feeding to prevent aspiration pneumonia. Lancet 1996;348(9039):1421–1424

Gottlieb D, Kipnis M, Sister E, Vardi Y, Brill S. Validation of the 50 ml3 drinking test for evaluation of post-stroke dysphagia. Disabil Rehabil 1996;18(10):529–532

Langmore SE, Schatz K, Olsen N. Fiberoptic endoscopic examination of swallowing safety: a new procedure. Dysphagia 1988; 2(4):216–219

Logemann JA, Rademaker AW, Pauloski BR, Kahrilas PJ. Effects of postural change on aspiration in head and neck surgical patients. Otolaryngol Head Neck Surg 1994;110(2):222–227

Matsuse T, Oka T, Kida K, Fukuchi Y. Importance of diffuse aspiration bronchiolitis caused by chronic occult aspiration in the elderly. Chest 1996;110(5):1289–1293

Mendelsohn M. A guided approach to surgery for aspiration: two case reports. J Laryngol Otol 1993;107(2):121–126

Montgomery WW, Hillman RE, Varvares MA. Combined thyroplasty type I and inferior constrictor myotomy. Ann Otol Rhinol Laryngol 1994;103(11):858–862

Murry T, Wasserman T, Carrau RL, Castillo B. Injection of botulinum toxin A for the treatment of dysfunction of the upper esophageal sphincter. Am J Otolaryngol 2005;26(3):157–162

Muz J, Mathog RH, Nelson R, Jones LA Jr. Aspiration in patients with head and neck cancer and tracheostomy. Am J Otolaryngol 1989;10(4):282–286

Rasley A, Logemann JA, Kahrilas PJ, Rademaker AW, Pauloski BR, Dodds WJ. Prevention of barium aspiration during videofluoroscopic swallowing studies: value of change in posture. AJR Am J Roentgenol 1993;160(5):1005–1009

Shapiro J, Martin S. Disorders of the upper esophageal sphincter. In: Fried MP, ed. The Larynx, a Multidisciplinary Approach. Philadelphia, PA: Mosby–Year Book; 1996:337–356

Silver KH, Van Nostrand D, Kuhlemeier KV, Siebens AA. Scintigraphy for the detection and quantification of subglottic aspiration: preliminary observations. Arch Phys Med Rehabil 1991; 72(11):902–910

Stein M, Williams AJ, Grossman F, Weinberg AS, Zuckerbraun L. Cricopharyngeal dysfunction in chronic obstructive pulmonary disease. Chest 1990;97(2):347–352

St Guily JL, Périé S, Willig TN, Chaussade S, Eymard B, Angelard B. Swallowing disorders in muscular diseases: functional assessment and indications of cricopharyngeal myotomy. Ear Nose Throat J 1994;73(1):34–40

Warwick-Brown NP, Richards AES, Cheesman AD. Epiglottopexy: a modification using additional hyoid suspension. J Laryngol Otol 1986;100(10):1155–1158

58 Diagnosis and Management of Dysarthria

■ Introduction

Up to 51% of adults with acquired communication disorders demonstrate motor speech impairments, of which dysarthria is most common. Dysarthria represents any generalized neuromuscular impairment affecting speech production. In this context, *generalized* means that the motor system is dysfunctional for nonspeech as well as speech activity. Nonspeech activities include mastication and swallowing, and, depending on the neurological insult, even respiration.

Underlying muscular deficiencies associated with dysarthria include impaired muscular tone, strength, speed, range, and accuracy of movement. On this basis, dysarthria is differentiated diagnostically from other speech-specific disorders, including stuttering, apraxia of speech, and functional articulation impairment or developmental phonological disorder. Dysarthria is a problem with the execution of speech due to paralysis, weakness, or loss of coordination of speech musculature, rather than the planning of sensorimotor commands resulting in muscle movements and positioning of musculature needed for speech. Dysarthria is also differentiated from aphasia and other acquired neurogenic language problems and from peripheral musculoskeletal disorders, such as cleft palate or macroglossia, which may also impede speech.

Although the base term *arthric* seems to imply a disorder of articulation, in common clinical usage the meaning of *dysarthria* has been extended to include neuromuscular impairments of all component processes of speech production, including respiration, phonation, articulation, resonance, and prosody. In practice, most individuals with dysarthria tend to exhibit impairments in all or most of these components; however, it is possible to observe isolated impairments (e.g., speech breathing difficulty secondary to spinal cord injury), which are also properly considered dysarthria if speech intelligibility and naturalness are compromised to some extent.

Normal Speech and Dysarthria

Normal speech production requires use of respiratory outflow as the driving energy for sound production, which is transduced into sound by muscular valving either at the level of the vocal folds (for voice production) or at various points of constriction in the pharynx, oral cavity, and velum (for vowel and consonant production). In addition, the resonating properties of both voiced and unvoiced sounds are modified by the shaping and coupling of the pharyngeal, oral, and nasal cavities. Normal speech production uses the structures and functions of the upper aerodigestive pathway, which are common to swallowing and respiration; however, speech production is said to be overlaid upon these more basic, phylogenetically older functions. For example, a decerebrate animal is able to breathe, masticate, and swallow sufficiently for self-maintenance; however, humans require a cerebrum to speak. Thus phylogenetically newer systems, including the cortical motor pathways and the basal ganglia, interact with and regulate the activities of phylogenetically older systems, such as the cerebellum and lower motor neuron levels, during speech production.

The exquisitely precise and rapid bilateral coordination of spinally and cranially innervated musculature of the thorax, larynx, pharynx, and oral cavity exhibited during normal speech production attests to this complex interplay among higher- and lower-level central nervous system (as well as peripheral nervous system) structures. Unfortunately, it also leaves the speech production process peculiarly vulnerable to a wide variety of neuromotor impairments at various levels of the nervous system, all of which may result in some type of dysarthria.

Normal age-related changes occur in several of the structures required for normal speech. Specific changes occur in the lingual musculature, which impact speech, swallowing, and respiratory activity. These include sarcopenia, or muscle fiber loss, with an increase in fatty and connective tissue, and amyloid blood vessel deposits in the muscle and subepithelial layers. Tongue mobility and strength (lingual suction pressure) are also reduced, as well as the isometric pressures in the tongue, and there is decreased overall thickness of the tongue. The balance of muscle fiber to motor neuron changes, with more muscle fibers per motor unit, leading to smaller overall lingual forces. However, the tongue is not affected in isolation because most of the head and neck muscles undergo sarcopenia with aging. This may also underlie the higher susceptibility to motor speech disorders, as well as obstructive sleep apnea, in which the tongue can play a central role.

Dysarthria may be subclassified on the basis of age at onset (e.g., developmental dysarthria is associated with cerebral palsy), by the musculature or nerves affected, or by specific etiology. However, the most widely used classification scheme remains that promulgated by researchers at the Mayo Clinic. This scheme classifies dysarthrias on the basis of the nature of the underlying neuromuscular impairment (i.e., flaccid, spastic, ataxic, hypokinetic, hyperkinetic, and mixed) as a consequence of damage or dysfunction of specific neuromotor subsystems. For example, ataxic dysarthria is ascribed to the cerebellum or its input and output pathways, whereas flaccid dysarthria is ascribed to the lower motor neuron system or final common pathway. By understanding these relationships and their associated symptoms, one can potentially identify a culprit neurological site and better target therapy for the patient. Although distorted speech is indeed the hallmark of dysarthria symptomatology, it is clear that a multiplicity of specific symptoms accounts for this global attribute, and that the symptoms vary markedly across speakers with dysarthria (**Table 58.1**).

■ Evaluation and Diagnosis of Dysarthria

Diagnostic assessment of dysarthria involves a variety of formal and informal clinical and instrumental tests. Because the diagnosis pertains to the effects of a primary physical deficit upon the production of speech, a speech-language pathologist is typically consulted. According to Darley et al, the diagnosis of

Table 58.1 Symptoms of dysarthria

Type of dysarthria	Site of lesion	Neuromuscular deficit	Perceptual characteristics
Flaccid (myasthenia, bulbar palsy)	Lower motor neuron or peripheral motor neuron	Weakness and low muscle tone	Hypernasality, imprecise consonant productions, breathy voice
Spastic (pseudobulbar palsy)	Pyramidal or extrapyramidal	Increased muscle tone, reduced ROM, strength, speed	Imprecise articulation, hypernasality, strained, strangled, harsh voice monotonous pitch and loudness
Ataxic	Cerebellum	Inaccurate range, timing direction; low muscle tone; decreased speed of movement	Imprecise, irregular and slow articulation, rhythm disturbance excess and equal stress and loudness
Hypokinetic (Parkinsonism)	Basal ganglia/ extrapyramidal	Significantly decreased ROM and speed of movement, muscle rigidity, resting tremors	Monopitch/monoloudness, long, inappropriate pauses, accuracy fluctuates widely
Hyperkinetic (Huntington, Tourette chorea, athetosis, dystonia, dyskinesia, voice tremor, myoclonus)	Basal ganglia/ extrapyramidal	Rapid, jerky, uncontrolled movements or slow writhing postures	Coprolalia, echolalia abrupt grunting/ barking (rest as above), harsh voice phonatory breaks
Mixed (ALS, MS, Wilson disease)	Multiple motor systems	Muscle weakness, reduced ROM and speed, intention tremors	ALS—defective articulation, hypernasal, harsh, prosodic disturbances MS—harsh voice, inconsistent articulatory precision and rate Wilson—similar to hypokinetic dysarthria

Abbreviations: ALS, amyotrophic lateral sclerosis; MS, muscular sclerosis; ROM, range of motion.
Data from Robbins J. Upper aerodigestive tract neurofunctional mechanisms: lifelong evolution and exercise. Head Neck 2011; 33(Suppl 1):S30–S36.

dysarthria is largely a perceptual judgment. That is, a primary neuromuscular impairment (e.g., spasticity) may be considered dysarthrogenic only if it has a perceptible effect on speech. Hence, there has been particular emphasis on perceptual methodology in the clinical evaluation of dysarthria.

In the Mayo Clinic framework, the examiner rates 40 specific attributes using a five-point ordinal scale (i.e., normal, mild, moderate, severe, or profound degree of impairment) pertaining to different aspects of respiration, phonation (i.e., pitch and loudness), articulation, resonance, and prosody. These aspects are examined in the context of a connected speech sample, sustained vowels, and syllable repetitions. As seen in **Table 58.1**, various attributes can be associated with particular neurological site lesions.

An overall judgment of dysarthric severity is typically based on ratings of the more global attributes of intelligibility and naturalness of connected speech. *Intelligibility* refers to the extent to which the patient's speech is understood by normal listeners, whereas *naturalness* aptly pertains to how natural speech sounds to others. Naturalness is largely determined by prosody, or the rhythms and melodies of connected speech. Although impairments of intelligibility and naturalness are often correlated, this is not necessarily the case. Moreover, during rehabilitation it may be necessary to make significant compromises in the naturalness dimension to achieve a functional level of intelligibility needed for everyday communication.

To supplement these clinical perceptions, other procedures, including measurement of alternating motion rates for syllable production (diadochokinesis), maximum phonation times, quantification of the exact percentage of intelligibility (words actually understood by listeners), as well as acoustic, aerodynamic, fiberoptic, and fluoroscopic analyses, may be employed both to support the initial diagnosis and to monitor the effects of various forms of treatment. The Frenchay Dysarthria Assessment-2, published in 2008, is a very thorough perceptual assessment tool for dysarthria, with relatively high interrater reliability in measuring intelligibility on several levels. In addition, quality of life can be greatly impacted by dysarthria, and there are several more recent efforts to quantify the impact on affected patients.

In addition to perceptual assessment of dysarthric speech symptoms, evaluation of dysarthria incorporates a detailed examination of the upper aerodigestive mechanism to assess the structure and function of the musculature at rest and during execution of nonspeech motor activity. Attention is given to noting facial symmetry and evaluating tone, sensation, and strength of the lips, tongue, cheeks, jaw, and velum. While recognizing that aerodigestive structures may be impaired in the absence of other neuromuscular dysfunction, it is also of interest to explore for confirmatory signs of neuromuscular impairment external to the vocal tract via observation of station and gait or upper extremity movements (e.g., finger–nose test).

New devices that are primarily of research interest may shed further light on articulatory dynamics, such as three-dimensional (3D) electropalatography, which records real-time tongue-to-palate contacts during speech, and 3D electromagnetic articulography, which records and is able to help quantify real-time movements of the tongue, lips, and jaw during speech. These devices have the potential to be used as biofeedback tools for treatment in the future.

◼ Management of Dysarthria

Dysarthria management is a multifaceted and interdisciplinary endeavor, in which various strategic approaches are used to enhance the comprehensibility of the distorted speech. Rather than attempting to restore the premorbid speech patterns, which is difficult in most neuromuscular pathology, a primary goal of dysarthria management is "compensated intelligibility," enabling patients to make themselves understood in spite of the deficit. Secondary goals include improving speech naturalness and, where necessary, providing alternative systems for functional communication. To accomplish these objectives, a variety of nonbehavioral (medical) and behavioral therapeutic interventions may be considered. Yorkston et al conceptualize the combined application of various procedures as "weights" that may be employed collectively to offset the magnitude of the intelligibility impairment.

Medical and Surgical Interventions

Many interventions are of a more general nature, such as the administration of oral medications (e.g., physostigmine for myasthenia gravis). Neurosurgical procedures, such as thalamotomy, pallidotomy, and deep brain stimulation, have produced only mixed results in the improvement of speech for patients with Parkinson disease, in some cases worsening intelligibility. Other procedures, however, are indicated specifically for the amelioration of the speech disorder.

Medical interventions specifically targeting dysarthria involve a variety of surgical and pharmacological procedures that aim, in whole or in part, to restore speech motor function. The deficient physiology is modified to provide increased physiological support for speech production. An effective pharyngeal flap or veloplasty enables a flaccid dysarthric patient who lacks adequate range of velar movement to close the velopharyngeal portal to prevent nasal escape of airflow during speech production. Patients can also benefit from surgical procedures, such as lateral palatopharyngeal wall narrowing to improve intelligibility. In cases involving laryngeal hyperkinesia, botulinum toxin injection of the vocal folds helps to minimize the effects of intermittent bursts of increased laryngeal muscle tone, thereby improving speech fluency and voice quality, which in turn enhances intelligibility and naturalness. Implantation of a phrenic nerve pacer is an example of a surgical intervention to improve speech production in a case of high cervical spinal cord injury. Patients with ankyloglossia (typically children) benefit from surgical correction by frenulotomy, Z-plasty, and possibly genioglossus myotomy.

The judicious application of such procedures to appropriate candidates should not be overlooked as part of an overall dysarthria rehabilitation plan. The level of evidence for medical and surgical treatments for dysarthria is largely level C given the lack of controlled studies and the plethora of individual case reports or small case series. It is clear that, given the complex pathophysiology of dysarthria, a tailored treatment plan that may or may not include surgery is warranted.

Prosthetic and Augmentative Devices

Several prosthetic devices have been developed to enhance dysarthric speech production. Some of these techniques compensate for impaired physiology by replacing or augmenting the function of the deficient structure(s). For example, for a patient with reduced range of anterior tongue movement, a maxillary pseudopalate effectively lowers the palatal arch and, therefore, may make the difference between production of accurate versus distorted lingua-palatal consonants. Beneficial effects of palatal prostheses for velopharyngeal incompetence have also been reported. An artificial larynx may provide an alternative voice source for cases of dysarthria in which phonation is absent or severely diminished. Rosenbek reports using a "wheelchair paddle" or flat surface attached to a wheelchair, so that patients with respiratory weakness may lean their abdomen against the paddle to enhance exhalatory support for speech production.

Other more generic types of assistive devices include such items as the "pacing board" for individuals with impaired speech rhythm or timing. However, these boards are not universally beneficial, with some studies showing no improvement with simple reduction of speech rate independent of other techniques. A simple portable amplifier can be used to counteract reduced loudness in hypofunctional cases. A new device, the voice-input voice-output communication aid (VIV-OCA), appears promising for dysarthric patients, given its enhanced ability to produce intelligible speech, even

with significantly disordered speech input, improving intelligibility by 67%. These types of speech synthesis technologies are ideal for a patient with severe speech impairments not amenable to treatment.

Behavioral Interventions

Behavioral interventions for dysarthria, typically administered by a speech-language pathologist, include the use of rehabilitative exercise regimens, training of compensatory speaking strategies, and the use of augmentative communication techniques. The premise underlying physical exercise approaches is that, following neurological injury, the functioning of deficient musculature is amenable to some degree of retraining, albeit probably not to the premorbid level of functioning. Dworkin has provided the most fully elaborated exercise program for dysarthria, which addresses underlying neuromuscular deficiencies with exercises targeting the respiratory, resonatory, phonatory, articulatory, and prosodic subsystems for speech production. Such "physical therapy of the vocal tract" has face validity and provides a highly structured drill and practice framework that lends itself readily to detailed documentation of treatment-related change. However, there is a danger that, in structuring such a treatment sequence, clinicians may fail to make the transition between exaggerated nonspeech movements and the movements actually needed for speech production. Recent evidence-based systematic reviews of oral motor exercises using nonspeech tasks have shown equivocal results in improvement of dysarthria. These exercises may include the use of myofunctional therapy, oral stimulating plates, range-of-motion exercises, strengthening exercises, sensory stimulation, and blowing/sucking exercises. In addition, incentive spirometry can teach a patient to use breathing effectively to support speech production by using biofeedback. Ultimately, having improved the underlying physiology to a reasonable extent, it is necessary to instruct a patient in ways of speaking more effectively in functionally meaningful situations.

Retraining the production of specific speech sounds in dysarthria typically involves identifying the distorted sounds and sound patterns associated with particular muscular impairments and exploring compensatory production strategies. For example, a patient with bilabial flaccidity (but relatively intact jaw movement) may not be able to effect a seal needed to produce a bilabial pressure consonant /b/ or /p/, and consequently produces something that sounds more like a weak, distorted /v/ or /f/. With instruction, feedback, and practice, this patient may be able to acquire a labiodental contact sufficient to allow a nonstandard production that is not perceptibly differentiable from the intended sounds. This type of sound-by-sound, or valve-by-valve, orientation, known as a componential approach, is useful in some cases or for specific sounds. However, it may be inefficient for cases in which multiple classes of speech sounds have become distorted.

In contrast to the componential approach, a more global strategy, typically involving a simple modification of the patient's customary production plan, may result in widespread beneficial effects that reverberate throughout the speaking system. One such strategy that has been well documented in recent literature is the Lee Silverman Voice Treatment for Parkinson disease and other types of neurogenic hypofunction, including stroke. In this method, the patient is instructed to increase vocal effort and "think loud," along with other facilitators, such as pushing or bearing down while phonating. Although this effortful mode of speech production may initially seem strange and uncomfortable to the speaker, the resultant acoustic output more closely resembles normal intelligibility and naturalness than does hypokinetic speech.

Speech is not the only facet of communication. Other facets, such as facial expression, body language, and nonverbal gestures, are equally important and can be maximized in the form of augmentative or compensatory strategies for the speech-impaired patient and enhance listeners' intelligibility. A simple alphabet chart can significantly increase listeners' comprehensibility of distorted speech, with the speaker pointing to the first letter of each spoken word. Similarly, the use of naturalistic communicative or pantomimic gestures while talking provides contextualizing information that significantly increases comprehensibility. A communication notebook containing printed words, such as favorite places or the pictures of family members, used while speaking, provides a helpful "low-tech" augmentative solution in some situations.

Multiple Treatment Modalities

Finally, it should be recognized that, in most real-life cases of dysarthria, some combination of medical and behavioral treatments, as well as augmentative techniques, will each contribute to some degree of improved intelligibility and will need to be optimized for improved communicative function. Further, these combinations will vary, depending on the communicative needs of the individual, the functional outcome expectations or prognosis, and the patient's overall physical and cognitive status. Modest gains attained as a result of one treatment modality should not be taken as a sign that treatment is unwarranted. Rather, the cumulative effects of multiple treatment modalities should be regarded as the ultimate goal. The data are clear that approximately two-thirds of adults with central nervous system diseases who are unintelligible at the outset of outpatient speech pathology services (involving multiple modalities) can progress to a significantly improved level of intelligibility after treatment. A higher intensity of treatment is also a key determinant of a greater level of success in the production of intelligible speech in a dysarthric patient.

■ Conclusion

The upper aerodigestive tract and its neurological innervation are responsible for normal speech production. Damage to either the mechanism or the nervous system can result in speech and/or swallowing disorders. Speech disorders are usually treated behaviorally by speech-language pathologists. Otolaryngologists also play an important role in the diagnosis and medical and/or surgical management of dysarthria.

Diagnosis of dysarthria is mainly a perceptual endeavor, with speech intelligibility and naturalness the primary variables of interest. Although mechanistic aspects of neuromuscular dysfunction are initially addressed (via surgery, pharmacology, prosthetics, or physical exercise), there remains in dysarthria a phonetic overlay that exists largely in the ear of the listener. Compensated intelligibility and increased prosodic naturalness, leading to functional communication, are the ultimate goals achieved through intensive behavioral therapy.

■ Suggested Reading

Anderson M, Anzalone J, Holland L, Tracey E. Treatment of language, motor speech impairments, and Dysphagia. Continuum (Minneap Minn) 2011;17(3 Neurorehabilitation):471–493

Bass NH, Morell RM. The neurology of swallowing. In: Groher ME, ed. Dysphagia: Diagnosis and Management. 2nd ed. Stoneham, MA: Butterworth Heinewana; 1992:1–29

Beukelman DR, Garrett KL, Yorkston KM. Augmentative Communication Strategies for Adults with Acute or Chronic Medical Conditions. Baltimore, MD: Paul H. Brookes; 2007

Beukelman DR, Yorkston K. A communication system for the severely dysarthric speaker with an intact language system. J Speech Hear Disord 1977;42(2):265–270

Brookshire RH. Introduction to Neurogenic Communication Disorders. St. Louis, MO: Mosby; 2007

Buder EH, Kent RD, Kent JF, Milenkovic P, Workinger M. Formoffa: an automated formant, moment, fundamental frequency, amplitude analysis of normal and disordered speech. Clin Linguist Phon 1996;10(1):31–54

Bunton K. Speech versus nonspeech: different tasks, different neural organization. Semin Speech Lang 2008;29(4):267–275

Cannito MP, Marquardt TP. Ataxic dysarthria. In: McNeil M, ed. Clinical Management of Sensorimotor Speech Disorders. New York, NY: Thieme; 1997:217–248

Choi YS, Lim JS, Han KT, Lee WS, Kim MC. Ankyloglossia correction: Z-plasty combined with genioglossus myotomy. J Craniofac Surg 2011;22(6):2238–2240

Darley FL, Aronson AE, Brown JR. Motor Speech Disorders. Philadelphia, PA: WB Saunders; 1975

DeWalt DA, Rothrock N, Yount S, Stone AA; PROMIS Cooperative Group. Evaluation of item candidates: the PROMIS qualitative item review. Med Care 2007;45(5, Suppl 1):S12–S21

Donovan NJ, Kendall DL, Young ME, Rosenbek JC. The communicative effectiveness survey: preliminary evidence of construct validity. Am J Speech Lang Pathol 2008;17(4):335–347

Duffy JR. Motor Speech Disorders: Substrates, Differential Diagnosis, and Management. St. Louis, MO: Mosby–Year Book; 1995

Dworkin JP. Motor Speech Disorders: A Treatment Guide. St. Louis, MO: Mosby–Year Book; 1991

Enderby P, Palmer R. FDA-2: Frenchay Dysarthria Assessment, Examiner's Manual. 2nd ed. Austin, TX: Pro-Ed; 2008

Garcia JM, Cannito MP. Influence of verbal and nonverbal contexts on the sentence intelligibility of a speaker with dysarthria. J Speech Hear Res 1996;39(4):750–760

Hawley MS, Cunningham SP, Green PD, et al. A voice-input-voice-output communication aid for people with severe speech impairment. IEEE Trans Neural Syst Rehabil Eng 2013;21(1):23–31

Hoit JD, Shea SA. Speech production and speech with a phrenic nerve pacer. Am J Speech Lang Pathol 1996;5:53–60

Johns DF, Cannito MP, Rohrich RJ, Tebbetts JB. The self-lined superiorly based pull-through velopharyngoplasty: plastic surgery-speech pathology interaction in the management of velopharyngeal insufficiency. Plast Reconstr Surg 1994;94(3):436–445

Jones HN, Donovan NJ, Sapienza CM, Shrivastav R, Fernandez HH, Rosenbek JC. Expiratory muscle strength training in the treatment of mixed dysarthria in a patient with Lance-Adams syndrome. J Med Speech-Lang Pathol 2006;14:207–217

Klostermann F, Ehlen F, Vesper J, et al. Effects of subthalamic deep brain stimulation on dysarthrophonia in Parkinson's disease. J Neurol Neurosurg Psychiatry 2008;79(5):522–529

Kolb B, Wishaw IQ. Fundamentals of Human Neuropsychology. 4th ed. New York, NY: W.H. Freeman; 1996.

Larson C. Neurophysiology of speech and swallowing. Semin Speech Lang 1985;6:275–291

Maas E, Robin DA, Austermann Hula SN, et al. Principles of motor learning in treatment of motor speech disorders. Am J Speech Lang Pathol 2008;17(3):277–298

Mahler LA, Ramig LO. Intensive treatment of dysarthria secondary to stroke. Clin Linguist Phon 2012;26(8):681–694

McCauley RJ, Strand E, Lof GL, Schooling T, Frymark T. Evidence-based systematic review: effects of nonspeech oral motor exercises on speech. Am J Speech Lang Pathol 2009;18(4):343–360

Murdoch BE. Physiological investigation of dysarthria: recent advances. Int J Speech-Language Pathol 2011;13(1):28–35

Murdoch BE. Surgical approaches to treatment of Parkinson's disease: Implications for speech function. Int J Speech-Language Pathol 2010;12(5):375–384

Netsell R, Daniel B. Dysarthria in adults: physiologic approach to rehabilitation. Arch Phys Med Rehabil 1979;60(11):502–508

Netsell R, Lotz W, Barlow SM. A speech physiology examination for individuals with dysarthria. In: Yorkston KR, Beukelman DR, eds. Recent Advances in Clinical Dysarthria. Boston, MA: Little, Brown; 1989:3–37

Ramig LO, Bonitati CM, Lemke JH, Horii Y. Voice therapy for patients with Parkinson's disease: development of an approach and preliminary efficacy data. J Med Speech-Lang Pathol 1994;2:191–210

Ramig LO, Pawlas AA, Countryman S. The Lee Silverman Voice Treatment: A Practical Guide for Treating the Voice and Speech Disorders in Parkinson's Disease. Iowa City, IA: The National Center for Voice and Speech; 1995

Robbins J. Upper aerodigestive tract neurofunctional mechanisms: lifelong evolution and exercise. Head Neck 2011;33(Suppl 1):S30–S36

Rosenbek JC. Selected alternatives to articulation training for the dysarthric adult. In: Winitz H, ed. Treating Articulation Disorders: For Clinicians by Clinicians. Austin, TX: Pro-Ed; 1984.

Rosenbek JC, LaPointe L. The dysarthrias: description, diagnosis and treatment. In: Johns DF, ed. Clinical Management of Neurogenic Communicative Disorders. Boston, MA: Little, Brown; 1985:97–152

Van Nuffelen G, De Bodt M, Wuyts F, Van de Heyning P. The effect of rate control on speech rate and intelligibility of dysarthric speech. Folia Phoniatr Logop 2009;61(2):69–75

Yorkston KM. Treatment Efficacy Summary: Dysarthria (Neurologic Motor Speech Impairment). American Speech-Language Hearing Association Web site. http://www.asha.org/

Yorkston K, Beukelman D. Assessment of Intelligibility of Dysarthric Speech. Austin, TX: Pro-Ed; 1981

Yorkston KM, Hakel M, Beukelman DR, Fager S. Evidence for effectiveness of treatment of loudness, rate or prosody in dysarthria: a systematic review. J Med Speech-Lang Pathol 2007;15(2):xi–xxxvi

Yorkston KM, Strand EA, Kennedy RT. Comprehensibility of dysarthric speech: implications for assessment and treatment planning. Am J Speech Lang Pathol 1995;5:55–66

59 Recurrent Respiratory Papillomatosis

■ Introduction

Papilloma is the most common benign laryngeal neoplasm. Although this lesion has a particular predilection for the larynx, the entire upper respiratory tract—from the nasal vestibule to the peripheral lung—is at risk. The lesions are histologically benign; however, rapid growth may threaten airway patency, and repeated surgical excisions may be needed.

Although historically known by different names, the preferred term for this disease, *recurrent respiratory papillomatosis* (RRP), refers to both the juvenile and the adult disorders and describes the widespread extent of disease and its tendency for repeated regrowth. Approximately half of RRP cases are designated *juvenile onset* (JO)—that is, initial lesions appear from early infancy up through age 12 years. *Adult onset* (AO) RRP includes patients in whom initial diagnosis occurs as late as the seventh or eighth decade of life, although the peak incidence is during the third and fourth decades. Initial presentation of papilloma between ages 12 and 20 years is less common.

JO-RRP typically presents with hoarseness attributable to vocal fold lesions that interfere with phonation. The smaller size of the infant and pediatric larynges predisposes to upper airway obstruction in the face of rapid growth of the papilloma. Among patients with JO-RRP, males and females are afflicted in equal numbers. AO-RRP is histologically indistinguishable from JO-RRP. Clinically, the lesions are more often solitary. Upper airway obstruction occurs less frequently in AO-RRP because of the larger adult laryngotracheal dimensions. In contrast to JO-RRP, there is a distinct male predominance among AO-RRP patients.

Etiology

Human papillomavirus (HPV) types 6 and 11 have been identified in respiratory papillomata and genital warts. This double-stranded deoxyribonucleic acid (DNA) virus infects cells within the basal layer of the mucosa. Although more than 100 serotypes of the HPV virus have been identified, types 6 and 11 are the most commonly found in RRP. The serotypes 16 and 18, though less common, are thought to have a greater malignant potential than 6 and 11.

Epidemiology

In the United States, the incidence rate of JO-RRP is 4.3 per 100,000 people and 1.8 per 100,000 for AO-RRP. A history of maternal condyloma is elicited in 30 to 50% of patients with JO-RRP. Transmission of HPV infection is presumed to occur during passage of the newborn through an HPV-infected birth canal. The prevalence of genital condyloma in women of child-bearing age far exceeds the reported number of new cases of respiratory papillomatosis. Between 1 per 230 to 400 children born via vaginal delivery to a mother with active condylomata will develop RRP. However, transmission has occurred even after Caesarian section delivery, suggesting a possible in utero mechanism. In addition, while HPV has been found in 30% of nasopharyngeal secretions of infants exposed to HPV in the birth canal, only a small percentage of these children develop RRP.

AO-RRP has been presumed to occur on the basis of sexual contact, mainly oral-genital exposure. AO-RRP subjects report more lifetime sex partners and higher frequency of oral sex than adult controls. Some cases of AO-RRP have a lifelong history of hoarseness, which suggests the alternative possibility that initial viral transmission and infection had occurred at childbirth, but that the infection remained dormant until diagnosis in adulthood. Transmission of HPV infection through oropharyngeal secretions is rare. There has been no documented case of RRP occurring among siblings, marital partners, or family members who are constantly exposed to secretions from papillomatosis patients.

■ Evaluation

Clinical Manifestations

Childhood

Inasmuch as the vocal fold is usually the first and predominant site of a papilloma lesion, hoarseness is the cardinal symptom in JO-RRP and AO-RRP. In JO-RRP, it is not unusual for family members to remark that the voice was hoarse or "weak" from the time of initial vocal utterance. JO-RRP is most commonly diagnosed between the ages of 2 and 4, and 75% of patients with JO-RRP are diagnosed by the age of 5.

Upper airway obstructive symptoms of varying severity often worsen during upper respiratory tract infection. In preschool children, whose airway dimensions are small, the initial presentation may occur as a sudden airway crisis, accompanying an otherwise routine respiratory tract infection.

Adolescence

The severity of symptoms often diminishes at puberty, when the adult-sized larynx is developed. Coincident with this lessening in clinical severity, the intervals between operations lengthen. The symptoms may diminish to the point that the patient ceases to consult the otolaryngologist, although active papillomatous lesions may remain. An undetermined proportion of patients may achieve spontaneous remission from papilloma regrowth, but the belief that JO-RRP always undergoes spontaneous remission at puberty is unwarranted: numerous adults have persistent papillomatosis, whose childhood onset is well documented.

Adulthood

Due to the larger size of the larynx, papillomatosis in adulthood is not usually as severe as in younger patients. The growth rate is slower than that occurring in JO-RRP. In women, accelerated regrowth of papilloma occurs during pregnancy, particularly during the third trimester. Respiratory papillomas have widespread anatomical distribution. The nasal vestibule, the nasopharyngeal surface of the soft palate, the midzone on the laryngeal surface of the epiglottis, the immediate undersurface of the vestibular fold, the upper- and undersurface of the vocal folds, the carina, and the bronchial spurs are sites where the papillomas commonly occur. It has been observed that the ciliated respiratory epithelium meets squamous epithelium at these sites. The squamociliary junction has been suggested as a particular site of predilection for papilloma lesions. Iatrogenic squamociliary junctions may be produced after procedures, such as tracheostomy, where the metaplastic squamous epithelium in a tracheostomy tract meets the ciliated epithelium of the trachea.

Intraoral papilloma have been identified on the soft palate, uvula, tonsils, and tonsillar fossae, as well as on the alveolar mucosa and tongue. Oral lesions have an association with a wider range of HPV types. The larynx is the most commonly affected site. The subglottic larynx and tracheobronchial tree are rarely, if ever, the site of disease in the absence of laryngeal lesions. Tracheal, bronchial, and pulmonary papillomatosis occurs in a stepwise fashion. Papillomas are rarely observed at these sites at initial presentation. The history of tracheotomy is present in a high proportion of patients with tracheobronchial spread of papilloma and underscores the importance of atraumatic instrumentation and avoidance of tracheotomy.

Pulmonary papilloma usually presents initially as an asymptomatic noncalcified nodule in the pulmonary parenchyma; slow enlargement and central cavitation occur late. Pulmonary lesions may have widespread distribution, and the radiographic picture is alarming. The clinical course is slowly progressive; pulmonary dysfunction may be surprisingly mild, but respiratory failure and death ultimately occur. Detailed histological examination of pulmonary lesions may reveal sites of squamous metaplasia and unsuspected squamous cell carcinoma.

The malignant transformation of respiratory papillomata squamous carcinoma is unusual and occurs in less than 5% of cases. These malignancies most often occur in the larynx or lung. Neither adult nor childhood cases appear to be disproportionately at risk. Irradiation therapy and tobacco use have long been thought to be factors that increase the risk for this malignant transformation.

Pathology

The typical clinical appearance of a papilloma is that of a multinodular growth, which may present as a solitary exophytic lesion arising from a narrow or broad-based stalk, or as a velvety, sheetlike abnormality mimicking an inflammatory reaction, rather than a benign neoplasm. This latter type of lesion is most frequently encountered on the vocal fold, where the confluent growth spreads to involve the entire epithelium. In its most severe form, particularly in childhood, the tumor may resemble a cauliflower firmly impacting the laryngeal aperture, with near-total obliteration of the airway.

The exophytic and sessile types of papilloma also occur in the tracheobronchial tree. The earliest lesions may appear as small, pale, buttonlike lesions, with a central vascular tuft being the telltale feature identifying these as early papilloma.

Histologically, the papilloma consists of stratified, squamous epithelium with a vascularized connective tissue stroma. There is increased proliferation of epithelial cells with abnormal differentiation, including nuclear retention in the superficial layers. The presence of cells with hyperchromatic nuclei surrounded by a large, clear transparent space (a koilocyte) is regarded as a histological feature implicating a viral etiology.

HPV DNA has been documented in normal-appearing epithelium in RRP patients during complete clinical remission. Although the implication of this viral presence is not known, documentation of widespread distribution of HPV DNA may partially explain the relapses that may occur after complete remission of variable duration and the susceptibility of traumatized epithelium to form new papilloma lesions.

■ Treatment

The clinical course of RRP is predictably unpredictable. The cornerstone of papilloma management is endoscopic excision under magnified visualization. Total disease elimination is *not* the objective at every surgical intervention, particularly if there is risk of damage to normal laryngotracheal anatomy and function. Because there is a known risk for malignant transformation, biopsy is recommended at the time of surgical intervention.

Endoscopic excision is accomplished most commonly through microlaryngeal techniques, often using laser or microdebrider instruments. Numerous lasers have been used in the treatment of RRP, including the carbon dioxide (CO_2), potassium-titanyl-phosphate (KTP), and pulse-dyed lasers. These latter two lasers are also amenable to in-office, unsedated technique and are associated with less injury to the laryngeal epithelium.

The microdebrider has also been used with success. One study comparing CO_2 versus microdebrider found that, for disease of equal severity, the microdebrider was associated with an equal pain score 24 hours postoperatively, the microdebrider group rated better voice quality 24 hours postoperatively, and the microdebrider had shorter procedure times and lower procedure costs.

Tracheostomy is reserved for extreme cases with impending airway loss because this operation may result in the papilloma spreading into the tracheobronchial system. More than half of RRP children with a tracheostomy had tracheal papilloma. Irradiation therapy is generally not recommended for treatment of histological benign papillomatosis and is used only in exceptional circumstances.

Nonsurgical Treatment Adjuvants

While surgery is the main treatment modality for RRP, adjuvant medical therapy may be used in select patient populations to help control the disease. An RRP task force has generated consensus recommendations on when to use adjuvant therapy. These indications include more than four surgical procedures per year, rapid growth of papilloma with airway compromise, and distal multisite spread of disease.

Antivirals are the most commonly used adjuvant therapy for RRP. Multiple antivirals have been used in patients with RRP with mixed results. Although many case reports and case series support the use of antivirals as adjuvant therapy, a recent Cochrane review evaluating the effectiveness of antivirals in treatment of RRP determined there is insufficient evidence to support the efficacy of antivirals as adjuvant therapy to manage RRP.

Cidofovir is the most commonly used adjuvant antiviral medication in children with RRP. Of note, this cytosine nucleoside analogue is only approved by the U.S. Food and Drug Administration (FDA) for the treatment of cytomegalovirus retinitis. Cidofovir has been used for many years as an intralesional injection adjuvant treatment for RRP and, more recently, has been introduced as an inhalational form. Multiple case reports and case series support the use of intralesional cidofovir, with both short- and long-term responses that increase the time between surgeries for patients with RRP. There is a reported risk of carcinogenicity with cidofovir demonstrated in animal studies, and a case report of dysplasia in patients with RRP treated with cidofovir, so careful informed consent should be performed prior to treatment with this medication.

Other antiviral medications, including a-interferon, ribavirin, and acyclovir, are also used as adjuvant treatment in complicated RRP patients. Multiple case reports and case series exist that mention decreased intervals between surgeries with the use of these medications in patients with RRP; however, their use is limited due to their systemic side effects.

Another adjuvant treatment for patients with RRP is indole-3-carbinol, a dietary supplement found in leafy green vegetables. RRP lesions have been demonstrated to increase estrogen binding, and indole-3-carbinol use in mice has been shown to decrease estrogen metabolism and reduce the formation of HPV-induced papilloma. Rosen and Bryson performed a multicenter phase 1 clinical trial on 18 patients with RRP and found that, after complete surgical removal of papilloma and then treatment with indole-3-carbinol, one-third of patients had no further papilloma growth, one-third had decreased papilloma growth, and one-third had no response. More complete studies are needed to evaluate the effectiveness of this therapy for RRP patients.

Although the traditional therapies already mentioned are used as adjuvant treatment for RRP patients, a few emerging treatment options are promising as adjuvant therapy. The FDA has recently approved two HPV vaccines for use. Gardasil (Merck, Whitehouse Station, NJ), a quadrivalent HPV vaccine against HPV types 6, 11, 16, and 18, is FDA approved for use in females ages 9 to 26 for prevention of vulvar, vaginal, and uterine cancer and prevention of genital warts and in males ages 9 to 26 for prevention of genital warts. Cervarix (GlaxoSmithKline, Philadelphia, PA), a bivalent HPV vaccine against HPV types 16 and 18, is FDA approved for use in females ages 9 to 25 for prevention of cervical cancer. There are multiple ongoing studies in the literature of these vaccines' effectiveness in prevention of these diseases. Given the short period of time these products have been on the market, more studies with longer follow-up are needed to determine their effectiveness.

Derkay and colleagues recently introduced the use of another form of HPV-specific immunotherapy, HSP-E7, for RRP patients. Heat-shock protein (Hsp)E7 is a recombinant fusion protein derived from *Mycobacterium bovis* bacillus Calmette-Guérin Hsp65, fused to the E7 protein of HPV 16. The effectiveness of this vaccine has been demonstrated by inducing lesion regression in women with high-grade cervical intraepithelial neoplasia. Derkay and colleagues performed an open-label, single-arm, muilticenter interventional study to evaluate the effect of HspE7 on 27 total patients with RRP. After baseline debulking of papilloma lesions, the patients received subcutaneous injections of HspE7 every 28 days for a total of three doses. Overall, patients demonstrated increased intersurgical intervals and decreased number of surgeries with the use of HspE7. More detailed studies are needed to confirm these results.

Sublesional injection of bevacizumab has recently been introduced as a potential adjuvant treatment modality for RRP in combination with KTP laser excision. Bevacizumab is a monoclonal antibody that blocks vascular endothelial growth factor, preventing angiogenesis. Zeitels and colleagues analyzed 20 adult patients with bilateral laryngeal RRP. They performed bevacizumab sublesional injection on one side of each patient and saline injection on the contralateral side and then debulked the papilloma with KTP laser. They found that 3 of the 20 patients had complete resolution of disease, 16 had less disease, and 1 had more disease on the bevacizumab-injected side. A larger number of patients is needed to evaluate the usefulness of this medication in RRP patients.

■ Suggested Reading

Armstrong LR, Derkay CS, Reeves WC. Initial results from the national registry for juvenile-onset recurrent respiratory papillomatosis. RRP Task Force. Arch Otolaryngol Head Neck Surg 1999;125(7):743–748

Chadha NK, James A. Adjuvant antiviral therapy for recurrent respiratory papillomatosis. Cochrane Database Syst Rev 2010;(1):CD005053

Chadha NK, James AL. Antiviral agents for the treatment of recurrent respiratory papillomatosis: a systematic review of the English-language literature. Otolaryngol Head Neck Surg 2007;136(6):863–869

Cohn AM, Kos JT II, Taber LH, Adam E. Recurring laryngeal papillopa. Am J Otolaryngol 1981;2(2):129–132

Derkay C; Multi-Disciplinary Task Force on Recurrent Respiratory Papillomas. Cidofovir for recurrent respiratory papillomatosis (RRP): a re-assessment of risks. Int J Pediatr Otorhinolaryngol 2005;69(11):1465–1467

Derkay CS. Recurrent respiratory papillomatosis. Laryngoscope 2001;111(1):57–69

Derkay CS. Task force on recurrent respiratory papillomas. A preliminary report. Arch Otolaryngol Head Neck Surg 1995;121(12):1386–1391

Derkay CS, Smith RJ, McClay J, et al. HspE7 treatment of pediatric recurrent respiratory papillomatosis: final results of an open-label trial. Ann Otol Rhinol Laryngol 2005;114(9):730–737

Donne AJ, Hampson L, Homer JJ, Hampson IN. The role of HPV type in recurrent respiratory papillomatosis. Int J Pediatr Otorhinolaryngol 2010;74(1):7–14

Freed GL, Derkay CS. Prevention of recurrent respiratory papillomatosis: role of HPV vaccination. Int J Pediatr Otorhinolaryngol 2006;70(10):1799–1803

Kashima H, Mounts P, Leventhal B, Hruban RH. Sites of predilection in recurrent respiratory papillomatosis. Ann Otol Rhinol Laryngol 1993;102(8 Pt 1):580–583

Kashima HK, Shah F, Lyles A, et al. A comparison of risk factors in juvenile-onset and adult-onset recurrent respiratory papillomatosis. Laryngoscope 1992;102(1):9–13

Koss LG, Durfee GR. Unusual patterns of squamous epithelium of the uterine cervix: cytologic and pathologic study of koilocytotic atypia. Ann N Y Acad Sci 1956;63(6):1245–1261

Ksiazek J, Prager JD, Sun GH, Wood RE, Arjmand EM. Inhaled cidofovir as an adjuvant therapy for recurrent respiratory papillomatosis. Otolaryngol Head Neck Surg 2011;144(4):639–641

Mounts P, Shah KV, Kashima H. Viral etiology of juvenile- and adult-onset squamous papilloma of the larynx. Proc Natl Acad Sci U S A 1982;79(17):5425–5429

Newfield L, Goldsmith A, Bradlow HL, Auborn K. Estrogen metabolism and human papillomavirus-induced tumors of the larynx: chemo-prophylaxis with indole-3-carbinol. Anticancer Res 1993;13(2):337–341

Pasquale K, Wiatrak B, Woolley A, Lewis L. Microdebrider versus CO2 laser removal of recurrent respiratory papillomas: a prospective analysis. Laryngoscope 2003;113(1):139–143

Quick CA, Watts SL, Krzyzek RA, Faras AJ. Relationship between condylomata and laryngeal papillomata. Clinical and molecular virological evidence. Ann Otol Rhinol Laryngol 1980;89(5 Pt 1):467–471

Roman LD, Wilczynski S, Muderspach LI, et al. A phase II study of Hsp-7 (SGN-00101) in women with high-grade cervical intraepithelial neoplasia. Gynecol Oncol 2007;106(3):558–566

Rosen CA, Bryson PC. Indole-3-carbinol for recurrent respiratory papillomatosis: long-term results. J Voice 2004;18(2):248–253

Schraff S, Derkay CS, Burke B, Lawson L. American Society of Pediatric Otolaryngology members' experience with recurrent respiratory papillomatosis and the use of adjuvant therapy. Arch Otolaryngol Head Neck Surg 2004;130(9):1039–1042

Silverberg MJ, Thorsen P, Lindeberg H, Grant LA, Shah KV. Condyloma in pregnancy is strongly predictive of juvenile-onset recurrent respiratory papillomatosis. Obstet Gynecol 2003;101(4):645–652

Smith EM, Pignatari SS, Gray SD, Haugen TH, Turek LP. Human papillomavirus infection in papillomas and nondiseased respiratory sites of patients with recurrent respiratory papillomatosis using the polymerase chain reaction. Arch Otolaryngol Head Neck Surg 1993;119(5):554–557

Steinberg BM, Topp WC, Schneider PS, Abramson AL. Laryngeal papillomavirus infection during clinical remission. N Engl J Med 1983;308(21):1261–1264

Syrjänen SM, Syrjänen KJ, Happonen RP. Human papillomavirus (HPV) DNA sequences in oral precancerous lesions and squamous cell carcinoma demonstrated by in situ hybridization. J Oral Pathol 1988;17(6):273–278

Tasca RA, Clarke RW. Recurrent respiratory papillomatosis. Arch Dis Child 2006;91(8):689–691

Valdez TA, McMillan K, Shapshay SM. A new laser treatment for vocal cord papilloma—585-nm pulsed dye. Otolaryngol Head Neck Surg 2001;124(4):421–425

Walsh TE, Beamer PR. Epidermoid carcinoma of the larynx occurring in two children with papilloma of the larynx. Laryngoscope 1950;60(11):1110–1124

Weiss MD, Kashima HK. Tracheal involvement in laryngeal papillomatosis. Laryngoscope 1983;93(1):45–48

Wemer RD, Lee JH, Hoffman HT, Robinson RA, Smith RJ. Case of progressive dysplasia concomitant with intralesional cidofovir administration for recurrent respiratory papillomatosis. Ann Otol Rhinol Laryngol 2005;114(11):836–839

Zeitels SM, Akst LM, Burns JA, Hillman RE, Broadhurst MS, Anderson RR. Office-based 532-nm pulsed KTP laser treatment of glottal papillomatosis and dysplasia. Ann Otol Rhinol Laryngol 2006;115(9):679–685

Zeitels SM, Barbu AM, Landau-Zemer T, et al. Local injection of bevacizumab (Avastin) and angiolytic KTP laser treatment of recurrent respiratory papillomatosis of the vocal folds: a prospective study. Ann Otol Rhinol Laryngol 2011;120(10):627–634

60 Diagnosis and Management of Oropharyngeal Dysphagia

■ Introduction

The upper aerodigestive tract, which consists of the oral, pharyngeal, and nasal cavities, as well as the larynx, serves three functions: swallowing, speech, and respiration. The adult human is the only species in which the larynx assumes a lower position in an elongated pharynx, so the base of the tongue makes up the anterior wall of the oropharynx. This anatomical configuration, which enables humans to speak, yields a bending of the vocal tract that is an important characteristic of the sound-producing apparatus in humans; however, it is not an efficient system for swallowing. The lowered position of the larynx can result in increased risk of choking or aspiration in a patient who has neurological damage or alteration of anatomical structures (e.g., ablative surgery for head and neck cancer). Furthermore, the neurological system controlling the musculature of the upper aerodigestive tract is intricate and complex. Thus, when neurological damage occurs, both swallowing and speech may be affected.

Swallowing dynamics patterned in the brainstem are expressed by the oropharyngeal musculature and are modulated via cortical and reflexogenic influences traveling the trigeminal nerve, facial nerve, last four cranial nerves, and cervical plexus. Sympathetic and parasympathetic control of salivary flow and viscosity ensures appropriate lubrication of the oropharyngeal path. During the oral stage of deglutition, the bolus, prepared by mastication, is squeezed toward the faucial isthmus. The pharyngeal stage starts with tongue base down-thrusting as elevation of the soft palate prevents nasal regurgitation. With anterosuperior laryngeal pull from the suprahyoid muscles, the hypopharynx receives the descending bolus, while the relaxed upper esophageal sphincter (UES) opens for food passage through the cricopharyngeal inlet. Lung protection is further secured by glottic seal supplemented with posterior epiglottic tilt.

Dysphagia is defined as impaired swallowing, which can occur anywhere from the mouth to the stomach, resulting from impaired function of the jaw, lips, tongue, velum, larynx, pharynx, UES, or esophagus. More specifically, *oropharyngeal dysphagia* refers to swallowing disorders involving the oral and pharyngeal cavities, which are distinguished from primary esophageal disorders. Before one can begin to diagnose and treat dysphagia, a comprehensive knowledge of the various aspects of normal swallowing is essential. Any dysfunction of cranial nerves V, VII, IX, X, and XII and corticobulbar pathways can lead to a disordered swallow.

Normal Swallowing

Swallowing can be divided into four stages: (1) oral preparatory, (2) oral, (3) pharyngeal, and (4) esophageal.

Oral Preparatory Stage

The oral preparatory stage involves mastication of semisolid or solid food and formation of a bolus, which renders the food into an appropriate consistency for swallowing, with the bolus being lubricated and chemically altered by being mixed with saliva. This first stage involves lip closure, rotary and lateral motion of the jaw, buccal or facial tone, rotary and lateral motion of the tongue, and anterior bulging of the soft palate. Soft palate bulging prevents premature spillover of food into the pharynx.

Oral Stage

During the oral stage, the bolus of food is transported to the posterior area of the oral cavity. Initially, the tongue tip contacts the anterior portion of the hard palate. The tongue is grooved as its dorsum gradually presses the hard palate and "strips" the bolus back into the oral pharynx. Two distinct patterns of tongue movement during the oral stage have been identified: the "tipper" and the "dipper." The tipper occurs when the bolus is positioned on the dorsum of the tongue, with the tongue tip pressed against the posterior surface of the maxillary incisors. The dipper occurs when the bolus is in the anterior sublingual sulcus, which requires the tongue to elevate the bolus to a supralingual position. Physiologically, four events signal the onset of either the tipper- or the dipper-type swallow: tongue-tip movement, tongue-base movement, superior hyoid movement, and submental movement (electromyographic [EMG] activity).

Pharyngeal Stage

Once an actual swallow is triggered, the pharyngeal stage has begun. The pharyngeal stage guides the bolus through the pharynx into the esophagus, without penetrating into the nasopharynx or larynx, and is an automatic phase governed by the brainstem. Normal pharyngeal swallowing involves palatal closure, bolus transport through the pharynx, glottal closure to prevent aspiration, UES opening and transsphincteric fluid flow, and base of tongue propulsion to the posterior pharyngeal wall. The bolus is transported through the pharynx mainly by the pressure applied by the tongue base directly onto the bolus in the oropharynx. The anatomical and neurological integrity of the tongue plays an important role in bolus transport during both the oral and the pharyngeal stages of swallowing.

The pharyngeal stage is a swallowing response (as opposed to a swallowing reflex) that varies with changes in bolus volume and/or viscosity. For example, there is a progressive increase in the magnitude of superior hyoid movement with increases in the size of the bolus up to a volume of 10 mL. The upward motion of the cricopharyngeus or UES increases with enlarging volumes of liquid. In addition, the diameter and duration of UES opening also increase with larger volumes swallowed. In a barium swallow, increasing the viscosity of barium to a high-density paste results in a greater magnitude of anterior hyoid movement and greater diameter and duration of UES opening, as compared with the same volume of a low-density liquid barium.

Research during the past decade has focused on the mechanism of cricopharyngeal or UES opening. The interrelationship between hyoid/laryngeal movement and UES opening has been established. Anatomically, the cricoid cartilage is linked to the hyoid by muscular and ligamentous connections; it is an insertion point for the cricopharyngeus muscle

as well. As the hyoid moves superiorly and anteriorly during the swallow, the larynx also elevates, which in turn elevates and opens the cricopharyngeus muscle (UES). As a result, in a barium swallow the passage of barium across the UES occurs while the hyoid is at its highest and most anterior point.

In addition to the upward and forward movements of the hyoid and larynx, there is a three-tier protective adduction of the laryngeal structure during the swallow. From a superior to inferior anatomical location, the first level of adduction involves the approximation of the aryepiglottic folds to cover the superior inlet of the larynx. The downward and backward movement of the epiglottis completes this level of closure, preventing food and liquid from entering the laryngeal vestibule. The second layer of adduction is the false vocal folds. The final and most important layer is a forceful adduction at the level of the true vocal folds.

Mechanoreceptors send afferent fibers through the internal branch of the superior laryngeal nerve (SLN) to supply the supraglottic larynx, epiglottis, pyriform sinuses, and base of the tongue. The internal branch of the SLN (ISLN) exhibits both tonic activity and bursts of activity in early and late phases of the swallow cycle. The act of swallowing temporarily halts respiratory airflow at a central level while resetting the respiratory rhythm. As a result, there is a partitioning between bolus transit across the laryngeal opening and inspiratory airflow into the lungs. This naturally aids in protection of the larynx from aspiration. In experiments in which the ISLN afferent function is blocked by lidocaine injection, symptoms include effortful swallow, globus sensation, and loss of airway protection because of poor closure of the larynx during swallowing.

Esophageal Stage

The esophageal stage of swallowing is a reflex that involves the descent of the bolus of food down the esophagus. The evaluation and management of swallowing detailed here will deal with dysphagia in only the first three stages of swallowing—that is, oropharyngeal dysphagia.

◾ Evaluation

Whatever the cause of dysphagia, clinical evaluation begins with a complete history and physical examination that must include a full head and neck evaluation and the assessment of nutritional and respiratory status. Current evaluation includes flexible nasopharyngolaryngoscopy for dynamic examination of the swallowing apparatus. With the history and physical examination as a guide, imaging, such as plain cervical films, computed tomography (CT), and/or magnetic resonance imaging (MRI), can add to diagnostic acuity, especially in the case of neurological or structural anomalies.

The swallowing process already described is complex and cannot be clinically observed without instrumentation. Because anatomical or neurological deficits can affect any or all stages of swallowing, and oropharyngeal dysphagia can have severe side effects, including malnutrition, dehydration, and complications of aspiration, it is extremely important that the parameters that impair swallowing be diagnosed effectively and accurately.

Diagnostic Methods

Swallowing is a rapidly moving process that is best assessed with a dynamic instrumental technique. Among the several methods proposed for examining the oropharyngeal swallowing mechanism, videofluoroscopy is most frequently employed. Other dynamic methods include flexible endoscopic examination of swallowing (FEES) and ultrasonography. Additional methods have been used for research purposes or to assess a specific aspect of swallowing; however, they have not been used widely as standard clinical tools. Such methods include X-ray microbeam, scintigraphy, and air pulse quantification. Some instrumental techniques have been combined with fluoroscopy and used clinically and for research (e.g., manofluorography and EMG and fluoroscopy).

Flexible Endoscopic Evaluation of Swallowing

FEES consists of passing an endoscope transnasally to view the larynx and pharynx while the patient swallows measured volumes of food and liquid dyed with food coloring. The advantages of FEES are (1) the procedure can be done at bedside, (2) real food is used, (3) there is no radiation exposure, and (4) flexible endoscopes are available in medical settings. The disadvantages of FEES include (1) the oral phase of swallowing cannot be viewed, (2) the deflection of the epiglottis covering the laryngeal introitus obstructs visualization of pharyngeal response, (3) there is no visualization of the cervical esophageal stage of swallowing, and thus (4) it is sometimes difficult to diagnose the parameters that cause dysphagia (e.g., identifying the underlying cause of aspiration).

Manofluorography

Manofluorography allows for the simultaneous presentation of fluoroscopy and manometry, thus permitting the study of pharyngeal pressure generation and its relationship to bolus transport. In the past, manofluorography could not be used routinely because of difficulties passing the strain gauges transnasally and because catheter movement can cause erroneous pressure measurements. However, there have been recent improvements of manofluorography technology with validation studies using high-resolution, solid-state technology and circumferential sensor placement. The addition of manometry is helpful in identifying the function of muscular components of the oropharyngeal swallow.

Videofluoroscopy or Modified Barium Swallow

Videofluoroscopy has been cited as the best available method for assessing the dynamic process of swallowing. Usually referred to as a modified barium swallow (MBS), videofluoroscopy studies the anatomy and physiology of the oral preparatory, oral, pharyngeal, and cervical esophageal stages of swallowing. It documents the sequential occurrences of tongue loading, pulsion, nasopharyngeal closure, UES opening, airway protection, and pharyngeal clearance and can recognize patients at risk for aspiration pneumonia. By identifying abnormalities that can cause aspiration or pharyngeal residue, the clinician can develop potential management strategies to improve swallowing.

Manometry

Though evaluation and treatment of laryngopharyngeal reflux (LPR) are discussed elsewhere in this manual, LPR deserves mention as a notable cause of dysphagia. As mentioned previously, the use of manometry is becoming more widespread with better technology available, including multichannel impedance manometry with ambulatory pH testing to evaluate acid and nonacid reflux disease, and high-resolution manometry.

GOOSE

The combination of transnasal esophagoscopy with the FEES technique has culminated in a new diagnostic modality—guided observation of swallowing in the esophagus (GOOSE). GOOSE may be helpful in cases of a normal FEES but persistent dysphagia. With GOOSE, the food bolus is followed through the esophagus and the lower esophageal sphincter (LES). Any residue left in the esophagus after 13 seconds would be an indication of delayed motility in the esophagus.

■ Management

Important Patient Factors

Two important factors must be considered when managing dysphagia: (1) whether the patient can swallow safely with or without therapeutic strategies, and (2) whether the patient can consume adequate calories orally to maintain or improve nutritional status. Several patient factors in addition to the underlying swallowing disorder may influence how the clinician approaches management.

First, the patient's level of alertness will determine how dysphagia is managed. Patients should be fed only when they are awake and alert. Although this seems intuitive, many neurological or chronically ill patients experience periods where their level of alertness is diminished. Nursing staff, aides, families, and other hospital personnel should be instructed not to feed patients during nonalert periods.

Second, patients must have adequate cognitive ability and receptive language skills to perform the recommended therapeutic strategy. Therapeutic intervention can be direct or indirect. Direct intervention involves techniques the patient must perform when swallowing. Indirect intervention involves environmental modifications, such as alterations in viscosity, temperature, or texture of food that can be controlled for the patient. Such techniques are usually the only option for patients with poor cognitive or receptive language skills. The National Dysphagia Diet is a guide for clinicians and caregivers in determining appropriate consistencies for patients. A Dysphagia 1 diet is a pureed consistency, a Dysphagia 2 diet is a soft mechanical diet (mechanically altered characteristics), and a Dysphagia 3 diet is considered advanced.

Finally, the etiology of the swallowing disorder or underlying disease process must also be considered in approaching management. For example, swallowing function may improve with oral exercises in a patient recovering from a cerebrovascular accident (CVA, e.g., stroke); however, improvement is not likely in the face of a degenerative neurological disease.

Focus on the Swallowing Disorder

Management of oropharyngeal dysphagia is possible only after the pathophysiology of the swallowing mechanism is diagnosed. Many clinicians refer to aspiration and material in the pharynx after the swallow (pharyngeal residue) as the swallowing disorder. Aspiration and pharyngeal residue are merely symptomatic of a swallowing problem. Treatment must focus on the swallowing disorder itself, rather than just the management of aspiration.

For example, if a patient with a unilateral pharyngeal paresis aspirates from the weaker side of the pharynx, then having the patient turn the chin to the weak side, thereby closing off that pyriform sinus, would improve the swallow and eliminate the aspiration. Pharyngeal residue may be aspirated after the swallow or even during the next swallow. However, the residue is usually symptomatic of inadequate base-of-tongue propulsion; therefore, improving base-of-tongue propulsion via exercises will reduce pharyngeal residue and decrease the risk of aspiration.

Surgical Management

Management of a swallowing problem can be either surgical or behavioral. The most common surgical procedure has been the cricopharyngeal myotomy. Indications for a myotomy are found in patients who present with bolus obstruction at the level of the UES. Botulinum A toxin of the cricopharyngeal muscle has been proposed as an alternative to the myotomy.

Cricopharyngeal myotomy has been used with mixed success in patients with Zenker diverticulum, stenotic esophageal inlet or web, neuromuscular disease, cricopharyngeal achalasia, and dysphagia of unknown cause. However, swallowing involves the oral cavity, oropharynx, and pharyngolarynx; any dysfunction at these levels may contribute to dysphagia and may respond to surgical intervention. Oral-labial incompetence may require reestablishment of the orbicularis oris or release of oral contractures that may cause the incompetence. Soft palate weakness or deficiency can cause nasopharyngeal regurgitation or premature bolus spillage into the pharynx, for which a palatoplasty may be helpful. By the same token, tongue or base of tongue deficiency can cause difficulty in transitioning/propulsion of the bolus from the oral cavity to the oropharynx and/or cause premature pharyngeal spillage.

Reconstruction of defects with locoregional or free flaps can restore some competence to the oropharyngeal valve. Vocal fold paralyses or pareses disrupt the glottis valve, which impairs the buildup of subglottic pressure necessary to generate the force needed for deglutition. In addition, the patient with a vocal fold paralysis is more at risk for aspiration due to both anatomical and sensory deficits. Treatment of this glottal insufficiency is important in reestablishing subglottic pressure in the glottis valve and in lessening (though not eliminating) the risk for aspiration.

Finally, in the event of refractory aspiration, options include tracheotomy, narrow field laryngectomy, laryngotracheal separation, or diversion. It is critical to identify the appropriate site of a structural or anatomical abnormality contributing to dysphagia to ensure an improvement in the patient's swallowing.

Behavioral Management

Behavioral treatment techniques often provide a lower risk, are less costly, and are a more effective alternative to surgery in the treatment of dysphagia. Commonly used behavioral treatment techniques and their physiological effects on swallowing are listed in **Table 60.1**. Nonsurgical management techniques can be divided into the following categories based on function: (1) postural variations, (2) maneuvers to protect the airway or improve bolus clearance (compensatory), (3) increases in sensory input, and (4) exercises to improve function (restor-

ative). More than one technique may be effective in improving swallowing disorders, and techniques may also be combined (e.g., chin tuck with head turn) for maximum effectiveness.

One specific treatment, called the McNeill Dysphagia Therapy Program, can be considered analogous to Lee Silverman Voice Treatment (LSVT) in Parkinson disease (PD). This short-duration, intensive program incorporates exercises that push the patient's swallowing mechanism to a point of fatigue to strengthen the musculature. It has been shown to be effective in both head and neck cancer patients and neurologically impaired patients. Thermal-tac-

Table 60.1   Common management techniques for dysphagia (nonsurgical)

Category	Technique	Physiological effect on swallowing
Postural variations	Chin down or tuck (may also be considered a maneuver to protect airway	Improves airway protection by posterior shift in anterior pharyngeal structures narrowing the laryngeal entrance
	Chin up	Facilitates posterior movement of food in oral cavity using gravity
	Rotating head to weaker side	Bolus moves down more functional side; diminished resistance at the pharyngoesophageal segment
	Tilting head to stronger side	Directs material down stronger side in both the oral cavity and pharynx
Maneuvers		
Protect the airway	Super-supraglottic swallow	Closes the entrance of the airway before and during the swallow by patient holding breath and bearing down before and during the swallow
Improved bolus clearance	Dry or repeated swallows	May clear some residue
	Washing food through pharynx	Alternating solids and liquids may clear residue of thicker materials
	Effortful swallow	Improves tongue base movement posteriorly
	Mendelsohn maneuver	Prolongs laryneal elevation at mid-swallow thus augmenting opening of the UES
	Tongue-hold maneuver	Holding tongue tip between anterior dentition may increase posterior pharyngeal wall bulging
Increasing sensory input	Thermal-tactile stimulation	Cold contact to base of anterior facial arches sensitizes and improves triggering of the pharyngeal response
	Larger bolus Thicker bolus Textured bolus	May improve triggering of the pharyngeal swallow
Exercises to improve function	Pushing exercises	Increase adduction at top of airway
	Oral exercises	Improve strength and function over time

tile sensory stimulation using a cold probe to various locations in the oropharyngeal mucosa is especially helpful in a patient demonstrating a delayed or absent pharyngeal swallow trigger.

Neuromuscular electrical stimulation (NMES) involves delivery of small electrical impulses to swallowing muscles in the throat through skin electrodes. The most common NMES device in use is the VitalStim Therapy System (Empi, Inc., St. Paul, MN), which aims to strengthen the muscles (primarily hyolaryngeal) through constant, high-intensity stimulation. Although several studies of the device indicate promising results, most of these studies are not blinded or controlled. Therefore, the results are difficult to interpret.

Sensory NMES to the palate, faucial pillars, pharynx, and neck using catheter-based electrodes also appears to have some initially encouraging results in patients with delayed or absent swallow triggers, though much more research is needed in this area. Transcranial magnetic stimulation and direct current stimulation are two modalities on the horizon that take advantage of dominant pharyngeal motor representation in the dominant cortex. These techniques have been shown to help reduce swallowing reaction times and may have applications for swallowing rehabilitation in the future.

Initially, regardless of their etiologies, most cases of pharyngeal dysphagia may be conservatively managed based on the flexibility of the swallowing mechanisms. Exercises may be used to enhance the swallowing reflex, alter muscle tone, and improve voluntary function. However, controlling aspiration to safe levels and ensuring adequate nutritional intake may necessitate long-term enteral nutrition and selected surgical procedures. Although even small nasogastric tubes are not always well tolerated and have a high extrusion rate, percutaneous endoscopic gastrostomy (PEG) is usually safe and effective. Locally, although mild aspiration may decrease with time or be handled through vocal cord medialization, complete airway and foodway separation may be impossible.

■ Etiologies

The pathologies that may affect swallowing biomechanics to produce dysphagia require specific management. Clinically, the problems are usually encountered under a series of well-defined circumstances (**Table 60.2**).

Table 60.2 Etiologies of oropharyngeal dysphagia

Neurological diseases	Cerebrovascular accident Parkinson disease Multiple sclerosis Brain neoplasm Polio and postpolio system Alzheimer disease Huntington disease
Myopathic diseases	Myositis Dermatomyositis Myasthenia gravis Muscular dystrophies
Metabolic diseases	Hyperthyroidism
Inflammatory/ autoimmune diseases	Amyloid Sarcoidosis Systemic lupus erythematosus
Infectious diseases	Meningitis Diphtheria Botulism Lyme disease Syphilis Vira l (coxsackie virus, herpes virus, cytomegalovirus)
Structural diseases	Inflammatory (pharyngitis, abscess, tuberculosis Congenital webs Plummer–Vinson syndrome Neoplasm Cricopharyngeal bar Zenker diverticulum Extrinsic compression (osteophytes, goiter, lymphadenopathy) Bullous skin diseases Poor dentition
Iatrogenic diseases	Medical side effects (neuroleptics) Surgical resection Radiation induced Corrosive
Neuromuscular disorders	Achalasia Diffuse esophageal spasm Scleroderma Gastroesophageal reflux
Structural lesions (intrinsic)	Benign peptic stricture Esophageal rings and webs Esophageal diverticula Foreign bodies Esophageal carcinoma Medication-induced lesions
Structural lesions (extrinsic)	Vascular compression Mediastinal lesions Cervical osteoarthritis

Dysphagia Resulting from Neurological Causes

Because diverse neurological conditions affect the swallowing mechanism by confusing sensory and/or motor traffic in the central nervous system (CNS), the otolaryngologist–head and neck surgeon is often consulted to determine the effect of a neurological condition on soilage of the lungs.

Infants

In infants, antenatal problems, prematurity, and associated anomalies will often alert a practitioner, but because swallowing follows suckling and precedes respiration, the pattern of response to feeding attempts is often the key to correct diagnosis. Difficulties in initiating a swallow or incomplete UES relaxation with coughing and choking are often temporary, but silent aspiration must not be missed. Usually self-limited in *unilateral recurrent laryngeal nerve (RLN) paralysis* (e.g., from birth trauma), stridor, aspiration, and cyanosis are worse with *bilateral* paralysis (e.g., from hydrocephalus) and require tracheostomy and neurosurgical decompression. In the untreated *Arnold-Chiari malformation*, nasal regurgitation, UES incoordination, and failure to relax reflect increased intracranial pressure and are satisfactorily treated with a shunt. In *cerebral palsy*, aspiration pneumonia may be predicted by poor head and trunk control, slow oral intake, drooling, and inability to feed independently. Unfortunately, sensorimotor therapy often fails in children who aspirate.

Stroke

Dysphagia with aspiration in CVAs (or stroke) is associated with an increased risk of death. The incidence of dysphagia in stroke patients is 19 to 81%. Bedside assessment must be supplemented by instrumental examinations that can predict pneumonia by showing specific pharyngeal transit times to be prolonged in severely aspirating patients. Manometry confirms longer pharyngeal delays but also demonstrates shorter laryngeal closure, cricopharyngeal opening, and laryngeal elevation times in stroke patients when compared with normal subjects, indicating discoordination of pharyngeal musculature. Increased pharyngeal contraction amplitudes and reduced pharyngoesophageal wave durations with associated central RLN paralysis suggest that the problem is not limited to laryngeal dysfunction. There may be sensory deficits involved as well, which can cause delay in the swallow trigger. There are notable changes in swallow-respiration patterns in stroke patients, though the clinical significance of these changes is unclear.

A clinical bedside evaluation should be ordered within the first week after the stroke. Findings that would necessitate further dynamic swallowing studies (FEES and/or MBS) include the development of aspiration pneumonia, cough and "wet lung" or "wet voice" postswallow, and difficulty maintaining oral nutrition and hydration. The management of aspiration through patient and family instruction is often as effective as when the therapist is directly involved, because aspiration will often stop after 6 weeks. In severe forms, however, early gastrostomy is preferred to nasogastric tube feeding, although there is no consensus on optimal timing of PEG placement.

Parkinson Disease

The multifactorial nature of PD entails various degrees of cognitive and psychological changes with anomalies of the extrapyramidal and autonomic nervous systems. Incomplete UES relaxation and reduced opening associated with high intrabolus pressures impair pharyngeal bolus transport, though there is no correlation between the presence or severity of dysphagia and prepharyngeal anomalies (e.g., jaw rigidity, impaired head and neck posture during meals). There is some hesitation in initiating the oral stage, and the lack of adaptation between bolus volume and hyoid excursion further reduces pharyngeal contraction, with increased residue and drooling in spite of repetitive tongue pumping. Drooling occurs due to decreases in spontaneous swallows; in fact, more patients with PD complain of xerostomia. Management is supportive and has improved using new drugs (selegiline hydrochloride [Eldepryl, Orion Pharma, Berkshire, UK], carbidopa-levodopa [Sinemet, Merck, Whitehouse Station, NJ], pergolide mesylate [Permax]), synthetic saliva, and cricopharyngeal myotomy in selected cases of UES dysfunction. Therapy is of benefit in patients who have maintained cognitive abilities. LSVT used for PD-related dysphonia has actually had some positive effects on swallowing function by improving oral tongue bolus control and tongue base function and oropharyngeal swallow efficiency.

Lower Motor Neuron Deficits

Lower motor neuron deficits may affect any location between the nuclei and neuromuscular junctions. By preventing the release of acetylcholine at the motor end plate, *myasthenia gravis* causes swallowing hesitancy and fatigability, progressively leading to hypotonia. The diagnosis is suspected in patients with early symptoms, such as diplopia or subtle voice changes, and it is confirmed by therapeutic administration of edrophonium, anticholinesterases, prednisone, and plasmapheresis, when necessary, to clear the circulating antibodies targeted against acetylcholine. Thymectomy is indicated in the absence of response, especially in females with a hyperplastic gland and high antibody titers or in the presence of a thymoma. The clinically similar *Eaton Lambert syndrome*, occurring in the setting of oat cell carcinoma of the lung, may be alleviated by guanidine hydrochloride, which increases release from the nerve terminals. By contrast, the progressive motor deficits caused by *amyotrophic lateral sclerosis* are irreversible, and as motor neuron depopulation progresses, atonia of the swallowing mechanism may require surgical protection of the lungs. Finally, the unpredictability of dysphagia in *multiple sclerosis* follows the erratic demyelinization course characterizing this disease, although almost half of the patients show some degree of swallowing difficulties.

Iatrogenic Conditions

Iatrogenic causes of dysphagia are more frequent than suspected. *Surgery for base of skull tumors* may cause significant pharyngoesophageal dysphagia if cranial nerves IX, X, and XII are sacrificed. If a single nerve is damaged, particularly in a younger patient, this may improve after 2 weeks of tube feedings.

Dysphagia after *pharyngeal plexus injury* from such procedures as carotid endarterectomy, cervical fusion, and ventral rhizotomy for torticollis has often been overlooked. Dysphagia is a very common problem after *anterior cervical spine surgery*, with incidences ranging from 47 to 66% in the first postoperative week. Multilevel fusion is associated with a higher risk of dysphagia. This dysphagia is multifactorial: causes include pharyngeal and esophageal edema and ischemia from intraoperative retraction, prevertebral edema, and possible denervation of multiple cranial nerves, particularly the RLN. Because of the myriad causes, dysphagia after anterior cervical spine surgery can be prolonged.

The diagnosis of *SLN paralysis* is suspected on persistent cough and subtle voice changes. It is confirmed by laryngoscopy showing the ipsilateral true vocal cord shifted posteriorly toward the involved side (though this is not a consistent finding), and laxity of the involved vocal fold, unless only the ISLN has been injured. As with unilateral RLN paralysis recognized by the paramedian position of the ipsilateral vocal cord, aspiration is most often transient. When necessary, medialization laryngoplasty or temporary vocal fold injection augmentation may be employed. Although rare, *bilateral combined SLN/RLN paralysis* may cause aspiration because the cords remain unable to adduct and the larynx is without sensation. Finally, unexplained dysphagia with negative

imaging occurring after *cardiac surgery* may be due to embolism or hypotension.

Medications potentially affect swallowing at all levels of the nervous system. CNS depressants aggravate already impaired swallowing by combining their effects with the underlying neurological disorder, although certain drugs (e.g., nitrazepam [Mogadon]) have similar effects without decreasing arousal. Neuroleptics, antiemetics, metoclopramide, and other dopamine antagonists should also be used with caution because of the extrapyramidal reactions, dyskinesia, dystonia, and Parkinsonism they occasionally induce. The peripheral nervous system may be affected by neuromuscular junction blockade. Aminoglycosides, certain tetracyclines, succinylcholine, muscle relaxants, and immunosuppressants may induce pharyngeal muscle weakness in a dose-dependent fashion. Anticholinergic drugs, tricyclic antidepressants, and antihistamines can make swallowing difficult by increasing salivary viscosity or causing xerostomia. Conversely, while excessive secretion may indicate only the inability to swallow normal salivary volumes, it may also be due to the administration of cholinergic antagonists and anticholinesterases. Dysphagia may also develop after the administration of quinidine, propanolol, and lithium, or from seepage or overdosage of botulinum toxin after injections for spasmodic torticollis. Finally, topical anesthetics and cough suppressants should be used with caution, because the oropharyngeal sensory deficits they may induce encourage silent aspiration.

The Elderly

Recent evidence shows that pharyngolaryngeal sensory discrimination may decrease with age and potentially lead to silent aspiration. Also, slower reactions delay swallowing function; the elderly take more time and use smaller volumes. Chewing may be compromised (even with dentures) as part of overall weakness and decreased lingual force obliges patients to work harder to produce adequate pharyngeal pressures. New research demonstrates that natural capsaicinoids can improve laryngeal vestibular closure time, pharyngeal residue, upper esophageal sphincter opening, and maximal hyolaryngeal displacement in older patients.

Dysphagia Resulting from Structural Anomalies

In cases of dysphagia resulting from structural anomalies, the pharyngeal path is directly affected and the swallowing dynamics may be worsened by accompanying sensory damage. The primary cervical etiologies of the following conditions underscore the pivotal role of the otolaryngologist–head and neck surgeon in their early detection and treatment.

Congenital Anomalies

Congenital anomalies expressed above the cricopharyngeus are mostly craniofacial in origin and produce obstructive apneic episodes during feedings because those infants are still obligate nasal breathers. Oropharyngeal obstruction from altered mandible–hyoid relationship, as seen in Pierre Robin syndrome, may be alleviated by feeding in the prone position or nasopharyngeal intubation. However, other cases of midfacial hypoplasia, such as Apert, Treacher Collins, and Crouzon syndromes, may require craniofacial surgery. Cleft palate/lip, choanal atresia, and septal anomalies are less dramatic, and obstacles along the pharyngeal path, such as webs, are rarely encountered.

Trauma

Trauma may impair oropharyngeal transit directly or by creating neurological deficits. Isolated *head contusions* alter coordination in a very diffuse and poorly explained manner. The *traumatic pontomedullary syndrome* from stretch injury after cervical hyperextension is characterized by spastic quadriparesis, dysarthria, and dysphagia, but neuroimaging is normal, and supportive treatment is usually sufficient. Although the mechanism of dysphagia in a *gunshot or blade wound* is usually self-explanatory, possible tenth and twelfth nerve palsies must not be missed in *fractures of the odontoid process.*

Surgical Iatrogenic Conditions

Surgical iatrogenic conditions are often due to *tracheostomy,* which impairs deglutitive ascent of the larynx by anchoring the airway to skin and strap muscles. Aspiration also relates to timing discrepancies within the swallowing cascade and shorter (albeit complete) closure of the desensitized larynx. Use of a Passy-Muir Tracheostomy and Ventilator Swallowing and Speaking Valve (Passy-Muir, Inc., Irvine, CA) in addition to cuff deflation of the tracheotomy tube can assist in swallowing by helping reestablish adequate subglottic pressure for the swallow. Oronasotracheal *intubation* affects deglutition from prolonged inactivity of skeletal muscles and neuromuscular blocking agents.

Head and Neck Neoplasia

The surgeon must expect that procedures on the *oral cavity* usually produce chewing difficulties and decreased tongue movement, limiting the initiation of the oral stage. Compromise of the pharyngeal stage occurs with reduced oropharyngeal thrust, and repeated swallows are usually necessary to propel the bolus. With mandible disarticulation or resection, the inability of the resected submandibular muscles to elevate the larynx may result in aspiration, potentially aggravated by resection of the oropharyngeal receptors.

The increased resistance to bolus transfer from a *hypopharyngeal resection* and circular defects may not be as clinically significant if the tongue base has remained untouched. The missing tongue bulk can be restored with a myocutaneous flap, but since the UES lacks the disparity between a wide pharynx and a narrow esophagus, a softer and smoother myofascial flap is indicated in this area.

Pharyngeal transit after *total laryngectomy* is prolonged due to an increased resistance from the decreased hypopharyngeal suction pump with the UES. The problem is compounded by the collapse of the pharyngeal lumen following hyoid bone and thyroid cartilage resection and possible stricture and stenosis after pharyngectomy and radiation.

Aspiration after *supraglottic laryngectomy* is due to the combined effects of supraglottic sensory denervation, incomplete motion of the tongue base toward the posterior pharyngeal wall, restricted anterior arytenoid tilting to close the airway, and delays in bolus propulsion from closure of the airway at the laryngeal inlet. The respective contributions of surgical laryngeal suspension, cricopharyngeal myotomy, and compensatory maneuvers to prevent aspiration have not been firmly established, but clinically may provide assistance and should be considered.

Dysphagia Resulting from Composite Mechanisms

Several causes of dysphagia fit into less well defined categories. Such conditions may not be necessarily referred to the head and neck specialist when they do not express dysphagia, their common denominator.

Radiation Therapy

Radiation therapy induces decreased salivary flow, edema, myositis, and eventual fibrosis, which impair swallowing by reducing pressure gradients over the bolus. While sialogogues (pilocarpine hydrochloride [Silalagen]) alleviate dryness, the best prevention is a treatment schedule sufficiently delayed from the inflammatory responses of the original surgery. The quandary is that NMES, which could be a helpful adjunct to traditional therapy for these patients, should not be so delayed that significant radiation-induced muscular fibrosis has occurred.

Inflammatory Diseases

Among inflammatory diseases affecting deglutition, the most outstanding causes of *pharyngitis* are rhinovirus (common cold), influenza, adenovirus (pharyngoconjunctival fever), herpes simplex, Coxsackie virus (herpangina), Epstein-Barr virus (EBV, infectious mononucleosis), human immunodeficiency virus (HIV), acquired immunodeficiency syndrome (AIDS), *Streptococcus pyogenes,* anaerobic bacteria, and spirochetes (Vincent angina). Deep neck abscesses and Ludwig angina exacerbate the effects of pain and airway/foodway compression with dehydration. Exudates are usually observed with bacterial diseases, adenoviruses, and herpes simplex and EBV. Penicillin is the treatment of choice for streptococcal disease.

Infectious mononucleosis is suspected if the patient has protracted fatigue, splenomegaly, and elevated lymphocytes with atypical forms. This is confirmed by heterophil antibodies noted in the serum as early as the first week of illness. Supportive treatment usually suffices in the mild forms. Epidemiological factors will help diagnose rarer forms of pharyngitis. In diphtheria, neurotoxins can also affect the soft palate (with nasal regurgitation) and the pharyngolarynx in addition to pseudomembranes. Spasm, hydrophobia, and hypersalivation may be fatal in rabies and tetanus where dysphagia can even be the presenting symptom. Vaccination is preventive.

The consequences of *AIDS* on deglutition are indirect from opportunistic infections, such as actinomycosis, cryptosporidium, atypical *Mycobacterium,* and *Candida albicans,* which appears as white oral or pharyngeal confluent pseudomembranous plaques with pseudohyphae on the smear. Topical nystatin (Mycostatin, Bristol-Myers Squibb, New York, NY) or clotrimazole (Canesten, Bayer HealthCare, Whippany, NJ) may alleviate the burning sensation. Cytomegalovirus, herpes simplex, and *Mycobacterium avium intracellulare* present as discrete ulcerations on a normal mucosal background as compared with the well-circumscribed ulcer craters from the HIV virus itself. The diagnosis is established by serum antibodies and electronmicroscopy of the biopsy specimens. The optimal management of this disease has not yet been defined.

Dysphagia of several *inflammatory myopathies* may be linked to identifiable autoimmune diseases, when recognized. In scleroderma, decreased sensation in the oral cavity may be complicated by the sicca syndrome (lack of saliva production) and may depress the gag reflex. Dermatomyositis (DM), polymyositis (PM), and inclusion body myositis (IBM) produce vallecular and piriform sinus retention with penetration, aspiration, and nasopharyngeal regurgitation. Therefore, the pharyngeal phase is the most affected in these disorders. The dysphagia associated with DM and PM responds better to immunosuppressive treatment, whereas IBM responds better to cricopharyngeal myotomy and/or pharyngoesophageal dilation. In systemic lupus erythematosus, dysphagia and xerostomia from secondary Sjögren syndrome also feature prolonged VFE pharyngeal transit times.

Sarcoidosis may be locally symptomatic through epiglottic enlargement or granulomatous myositis and cranial nerve involvement. It is resistant to treatment with corticosteroids, but like other forms of myopathy without neurological anomalies, sarcoidosis is alleviated by cricopharyngeal myotomy.

Hematologic Diseases

Hematologic diseases include *amyloid infiltration* of the salivary glands and the tongue, which may have to be partially resected when macroglossia compromises swallowing. Pharyngolaryngeal involvement may result in poor contraction, with stasis and penetration or aspiration from defective vocal cord apposition.

Postcricoid dysphagia associated with iron deficiency anemia and lingual, pharyngeal, and cervical esophageal atrophy has been attributed to the *Plummer–Vinson* syndrome. The importance of this uncertain condition relates to its possible association with postcricoid carcinoma.

Rheumatologic and Connective Tissue Diseases

In *rheumatoid arthritis*, dysphagia should trigger a workup for bulbar pharyngeal paralysis, medullary compression by the odontoid process, or vertical subluxation of the axis, cervical myopathy, and all local factors potentially interfering with normal suspension and elevation of the laryngopharynx. Cricoarytenoid and cricothyroid joint inflammation may also produce tenderness, swelling, and odynophagia. *Degenerative changes* in the cervical spine can produce osteophytes, which impair bolus flow through the pharynx.

Guillain-Barré syndrome is an acute, progressive polyradiculoneuropathy. Though triggered by an infectious process, it is considered an autoimmune disease because of antibodies directed against peripheral nerve myelin sheaths. The severity of dysphagia varies and can range from mild oromotor weakness to severe oropharyngeal dysphagia. Other symptoms include respiratory failure, autonomic dysfunction, and gastrointestinal complications. Treatment consists of a combination of immunotherapy and plasma exchange. Most patients will ultimately recover from the dysphagia.

Miscellaneous Diseases

Blistering diseases, such as pemphigus vulgaris, cicatricial pemphigoid, Stevens–Johnson syndrome, and Behçet disease, may be differentiated on the basis of immunofluorescence tests. *Zenker diverticula* rarely produce aspiration, but their occasional association with upper esophageal carcinoma should not be missed. The effects of diverticulotomy and cricopharyngeal myotomy have been difficult to evaluate due to a lack of correlation between postoperative symptoms and objective radiographic abnormalities.

Psychogenic and Globus Etiologies

These etiologies do not affect patients with psychological profiles different from those of patients with dysphagia due to organic causes. In cases of schizophrenia, dysphagia may occur secondary to the side effects of medications, but salivary flow may be affected in depressive psychoses and high states of anxiety. *Globus pharyngeus* is found more often in middle-aged women who complain of a feeling of something stuck in their throat, discomfort or irritation, and the need to swallow all the time. Although symptoms usually regress after long-term follow-up, there are no reliable prognostic indicators for this problem. The main point is to rule out another pathological condition.

■ Suggested Reading

Alagiakrishnan K, Bhanji RA, Kurian M. Evaluation and management of oropharyngeal dysphagia in different types of dementia: a systematic review. Arch Gerontol Geriatr 2013;56(1):1–9

Ashford J, McCabe D, Wheeler-Hegland K, et al. Evidence-based systematic review: Oropharyngeal dysphagia behavioral treatments. Part III—impact of dysphagia treatments on populations with neurological disorders. J Rehabil Res Dev 2009;46(2):195–204

Belafsky PC, Rees CJ. Emerging technology in dysphagia assessment. In: Leonard R, Kendall K, eds. Dysphagia Assessment and Treatment Planning—A Team Approach. San Diego, CA: Plural Publishing; 2008:193–200

Bulow M. Psychogenic dysphagia. In: Shaker R, Belafsky PC, Postma GN, Easterling C, eds. Principles of Deglutition. New York, NY: Springer; 2013:771–776

Chalela JA. Pearls and pitfalls in the intensive care management of Guillain-Barré syndrome. Semin Neurol 2001;21(4):399–405

Clark H, Lazarus C, Arvedson J, Schooling T, Frymark T. Evidence-based systematic review: effects of neuromuscular electrical stimulation on swallowing and neural activation. Am J Speech Lang Pathol 2009;18(4):361–375

Crary MA, Carnaby GD, LaGorio LA, Carvajal PJ. Functional and physiological outcomes from an exercise-based dysphagia therapy: a pilot investigation of the McNeill Dysphagia Therapy Program. Arch Phys Med Rehabil 2012;93(7):1173–1178

Doeltgen SH, Huckabee ML. Swallowing neurorehabilitation: from the research laboratory to routine clinical application. Arch Phys Med Rehabil 2012;93(2):207–213

El Sharkawi A, Ramig L, Logemann JA, et al. Swallowing and voice effects of Lee Silverman Voice Treatment (LSVT): a pilot study. J Neurol Neurosurg Psychiatry 2002;72(1):31–36

Frempong-Boadu A, Houten JK, Osborn B, et al. Swallowing and speech dysfunction in patients undergoing anterior cervical discectomy and fusion: a prospective, objective preoperative and postoperative assessment. J Spinal Disord Tech 2002;15(5):362–368

Humbert IA, Michou E, MacRae PR, Crujido L. Electrical stimulation and swallowing: how much do we know? Semin Speech Lang 2012;33(3):203–216

Jones HN, Rosenbek JC, eds. Dysphagia in Rare Conditions: An Encyclopedia. San Diego, CA: Plural Publishing; 2010

Krisciunas GP, Sokoloff W, Stepas K, Langmore SE. Survey of usual practice: dysphagia therapy in head and neck cancer patients. Dysphagia 2012;27(4):538–549

Leonard R, Kendall K, McKenzie S, Goodrich S. The treatment plan. In: Leonard R, Kendall K, eds. Dysphagia Assessment and Treatment Planning—A Team Approach. San Diego, CA: Plural Publishing; 2008:295–336

Loren B. Nutritional concerns and assessment in dysphagia. In: Leonard R, Kendall K, eds. Dysphagia Assessment and Treatment Planning—A Team Approach. San Diego, CA: Plural Publishing; 2008

Mandl T, Ekberg O. Dysphagia in systemic disease. In: Ekberg O, ed. Dysphagia: Diagnosis and Treatment. New York, NY: Springer; 2012:155–163

Martino R, Foley N, Bhogal S, Diamant N, Speechley M, Teasell R. Dysphagia after stroke: incidence, diagnosis, and pulmonary complications. Stroke 2005;36(12):2756–2763

Matthews CT, Coyle JL. Reducing pneumonia risk factors in patients with dysphagia who have a tracheostomy: what role can SLPs play? May 18, 2010. http://www.asha.org/Publications/leader/2010/100518/Reducing-Pneumonia-Risk-Factors.htm

McCabe D, Ashford J, Wheeler-Hegland K, et al. Evidence-based systematic review: Oropharyngeal dysphagia behavioral treatments. Part IV—impact of dysphagia treatment on individuals' postcancer treatments. J Rehabil Res Dev 2009;46(2):205–214

Murphy BA, Gilbert J. Dysphagia in head and neck cancer patients treated with radiation: assessment, sequelae, and rehabilitation. Semin Radiat Oncol 2009;19(1):35–42

Nativ-Zeltzer N, Kahrilas PJ, Logemann JA. Manofluorography in the evaluation of oropharyngeal dysphagia. Dysphagia 2012;27(2):151–161

Paydarfar D. Protecting the airway during swallowing: what is the role for afferent surveillance? Head Neck 2011;33(Suppl 1):S26–S29

Rofes L, Arreola V, Martin A, Clavé P. Natural capsaicinoids improve swallow response in older patients with oropharyngeal dysphagia. Gut 2013;62(9):1280–1287

Setzen M, Cohen MA, Mattucci KF, Perlman PW, Ditkoff MK. Laryngopharyngeal sensory deficits as a predictor of aspiration. Otolaryngol Head Neck Surg 2001;124(6):622–624

Shaker R, Belafsky PC, Postma GN, Easterling C, eds. Principles of Deglutition: A Multidisciplinary Text for Swallowing and Its Disorders. New York, NY: Springer; 2013

VI

Otology and Neurology

61 Contemporary Auditory and Vestibular Testing

◼ Introduction

Audiometric and vestibular testing is critical in the evaluation of patients with hearing or balance complaints. Audiometric testing provides quantitative information on the magnitude and type of the hearing loss and can help determine the site of the lesion. A wide range of audiometric tests is used to provide a complete picture of the function of the auditory system. The auditory system has many parts in which pathology can arise, so testing must be designed to investigate the pathway of sound conduction from the ear canal to the brain. Similarly, vestibular testing can provide objective measures of vestibular system function through a wide range of physiological parameters. Like the auditory system, the vestibular system has several components along the pathway from the inner ear to the brainstem, cerebellum, and higher centers in the brain. Vestibular testing is designed to test these various sites.

It is incumbent upon clinicians to have a working knowledge of the audiometric and vestibular tests they order. Without understanding the basic testing procedures, the clinician is not able to make rational use of the data they provide.

Auditory Tests

The human ear has a wide dynamic range over which it can respond. Tests of auditory function need to be designed to describe and measure a behavioral or physiological response to sound. The unit of measure for sound in hearing tests is the decibel (dB), which is a logarithmic scale to the base 10 of the ratio between a reference sound intensity (I_0) and the sound relative to the reference (I_1). This provides a ratio measurement of pressure, not an absolute measure of intensity. Sound level measurements can use different reference levels to provide an absolute measure of intensity. One commonly used reference is sound pressure level (SPL), which designates 0 dB as a spe-

cific amount of force. For hearing measurements, it is more desirable to measure a patient's thresholds relative to a "normal" hearing threshold. The standard measurement level is dB hearing level (HL).

Pure-Tone Audiometry

Two standard components of audiometric testing are determining air conduction and bone conduction thresholds. Air-conduction thresholds are determined at various frequencies ("pitches") using earphones or ear inserts. This tests the integrity of the entire auditory pathway from the ear canal to the cochlea and higher brain centers. Bone-conduction thresholds are obtained by the use of a bone oscillator on the mastoid. Bone-conduction hearing occurs by three mechanisms:

1. Sound energy from vibration of the bony ear canal radiating to the eardrum
2. Inertial properties of the ossicles moving relative to the vibrating skull
3. Vibration of the cochlear fluids causing compression and rarefaction of the inner ear spaces

Therefore, bone conduction bypasses the conductive mechanisms of the ear canal and middle ear and approximates true sensorineural thresholds. Thresholds for air and bone conduction should be equal in a normally functioning auditory system or in a patient with purely sensorineural hearing loss. A difference between the air conduction and bone conduction, or air–bone gap, is a measure of the amount of hearing loss attributable to the conductive (ear canal and middle ear) mechanisms.

The interaural attenuation when using a bone oscillator is negligible, so a sound presented anywhere on the skull can be detected equally by both cochleas. During bone-conduction testing, a masking stimulus, typically a narrowband noise, is presented to the nontest ear via air conduction to prevent sound presented to the test ear from being perceived in the nontest ear. A masking dilemma occurs when it is not possible to mask the nontest ear without stimulating the test ear. The most common scenario for a masking dilemma is in patients with severe bilateral conductive losses with near normal sensorineural, or bone conduction, thresholds.

Speech Discrimination Testing

Speech is the primary mode of communication, so testing the ability to hear and understand speech is an important component of audiological testing. Speech reception threshold (SRT) is the level in decibels in which a subject can correctly repeat 50% of a list of two-syllable words. SRT correlates highly with the pure-tone average, and the two measurements should not differ by > 10 dB. Word-recognition testing is also routinely administered and is obtained by presenting a list of monosyllabic words at a relatively moderate intensity, usually 40 dB above SRT. Word-recognition scores are expressed as a percentage of words correct and provide information regarding how well the patient can identify words at a suprathreshold level.

Impedance Testing

Tympanometry measures the compliance of the eardrum and the middle ear sound conducting system. The examiner places a probe in the ear canal to create an airtight seal. A tone (226 Hz) is delivered to the eardrum as the air pressure in the ear canal is varied (+200 to −400 decapascals). The compliance of the system is recorded as the air pressure is changed, and the peak compliance is the pressure at which the pressure in the ear canal equals that in the middle ear—the point of maximum compliance of the eardrum. A classification system for the measured response is widely used and correlates with middle ear pathology (**Fig. 61.1**).

Acoustic reflex testing seeks to find the softest sound (threshold) that will elicit reflex contraction of the stapedius muscle. The reflex arc includes the ear canal, middle ear, cochlea and eighth nerve to the ventral cochlear nucleus (afferent pathway) to the ipsilateral medial superior olive and then the facial (seventh nerve) motor nucleus, and crossing the trapezoid body to the contralateral medial superior olive to the contralateral facial nerve nucleus. From the facial motor nuclei, the signal courses along the ipsilateral and contralateral facial nerves to the stapedius muscle (efferent pathway) where a stimulus of adequate intensity (generally in the range of 70–100 dB SPL) will elicit contraction of the muscle, which can be recorded as a change in compliance in the middle ear system.

The testing is done with the probe tone in one ear and the recording probe either in the same ear (ipsilateral) or opposite (contralateral) ear. Four testing protocols are evaluated: stimulate and record ipsilateral (right and left ears); stimulate ipsilateral and record contralateral (right and left ears). The softest tone (usually tested at 500, 1,000, 2,000, and 4,000 Hz) that elicits a change in middle ear compliance (contraction of the stapedius muscle) is identified as threshold.

Elevated or absent acoustic reflex thresholds may give some indication as to the site of a lesion. A unilateral, stiff middle ear system (glue ear, otosclerosis) will elevate (or the acoustic reflex will be absent) the reflex threshold in three of the protocols: stimulus and recording probe ipsilateral, stimulus ipsilateral and recording contralateral (sound can't get in), and stimulus contralateral and recording probe ipsilateral (no contraction from the stiff middle ear system). A retrocochlear lesion (e.g., vestibular schwannoma) will elevate (or the acoustic reflex will be absent) the reflex threshold when the stimulus and recording probe are ipsilateral to the lesion, and when the stimulus is ipsilateral and the recording is contralateral (sound can't get in—afferent pattern). In this instance, stimulus and recording contralateral to the lesion and stimulus contralateral and recording ipsilateral should be normal unless the tumor has affected the facial nerve (rare). Facial nerve pathology will show a pattern where all recordings ipsilateral to the lesion (stimulus ipsilateral and contralateral) will be absent or elevated, and recordings contralateral to the lesion will be normal (efferent pattern).

Electrocochleography (ECochG)

ECochG provides electrophysiological, diagnostic assessment of the cochlea and auditory nerve. The response is thought to be generated by the cochlea (endocochlear potentials) and the eighth cranial nerve. ECochG is performed with either an extratympanic or a transtympanic electrode. Theoretically, the transtympanic electrode should provide a stronger signal by directly recording from the cochlea, resulting in a more robust response. A prospective controlled study of normal volunteers, however, failed to find a significant difference between canal-extratympanic and transtympanic electrode responses. The ECochG response consists of a summating potential (SP) and an action potential (AP), with the most clinically useful feature being the amplitude and latency of the two potentials. Most centers consider an SP:AP ratio (with regard to response amplitude) of 40 to 50% or greater as significant (abnormal). An abnormal ECochG result may suggest an increased volume or pressure of endolymph or decreased volume or pressure of perilymph.

Type A = Normal

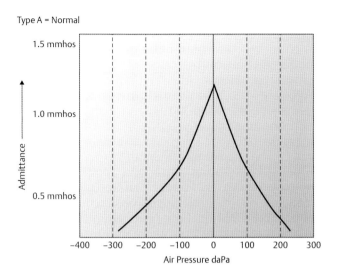

Type B = Flat (Tympanic membrane perforation [elevated ear canal volume]; middle ear fluid; patent ventilation tube)

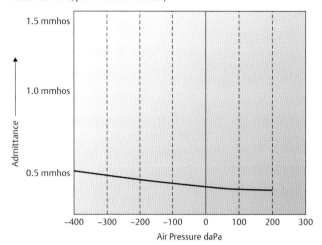

Type A_S = Shallow (Otosclerosis; ossicular stiffness; can be glue ear)

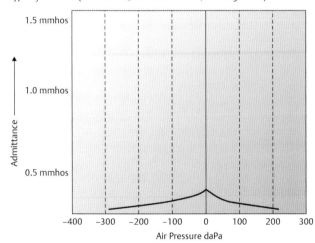

Type C = Left shift (Eustachian tube dysfunction with negative middle ear pressure)

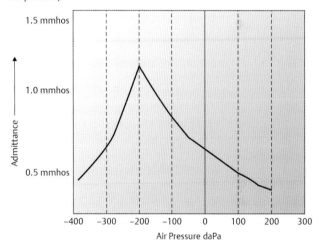

Type A_D = Deep (Ossicular discontinuity)

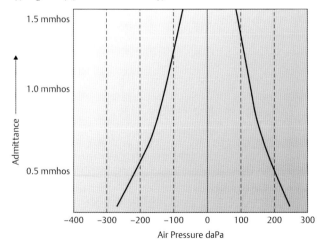

Fig. 61.1   Classification for impedance audiometry. Used with permission from Medscape Reference (http://emedicine.medscape .com/), 2014, available at: http://emedicine.medscape.com/article/1831254-overview.

ECochG can be used to do the following:

1. Identify and monitor endolymphatic hydrops
2. Identify wave I when not evident in brainstem auditory-evoked potential testing (especially important to measure interwave intervals when the patient has a hearing loss)
3. Monitor hearing when used intraoperatively

Auditory Brainstem Response (ABR)

Auditory brainstem response (ABR) testing is perhaps the most popular approach to assessing the auditory nervous system for dysfunction at the level of the eighth cranial nerve, pons, or midbrain (the exact origins of potentials within the brainstem are still uncertain and controversial). ABR is also used for young children who cannot perform behavioral testing, for infant hearing screening, as a possible screening tool for retrocochlear lesions (e.g., vestibular schwannoma), and for evaluating potential candidates for pediatric cochlear implantation. The ABR test result in a normal listener will show seven distinct peaks, with the first, third, and fifth peaks considered the most stable and most critical in making measurements. Testing protocol involves placing a small speaker probe in the patient's ear and, using surface electrodes on the scalp and mastoid, recording the evoked auditory potentials along the cochlear nerve and brainstem and midbrain auditory pathway. Threshold is identified as the lowest sound intensity that reliably and repeatedly elicits a waveform, usually recorded as a wave V. Other variables measured include latency and amplitude, which are compared within the same ear (intra-aural; e.g., I–III vs. III–V latency) and between ears (interaural).

Central Auditory Assessment

The current primary focus of central auditory testing is to describe functional disorders of communication. These disorders of listening and understanding are called central auditory processing disorders (CAPDs), which result from abnormal interaction and/or incomplete maturation of central auditory pathways in the brainstem and cortex.

Pure-tone and speech testing usually cannot reveal CAPDs. Only tests of reduced acoustic redundancy (distorted speech materials, i.e., sensitized speech tests) are sufficiently challenging to the auditory system to identify CAPDs. Sensitized speech tests can be created by increasing background noise, interrupting the speech at different rates, and increasing the rate of presentation. Under these test conditions, when a central auditory disorder is present, speech intelligibility is poor.

CAPDs traditionally have been associated with central nervous system disease, head injury, and stroke in adults; however, attention is now focused on chronic/recurrent middle ear disease of childhood as a contributing cause of auditory–language learning problems. Most children affected with CAPDs are male, have normal pure-tone audiograms, have short attention spans, and distract easily. In addition, many have reading or writing problems and articulation or language disorders. These children can be helped by enhancing the speech signal, reducing background noise, and applying learning auditory strategies. Preferential seating in school, frequency-modulation assistive-listening devices, sound-field amplification, language therapy, focusing of auditory attention, and vocational and/or college planning are examples of treatment strategies that can help these individuals lead normal, productive lives.

Otoacoustic Emissions (OAEs)

Otoacoustic emissions (OAEs) are low-level, inaudible sounds generated actively by the outer hair cells (OHCs) of the cochlea. OAEs can be measured by a sensitive microphone in the external auditory canal. They are a by-product of fine tuning the traveling wave within the cochlea. As the mechanical traveling wave displaces the basilar membrane, a change in OHC intracellular voltage is produced by cell shortening (depolarization) and elongation (hyperpolarization), which increase the amplitude and sharpen the peak of the wave at the point of maximal displacement. Together, the OHC motility process and its consequences are called the cochlear amplifier. This OHC physiology helps explain the fine tuning known to occur in the cochlea.

Spontaneous OAEs occur in 35 to 50% of healthy ears but are absent in hearing loss > 40 dBHL. Transient-evoked OAEs can be click- or tone-pip-evoked and are present in 90% of normal ears. Other OAEs can be evoked by continuous pure tones (stimulus-frequency OAEs) or generated by two stimuli presented simultaneously (distortion-product OAEs).

Transient-evoked OAEs are clinically useful because they are present in > 90% of normal ears (infancy through adulthood) and are usually easily generated with only moderately intense stimuli. Generally, any hearing loss > 30 dB inhibits transient-evoked OAEs; hearing loss > 50 dB inhibits distortion-product OAEs; and middle ear disease inhibits all OAEs, even if the hearing loss is < 30 dB, because of faulty retrograde transmission of the response from the cochlea through the abnormal middle ear. Thus, when the middle ear is normal, measurable transient-evoked OAEs suggest that hearing sensitivity is no worse than 30 dBHL in the test ear.

OAEs can be used clinically to screen hearing in infants, in difficult-to-test (aphasic, demented, or developmentally disabled) adults, and in pseudohypoacoustic (functional) patients. They can be used to monitor potential hearing changes, for example, in patients receiving ototoxic medications. Also, OAEs can occasionally be used to differentiate sensory (cochlear) from neural (retrocochlear) hearing loss because they are produced solely by OHCs of the cochlea.

■ Vestibular Tests

A comprehensive evaluation of the patient with dizziness requires a careful history, physical exam, and vestibular testing. The patient history is the most revealing part of the evaluation, but vestibular testing can help clarify the diagnosis and provide the site and degree of the lesion. Vestibular testing can be divided into clinical and laboratory tests. Clinical tests are performed in an office examination room or at the patient's bedside. Laboratory tests include traditional electronystagmography (ENG) or videonystagmography (VNG), rotational chair testing, vestibular-evoked myogenic potential (VEMP), and posturography.

Bedside Vestibular Tests

Dynamic visual acuity tests are a frequently used bedside test. Bilateral severely reduced or absent inner ear vestibular function will prevent the patient from visually fixating during head movement, because inner ear function, or vestibulo-ocular reflex (VOR), is required for visual–vestibular interaction to maintain foveation at frequencies > 2 Hz. For example, the patient cannot read print while randomly moving the head vertically and horizontally. Visual acuity with random head motion is useful for patients with suspected ototoxicity.

The head-shaking test is easy to perform and objectively identifies abnormalities of the vestibular system. Head shaking back and forth, twice each second for 20 seconds, elicits latent nystagmus caused by asymmetric peripheral (inner ear) input. The head-thrust test is sensitive to unilateral and bilateral canal paresis. The clinician rapidly thrusts the head to the left and then to the right and observes a "catch-up" saccade as the head is turned toward the affected ear. The Fukuda stepping test is a useful tool for assessing patients with acute vestibular loss, although it may not be as accurate a predictor of unilateral vestibular function in chronically dizzy patients. The patient is asked to march in place. Once marching, the patient is asked to close the eyes. In the presence of a unilateral vestibular loss, the patient will turn to the side of the loss. The patient will be able to maintain a straight, forward gaze with normal vestibular function.

Positional and positioning (Dix–Hallpike) tests are performed in the standard head and body left, right, and center positions using Frenzel glasses or infrared goggles. The acceleration–deceleration from sitting to lying flat is sufficient stimulus to elicit benign paroxysmal positional vertigo (BPPV). BPPV is caused by free-floating otoconia, most often affecting the posterior semicircular canal. Posterior canal BPPV is characterized by transient, upbeating, and rotatory nystagmus with the fast phase of the rotatory component toward the down ear. Positioning nystagmus is latent, paroxysmal, reversible, and fatigable; however, not all characteristics are present in all patients.

Laboratory Tests

Traditional ENG and computerized VNG are well accepted tests of both peripheral and central vestibular function and the VOR. The saccadic, gaze, pursuit, positional, positioning, and caloric test techniques may vary somewhat between laboratories but generally follow well-standardized protocols.

Most types of gaze nystagmus are caused by brainstem or cerebellar lesions. Bilateral slow or absent saccadic eye movements, dysconjugate saccades, and dysmetria reflect ocular motor dysfunction, often caused by central lesions in the parapontine gaze centers, medial longitudinal fasciculus, and/or cerebellum. Thus abnormalities of ocular motor function imply central vestibular dysfunction.

The positional test is the most important test in evaluating symptoms of positional dizziness or vertigo. Traditionally, direction-fixed positional nystagmus is attributed to peripheral dysfunction, whereas direction-changing positional nystagmus is attributed to central dysfunction. More important, vigorous nystagmus (> 10 deg/s), despite minimal symptoms of dizziness, is more likely caused by central dysfunction, even if positional nystagmus is direction-fixed.

The caloric exam is the single-most sensitive measure of peripheral vestibular weakness in the VNG battery. It is performed by irrigating the ear canal with warm and cool water or air. The temperature change creates current flow in the lateral semicircular canal; therefore, it is an assessment of horizontal canal and superior vestibular nerve function. The maximal slow-phase velocity of the nystagmus is recorded and the two ears are compared. A unilateral weakness is present when there is a > 20 to 30% difference between the two ears. The full test includes bilateral testing and bithermal (cold and warm) irrigations, although monothermal testing is acceptable if there is a small difference in slow-phase velocity between the ears.

The clinical significance of residual inner ear vestibular function depends on whether it is stable (static) or unstable (dynamic). Stable function promotes central compensation; dizziness usually resolves. Unstable (irritative) function resists central compensation; dizziness may persist.

Failure of fixation suppression is present when the peak of caloric-induced nystagmus cannot be suppressed at least 50% with visual fixation and results usually from cerebellar disease. The test requires intact visual acuity.

Rotary Chair Test

The most common rotary chair test is sinusoidal harmonic acceleration (SHA), which evaluates low-frequency (0.64–1 Hz) VOR. The principle of SHA is that angular acceleration and deceleration generate nystagmus in the same and opposite directions, respectively. These tests are fundamentally different from calorics in several ways. Rotational chair testing stimulates and tests both ears simultaneously for a true binaural response. It also tests head movements through a slow and more "physiological" speed of movement than calorics.

Head and eye velocity signals are correlated to calculate VOR gain, latency, and asymmetry. Gain is a measure of VOR sensitivity, calculated as peak eye velocity/peak head velocity. Gain can be absent, normal, or hyperactive. Reduced or absent gain results from decreased or absent vestibular function, respectively. Elevated gain reflects VOR hyperactivity, which is commonly seen in cerebellar degeneration and motion sickness (motion intolerance). Phase measurements reflect the time difference between head and eye velocity. Phase is prolonged in both peripheral and central dysfunction and remains abnormal with minimal change over time. Asymmetry is a measure of vestibular compensation and is calculated as the difference between velocities of left- and right-beating nystagmus. Asymmetry is correlated with the patient's symptoms and helps monitor VOR compensation (i.e., as asymmetry decreases, subjective dizziness decreases).

The advantages of rotary chair testing compared with conventional VNG are (1) angular acceleration is a more natural, physiological stimulation than caloric irrigation; (2) results provide an objective measure of recovery (compensation) following vestibular injury; (3) high-frequency SHA testing can be used to determine whether residual vestibular function is present; and (4) exact visual–vestibular interaction can be studied. Disadvantages are relatively high cost, need for technical support, and nonreimbursement by insurance companies.

Vestibular-Evoked Myogenic Potential

VEMP is a test of peripheral vestibular function not generated by the VOR. It is a test of the vestibulocollic reflex through the function of the saccule and inferior vestibular nerve, which is a response to a high-intensity, low-frequency sound stimulus. A sound is put in the testing ear at ~ 90 dB, and the myogenic response is recorded from the ipsilateral sternocleidomastoid muscle. This is the only test available for the evaluation of the saccule and inferior vestibular nerve. Measured parameters include threshold for inducing the response, amplitude of the response, and latency. VEMPs have been useful in diagnosing third windows, such as dehiscence of the superior semicircular canal, which shows a reduced threshold, elevated amplitude pattern when compared with the contralateral ear.

Computerized Dynamic Posturography (CDP)

Commercially available since 1985, computerized dynamic posturography (CDP) is a computer-controlled platform and visual booth used to evaluate both sensory and motor components of balance. The test protocol is divided into a motor control test (MCT) and a sensory organization test (SOT). The MCT evaluates postural reflexes for both feet when the body is perturbed forward and backward. MCT should take into account orthopedic and age-related decrease in motor strength and coordination of the lower extremities.

Both MCT and SOT can be used to identify an aphysiological sway pattern in which there is excessive and intentional sway, commonly seen in nonphysiological dizziness. The aphysiological sway pattern can be associated with the vestibular loss pattern; however, in isolation, aphysiological sway is psychogenic or intentional and can be very helpful in assessing symptoms in worker's compensation and medicolegal cases.

The SOT evaluates postural control under six different test conditions in which visual and proprioceptive inputs are altered statically, dynamically, or both, to challenge the vestibular system. In general, abnormal sensory patterns reflect the relative contributions of the visual, vestibular, and proprioceptive systems. The SOT also measures the patient's ability to differentiate between "stable" and "unstable" visual and proprioceptive references.

SOT results can be adaptive or nonadaptive. Adaptive patterns are evident when test scores improve with repeated trials. Patients with adaptive patterns have a better prognosis with vestibular rehabilitation.

CDP cannot diagnose a specific vestibular disorder, but it can do the following:

1. Evaluate sensory integration of vestibular, visual, and proprioceptive input
2. Identify optimal candidates for vestibular rehabilitation
3. Document aphysiological sway

Thus CDP provides unique information and supplements ENG and rotational chair testing.

■ Suggested Reading

Dirks D, Ahlstrom J, Morgan D. Auditory sensitivity: air and bone conduction. In: Rinaldo R, Lamber P, eds. The Ear: Comprehensive Otology. Philadelphia, PA: Lippincott Williams and Wilkins; 2000:197–209

Dubno J, Dirks D. Measures of auditory function using speech stimuli. In: Rinaldo R, Lamber P, eds. The Ear: Comprehensive Otology. Phialdelphia, PA: Lippincott Williams and Wilkins; 2000:211–221

Halmagyi GM, Curthoys IS. A clinical sign of canal paresis. Arch Neurol 1988;45(7):737–739

Hamid M. Clinical and laboratory tests of vestibular and balance function. In: Hughes G, Pensak M, eds. Clinical Otology. New York, NY: Thieme; 1997:111–129

Hamid M. Clinical patterns of dynamic posturography. In: Arenberg I, ed. Dizziness and Balance Disorders: An Interdisciplinary Approach to Diagnosis, Treatment and Rehabilitation. Amsterdam, Netherlands: Kugler Press; 1993

Hamid MA, Hughes GB, Kinney SE, Hanson MR. Results of sinusoidal harmonic acceleration test in one thousand patients: preliminary report. Otolaryngol Head Neck Surg 1986;94(1):1–5

Honaker JA, Boismier TE, Shepard NP, Shepard NT. Fukuda stepping test: sensitivity and specificity. J Am Acad Audiol 2009;20(5):311–314, quiz 335

Hotz MA, Harris FP, Probst R. Otoacoustic emissions: an approach for monitoring aminoglycoside-induced ototoxicity. Laryngoscope 1994;104(9):1130–1134

Huynh MT, Pollack RA, Cunningham RA. Universal newborn hearing screening: feasibility in a community hospital. J Fam Pract 1996;42(5):487–490

Kaylie D, Garrison D, Tucci DL. Evaluation of the patient with recurrent vertigo. Arch Otolaryngol Head Neck Surg 2012;138(6):584–587

Keith R. Central auditory assessment. In: Hughes G, Pensak M, eds. Clinical Otology. New York, NY: Thieme; 1997:101–108

Keith RW, Pensak ML. Central auditory function. Otolaryngol Clin North Am 1991;24(2):371–379

Kemp DT. Evidence of mechanical nonlinearity and frequency selective wave amplification in the cochlea. Arch Otorhinolaryngol 1979;224(1-2):37–45

Kemp DT. Stimulated acoustic emissions from within the human auditory system. J Acoust Soc Am 1978;64(5):1386–1391

Menyuk P. Relationship of otitis media to speech processing and language development. In: Katz J, Stecker N, Henderson D, eds. Central Auditory Processing: A Transdiciplinary View. St. Louis, MO: Mosby–Year Book; 1992

Musiek FE, Pinheiro ML. Frequency patterns in cochlear, brainstem, and cerebral lesions. Audiology 1987;26(2):79–88

Nodar R. Diagnostic audiology. In: Hughes G, Pensak M, eds. Clinical Otology. New York, NY: Thieme; 1997:98–100

Roland PS, Yellin MW, Meyerhoff WL, Frank T. Simultaneous comparison between transtympanic and extratympanic electrocochleography. Am J Otol 1995;16(4):444–450

Rosengren SM, Welgampola MS, Colebatch JG. Vestibular evoked myogenic potentials: past, present and future. Clin Neurophysiol 2010;121(5):636–651

Schwaber M, Hall JW, Zealor DL. Intraoperative monitoring of the facial and cochleovestibular nerves in otologic surgery: Part II. Insights Otolaryngol 1991;6:108

62 Diagnostic Imaging Techniques in Otology

■ Introduction

In the field of otology, imaging plays a prominent role in patient evaluation and management. Imaging techniques have evolved over the years. Currently, the most frequently used techniques are magnetic resonance imaging (MRI) and high-resolution computed tomography (HRCT) scanning (**Fig. 62.1**). On occasion, magnetic resonance angiography (MRA), magnetic resonance venography (MRV), CT angiography (CTA), conventional angiography, and nuclear medicine studies are employed.

This chapter addresses many common otologic and neurotologic diagnoses and the role imaging plays in the diagnosis and management of these conditions.

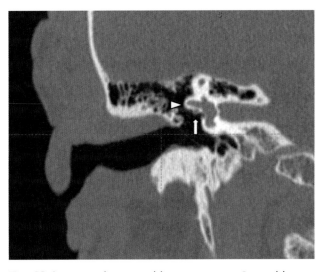

Fig. 62.1 Normal temporal bone anatomy. Coronal bone–windowed computed tomography of a normal right ear through the level of the middle ear. Midtympanic segment of the facial nerve (*small white arrow*), lateral semicircular canal (*white arrowhead*).

Chronic Otitis Media

Imaging studies help in the management of chronic otitis media by determining the extent of the disease, any associated complications of the disease (e.g., lateral semicircular canal fistula), and pneumatization of the mastoid. Some clinicians advocate routine CT scanning for operative cases to help plan the surgery, whereas others limit imaging studies to those patients in whom a complication of chronic otitis media is suspected or when surgery is planned on an only-hearing ear. Many clinicians believe that the diagnosis of cholesteatoma is a clinical diagnosis based on binocular microscopic examination of the patient, whereas others rely on imaging studies to establish that diagnosis. Preoperative knowledge of the extent of mastoid pneumatization can help in making an early decision to perform a canal-wall-down procedure, particularly in ears with poorly pneumatized mastoids.

Some clinicians have advocated routine imaging, instead of a "second-look" procedure, to assess a patient for possible residual cholesteatoma, particularly after canal-wall-up surgery. Traditional CT or MRI is often unreliable in this application because it cannot differentiate between mural cholesteatoma lining the mastoid cavity and normal mucosal lining. However, newer imaging techniques, such as non-echo-planar diffusion-weighted MRI, have been shown to be highly sensitive and specific for detecting cholesteatomas down to 3 mm in size. This imaging modality can be a useful adjunct in determining the presence of residual or recurrent cholesteatoma and has been advocated as a possible alternative to second-look surgery (**Fig. 62.2**). It is also useful when a cartilage tympanoplasty has been performed and the presence of cholesteatoma in the middle ear medial to the cartilage graft is difficult to determine on physical examination.

One of the most common complications of chronic otitis media is lateral canal fistula (**Fig. 62.3**).

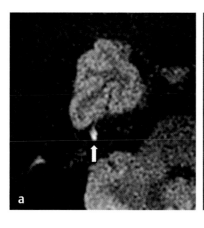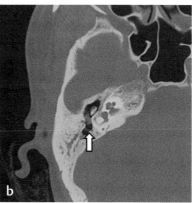

Fig. 62.2 Imaging of cholesteatoma. (**a**) A non-echo-planar diffusion-weighted magnetic resonance imaging scan (HASTE protocol) with a bright area of diffusion restriction, suggestive of cholesteatoma (*arrow*). (**b**) A noncontrast temporal bone computed tomographic (CT) scan of the same patient showing opacification in the antrum. The CT imaging alone would not allow a clinician to differentiate between residual disease versus postoperative fibrosis, mucosal edema, or fluid.

In 50% of lateral canal fistula cases, the facial nerve is also involved by cholesteatoma. Preoperative HRCT helps alert a surgeon to the presence of these complications.

Other complications of chronic otitis media may be best evaluated by MRI or by a combination of CT and MRI. Sigmoid sinus thrombosis can be seen on MRI (**Fig. 62.4**), although in some patients with a patent sinus and slow or turbulent blood flow, conventional MRI scans may erroneously suggest sinus thrombosis. Sigmoid sinus thrombosis should be diagnosed only when all images suggest a mural thrombus and absence of venous flow. In some cases, MRV may be helpful to establish the diagnosis of sigmoid sinus thrombosis. Other intracranial complications include meningitis, encephalitis, and brain abscess (**Fig. 62.5**) and are best imaged on MRI.

Apical petrositis (Gradenigo syndrome) (**Fig. 62.6**) is an example of a complication of chronic otitis media that can be diagnosed radiologically through a combination of HRCT and MRI. CT scan shows a destructive petrous apex lesion, and MRI demonstrates leptomeningeal enhancement, which suggests an infectious etiology.

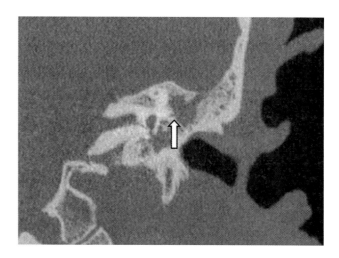

Fig. 62.3 Acquired cholesteatoma with lateral canal fistula. This coronal computed tomographic scan of the left ear shows a large soft tissue mass (cholesteatoma) filling the mastoid and eroding through the bone of the lateral semicircular canal (*arrow*).

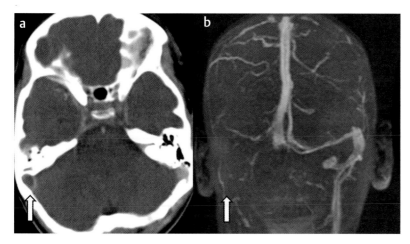

Fig. 62.4 Sigmoid sinus and jugular bulb thrombosis secondary to mastoiditis. Absence of contrast flow in right sigmoid sinus seen on axial, postcontrast head computed tomographic scan (*arrow*, **a**) and magnetic resonance venography (*arrow*, **b**).

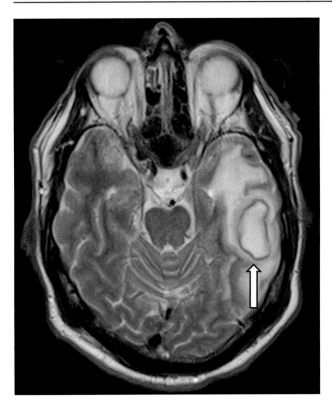

Fig. 62.5 Temporal lobe abscess. This T2-weighted axial magnetic resonance imaging scan shows a left temporal lobe abscess (*arrow*) with adjacent brain edema. The patient had chronic otitis media and cholesteatoma in the ipsilateral ear.

Congenital Aural Atresia

Imaging studies (specifically HRCT) are critical in the evaluation of a patient's candidacy for aural atresia surgery and help provide the following information in these patients:

- Feasibility of reconstruction
- Anatomical information to facilitate surgery
- Presence of coexisting congenital cholesteatoma

Jahrsdoerfer and others have shown that hearing results after atresia repair correlate with the development of specific anatomical features of the temporal bone, as evaluated by HRCT (**Fig. 62.7**): the presence of stapes, malleus/incus complex, incus–stapes connections, round window, patent oval window, middle ear space, mastoid pneumatization, and facial nerve in favorable location.

With children it is usually best to delay imaging tests until a child is old enough to cooperate with the test procedure without requiring sedation. Typically, this is at age 5 to 6 years, which is also usually the age that reconstructive surgery is contemplated.

Imaging can also be helpful in children with an unexplained conductive hearing loss in the presence of a normal-appearing tympanic membrane. Clinicians can assess the patency of the oval window, other congenital ossicular anomalies, congenital cholesteatoma, or enlarged vestibular aqueduct and be alerted to associated facial nerve anomalies. HRCT is the study of choice in children with an unexplained conductive hearing loss.

Pediatric Sensorineural Hearing Loss

For purposes of imaging, pediatric sensorineural hearing loss (SNHL) can be categorized as progressive and nonprogressive. However, the inherent difficulties of audiometric testing of young children can, at times, make the determination of true progression difficult.

Reviews suggest that temporal bone imaging is cost-effective for evaluating SNHL in pediatric patients. In patients with stable congenital SNHL, inner ear anomalies shown on imaging studies provide a diagnosis for the child (and especially the parents), but do not usually change the treatment.

However, in patients with progressive SNHL, imaging studies may provide information that alters therapy. Perilymphatic fistula repair has fallen out of favor in the setting of a progressive SNHL and inner ear anomalies demonstrated on imaging studies. The

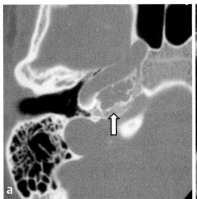
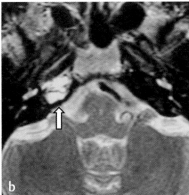

Fig. 62.6 Apical petrositis (Gradenigo syndrome). (**a**) Computed tomography demonstrates a destructive lesion of the pneumatized portion of the right petrous apex (*arrow*). (**b**) T2-weighted magnetic resonance imaging shows fluid in right petrous apex (*arrow*). These radiographic findings along with clinical symptoms of retro-orbital pain, otorrhea, and abducens nerve palsy would be consistent with Gradenigo syndrome.

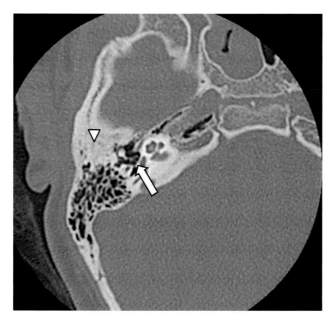

Fig. 62.7 Congenital external auditory canal atresia. Axial high-resolution computed tomography through the expected location of the right external auditory canal (*arrowhead*). Note the dysplastic incus and malleus have formed a "fusion mass," but a stapes is present (*arrow*). The mastoid and middle ear are well aerated.

detection of a large vestibular aqueduct (**Fig. 62.8**) may lead to restrictions of physical activity or any activity that could predispose to head trauma. Finally, in the older child, a retrocochlear lesion can be detected, particularly a vestibular schwannoma associated with neurofibromatosis type 2.

High-resolution CT scanning is usually recommended for evaluating a young child and prior to surgery for any congenital conductive hearing loss. Abnormalities of inner ear morphology are the primary concerns in this patient group (**Fig. 62.9**). In patients with congenital conductive hearing loss, abnormalities such as oval window atresia, anoma-

lous facial nerve over the oval window, and enlarged vestibular aqueduct (which can cause a conductive loss) would all be reasons not to operate. T2-weighted fast spin-echo (FSE) MRI is used by some clinicians for children with SNHL and may have some advantage in detection of defects of the membranous labyrinth.

In older children, if there is suspicion of a vestibular schwannoma associated with neurofibromatosis type 2, a gadolinium-enhanced MRI scan is indicated. In these patients, multiple cranial nerve tumors may also be evident.

Precochlear implant imaging provides important surgical information, including the patency of the cochlea, the presence of cochlear malformations, associated facial nerve anomalies, and the presence of the cochlear nerve. HRCT is a commonly used preoperative imaging technique, but it may underestimate cochlear lumen occlusion, particularly with a history of otosclerosis or meningitis (**Fig. 62.10**). High-resolution T2-weighted MRI with a sagittal view of the internal auditory canal OHC) provides excellent definition of the nerves of the IAC to verify the presence of a cochlear nerve (**Fig. 62.11**). The use of MRI in the precochlear implant screening of children with profound congenital SNHL has the additional benefits of identifying other central nervous system (CNS) abnormalities and not delivering radiation to the patient, who may be a young child.

Pulsatile Tinnitus and Vascular Tympanic Membrane

When confronted with a patient with unilateral pulsatile tinnitus, the extent of imaging is dependent on the physical findings and the degree of clinical suspicion.

Patients with an obvious vascular middle ear mass require imaging with HRCT scan. Although MRI/MRV can image intratemporal vascular structures, it can be difficult to see these structures on

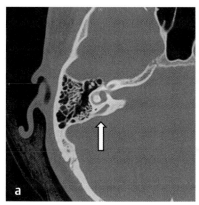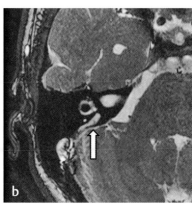

Fig. 62.8 Large vestibular aqueduct syndrome. (**a**) High-resolution bone-only computed tomography through the temporal bone demonstrates enlargement of the osseous vestibular aqueduct (*arrow*). (**b**) T2-weighted high-resolution magnetic resonance imaging source images demonstrate enlarged endolymphatic duct/sac (*arrow*).

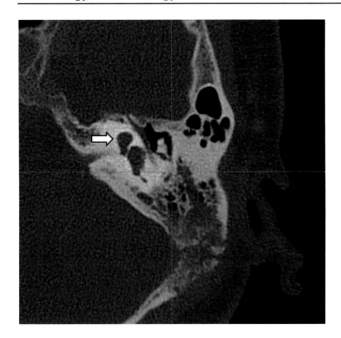

Fig. 62.9 Congenital inner ear dysplasias. Axial bone-only computed tomography of the left ear demonstrating cochlear dysplasia, without development of the normal full two-and-one-half turns and identification of a cystic cochlea and vestibule (*arrow*).

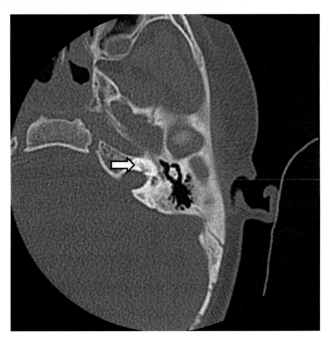

Fig. 62.10 Cochlear ossification. Axial computed tomography (CT) of the left temporal bone of a patient with previous meningitis and subsequent development of bilateral sensorineural hearing loss shows obliteration of much of the cochlear lumen (*arrow*). The CT diagnosis of labyrinthine ossification is made when the normal membranous labyrinth fluid space is compromised by bony deposition. Any area of the membranous labyrinth may be involved.

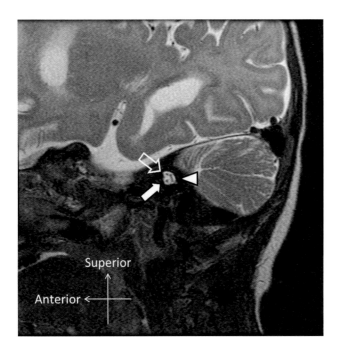

Fig. 62.11 Sagittal high-resolution T2-weighted magnetic resonance imaging showing a cross-sectional view of the internal auditory canal (IAC). In the normal anatomical state, each of the four nerves within the IAC can be identified—cochlear (*solid arrow*), facial (*outlined arrow*), and superior and inferior vestibular nerves (*arrowhead*).

MRI because of the juxtaposition of low-signal bone and the low natural contrast of air and flowing blood. However, HRCT remains a good choice because of its ability to depict fine bony detail. In cases of an aberrant carotid artery, dehiscent or high jugular bulb (**Fig. 62.12**), or paraganglioma (glomus tumor) confined to the temporal bone, no further imaging studies are required. For paragangliomas with suspected jugular bulb involvement, or intracranial extension, contrast-enhanced MRI can further delineate tumor margins. In large glomus tumors, a characteristic "salt and pepper" appearance (**Fig. 62.13**) will be seen on the unenhanced T1 MRI scans. The "salt" is thought to be secondary to the subacute hemorrhage with the tumor. The "pepper" results from channel voids of the tumor vessels. MRI with the use of contrast will clarify the size and extent of the tumor, and unenhanced bone window axial and coronal CT will identify the precise bony surgical landmarks. However, some clinicians have suggested that CTA is superior at differentiating between glomus tumors and jugular foramen schwannomas. CTA also provides important information about arterial supply to the tumor and flow status of the jugular vein. Glo-

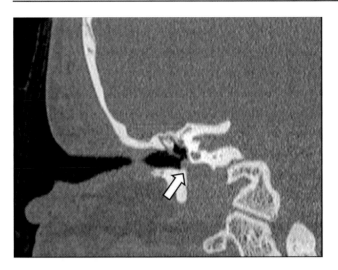

Fig. 62.12 Dehiscent high jugular bulb. Coronal computed tomographic image reveals a high, laterally bulging jugular bulb. The bulging vein abuts the inferior tympanic membrane marked by its inferior bony attachment, the tympanic annulus (*arrow*).

mus jugulare tumors usually require angiography, but primarily for preoperative embolization, rather than diagnostic imaging.

Patients without an obvious middle ear mass, but with a strong clinical suspicion (such as objective pulsatile or pulse-synchronous tinnitus), most likely require additional imaging. Modalities such as CT/CTA or MRI/MRA are good choices for initial evaluation of these patients. These modalities can detect a paraganglioma not visible on clinical exam. They can also demonstrate a dural arteriovenous malformation or internal carotid artery stenosis. Although MRA can detect small arteriovenous malformations, it can miss very small lesions. If sufficient concern exists, the patient should undergo diagnostic angiog-

raphy, with concomitant therapeutic embolization planned if an arteriovenous malformation is found (**Fig. 62.14**). Sigmoid sinus dehiscence/diverticulum (SSDD) can also present with objective, pulse-synchronous tinnitus. SSDD is diagnosed on HRCT as loss of bone overlying the sigmoid sinus or diverticulum from the sinus.

Other tumors of the jugular foramen include meningiomas (**Fig. 62.15**) and lower cranial nerve schwannomas (**Fig. 62.16**). These lesions are best demonstrated on enhanced MRI scans. HRCT shows erosive changes in the jugular foramen and provides bony detail to aid in surgical planning. On casual inspection, because of the obvious intratemporal extension, these lesions may be confused with acoustic tumors. However, the intratemporal extension is seen inferior to the level of the IAC.

Facial Nerve Tumor

Facial nerve imaging is required when a tumor involving the nerve is suspected. The most common clinical setting in which this occurs is a patient with an acute facial paralysis thought to be Bell palsy. Most clinicians agree that patients with Bell palsy do not require immediate imaging. Patients who should be imaged (MRI with and without gadolinium) are atypical in presentation, such as in the following cases:

1. Recurrent ipsilateral paralysis
2. Slowly progressive paralysis
3. No recovery after 6 months
4. Palsy associated with twitching

High-resolution contrast-enhanced MRI from the brainstem through the parotid is required in most cases of suspected tumors. It is important to differentiate tumors from viral etiologies, because enhancement and thickening of the nerves can be

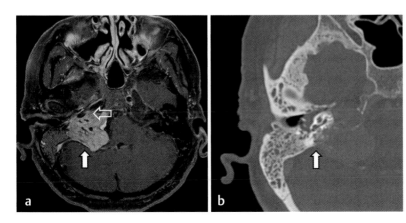

Fig. 62.13 Intra- and extracranial glomus jugulare invading inferiorly into the internal jugular vein. (**a**) An axial, postcontrast T1-weighted magnetic resonance imaging scan showing a tumor centered in the jugular foramen with cerebellopontine angle (CPA) extension and brainstem compression (*white arrow*). The tumor abuts the petrous segment of the carotid artery (*open arrow*). The dark flow voids within the tumor reveal the typical highly vascularized nature of glomus tumors. (b) An axial temporal bone computed tomographic scan. This tumor has caused significant otic capsule and temporal bone erosion (*solid arrow*).

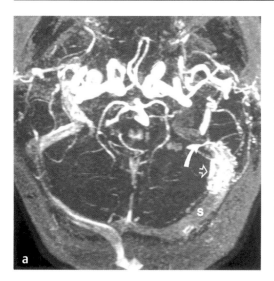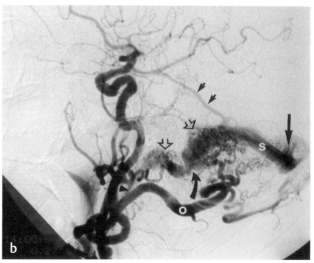

Fig. 62.14 Dural arteriovenous fistula (AVF) in a patient with objective left ear pulsatile tinnitus. (**a**) Basal magnetic resonance angiography reconstruction shows a dural AVF involving the left distal transverse sinus (S). The many high-signal dots and lines (*open arrow*) at the site of the fistula represent the multiple microfistulas seen in these lesions. The *curved arrow* marks a site of stenosis of the venous sinus at the junction of the transverse and sigmoid sinus. (**b**) Lateral view of a left common carotid angiogram better delineates the nature of this dural AVF. The microfistulas (*open arrows*) are most densely concentrated in the area of the distal transverse sinus (S). There is retrograde flow in the transverse sinus to the level of the torcular herophili (*long black arrow*) and in the vein of Labbé (*short black arrows*). The two main feeding arteries are the occipital artery (O) and the ascending pharyngeal artery (*arrowhead*). Again, notice the stenosis of the venous sinus at the junction of the transverse and sigmoid sinuses (*curved arrow*). The retrograde venous flow in the transverse sinus and vein of Labbé seen on the angiogram indicates the more serious nature of this dural AVF, which is the type that will often develop intracranial hypertension. Definitive intravascular occlusion of this lesion is highly recommended.

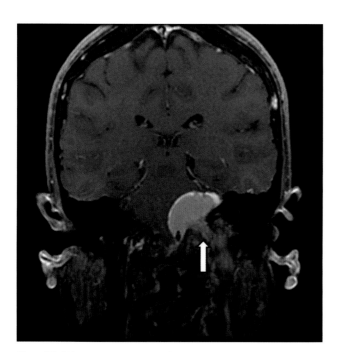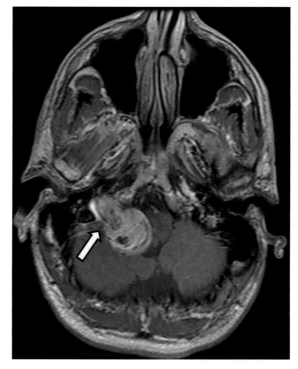

Fig. 62.15 Meningioma with jugular foramen involvement. Coronal T1-weighted postcontrast magnetic resonance imaging shows a left meningioma in the cerebellopontine angle with tumor extension through the jugular foramen (*arrow*).

Fig. 62.16 Large jugular foramen lower cranial nerve schwannoma. Axial T1-weighted postcontrast magnetic resonance imaging demonstrating a right jugular foramen schwannoma of one of the lower cranial nerves with intracranial extension into the cerebellopontine angle and widening of the jugular foramen (*arrow*).

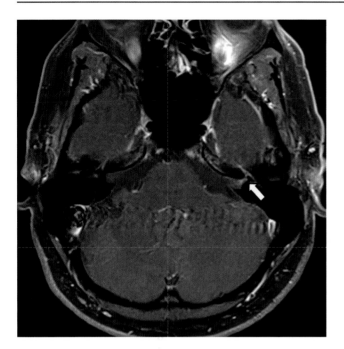

Fig. 62.17 Magnetic resonance imaging (MRI) findings in Bell palsy. Right axial enhanced T1 MRI demonstrates typical findings of Bell palsy, including enhancement at the fundus of the internal auditory canal (*arrow*), and along the labyrinthine, geniculate, and tympanic segments of the facial nerve. Note that the enhancement pattern is uniform and that the nerve is minimally and linearly enlarged without nodularity. This important feature helps differentiate Bell palsy from perineural neoplasm along the course of the facial nerve. Abnormal enhancement may persist well beyond clinical improvement, and has been observed for as long as 13 months following initial diagnosis.

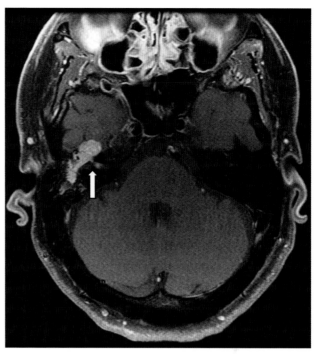

Fig. 62.18 Facial nerve schwannoma. Axial enhanced T1-weighted magnetic resonance imaging (MRI) at the level of the internal auditory canal shows an avidly enhancing mass at the labyrinthine segment (*arrow*). The mass is centered in the geniculate ganglion and extends along the distal course of the facial nerve. Although bone-windowed computed tomographic images are often helpful to the surgeon in planning extensive temporal bone or skull base surgery, it is the soft tissue details available from MRI that often make the radiological diagnosis.

seen on MRI (**Fig. 62.17**) in cases of Bell palsy and herpes zoster oticus.

The most common intrinsic facial nerve tumors are facial nerve schwannomas and hemangiomas. Facial nerve schwannomas (**Fig. 62.18**) produce symptoms when large, enhance homogeneously and intensely on MRI, and produce smooth bony margins when viewed on CT scan. Facial nerve hemangiomas (**Fig. 62.19**) produce severe deficits when small, and they enhance intensely but not always in a uniform pattern on MRI. When viewed on CT, hemangiomas have irregular bone margins and may have intratumoral calcifications. Malignant parotid tumors (**Fig. 62.20**), such as adenoid cystic carcinoma, may also track up the facial nerve via perineural spread and may present with intratemporal involvement of the nerve. Therefore, it is important to image the parotid gland in a patient with an unresolved or progressive facial paresis/paralysis.

Patients with temporal bone fractures do not need acute imaging unless they have a facial nerve injury that will require surgical intervention. Most patients with facial trauma will undergo a maxillofacial CT scan, which is often adequate if the patient

is awake enough to get a reliable facial nerve exam. Temporal bone fractures (**Fig. 62.21**) are generally classified as longitudinal (parallel to the long axis of the temporal bone); transverse (perpendicular to the long axis of the temporal bone, often involving the labyrinth); and mixed types. In the setting of a temporal bone fracture with facial nerve paralysis, HRCT is helpful in defining the location and severity of the injury and associated injuries such as involvement of the labyrinth, ossicles, or vascular structures. Should a petrous carotid artery injury be suspected, a CTA may be indicated.

The radiological investigation of patients with hemifacial spasm seems to answer two principal questions: (1) Is there a lesion other than a vascular loop causing this problem? and (2) Can the offending redundant vascular loop be identified?

MRI/MRA is often used for evaluating patients with hemifacial spasm because of its inherent ability to visualize the relationships of the structures of the CPA cistern and to evaluate the facial nerve from pons to parotid. High-resolution T2 MRI scans (constructive interference into steady state [CISS] or fast imaging employing steady-state acquisition [FIESTA]

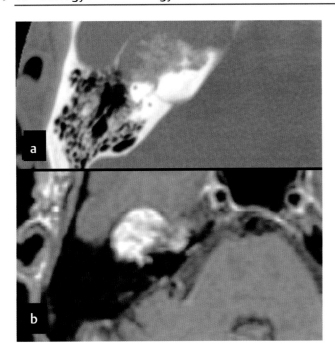

Fig. 62.19 Facial nerve hemangioma. (**a**) Right axial computed tomographic (CT) image demonstrates a large ossifying hemangioma centered in the geniculate fossa, with numerous intrinsic spicules of bone and permeative changes. Extension into the labyrinthine segment of the facial nerve canal can be seen. (**b**) Right axial enhanced T1-weighted magnetic resonance imaging (MRI) shows intense enhancement of the hemangioma. The intense lesion enhancement tracking along the facial nerve on the MRI suggests the diagnosis, but facial nerve schwannoma and meningioma would also have to be considered. The ossifying matrix of the tumor, seen well by CT, is characteristic of an ossifying hemangioma.

sequences) also show excellent neurovascular definition and can identify the relationships of vascular loops to the cranial nerves (**Fig. 62.22**).

Retrocochlear

Perhaps the most common indication for imaging in an otologic practice is evaluation of patients suspected of having a vestibular schwannoma or other retrocochlear lesion. These patients may present with a variety of unilateral auditory symptoms, including progressive SNHL, sudden SNHL, tinnitus, and dizziness. The evaluation methods for such patients have evolved over the years, and many tests used in the past, such as site-of-lesion audiometric tests or air contrast CT cisternography, are no longer used.

There has been recent concern over the poor accuracy of auditory brainstem response (ABR) measures in detecting small acoustic tumors. However, contrast-enhanced MRI has such high sensitivity to detect a lesion, this imaging modality has become the primary diagnostic test to evaluate for vestibular schwannomas. It is important to note that a noncontrast CT scan is insensitive to the detection of vestibular schwannomas. Even contrast-enhanced CT scans will rarely detect intracanalicular lesions. In the past, air-contrast CT cisternography was used to evaluate patients for possible intracanalicular lesions. This evaluation method has been replaced by contrast-enhanced MRI scans, except in the rare patient who is unable to undergo MRI.

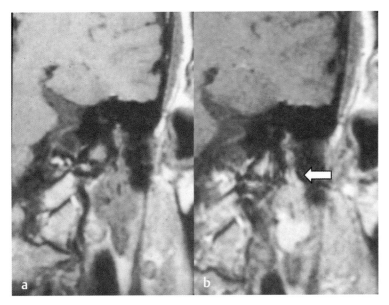

Fig. 62.20 Perineural tumor spread along the facial nerve from parotid malignancy. Parotid mucoepidermoid carcinoma spreading in a perineural fashion along the mastoid segment of the left facial nerve. (**a**) A coronal T1-weighted precontrast magnetic resonance imaging (MRI) scan of the parotid and left ear. (**b**) Coronal postcontrast T1-weighted MRI reveals the parotid mucoepidermoid carcinoma spreading into the temporal bone along the mastoid segment of the facial nerve (*arrow*) to the level of the posterior or second genu. The original presenting symptom in this patient's case was hemifacial spasm. Over a 2-year period, the patient underwent two MRI scans focused to the cerebellopontine angle without a diagnosis being made. The symptom progressed to peripheral facial nerve paralysis before an MRI scan was completed that included the parotid tumor in its field of view. Imaging of the extracranial facial nerve is critical in all cases of peripheral facial nerve paralysis where an isolated motor facial neuropathy is present with sparing of the three special functions of the facial nerve. Conversely, when an infiltrating malignancy of the parotid gland with facial nerve findings is identified, imaging of the intratemporal facial nerve is critical.

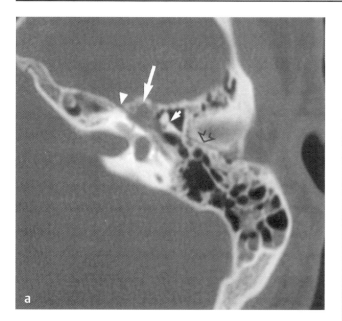

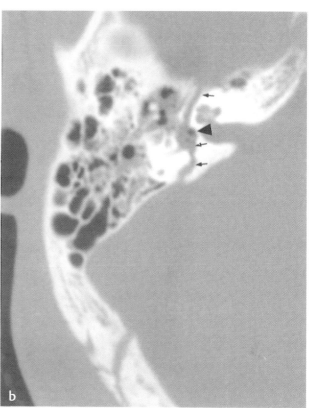

Fig. 62.21 Temporal bone fracture. (**a**) Left axial computed tomography (CT) shows a longitudinal temporal bone fracture (*open arrow*) involving the area of the geniculate ganglion (*arrowhead*). Blood in the geniculate fossa (*long arrow*) and ossicular dislocation (*short arrow*) are also seen involving the bony labyrinth (*arrow*). (**b**) Right axial CT shows a transverse temporal bone fracture (*small arrows*) through the vestibule with evidence of pneumolabyrinth (*arrowhead*).

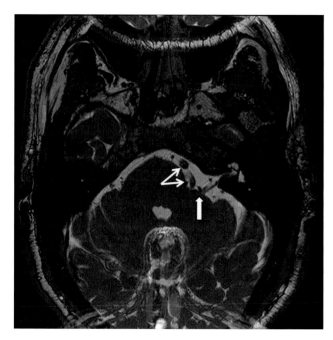

Fig. 62.22 Magnetic resonance imaging (MRI) in hemifacial spasm. This axial high-resolution T2-weighted MRI scan shows the root entry zone of the left facial nerve being compressed by a vascular loop of the anteroinferior cerebellar artery (*white arrow*). This patient also had asymmetry of the vertebral arteries with both on the left side of the brainstem before their anastomosis to become the basilar artery.

Vestibular schwannomas (**Fig. 62.23**) are the most common extra-axial mass lesion of the cerebellopontine angle (CPA). They enhance intensely and uniformly on MRI (**Table 62.1**) although there may be a cystic component in up to 15% of these tumors. On precontrast T1 MRI scans, neuromas are usually isointense to the brain, whereas on T2 MRI scans, they are mildly hyperintense to the brain. Enhanced T1 MRI features that define an IAC-CPA cistern lesion as a vestibular schwannoma include a uniformly enhancing mass centered in the CPA over the porus acusticus, with an IAC component having an "ice cream cone" appearance or being entirely within the IAC. For patients with unilateral audiovestibular symptoms, care should also be taken to evaluate the inner ear in postcontrast MRI for an isolated intralabyrinthine or intracochlear schwannoma.

Meningiomas (**Fig. 62.24**) also enhance on MRI scan and may have an associated enhancing dural "tail." The most important imaging criteria for diagnosing a CPA meningioma are lesion location and shape. The pertinent anatomical information regarding an IAC-CPA mass includes whether the lesion is intra-axial or extra-axial and where the lesion is centered relative to the IAC. Characteristics of meningiomas include an extra-axial dural-based location off center from the IAC. Unlike vestibular schwannomas, meningiomas typically have a sessile growth pattern

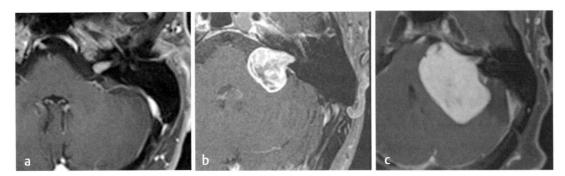

Fig. 62.23 Typical magnetic resonance imaging (MRI) scans of vestibular schwannomas. (**a**) T1-weighted axial MRI with gadolinium enhancement demonstrating small intracanalicular, (**b**) medium-sized, and (**c**) very large vestibular schwannomas.

Table 62.1 Posterior fossa masses: imaging characteristics

Lesion	T1[a]	T2[a]	Enhancement
Acoustic neuroma	Isointense	Mildly hyperintense	Yes
Meningioma	Isointense	Hypohyperintense (depends on calcium content)	Yes
Epidermoid	Hypointense (slightly greater than cerebrospinal fluid)	Hyperintense	No, or mild rim enhancing only if inflammatory response is present
Arachnoid cyst	Hypointense	Hyperintense	No
Lipoma	Hyperintense	Intermediate	No

[a] For acoustic neuroma and meningioma, comparisons are relative to brain; for the remainder, comparisons are relative to cerebrospinal fluid.

and form an obtuse angle with the temporal bone and rarely extend into the IAC. Calcification and hyperostosis help suggest the diagnosis of meningioma when present. Occasionally, a meningioma may arise from the dura of the internal auditory canal and present as an intracanalicular mass.

Facial nerve neuromas may arise in the cerebellopontine angle, and in some cases may be differentiated from vestibular schwannomas on imaging only by the extension of enhancement on MRI along the course of the labyrinthine segment of the facial nerve (**Fig. 62.18**). Other findings that suggest a facial nerve origin include erosion of the superior margin of the IAC, expansion of the labyrinthine facial nerve canal, erosion of the region of the geniculate fossa, and eccentricity of the CPA portion of the tumor relative to the porus of the IAC. The most important evidence that an IAC-CPA mass is a facial nerve neuroma is extension along the labyrinthine segment of the facial nerve. This labyrinthine segment "tumor tail" must be carefully looked for in all cases of suspected vestibular schwannomas to dif-

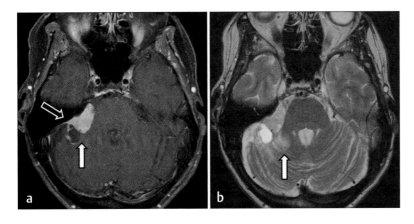

Fig. 62.24 Meningioma of the cerebellopontine angle. The left panel of an axial, postcontrast T1-weighted magnetic resonance imaging (MRI) scan shows a meningioma of the right cerebellopontine angle (CPA) with a posterior cystic component (*white arrow*). A typical dura tail is seen on the petrous face (*open arrow*). The right panel shows an axial T2-weighted MRI at the same level highlighting the adjacent peduncular edema (*white arrow*), suggestive of "vascular steal" from the tumor.

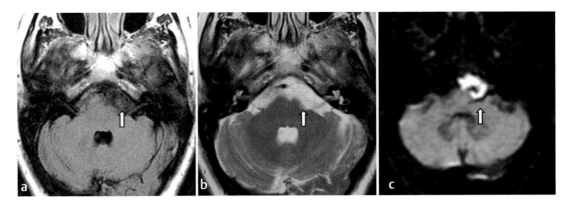

Fig. 62.25 Posterior fossa epidermoid. (**a**)T1-weighted axial magnetic resonance imaging (MRI) showing low signal mass in the left cerebellopontine angle and prepontine space (*arrow*). (**b**) On T2-weighted MRI, this was slow high signal, consistent with posterior fossa epidermoid. (**c**) Diffusion-weighted imaging showing diffusion restriction (bright signal) in the area of the mass, suggesting that this is an epidermoid.

ferentiate the facial from vestibular schwannomas preoperatively.

Other less common lesions in the cerebellopontine angle include epidermoid cysts (**Fig. 62.25**), which are typically irregularly shaped and do not enhance on MRI scan. These lesions most commonly have a low signal on T1 and high signal on T2. The hallmark of an arachnoid cyst (**Fig. 62.26**) is lack of enhancement and signal intensity that follows cerebrospinal fluid (CSF) on all sequences. Additionally, the fluid in the cyst should not demonstrate any flow-related phenomena as may be seen in the adjacent

CSF. Arachnoid cysts can demonstrate mass effect. Imaging distinction from an epidermoid cyst is on the basis of signal characteristics and displacement of, rather than insinuation into, the adjacent brainstem. Diffusion-weighted imaging (DWI) sequences on MRI can differentiate an epidermoid cyst, which will be diffusion-restricted (bright on DWI), from an arachnoid cyst.

On MRI scan, lipomas (**Fig. 62.27**) in the cerebellopontine angle or IAC will appear bright on T1, but lose signal on T2 MRIs and fat-saturated sequences. Lipomas or lipomatous hamartomas occur less fre-

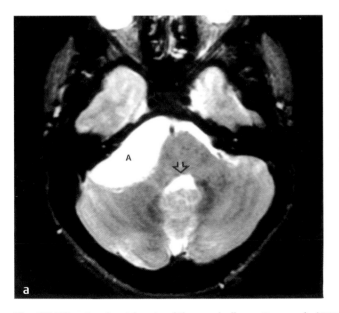

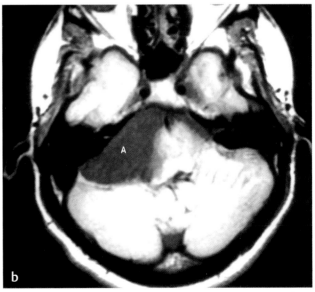

Fig. 62.26 Arachnoid cysts of the cerebellopontine angle (CPA) cistern. (**a**) Axial T1-weighted magnetic resonance imaging (MRI) demonstrates the cyst (A) displacing the brainstem to the left and indenting the right cerebellar hemisphere (*open arrow*). Unlike the epidermoid, the signal of this lesion is identical to that of normal cerebrospinal fluid (CSF) in the cisterna magna. (**b**) Axial T2-weighted MRI shows T2 hyperintensity of the cyst (A), which matches the signal of CSF in the fourth ventricle.

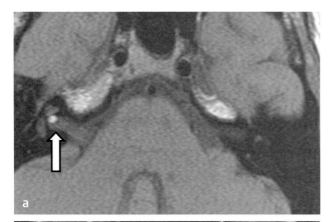

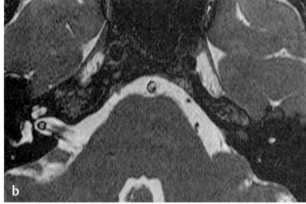

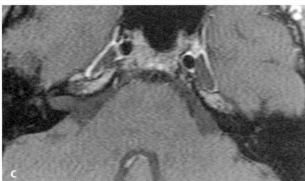

these reliable signal characteristics, clinicians can accurately predict the histology of lipomas on MRI scanning, which gives important information regarding treatment.

CNS hemosiderosis can cause a progressive SNHL and can be detected on MRI. This disease is usually caused by chronic bleeding in the subarachnoid space. Superficial siderosis can be seen in association with intracranial tumors, a history of trauma, vascular malformations, or aneurysms, though the source of the bleed is often unknown (**Fig. 62.28**). On MRI scan, hemosiderosis appears as a dark lining on T2-weighted images of the arachnoid membranes on the surface of the brainstem and cerebellum.

Screening techniques for imaging vestibular schwannomas include FSE MRI. This technique does not require gadolinium, provides submillimeter resolution, and has a low cost that approaches that of ABR. It provides very detailed anatomy of the IAC and CPA but is less sensitive to intra-axial or intratemporal pathology.

Fig. 62.27 Internal auditory canal (IAC) lipoma. (**a**) Axial precontrast T1-weighted magnetic resonance imaging (MRI) shows an inherently bright lesion in the right lateral IAC. (**b**) High-resolution axial T2-weighted MRI shows the same lesion with a dark rim around it, typical of adipose tissue. (**c**) Axial, postcontrast T1-weighted MRI with fat saturation protocol eliminates the signal from the lesion, confirming the radiographic diagnosis of an IAC lipoma. These lesions can also be multifocal and are occasionally seen within the vestibule.

quently in the CPA cistern than epidermoid and arachnoid cysts. Rarely, they may also be found in the IAC or within the membranous labyrinth or vestibule. Imaging findings are characteristic with fat density on CT and fat signal on MRI. Lipomas typically surround neurovascular structures. Because of

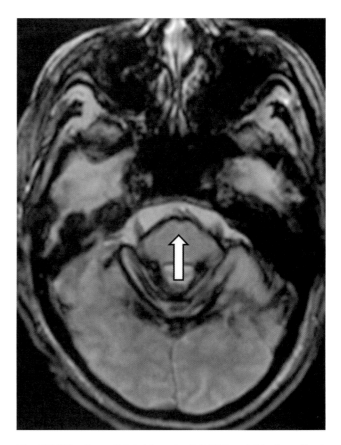

Fig. 62.28 Superficial siderosis. Axial T2-weighted gradient-echo magnetic resonance imaging shows a dark layering on the brainstem (*arrow*), cranial nerves, and cerebellum. This imaging finding is consistent with superficial siderosis.

Petrous Apex

Cholesterol granuloma is the most common surgical lesion confined to the petrous apex. On MRI, it usually appears bright on both T1- and T2-weighted sequences. Cholesterol granuloma does not enhance on MRI and has an expansile appearance (**Fig. 62.29**). On HRCT scan, there will be loss of bony septation in the petrous apex and pushing margins. The opposite petrous apex may be well pneumatized.

The differential diagnosis of petrous apex lesions includes cholesteatoma, mucocele, trapped sterile fluid (effusion), and asymmetrical pneumatization/bone marrow. The signal characteristics are detailed in **Table 62.2**.

It is important to identify nonpathological lesions of the petrous apex because they may appear similar to cholesterol granuloma. Generally, these lesions can be differentiated by their radiological signal characteristics using a combination of MRI and HRCT scans.

Asymmetrical pneumatization can appear as a bright petrous apex lesion (**Fig. 62.30**). On MRI, petrous apex yellow or fatty bone marrow in the nonpneumatized side can appear bright on T1, and intermediate signal on FSE T2, but HRCT shows a nonexpansile, nonpneumatized, marrow-filled petrous apex.

"Trapped fluid" or a meningocele/arachnoid cyst in petrous apex air cells (**Fig. 62.31**) can be confused with a pathological condition but can be differentiated by the imaging characteristics. T2 MRI demonstrates bright signal in the petrous apex air cells, with T1 signal being variable. HRCT shows characteristic nonexpansile opacification of petrous apex air cells. DWI will not show any diffusion restriction in the area of interest. Trapped fluid, petrous apex meningoceles/arachnoid cysts, and asymmetrical pneumatization constitute "leave me alone" lesions of the petrous apex and generally should not be managed surgically, though clinicians must use their judgment if a patient is symptomatic.

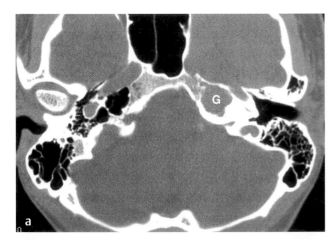

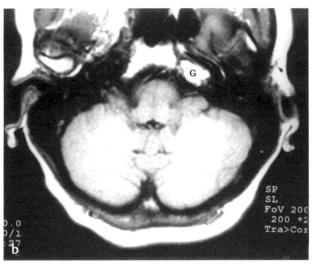

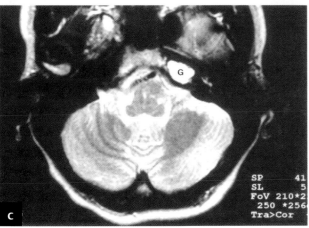

Fig. 62.29 Cholesterol granuloma. (**a**) Computed tomography demonstrates an expansile lesion (G) of the pneumatized left petrous apex. Magnetic resonance imaging shows a high signal intensity on both (**b**) T1- and (**c**) T2-weighted images. G, cholesterol granuloma.

Table 62.2 Petrous apex lesions: imaging characteristics

Lesion	Computed tomography	Magnetic resonance imaging		
		T1	T2	Enhancement
Cholesterol granuloma	Air cell trabecular breakdown, expansile	Hyperintense	Hyperintense	No
Cholesteatoma	Air cell trabecular breakdown, expansile	Hypointense	Hyperintense	No
Trapped fluid (effusion)	Air cell trabecular preservation, nonexpansile	Hypointense, isointense, or hyperintense	Hyperintense	No
Mucocele	Air cell trabecular breakdown, expansile	Hypointense	Hyperintense	Rim enhancement

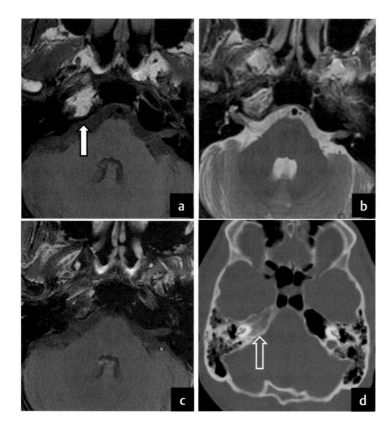

Fig. 62.30 Asymmetric pneumatization of petrous apex. (**a**) Axial magnetic resonance imaging (MRI) demonstrates high signal intensity (*white arrow*) in the right petrous apex on (**a**) precontrast T1- and (**b**) T2-weighted images that follows clival and scalp fat signal intensity. (**c**) A postcontrast MRI scan with fat saturation that eliminates the signal in the petrous apex, suggestive of a fatty marrow signal. (**d**) Computed tomography confirms a normal pneumatized left petrous apex and a nonexpansile, nonpneumatized right petrous apex with opacification suggestive of fatty marrow (*open arrow*).

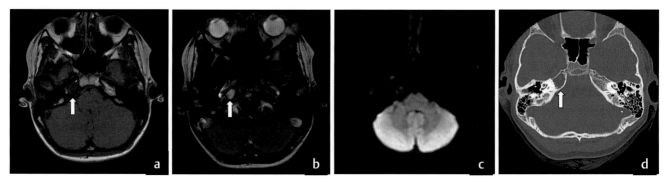

Fig. 62.31 Petrous apex meningocele/arachnoid cysts. (**a**) Magnetic resonance imaging shows low signal intensity abnormality in the right petrous apex (*arrow*) on the T1-weighted image and (**b**) high signal intensity on the T2-weighted image consistent with uncomplicated fluid (*arrow*). (**c**) Diffusion-weighted imaging does not show an area of bright diffusion restriction. (**d**) Computed tomography (CT) demonstrates nonexpansile low-attenuation fluid opacification (*arrow*) of the pneumatized left petrous apex. The absence of expansile changes on CT in conjunction with the low signal intensity on T1- and high signal intensity on T2-weighted images is highly suggestive of the diagnosis of trapped fluid in the petrous apex air cells.

Otosclerosis

Otosclerosis involving the otic capsule can be detected by CT scan using a bone marrow algorithm. Typically, the dense bone of the otic capsule is demineralized, sometimes appearing as an "extra turn" of the cochlea. Whether HRCT can diagnose less severe forms of cochlear otosclerosis has not been established. Far-advanced or cochlear otosclerosis develops when abnormal otospongiotic bone involves the otic capsule. When this occurs, a "halo" sign can often be seen around the cochlea (**Fig. 62.32**). Imaging in these patients may have implications for optimal management of hearing rehabilitation, including cochlear implantation.

Skull Base Osteomyelitis

Skull base osteomyelitis, or malignant otitis externa, usually develops in diabetic or other immunocompromised patients. This condition causes severe otalgia and granulation tissue at the bony–cartilaginous junction of the external auditory canal. The causative organism is typically *Pseudomonas aeruginosa.*

In these patients, CT scanning becomes abnormal in late cases and may be normal early in the course of the disease. The evaluation of patients is usually by nuclear medicine scans, with patients first undergoing technetium (bone) scan, which helps establish the diagnosis and extent of disease. However, once positive, the changes of technetium scan lag behind the resolving clinical condition and will remain abnormal even after the infection has cleared. To assess the response to treatment, serial gallium (tagged white blood cell) scans are obtained. Treatment is usually continued until the gallium scans normalize. Positron-emission tomography with coregistered CT scans has been reported for use in evaluating skull base osteomyelitis. MRI can also be useful to determine the extent of soft tissue involvement seen on postcontrast T1 images (**Fig. 62.33**). Precontrast T1 images can also be useful to determine if the infection has involved the marrow spaces of the clivus and skull base.

Superior Canal Dehiscence

Imaging of the temporal bone plays a large role in the diagnosis of superior semicircular canal dehiscence (SSCD). Superior canal dehiscence occurs when bone is missing over the superior semicircular canal,

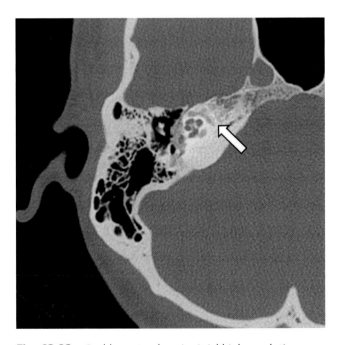

Fig. 62.32 Cochlear otosclerosis. Axial high-resolution computed tomography shows demineralization of the right otic capsule (*arrow*) and exuberant bone deposition around the oval window associated with far-advanced (cochlear) otosclerosis.

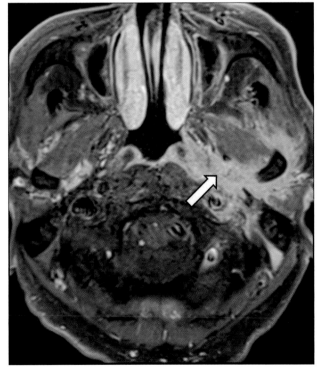

Fig. 62.33 Skull base osteomyelitis. This axial T1-weighted postcontrast magnetic resonance imaging scan shows diffuse enhancement of the soft tissues surrounding the left skull base in an elderly diabetic patient with skull base osteomyelitis. Enhancement is seen in the pterygoid space (*arrow*), and surrounding the mandible.

exposing the membranous labyrinth of the inner ear and creating a "third window" phenomenon. This condition has been termed the great otologic mimicker because it can cause nearly any ear-related symptom—conductive and sensorineural hearing loss, aural fullness, tinnitus, and vertigo. More specific symptoms include autophony and sound- or pressure-induced vertigo. For patients with these symptoms, HRCT can show a dehiscence over the superior canal, which is best seen on sagittal oblique reformatted images that can show the entire course of the superior canal in one image (**Fig. 62.34**). Often, contralateral SSCD or tegmen dehiscence will also be seen on HRCT.

◼ Summary

With refinements in technique and image quality, temporal bone imaging now plays a more critical role in the evaluation and management of patients with hearing loss, dizziness, chronic ear disease/cholesteatoma, aural atresia, pulsatile tinnitus, and facial nerve symptoms. In general, HRCT, with its ability to resolve the bony–soft tissue interface, is the modality of choice for the evaluation of the middle ear and conductive hearing loss, whereas MRI, better at resolving soft tissue and fluid planes, is better for evaluating retrocochlear pathology. Vascular imaging

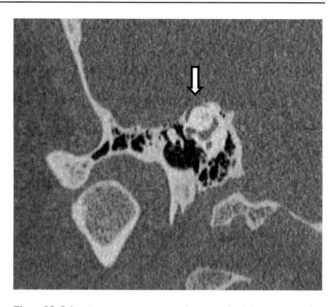

Fig. 62.34 Superior semicircular canal dehiscence. This temporal bone computed tomographic image reformatted in the sagittal oblique view shows absence of bone overlying the superior semicircular canal (*arrow*).

of the temporal bone, including CT/CTA, MRI/MRA, and conventional angiography must be chosen based on the patient's symptoms and signs and based on clinical outcomes that will assist the practitioner in pursuing the optimal imaging study.

◼ Suggested Reading

Christie A, Teasdale E. A comparative review of multidetector CT angiography and MRI in the diagnosis of jugular foramen lesions. Clin Radiol 2010;65(3):213–217

Dempewolf R, Gubbels S, Hansen MR. Acute radiographic workup of blunt temporal bone trauma: maxillofacial versus temporal bone CT. Laryngoscope 2009;119(3):442–448

Harnsberger HR, Dahlen RT, Shelton C, Gray SD, Parkin JL. Advanced techniques in magnetic resonance imaging in the evaluation of the large endolymphatic duct and sac syndrome. Laryngoscope 1995;105(10):1037–1042

Harnsberger HR, Glastonbury CM, Michel MA, Koch BL. Diagnostic Imaging: Head and Neck. Philadelphia, PA: Lippincott; 2010

Jackler RK, Parker DA. Radiographic differential diagnosis of petrous apex lesions. Am J Otol 1992;13(6):561–574

Jahrsdoerfer RA, Yeakley JW, Aguilar EA, Cole RR, Gray LC. Grading system for the selection of patients with congenital aural atresia. Am J Otol 1992;13(1):6–12

Kumar N. Superficial siderosis: associations and therapeutic implications. Arch Neurol 2007;64(4):491–496

Lalwani AK, Jackler RK. Preoperative differentiation between meningioma of the cerebellopontine angle and acoustic neuroma using MRI. Otolaryngol Head Neck Surg 1993;109(1):88–95

Li PM, Linos E, Gurgel RK, Fischbein NJ, Blevins NH. Evaluating the utility of non-echo-planar diffusion-weighted imaging in the preoperative evaluation of cholesteatoma: a meta-analysis. Laryngoscope 2013;123(5):1247–1250

Lin JW, Chowdhury N, Mody A, et al. Comprehensive diagnostic battery for evaluating sensorineural hearing loss in children. Otol Neurotol 2011;32(2):259–264

Mattox DE, Hudgins P. Algorithm for evaluation of pulsatile tinnitus. Acta Otolaryngol 2008;128(4):427–431

Minor LB. Clinical manifestations of superior semicircular canal dehiscence. Laryngoscope 2005;115(10):1717–1727

Minor LB, Solomon D, Zinreich JS, Zee DS. Sound- and/or pressure-induced vertigo due to bone dehiscence of the superior semicircular canal. Arch Otolaryngol Head Neck Surg 1998;124(3):249–258

Nadaraja GS, Gurgel RK, Fischbein NJ, et al. Radiographic evaluation of the tegmen in patients with superior semicircular canal dehiscence. Otol Neurotol 2012;33(7):1245–1250

Salzman KL, Childs AM, Davidson HC, Kennedy RJ, Shelton C, Harnsberger HR. Intralabyrinthine schwannomas: imaging diagnosis and classification. AJNR Am J Neuroradiol 2012;33(1):104–109

Shelton C, Luxford WM, Tonokawa LL, Lo WW, House WF. The narrow internal auditory canal in children: a contraindication to cochlear implants. Otolaryngol Head Neck Surg 1989;100(3):227–231

Som PM, Curtin HD. Head and Neck Imaging. St. Louis, MO: Mosby–Year Book, 1996

Swartz JD, Harnsberger HR. Imaging of the Temporal Bone. New York, NY: Thieme; 1992

Valvassori GM, Mafee MF, Carter BC. Imaging of the Head and Neck. New York, NY: Thieme; 1995

63 Otosclerosis: Diagnosis and Management

■ Introduction

Otosclerosis is a disorder of bone remodeling in the otic capsule, causing progressive hearing loss. The hearing loss is most often conductive, sometimes mixed and, on rare occasions, purely sensorineural. The degree of hearing loss varies among patients and can progress to complete deafness. Two thirds of patients are women. The prevalence of otosclerosis varies among races; it is more common in Caucasians (~ 0.3%) and rare in African Americans, Asians, and Native Americans.

Histopathology

Otosclerosis is characterized by abnormal bone remodeling in the otic capsule, which normally has very little bone turnover. The early otosclerotic lesion exhibits both increased bone absorption by osteoclasts and new bone deposition by osteocytes. The osteocytes are found at the advancing edge of the lesion, which extends into the otic capsule in finger-like projections. The new bone formation is hypervascular at first and sclerotic later, but it remains disorganized. An early lesion is typically found anterior to the oval window at the fissula ante fenestram. As the disease progresses, the lesion may spread across the stapedial annular ligament, causing fixation of the stapes and conductive hearing loss. The lesion may also spread medially to the endosteum of the cochlea, causing sensorineural hearing loss (SNHL).

Genetic and Environmental Factors

Otosclerosis can be inherited in an autosomal-dominant fashion, with incomplete penetrance. About half of otosclerosis patients do not have a family history of the disease. Genetic analyses in large families have linked otosclerosis with 10 loci on various chromosomes, although no specific mutations have been identified. Genetic analyses in large groups of unrelated patients and control populations have associated otosclerosis with various genes involved in bone metabolism, hormonal regulation, and immune response. In addition, measles virus and other environmental factors might play a role in the pathogenesis of otosclerosis in some patients.

■ Evaluation

History

Patients with otosclerosis commonly present with gradual, progressive hearing loss over several years. Women frequently report significant progression of hearing loss during or after pregnancy. Hearing loss is present in both ears in 70% of patients, and about half of these patients have a positive family history.

Examination

The otomicroscopic examination is typically normal in otosclerosis. At times a red blush is seen over the promontory (Schwartze sign), due to increased blood flow in the otosclerotic (otospongiotic) lesion. Tuning forks are an important part of the evaluation. In the Weber test, a 512 Hz tuning fork is placed on the bridge of the patient's nose or forehead. The sound will lateralize to the ear that has the greater conductive hearing loss, with as little as 5 dB difference. In the Rinne test, a tuning fork is placed in contact with the mastoid behind the ear and alternately in the air ~ 2 to 3 cm from the external ear canal. With a 512 Hz tuning fork, bone conduction is louder than air conduction when there is at least 15 dB of conductive loss at that frequency. With a 1,024 Hz fork, bone conduction is louder when there is at least 25 dB of conductive loss at that frequency.

Audiometry

Routine audiometric evaluation includes air conduction, bone conduction, and speech audiometry. Because otosclerosis may cause a unilateral conductive hearing loss, masking the contralateral ear is important. In patients with bilateral conductive hearing loss, a masking dilemma exists where the examiner does not know from which ear the patient is "hearing" when doing bone conduction testing. The sensorineural acuity level test can differentiate bone conduction thresholds for each individual ear. In many otosclerosis patients, an artificial diminution in the bone conduction thresholds surrounding 2,000 Hz may be identified. This "Carhart notch" often returns to normal after stapes surgery. Tympanometry can be helpful in the differential diagnosis. For example, normal impedance and absent acoustic reflex are supportive of otosclerosis, whereas the presence of acoustic reflex in spite of conductive hearing loss suggests superior semicircular canal dehiscence.

Vestibular Tests

Vestibular function tests are not routinely considered in the workup of otosclerosis, but they can be helpful when a vestibular disorder is suspected. For example, vestibular-evoked myogenic potential is hyperactive (low threshold, high amplitude) in superior semicircular canal dehiscence, whereas it is absent in otosclerosis due to the middle ear conduction block. In a patient with a high index of suspicion for vestibular hypofunction in the contralateral ear, electronystagmography (ENG) or videonystagmography (VNG) may be obtained to investigate this potential contraindication to stapedectomy.

Imaging Studies

Temporal bone computed tomography (CT) is not required for the diagnosis of otosclerosis. However, because CT may show evidence of cochlear otosclerosis or superior semicircular canal dehiscence, it can be helpful when there is appropriate clinical suspicion. In advanced cochlear otosclerosis, high-resolution temporal bone CT imaging may show a "double ring" or "halo sign" around the cochlea suggestive of active otosclerotic foci surrounding the otic capsule bone of the cochlea.

Differential Diagnosis/Diagnosis

Otosclerosis is the leading differential diagnosis for conductive hearing loss in a normal-appearing ear under otomicroscopy. Fixation of the malleus or incus is much rarer. Ossicular discontinuity is not expected without a history of trauma to the ear. Peculiar symptoms, such as noise-induced or pressure-induced dizziness, autophony, conductive hyperacusis, or a history of failed stapedectomy, should raise suspicion of superior semicircular canal dehiscence.

Paget disease and osteogenesis imperfecta are also in the differential diagnosis and can be diagnosed on temporal bone CT imaging. The demineralization of bone in Paget disease results in a diffuse, washed-out appearance of the temporal bone, often referred to as cotton wool.

■ Management

Patients with otosclerosis have several options for hearing rehabilitation. If the hearing loss is unilateral, they may do very well without treatment. Conventional hearing aids can be offered to patients who want to improve their hearing. Bone conduction hearing devices, osseointegrated implants, and middle ear surgical exploration are also viable options discussed here. Oral fluoride may be offered for progressive SNHL, although the evidence supporting its efficacy is not strong.

Hearing Aids

Patients should be informed of the option of hearing aids in addition to surgical treatment. Hearing amplification is particularly suitable for patients with mixed conductive and sensorineural hearing loss because only the conductive component is correctible with stapedectomy. Various types of air-conduction hearing aids can be used, depending on the degree of hearing loss. Some hearing aids can be fitted completely in the canal, near or on the tympanic membrane. A new device combining an ear-level microphone and transmitter with an intraoral sound transducer in contact with teeth (SoundBite, Sonitus Medical, San Mateo, CA) offers yet another nonsurgical option to bypass the middle ear conduction block.

Osseointegrated Implants

Osseointegrated implants, such as the Baha System (Cochlear Americas, Centennial, CO), Oticon (Oticon Medical, Somerset, NJ), or Sophono (Sophono Inc., Boulder, CO), make use of direct bone conduction of sound to bypass the middle ear conductive hearing loss. Depending on the configuration, some of these systems have adequate amplifying power for even severe mixed hearing losses. Although placement of these devices requires surgery, the procedure does not expose patients to the risks of SNHL, dizziness, or taste disturbance that stapedectomy does.

Stapedectomy

Stapedectomy reestablishes sound conduction in the ossicular chain through a prosthesis from the incus into the inner ear. Patients who contemplate stapedectomy should be informed of the risks of SNHL, dizziness, and taste disturbance. Because the sole objective of stapedectomy is improvement of hearing, surgeons should quote their own statistics of success and failure in stapedectomy to their patients. Experienced surgeons have reported success rates in excess of 90%, further hearing loss rates of less than 2%, and incidence of total SNHL rates of far less than 1%. Patients with tinnitus should be advised that tinnitus often improves with hearing gain, but it may persist, nonetheless.

A suitable candidate for surgery is a patient who has an air–bone gap of > 20 dB, who "reverses" at least the 512 Hz tuning fork, whose overall hearing level is worse than 35 dB, and whose acoustic reflexes are absent in the affected ear. Surgery is contraindicated in (1) the only-hearing ear or the better-hearing ear, (2) the presence of an infection or significant perforation, and (3) an ear with active Ménière disease. An additional relative contraindication is a vestibular problem in the contralateral ear. If there is a high index of suspicion for this problem, ENG or VNG may be done to rule out vestibular hypofunction in the contralateral ear.

Medical Therapeutics

When there is progressive SNHL from cochlear otosclerosis, oral fluoride may be offered in an attempt to stabilize hearing, although the evidence supporting its efficacy is not strong. A typical fluoride regimen is Florical (Mericon Industries, Peoria, IL) or Monocal (Mericon), one tablet three times daily for a year.

Cochlear Implant

Patients with advanced otosclerosis, who do not derive adequate benefit from stapedectomy and/or hearing amplification, are candidates for cochlear implant (CI) and are capable of achieving excellent speech comprehension with CI. High-resolution CT imaging is important to document patency or the status of the round window and basal turn of the cochlea in the preoperative evaluation.

Description of Stapedectomy

The following is a brief description of stapedectomy. The procedure has many variations adopted by individual surgeons. The surgery is performed in an outpatient setting under local or general anesthesia. Local anesthesia is preferred by some surgeons because it allows the patient to report if vertigo occurs and report their hearing status, and it avoids the risks and cost of general anesthesia. Even if general anesthesia is used, local anesthesia is also provided with injections of 1 or 2% xylocaine with epinephrine 1:100,000 under the ear canal skin and into the vascular strip.

The procedure is performed through an ear speculum with or without a speculum holder. A tympanomeatal incision is made, and the flap is elevated until the middle ear is entered. Care is taken to preserve the chorda tympani nerve. Some of the scutum is removed with a curette or a drill until the facial nerve is seen superiorly and the pyramidal process is seen posteriorly. The ossicular chain is palpated to confirm fixation of the stapes and to rule out fixation of the malleus or incus.

The distance from the incus to the stapes footplate is measured. The usual distance from the lateral surface of the incus to the footplate is 4.5 mm. Because stapes piston prostheses are measured from the end of the piston to the medial surface of the incus, the correct size for the prosthesis is determined by subtracting 0.25 mm from the lateral surface measurement (subtracting 0.5 mm for the thickness of the incus and adding 0.25 mm for the insertion depth). The most commonly used piston size is 4.25 mm.

At this point, some surgeons remove the stapes superstructure entirely before fenestration of the footplate; others make a small "control hole" in the stapes footplate before removing the superstructure, and others leave attached all or part of the superstructure until after they have placed and crimped the prosthesis. Although minor modifications to the procedure can be made, surgeons should essentially stick with one technique that works and that they find technically sustainable.

The creation of the fenestra is accomplished with a drill, a laser, both, or a small straight pick and footplate hook to remove a portion of the footplate. A diamond bur can be used to make a 0.7 mm diameter opening in the footplate. Care is taken to let the bur create the fenestra, without pressing hard lest the footplate be cracked or mobilized. A potassium-titanyl-phosphate, argon, or carbon dioxide laser can also be used to create the fenestra. Typically, the laser is directed to make a rosette pattern on the footplate, and a fine pick is used to smooth out the edge of the opening. Alternatively, a diamond bur can be used to finish off the stapedotomy after lasering.

Once the fenestra has been created, a 0.6 mm diameter piston with appropriate length (usually 4–4.5 mm) is inserted and crimped onto the incus. Any remaining stapes superstructure can be removed at this time. The mobility of the prosthesis is tested with gentle pressure on the incus while observing for a round window reflex. If general anesthesia is not used, the patient may be asked to report any vertigo with this maneuver. If vertigo is reported, the prosthesis is too long and should be replaced with another 0.25 mm shorter. Anterior-posterior stability of the prosthesis is tested with gentle pressure on the piston. If the piston is well seated into the fenestra, there should be no anterior-posterior displacement.

For those performing stapedectomy with removal of half or more of the footplate, an oval window tissue seal, usually temporalis fascia or tragal perichondrium, is needed. With this technique, surgeons often use a bucket handle prosthesis placed down into the oval window niche and fenestration over the tissue graft. The bucket is tipped so that the lenticular process of the incus rests in the bucket well, and the bale is delivered over the long arm of the incus.

The tympanomeatal flap is returned to its normal position and packed in place with Gelfoam. A cotton ball is placed in the meatus, and a Band-Aid is applied to the ear.

Postoperative Care

The patient is advised to avoid strenuous exercise, lifting heavy objects, blowing the nose, or flying in the first week after the operation. The ear is kept dry for the first 3 weeks or until the patient returns for the first postoperative visit. Hearing may be tested at 3 weeks. Patients who resume scuba diving or skydiving after 3 weeks do not appear to have increased risk of inner ear barotrauma.

Postoperative Complications

If postoperative SNHL is suspected and confirmed with an audiogram, immediate treatment with oral prednisone, 60 mg daily for 10 to 14 days, is recommended. About 5% of patients experience mild and transient postoperative dizziness or vertigo. If the dizziness is significant and prolonged, it may be due to vestibular damage or perilymph fistula. If there is a high suspicion for fistula, reexploration may be undertaken. Acute management of vertigo may include vestibular suppressant, antiemetic, and oral corticosteroid. Long-term compensation benefits from vestibular rehabilitation. Postoperative taste disturbance occurs in ~ 9% of patients and usually subsides in a few weeks to a few months.

■ Suggested Reading

Bretlau P, Salomon G, Johnsen NJ. Otospongiosis and sodium fluoride. A clinical double-blind, placebo-controlled study on sodium fluoride treatment in otospongiosis. Am J Otol 1989;10(1):20–22

Derks W, De Groot JA, Raymakers JA, Veldman JE. Fluoride therapy for cochlear otosclerosis? an audiometric and computerized tomography evaluation. Acta Otolaryngol 2001;121(2):174–177

House JW, Cunningham CD. Otosclerosis. In: Flint PW, Haughley BH, Lund VJ, Niparko JK, et al., eds. Cummings Otolaryngology—Head and Neck Surgery. Philadelphia, PA: Mosby Elsevier; 2010:2028–2035

House JW, Toh EH, Perez A. Diving after stapedectomy: clinical experience and recommendations. Otolaryngol Head Neck Surg 2001;125(4):356–360

Linthicum FH Jr. Histopathology of otosclerosis. Otolaryngol Clin North Am 1993;26(3):335–352

Mikulec AA, McKenna MJ, Ramsey MJ, et al. Superior semicircular canal dehiscence presenting as conductive hearing loss without vertigo. Otol Neurotol 2004;25(2):121–129

Murray M, Miller R, Hujoel P, Popelka GR. Long-term safety and benefit of a new intraoral device for single-sided deafness. Otol Neurotol 2011;32(8):1262–1269

Schrauwen I, Van Camp G. The etiology of otosclerosis: a combination of genes and environment. Laryngoscope 2010;120(6):1195–1202

Schrauwen I, Weegerink NJ, Fransen E, et al. A new locus for otosclerosis, OTSC10, maps to chromosome 1q41-44. Clin Genet 2011;79(5):495–497

Semaan MT, Gehani NC, Tummala N, et al. Cochlear implantation outcomes in patients with far advanced otosclerosis. Am J Otolaryngol 2012;33(5):608–614

Snik AFM, Mylanus EAM, Proops DW, et al. Consensus statements on the BAHA system: where do we stand at present? Ann Otol Rhinol Laryngol Suppl 2005;195:2–12

64 Benign and Malignant Lesions of the Ear and Skull Base

■ Introduction

Tumors of the ear and temporal bone are uncommon lesions, but they merit review by the practicing otolaryngologist (**Table 64.1**). This concise review emphasizes recent conceptual and technological advances that have influenced contemporary diagnostic and management strategies.

■ Tumors of the Auricle

The most frequent malignant tumors of the pinna are all actinic: basal cell carcinoma, squamous cell carcinoma, and melanoma. The vast majority of basal and squamous tumors occur in Caucasian men more than 60 years old. Involvement of the helix is most common, followed by the posterior pinna surface. The lobule and concha are least frequently involved. Tragal and pretragal tumors have a particular tendency to invade the anterior aspect of the ear canal.

Basal Cell Carcinomas

Basal cell carcinomas are locally infiltrating nodular growths with rolled borders and central crusting ulcers. When completely excised, basal cell carcinomas have little tendency to recur, except for those with morphea elements, which infiltrate along deep-tissue planes and can remain undetected until far advanced. Basal cell carcinomas do not metastasize but can be locally invasive and aggressive.

Squamous Cell Carcinomas

Squamous cell carcinomas are scaly, irregular, indurated maculopapular lesions that often ulcerate or crust. They are more aggressive than basal cell carcinomas, with a 25% recurrence rate after simple excision. Mohs micrographic surgery offers a superior chance of primary tumor control in complex lesions. Recurrence in the parotid or cervical lymphatics occurs in up to 10% of patients. Most surgeons advocate neck dissection when palpable or radiographically apparent adenopathy exists, as well as for large and deeply invasive lesions. Adjunctive radiotherapy should be considered for recurrent or deeply invasive lesions. Squamous cell carcinoma is the most common malignant neoplasm of the temporal bone.

Melanoma

Melanoma of the pinna can present as superficial spreading melanoma, which is a flat, deeply pigmented, irregular, rapidly growing lesion that ulcerates either as nodular melanoma, which is an aggressive nodular pigmented lesion, or as lentigo maligna, which is a pigmented macular growth with a prolonged radial growth phase. Because depth of invasion correlates with risk of local and distant metastases, tumor thickness is a valuable guide to surgical management. Surgical excision with a 1 cm margin is recommended for lesions < 2 mm thick, and a 2 cm margin is recommended for deeper lesions. Sentinel node mapping and sampling using preoperative lymphoscintigraphy and intraoperative intradermal injection of marker dye and radioactive isotope are recommended for patients with a clinically negative neck but lesion thickness > 0.75 mm. Neck dissection and parotidectomy for clinically positive necks may not improve survival but are often used to provide locoregional control.

■ Tumors of the Ear Canal

Benign Tumors

Benign tumors of the external auditory canal (EAC), with the exception of exostoses and osteomata, are uncommon. Benign osseous lesions require peri-

Table 64.1 Predominant neoplasms of the ear and temporal bone

Neoplasms	Benign	Malignant
Auricle	Nevus Hemangioma Keloid	Squamous cell carcinoma Basal cell carcinoma Melanoma
Ear canal	Osteoma Exostoses Neurofibroma	Squamous cell carcinoma Glandular adenocarcinoma
Middle ear and mastoid	Mucosal adenoma Paraganglioma (glomus tympanicum)	Squamous cell carcinoma
Inner ear	Intralabyrinthine schwannoma	Papillary adenoma (endolymphatic sac tumor)[a]
IAC and CPA	Vestibular schwannoma Meningioma	Metastasis Exophytic parenchymal tumors (e.g., ependymoma, glioma)

Facial nerve	Schwannoma
	Geniculate hemangioma
		Primary (exceedingly rare)
		Secondary
		    Adenocystic carcinoma
		    Squamous cell carcinoma

Petrous apex	Fibrous dysplasia	Primary
		    Chondrosarcoma
		Secondary
		    Chordoma
		    Metastasis (esp. breast, prostate)

Jugular foramen	Paraganglioma Meningioma Lower cranial nerve schwannoma	Rare
Temporal bone tumors in children	Eosinophilic granuloma	Rhabdomyosarcoma

Abbreviations: CPA, cerebellopontine angle; IAC, internal auditory canal.

[a] Endolymphatic sac tumors have a benign histology, but a malignant clinical course.

odic cleaning and water avoidance, unless they have become severely obstructive or stubbornly infected or are generating pain. Another benign lesion, periauricular plexiform neurofibromas associated with neurofibromatosis type 1, can impinge on the EAC. Excision of these lesions is usually incomplete, with debulking performed to maintain EAC patency. The facial nerve is often engulfed in these tumors, which typically originate from small cutaneous sensory nerves.

Squamous Cell Carcinoma

Squamous cell carcinoma is the most common malignant tumor arising in the EAC. It often arises in the setting of chronic inflammation due to either chronic otitis externa or habitual self-excoriation. Early biopsy is indicated for chronic ulcerative or granular ear canal conditions that do not promptly respond to routine medical management. Accurate staging of squamous cell carcinoma of the EAC is an essential prelude to treatment planning (**Table 64.2**). Computed tomographic (CT) scans, which depict osseous destruction, often fail to reveal the true extent of disease. Magnetic resonance imaging (MRI) and positron-emission tomography/CT imaging are commonly used to improve staging accuracy and guide treatment.

Treatment includes wide surgical excision and aggressive radiotherapy. The minimal surgical procedure is lateral temporal bone resection. This consists of an en bloc resection of the entire osseous and cartilaginous portions of the canal along with the tympanic membrane, malleus, and incus. Involvement of the medial wall of the middle ear mandates excision of the inner ear. Currently, most practitioners accomplish this piecemeal through drill exenteration, rather than by en bloc resection of the medial petrous bone. Most surgeons resect the facial nerve only when it is grossly involved by tumor. Following more extensive resection, closure of the meatus and flap obliteration of the cavity are indicated because a large open cavity predisposes to osteoradionecrosis. Neck dissection is performed for clinical and radiographic evidence of nodal metastases.

Table 64.2   Familial tumor syndromes with otologic manifestations

	Neurofibromatosis type 2	**Multiple paragangliomas**	**Von Hippel-Lindau**
Inheritance	Autosomal dominant	Autosomal dominant (with genomic imprinting)	Autosomal dominant
Locus	Chromosome 22	Chromosome 11	Chromosome 3
Tumor types	Schwannoma Meningioma Rare CNS parenchymal lesions	Paraganglioma Pheochromocytoma	Papillary adenoma Hemangioblastoma Renal cell carcinoma Pheochromocytoma
Sites	Internal auditory canal Cerebellopontine angle Other intracranial sites	Middle ear (tympanicum) Jugular foramen (jugulare) Upper neck (vagale) Carotid bifurcation (carotid body)	Endolymphatic sac Cerebellum Retina Kidney Adrenal
Common manifestations	SNHL, disequilibrium Myriad others	Pulsatile tinnitus Hearing loss (CHL or SNHL) Lower cranial neuropathies	Hearing loss Vertigo

Abbreviations: CNS, central nervous system; CHL, conductive hearing loss; SNHL, sensorineural hearing loss.

Radiotherapy is considered as an alternative to surgery for stage I disease and is recommended as combined treatment for more advanced disease. Little prospect for cure exists when the tumor invades the petrous apex, surrounds the intrapetrous carotid artery, or involves the dura. The same strategies are used to treat malignant adenomatous tumors (adenocarcinoma and adenoid cystic carcinoma) of the external ear canal.

■ Tumors of the Middle Ear and Mastoid

The most common primary tumor of the middle ear is the glomus tympanicum (tympanic paraganglioma), which originates from paraganglia on the promontory located along the course of the Jacobson and Arnold nerves. As these tumors grow to occupy the tympanic cavity, they produce pulsatile tinnitus, and as they impinge upon the ossicles, conductive hearing loss occurs. The otoscopic appearance is characteristic, with a violaceous, cherry-red retrotympanic mass that, upon microscopic inspection, can often be observed to pulsate.

There are several primary differential diagnoses:

1. Glomus tumor
2. High jugular bulb
3. Aberrant carotid artery

High-resolution CT can distinguish a glomus tympanicum from a glomus jugulare tumor by evaluating the integrity of the bony septation that separates the dome of the jugular bulb from the hypotympanum.

CT is also the best means of screening for congenital vascular malpositions. Traditionally, the characteristic flow voids described as salt-and-pepper patterns that are seen on MRI have been used to diagnose these lesions. However, new data suggest that computed tomography angiography (CTA) may be superior to MRI.

Treatment for small tumors is surgical excision via tympanotomy. Extension into the posterior tympanic spaces (sinus tympani, facial recess) may necessitate a supplemental transmastoid exposure. More extensive disease requires infratemporal fossa exposure with or without facial nerve transposition. Additionally, stereotactic radiosurgery now plays an important role as primary treatment and as treatment for residual or recurrent disease.

Mucosal adenomas arising in the middle ear or mastoid are not common lesions. They are characterized by slow growth, conductive hearing loss due to ossicular envelopment, and a modest degree of smoothly marginated bone erosion. Treatment requires simple surgical excision. Adenomas with a papillary growth pattern are a special case (see Papillary Adenoma of the Endolymphatic Sac).

Primary malignant tumors of the middle ear and mastoid are rare. Although squamous cell carcinoma may hypothetically originate in these areas, particularly in the setting of long-standing chronic otitis media, its occurrence is extremely rare and thought to be the result of squamous metaplasia. Primary adenocarcinomas of the middle ear and mastoid are also exceptionally uncommon. Identification of such a lesion in this location should raise suspicion of metastatic disease or secondary spread from a salivary source.

■ Tumors of the Inner Ear

Only two tumors are considered to take their origin from the inner ear: papillary adenoma of the endolymphatic sac (ELS) and intralabyrinthine schwannoma.

Papillary Adenoma of the Endolymphatic Sac

In contrast to the indolent mucosal adenoma, which arises from the lining of the middle ear and mastoid, papillary adenomas of the ELS can be highly aggressive. Anatomically, small lesions have been observed to be localized to the region of the ELS on high-resolution CT, but most tumors have invaded the temporal bone and posterior cranial fossa by the time they are diagnosed. For extensive tumors, MRI can identify cystic components and vascular flow voids. Bilateral ELS tumors have been seen in association with von Hippel-Lindau disease.

Although papillary adenomas are histologically benign, they have an aggressive clinical course. Erosion of the otic capsule and facial nerve are frequent, as is spread into the posterior cranial fossa. Widespread destruction of the cranial base may evolve. Although these adenomas have not been shown to have a metastatic potential, some authors have considered them to be a form of low-grade adenocarcinoma, rather than adenoma. Clinically, early ELS tumors present nonspecifically with hearing loss and vertigo and may even present similarly to Ménière disease. More advanced lesions may present with facial paralysis or a mass behind an intact tympanic membrane. In the latter scenario, a lesion may simulate the clinical and radiographic appearance of a glomus jugulare tumor.

Treatment requires radical surgical excision (usually transmastoid/translabyrinthine), often with a combined intra- and extracranial approach and preoperative embolization. Radiotherapy appears to play a role in treatment, but it is difficult to evaluate, given the paucity of data. Radical surgery has resulted in a 90% long-term control rate, whereas subtotal removal followed by radiotherapy controlled only ~ 50%.

Intralabyrinthine Schwannoma

Schwannoma within the inner ear may result from either lateral extension of an internal auditory canal tumor via the fundus, or origination within the inner ear itself. Primary intralabyrinthine schwannoma is a rare, but distinctive, lesion. Typically, the vestibule is involved with a variable degree of cochlear and semicircular canal penetration.

The clinical manifestations of intralabyrinthine schwannoma simulate those of small vestibular schwannomas (acoustic neuromas): sensorineural hearing loss (SNHL), and occasionally vertigo. The customary means of detecting these lesions is enhanced MRI scanning, although noncontrast high-resolution T2-weighted images may demonstrate a segmental absence of inner ear fluid. The site of origin is controversial but is most likely from the terminal filaments of the vestibular nerves. A few have been described as originating in the modiolus, presumably from auditory fibers.

Because surgical removal invariably results in deafness in the operated ear, a conservative approach to small lesions is reasonable given that these lesions tend to grow very slowly. Surgical removal (translabyrinthine) may be undertaken when growth is evident on serial imaging studies or when troublesome vestibular symptoms require it.

■ Tumors of the Facial Nerve

Facial nerve schwannomas and facial nerve hemangiomas are uncommon lesions, but they require the attention of an astute clinician when patients present with facial palsy. Schwannomas are fusiform lesions, which are typically elongated to involve more than one segment of the nerve. They cause a smooth-walled expansion of the fallopian canal that is demonstrated on high-resolution CT. The predominant pattern of involvement may be geniculate-tympanic, vertical-stylomastoid, or internal auditory canal–cerebellopontine angle (IAC-CPA).

Osseous hemangiomas are not tumors of the facial nerve itself but rather appear to arise from a vascular plexus located in the region of the geniculate ganglion. In contrast to schwannomas, hemangiomas irregularly erode the perigeniculate bone, often leaving small, calcified flakes within the substance of the tumor. Although primary malignant tumor of the facial nerve (neurofibrosarcoma) is exceedingly rare, secondary involvement by regional malignancy is not uncommon. Frequent among these are parotid neoplasms (especially adenocystic carcinoma) and squamous cell carcinoma originating in the ear canal.

Evaluation

Radiographic screening for a suspected facial nerve tumor varies according to the clinical circumstance. In a patient undergoing imaging for facial dysfunction (weakness or twitch), enhanced MRI is the preferred initial study. This permits identification of lesions in the parotid and infratemporal fossa region, as well as the IAC, CPA, and brainstem. MRI is also an excellent screen for intratemporal lesions, although it is essential that the imaging sequences be of high resolution and thinly spaced. When an intratemporal lesion is suspected (e.g., middle ear mass, conductive hearing loss), then CT is superior because it is more sensitive than MRI for small lesions with subtle osseous erosion. In proven tumors, both CT and MRI are obtained because they provide complementary and surgically relevant information.

Contrary to what common sense might dictate, tumors of the facial nerve do not invariably present with facial weakness. In fact, many patients have normal facial nerve function and present with conductive hearing loss. When they have facial nerve dysfunction, it often manifests as hyperfunction, such as a limited regional twitch or a full hemifacial spasm. When facial nerve tumors present with weakness, the course is usually slowly progressive. However, an occasional tumor will result in recurrent episodes of acute palsy, with partial or even complete recovery. This is particularly true for hemangiomas, which may have a dynamic vascular component. Patients may also present with hearing loss and dizziness when tumor invades the labyrinth adjacent to the tympanic segment of the facial nerve or involves the intracanalicular segment in the internal auditory canal. Some patients are asymptomatic when they present with an incidental retrotympanic mass during routine examination. It is axiomatic that the patient with facial palsy deserves a comprehensive head and neck examination to detect subtle signs of tumor in the ear as well as in the facial and parotid regions.

Management

Arriving at the optimal management strategy for facial nerve schwannomas and hemangiomas requires considerable judgment. From a functional perspective, surgical excision seldom improves preoperative facial mimetic status and usually worsens it. Yet experience shows that, if surgery is delayed until facial function is lost, results from nerve repair or nerve grafting are much poorer. For this reason, surgery for facial nerve schwannoma is considered for patients with House–Brackmann grade III palsy and recommended for patients with grade IV palsy. Facial nerve hemangiomas, on the other hand, can often be removed leaving the nerve intact. Therefore, these lesions might be addressed earlier in their clinical course to improve the chance of facial nerve preservation. Variance from these principles is at the surgeon's discretion when tumors are large or when patients are deemed poor surgical candidates.

Selection of surgical approach for tumor removal depends on anatomy (e.g., mastoid approach for vertical segment lesions) and function (e.g., geniculate lesions are approached via the middle fossa when hearing is intact and via the translabyrinthine route

when it is absent). Interposition nerve grafting has a high probability of success, but a limited potential for recovery (at best grade III/VI with synkinesis). Nevertheless, facial nerve grafting produces results superior to those from crossover anastomosis (e.g., XII–VII) or other modalities of reanimation.

■ Tumors of the Internal Auditory Canal and Cerebellopontine Angle

Schwannoma of the eighth cranial nerve is the most common tumor of the temporal bone. In the vast majority of cases, it arises from the vestibular nerve. Therefore, it is most appropriately called vestibular schwannoma (VS), although the older and less accurate term *acoustic neuroma* is still widely used.

Evaluation

Clinical studies have documented a surprisingly high incidence of atypical clinical presentations. The classical description of a slowly progressive unilateral or asymmetrical hearing loss accompanied by a loss of speech discrimination out of proportion to the pure-tone loss is far from universal. For example, a high fraction of VS patients have a sudden loss at some point during their clinical course. In this MRI era, quite a few tumors are being detected with minimally asymmetric or even normal hearing thresholds. Episodic vertigo is uncommon for VS, whereas a continuous sense of dysequilibrium is frequent. Trigeminal symptoms, particularly midfacial tingling or hypesthesia, herald the presence of a large tumor.

Although auditory brainstem response (ABR) screening is still in widespread use for VS, an increasing body of evidence has demonstrated an alarmingly high false-negative rate (especially for smaller tumors) and a high false-positive rate. In many medical centers, ABR is bypassed in favor of the current gold standard for evaluation: gadolinium-enhanced MRI. MRI reliably visualizes vestibular schwannomas as small as 1 to 2 mm in diameter. Recent efforts have attempted to reduce the cost of VS screening MRI sequences by avoiding the use of contrast. High-resolution T2-weighted images (e.g., fast spin-echo) use the bright signal of cerebrospinal fluid in the IAC to outline the audiovestibular and facial nerves; this may offer a cost-effective screening alternative. CT is currently used for patients with metallic implants (e.g., pacemakers, aneurysm clips), which preclude MRI use. It is also an acceptable screen in elderly patients in whom the detection of small tumors is not a priority.

Management

Management options for patients with VS include observation, microsurgical removal, and stereotactic radiosurgery. Deciding which option is most appropriate can be complex when considering such factors as the size and location of the tumor, hearing status, patient age and health status, growth rate demonstrated on sequential imaging studies, and patient preference for treatment. Because recent trends stress functional preservation, observation and radiosurgery have played a greater role in the management of small and medium-sized tumors.

Three surgical approaches are in widespread use: translabyrinthine, middle fossa, and retrosigmoid. Most large medical centers use a variety of approaches, selecting the optimal technique according to the tumor's size, location, and residual hearing. A middle fossa technique offers the highest probability of hearing conservation (as much as 50–70% in the most favorable circumstances) for patients with intracanalicular tumors. For some patients with substantial CPA components (up to 1.5 cm), an extended middle fossa approach can be employed to preserve hearing. A translabyrinthine approach is used by most neurotologists, but it has the disadvantage of sacrificing hearing. A retrosigmoid approach is still popular, especially in the neurosurgical community, because it allows rapid access to tumors with a large intracranial component.

Stereotactic radiosurgery now plays a major role in the care of patients with VS. For patients with small and medium-sized tumors, a conformal radiation treatment plan is created using imaging data with a localizer in place (stereotactic frame for gamma knife). Advantages are that treatment is performed on an outpatient basis, and patients can usually return to their regular activities within a few days. Controversy regarding hearing preservation rate with single-dose versus fractionated radiosurgery remains, but 20 year data show that control rates using radiosurgery (tumor shrinkage or no growth) are ~ 95%. Some concern about the long-term effects of high-dose radiotherapy for benign lesions remains when treating patients 65 years or younger.

Traditionally, observation was the best choice for management of patients with smaller tumors who have a limited life expectancy. However, recent clinical studies have shown that 60% of schwannomas remain stable or involute during an average of 4 years of follow-up. This information suggests that, especially in patients with small or medium-sized tumors who have no residual hearing, observation should be considered before recommending microsurgery or radiosurgery. In such cases, MRI scans are obtained every 6 months to establish the tumor's growth rate. If no growth is seen after 1 year and the patient remains asymptomatic, MRI scans can be repeated every 1 to 2 years.

Many other benign tumors affect the IAC and CPA. The most common among these are meningioma, epidermoid, and lipoma. Meningiomas of the posterior fossa tend to originate along the venous sinuses, or in neural foramina at the base of the skull, particularly the IAC, Meckel cave, jugular foramen, and foramen magnum. They typically spread across dural surfaces with an *en plaque* growth pattern. Audiovestibular dysfunction is similar to that of VS. Fortunately, hearing conservation rates with these lesions are, in general, superior to those obtained for VS.

Epidermoids are analogous to congenital cholesteatoma in that they originate from ectopic squamous epithelium. Surgical management usually entails debulking of the accumulated keratin debris. Radical excision is usually not feasible due to the intimate adherence of the matrix to the pial surface of the cranial nerves and the brainstem. Neural preservation is nearly always possible in epidermoid surgery, at the expense of probable long-term recurrence.

Unlike other IAC and CPA tumors, lipomas usually require no treatment. They have little penchant for producing progressive brainstem compression over time. Some clinicians have suggested weight loss as a means of encouraging the lesion to shrink. At surgery (which is ordinarily ill advised), cranial nerves typically traverse within the tumor's substance, and dissection can be difficult and tedious with a high risk of nerve injury.

■ Tumors of the Petrous Apex

Although the petrous apex is involved by a variety of nonneoplastic processes (e.g., infection, cholesteatoma, cholesterol granuloma), tumor involvement is uncommon. Perhaps the most frequent neoplasm of the medial petrous bone is metastasis to the apical marrow space. Among the more prevalent primary sites are breast, lung, kidney, and gastrointestinal tract. Primary benign tumors of the petrous apex are exceedingly rare. Benign chondroma has been reported in a few cases. Primary malignant tumors are somewhat more often seen, particularly chondrosarcoma, which arises at the petroclival junction from the fibrocartilage of the foramen lacerum. Chordoma arises from notochordal remnants in the clivus and can spread laterally to erode the petrous apex. Both lesions most commonly present with constant, dull headache. Dysfunction of cranial nerves V (facial sensory disturbance) and VI (diplopia) is frequent because these nerves traverse the superior surface of the medial petrous bone.

Surgery of apical tumors is usually conducted through an anterolateral approach (subtemporal or infratemporal). Clival tumors with lateral extension into the apex are customarily approached anteriorly (e.g., transoral, transnasal/transsphenoethmoidal). True lateral approaches (e.g., transcochlear) provide limited access to the petroclival junction due to the interposition of the petrous segment of the carotid artery. They become important only when the otic structures are involved or when there is transdural involvement of the posterior fossa.

Tumors of the Jugular Foramen

The vast majority of tumors of the jugular foramen are benign, with paraganglioma (glomus), meningioma, and schwannoma predominating. Although primary malignant tumors are exceedingly rare, secondary involvement by upward spread of neck disease (e.g., squamous cell carcinoma) is not infrequent. The manifestations of jugular foramen disease are primarily related to dysfunction of the lower cranial nerves (IX–XI): hoarseness, dysphagia, and shoulder weakness. Extensive destruction of this region of the cranial base also comes to involve the twelfth nerve, with resultant unilateral tongue paralysis. Superior spread to the tympanic cavity may lead to conductive hearing loss. Although glomus tumors and meningiomas have a tendency to possess a middle ear component (the former red-violet, the latter pale), schwannomas do not. Glomus tumors, due to their rich vascularity, have a tendency to cause pulsatile tinnitus. Inner ear, IAC, or CPA involvement may lead to SNHL.

Evaluation

Because the facial nerve lies just lateral to the jugular bulb, it too may be invaded by larger tumors. MRI and high-resolution CT of the skull base are complementary studies and help to diagnose these lesions; these studies are recommended for unexplained lower cranial nerve dysfunction, pulsatile tinnitus, or middle ear mass identified on otomicroscopy.

CT is sensitive to detecting erosion of the osseous margin of the foramen, a reliable sign of neoplastic disease. MRI has the important advantage of identifying any cervical or intracranial tumor component. Once a tumor has been identified, CT and MRI provide complementary information and should both be obtained for surgical planning.

It is important to note that formal intravascular angiography should not be done in jugular foramen tumors as a diagnostic exercise until shortly before surgical removal. Preoperatively, angiography serves both a diagnostic as well as a therapeutic role through its ability to permit tumor embolization. Embolization is now widely practiced, particularly in glomus tumors and vascular meningiomas, because it markedly reduces blood loss and facilitates orderly microsurgical technique.

Recently, CTA, magnetic resonance angiography, and magnetic resonance venography have proved useful as noninvasive means of visualizing the vascular supply and relationships of these tumors. Although these methods do not obviate the need for intravascular angiography for the purposes of embolization, they can assess patency of the sigmoid sinus and jugular vein as well as delineate the extent of their involvement by tumor. Preoperative preparation for glomus tumors includes screening for tumor endocrine function if patients have any history of hypertension, diaphoresis, and palpitations. Most medical centers obtain a quantitative 24-hour urine measurement of vanillylmandelic acid and metanephrines.

Management

The management of glomus jugulare tumors is controversial. The natural history is one of slow growth with gradual evolution of neuropathies. Although intracranial spread may occur, sometimes to an impressive degree, it is not inevitable. Thus observation alone, especially in individuals with a limited predicted lifespan and minimal symptoms, is sometimes the wisest course.

Analogous to the conservative management of VS, serial imaging studies can be obtained to delineate the tumor's rate of growth. Most tertiary care centers offer both microsurgical removal and stereotactic radiosurgery for glomus tumors. Since the advent of modern skull base surgery, fostered in large part by the availability of high-resolution imaging studies and preoperative embolization, operative morbidity and mortality have been greatly reduced. Curative resection is usually possible, but there is substantial risk of creating new neuropathies, particularly in large lesions associated with functioning lower cranial nerves. For this reason, there is a trend toward subtotal resection, with or without radiosurgery. Additionally, because the 10- to 15-year data are favorable, more patients are receiving radiosurgery as primary therapy.

Management of meningiomas and schwannomas of the jugular foramen is similar to that of glomus tumors, except that intracranial components are more common. Neural preservation is usually more favorable in schwannoma than it is with meningiomas, which have a more infiltrative nature. Single-stage removal of both intra- and extracranial components is now practiced in most medical centers.

Temporal Bone Tumors in Children

Characteristic benign tumor of the temporal bone in childhood is eosinophilic granuloma. Langerhans cell histiocytosis, of which eosinophilic granuloma is the mildest variety, may occur in solitary or multiple forms.

Clinically, temporal bone lesions present with sagging of the posterior ear canal wall, often with ear canal granulations, in an appearance that may simulate an infectious process. Although conductive hearing loss is common, sensorineural impairment and facial palsy are infrequent. Imaging studies reveal an irregular erosive lesion, most commonly centered in the mastoid region. The clinical presentation and radiographic appearance of these lesions commonly lead to the diagnosis of mastoiditis. Only at surgery, where a soft, red, friable mass is encountered, is the actual diagnosis made. Histologically, these are rich in histiocytes, eosinophils, and multinucleated giant cells. Treatment is by conservative curettage. Low-dose radiotherapy should be considered for complex or recurrent tumors. Prognosis is excellent in solitary lesions, but more guarded for the disseminated variety (Letterer–Siwe disease and Hand–Schüller–Christian disease).

The most common malignant tumors of the temporal bone in childhood are sarcomas, with rhabdomyosarcoma and osteogenic sarcoma predominating. Most lesions are advanced when first discovered. Common presentations include otorrhea and cranial neuropathies, often multiple. The prognosis for temporal bone lesions, as with other parameningeal locations, is less favorable than for other sites. Combined therapy, including surgery, radiation, and aggressive chemotherapy, offers the best chance for cure.

■ Suggested Reading

Ahmad Z, Brown CM, Patel AK, Ryan AF, Ongkeko R, Doherty JK. Merlin knockdown in human Schwann cells: clues to vestibular schwannoma tumorigenesis. Otol Neurotol 2010;31(3):460–466

Arthurs BJ, Fairbanks RK, Demakas JJ, et al. A review of treatment modalities for vestibular schwannoma. Neurosurg Rev 2011;34(3):265–277, discussion 277–279

Bigelow DC, Eisen MD, Smith PG, et al. Lipomas of the internal auditory canal and cerebellopontine angle. Laryngoscope 1998;108(10):1459–1469

Chapman DB, Lippert D, Geer CP, et al. Clinical, histopathologic, and radiographic indicators of malignancy in head and neck paragangliomas. Otolaryngol Head Neck Surg 2010;143(4):531–537

Christie A, Teasdale E. A comparative review of multidetector CT angiography and MRI in the diagnosis of jugular foramen lesions. Clin Radiol 2010;65(3):213–217

Cioffi JA, Yue WY, Mendolia-Loffredo S, Hansen KR, Wackym PA, Hansen MR. MicroRNA-21 overexpression contributes to vestibular schwannoma cell proliferation and survival. Otol Neurotol 2010;31(9):1455–1462

Cochran AJ, Ohsie SJ, Binder SW. Pathobiology of the sentinel node. Curr Opin Oncol 2008;20(2):190–195

Dong F, Gidley PW, Ho T, Luna MA, Ginsberg LE, Sturgis EM. Adenoid cystic carcinoma of the external auditory canal. Laryngoscope 2008;118(9):1591–1596

Fish JH, Klein-Weigel P, Biebl M, Janecke A, Tauscher T, Fraedrich G. Systematic screening and treatment evaluation of hereditary neck paragangliomas. Head Neck 2007;29(9):864–873

Gloria-Cruz TI, Schachern PA, Paparella MM, Adams GL, Fulton SE. Metastases to temporal bones from primary nonsystemic malignant neoplasms. Arch Otolaryngol Head Neck Surg 2000;126(2):209–214

Heffner DK. Low-grade adenocarcinoma of probable endolymphatic sac origin A clinicopathologic study of 20 cases. Cancer 1989;64(11):2292–2302

Heth J. The basic science of glomus jugulare tumors. Neurosurg Focus 2004;17(2):E2

Ivan ME, Sughrue ME, Clark AJ, et al. A meta-analysis of tumor control rates and treatment-related morbidity for patients with glomus jugulare tumors. J Neurosurg 2011;114(5):1299–1305

Jackler RK, Driscoll CLW. Tumors of the Ear and Temporal Bone. Philadelphia, PA: Lippincott Williams & Wilkins; 2000

Koopmans KP, Jager PL, Kema IP, Kerstens MN, Albers F, Dullaart RP. 111In-octreotide is superior to 123I-metaiodobenzylguanidine for scintigraphic detection of head and neck paragangliomas. J Nucl Med 2008;49(8):1232–1237

Kramer F, Stöver T, Warnecke A, Diensthuber M, Lenarz T, Wissel K. BDNF mRNA expression is significantly upregulated in vestibular schwannomas and correlates with proliferative activity. J Neurooncol 2010;98(1):31–39

Lonser RR, Kim HJ, Butman JA, Vortmeyer AO, Choo DI, Oldfield EH. Tumors of the endolymphatic sac in von Hippel-Lindau disease. N Engl J Med 2004;350(24):2481–2486

Lustig LR, Sciubba J, Holliday MJ. Chondrosarcomas of the skull base and temporal bone. J Laryngol Otol 2007;121(8):725–735

Markou K, Karasmanis I, Goudakos JK, Papaioannou M, Psifidis A, Vital V. Extramedullary plasmacytoma of temporal bone: report of 2 cases and review of literature. Am J Otolaryngol 2009;30(5):360–365

Martin TPC, Irving RM, Maher ER. The genetics of paragangliomas: a review. Clin Otolaryngol 2007;32(1):7–11

Moody SA, Hirsch BE, Myers EN. Squamous cell carcinoma of the external auditory canal: an evaluation of a staging system. Am J Otol 2000;21(4):582–588

Murphy ES, Suh JH. Radiotherapy for vestibular schwannomas: a critical review. Int J Radiat Oncol Biol Phys 2011;79(4):985–997

Phan GQ, Messina JL, Sondak VK, Zager JS. Sentinel lymph node biopsy for melanoma: indications and rationale. Cancer Contr 2009;16(3):234–239

Ravin AG, Pickett N, Johnson JL, Fisher SR, Levin LS, Seigler HF. Melanoma of the ear: treatment and survival probabilities based on 199 patients. Ann Plast Surg 2006;57(1):70–76

Sbeity S, Abella A, Arcand P, Quintal MC, Saliba I. Temporal bone rhabdomyosarcoma in children. Int J Pediatr Otorhinolaryngol 2007;71(5):807–814

Semaan MT, Slattery WH, Brackmann DE. Geniculate ganglion hemangiomas: clinical results and long-term follow-up. Otol Neurotol 2010;31(4):665–670

Shpitzer T, Gutman H, Barnea Y, et al. Sentinel node-guided evaluation of drainage patterns for melanoma of the helix of the ear. Melanoma Res 2007;17(6):365–369

Simon M, Boström JP, Hartmann C. Molecular genetics of meningiomas: from basic research to potential clinical applications. Neurosurgery 2007;60(5):787–798, discussion 787–798

Suryanarayanan R, Ramsden RT, Saeed SR, et al. Vestibular schwannoma: role of conservative management. J Laryngol Otol 2010;124(3):251–257

Verma S, Quirt I, McCready D, Bak K, Charette M, Iscoe N. Systematic review of systemic adjuvant therapy for patients at high risk for recurrent melanoma. Cancer 2006;106(7):1431–1442

Wenig BM. Atlas of Head and Neck Pathology. 2nd ed. Philadelphia, PA: Saunders Elsevier; 2007

Zada G, Pagnini PG, Yu C, et al. Long-term outcomes and patterns of tumor progression after gamma knife radiosurgery for benign meningiomas. Neurosurgery 2010;67(2):322–328, discussion 328–329

65 Assessment and Management of Patients with Severe-to-Profound Sensorineural Hearing Loss

■ Introduction

Severe-to-profound sensorineural hearing loss (SNHL) is a significant impediment to an individual's ability to communicate successfully. If hearing loss occurs prior to the development of speech, additional reading and language difficulties confront the individual. Although postlingual hearing loss does not necessarily affect speech and language development, it can also have a profoundly negative impact on a person's ability to function. The successful application of cochlear implantation in children and adults with severe-to-profound SNHL has been pivotal in helping overcome these functional deficits. This chapter reviews various etiologies of severe-to-profound SNHL, highlights aspects involved in patient evaluation, and discusses potential management options for rehabilitation. Particular focus is given to the role of cochlear implants in the management of patients with severe-to-profound SNHL.

Pathophysiology

With the early work of Hermann von Helmholtz and subsequent work of Georg von Bekesy on the mechanics of the basilar membrane and the traveling wave theory of cochlear stimulation, our understanding of cochlear physiology has grown considerably over the last century. Inner hair cells within the cochlea are responsible for transduction of sound energy into electrical signals carried by fibers of the auditory nerve, while outer hair cells are believed to play a role in altering this process of mechanoelectrical transduction.

Much of our understanding of the pathophysiology of SNHL arises from studies of human temporal bone specimens, which allow correlation of these delicate inner ear structures with clinical characteristics of the affected individual. Pathophysiological correlates of SNHL include loss of hair cells as well as loss of spiral ganglion neurons and atrophy of the stria vascularis.

In clinical practice, severe-to-profound SNHL may best be classified as either prelingual or postlingual, depending on whether the loss develops before or after the critical period of speech and language development in the brain, generally regarded as being between 0 and 7 years of age. Prelingual SNHL may be congenital, stemming from various genetic etiologies, developmental anomalies, intrauterine and perinatal infections such as cytomegalovirus (CMV), or neurodegenerative disorders. Additionally, acquired prelingual SNHL may occur as a result of prematurity, hypoxia, trauma, ototoxicity, hyperbilirubinemia, meningitis, or other systemic infections. Postlingual SNHL may be genetic in nature (delayed-onset), though it may also arise from ototoxic drug exposure, immune-mediated inner ear disease, trauma, noise exposure, infection (including meningitis), and aging. In many patients with severe-to-profound SNHL, an exact cause may not be identifiable. Although the incidence of children born with significant hearing loss is thought to be ~ 1 in 1.000, more than 30 million adult Americans have SNHL, of which as many as 3% may have severe-to-profound SNHL.

■ Evaluation

Clinical Findings: Prelingual Severe-to-Profound Sensorineural Hearing Loss

Evaluation of prelingual children with suspected severe-to-profound SNHL begins with a comprehensive history and physical examination. Particular emphasis is placed on the pregnancy and birth histories for infants and young children suspected of having SNHL. Newborn hearing screening is now mandated in most states and has been successful in helping provide early identification of hearing loss. However, some hospitals may still not offer newborn hearing screening, families may refuse screening or miss screening opportunities, and false-negative tests are possible, highlighting the need for continued diligence by parents, families, teachers, and medical professionals.

High-risk factors for congenital hearing impairment include a family history of congenital hearing loss or delayed-onset SNHL in childhood, a maternal history of infection during pregnancy (i.e., toxoplasmosis, rubella, CMV, syphilis, herpes, and human immunodeficiency virus [HIV]), severe hypoxia (low APGAR [appearance, pulse, grimace, activity, respiration] scores), prematurity, hyperbilirubinemia requiring phototherapy or exchange transfusion, and a need for neonatal intensive care unit admission. A history of maternal use of alcohol or illicit drugs, gestational diabetes or pregnancy-induced hypertension, and any other complications during pregnancy should also be sought. Additionally, a history of postnatal infection treated with potentially ototoxic drugs (e.g., gentamicin) or systemic infections, including meningitis or sepsis, should be elicited.

A complete physical examination is also critical for identifying potential syndromic causes of SNHL as well as other associated anomalies in children. Special emphasis should be placed on the head and neck examination, with particular emphasis on craniofacial features. A basic neurological examination, including an assessment of vision, muscle tone, and developmental behavior, is also imperative. Although most genetic causes of SNHL are nonsyndromic, autosomal recessive in nature, there are also several autosomal-dominant conditions, many of which may be discovered by a careful family history. Autosomal-dominant disorders associated with hearing loss include Waardenburg syndrome, Stickler syndrome, branchiootorenal syndrome, Treacher Collins syndrome, and neurofibromatosis type 2. Many of these syndromes have fairly classic features that are readily identifiable on physical examination, but additional studies may be indicated to further evaluate for the presence of associated abnormalities. Syndromic autosomal-recessive disorders associated with SNHL include Pendred syndrome, Usher syndrome, and Jervell and Lange-Nielsen syndrome. Sex-linked syndromes associated with SNHL include Norrie disease, otopalatodigital syndrome, Wildervanck syndrome, and Alport syndrome.

Special Investigations: Prelingual Severe-to-Profound Sensorineural Hearing Loss

After the clinical history and physical examination, audiometric evaluation of a patient with suspected severe-to-profound SNHL is the next most important investigation. Following failure of a newborn hearing screening exam or if there is a suspicion of hearing loss in an infant, diagnostic audiometry should be initiated through the use of threshold auditory brainstem response (ABR) testing. Both air- and bone-conduction ABR testing should be performed to confirm a sensorineural (rather than conductive or mixed) hearing loss. Auditory steady-state response testing may also be used to help distinguish between severe and profound SNHL. In cases with absent ABRs, otoacoustic emission (OAE) testing should be performed to rule out the possibility of auditory neuropathy. For older children with suspected severe-to-profound SNHL, visual reinforcement audiometry, play audiometry, and standard pure-tone audiometry are used to help aid in the assessment of hearing loss.

In the past, evaluation of children suspected of having severe-to-profound SNHL often involved a battery of blood tests and ancillary studies aimed at identifying a possible cause. Although a comprehensive history and physical examination can in fact provide a great deal of information about possible causes of prelingual SNHL, additional studies are occasionally necessary and still play an important role in many cases. Electroretinography is still recommended to assess for the presence of Usher syndrome if there is any suspicion of vestibular dysfunction or visual problems in a child with SNHL. Similarly, many clinicians believe electrocardiography is still a cost-effective test to perform in children with SNHL and any questionable history of syncope to evaluate for Jervell and Lange-Nielsen syndrome. Thyroid function testing is not useful in Pendred syndrome, though genetic testing may be useful if this is suspected. Genetic testing is also available for connexin-related SNHL, which is responsible for most cases of nonsyndromic genetic deafness.

Imaging studies are also often employed in the assessment of patients with prelingual severe-to-profound SNHL. High-resolution computed tomographic (CT) scan of the temporal bone is a fairly low-cost, rapid test to examine the anatomy of the petrous bone. The detailed bony anatomy seen with a high-resolution CT scan allows for the identification of developmental anomalies of the inner ear. Specific radiographic inner ear abnormalities associated with SNHL include complete absence of the labyrinth (Michel deformity), common cavity or cystic deformity, hypoplastic abnormalities, and incomplete partition. Classic Mondini deformity includes an enlarged vestibular aqueduct, dilated vestibule, and incomplete partition of the cochlea. Enlargement of the vestibular aqueduct, narrowing of the internal auditory canal, and cochlear aperture abnormalities may also be seen with a high-resolution CT scan and may occur in isolation or as part of a larger syndrome.

Magnetic resonance imaging (MRI) may also be employed in the evaluation of prelingual severe-to-profound SNHL. MRI has become the study of choice at some centers (and has superseded high-resolution CT scans), whereas others use it to complement the evaluation provided by the CT scan. High-resolution T2-weighted MRI sequences available today allow for careful examination of inner ear anatomy, including assessment of the shape, size, and patency of the cochlea and labyrinthine structures. These sequences also allow for assessment of the internal auditory canal and the cochleovestibular nerve complex. As a result of these sequences, MRI (unlike CT) is able to identify fibrosis within the cochlea or labyrinth, as well as cochlear nerve aplasia or deficiency. This is particularly important in the assessment of recent cases of meningitis-induced hearing loss, which may demonstrate fibrosis but not ossification of the cochlear lumen, and in children with profound SNHL who may lack a cochlear nerve. MRI also has the advantage of being radiation-free.

Clinical Findings: Postlingual Severe-to-Profound Sensorineural Hearing Loss

As with infants and children, evaluation of patients with postlingual SNHL should begin with a complete history and physical examination. In addition to the standard components of a clinical history, several specific questions should be asked when evaluating a patient with suspected severe-to-profound SNHL. A history of potential ototoxic medication use, such as intravenous antibiotics or diuretics, chemotherapeutic drugs, and certain pain medications, should be sought. A detailed noise history, a history of chronic ear infections, a history of direct head or ear trauma, and any prior ear, skull base, or intracranial surgery should also be questioned. A family history of hearing loss, a history of meningitis or other possible viral infections in childhood, autoimmune disorders, otosclerosis, Ménière disease, or other fluctuating or progressive hearing loss symptoms should also be routinely questioned. In children and adolescents, a perinatal history should be obtained because some congenital hearing losses may be progressive or delayed in onset.

Physical examination should focus on the head and neck and neurotologic exam. Evidence of prior ear surgery or prior trauma to the head may be identified. Many autoimmune conditions may have other head and neck manifestations, including visual, nasal, and vestibular manifestations. Tuning fork examination should be performed to confirm an SNHL, rather than a conductive or mixed hearing loss.

Special Investigations: Postlingual Severe-to-Profound Sensorineural Hearing Loss

Standard pure-tone audiometry is used to help delineate the specific type, pattern, and degree of hearing loss in individuals with suspected hearing loss. Word-recognition testing is also included in the assessment of these patients. OAE testing may be helpful if there is a question of test reliability or to help rule out auditory neuropathy. ABR testing may be used similarly or if there is a suspicion for retrocochlear pathology.

In certain situations, blood testing may be helpful. Thyroid studies, autoimmune markers (e.g., rheumatoid factor, antinuclear antibody [ANA], cytoplasmic antineutrophil cytoplasmic antibodies [c-ANCA], and erythrocyte sedimentation rate [ESR]); fluorescent treponemal antibody absorption (FTA-Abs) test (for syphilis), and human immunodeficiency virus (HIV) testing may be indicated if the clinical suspicion exists. In older children and adolescents, genetic screening may be indicated because certain diseases may be delayed in onset or progressive in nature.

Imaging studies may be helpful if there is a history of trauma, ear surgery, meningitis, or ear infections. High-resolution CT scan of the temporal bone can identify cochlear or labyrinthine ossification but may miss fibrosis. MRI may be useful if there is a suspicion for internal auditory canal lesions and to assess cochlear patency in cases of recently diagnosed meningitis.

■ Management

Nonsurgical Management and Candidacy

In patients with prelingual severe-to-profound SNHL, the educational environment in which they are raised has a significant impact on their spoken speech and language skills. Three basic educational approaches have been described: (1) auditory-oral, (2) bilingual/bicultural, and (3) total communication (TC). All three have a common goal of developing functional language.

The auditory-oral approach emphasizes only spoken language for communication. For children who are severely to profoundly hearing impaired, this strategy is usually selected in conjunction with cochlear implantation.

The bilingual/bicultural strategy teaches American Sign Language (ASL) as the primary method of communication. Reading and writing the English language are taught secondarily. Advocates of this methodology contend that ASL is a natural and complete language that is totally visual and therefore accessible to the deaf child. Proponents of bilingual education align themselves with the deaf community, which recognizes deafness as a cultural difference rather than a disability. The success of this approach depends on ASL proficiency. ASL has an entirely different grammatical structure from English; therefore, the task of learning ASL for a normal-hearing individual is challenging and limited to those who are closely associated with a deaf individual.

The TC approach is the most common educational method used in the United States. TC employs all communication modalities, including speech, signs, gestures, finger spelling, speech reading, reading, and writing. The objective is to develop a communication strategy that maximizes the residual auditory information a child can access. The most common implementation of TC incorporates simultaneous speech and signed English because ASL cannot be correlated with spoken language. Advocates of the TC school strongly believe that such a combined code will lead to better competence with the English language.

Otolaryngologists, audiologists, speech therapists, and educators serve a vital function in helping families make decisions about the most appropriate communication strategy for an individual child. If a cochlear implant is to be considered as part of the child's rehabilitation, the earliest possible application with hearing aids must be strongly encouraged. Auditory-oral and TC education with a strong aural–oral emphasis are suggested for families who want to emphasize spoken language for a child's future communication strategy.

For any patient with severe-to-profound SNHL, nonsurgical management options are available for rehabilitation. Appropriately fitted hearing aids may provide some benefit to patients and should be initiated as early as possible after the hearing loss is identified. Speech reading, visual cues, written communication, cued speech, and ASL may be useful for some individuals. However, if there is a desire to develop spoken language (if prelingual SNHL) or restore auditory function (pre- and postlingual SNHL), application of the cochlear implant has become the preferred management option.

The criteria used to determine cochlear implant candidacy have evolved fairly rapidly over the past several years. At present, pure-tone averages should exceed 70 dB sound pressure level, whereas word-recognition scores should be less than 50% in the best-aided condition using the Hearing in Noise Test or comparable testing methods. As discussed, a trial of appropriate amplification should be undertaken before using a cochlear implant. Additional criteria include inner ear anatomy amenable to receiving a cochlear implant, a lack of medical contraindications, appropriate patient/family expectations and support, ear free of active infection, and age older than 12 months. As implant technology improves, indications for cochlear implantation will expand to include those with better residual hearing.

Although CT and/or MRI may be used to aid in the evaluation of patients with severe-to-profound SNHL, one of these modalities is required to confirm the presence of an adequate cochlear lumen prior to cochlear implant surgery. Preimplant vestibular testing is also often performed in patients with suspected vestibular dysfunction or in elderly individuals and may aid in determining the side of implantation.

Surgical Management

Surgical Considerations

Candidates displaying significant labyrinthine ossification should undergo preoperative electrical stimulation testing using a round-window (evoked ABR) or promontory-stimulating paradigm to determine whether they perceive sound. Lack of response is not an absolute contraindication for implantation, but it may indicate limited auditory information transfer with an implant. Similarly, a history of temporal bone fracture, intracranial surgery, or head trauma causing profound deafness may also require preoperative electrical stimulation to determine whether the auditory nerve is intact.

A diagnosis of otosclerosis should alert the surgeon to the possibility of distortion of cochlear anatomy with bony obliteration of the round window. Patients with otosclerosis may be more prone to facial nerve stimulation when the implant is activated due to demineralization of the otic capsule. A history of deafness following stapedectomy or iatrogenic labyrinthine injury could also result in intracochlear fibrosis that may be encountered during implantation. Intracochlear fibrosis is not seen on CT scans but may be identified with preoperative MRI, as previously discussed. Intracochlear fibrosis and/or ossification can be removed through a routine surgical approach if confined to the most basal portion of the basal turn. However, complete electrode insertion may be difficult in such cases. Extensive ossification requires more radical surgery, including the use of split electrodes and alternative electrode placements.

In patients with a mastoid cavity seeking a cochlear implant, ear canal closure with removal of all skin is recommended as a first stage. Silastic may be left within the cavity and over the region of the promontory to aid in identification of this area during the implant surgery.

Cochlear Implant Devices

Cochlear implant devices are continually undergoing modification and upgrades. However, the basic components of these devices are unchanged. Cochlear implants attempt to replace the transducer function of damaged inner ear hair cells. In most causes of neurosensory deafness, injury to the hair cells rather than auditory nerve fibers results in severe-to-profound SNHL.

The basic components of a cochlear implant include the following:

1. A microphone to pick up auditory information
2. A speech processor that changes the mechanical acoustic sound energy into an electrical signal
3. A transmitter coil to send the information via radiofrequency through the skin
4. An implanted receiver/stimulator that interprets the electrical signal sent by the speech processor
5. An intracochlear electrode array that distributes the electrical sound information to the auditory nerve (**Fig. 65.1**)

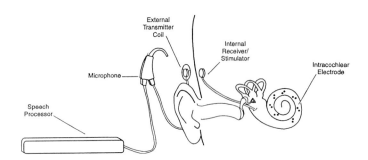

Fig. 65.1 The basic components of a cochlear implant.

Innovative methods of processing speech have been developed by many independent research programs and cochlear implant manufacturers. Most cochlear implants use a band-pass filter system to separate the acoustic signal into discrete frequency bands that can be delivered to the appropriate frequency regions of the cochlea, providing spectral information about the speech signal. Temporal and intensity cues are delivered by varying the rate of stimulation and the amount of stimulating current. Most implant systems use a nonsimultaneous stimulation paradigm that prevents stimulation of more than one channel at a time and eliminates channel interaction because it can induce excessive current loads from overlapping signals. Changes in speech-processing strategies will continue as the technology advances. It is fortunate that new implant systems are being designed to enable adoption of a broad array of speech-processing software changes without requiring surgical hardware reimplantation.

Cochlear Implant Surgery

Standard cochlear implant surgery involves a post-auricular approach that accesses the middle ear through a mastoid-facial recess approach (posterior tympanotomy) with the use of facial nerve monitoring. Incision styles, methods of flap development, and techniques for securing the processor vary considerably. Depending upon surgeon preference, anatomical features, and preoperative audiometric factors, cochleostomy or direct round-window insertion techniques may be used. Various electrode designs are now available that allow the surgeon to tailor surgery for the patient's specific anatomy.

Implants are normally placed in the scala tympani, though in rare situations, the scala vestibuli may be used. With children, special attention must be given to skull thickness and position of the facial nerve and mastoid cortex, but the remainder of the anatomy in the mastoid, facial recess, and cochlea is similar to that of an adult. Patients with inner ear abnormalities (e.g., Mondini deformity, cystic cochlea, cochlear aperture deficiency) may require modifications to the standard surgical technique. Shorter, noncurved electrodes (with circumferential contacts) are often employed in such cases, and fluoroscopy may be used to ensure proper placement. Eustachian tube obliteration and packing of the middle ear may be required in these patients if perilymphatic gusher or cerebrospinal fluid leakage is encountered.

Awareness of the potential complications of cochlear implant surgery is critical and should be thoroughly discussed during the informed consent process. Facial paralysis, implant extrusion, implant failure, and meningitis are serious complications that can occur following cochlear implant surgery. Preoperative vaccination against *Streptococcus pneumoniae* and early treatment of infections are important means of avoiding meningitis and device-related infections or failure.

Cochlear Implant Outcomes

Although it is beyond the scope of this chapter to discuss the extensive literature that is available in terms of cochlear implant user outcomes, it is important to recognize that the use of cochlear implants has been transformational. Within the pediatric population, early use of cochlear implants has allowed language development equivalent to that of hearing children and has provided hearing-impaired children an opportunity to participate and thrive in mainstream educational settings. Certainly, there is great individual variability among cochlear implant users, and it is difficult to prognosticate expected outcomes for any one potential candidate. Nevertheless, there is growing evidence that the average cochlear implant user will benefit greatly from the use of this device.

Criteria for Cochlear Implant Candidacy

With advances in speech processing and electrode technology as well as improvement in patient outcomes, criteria for cochlear implant candidacy are continuing to broaden. Hybrid cochlear implants provide a means of delivering electrical and acoustic stimulation to a single ear by inserting a shortened electrode into the more basal aspects of the cochlea. In combination with "soft" surgical techniques, this technology aims to preserve low-frequency residual hearing, which can subsequently be used in conjunction with "electrical" stimulation of the higher frequencies encoded along the basal turn, provided by the implant.

Cochlear implants are also being explored in cases of single-sided deafness and tinnitus. Preliminary data are limited, but this technology may help improve listening for these individuals in a variety of situations, particularly when compared with the nonimplant and contralateral routing of sound (CROS)-aided conditions.

■ Suggested Reading

Adunka OF, Teagle HFB, Zdanski CJ, Buchman CA. Influence of an intraoperative perilymph gusher on cochlear implant performance in children with labyrinthine malformations. Otol Neurotol 2012;33(9):1489–1496

Arndt S, Aschendorff A, Laszig R, et al. Comparison of pseudobinaural hearing to real binaural hearing rehabilitation after cochlear implantation in patients with unilateral deafness and tinnitus. Otol Neurotol 2011;32(1):39–47

Chau JK, Cho JJ, Fritz DK. Evidence-based practice: management of adult sensorineural hearing loss. Otolaryngol Clin North Am 2012;45(5):941–958

Eisenberg L, ed. Clinical Management of Children with Cochlear Implants. San Diego, CA: Plural Publishing; 2009

Niparko J, ed. Cochlear Implants: Principles and Practice. Philadelphia, PA: Lippincott Williams and Wilkins; 2009

66 Tinnitus

■ Introduction

Tinnitus is a common symptom that has many causes; it may present diagnostic and management dilemmas to the otolaryngologist. Because of poor understanding in the past, many tinnitus patients have had to live with this disturbing symptom for the rest of their lives. Recent developments in tinnitus research, however, have led to a more optimistic approach to the management of these patients. Because nonpulsatile tinnitus has a very different pathophysiology and management from pulsatile tinnitus, these two entities are discussed separately.

■ Nonpulsatile Tinnitus

Introduction

Incidence and Epidemiology

Nonpulsatile tinnitus is more common than pulsatile tinnitus and has a complex pathophysiology. Nonpulsatile tinnitus (henceforth referred to as tinnitus) is more prevalent in patients between the ages of 40 and 70 years, although it can occur in children, and has equal distribution among males and females. It is estimated that 10 million people in the United States have tinnitus, and in 2 million of them, tinnitus is debilitating to the extent of affecting their quality of life. The majority of tinnitus sufferers have an associated otologic pathology; however, many other factors and medical conditions are responsible for this symptom. In a study of tinnitus patients, 75% of them had an average of a 30 dB hearing loss between 3,000 and 8,000 Hz. Usually the pitch of reported tinnitus corresponds to the frequency range of hearing loss.

Etiology

Noise trauma and presbycusis are the two most common etiologies of tinnitus. Other disease processes, such as Ménière disease, immune-mediated cochleovestibular disorders, chronic otitis, otosclerosis, acoustic neuromas, and temporomandibular joint (TMJ) dysfunction should be considered. Tinnitus in TMJ disorders can be associated with aural fullness, dizziness, pain/discomfort, and tenderness over the involved joint and pterygoid muscles. Ototoxic agents, including common over-the-counter medications such as aspirin (in high doses), can cause tinnitus. Potential exposure to such ototoxic agents or suspect medications should be discussed. Therefore, it is very important to thoroughly review all patient medications—both prescription and over-the-counter intake. Many patients are unaware that they are taking a product containing aspirin, which can induce tinnitus at doses as low as 1.5 g.d. **Tables 66.1** and **66.2** summarize the various medications and aspirin-containing compounds associated with tinnitus.

Psychological factors, such as depression and anxiety, can be related to tinnitus. It has been estimated that up to 50% of tinnitus sufferers are clinically depressed. The otolaryngologist should determine whether depression or anxiety is playing a significant role in a patient's tinnitus. **Table 66.3** summarizes the common etiologies and medical conditions associated with tinnitus.

Pathophysiology

Studies have revealed that tinnitus may arise not only from pathophysiological processes of the ear and cochlear nerve but also from processes affecting the central auditory pathways. These abnormalities may consist of synchronous discharge of hair cells, increased random spontaneous activity in cochlear nerve fibers, and elevated discharge patterns of auditory nuclei cells. Abnormalities of auditory nuclei may develop over time as a result of decreased or increased input from the peripheral auditory system, resulting in increased activity. Primary disease process of the auditory nuclei may also cause tinnitus in the absence of any peripheral auditory pathology. Involvement of the prefrontal cortex has also been implicated in cases of tinnitus.

Table 66.1 Medications associated with tinnitus

Aminoglycoside antibiotics
Streptomycin
Neomycin
Gentamicin
Tobramycin
Amikacin
Cisplatin
Furosemide
Nonsteroidal anti-inflammatory drugs
Quinidine
Quinine
Salicylates (aspirin)
Other antibiotics
Vancomycin
Polymyxins
Erythromycin (intravenous)

Table 66.2 Aspirin-containing compounds

Alka-Seltzer	Midol
Empirin compound	Darvon compound
Asper-Gum	Dristan
Exedrin	Ecotrin
Bufferin	Pepto-Bismol
Fiorinal	Theracin
Coricidin	Trigesic

Table 66.3 Common etiologies and medical conditions associated with nonpulsatile tinnitus

Central nervous system disorders
Closed head injury
Temporal bone fracture
Multiple sclerosis
Postmeningitis
Vascular loop compression
Depression/anxiety
Metabolic
Hyperlipidemia
Diabetes mellitus
Otologic
Noise-induced hearing loss
Presbycusis
Ménière disease
Labyrinthitis
Chronic otitis
Otosclerosis
Acoustic neuroma
Cerumen impaction
Temporomandibular joint disorders

Evaluation

History

Obtaining a thorough history is of utmost importance in the evaluation of tinnitus patients. The time of onset and any possible causative events, such as exposure to noise, viral infections, or head trauma, should be elicited. Other important information should include localization of the tinnitus (unilateral, bilateral, centered in the head); composition (ring, buzz, hiss, roar, cricket sounds, multiple sounds); loudness; annoyance; and pitch (high or low). According to the Nodar classification system, tinnitus can be classified using two simple mnemonics A-B-C, and C-C-L-A-P, as depicted in **Table 66.4**. The psychological impact of tinnitus should also be determined by seeking symptoms of depression, anxiety, sleep disturbances, and inability to concentrate. Important questions to ask include, Does the tinnitus keep you awake at night? Does it wake you from sleep? Can you ignore it during the day?

Physical Examination

The neurotologic evaluation includes otoscopy, tuning fork testing, palpation of the neck and TMJs, and cranial nerve testing.

Audiological and Electrophysiological Testing

Comprehensive audiologic testing may be performed in any patient with tinnitus. Prompt audiologic examination should be ideally obtained within 4 weeks of initial patient presentation in patients with perceived hearing difficulties and those with persistent or unilateral tinnitus. Assessment of auditory function should include the following:

1. Pure-tone (air and bone thresholds) and speech audiometry
2. Tympanometry
3. Acoustic reflexes
4. Acoustic reflex decay

Table 66.4 Nodar tinnitus classification system

A	Aurium (unilateral)
B	Binaural (bilateral)
C	Cerebri (centered in the head)
C	Cause (i.e., noise, presbycusis, acoustic neuroma, idiopathic)
C	Composition (ring, buzz, hiss, roar, crickets, multiple sounds)
L	Loudness (1–10; 10 being very loud)
A	Annoyance (1–10; 10 being very annoying)
P	Pitch (high or low)

Data from Nodar RH. "C.A.P.P.E. "–A Strategy for Counselling Tinnitus Patients. Int Tinnitus J 1996;2(2):111–113

Auditory brainstem responses (ABRs), electrocochleography, and otoacoustic emissions should be considered in selected cases only, such as suspected acoustic neuromas, endolymphatic hydrops, or ototoxicity. Electronystagmography (ENG) could be considered for patients with associated vestibular symptomatology.

Radiological Evaluation

Head magnetic resonance imaging (MRI) with gadolinium enhancement should be considered for patients with the following:

1. Unilateral unexplained tinnitus with or without hearing loss
2. Bilateral symmetrical or asymmetrical hearing loss suspicious of retrocochlear origin (poor discrimination, absent acoustic reflexes, acoustic reflex decay, abnormal ABR)

Computed tomography (CT) of the temporal bones should be considered when otic capsule pathology is suspected (otosclerosis, Paget disease, marble bone disease).

Metabolic and Allergy Testing

Metabolic testing should be performed in selected cases and may include complete blood count, serum lipids, fasting blood sugar, sedimentation rate, antinuclear antibody, rheumatoid factor, thyroid function tests, fluorescent treponemal antibody absorption (FTA-abs), and Western blot tests. Allergy workup could be considered in selected cases.

Tinnitus Analysis

Tinnitus analysis should be considered, especially when tinnitus is severe and disabling. This evaluation may include the following:

1. *Pitch matching* This can be achieved in the majority of patients by using pure tones for tonal tinnitus or white, narrow, or speech noise for complex tinnitus.
2. *Loudness matching* This test may predict which patients will respond to masking. With this technique, tinnitus is matched first by pitch and then by increasing the masking level from threshold to a level that is equal to the intensity of the tinnitus. In the majority of patients, the "sensation level" is < 7 dB. Psychological factors should be considered in patients with a < 2 dB sensation level of loudness.
3. *Minimum masking level* In this test, the level and frequency of sound required to barely mask the tinnitus are determined. This test is also helpful in predicting patients who may benefit from masking.
4. *Residual inhibition* This phenomenon is characterized by decreased or absent tinnitus following exposure to a masking tone for 1 minute. Patients with residual inhibition are good candidates for masking.

Management

In managing tinnitus, it is crucial for the otolaryngologist to gauge the impact of the tinnitus on the patient's quality of life and to have a very positive and empathetic attitude. Negative statements by the physician, such as, "There is nothing much that can be done, you just have to live with it," are strongly condemned. The astute otolaryngologist should detect symptoms of anxiety or depression early on in treating tinnitus patients, and should address them properly. Psychiatric evaluation should be obtained for severely depressed patients.

Management should begin by giving the patient a detailed report of the audiogram and other evaluation results. An outline of the anatomy and function of the auditory system should be given to the patient. It is speculated that in patients with tinnitus a "vicious cycle" exists between tinnitus and fear/anxiety, and the latter can enhance the perception level and duration of awareness of tinnitus. Reducing fear and anxiety by reassuring the patient goes a long way toward helping patients cope with tinnitus.

Once serious pathology has been eliminated, the patient should be appropriately informed. The majority of tinnitus patients respond well to explanation of their problem and reassurance. Many patients are concerned that they may have a brain tumor, or are going deaf, or are becoming insane. Others are afraid that they will not be able to sleep or concentrate and may lose their job as a result of their tinnitus.

Intake of aspirin-containing medications and nonsteroidal anti-inflammatory drugs should be avoided. Home-masking techniques, such as listening to music or a fan, or broadband masking by tuning the radio between AM stations, are very helpful. They are also informed that tinnitus may increase in intensity in a very small number of patients or may temporarily increase from time to time. The participation of an audiologist with expertise in tinnitus evaluation and full understanding of the patient's needs is very important.

For patients with severe, disabling tinnitus, the following management modalities are available: sound therapy, habituation, cognitive behavior therapy, medication, and surgery.

Sound Therapy

Masking is effective for patients with low masking levels and can be accomplished with various devices. *Hearing aids* are probably the most commonly used masking devices and have been reported to provide significant improvement of tinnitus in 25 to 70% of patients. The *tinnitus instrument*, a combination of a hearing aid and a masker, has been reported to obtain long-term benefits in 55% of patients. The masker component of the tinnitus instrument is capable of producing a 1,500 to 8,000 Hz tone, and has individual volume controls for both the hearing aid and the masker components. This allows the patient to adjust the devices for maximum comfort and benefit. The tinnitus masker is a device indicated for tinnitus sufferers with normal or near-normal hearing. Thirty percent of patients find this device helpful.

Habituation

Habituation to tinnitus perception is a process by which tinnitus patients, by using specific protocols, can reach a state of being unaware of the presence of tinnitus, except when they deliberately concentrate their attention on it. Habituation is a different technique from masking and is basically a reconditioning of connections within subcortical centers. Popularized by Dr. Pawel Jastreboff at Emory University School of Medicine, this technique involves extensive counseling and use of binaural broadband noise generators (Viennatone maskers). These noise generators allow smooth increase of the sound volume and are used for at least 6 hours a day, particularly when the patient is in a quiet environment. Tinnitus habituation requires at least 12 months, and it is rec-

ommended that patients continue for an additional 6 months.

Significant improvement of tinnitus has been reported in 83% of patients treated with this method. Newer devices, such as Neuromonics and combination hearing aids, have been developed recently that provide masking and habituation. These devices will require further investigation to determine their efficacy and benefit to patients.

Electrical Stimulation

Electrical stimulation for tinnitus has recently regained attention; however, it continues to be investigational. Although some studies have shown prolonged relief of tinnitus after transcutaneous electrical stimulation, randomized controlled trials and systematic reviews have not demonstrated long term reduction of tinnitus or improvements in patient quality of life.

Cognitive Behavioral Therapy

Cognitive behavioral therapy (CBT) should be considered for patients with persistent and bothersome tinnitus who have failed sound therapy, those with normal hearing, and those with associated anxiety and stress, tension headaches, and depression. CBT is a type of psychotherapeutic treatment that provides patients with the necessary skills to understand negative thoughts that influence behaviors. The treatment also helps patients change the destructive or disturbing thought patterns and redirect them to more accurate and helpful thoughts. Cooperation among the patient, therapist, and psychologist is necessary.

Medical Treatment

Antidepressant medications, such as nortriptyline (Pamelor, Mallinckrodt, Inc., Hazelwood, MO) and amitriptyline (Elavil), have been found useful for tinnitus patients who have concomitant depression or sleep difficulty. If antidepressant medications are to be used, psychiatric consultation may be in order.

Alprazolam (Xanax, Pfizer, New York, NY) and diazepam (Valium, Roche, Branchburg, NJ) have a beneficial effect on tinnitus; however, their use should be limited because of their addictive properties.

Anticonvulsive medications, such as primidone (Mysoline, Valeant Pharmaceuticals International, Aliso Viejo, CA), phenytoin (Dilantin, Pfizer, New York, NY), and carbamazepine (Tegretol), have been used for treating tinnitus without any significant success.

Intratympanic injection of gentamicin in patients with Ménière disease has been reported to reduce severe tinnitus in 65% of patients with this disease.

Nimodipine, an L-type calcium channel antagonist, has been reported to provide relief to a small number of patients with tinnitus.

The effectiveness of medications with gamma-aminobutyric acid (GABA) or GABA-like effects, such as baclofen, are promising; however, they remain investigational. Gabapentin has not been shown to be beneficial.

Table 66.5 summarizes medications reported in the tinnitus treatment literature. The effectiveness of these medications, however, is either anecdotal or lacks rigorous scientific evidence.

Surgical Treatment

Relief of tinnitus following labyrinthectomy and translabyrinthine section of the eighth nerve has been reported in up to 70% of patients. These procedures, however, are limited to patients with profound hearing loss.

Improvement or relief of tinnitus has been reported in 31% of patients with vertigo who have undergone retrolabyrinthine section of the vestibular nerve and in 31% of patients who have had retrosigmoid vestibular nerve section. It has been speculated that the beneficial effect of vestibular nerve section in these patients may be secondary to sectioning the cochlear efferent bundle, which is in proximity to the vestibular nerve.

For patients with vascular compression syndrome, tinnitus has been totally eliminated or improved in 40 to 78% of cases after microvascular decompression of the auditory nerve.

Tinnitus following surgery for acoustic neuroma has been reported to decrease in 40 to 50% of patients. In 50% of these patients, however, tinnitus has been reported to be worse after surgery.

Table 66.5 Medications reported for tinnitus treatment (without scientific documentation)

Betahistine hydrochloride (SERC)	Hydergine
	Lecithin
Caroverine	Meclizine
Ginkgo biloba	Niacin
Glutaminic acid diethyl ester	Vincamine
Histamine	Vinpocetine

Relief of tinnitus has been reported in 40% of patients with otosclerosis following successful stapedectomy.

■ Pulsatile Tinnitus

Introduction

Pulsatile tinnitus (PT) is a less common type of tinnitus. In the majority of patients, PT is associated with a treatable underlying etiology. Accurate diagnosis is crucial because in some patients this symptom can be associated with a life-threatening pathology.

Pathophysiology and Classification

PT can originate from vascular structures within the cranial cavity, head and neck region, and thoracic cavity and can be transmitted to the cochlea via bony structures, blood vessels, and the bloodstream. PT arises from either increased flow volume or stenosis of the vascular lumen.

Vascular PT can be classified as *arterial* or *venous,* according to the vessel of origin. The venous type can originate not only from primary venous pathology but also from conditions causing increased intracranial pressure by transmission of arterial pulsations to the dural venous sinuses. PT originating from other nonarterial/venous structures is classified as *nonvascular.* PT is called *objective* or *subjective* according to whether it is audible to both patient and examiner (objective) or patient only (subjective).

Evaluation

Patient History

The patient's history is the most important part of PT evaluation and must include onset, laterality, associated symptoms, exacerbating/relieving factors, intensity, and pulse-synchronicity. Associated symptoms of hearing loss, dizziness, aural fullness, headaches, and visual disturbances (blurred vision, visual loss, and visual obscurations) are highly suggestive of benign intracranial hypertension (BIH) syndrome.

Older PT patients with a previous history of cerebrovascular accident, transient ischemic attacks, hypertension, hyperlipidemia, diabetes mellitus, and smoking should be suspected of atherosclerotic carotid artery disease (ACAD). Females with associated headaches, dizzy spells, fatigue, syncope, and lateralizing neurological deficits should be suspected for fibromuscular dysplasia (FMD). Sudden onset of PT in association with cervical or facial pain, headache, and symptoms of cerebral ischemia is highly suggestive of extracranial or intrapetrous carotid artery dissection. Association with noise-induced or pressure-induced dizziness may lead to the consideration of superior canal dehiscence. Vascular PT that varies with position or neck compression is suggestive of dehiscence of the sigmoid sinus or sigmoid sinus diverticulum.

Nonvascular etiologies include middle ear muscle myoclonus, palatal myoclonus, and patulous eustachian tube.

Examination

Young and morbidly obese females with unilateral PT should be suspected of suffering from BIH syndrome. Meticulous micro-otoscopy is essential for detection of any middle ear pathology, such as a high or exposed jugular bulb, glomus tumor, aberrant carotid artery, or Schwartze sign.

A palpable thrill may be present in cervical arteriovenous malformations. Myoclonic contractions of the soft palate can be seen in patients with palatal myoclonus.

Auscultation of the ear canal, periauricular region, orbits, cervical region, and chest is essential for detecting objective PT, bruits, and heart murmurs. This should be performed in a sound-treated room, preferably with a modified electronic stethoscope (Auscultear, Starkey ST3). Auscultation with this instrument is more sensitive than with the Toynbee tube for detection of PT. The effect of light digital pressure over the ipsilateral internal jugular vein (IJV) should be checked. PT of venous origin, which typically is present in patients with BIH syndrome, decreases or completely subsides with this maneuver. In patients with arterial PT such as ACAD, arteriovenous fistulas (AVFs), and arteriovenous malformations (AVMs), this maneuver results in no change in tinnitus intensity. In patients with dural AVMs/AVFs, a loud retroauricular bruit is present. Complete neurotologic examination and funduscopy should be included in the examination, including pressure- and noise-induced nystagmus evaluation. Papilledema is suggestive of BIH syndrome. Tinnitus characteristics in various pathologies are summarized in **Table 66.6**.

Consultation with Other Specialties

When clinical evaluation suggests BIH syndrome, consultation with a neuro-ophthalmologist is imperative. Funduscopic examination for detection of papilledema, tonometry to measure intraocular pressure, and measurement of visual acuity and visual fields are essential. Although the presence of papilledema is highly suggestive of BIH syndrome, its absence does not rule out this entity. Diagnosis of this condition is established by lumbar puncture and

Table 66.6 Characteristics of pulsatile tinnitus

	BIH syndrome	ACAD	Glomus tumors	AVM/AVF
Age	< 40 years	> 50 years	40 years, average	40 years, average
Sex	Females mainly	More common in females	More common in females	NR
Weight	Obese	NR	NR	NR
Retrotympanic mass	–	–	+	–
Objective PT	+	+	–	+
Arterial PT	–	+	+	+
Venous PT	+	–	–	–
Head bruit	–	–	–	+
Neck bruit	–	+	–	–
Papilledema	Common	–	–	–

Abbreviations: ACAD, atherosclerotic carotid artery disease; AVF, arteriovenous fistula; AVM, arteriovenous malformation; BIH, benign intracranial hypertension; NR, not relevant; PT, pulsatile tinnitus documentation of elevated cerebrospinal fluid (CSF) pressure (> 200 mm of water).

For patients suspected of ACAD, consultation with a neurologist, vascular surgeon, or neurosurgeon should be considered.

Audiological and Electrophysiological Testing

Pure-tone (air and bone conduction) and speech audiometry should be performed in all PT patients. When hearing loss of 20 dB or more is detected, a repeat audiogram should be obtained while the patient is applying light digital pressure over the ipsilateral IJV. This maneuver typically results in normalization or improvement of pure tones in patients with venous PT, such as BIH syndrome or sigmoid sinus dehiscence (which may be related to BIH), due to elimination of the masking effect of the tinnitus. Discrimination is typically excellent in these patients.

Tympanometry should be obtained in patients suspicious for tensor tympani myoclonus for detection of any abnormal movements of the tympanic membrane. ABRs should be considered in patients suspected of BIH syndrome. Abnormalities of this test, consisting mainly of prolonged interpeak latencies, have been detected in one third of BIH patients.

ENG should be considered in patients with associated vestibular symptoms.

Metabolic Evaluation

Complete blood count will exclude anemia in patients suspected of increased cardiac output syndrome. Vitamin A level and thyroid function should be tested in patients suspected for BIH syndrome. Hypothyroidism alone can cause PT. Serum lipid profile and fasting blood sugar should be performed in patients with ACAD.

Ultrasound Studies

Duplex carotid ultrasound and echocardiography are obtained for patients suspected of ACAD or cardiac murmurs, respectively. These tests should be performed prior to any radiological evaluation, because they may be the only evaluation required to establish diagnosis.

Radiological Evaluation

Radiological evaluation needs to be individualized according to the clinical presentation, physical findings (retrotympanic mass, objective PT, bruit, papilledema), and audiometric and electrophysiological results. **Fig. 66.1** depicts an algorithm for evaluating PT patients.

The following represents a recommended radiological protocol.

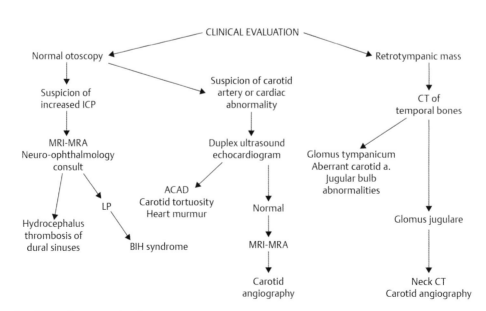

Fig. 66.1   Algorithm for evaluating pulsatile tinnitus patients.

Normal Otoscopy

For patients with normal otoscopy, screening with high-quality magnetic resonance angiography (MRA), in conjunction with brain MRI, should be performed. Small ventricles and/or empty sella are findings often seen in patients with BIH syndrome. MRI demonstration of dilated cortical veins is suggestive of a dural AVM. Neither the arterial supply nor the nidus of an AVM may be detectable on MRI. Dural venous sinus thrombosis can also be diagnosed with MRA. For patients with normal MRI/MRA studies, four-vessel cerebral angiography should be considered, especially when PT is objective and/or an associated head bruit is present, to exclude small dural AVFs or AVMs. At present, MRA should not be considered a substitute for conventional angiography. Another initial study that may be considered is CT with CT angiography (CTA) for evaluation of vascular anomalies and superior canal dehiscence.

Retrotympanic Mass

Patients with a retrotympanic mass should have a high-resolution temporal bone CT as their initial evaluation. If a glomus tympanicum, jugular bulb abnormalities, sigmoid sinus dehiscence or diverticulum, or aberrant internal carotid artery is diagnosed, no other imaging studies are needed. For patients with glomus jugulare tumors, CT examination of the neck should also be obtained to detect any possible synchronous chemodectomas along the carotid arteries. Carotid angiography is indicated only for prospective surgical cases to evaluate the collateral circulation of the brain (arterial and venous) in anticipation of possible vessel ligation and/or preoperative tumor embolization.

Arterial Etiologies

ACAD has been the most common reported cause of PT in patients over 50 years of age, especially when associated risk factors for atherosclerosis are present (hypertension, angina, hyperlipidemia, diabetes mellitus, smoking). Objective PT can be the first manifestation of ACAD in some of these patients. PT in ACAD is secondary to bruits produced by turbulent blood flow at the stenotic segment(s) of the carotid artery system. Diagnosis can be confirmed by duplex ultrasound studies. Dural AVFs/AVMs are less common causes of arterial PT; however, they should always be included in the differential diagnosis, especially when a retroauricular or orbital bruit is present. The majority of AVF/AVM patients present with PT.

Venous Etiologies

BIH syndrome has been reported as a common etiology of venous PT. This syndrome is characterized by increased intracranial pressure without focal signs of neurological dysfunction, except for occasional sixth and seventh cranial nerve palsies. Synonyms for this disorder are pseudotumor cerebri and idiopathic intracranial hypertension. BIH syndrome is diagnosed by exclusion of lesions producing intracranial hypertension, such as obstructive hydrocephalus, mass lesions, chronic meningitis, and hypertensive and pulmonary encephalopathy. This syndrome is usually idiopathic; however, it may be associated with various medical conditions, disorders, and intake of medications.

Table 66.7 summarizes the medical conditions, disorders, and medications associated with BIH syndrome. In the majority of patients, this syndrome has a benign and self-limiting course; however, in 25% of patients it may become chronic. The exact

Table 66.7 Medical conditions, disorders, and medications associated with benign intracranial hypertension syndrome

Condition or disorder	Medications
Cushing syndrome and disease	Indomethacin
Hyperthyroidism	Nalidixic acid (antibiotic)
Iron-deficiency anemia	Nitrofurantoin
Vitamin D deficiency	Oral contraceptives (without sinus thrombosis)
Menstrual irregularities	Tetracycline
Obesity	Vitamin A (excessive intake, deficiency)
Pregnancy and postpartum (without sinus thrombosis)	
Hypothyroidism	

pathophysiology of BIH syndrome remains unclear; however, an increase in resistance to CSF absorption resulting in interstitial brain edema is strongly suspected. It has been postulated that BIH syndrome in morbidly obese patients is due to increased intra-abdominal pressure and associated elevation of the diaphragm, resulting in increased pleural pressure and decreased venous return from the brain.

The majority of patients with BIH syndrome are female and morbidly obese (more than 100 lb above their ideal weight). Although papilledema is present in many of these patients, its absence does not exclude BIH syndrome. Head CT or MRI is normal in the majority of these patients, although an empty sella and/or small ventricles may be present. Diagnosis should be established in all patients with lumbar puncture and documentation of elevated CSF pressure (> 200 mm of water).

PT in BIH syndrome, usually unilateral, is believed to result from systolic pulsations of the CSF, originating mainly from the arteries of the circle of Willis. These pulsations are transmitted to the medial aspect of the dural venous sinuses (transverse, sigmoid), compressing their walls synchronously with the arterial pulsations. These periodic compressions convert the normal laminar blood flow in the smooth-walled dural venous sinuses to turbulent blood flow, thus producing a low-frequency PT. The low-frequency sensorineural hearing loss, found in many of these patients, is believed to result from the masking effect of the PT. This is supported by the fact that, in most of these patients, light digital compression over the ipsilateral IJV results in cessation of the tinnitus and immediate improvement or normalization of hearing. Stretching or compression of the cochlear nerve and brainstem, caused by the intracranial hypertension and/or primary edema due to the BIH syndrome itself, can also play a role in the hearing loss encountered in these patients. This is supported by abnormal auditory-evoked responses present in one third of these patients.

Idiopathic or *essential PT* and *venous hum* are terms used interchangeably to describe patients with PT of unknown etiology. The most common age of patients with idiopathic PT is between 20 and 40 years, and there is a marked female preponderance. A possible cause of idiopathic PT is believed to be turbulent blood flow produced in the IJV as it curves around the lateral process of the atlas. This condition should be diagnosed only after appropriate evaluation and elimination of other disorders, such as BIH syndrome. Associated symptoms of headaches and blurred vision, especially in morbidly obese female patients, should alert the otolaryngologist to BIH syndrome.

Tables 66.8, 66.9, and **66.10** summarize the various causes of PT.

Table 66.8 Arterial etiologies of pulsatile tinnitus

Intra- and extracranial arteriovenous malformations
Dural arteriovenous fistulas and aneurysms
Atherosclerotic carotid artery disease
Atherosclerotic subclavian artery disease
Atherosclerotic occlusion of the contralateral common carotid artery
Fibromuscular dysplasia of the carotid artery
Extracranial carotid artery dissection
Intrapetrous carotid artery dissection
Brachiocephalic artery stenosis
External carotid artery stenosis
Ectopic intratympanic carotid artery
Persistent stapedial artery
Aberrant artery in the stria vascularis
Vascular compression of the eighth nerve
Increased cardiac output (anemia, thyrotoxicosis, pregnancy)
Aortic murmurs
Paget disease
Otosclerosis
Hypertension-antihypertensive agents (enalapril maleate, verapamil hydrochloride)
Vascular neoplasms of skull base and temporal bone

Table 66.9 Venous etiologies of pulsatile tinnitus

Abnormal condylar and mastoid emissary veins
Abnormalities of dural venous sinuses
Stenosis
Aneurysmal dilatation
Benign intracranial hypertension
Hydrocephalus associated with stenosis of the sylvian aqueduct
Idiopathic or essential tinnitus
Increased intracranial pressure associated with Arnold–Chiari malformation
Jugular bulb abnormalities
Megabulb
High/dehisced bulb

Table 66.10 Nonvascular etiologies of pulsatile tinnitus

Palatal myoclonus

Stapedial myoclonus

Tensor tympani muscle myoclonus

Management

Management of patients' PT should be directed toward treating any underlying etiology. Explaining the exact nature of the problem to the patient and reassurance are essential. The following sections describe management for the most common etiologies of PT.

Atherosclerotic Vascular Disease

Carotid endarterectomy for patients with 70 to 99% reduction in luminal diameter has resulted in a reduced 5-year risk of ipsilateral stroke. Management of the risk factors is essential for these patients. Objective PT secondary to atherosclerotic involvement of the subclavian artery has been relieved by angioplasty.

Dural Arteriovenous Malformations and Fistulas

In the past decade, selective endovascular embolization of AVMs/AVFs has gained popularity in treating these lesions, and excellent results with minimal complications have been reported. Stereotactic radiosurgery with focused gamma-beam irradiation has also achieved excellent results with no mortality and very low morbidity.

Carotid–Cavernous Fistulas (CCFs)

The majority of carotid–cavernous fistulas (CCFs) can be treated very effectively with intra-arterial balloon occlusion. This approach has been successful in 95% of cases. Transvenous occlusion, through the cavernous sinus, can also be achieved through the inferior petrosal or the superior orbital vein. Direct surgical exposure of the cavernous sinus should be performed only when intravascular techniques have failed.

Fibromuscular Dysplasia (FMD)

Isolated cervical and cerebral fibromuscular dysplasias (FMDs) are considered relatively benign disorders and rarely result in ischemic symptoms. Surgical management, therefore, should be reserved for patients with significant clinical symptomatology. Management includes transcutaneous angioplasty or open balloon dilation of the internal carotid artery.

BIH Syndrome

Participation of a neuro-ophthalmologist in the management of BIH patients is imperative. These patients should be treated for any possible associated disorders. PT secondary to idiopathic BIH syndrome responds well to weight reduction and medical management with acetazolamide (Diamox), 250 mg three times a day. Furosemide (Lasix), 20 mg twice a day, should be considered for refractory cases. Both

of these medications are thought to reduce CSF production. Lumbar-peritoneal shunt has been recommended in the past for patients with progressive deterioration of vision, chronic BIH syndrome, and disabling PT. In morbidly obese patients with BIH syndrome, however, this procedure is often complicated by occlusion of the shunt, probably due to increased intra-abdominal pressure, commonly present in these patients. Recently, it has been reported that gastric surgery for obesity (gastroplasty, gastric bypass) is helpful in eliminating PT in these patients.

Sigmoid sinus dehiscence or diverticulum may be an anatomical correlate of BIH syndrome. Diagnosis is made by high-resolution temporal bone CT imaging. Surgical resurfacing of the sinus can be an effective treatment.

Other Etiologies

Vascular neoplasms are treated surgically in the majority of patients. Repair of a symptomatic high-dehisced jugular bulb has been reported by using pieces of mastoid cortical bone and septal, conchal, or tragal cartilage. PT secondary to otosclerosis may respond to stapedectomy. Botox (Allergan, Irvine, CA) injection or section of the levator veli palatini muscle has been reported for treating palatal myoclonus. Tensor tympani and stapedial myoclonus may respond to section of the respective muscles via tympanotomy. Palatal myoclonus may respond to anticonvulsive medications or local injection with botulinum toxoid. Finally, PT secondary to the antihypertensive medications enalapril maleate and verapamil hydrochloride subsides soon after discontinuation of these agents.

Idiopathic (Essential) Pulsatile Tinnitus

Ligation of the ipsilateral IJV has been recommended in the literature for patients with idiopathic PT. However, the results of this procedure have been very inconsistent and poor overall. In a series of 13 patients with essential PT, 3 underwent ligation of the ipsilateral IJV and only 1 benefited permanently. The other 2 patients experienced return of their PT within a few days. This procedure has also been recommended for patients with abnormalities of the jugular bulb (high or large bulb). It is strongly recommended that IJV ligation be considered only after careful elimination of any other causes of PT, especially BIH syndrome and sigmoid sinus dehiscence/diverticulum. The validity of this procedure remains very questionable.

■ Controversial Issues

The pathophysiology of nonpulsatile tinnitus is still elusive, making accurate, evidence-based research difficult. Treatment recommendations at this time mostly focus on mitigating the reactionary symptoms, such as anxiety, depression, or sleep deprivation, rather than the actual cause of the tinnitus.

■ Clinical Practice Guidelines, Consenus Statements, and Measures

AAO-HNS Clinical Practice Guideline: Tinnitus
Otolaryngology -- Head and Neck Surgery 2014 151: S1

Phillips, Shannon K. Robinson, Malcolm B. Taw, Richard S. Tyler, Richard Waguespack and Elizabeth J. Whamond Hollingsworth, Fawad A. Khan, Scott Mitchell, Ashkan Monfared, Craig W. Newman, Folashade S. Omole, C. Douglas Cunningham, Jr, Sanford M. Archer, Brian W. Blakley, John M. Carter, Evelyn C. Granieri, James A. Henry, Deena David E. Tunkel, Carol A. Bauer, Gordon H. Sun, Richard M. Rosenfeld, Sujana S. Chandrasekhar, Eugene R.

■ Suggested Reading

Brookes GB. Vascular-decompression surgery for severe tinnitus. Am J Otol 1996;17(4):569–576

Catalano PJ, Post KD. Elimination of tinnitus following hearing preservation surgery for acoustic neuromas. Am J Otol 1996; 17(3):443–445

Chouard CH, Meyer B, Maridat D. Transcutaneous electrotherapy for severe tinnitus. Acta Otolaryngol 1981;91(5-6):415–422

Davies E, Knox E, Donaldson I. The usefulness of nimodipine, an L-calcium channel antagonist, in the treatment of tinnitus. Br J Audiol 1994;28(3):125–129

Hobson J, Chisholm E, El Refaie A. Sound therapy (masking) in the management of tinnitus in adults. Cochrane Database Syst Rev 2012;11:CD006371

House JW, Brackmann DE. Tinnitus: surgical treatment. In: Tinnitus (Ciba Foundation Symposium 85). London, UK: Pitman Books, Ltd.; 1981

Jastreboff PJ, Gray WC, Gold SL. Neurophysiological approach to tinnitus patients. Am J Otol 1996;17(2):236–240

Kaasinen S, Pyykkö I, Ishizaki H, Aalto H. Effect of intratympanically administered gentamicin on hearing and tinnitus in Ménière's disease. Acta Otolaryngol Suppl 1995;520(Pt 1):184–185

McKerrow WS, Schreiner CE, Snyder RL, Merzenich MM, Toner JG. Tinnitus suppression by cochlear implants. Ann Otol Rhinol Laryngol 1991;100(7):552–558

Moller AR. Tinnitus. In: Jackler RK, Brackmann DE, eds. Neurotology. St. Louis, MO: Mosby–Year Book; 1994:153–165

Møller MB, Møller AR, Jannetta PJ, Jho HD. Vascular decompression surgery for severe tinnitus: selection criteria and results. Laryngoscope 1993;103(4 Pt 1):421–427

Nodar RH. Tinnitus reclassified; new oil in an old lamp. Otolaryngol Head Neck Surg 1996;114(4):582–585

Nodar RH, Sahley TL. Nonpulsatile tinnitus. In: Hughes GB, Pensak ML, eds. Clinical Otology. 2nd ed. New York, NY: Thieme; 1997:461–463

Pulec JL. Tinnitus: surgical therapy. Am J Otol 1984;5(6):479–480

Schleuning AJ II. Tinnitus. In: Gates GA, ed. Current Therapy in Otolaryngology–Head and Neck Surgery. 5th ed. St. Louis, MO: Mosby–Year Book; 1994:91–97

Shulman A. Tinnitus: Diagnosis/Treatment. Philadelphia, PA: Lea & Febiger; 1991

Sismanis A. Pulsatile tinnitus. In: Hughes GB, Pensak ML, eds. Clinical Otology. 2nd ed. New York, NY: Thieme; 1997:461–463

Sismanis A, Smoker WRK. Pulsatile tinnitus: recent advances in diagnosis. Laryngoscope 1994;104(6 Pt 1):681–688

Sullivan M, Katon W, Russo J, Dobie R, Sakai C. A randomized trial of nortriptyline for severe chronic tinnitus: effects on depression, disability, and tinnitus symptoms. Arch Intern Med 1993;153(19):2251–2259

Vernon JA, Moller AR, eds. Mechanisms of Tinnitus. Boston, MA: Allyn & Bacon; 1995

67 Assessment and Management of the Vertiginous Patient

■ Introduction

The balance system, often referred to as a three-legged stool, is composed of three sensory systems—vestibular sense, proprioceptive sense, and visual sense—all sending information to the brain. Central nervous system (CNS) centers (including the spinal cord, brainstem, cerebellum and cerebellar peduncles, and sensory and motor cortices) integrate this information to maintain balance, stabilize the head on the neck, stabilize the body, prevent falls, maintain the gaze in a stable plane despite head or body movements, and prevent dizziness. Any of the following can cause dizziness:

1. Dysfunction in any one or combinations of these sensory systems
2. Poor integration of this peripheral information in the CNS
3. Orientationally incorrect sensory input (the seasick model—vestibular and proprioceptive senses feel the boat rocking, yet eyes looking within the boat do not detect motion)
4. Faulty motor signal or muscle response

Taken together, most patients with dizziness can be placed into either of the first two categories. The patient's history will be the most important diagnostic tool to identify the underlying etiology.

Vestibular System

The vestibular system is designed to maintain our gaze on a fixed object, despite head or body movements (Newlands and Wall provide a more detailed discussion). The system detects head and body motion and converts these sensed motions into signals useful to the brain. The vestibular system is also an antigravity system, designed to detect and oppose the force of gravity to allow us to maintain an upright posture. To accomplish these functions, the vestibular system is composed of three paired semicircular canals (superior, lateral, and posterior) that detect angular acceleration and two paired otolithic organs (saccule and utricle) that detect linear acceleration.

Pitch refers to movement of the head in the vertical axis up and down on the neck, mediated by a superior canal on one side and its oppositely oriented posterior canal on the contralateral side. *Yaw* is horizontal (side-to-side) motion of the head on the neck and is mediated by the paired lateral (horizontal) semicircular canals. *Roll* describes putting the ear to the shoulder as though reading book titles on a shelf and is mediated again by a paired superior canal with a posterior canal. The otolithic organs are gravity detectors—the saccule is oriented at a right angle to the utricle and detects up-and-down (e.g., elevator) motion, whereas the utricle detects side-to-side/forward–backward motion (e.g., accelerating in an airplane).

The paired vestibular organs act as a "push-pull" system—when one set of organs is stimulated (the right lateral canal with right head turn), its contralateral partner (left lateral canal) is inhibited. Stimulation or excitation of a semicircular canal results in deflection of the cupula located in the ampulla, a dilated area at the end of the canal. Hair cells project up into the cupula and are deflected as the cupula is suspended in endolymphatic fluid. When the head moves, the fluid has inertia and tends to oppose the motion causing deflection of the cupula and the hair cells within. This deflection causes a depolarization of the hair cell, which increases the baseline firing rate of the vestibular nerve. (Depending on the direction of the motion, ampullopetal is fluid flow toward the ampulla, which is excitatory in the lateral canals but is inhibitory in the superior/posterior canals.)

The otolithic organs contain calcium carbonate crystals (otoconia) resting on a gelatinous matrix. The crystals have mass, and when the head or body moves, the crystals oppose the motion and cause deflection of the underlying hair cells. The excitatory response of the hair cell depends on its vector and orientation within the otolithic organ. The otolithic organs are sensitive to linear motion in multiple vectors. The superior vestibular nerve innervates the lateral and superior semicircular canals, the utricle, and a portion of the saccule. The inferior vestibular nerve innervates the posterior canal and the saccule.

The vestibulo-ocular reflex (VOR) ensures that eye position is maintained, despite movement of the head or body. When the head moves right, the vestibular system senses this rightward motion and sends signals, through the medial longitudinal fasciculus, to the extraocular muscles of the eye to turn the eyes in the opposite direction of the head turn. Through the vestibulocollic and vestibulospinal pathways, the vestibular system senses gravity and activates, in general, extensor/antigravity muscle groups for coordinated movements to oppose gravity, to maintain posture and stability with the head and body upright.

Prevalence

Approximately 20 to 30% of the U.S. population is affected by dizziness or vertigo. In the pediatric population, estimates of the prevalence of dizziness range from 1 to 6%. In the elderly population, prevalence rates of dizziness increase to nearly 50%, with 25 to 33% of the population older than 65 experiencing some form of dizziness. Seven percent of all primary care visits for patients older than 65 are for dizziness, and dizziness is the most common complaint of patients older than 75. Data from the U.S. National Health and Nutrition Examination Survey indicate that the prevalence of vestibular dysfunction for individuals in the seventh decade of life, eighth decade of life, and older was 49.4, 68.7, and 84.8%, respectively.

Pathogenesis/Pathology

All vertigo is dizziness, but not all dizziness is vertigo. The statement underscores the importance of taking the history of the patient presenting with dizziness. Dizziness can also be described as a floating, lightheaded, woozy, weird, off, or tired sensation. No understanding of the diagnosis or pathology can be realized without a clear picture of the patient's symptomatology. Vertigo is the sensation of the room or the world moving, usually a spinning sensation, much like a child who turns round and round only to stop and see the world turning or spinning. The pathogenesis and pathology of many conditions that cause dizziness and vertigo will be discussed later in this chapter under the individual diagnoses of dizziness and vertigo.

Evaluation

History

Taking the history of the patient with dizziness is both an art and a science. An easy, straightforward question to start with and to get patients thinking about their symptoms is to ask when the dizziness started. Perhaps the most important question is to ask whether the dizziness comes in discrete spells or episodes or whether the patient feels dizzy all the time. Episodic dizziness puts the differential diagnosis in an entirely separate category from the continuous dizziness. If episodic, the examiner will want to know how long the episodes last, their frequency, and the time of the last episode. Sometimes, the diagnosis can be made simply on the temporal pattern of the dizziness:

- *Seconds* Benign paroxysmal positional vertigo (BPPV), postural hypotension
- *Minutes* Transient ischemic attacks
- *Hours* Ménière disease
- *Days* Viral labyrinthitis
- *Constant* Metabolic, psychogenic, toxic or drug side effect (unlikely to be vestibular)

The next critical step is to try to understand the character of the dizziness: "Without using the word 'dizzy,' describe the sensation you get when you feel dizzy." Numerous words in the English language describe dizziness, but helpful hints include wooziness, feeling "off," room spinning, lightheaded, rocking/swaying as if on a boat, and imbalance/disequilibrium. Associated symptoms to query include nausea, vomiting, headache and its nature, syncope, hearing loss, aural fullness, associated tinnitus, and neck/musculoskeletal pain.

Several factors can precipitate dizziness. Eliciting this information can often point to an underlying pathology. Specific events that should be explored in this context include food ingestion, sudden head movement, turning over in bed, coughing or sneezing, loud noise, postural change, and exercise.

Ingestion of large amounts of sodium can precipitate an attack of Ménière disease in some individuals. Other patients with this diagnosis can experience dizziness after eating certain foods, as though the attack were triggered by allergy.

Vertigo of short duration (< 1 min), precipitated by sudden head movement or turning over in bed, strongly suggests BPPV. However, any type of sudden head or body movement places significant demands on the vestibular system and, therefore, can exacerbate vertigo occurring from a variety of vestibular lesions.

Dizziness caused by coughing or sneezing could be due to dehiscence of the superior semicircular canal, a perilymph fistula, or CNS pathology causing increased intracranial pressure. Fibrosis within the vestibule secondary to Ménière disease or syphilis or dehiscence of the superior semicircular canal can produce dizziness in response to loud sound (Tullio phenomenon). Dizziness precipitated by posture change or exercise suggests a cardiovascular problem, such as postural hypotension or cardiac disease. The prevalence of orthostatic dizziness has been reported to be as high as 10 to 15%.

A patient's current medications as well as those used in the recent past, including those used in hospitalizations (especially intravenous antibiotics, e.g., aminoglycosides), should be reviewed. In a study of patients presenting to the emergency room with the chief complaint of dizziness, medications were found to be the cause in 10% of cases; in patients older than 60 years, the incidence was 20%. Drugs may cause orthostatic hypotension (e.g., antihypertensives); central vestibular dysfunction resulting in nonspecific disequilibrium (e.g., antidepressants, sedatives, antihistamines); and direct damage to vestibular sensory cells (e.g., aminoglycoside antibiotics). Shoair et al provide an excellent review.

Physical Examination

Physical examination includes the ear and peripheral vestibular system, the vascular system, eyes and extraocular motility, and the neurological system. Careful otoscopic examination will reveal an occult cholesteatoma, middle ear fluid, or an inflammatory or neoplastic process that may be the source of dizziness. Fistula test to identify the presence of a third window, either a perilymphatic fistula or superior semicircular canal dehiscence syndrome, is performed using pneumatic otoscopy to apply pressure to the tympanic membrane into the external canal. The clinician observes for nystagmus or complaints of a sensation that the world is tilting or moving to one side. Tuning fork exam will help clarify hearing status (and if loud enough, may cause a Tullio phenomenon suggestive of syphilis or a third window).

Because nystagmus is the only objective sign of vertigo, the examination initially focuses on the presence or absence of this abnormality. If present, nystagmus should be defined by the following parameters: direction, plane, intensity, and evoking maneuvers. Frenzel glasses should be used to prevent nystagmus suppression by visual fixation. **Table 67.1** outlines features of peripheral versus central nystagmus.

Gaze-paretic nystagmus, a common type of central nystagmus, is characterized by an inability to maintain lateral gaze, so that right gaze causes a right-beating nystagmus, and left gaze causes a left-beating nystagmus. The most common causes for this type of nystagmus are ingestion of drugs (e.g., alcohol, diazepam, or anticonvulsants) and specific CNS lesions, including multiple sclerosis, cerebellar atrophy, and large acoustic tumors.

The physical examination should also include postural blood pressure measurements, auscultation of the neck and chest, and the neurological examination. The neurological examination should evaluate the cranial nerves and cerebellar function with tests of rapidly alternating movement and finger-to-nose/finger-to-finger coordination to evaluate for disdiadochokinesia or dysmetria. Midline or vermis lesions of the cerebellum can cause ataxia (especially truncal) and intention tremor, whereas hemispheric lesions affect fine motor control (disdiadochokinesia and dysmetria). Ataxia is assessed by having the patient walk with a tandem gait.

Table 67.1 Peripheral versus central nystagmus

Spontaneous nystagmus	
Peripheral	**Central**
Horizontal rotary	Any direction, including vertical
Direction fixed	Direction fixed or changing
Intensity diminished by visual fixation	No change with visual fixation
Increased by gaze in direction of fast phase (Alexander's law)	Gaze has little or no effect on fast phase
Evoked nystagmus (Hallpike)	
Peripheral	**Central**
Latency 2–10 seconds	Immediate onset
Direction predominantly rotary	Any direction, including vertical
Duration < 30 seconds	Duration > 45 seconds
Fatigable	Not fatigable

Vestibulo-ocular Reflex

Electronystagmography (ENG) and rotary chair testing provide quantitative information on the VOR. On physical examination, the head-shaking test and dynamic visual acuity test can provide some qualitative information. With Frenzel glasses in place, the patient quickly shakes his or her head back and forth (horizontal plane) 15 to 20 times. The presence of nystagmus after head shaking suggests an imbalance in the VOR that has undergone partial compensation. The dynamic visual acuity test assesses visual acuity with the head at rest and in motion. The patient first reads a Snellen eye chart with the head stationary, and then with the head randomly rotated about the visual axis by the examiner. A drop in acuity of two lines or more indicates an abnormality within the VOR, usually bilaterally. A patient with a positive test will typically complain of oscillopsia. The head-thrust test is performed by rapidly thrusting the head from the midline 20 degrees (does not have to be high amplitude) to one side and looking for a refixation saccade. The presence of a refixation saccade is diagnostic of a unilateral vestibular loss to the side of the head thrust.

Vestibulo-ocular Control System

This system involves saccadic and smooth pursuit eye movements. Abnormal saccadic movement is characterized by overshooting or undershooting as the patient follows the examiner's finger, which is quickly moved from 30 degrees right to 30 degrees left of center. In smooth pursuit testing, the patient should be able to follow the examiner's finger across the visual field with smooth, pendular motion of the eyes without saccadic movements. Abnormalities in these tests suggest a central lesion.

Vestibulospinal Testing

The vestibulospinal system involves complex reflexes acting on many joints, adjusting antigravity muscle tension to maintain posture and body stability. Romberg and gait testing provide some qualitative information on the integrity of this system. The vestibulospinal reflexes are dependent on proprioceptive, visual, and vestibular input. Romberg testing with eyes closed eliminates the visual input and isolates the vestibular and proprioceptive systems. Proprioceptive input can be largely negated by having the patient stand on a 6 in foam mat while performing a Romberg test.

More quantitative information on the vestibulospinal system can be obtained with dynamic posturography testing. Vestibular-evoked myogenic potentials (VEMPs) are recorded from the sternocleidomastoid muscle (SCM) in response to loud sounds (vestibulocollic reflex). The reflex arc involves the saccule—inferior vestibular nerve, lateral vestibular nucleus, motor nucleus of the spinal accessory nerve—SCM muscle. Parameters recorded include the threshold for evoking the SCM muscle contraction (reduced in conditions, such as third window) and amplitude of the contraction (elevated in third-window conditions). Higher threshold with lower amplitudes (or absent VEMPs) have been seen in patients with Ménière disease and vestibular schwannoma.

Special Investigations

Comprehensive audiometry is recommended for all patients complaining of dizziness. Any asymmetry between ears should be investigated with a retrocochlear evaluation. Magnetic resonance imaging (MRI) with gadolinium contrast is the gold standard for diagnosing vestibular schwannoma. Most patients presenting with dizziness do not have a vestibular schwannoma, but an asymmetry in hearing may tip the balance toward pursuing an imaging study. The presence of sensorineural hearing loss (SNHL) with aging (presbycusis) may also indicate an underlying loss of vestibular function with aging (presbystasis) and will make explanation to the patient clearer.

Vestibular testing, including videonystagmography or ENG, rotary chair testing, platform posturography, and VEMP testing, is discussed in Chapter 61.

Imaging is rarely indicated in the patient with dizziness. However, the physical exam should be directed toward identifying other neurological findings that would necessitate imaging, such as a weakness of the face, ataxia, dysmetria, or other focal neurological deficit. The importance of the neurological exam and imaging is to rule out potentially dangerous or serious conditions, including stroke (brainstem or cerebellar hemorrhage or infarct), CNS neoplasm, CNS infection, or complicated otitis media (acute purulent otitis media or chronic otitis media with cholesteatoma).

Miscellaneous tests might include complete blood count for patients with lethargy or hypotension suspected of anemia or blood dyscrasia, lipid panel for patients suspected of vascular/cerebrovascular disease, thyroid panel, rheumatologic workup (or consultation) for patients suspected of an autoimmune disease, or neck ultrasound to evaluate carotid and vertebral arteries.

Differential Diagnosis

The following diagnoses and their discussions are meant to be neither exhaustive nor exclusive. Space constraints allow for including only the most prevalent diagnoses with limited discussions. Kesser and Gleason provide a more comprehensive review.

◼ Benign Paroxysmal Positional Vertigo

Pathophysiology

BPPV is thought to result from particles of inner ear debris (possibly degenerated otoconia from the utricular macula) that are either attached to the cupula of the posterior semicircular canal (cupulolithiasis) or free floating in the posterior canal (canalithiasis). Because the particles have a higher specific gravity than the surrounding endolymph, the displaced otoconia will produce abnormal cupular deflection with certain head movements, typically back and to one side. (The classic history is lying back in bed and rolling over or turning to one side.) A prior history of head trauma or viral labyrinthitis may be elicited in some patients, but the majority will have no obvious predisposing factors.

Evaluation

The typical patient describes sudden, fleeting (< 30 s) episodes of intense vertigo, precipitated by certain head or body motions. Nausea is possible, but the episodes are generally too brief to induce emesis. Dix–Hallpike testing will usually confirm nystagmus (rotary) with either the right or the left ear undermost. The undermost ear is usually the pathological ear.

Treatment

Various vestibular exercise programs have been described for BPPV. In most cases, this problem is self-limited. Of all the vestibular exercises, the particle repositioning maneuver, as described by Epley, appears to be the most efficacious. This maneuver rotates the patient's head from the provocative head hanging position to the opposite side with the head turned 45 degrees downward. The patient continues to rotate to a lateral decubitus position and then sits up. This maneuver is designed to promote gravity-assisted movement of the particles from the posterior semicircular canal through the common crus into the utricle, where they will no longer cause cupular deflection. Rarely, a singular neurectomy to denervate the posterior semicircular canal is necessary. Although this operation has a high degree of success, hearing loss can be a complication, and anatomical factors may preclude identification of the nerve. Most recently, surgical occlusion of the posterior semicircular canal through a transmastoid approach has been advocated. Large numbers of patients who have undergone this surgical procedure have not yet been reported, in part due to the high success of the particle-repositioning maneuver.

◼ Ménière Disease

Pathophysiology

An abnormality in endolymph fluid dynamics—possibly poor absorption—is still considered to be the underlying etiology of Ménière disease. Recent investigations have looked at immunologic factors, including allergy, and a small set of patients with Ménière disease exhibit autoimmune disorders.

Evaluation

The diagnosis of Ménière disease is based on a patient's history and the audiometric findings. Abnormal ENG (i.e., reduced caloric response) testing is seen in ~ 60% of patients but is not essential to making the diagnosis. Electrocochleography (ECochG) has been suggested as a physiological indicator of hydrops. In this test, a recording electrode is placed within the ear canal, or on the tympanic membrane, and in response to auditory stimulation (clicks or tone bursts) the summating potential (SP) and action potential (AP) are recorded. Patients with Ménière disease will often have an enlarged SP, resulting in an SP to AP ratio > 0.4. Recent studies have shown that this test is not as precise as initially anticipated, especially since the Ménière disease has to be active for the recordings to show an elevated SP:AP ratio. Approximately one third of patients with Ménière disease will have a normal ECochG response. The American Academy of Otolaryngology—Head and Neck Surgery has developed guidelines on the diagnosis of Ménière disease.

Treatment

The medical therapy of Ménière disease is centered on sodium restriction (< 1,500 mg/d), a diuretic, vestibular-suppressant medications, and occasional allergy management. In a small percentage of patients, a short course of steroids may be helpful for a sudden exacerbation in hearing loss or vertigo.

The mainstays of surgery are endolymphatic sac shunt or decompression, vestibular neurectomy, and labyrinthectomy. The shunt operation remains a viable, nonablative treatment of Ménière disease, with low morbidity and preservation of vestibular function. Ablative therapies, including intratympanic gentamicin therapy, tend to have higher control rates at the expense of vestibular ablation and a risk of SNHL. The titration method, where the number of injections is titrated to patients' complaints, has been accepted as the preferred method of delivery.

A standard protocol for the treatment of Ménière disease has not been agreed upon. Treatment must involve a discussion of options—both medical and surgical—between patient and physician, with the caveat that Ménière disease has no cure and that the symptoms of the disease are controlled by reducing the frequency, intensity, and duration of the attacks of vertigo. It is also important to point out that hearing, in general, cannot be restored (the disease manifests a fluctuating hearing loss) and that tinnitus can be helped but not "cured."

■ Migraine-Associated Dizziness (MAD)

Pathophysiology

The relationship between migraine and dizziness has been established in epidemiological studies, but the pathophysiology of migraine-associated dizziness (MAD) has yet to be determined. If migraine is caused by a hyperexcitable brain or by neurovascular dysregulation/vasospasm, it is possible that MAD could be caused by hyperexcitability of the vestibular system or spasm of vessels in the posterior circulation, resulting in temporary loss or intermittency of vestibular function.

Evaluation

When dizziness accompanies the migraine headache in the migraineur, the diagnosis is easily made. Episodic dizziness lasts minutes or even an hour but is not accompanied by hearing loss. Differentiating MAD from Ménière disease can be challenging because 50% of patients with Ménière disease meet the criteria for migraine. Although MAD patients often complain of aural fullness and pressure, it is typically bilateral. Risk factors should be screened and include childhood history of migraine or motion intolerance, family history of migraine, fluctuation of symptoms around the menstrual cycle, and triggers—dietary (e.g., chocolate, caffeine, red wine, aged cheese) and environmental (e.g., hormonal, stress, strong odors, chemicals, or pollutants). Physical exam is generally normal.

Treatment

Treatment of MAD centers around controlling the migraine component: control the migraine and the dizziness will come under better control. Environmental triggers should be explored, including dietary triggers already noted, stress, stress letdown, chemical sensitivity (e.g., odors, pollutants, strong perfumes), and hormonal changes in women. Avoidance

of possible triggers may bring the dizziness under control, even if it is not associated with migraine.

Migraine prophylaxis including a trial of a b-blocker (propranolol 10 mg orally twice a day) or topiramate (25 mg orally at bedtime) can be tried, but often referral to a neurologist for formal migraine evaluation and management is a safe and effective recommendation for these patients.

■ Labyrinthitis/Vestibular Neuritis

Pathophysiology

Bacteria, viruses, and spirochetes can all cause an inflammatory response within the labyrinth. Serous or purulent labyrinthitis develops as bacteria and/or their toxins diffuse across the round-window membrane, enter through a bony fistula, or traverse the cochlear aqueduct or internal auditory canal to access the vestibular labyrinth. Serous labyrinthitis can accompany a serous otitis media. Patients will complain of hearing loss (a conductive loss secondary to middle ear effusion but not a sensorineural loss) and dizziness/disequilibrium. These symptoms resolve with clearance of the middle ear pathology. Purulent labyrinthitis refers to a suppurative infection (bacterial) of the inner ear. Patients complain of severe vertigo with nausea and often vomiting with hearing loss (sensorineural) and vestibular loss that are permanent in the affected ear.

"Vestibular neuritis," "vestibular neuronitis," or "viral labyrinthitis" is more common than bacterial labyrinthitis, and has a very typical patient presentation (discussion follows). Although a viral etiology has not been demonstrated unequivocally, there are good epidemiological and histopathological data implicating an inner ear (or vestibular nerve) viral infection in this disorder.

Evaluation

The typical history of a patient with vestibular neuritis is the sudden onset of intense vertigo, lasting one to several days, accompanied by nausea and vomiting and requiring bed rest. Patients typically do not complain of hearing loss but may experience aural fullness. An ENG frequently will show a reduced caloric response in one ear. The intense vertigo resolves within 1 to several days and is followed by a motion-induced disequilibrium. Patients feel fine if not moving, but any turning or moving will cause dizziness and disequilibrium. The dizziness/disequilibrium gradually resolves over several weeks, although mild unsteadiness or positional vertigo may persist for several months. The diagnosis is made mostly based on the patient history.

Treatment

Vestibular suppressants are the mainstay of therapy during the acute and subacute phases of vestibular neuritis. Vestibular exercises or a formal, therapist-directed vestibular rehabilitation program are often helpful in expediting central compensation during the recovery phase. Patients typically make a full recovery.

■ Vestibular Schwannoma

Pathophysiology

A vestibular schwannoma (acoustic tumor) originates from the vestibular division of cranial nerve VIII. Because the tumor is slow growing, actual vertigo, or even dizziness, is uncommon, although mild disequilibrium can occur.

Evaluation

Patients usually complain of a gradual loss of hearing in one ear. Asymmetric SNHL, decreased corneal reflex, or hypesthesia or paresthesia of the ipsilateral face, and mild ataxia may be seen on the physical examination. An audiogram is important in the evaluation of the patient with dizziness to document any asymmetry between ears. The definitive diagnosis is made by gadolinium-enhanced MRI scan. Auditory brainstem response testing can be used as a screening tool, but it may miss 5 to 10% of tumors, particularly smaller ones.

Treatment

Depending on tumor size, the patient's health and age, surgical resection, observation, or radiation (gamma knife radiosurgery or fractionated stereotactic radiation) may be recommended. Observation simply involves monitoring tumor growth and hearing status with serial audiograms and MRI scans. Surgical approach (translabyrinthine, retrosigmoid/suboccipital, or middle fossa) depends on tumor size, hearing status, and tumor location (internal auditory canal, cerebellopontine angle). Gamma knife radiosurgery involves delivery of a single high-dose fraction of gamma radiation to the tumor. The beam accuracy of ~ 0.3 mm spares surrounding tissues from radiation effects. Recent studies show

excellent (> 85%) tumor control (no growth, possible tumor shrinkage) during follow-up periods of 10 to 15 years. Cranial nerve or other central complications are rare, with the exception that the majority of patients do lose hearing. The best treatment modality is a decision made between the patient and surgeon and takes many factors into account.

■ Vertebrobasilar Insufficiency (VBI)

Pathophysiology

Vertebrobasilar insufficiency (VBI) usually results from atherosclerosis involving the subclavian, vertebral, or basilar arteries and the posterior fossa circulation.

Evaluation

VBI is typically seen in patients older than 50 years of age and often with other signs and symptoms of vascular pathology, such as history of stroke, myocardial infarction, lower-extremity claudication, or peripheral vascular disease. Vertigo or disequilibrium is a common initial symptom of this disorder and usually lasts several minutes. It is brought on by or exacerbated by turning or craning the neck. The key to diagnosis is finding associated symptoms of posterior circulation ischemia, such as hoarseness/dysphagia, ataxia, hypesthesia/paresthesias of the ipsilateral face (and contralateral body, such as seen in Wallenberg or lateral medullary syndrome), and drop attacks.

Treatment

Treatment consists of controlling the atherosclerosis risk factors and the use of antiplatelet medication.

■ Presyncopal Lightheadedness

Pathophysiology

Decreased cerebral perfusion on a global, rather than a focal, basis can cause lightheadedness or dizziness. Common disorders precipitating central ischemia include postural hypotension; cardiac disease, especially aortic stenosis; vasovagal attacks; hyperventilation; panic attack; dehydration; and autonomic dysfunction, such as seen in patients with postural orthostatic tachycardia syndrome.

Evaluation

Factors that can contribute to postural hypotension include antihypertensive medications, hypovolemia, or diabetes (and secondary autonomic dysfunction). One must also be alert, however, to the possibility that lightheadedness is the presenting symptom of an arrhythmia or other cardiac abnormality, such as aortic stenosis, especially in the elderly. The physical examination may show an irregular pulse or heart murmur. A history of fear or anxiety can often be elicited from patients experiencing psychogenic lightheadedness. The diagnosis is confirmed by finding symptoms associated with hyperventilation, such as circumoral numbness, paresthesias of the fingers, or air hunger. The diagnosis can be confirmed during the physical examination if hyperventilation for 1 or 2 minutes reproduces the patient's dizziness. Taking orthostatic vital signs can be the key to diagnosing this type of dizziness.

■ Inner Ear Fistula

Pathophysiology

A perilymph fistula is an abnormal communication between the inner ear fluids and the middle ear. A leak can result from trauma (e.g., penetrating injury, postsurgical, barotrauma), infection, or sudden change in cerebrospinal fluid pressure. Although rare, spontaneous perilymph fistulas can occur, usually secondary to developmental abnormalities of the inner ear (e.g., Mondini deformity).

Evaluation

Most clinicians consider inner ear fistula only if there is a clear history of a traumatic event or other predisposing cause. To date, there is no objective test for this abnormality with a high degree of specificity and sensitivity. Insufflating air into the ear canal by otoscope or impedance bridge and then examining for nystagmus (with ENG electrodes) or body sway (with platform posturography) are steps often taken, but they have not provided a definitive test.

Treatment

Most patients with a perilymph fistula will respond to bed rest and head elevation. Middle ear exploration with soft tissue packing around the oval and round windows may be necessary. Packing around the oval and round windows is advised, even if no leak is identified at the time of middle exploration.

■ Dehiscence of the Superior Semicircular Canal

Pathophysiology

Progressive thinning of the tegmen, the bone separating the middle and inner ear from the middle cranial fossa, may result in erosion of otic capsule bone overlying the membranous superior semicircular canal. Erosion of this bone (possibly related to elevated intracranial pressure, congenital thinning of the bone, trauma, or disease) results in a communication, or "third window," between the inner ear and dura, and gives rise to a constellation of both hearing and vestibular symptoms.

Evaluation

Presenting symptoms may include aural fullness, hyperacusis, autophony, hearing loss (conductive, sensorineural, or mixed), and imbalance exacerbated by loud noise, by coughing, by straining, or by any activity that elevates intracranial, intrathoracic, or intra-abdominal pressure. Patients report a feeling that the world is tilting or moving with increased pressure or with loud noise (Tullio phenomenon).

Otoscopic exam is normal in these patients, but examining the patient for nystagmus during pneumatic otoscopy (Hennebert sign) or with introduction of loud noise (Tullio phenomenon) is an important physical examination finding. Audiometric findings can be variable and include low-frequency conductive hearing loss, suprathreshold bone-conduction thresholds, and normal acoustic reflexes. Mixed and sensorineural hearing losses may also be present. Diagnosis is made by high-resolution computed tomographic scan; coronal and sagittal oblique (Pöschl view) reformatted images show the dehiscence well (**Fig. 67.1**).

Treatment

Patients can often be reassured that their dizziness is purely an anatomical problem and not a sign of anything more serious, such as a brain tumor. Patients can undertake trials of vestibular therapy, but the definitive therapy in patients with more debilitating symptoms is plugging the dehiscent canal through either a middle fossa craniotomy or a transmastoid approach. Resurfacing the dehiscent canal has a higher rate of recrudescence.

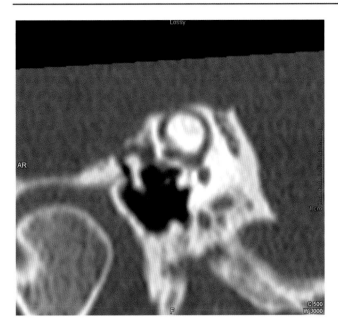

Fig. 67.1   Dehiscence of the superior semicircular canal.

■ Ototoxicity

Pathophysiology

Ototoxins, such as aminoglycosides, can damage the peripheral vestibular organs by injuring the hair cells. Of the aminoglycosides, gentamicin is preferentially vestibulotoxic and has been used successfully in Ménière disease to ablate the peripheral vestibular system to control the attacks of vertigo. Hydrocarbons, mercury, and possibly lead may affect the central vestibular system, including the cerebellum.

Evaluation

Because ototoxins affect vestibular function bilaterally, actual vertigo is uncommon. Significant unsteadiness, disequilibrium, and possible oscillopsia, ataxia, or SNHL are more typical. Reduced caloric responses are expected following aminoglycoside ototoxicity.

Treatment

Once damage has occurred, there is no specific therapy other than a vestibular rehabilitation program.

■ Disequilibrium of Aging (Presbystasis)

Pathophysiology

Changes to the peripheral and central vestibular systems because of aging include loss of hair cells and neurons, neurofiber degeneration, and accumulation of various inclusion bodies. Age-related changes in the vestibular system—in visual input, proprioceptive sense, and motor control—all contribute to loss of equilibrium with aging, or presbystasis.

Evaluation

Because peripheral vestibular aging changes may be compensated in large part by visual input, patients will often note more disequilibrium at night. Physical examination will show changes in gait and poor Romberg testing, especially with eyes closed or standing on foam. There are usually no localizing signs. Dynamic posturography can be helpful in identifying the various systems affected.

Screening for comorbidities, including peripheral neuropathy secondary to diabetes or other neurological deficit (proprioceptive); arthritis (proprioceptive); loss of vision, including macular degeneration; and any history of vestibular deficit is critical to identify, and possibly ameliorate, sources of disequilibrium.

Treatment

Simple solutions, such as installing a nightlight, using a walking stick or walker, sitting on the edge of the bed in the morning before arising, and arranging living quarters to minimize injury, can offer significant improvement and restore confidence. A formal program of therapist-directed vestibular rehabilitation offers the most help to patients with this problem.

■ Other Vertigo-Related Conditions

Many other rarer conditions, beyond the scope of this chapter, can cause dizziness. A few include mal de debarquement, polypharmacy, progressive supranuclear palsy, normal pressure hydrocephalus (characterized by ataxia, memory loss, and urinary incontinence), episodic ataxia (types 1 and 2), spinocerebellar ataxia, and cervicogenic vertigo. Cherchi provides a more detailed discussion.

■ Clinical Practice Guidelines, Consensus Statements, and Measures

AAO-HNS Clinical Practice Guideline: Benign paroxysmal positional vertigo doi: 10.1016/j.otohns.2008.08.022 Otolaryngol Head Neck Surg November 2008 vol. 139 no. 5 suppl S47-S81.

■ Suggested Reading

Alrwaily M, Whitney SL. Vestibular rehabilitation of older adults with dizziness. Otolaryngol Clin North Am 2011;44(2): 473–496, x

American Academy of Otolaryngology—Head and Neck Foundation, Inc. Committee on Hearing and Equilibrium guidelines for the diagnosis and evaluation of therapy in Ménière's disease. American Academy of Otolaryngology-Head and Neck Foundation, Inc. Otolaryngol Head Neck Surg 1995;113(3):181–185

Baloh RW, Honrubia V, Jacobson K. Benign positional vertigo: clinical and oculographic features in 240 cases. Neurology 1987; 37(3):371–378

Barin K, Dodson EE. Dizziness in the elderly. Otolaryngol Clin North Am 2011;44(2):437–454, x

Branstetter BF IV, Harrigal C, Escott EJ, Hirsch BE. Superior semicircular canal dehiscence: oblique reformatted CT images for diagnosis. Radiology 2006;238(3):938–942

Cherchi M. Infrequent causes of disequilibrium in the adult. Otolaryngol Clin North Am 2011;44(2):405–414, ix

Chi FL, Ren DD, Dai CF. Variety of audiologic manifestations in patients with superior semicircular canal dehiscence. Otol Neurotol 2010;31(1):2–10

Chien WW, Carey JP, Minor LB. Canal dehiscence. Curr Opin Neurol 2011;24(1):25–31

Derebery MJ. Allergic and immunologic features of Ménière's disease. Otolaryngol Clin North Am 2011;44(3):655–666, ix

Derebery MJ, Fisher LM, Berliner K, Chung J, Green K. Outcomes of endolymphatic shunt surgery for Ménière's disease: comparison with intratympanic gentamicin on vertigo control and hearing loss. Otol Neurotol 2010;31(4):649–655

Epley JM. The canalith repositioning procedure: for treatment of benign paroxysmal positional vertigo. Otolaryngol Head Neck Surg 1992;107(3):399–404

Furman JM, Raz Y, Whitney SL. Geriatric vestibulopathy assessment and management. Curr Opin Otolaryngol Head Neck Surg 2010;18(5):386–391

Humphriss RL, Hall AJ. Dizziness in 10 year old children: an epidemiological study. Int J Pediatr Otorhinolaryngol 2011;75(3): 395–400

Ishiyama G, Ishiyama A. Vertebrobasilar infarcts and ischemia. Otolaryngol Clin North Am 2011;44(2):415–435, ix–x

Katzenell U, Gordon M, Page M. Intratympanic gentamicin injections for the treatment of Ménière's disease. Otolaryngol Head Neck Surg 2010;143(5, Suppl 3):S24–S29

Kesser BW, Gleason AT, eds. Otolaryngology Clinics of North America: Dizziness and Vertigo Across the Lifespan. Philadelphia, PA: WB Saunders; 2011

Mathias CJ, Low DA, Iodice V, Owens AP, Kirbis M, Grahame R. Postural tachycardia syndrome—current experience and concepts. Nat Rev Neurol 2012;8(1):22–34

Minor LB. Clinical manifestations of superior semicircular canal dehiscence. Laryngoscope 2005;115(10):1717–1727

Monsell EM. New and revised reporting guidelines from the Committee on Hearing and Equilibrium. American Academy of Otolaryngology-Head and Neck Surgery Foundation, Inc. Otolaryngol Head Neck Surg 1995;113(3):176–178

Newlands SD, Wall C III. Vestibular function and anatomy. In: Bailey BJ, Johnson JT, eds. Head and Neck Surgery—Otolaryngology. 4th ed. Philadelphia, PA: Lippincott, Williams and Wilkins, 2006:1905–1917

O'Reilly RC, Morlet T, Nicholas BD, et al. Prevalence of vestibular and balance disorders in children. Otol Neurotol 2010;31(9): 1441–1444

Pullens B, van Benthem PP. Intratympanic gentamicin for Ménière's disease or syndrome. Cochrane Database Syst Rev 2011; (3):CD008234

Radtke A, Lempert T, Gresty MA, Brookes GB, Bronstein AM, Neuhauser H. Migraine and Ménière's disease: is there a link? Neurology 2002;59(11):1700–1704

Radtke A, Lempert T, von Brevern M, Feldmann M, Lezius F, Neuhauser H. Prevalence and complications of orthostatic dizziness in the general population. Clin Auton Res 2011;21(3):161–168

Rosengren SM, Welgampola MS, Colebatch JG. Vestibular evoked myogenic potentials: past, present and future. Clin Neurophysiol 2010;121(5):636–651

Shoair OA, Nyandege AN, Slattum PW. Medication-related dizziness in the older adult. Otolaryngol Clin North Am 2011;44(2): 455–471, x

Silverstein H, Wazen J, Van Ess MJ, Daugherty J, Alameda YA. Intratympanic gentamicin treatment of patients with Ménière's disease with normal hearing. Otolaryngol Head Neck Surg 2010;142(4):570–575

Syed I, Aldren C. Meniere's disease: an evidence based approach to assessment and management. Int J Clin Pract 2012;66(2): 166–170

Thanavaro JL, Thanavaro KL. Postural orthostatic tachycardia syndrome: diagnosis and treatment. Heart Lung 2011;40(6): 554–560

von Brevern M, Neuhauser H. Epidemiological evidence for a link between vertigo and migraine. J Vestib Res 2011;21(6): 299–304

Welgampola MS, Colebatch JG. Characteristics and clinical applications of vestibular-evoked myogenic potentials. Neurology 2005;64(10):1682–1688

Wuyts F. Principle of the head impulse (thrust) test or Halmagyi head thrust test (HHTT). B-ENT 2008;4(Suppl 8):23–25

68 Otologic Manifestations of Systemic Disease

■ Introduction

It is well established that numerous systemic diseases have accompanying otologic manifestations. The diseases include syndromic genetic disorders such as Usher syndrome, branchio-oto-renal syndrome, Pendred syndrome, Jervell and Lange-Nielsen syndrome, Treacher Collins syndrome, and many others. In addition, other systemic diseases are associated with hearing loss (e.g., osteogenesis imperfecta, Paget disease of bone, diabetes mellitus, renal disease, hypothyroidism, and others). Over the past 10 years, however, otologic disease has been newly noted to be associated with several inherited and acquired disorders. This chapter briefly discusses the more important of these.

■ Acquired Immunodeficiency Syndrome

Acquired immunodeficiency syndrome (AIDS) is caused by infection with a retrovirus called the human immunodeficiency virus (HIV). It is now well recognized that otologic manifestations are common in HIV infections. Further, as our understanding of the infectious disease process and its treatment has progressed, AIDS is increasingly being thought of as a chronic condition as opposed to a fatal one.

Most authors conclude that there are a variety of mechanisms by which HIV infection can result in otologic symptoms, and, in many cases, the HIV infection may not have progressed to AIDS. With a typical 10 year window between infection and the onset of symptoms with current treatment, HIV infection may be a possible etiologic factor in hearing and vestibular symptoms with or without other manifestations of HIV infection. The clinician should always keep HIV infection as part of the differential diagnosis of early-onset hearing loss or vestibular deficit.

Patients with AIDS are subject to systemic infections that may affect the inner and middle ear. Several cases of reactivation of otosyphilis have been documented. In addition, AIDS patients are subject to sudden sensorineural hearing loss (SNHL) due to cryptococcal meningitis. Further, *Pneumocystis carinii*, in addition to causing systemic disease and pneumonia, can cause otitis media. It has been demonstrated that recurrent otitis media is significantly more prevalent in HIV-infected children. Otomycosis has also been documented in this population. More serious infectious disorders, such as skull base osteomyelitis/malignant otitis externa caused by organisms including *Pseudomonas aeruginosa* and *Aspergillus fumigatus*, have been described.

There is evidence of a higher incidence of otovestibular abnormalities in AIDS patients than in the general population, and ~ 50% of HIV-positive patients, whether symptomatic or asymptomatic, have abnormalities on auditory and vestibular testing. Some of these abnormalities seem to indicate central auditory and vestibular system abnormalities.

Evaluation

Because contemporary chemotherapy has delayed the onset of AIDS symptoms in patients with HIV infection, otologic manifestations of the infection may occur prior to other symptoms. Thus awareness of the condition is paramount. The evaluation is dependent on the presenting condition, and for the most part, mirrors the evaluation of the condition in the absence of HIV. Audiological and radiological studies are guided by the presenting symptoms. Bloodwork, including CD4 cell counts, will help determine the degree of immunosuppression. For most patients, CD4 counts > 500/mm will not result in the opportunistic infections that are seen in the more severely immunosuppressed (i.e., < 200/mm).

Management

As with the evaluation, management is guided by the specific condition. Treatment of infectious processes includes directed antimicrobial therapy, which may be toward an unusual organism. Thus cultures of the infectious process are important.

◼ Immune-Mediated Inner Ear Disease

Introduction

In recent years it has been suggested that progressive hearing loss with and without vestibular symptoms may be related to the production of autoantibodies directed toward inner ear proteins. This concept has been supported by the fact that some patients with progressive hearing loss respond favorably to treatment with systemic steroids with significant improvements in hearing. Some of these patients may have other evidence of autoimmune disease, such as Cogan syndrome, rheumatoid arthritis, Wegener granulomatosis, Sjögren syndrome, or systemic lupus erythematosis. However, many patients have no other stigmata of autoimmune disease. Although it is widely recognized that some patients with progressive SNHL with and without vestibular symptoms may respond to corticosteroids, the exact mechanism of this syndrome is unclear. Most investigators feel that autoantibodies are produced and directed toward the inner ear. Although early studies identified a 68 kD protein as potentially being associated with a positive response to steroids in suspected cases, its unreliability as a clinical tool has led it to fall out of favor. Studies have demonstrated that elevated antibodies to inner ear structures can lead to SNHL in experimental animals, supporting the presumed autoimmune nature of this syndrome.

Evaluation

A rapid and progressive, and possibly fluctuating hearing loss, with or without associated vertigo, tips off the clinician to suspect an autoimmune etiology. The presence of other autoimmune disorders increases the suspicion. Associated conditions, including Cogan syndrome or relapsing polychondritis, should also be sought. Autoimmune screening laboratories, including antinuclear antibodies, rheumatoid factor, complement C3, and anti-DNA-ds antibodies should be ordered to evaluate for systemic disease. Audiological and radiological (computed tomography [CT] and/or magnetic resonance imaging [MRI]) studies are also indicated. If one suspects a central nervous system etiology, then a lumbar tap can identify an increased protein count in the cerebrospinal fluid.

Management

Management of autoimmune inner ear disease consists first of a course of steroids (typically prednisone 80 mg/kg/d for 10–14 days) with a slow taper. If symptoms persist despite appropriate doses of steroids, or if symptoms recur after tapering off steroids, options include a more lengthy course of steroids or other immunosuppressive medication, including methotrexate, Imuran, or CellCept (Roche, Branchburg, NJ). Coordinating care with a rheumatologist is highly recommended, with close audiological follow-up to document improvement in hearing. For patients who have lost all hearing, cochlear implantation can be considered.

Controversial Issues

There is ongoing uncertainty regarding the length of steroid administration, and what immunosuppressive medications are the most appropriate for this condition.

◼ Otosclerosis

Introduction

Until recently, otosclerosis has been regarded as a genetic disease without other systemic abnormalities. Histological otosclerosis is found in the temporal bones of up to 10% of autopsy specimens, and ~ 0.3% of the population has clinical otosclerosis. Several possible etiologies are now recognized that may contribute to the condition, including genetic, environmental factors (such as the use of fluorides in water), infectious agents (measles virus), as well as possible immune-mediated etiologic factors. Otosclerosis has been shown to be an autosomal dominant disease with variable penetrance in some families. Although generally thought to be a genetic disease, observers have been puzzled by the fact that ~ 50% of patients with otosclerosis have no family history of the disease. Early studies demonstrated measles antigens in osteoclasts in active otosclerosis lesions (otospongiosis), suggesting a measles etiology, further supported by the finding that several otosclerotic specimens demonstrated measles nucleocapsid gene. Linkage analysis studies of large families with otosclerosis have shown that T cell receptor b is one gene responsible for familial otosclerosis, implicating the immune system as an underlying etiology. Which of these factors plays the most important role in the genesis of otosclerosis remains to be determined.

Evaluation

Otosclerosis is suspected in a patient with a slowly progressive conductive or mixed hearing loss as documented by audiometry. There may be a characteristic "notch" at 2 kHz in the bone-conduction threshold line (i.e., the Carhart notch). As with other diseases causing a conductive hearing loss, acoustic reflexes are absent; the presence of an acoustic reflex implies a third mobile window syndrome (e.g., superior semicircular canal dehiscence). A CT scan may demonstrate otospongiotic changes surrounding the otic capsule. The disease may be unilateral or bilateral.

Management

There are several treatment options for otosclerosis: (1) observation, (2) conventional hearing aids, (3) bone-conduction hearing aids (e.g., Baha System, Cochlear Americas, Centennial, CO; Sophono, Sophono, Inc., Boulder, CO; SoundBite, Sonitus Medical, San Mateo, CA), and (4) stapedectomy or stapedotomy. Each of these options is associated with a variety of risks and benefits. There are also some early data suggesting that bisphosphonates can be used to treat SNHL associated with otosclerosis (cochlear otosclerosis). Clinical aspects and management of otosclerosis are further discussed in Chapter 63.

■ Osteogenesis Imperfecta

Introduction

Osteogenesis imperfecta (OI) in its various forms may manifest with ossicular abnormalities, including otosclerosis with stapes fixation. Osteogenesis imperfecta is a systemic, genetic disease affecting the entire skeleton. A majority of cases are due to mutations in the genes COL1A1 and Col1A2, coding for pro-a1 and -2 chains of type I collagen. It is inherited in an autosomal dominant pattern, and to date, over 1,500 mutations have been described. The disease consists of at least four subtypes (types I–IV). Type I is the most common; it is a dominantly inherited disorder and usually manifests later in life. Type IV also manifests later in life but is a recessive

characteristic. Types II and III manifest very early in life with multiple fractures and growth retardation. Although OI is a systemic skeletal disease, it often affects the ossicles of the middle ear, and about half of all patients with OI will develop some form of hearing loss. The conductive hearing loss seen in OI is correlated with fractures of the stapes, thinning of the stapes footplate, and fixation around the stapedial annulus. Cochlear degeneration has also been described. In advanced cases, a progressive SNHL occurs in OI patients with or without surgical intervention, similar to cochlear otosclerosis.

Evaluation

Evaluation of the patient with OI includes serial audiograms to document the degree and rate of hearing loss. In most cases genetic testing has been completed by the time the patient sees the otolaryngologist. CT scanning will often demonstrate otospongiotic changes of the otic capsule, causing a lucency surrounding the cochlea, often termed a halo effect.

Management

Management for OI is similar to otosclerosis, though the results of stapedectomy for OI have been disappointing. Although stapedectomy may correct many conductive losses, results tend not to be as good as in otosclerosis, with a higher risk of incus fracture with prosthesis placement. Some authors have shown that progressive SNHL occurs in OI patients with or without surgical intervention. In cases of severe to profound SNHL, cochlear implantation is an option.

■ Arnold–Chiari Malformation

Introduction

It is now recognized that vestibular and auditory abnormalities are extremely common in patients with Chiari I malformation. Chiari type I malformation leads to increased intracranial pressure. Unlike Chiari type II malformation, which usually manifests in infancy, Chiari I manifests later in life with recurrent headaches, weakness, vestibular abnormalities, and progressive hearing loss. Studies of a large series of patients with Chiari I malformation showed that eighth nerve symptoms were due to traction on the eighth cranial nerve. Although many of the patients identified with Chiari I malformation had central types of neurotologic findings, many had symptoms suggestive of a peripheral loss.

Evaluation

Hearing may be followed with serial audiometry. Patients with central or peripheral otologic symptoms who demonstrate symptoms consistent with Chiari I malformation (headaches, oculomotor deficits, and other cranial nerve deficits) should have an MRI scan. Tonsillar herniation is seen with Chiari malformations with or without hydrocephalus.

Management

Management includes referral to neurosurgery for repair.

■ Suggested Reading

Baisden J. Controversies in Chiari I malformations. Surg Neurol Int 2012;3(Suppl 3):S232–S237

Bovo R, Ciorba A, Martini A. The diagnosis of autoimmune inner ear disease: evidence and critical pitfalls. Eur Arch Otorhinolaryngol 2009;266(1):37–40

Buniel MC, Geelan-Hansen K, Weber PC, Tuohy VK. Immunosuppressive therapy for autoimmune inner ear disease. Immunotherapy 2009;1(3):425–434

Cohen HS, Cox C, Springer G, et al. Prevalence of abnormalities in vestibular function and balance among HIV-seropositive and HIV-seronegative women and men. PLoS ONE 2012;7(5):e38419

Cruise AS, Singh A, Quiney RE. Sodium fluoride in otosclerosis treatment: review. J Laryngol Otol 2010;124(6):583–586

Cureoglu S, Baylan MY, Paparella MM. Cochlear otosclerosis. Curr Opin Otolaryngol Head Neck Surg 2010;18(5):357–362

Greco A, Gallo A, Fusconi M, et al. Cogan's syndrome: an autoimmune inner ear disease. Autoimmun Rev 2013;12(3):396–400

Karosi T, Sziklai I. Etiopathogenesis of otosclerosis. Eur Arch Otorhinolaryngol 2010;267(9):1337–1349

Laske RD, Röösli C, Chatzimichalis MV, Sim JH, Huber AM. The influence of prosthesis diameter in stapes surgery: a meta-analysis and systematic review of the literature. Otol Neurotol 2011; 32(4):520–528

Levo H, Tapani E, Karppinen A, Kentala E. Chiari Malformation in otology practice. Auris Nasus Larynx 2010;37(1):95–99

Malik MU, Pandian V, Masood H, et al. Spectrum of immune-mediated inner ear disease and cochlear implant results. Laryngoscope 2012;122(11):2557–2562 doi: 10.1002/lary.23604

Merkus P, van Loon MC, Smit CF, Smits C, de Cock AF, Hensen EF. Decision making in advanced otosclerosis: an evidence-based strategy. Laryngoscope 2011;121(9):1935–1941 doi: 10.1002/lary.21904

Pillion JP, Vernick D, Shapiro J. Hearing loss in osteogenesis imperfecta: characteristics and treatment considerations. Genet Res Int 2011;2011:983942

Prasad HK, Bhojwani KM, Shenoy V, Prasad SC. HIV manifestations in otolaryngology. Am J Otolaryngol 2006;27(3):179–185

Quesnel AM, Seton M, Merchant SN, Halpin C, McKenna MJ. Third-generation bisphosphonates for treatment of sensorineural hearing loss in otosclerosis. Otol Neurotol 2012;33(8):1308–1314

Santos F, McCall AA, Chien W, Merchant S. Otopathology in Osteogenesis Imperfecta. Otol Neurotol 2012;33(9):1562–1566

Schrauwen I, Van Camp G. The etiology of otosclerosis: a combination of genes and environment. Laryngoscope 2010;120(6): 1195–1202

Sperling NM, Franco RA Jr, Milhorat TH. Otologic manifestations of Chiari I malformation. Otol Neurotol 2001;22(5):678–681

Swinnen FK, De Leenheer EM, Coucke PJ, Cremers CW, Dhooge IJ. Stapes surgery in osteogenesis imperfecta: retrospective analysis of 34 operated ears. Audiol Neurootol 2012;17(3):198–206

Swinnen FK, De Leenheer EM, Goemaere S, Cremers CW, Coucke PJ, Dhooge IJ. Association between bone mineral density and hearing loss in osteogenesis imperfecta. Laryngoscope 2012;122(2): 401–408 10.1002/lary.22408

Wiet RJ, Battista RA, Wiet RM, Sabin AT. Hearing outcomes in stapes surgery: a comparison of fat, fascia, and vein tissue seals. Otolaryngol Head Neck Surg 2013;148(1):115–120

69 Facial Nerve Paralysis: Diagnosis, Evaluation, and Management

■ Introduction

In the early 1800s, Charles Bell showed that the seventh nerve was responsible for motor innervation of the face. Since that time, many etiologies of facial paresis or paralysis have been identified; controversy still exists, however, over the etiology, diagnostic methods, and treatment of acute facial paralysis.

■ Embryology

The facial nerve begins developing around week 3 of gestation with a collection of neural crest cells called the acousticofacial primordium that forms the acoustic and facial nerves. The facial nerve develops within the second branchial arch. By week 8, the terminus branches have developed, and the facial muscles develop by week 12. The facial nerve fully develops by age 4.

■ Anatomy

The facial nucleus fibers extend to the precentral gyrus (motor cortex) of the cerebral cortex. The facial nucleus is in the ventrolateral aspect of the pons. The fibers of the facial nucleus extend dorsally around the sixth (abducens) cranial nerve nucleus. They emerge from the lower pons between the olive and the restiform body.

The facial nerve is divided into five segments: the intracranial, intracanalicular, labyrinthine, tympanic, and mastoid. The nerve receives its blood supply from the anterior inferior cerebellar artery, the middle meningeal artery, and the stylomastoid branch of the postauricular artery. The facial nerve contains four types of fibers:

1. Branchial or somatic motor (special visceral) efferents innervate the muscles of facial expression, stylohyoid, posterior belly of the digastric, and stapedius.
2. Visceral motor (general visceral) efferents innervate the lacrimal, nasal, submandibular, and sublingual glands as well as the mucous membrane of the nose and hard and soft palate.
3. Special sensory afferent fibers innervate the anterior two thirds of the tongue via the chorda tympani nerve.
4. General (somatic) sensory afferent fibers innervate the posterior ear canal and conchum cavum.

■ Incidence

Acute facial paresis/paralysis is one of the most common neuropathies, with an incidence of 15 to 40 per 100,000. This condition is usually diagnosed and managed by multiple specialists. Facial paresis can be due to infectious, ischemic, neoplastic, or autoimmune processes. Acute facial paresis of unknown etiology is termed Bell palsy and is thought to be viral in origin. It is uncommon in young patients, but the incidence increases with age. There is some thought that diabetes mellitus and pregnancy can be aggravating factors in the development of Bell palsy.

■ Pathogenesis

As already noted, it is important to realize that there are a multitude of etiologies for acute facial paralysis. Etiologies include congenital, traumatic, infectious, neoplastic, genetic, neurological, vascular, idiopathic, toxic, and iatrogenic.

Congenital causes include Möbius syndrome and myotonic dystrophy. Because the facial nerve is exposed near the stylomastoid foramen because the mastoid tip is not developed at birth, delivery trauma, such as forceps use, can be associated with facial paralysis.

Trauma to the skull base can lead to facial paralysis. Transverse fractures of the temporal bone, which usually involve the labyrinth, have a high incidence of facial nerve impingement, injury, or laceration. Penetrating injuries of the face, middle ear, or cranium can cause facial nerve injury. Barotrauma can also lead to facial paralysis.

Infections can lead to an inflammatory response around the nerve. Given that roughly 50% of patients have natural dehiscence of the fallopian canal, this loss of bone can lead to perineural involvement of an inflammatory process. Infections of the bony ear canal, mastoid, middle ear, or parotid are common causes. Multiple viral infections, including varicella, Herpesviridae, human immunodeficiency virus, coxsackievirus, influenza, polio, and mononucleosis can lead to facial paresis/paralysis as well. Encephalitis and meningitis can also lead to facial paralysis. It is important to review for any patient history of tuberculosis, Lyme disease, or botulism.

Skull base osteomyelitis (malignant otitis externa) is a bony infection of the temporal bone usually caused by *Pseudomonas aeruginosa* and seen in diabetics and immunocompromised patients. Patients present with severe otalgia, often worse at night, otorrhea, and granulation tissue along the floor of the ear canal at the bony–cartilaginous junction. Treatment centers around local debridement, intravenous and topical antibiotics directed toward *Pseudomonas* (fluoroquinolone), and diabetic control. Milder infections can occasionally be treated with oral antibiotics.

Neoplastic causes include facial nerve neuromas, hemangiomas, or schwannomas. Tumors of the cerebellopontine angle, such as acoustic neuroma and glomus tumors, can also lead to facial paralysis, although facial paresis in the setting of acoustic neuroma is rare. Malignant brainstem tumors or metastatic carcinomas can affect facial nerve function as well.

Unusual and idiopathic causes such as Melkersson–Rosenthal syndrome, thrombotic thrombocytopenic purpura, Guillain–Barré syndrome, multiple sclerosis, and myasthenia gravis need to be considered. Uncommon illnesses such as sarcoidosis, Wegener granulomatosis, and eosinophilic granuloma are also potential etiologies.

Iatrogenic causes most commonly occur during otologic surgery in the tympanic segment. Injury to the mastoid segment is the next most common site. Iatrogenic injuries most commonly occur when the nerve has not been clearly identified. Before any intervention is done on a patient with an immediate postoperative facial paralysis, the patient should be observed to make sure that this is not a lidocaine-induced paralysis. If the paralysis persists, intervention should be initiated immediately. Facial nerve

monitoring during surgery may help with early recognition of injury, and stimulation may enhance the ability to identify the nerve. However, this is not a substitute for surgical skill and knowledge of the anatomy and its variations.

Pathophysiology of facial nerve injury has been classified under two systems—Seddon's (1943) and Sunderland's (1951)—based on site of lesion. These systems do have prognostic value when considering outcomes of facial nerve injury (**Table 69.1**).

◼ Evaluation

Important details of the history that should be investigated include the time of onset of paresis, the speed of progression, any precipitating factors, and any associated symptoms, such as pain, hearing loss, taste disturbance, tinnitus, otorrhea, or systemic illnesses. These details are important in helping to develop a differential diagnosis.

Examination involves careful observation of the face. It is important to describe the face at rest, noting if there is any asymmetry at rest. Also, one should observe for any signs of synkinesis, or mass movement (e.g., when the patient is asked to close the eyes tightly, the corner of the mouth draws up). There should be a careful examination of the ears, looking for infections, granulation tissue, cholesteatoma, or masses that might lead to a paralysis. It is also important to note any signs of vesicular lesions that are around the auricle or on the face, consistent with Ramsay Hunt syndrome.

The House–Brackmann scale is used to describe the degree of facial weakness and the level of recovery. This grading system uses a scale of I to VI with the grades described briefly as follows:

- I—Normal movement
- II—Minimal weakness with symmetry at rest, possibly with mild synkinesis
- III—Mild to moderate weakness, with eye closure and symmetry at rest
- IV—Symmetry at rest with some movement and incomplete eye closure
- V—No asymmetry or mild asymmetry at rest with no movement
- VI—No movement and gross asymmetry at rest

◼ Special Investigations

Nearly 70% of facial paresis can be attributed to Bell palsy. In patients where there is a suspicion of other possible etiologies based on history and physical exam, additional testing may be warranted. Further

Table 69.1 Classification of facial nerve injury

Seddon classification	Name	Site of lesion	Characteristics
Class I	Neuropraxia	Conduction block	Intact nerve; temporary; no Wallerian degeneration; full recovery
Class II	Axonotmesis	Axon/myelin sheath	Preservation of endo-, peri-, and epineurium; Wallerian degeneration occurs; recovery overall good but may be incomplete
Class III	Neurotmesis	Transection	Total disruption; Wallerian degeneration; recovery poor without surgery
Sunderland classification			
1st degree (Class I)	Neuropraxia	Conduction block	Intact nerve; temporary; no Wallerian degeneration; full recovery
2nd degree (Class II)	Axonotmesis	Axon/myelin sheath	Preservation of endo-, peri-, and epineurium; Wallerian degeneration occurs; recovery overall good but may be incomplete
3rd degree (Class II)	Axonotmesis	Axon + endoneurium	Peri- and epineurium intact; recovery possible, may be incomplete
4th degree (Class II)	Axonotmesis	Axon, endo- and perineurium	Epineurium intact; recovery incomplete; surgery advised
5th degree (Class III)	Neurotmesis	Transection	Recovery poor without surgery

investigation may include an audiogram. It is important to document any type of hearing loss. It is helpful to note if the stapedius reflex is intact.

Patients with Lyme disease may present with recurrent or bilateral paralysis. There are several blood tests that may be helpful if there is a possibility of Lyme disease exposure, including a serum Lyme titer, a complete blood count, sedimentation rate, glucose testing, and angiotensin-converting enzyme level testing.

Imaging can play an important role in the workup of facial paralysis. The test of choice is magnetic resonance imaging with gadolinium. It is important that this test is protocoled to encompass all segments of the facial nerve, including the parotid gland. Imaging is not recommended in the acute presentation of facial paresis/paralysis. Imaging should be considered when a Bell palsy does not show any signs of recovery after 4 to 6 months, or if there is segmental paralysis. If there is a history of trauma, then a computed tomographic scan without contrast is the exam of choice to evaluate the bony anatomy.

One of the most helpful tests in facial nerve paralysis is electrical testing. Electromyography (EMG) and evoked EMG can evaluate motor unit potentials. This test is helpful if the patient is first being seen 10 to 14 days after the onset of the paralysis. The presence of motor unit potentials shows that the nerve is still innervating the muscle. Multiphasic action potentials indicate that the nerve is beginning to reinnervate the muscle, another good prognostic sign. Fasciculations are a poor prognostic sign for recovery. EMG is not necessary for patients with incomplete paresis (House–Brackmann score I–V) because studies show these patients will enjoy good recovery of function.

Electroneuronography (ENoG) is very important in the early stages of a complete paralysis. The test is very helpful to determine the degree of degeneration of the nerve compared with the contralateral, normal side. This test is ideally performed within the first 2 weeks of the onset of a paralysis and can be performed 72 hours after the onset. If the test suggests > 90% weakness compared with the normal side, then surgical decompression should be considered.

■ Management

Treatment of acute facial paralysis always includes steroids unless there are contraindications, such as poorly controlled diabetes. Typical steroid dosing is 1 mg/kg/d of prednisone in a single dose on a full stomach in the morning tapered over 2 to 3 weeks. Other considerations for treatment include antiviral regimens (e.g., oral valacyclovir or famciclovir 500 mg three times a day).

One very important consideration is eye care. The inability to close the eye can lead to corneal inflammation and scarring. Patients should be instructed on the use of artificial tears and ophthalmic ointments to keep the eye moist. Taping or patching the eye at night may also help. Moisture chambers for the eye are also available if the patient needs protection during the day. Eyeglasses or sunglasses are strongly encouraged to keep airborne debris out of the eye, especially on windy days.

Physical therapy may help with recovery. Patients are encouraged to try to move their face, even though they cannot see any movements. This allows the muscle to be stimulated with neurotransmitters to prevent atrophy. Electrical stimulation is also helpful in patients with a chronic or long-term paralysis and is thought to prevent muscle atrophy. These patients should continue their physical therapy.

■ Surgical Intervention

Surgical treatment of facial paralysis varies by etiology. It is widely accepted that iatrogenic injuries should be explored as soon as possible after allowing adequate time for any local anesthetic effect to wear off. In the case of acute trauma, exploration is usually performed in the setting of a complete (usually immediate-onset) paralysis. Surgical approach is generally through a combined transmastoid and middle fossa craniotomy. Any impingements should be removed and the facial nerve canal decompressed in the labyrinthine and perigeniculate regions. If an injury has caused more than 50% of the nerve to be transected, a reanastomosis or graft should be performed. If a segment is missing, then a graft should be considered. Facial nerve monitoring will be helpful in identifying the damaged nerve or its transected ends (as long as there has been no Wallerian degeneration, which occurs 72 hours after the injury). Even with a grafting procedure, the expected best recovery is a House–Brackmann grade III.

For patients with traumatic injuries, other common grafting procedures can be performed. The hypoglossal–facial transfer (XII–VII) is a very common procedure. The facial nerve is skeletonized and decompressed as medial as possible in the mastoid and is cut and transposed into the neck, where it is grafted to the hypoglossal nerve. Alternatively, the hypoglossal nerve can be partially transected and delivered up to the facial nerve trunk at the stylomastoid foramen. A cross-facial nerve (VII–VII) graft can also be performed.

In acute idiopathic facial nerve paralysis (Bell palsy), surgical decompression may be considered when the ENoG shows > 90% degeneration compared with the normal side. This surgery should be undertaken within 14 to 21 days of the onset of complete paralysis. There is controversy over whether the nerve, including the internal acoustic canal portion, can be decompressed through a mastoid approach. Usually, a total decompression is performed through a combination of middle fossa and transmastoid approaches.

Newer techniques are being developed to rehabilitate patients who regain little to no normal nerve function. Several procedures can be performed around the eye to aid in closure. A tarsorrhaphy can be performed to tighten the lower lid to prevent severe epiphora. The more common procedure performed around the eye is the placement of a gold weight in the eyelid to allow for closure of the lid when the third cranial nerve is relaxed.

There are many procedures to improve the appearance of the face. Static slings, rhytidectomy, blepharoplasty, and browlift can improve the resting tone and symmetry of the face. Newer procedures allow for active motion. The first is a temporalis transfer, which rotates slings of the temporalis muscle and attaches them to different areas of the face. Free gracilis muscle transfer has also shown some promise.

One of the unfortunate sequelae of recovery from a facial paralysis is synkinesis. When the peripheral fibers regenerate, their original directionality is lost. Therefore, fibers that should be innervating the perioral muscles may reinnervate the periorbital muscles. This commonly causes patients to wink their eye when they smile. Another sequela of recovery is spasm, which is typically seen after recovery of a facial paralysis after skull base surgery. In either circumstance, if synkinesis is severe, it can almost be as bothersome as the weakness itself. To lessen these side effects, botulinum toxin is usually targeted to the most affected muscle groups; however, overapplication of botulinum toxin may result in paresis.

■ Conclusion

Facial paralysis can be devastating to the patient. Prompt recognition of the etiology and intervention are vital. Steroid and antiviral therapy are the hallmarks of initial treatment. Controversies exist regarding the degree of ancillary testing needed and the type of surgical intervention. The American Academy of Otolaryngology–Head and Neck Surgery Foundation is currently working on a consensus statement regarding the management of acute facial paralysis.

■ Clinical Practice Guidelines, Consensus Statements, and Measures

AAO-HNS Clinical Practice Guideline: Bell's Palsy doi: 10.1177 /0194599813505967 Otolaryngol Head Neck Surg November 2013 vol. 149 no. 3 suppl S1-S27.

■ Suggested Reading

Berg T, Bylund N, Marsk E, et al. The effect of prednisolone on sequelae in Bell's palsy. Arch Otolaryngol Head Neck Surg 2012; 138(5):445–449

Berg T, Marsk E, Engström M, Hultcrantz M, Hadziosmanovic N, Jonsson L. The effect of study design and analysis methods on recovery rates in Bell's palsy. Laryngoscope 2009;119(10): 2046–2050

Cardoso JR, Teixeira EC, Moreira MD, Fávero FM, Fontes SV, Bulle de Oliveira AS. Effects of exercises on Bell's palsy: systematic review of randomized controlled trials. Otol Neurotol 2008;29(4): 557–560

Filipo R, Spahiu I, Covelli E, Nicastri M, Bertoli GA. Botulinum toxin in the treatment of facial synkinesis and hyperkinesis. Laryngoscope 2012;122(2):266–270 10.1002/lary.22404

Gantz BJ, Rubinstein JT, Gidley P, Woodworth GG. Surgical management of Bell's palsy. Laryngoscope 1999;109(8): 1177–1188

Greco A, Gallo A, Fusconi M, Marinelli C, Macri GF, de Vincentiis M. Bell's palsy and autoimmunity. Autoimmun Rev 2012;12(2): 323–328

House JW, Brackmann DE. Facial nerve grading system. Otolaryngol Head Neck Surg 1985;93(2):146–147

Kanazawa A, Haginomori S, Takamaki A, Nonaka R, Araki M, Takenaka H. Prognosis for Bell's palsy: a comparison of diabetic and nondiabetic patients. Acta Otolaryngol 2007;127(8):888–891

Kanerva M, Jonsson L, Berg T, et al. Sunnybrook and House-Brackmannsystems in 5397 facial gradings. Otolaryngol Head Neck Surg 2011;144(4):570–574

Kawaguchi K, Inamura H, Abe Y, et al. Reactivation of herpes simplex virus type 1 and varicella-zoster virus and therapeutic effects of combination therapy with prednisolone and valacyclovir in patients with Bell's palsy. Laryngoscope 2007;117(1):147–156

Korf ES, Killestein J. Prednisolone or acyclovir in Bell's palsy. N Engl J Med 2008;358(3):306–307, author reply 307

Mantsopoulos K, Psillas G, Psychogios G, Brase C, Iro H, Constantinidis J. Predicting the long-term outcome after idiopathic facial nerve paralysis. Otol Neurotol 2011;32(5):848–851

Marsk E, Bylund N, Jonsson L, et al. Prediction of nonrecovery in Bell's palsy using Sunnybrook grading. Laryngoscope 2012; 122(4):901–906

Smouha E, Toh E, Schaitkin BM. Surgical treatment of Bell's palsy: current attitudes. Laryngoscope 2011;121(9):1965–1970

Stjernquist-Desatnik A, Skoog E, Aurelius E. Detection of herpes simplex and varicella-zoster viruses in patients with Bell's palsy by the polymerase chain reaction technique. Ann Otol Rhinol Laryngol 2006;115(4):306–311

Takemoto N, Horii A, Sakata Y, Inohara H. Prognostic factors of peripheral facial palsy: multivariate analysis followed by receiver operating characteristic and Kaplan-Meier analyses. Otol Neurotol 2011;32(6):1031–1036

Yanagihara N, Honda N, Hato N, Murakami S. Edematous swelling of the facial nerve in Bell's palsy. Acta Otolaryngol 2000;120(5): 667–671

Yeo SG, Lee YC, Park DC, Cha CI. Acyclovir plus steroid vs steroid alone in the treatment of Bell's palsy. Am J Otolaryngol 2008;29(3):163–166

70 Rehabilitation of Hearing Loss and Balance Disorders

■ Introduction

This chapter outlines the appropriate diagnostic and rehabilitative modalities for hearing loss and balance disorders. As with all medical therapies, early detection and a precise diagnosis are mandatory before any treatments are initiated. The following discussion focuses on nonsurgical modalities because, with few notable exceptions, the majority of patients with cochlear and vestibular losses are not candidates for surgical intervention. Rather than being reparative, these strategies are designed to optimize patients' remaining hearing and balance function. Brief overviews of key interview and examination findings and relevant diagnostic testing are presented to lay the groundwork for understanding the theory and practice of rehabilitation of hearing loss and balance disorders.

■ Aural Rehabilitation

Evaluation

In the United States, 20% of the population suffers from unilateral or bilateral hearing loss. Common risk factors for developing sensorineural hearing loss (SNHL) include advancing age, noise exposure, ototoxicity, congenital and hereditary disorders, infection, and trauma. It is important to detect and rehabilitate SNHL early to avoid disability. Once a thorough head and neck examination and audiometric evaluation have determined the extent of hearing loss (**Fig. 70.1**) and reversible causes have been excluded, appropriate rehabilitation should be offered.

Newborn and Infant Screening

There is strong evidence that early detection and rehabilitation of hearing loss in infants are crucial to normal speech and language development. Imple-mentation of statewide newborn hearing screening protocols, as outlined by the Joint Committee on Infant Hearing, has led to earlier identification of children with significant hearing impairment. Today, hearing loss is commonly detected in children less than 12 months of age. Screening should not be limited to high-risk infants because this strategy will overlook approximately half of all cases of congenital severe-to-profound SNHL. Unilateral or bilateral hearing loss can be effectively screened at birth using automated otoacoustic emission (OAE) or auditory brainstem response (ABR) tests. For patients who do not pass initial screening, further testing should be performed, with the goal of identifying and treating the disorder before 6 months of age.

Audiometric Evaluation of Children

Behavioral audiometry requires that the patient be capable and cooperative during testing. In children, the complexity of testing must be matched with the patient's stage of development. Generally speaking, patients 4 years and younger can be tested with visual reinforcement or play audiometry, whereas patients 5 years and older (included in the following section on adults) can be evaluated using conventional pure-tone and speech audiometry. Objective testing, including OAE and ABR, may be helpful in very young children, children with limited interactive capacity, and children suspected of having functional hearing loss. In all cases, tympanometry should be performed to evaluate for mechanical/conductive causes of hearing loss, such as middle ear effusion and eustachian tube dysfunction.

Audiometric Evaluation of Adults

Most adults presenting with hearing loss can provide a detailed history of their condition, including laterality, onset, pattern, and duration of impairment. Associated symptoms, including tinnitus,

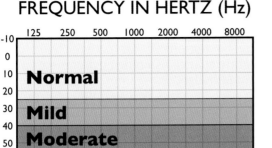

FREQUENCY IN HERTZ (Hz)

Fig. 70.1 Audiogram demonstrating progressive degrees of hearing loss.

aural fullness, vertigo, otorrhea, otalgia, and facial nerve disturbances, may provide important clues as to the underlying cause of hearing loss and should be addressed in the patient interview.

At a minimum, baseline audiometric evaluation should include air- and bone-conduction pure-tone audiometry (250–8,000 Hz), with masking, speech reception threshold, word recognition score (WRS), tympanometry, and stapedial reflex testing. Weber and Rinne testing should be performed, using a 512 Hz tuning fork to help confirm audiogram results. All patients with asymmetric SNHL (binaural difference in bone-conduction thresholds of > 10 dB at two consecutive frequencies, or > 15 dB at one frequency); patients with highly discrepant WRSs (binaural difference of > 15%); patients with sudden SNHL (30 dB hearing loss in three consecutive frequencies over a period of 3 days); and patients with abnormal reflexes and normal tympanometry warrant further investigation using gadolinium-enhanced magnetic resonance imaging to evaluate for retrocochlear pathology. Common causes of retrocochlear hearing loss include vestibular schwannomas, meningiomas, multiple sclerosis, and stroke.

Patient Psychological Assessment and Explanation of Treatment Options

Acknowledging hearing impairment and seeking medical attention are frequently difficult and emotional events. The evaluating team must be sensitive to the psychological aspects of counseling, and a thorough history should assess the impact hearing loss is having on a patient's life. Validated instruments, such as the Hearing Handicap Inventory for Adults and the Elderly, may be used to assess initial impairment and to gauge any improvements seen following therapy.

Once the audiometric evaluation is complete, it is critical that the physician take time to explain the characteristics of the patient's hearing loss and, more important, the full range of rehabilitative strategies outlined in this chapter. After being informed, patients must decide if their perceived disability warrants treatment. For example, patients with advanced unilateral or mild bilateral hearing loss that works in a quiet environment may not feel their hearing loss significantly interferes with their daily function. Furthermore, the timing of intervention should be considered. For patients with slowly progressive or stable hearing loss, treatment should be initiated early on, whereas patients with an acute insult (e.g., sudden SNHL, viral labyrinthitis, or active Ménière disease) may be observed for a period of time to determine their new audiometric baseline.

Etiology of Hearing Impairment

The exact cause of hearing loss should also be established because this will largely dictate initial management. Progressive hearing loss from "preventable" etiologies (e.g., ototoxicity, hypothyroidism, noise exposure, syphilis) should be first addressed to impede further progression. Many conditions associated with conductive hearing loss may be amenable to medical or surgical correction and should be discussed with the patient. Such processes include otosclerosis, tympanosclerosis, ossicular discontinuity, tympanic membrane perforation or retraction, middle ear effusion, and superior canal dehiscence, to name a few. Only after preventable and correctable conditions have been discussed and considered should rehabilitation begin.

Management

Choices for Aural Rehabilitation

The optimal method for aural rehabilitation depends on many factors: degree of loss, laterality (unilateral or bilateral), socioeconomic factors, physician expertise, and patient wishes. The practitioner must match the patient's needs with the most appropriate modality to ensure the best chance for success. Particular attention should be given to the pattern of pure-tone loss and WRS. Available resources for hearing rehabilitation include physician counseling, formal aural rehabilitation, assistive listening devices (ALDs), conventional hearing aids, implantable hearing aids, bone-conduction aids, and cochlear implantation.

Physician Counseling

The first step in aural rehabilitation is simply discussing the nature of the hearing loss and environmental and behavioral ways to improve hearing. Strategies such as manipulating the environment to reduce background noise (e.g., roll the windows up in the car, find the quietest table in the restaurant) and facing the person speaking seem self-evident, but they can be an invaluable and much appreciated means of counseling patients with any degree of hearing loss.

Formal Aural Rehabilitation

In patients with far-advanced hearing loss, conventional hearing aid amplification alone may be inadequate to restore satisfactory functional communication. In such cases, formal aural rehabilitation by specialty-trained audiologists and speech-language pathologists is desirable to perform a communication needs assessment and devise aural, verbal, and visual strategies aimed at enhancing communicate skills. Frequently, a hearing aid "failure" can be reversed by such methods and should be considered.

Assistive Listening Devices (ALDs)

ALDs go beyond conventional hearing aid amplification and seek to help hearing-impaired patients overcome difficulties related to the physical distance between the receiving microphone and the sound source. Nonauditory (vibrotactile and visual) alarm systems may alert the patient of an event, such as doorbell activation or an incoming telephone call. Auditory assisting devices are designed to optimize the signal-to-noise ratio of the sound source. A microphone system captures the desired signal, which is amplified and delivered to the listener through a hardwired system or wireless frequency modulation (FM), infrared, induction loop, or Bluetooth systems. Such devices work well for patients with mild-to-moderate losses during conferences, lectures, concerts, restaurants, and similar events. ALD input may be coupled to hearing aids through several wireless systems, may be connected to a direct audio input jack, or may function independently.

Hearing Aid Basics

Despite the tremendous number of commercially available hearing aid options, all devices share at least four essential ingredients: microphone, loudspeaker, power source, and electronics package. Hearing aids may be either analog or digital, with adjustable or programmable control. An adjustable analog con-figuration is the most economical option, but it provides the least flexibility. After initial fitting, the user is largely limited to volume adjustment. This option may be reasonable for patients who do not frequently change listening environments and are on a limited budget. Programmable analog devices allow the user to select between different programs that are optimized for various listening environments. Finally, digital platforms are now being used in the majority of, if not all, contemporary designs, offering many additional features over traditional analog systems. Beyond providing multiple programs, digital signal processors can selectively amplify certain frequencies, reduce acoustic feedback and background noise, automatically detect changes in listening environments to dynamically optimize signal, and offer enhanced connectivity to external sound sources.

One notable innovation in hearing aid design is the incorporation of directional microphone technology. Most conventional hearing aid models use an omnidirectional microphone, where sound from all directions is equally amplified and relayed to the listener. Directional microphones selectively amplify sounds located in front of the listener, thereby improving the signal-to-noise ratio. This technology assumes the device user is facing the sound source of interest. Adaptive directional microphones go one step further and are able to vary the direction of maximal amplification. Digital signal-processing strategies selectively target speech patterns and automatically maximize amplification in the direction of the detected speech source. Potential disadvantages of adaptive directional technology include interference from competing talkers and inadvertent targeting of background noise that mimics patterns of speech.

In-the-Canal (ITC) and Completely in-the-Canal (CIC) Hearing Aids

Patients with mild to moderate hearing losses benefit from miniaturized hearing aids that are contained entirely within the external auditory canal. Such devices are desirable to some patients because of their discreet profile and superior cosmesis. Additionally, in-the-canal (ITC) and completely-in-the-canal (CIC) hearing aids take advantage of the ear's innate shape, assisting with natural sound amplification and decreasing undesirable wind noise through pinna shielding.

However, patients should be counseled regarding potential disadvantages of these hearing aids, including power limitations, cerumen clogging, aural fullness and occlusion effect, difficult fit, fine-dexterity requirements, cost, and external canal irritation. ITC and CIC hearing aids are not recommended for patients with severe losses, given their limited amplification capacity and increased problems with feedback with higher gain.

In-the-Ear (ITE) Hearing Aids

Full-shell in-the-ear (ITE) hearing aids are designed to fit the conchal bowl and external auditory canal and deliver adequate sound to rehabilitate mild to moderately severe losses. ITE aids generally are more powerful and easier to manipulate than ITC and CIC models, but still require some manual dexterity for placement and volume control. Given their size and location, they are less discreet than ITC models.

Behind-the-Ear (BTE) Hearing Aids

Behind-the-ear (BTE) designs are the most popular and adaptable hearing aid option for patients with unilateral or bilateral moderately severe to severe hearing loss. They consist of a BTE electronics case coupled to an earmold or open-fit dome. These instruments are capable of delivering higher power, generally contain more signal-processing features, and are easier to handle than ITC or ITE devices in patients with poor manual dexterity. The modular design allows the mold to be easily reshaped, changed, or vented without disturbing the electronics package. Although early designs were often very bulky, newer-generation mini-BTE models incorporate smaller casing with an inconspicuous connecting tube and a nonocclusive earmold. In cases of progressive loss, BTE aids are often a good choice because of their flexibility, programmability, gain reserve, and enhanced connectivity with ALD systems.

A variation of the BTE aid is the contralateral routing of signal (CROS) aid for patients with unilateral severe-to-profound hearing loss and adequate contralateral hearing capacity. A microphone/transmitter captures sound from the unaidable ear and delivers it electronically to a receiver placed on the contralateral side. In instances where the better ear is impaired but remains aidable, a bilateral contralateral routing of signal (BiCROS) device with a microphone located on both sides delivers amplified sound to the better ear. The CROS and BiCROS aids assist in eliminating a "dead spot," but since sound is relayed to only one ear, they generally do not assist with sound localization.

Body Aids

In patients with bilateral severe to profound deafness, feedback problems occur with ear-level devices because of the proximity of the microphone to the receiver. This problem is overcome with the body aid, where the microphone is worn at a distant site from the amplifier, typically on a belt or in a pocket. The body aid devices provide sound awareness and limited closed-set speech recognition, but as a whole do not provide enough power and clarity to adequately rehabilitate profound deficits.

Bone-Conduction Hearing Aids (BCHAs) and Bone-Anchored Hearing Aids (BAHAs)

Patients with conductive hearing loss who cannot be fitted with a conventional aid (e.g., congenital aural atresia, canal wall down mastoidectomy, chronic otorrhea) and patients with unilateral deafness may benefit from bone-conduction hearing aids (BCHAs). BCHAs use mastoid vibration that bypasses the ear canal and middle ear sound-conducting mechanism and directly stimulates the ipsi- and contralateral cochleas. Conventional BCHAs incorporate a headband to hold the device tightly against the mastoid and are frequently used in children under the age of 5 with bilateral aural atresia.

BAHAs work by a similar principle, but they use a surgically implanted osseointegrated titanium implant (screw) to transmit vibration. BAHAs generally outperform conventional BCHAs by permitting higher gain.

Implantable Middle Ear Hearing Devices (IMEDs)

Implantable middle ear hearing devices (IMEDs) use either piezoelectric or electromagnetic platforms that transform sound signal into mechanical energy that is directly coupled to the ossicular chain, and in some instances the round window membrane. IMEDs were developed to overcome many of the limitations of conventional hearing aid designs, offering enhanced cosmesis, comfort, discrimination, and fidelity, while eliminating occlusion effect, minimizing feedback, and allowing increased gain. Additionally, totally implanted IMEDs permit amplification during swimming or bathing.

IMED candidates should be $\geq$ 18 years of age, should have moderate to severe SNHL, and should have tried conventional amplification prior to implantation. Patients with fluctuating or unstable hearing loss, poor WRS, and frequent recurrent or chronic otitis media should not be considered for IMED surgery. Several of the limitations and concerns regarding IMED include long-term device durability, battery capacity, technical difficulty of implantation, and expense. Currently, the semi-implantable Vibrant Soundbridge (MED-EL Corp. USA, Durham, NC) and the fully implantable Esteem (Envoy Medical Corp., St. Paul, MN) are the only two manufacturers with both U.S. Food and Drug Administration (FDA) approval and availability within the United Sates, although several other prototypes are under clinical trials.

Cochlear Implantation (CI)

Over the past several decades, cochlear implantation (CI) has undergone tremendous refinement and is now the preferred method of auditory rehabilitation in patients with severe-to-profound hearing loss and poor word understanding. CI involves placing an electrode, containing multiple channels, within the cochlea to provide electrical stimulation to surviving populations of spiral ganglion cells. Prolonged auditory deprivation and poor preoperative hearing capacity have been linked with poorer performance. However, the majority of implantees enjoy open-set capacity, and many are capable of using the telephone. Currently, CI candidacy is restricted to patients with bilateral severe-to-profound SNHL with no better than 50% word/sentence recognition scores in the ear to be implanted, and no more than 60% in the best-aided condition. Generally, CI should not be offered to patients with retrocochlear or unilateral SNHL, although several reports have demonstrated the benefits of implantation in carefully selected patients.

Application of Aural Rehabilitative Strategies

Unilateral SNHL

Unilateral SNHL is more aggressively treated in children than in adults because of the potential effects on language acquisition and educational needs. Parental counseling, preferential classroom seating, and an auditory trainer (FM system) are usually adequate for mild-to-moderate unilateral losses. For moderate-to-severe losses, ITE or BTE amplification is prescribed along with an auditory trainer, depending on a child's age and degree of loss.

As a general rule, rehabilitation of unilateral loss in adults depends on the status of the better-hearing ear, patient socioeconomic factors, and perceived disability. If the patient has a mild-to-moderate loss and the contralateral ear is normal, the patient may only require counseling regarding optimal seating in meetings, eye contact with speakers, and preferential ear use with the telephone. Moderate-to-severe losses can be aided with a variety of ITC, ITE, and BTE devices. Adults with bilateral asymmetric hearing loss who desire monaural amplification deserve special consideration. Instead of aiding the ear with the larger hearing deficit, patients may receive more benefit from optimizing the better ear, taking advantage of more favorable WDS and pure-tone thresholds.

Both children and adults with unilateral deafness may benefit from BCHAs, BAHAs, CROS, or BiCROS amplification, depending on the status of the better ear. Although BAHAs have been used in younger children, they are only approved by the FDA for use in children ≥ 5 years, to ensure sufficient bone stock. Additionally, CI for unilateral severe-to-profound hearing loss is not currently approved by the FDA, although limited reports demonstrate its potential benefit with regard to auditory rehabilitation and tinnitus modulation.

Bilateral Mild SNHL

Many patients in this category are unaware of their loss and frequently visit a doctor because an acquaintance has noticed a problem. Successful rehabilitation in these patients depends upon the characteristics of the hearing loss and the patient's social environment and motivation. Mild high frequency SNHL with intact word recognition in a patient who engages primarily in one-on-one, face-to-face, and phone conversation may only need visual rehabilitative strategies (eye contact, body positioning) and phone amplification. The busy executive who engages in a variety of complex listening tasks may benefit from ALDs or binaural aids, even when faced with a similar loss.

Bilateral Moderate-to-Moderately Severe SNHL

Patients with bilateral moderate-to-moderately severe SNHL and adequate WRS may experience the most benefit from conventional aural amplification. Binaural amplification restores the entire sound field, assisting in enhanced speech-in-noise understanding and sound localization; however, economic and physical considerations may dictate unilateral fitting.

Bilateral Severe-to-Profound SNHL

Given concurrent advances in CI technology and surgical refinement, the majority of patients with severe-to-profound hearing loss gain substantially more benefit from CI compared with conventional hearing aid use. Patients may undergo unilateral or bilateral (sequential or simultaneous) CI. Unilateral implantees may continue to use a hearing aid in the contralateral ear (bimodal mode), and a small subset may have residual hearing preserved in the implanted ear, permitting ipsilateral electroacoustic stimulation. Patients with severe-to-profound hearing loss who are not candidates for implantation may be fitted with BTE or body hearing aids with or without formal aural rehabilitation training. Additionally, manual communication (i.e., American Sign Language) or total communication strategies can be explored.

Conclusion

The options for hearing rehabilitation continue to expand. In many cases, the physician serves as a common entry point for patients seeking assistance with hearing impairment. Therefore, we must be aware of the various facets of the rehabilitative ladder and employ them in a timely and caring fashion. The most important aspect of the provider-patient interaction is the formulation of a customized, interdisciplinary rehabilitative strategy that the patient and family accepts and plays an active role in.

Vestibular Rehabilitation

An estimated 40% of all U.S. citizens will experience at least one episode of dizziness during their lifetime. One in five elderly patients reports problems with dizziness and balance within the last 12 months, and nearly half of them will seek medical evaluation. Unlike aural rehabilitation, the importance of formal therapy for vertigo and postural instability has only recently gained widespread recognition within the medical community, despite a high prevalence.

Akin to SNHL, currently there are no known medical or surgical interventions that can restore labyrinthine function after paretic injury. Current pharmacological treatments are either suppressive (e.g., meclizine) or ablative (e.g., intratympanic gentamicin), whereas "vestibular surgery" may, at best, turn an unstable deficit into a stable lesion, so that effective central compensation may begin. Superior semicircular canal dehiscence syndrome and perilymphatic fistulas should be reviewed separately. These two unique conditions cause vestibular dysfunction through increased inner ear compliance, resulting from a mobile third window within the labyrinth. Surgical repair, through occlusion of the pathological opening, may resolve patient symptoms and improve vestibular physiological function but possibly at the expense of a loss of ipsilateral superior semicircular canal function.

Broadly speaking, vestibular rehabilitation addresses two clinical conditions: (1) benign paroxysmal positional vertigo (BPPV) through canalith repositioning exercises, and (2) uncompensated stable vestibular dysfunction using balance retraining therapy (BRT), the latter being the focus of the remainder of this chapter. Although canalith repositioning techniques are often included under the umbrella of BRT, treatment does not depend on central compensation.

BRT is a specialized form of physical therapy focusing on the improvement of static and dynamic balance and gait, and promoting central vestibular compensation by taking advantage of the inherent plasticity of central balance pathways. Common strategies used during BRT include (1) the development of substitution strategies, taking advantage of alternate intact balance mechanisms that may compensate for specific deficits; (2) habituation maneuvers aimed at provoking episodes of imbalance to "fatigue" response; (3) adaptation exercises focusing on improving gaze stability and sharpening the vestibulo-ocular reflex (VOR); (4) gait stability exercises, using walking aids when indicated; (5) general conditioning; and (6) fall-prevention/reduction strategies, with advice about home environment modifications.

Clinical Basis for Balance Retraining Therapy

It has been known for many years that younger, more physically active patients tend to recover more quickly and fully from vestibular insults than their sedentary or elderly counterparts. Furthermore, it has been recognized that posture and gait instability can occur at multiple levels, given that both require an integrated process using multiple sensory inputs, rapid central processing and integration, and a coordinated motor response. Many studies have supported the efficacy of directed exercise therapy over general conditioning for patients with a variety of vestibular, proprioceptive, motor, and central nervous system (CNS) abnormalities.

In the initial phase of recovery following a peripheral vestibular insult, spontaneous nystagmus resolves, first with visual fixation then without, over a period of days to weeks. Static compensation occurs through a central adaptive process that rebalances tonic neural activity between vestibular nuclei, regardless of visual input or movement. The first phase of recovery may be prolonged, or impaired with the use of sedating and vestibular suppressive medications. Following recovery from the initial phase, patients are generally relieved from symptoms of spontaneous vertigo, but they often continue to experience general imbalance, disequilibrium, and motion-provoked unsteadiness.

The second phase of recovery, termed dynamic compensation, involves recalibrating brain and cerebellar reflex pathways in response to sensory conflicts occurring during head and eye movement. This process is dependent on the amount and nature of visual stimulation and proprioceptive input during activity. During the dynamic phase of recovery, subjects may experience incomplete compensation or may acquire maladaptive postural control strategies. It is during this phase that BRT exercises focusing on habituation, substitution, and adaptation are most beneficial.

Evaluation of the Balance-Disordered Patient

Patient Interview and History

An initial thorough clinical history is critical to establishing a correct diagnosis, selecting appropriate patients for rehabilitation, and designing tailored therapy. The exact character, severity, duration, quantity, and frequency of episodes as well as aggravating or relieving maneuvers should be well outlined. Particular attention should be given to identifying any inciting event(s), including otologic or neurological surgical procedures, head trauma, stroke, barotrauma, viral illness, boat cruise, stress, and new medications, to name a few. Furthermore, it is helpful to assess coinciding symptoms. For example, concurrent hearing loss or tinnitus may imply inner ear pathology, phono- or photophobia may implicate vestibular migraine, or chest palpitations or shortness of breath may indicate cardiopulmonary contribution. Comorbidities, including neurological disease (e.g., Parkinson disease, multiple sclerosis); psychiatric illness (e.g., anxiety and depression); conditions of peripheral neuropathy (e.g., diabetes, peripheral vascular disease); and musculoskeletal disorders should be considered. Finally, the severity of impairment and response to therapy may be assessed using a validated instrument, such as the Dizziness Handicap Inventory.

Physical Examination

A comprehensive physical examination of the dizzy patient must include an evaluation of all involved systems (see also Chapter 61). The clinician must be careful to avoid being distracted by a single obvious deficit when evaluating the patient, understanding that imbalance is often multifactorial and cumulative.

A cursory cardiovascular examination should evaluate for arrhythmia, murmur, carotid bruit, pronounced orthostatic blood pressure changes, or peripheral vascular disease. Neurological assessment should evaluate general cognitive function; trunk and extremity function (rigidity, ataxia, weakness, atrophy, and sensory loss); gait stability and discoordination (e.g., Parkinsonian syndrome; widebased, or cerebellar, ataxia); postural control (Romberg and sharpened Romberg test); and cerebellar function (finger-to-nose and heel-to-shin coordination revealing dysmetria and rapid alternating movements evaluating for dysdiadochokinesia). A complete cranial nerve examination should be performed to evaluate and localize any potential brainstem or skull base lesions.

A neurological examination should include otoscopy, fistula testing, and tuning fork examination (to confirm audiogram results). Evaluation of smooth pursuit, saccades, spontaneous nystagmus, and gaze nystagmus should be carefully performed. The sensitivity for detecting nystagmus may be greatly enhanced with the use of Frenzel goggles to remove the suppressing effects of gaze fixation. Unstable vestibular deficits manifest with spontaneous nystagmus. Patients with unstable peripheral lesions exhibit unidirectional horizontal rotary nystag-

mus (named in the direction of the fast phase) that becomes inhibited by visual fixation. The intensity will increase when the patient is gazing in the direction of the fast component (Alexander's law). Patients with central lesions may experience horizontal or vertical nystagmus that may alternate and that does not suppress with visual fixation. Disruption of smooth pursuit, with the observation of saccadic eye tracking, generally indicates CNS (cerebellar) origin. Head thrust testing, head shake maneuvers, and the Fukuda stepping test may help identify asymmetric vestibular hypofunction. Finally, positional nystagmus testing (e.g., Dix–Hallpike test) is helpful in identifying BPPV.

Formal Vestibular Testing

The primary goals of balance testing are to localize dysfunctional sensory, motor, and neural pathways and to determine the state (static or dynamic) and, to a lesser degree the completeness, of physiological compensation (see also Chapter 61). In particular, three commonly used tests may augment clinical history and physical exam findings. Electronystagmography (ENG) or videonystagmography (VNG) testing may provide helpful information regarding the laterality and degree of labyrinthine responsiveness (using bithermal caloric testing). Rotary chair testing analyzes the integrity of both labyrinths simultaneously and may provide additional information regarding the VOR and vestibular compensation not obtained from ENG/VNG. Finally, dynamic posturography assesses the patient's ability to detect and integrate appropriate visual, vestibular, and somatosensory input, and to initiate and execute corrective motor actions to maintain stable stance.

It is imperative to understand that, although balance testing may assist in lesion localization and severity determination, generally there is poor correlation between test results, patient symptomatology, and ability to perform demanding functional tasks. BRT candidacy determination and the selection of customized exercise regimens are largely based on patient-reported symptoms and physical examination findings, and to a lesser extent on formal balance testing. Observing the age-old adage, we must treat the patient, not the test.

Patient Selection

Appropriate patient selection is critical to a successful outcome. The process of central compensation, through methods of habituation and adaptation, requires consistent peripheral vestibular input and predictable responses. To this end, individuals with stable or indolent vestibular deficits with incomplete compensation receive the most benefit from BRT, whereas patients with unstable or fluctuating vestibular dysfunction are generally not candidates until their disease has stabilized. Patients with unstable deficits frequently complain of spontaneous vertigo, whereas those with a stable uncompensated condition often report imbalance with head turn (typically toward the side of lesion) and eye movement.

Realistic expectations should be outlined with the patient before commencing therapy. Patients with coexisting psychiatric illness, including depression and anxiety, as well as those with preexisting conditions affecting balance (multisensory dysfunction, musculoskeletal disorders, and neurological conditions) may have attenuated outcomes, although many still gain noticeable benefit. Patients taking antidepressants, tranquilizers, or other neurosuppressants may require significantly longer durations of therapy to achieve optimal outcomes. Finally, dependence on vestibular-suppressive medications may hinder vestibular compensation, resulting in less than maximal benefit.

Management

Application of Balance Rehabilitative Strategies

Unilateral Vestibular Dysfunction

Many individuals with isolated stable unilateral lesions are able to achieve adequate compensation through the course of everyday activities. However, if the patient continues to experience postural instability and symptoms of imbalance with head movement months after resolution of the initial phase of compensation, BRT may be used to augment remaining vestibular function and to stimulate appropriate sensory substitution with enhanced visual and proprioceptive cues. Exercises may include (1) progressive head turns with and without visual fixation to promote appropriate VOR responses, (2) tracking exercises to enhance smooth pursuit, (3) coordinated head–eye movements during refixation to suppress retinal slip, and (4) postural exercises with head movement under different visual and footing support surface conditions. Because vestibular input is intact on the opposite side, exercises that require vestibular input can be given, whereas in complete bilateral loss, such exercises would be unhelpful.

Bilateral Vestibular Dysfunction

BRT may provide great benefit for patients with bilateral vestibular hypofunction. In patients with total loss of bilateral vestibular input, the goal of BRT is to enhance sensory substitution and teach head and body movements that will minimize symptoms and prevent falls. Exercises that enhance smooth pursuit and predictive saccadic eye movements are used,

although the overall speed of head movement is reduced. During posture and gait exercises, head stabilization on the horizon and enhanced awareness of proprioceptive cues are emphasized. For these patients, modifications of the home environment are essential; elimination of irregular flooring, improvement of lighting, use of handrails, and providing appropriate nonskid footwear may help prevent falls.

Proprioceptive Dysfunction

Patients with diabetes, peripheral vascular disease, and other causes of distal sensory neuropathy have trouble sensing a support surface, often present with marked instability, and are prone to falls. For these patients, BRT is geared toward maximizing proprioceptive input by balance and strength exercises; changes in footwear; the use of assistance devices, such as a walker or cane; and an emphasis on using visual cues. Because gait and posture are heavily controlled by proprioception, these individuals experience variable improvement following BRT.

Sensory Integration Dysfunction

In many elderly and head trauma patients, motion-induced dizziness and postural instability stem from poor sensory integration within the CNS. Overreliance on incorrect sensory input leads to an inappropriate motor response. For these individuals, BRT consists of progressive exercises with varying combinations of visual and support surface alterations designed to make the patient quickly choose orientationally correct senses over misleading or destabilizing cues. This is an especially challenging problem in the elderly, who develop an overreliance on vision and are made unstable by visual cues (i.e., the supermarket syndrome).

Motion sensitivity syndrome is thought to be due to sensory conflict between vestibular cues and visual and somatosensory input. Although various centrally acting sedatives have been used, motion sickness remains a difficult problem. Exercise therapy has been used successfully in some cases of extreme motion sensitivity by applying progressively challenging visual environments during head movement in an attempt to desensitize the patient to similar conditions encountered in daily life.

Musculoskeletal Dysfunction

Regardless of the status of sensory input, difficulties with effective motor output may lead to instability. Focal or generalized muscle weakness, arthropathy, and spinal motor diseases all have an impact on the patient's ability to execute a correct response to a sensory challenge. In such cases, BRT must be adapted to fit the motor limitations of the patient. Strengthening exercises, flexibility training, and center-of-gravity exercises are used, along with assistive devices. In more severe cases, lifestyle modification for fall prevention should also be instituted.

Disequilibrium of Aging

Presbystasis is a term coined to describe the general balance difficulties of the elderly. In this condition, age-related decline in peripheral vestibular function, visual acuity, proprioception, and motor control has a cumulative effect on balance. Before BRT is initiated, individual system deficits must be quantified. Exercises are then tailored to optimize remaining sensory inputs and motor output, and lifestyle modifications are introduced to minimize sensory conflict and fall risk.

Neurological Diseases

The outcome of BRT for patients with central deficits may be less significant than for patients with isolated stable peripheral vestibular hypofunction. As a general rule, the benefit of BRT among patients with central or mixed (central and peripheral) deficits

is inversely proportional to the severity of the central neurological disease process. Nonetheless, BRT should not be withheld on these grounds because many such patients experience moderate improvements in balance function and enhanced quality of life.

Conclusion

BRT has broadened the armamentarium for the management of a wide variety of conditions associated with imbalance. The goals of BRT are to enhance balance function and prevent or at least limit falls, decrease symptoms of dizziness, and improve overall functional capacity and activity levels. The effectiveness of therapy hinges on an accurate assessment of the disease process, upfront counseling to gain patient commitment and establish realistic expectations, the appropriate selection of individuals with stable vestibular deficits, and a customized set of exercises aimed at rehabilitating specific balance deficits through substitution, adaptation, and habituation.

■ Suggested Reading

Agrawal Y, Carey JP, Della Santina CC, Schubert MC, Minor LB. Disorders of balance and vestibular function in US adults: data from the National Health and Nutrition Examination Survey, 2001-2004. Arch Intern Med 2009;169(10):938–944

Alrwaily M, Whitney SL. Vestibular rehabilitation of older adults with dizziness. Otolaryngol Clin North Am 2011;44(2): 473–496, x

Arlinger S. Negative consequences of uncorrected hearing loss—a review. Int J Audiol 2003;42(Suppl 2):S17–S20

Carlson ML, Driscoll CL, Gifford RH, McMenomey SO. Cochlear implantation: current and future device options. Otolaryngol Clin North Am 2012;45(1):221–248

Chien WW, Carey JP, Minor LB. Canal dehiscence. Curr Opin Neurol 2011;24(1):25–31

Christensen L, Smith-Olinde L, Kimberlain J, Richter GT, Dornhoffer JL. Comparison of traditional bone-conduction hearing AIDS with the Baha system. J Am Acad Audiol 2010;21(4):267–273

Cueva RA. Auditory brainstem response versus magnetic resonance imaging for the evaluation of asymmetric sensorineural hearing loss. Laryngoscope 2004;114(10):1686–1692

Cunningham M, Cox EO; Committee on Practice and Ambulatory Medicine and the Section on Otolaryngology and Bronchoesophagology. Hearing assessment in infants and children: recommendations beyond neonatal screening. Pediatrics 2003;111(2):436–440

Gomaa NA, Rubinstein JT, Lowder MW, Tyler RS, Gantz BJ. Residual speech perception and cochlear implant performance in postlingually deafened adults. Ear Hear 2003;24(6):539–544

Hall CD, Cox LC. The role of vestibular rehabilitation in the balance disorder patient. Otolaryngol Clin North Am 2009;42(1): 161–169, xi

Han BI, Song HS, Kim JS. Vestibular rehabilitation therapy: review of indications, mechanisms, and key exercises. J Clin Neurol 2011;7(4):184–196

Haynes DS, Young JA, Wanna GB, Glasscock ME III. Middle ear implantable hearing devices: an overview. Trends Amplif 2009;13(3):206–214

Hillier SL, McDonnell M. Vestibular rehabilitation for unilateral peripheral vestibular dysfunction. Clin Otolaryngol 2011;36(3): 248–249

Hillier SL, McDonnell M. Vestibular rehabilitation for unilateral peripheral vestibular dysfunction. Cochrane Database Syst Rev 2011; (2):CD005397

Jacobson GP, Newman CW. The development of the Dizziness Handicap Inventory. Arch Otolaryngol Head Neck Surg 1990;116(4):424–427

Jacobson GP, Shepard NT, eds. Balance Function Assessment and Management. San Diego, CA: Plural Publishing; 2007

Joint Committee on Infant Hearing; American Academy of Audiology; American Academy of Pediatrics; American Speech-Language-Hearing Association; Directors of Speech and Hearing Programs in State Health and Welfare Agencies. Year 2000 position statement: principles and guidelines for early hearing detection and intervention programs. Joint Committee on Infant Hearing, American Academy of Audiology, American Academy of Pediatrics, American Speech-Language-Hearing Association, and Directors of Speech and Hearing Programs in State Health and Welfare Agencies. Pediatrics 2000;106(4):798–817

Kileny PR, Zwolan TA. Diagnostic and rehabilitative audiology. In: Cummings C, Fredrickson J, Harker L, Krause CJ, Richardson M, Schueler DE, eds. Otolaryngology–Head and Neck Surgery. 4th ed. Philadelphia, PA: Elsevier Mosby; 2005;3483–3502

Kim HH, Barrs DM. Hearing aids: a review of what's new. Otolaryngol Head Neck Surg 2006;134(6):1043–1050

Krebs DE, Gill-Body KM, Riley PO, Parker SW. Double-blind, placebo-controlled trial of rehabilitation for bilateral vestibular hypofunction: preliminary report. Otolaryngol Head Neck Surg 1993;109(4):735–741

Lesner SA. Candidacy and management of assistive listening devices: special needs of the elderly. Int J Audiol 2003;42(Suppl 2): S68–S76

Lin FR, Niparko JK, Ferrucci L. Hearing loss prevalence in the United States. Arch Intern Med 2011;171(20):1851–1852

Lin HW, Bhattacharyya N. Balance disorders in the elderly: epidemiology and functional impact. Laryngoscope 2012;122(8): 1858–1861

Newman CW, Weinstein BE, Jacobson GP, Hug GA. The Hearing Handicap Inventory for Adults: psychometric adequacy and audiometric correlates. Ear Hear 1990;11(6):430–433

Niparko JK, Cox KM, Lustig LR. Comparison of the bone anchored hearing aid implantable hearing device with contralateral routing of offside signal amplification in the rehabilitation of unilateral deafness. Otol Neurotol 2003;24(1):73–78

Niparko JK, Tobey EA, Thal DJ, et al; CDaCI Investigative Team. Spoken language development in children following cochlear implantation. JAMA 2010;303(15):1498–1506

Priwin C, Granström G. The bone-anchored hearing aid in children: a surgical and questionnaire follow-up study. Otolaryngol Head Neck Surg 2005;132(4):559–565

Punte AK, Vermeire K, Hofkens A, De Bodt M, De Ridder D, Van de Heyning P. Cochlear implantation as a durable tinnitus treatment in single-sided deafness. Cochlear Implants Int 2011;12(Suppl 1): S26–S29

Ricketts T, Henry P. Evaluation of an adaptive, directional-microphone hearing aid. Int J Audiol 2002;41(2):100–112

Sabini P, Sclafani AP. Efficacy of serologic testing in asymmetric sensorineural hearing loss. Otolaryngol Head Neck Surg 2000; 122(4):469–476

Schow RL, Nerbonne MA. Introduction to Audiologic Rehabilitation. 5th ed. Boston, MA: Allyn & Bacon; 2006

Shepard NT, Telian SA, eds. Practical Management of the Balance Disorder Patient. San Diego, CA: Singular Publishing Group; 1996

Shepard NT, Telian SA. Vestibular rehabilitation. In: Cummings C, Fredrickson J, Harker L, Krause CJ, Richardson M, Schueler DE, eds. Otolaryngology–Head and Neck Surgery. 4th ed. Philadelphia, PA: Elsevier Mosby; 2005:3309–3318

Stachler RJ, Chandrasekhar SS, Archer SM, et al; American Academy of Otolaryngology-Head and Neck Surgery. Clinical practice guideline: sudden hearing loss. Otolaryngol Head Neck Surg 2012;146(3, Suppl):S1–S35

Tye-Murray N, ed. Foundations of Aural Rehabilitation: Children, Adults, and Their Family Members. 3rd ed. San Diego, CA: Singular Publishing Group; 1998

U.S. Department of Health and Human Services, National Institutes of Health. Early identification of hearing impairment in infants and young children. NIH Consensus Development Conference Statement. 1993 ;11(1):1–24

VII
Pediatric Otolaryngology

71 Otitis Media

■ Introduction

Incidence

Acute otitis media (AOM) is the most common childhood bacterial infection for which antibiotics are prescribed. It is pervasive in children, and high rates of disease are reported in both developed and emerging nations. Risk factors for the development of otitis media (OM) include male gender, young age, family history of recurrent OM (particularly in a sibling), low socioeconomic status, exposure to cigarette smoke, use of a pacifier, and daycare attendance. Malnutrition may also be an additional risk factor for chronic suppurative OM in developing countries.

Breast-feeding decreases the risk of OM. The 2013 American Academy of Pediatrics (AAP) Guideline on the Diagnosis and Management of Acute Otitis Media recommends exclusive breast-feeding for at least 6 months in an effort to reduce the incidence of AOM. The guideline also recommends that clinicians encourage avoidance of tobacco smoke exposure. In a limited number of studies, prophylactic frequent administration of xylitol in children in daycare can reduce the number of episodes of AOM. In the United States, racial disparities have been found in the treatment of OM, with higher rates of middle ear disease in African American children than Caucasian children. Caucasian children are more likely to undergo tympanostomy tube insertion, compared with African American or Hispanic children.

Viral upper respiratory tract infections, colonization of the nasopharynx, and eustachian tube dysfunction enable bacteria to invade the middle ear. A child's innate antibacterial defenses are the primary mechanism for preventing AOM. During the early years of life, the immune system is less robust and the eustachian tube dysfunction is more pronounced, leading to increased infections in the young.

Pathogenesis

Approximately 90% of episodes of AOM are associated with a concomitant viral upper respiratory tract infection. Children with AOM are typically colonized with bacterial otopathogens. The earlier in life and the more species they are colonized with, the more likely the children will develop AOM. It is hypothesized that the competition among otopathogens leads to an inflammatory response that causes increased eustachian tube dysfunction and consequent AOM. The most common bacterial pathogens responsible for AOM continue to be *Streptococcus pneumoniae* and nontypable *Haemophilus influenzae.* These two microorganisms are recovered in up to 80 to 90% of children with AOM. Less frequent causes of OM include *Moraxella catarrhalis,* group A streptococcus, *Staphylococcus aureus,* and gram-negative enteric bacteria. Viruses alone cause ~ 20% of AOM, with respiratory syncytial virus (RSV) being the most common virus recovered in AOM.

The microbiology of AOM has changed over the last decade as a result of routine pediatric immunization of the seven-valent pneumococcal conjugate vaccine (PCV7). This vaccine has been shown to reduce the number of pneumococcal AOM cases by ~ 30% and the overall incidence of AOM by ~ 7%. Consequently, there has been an increase in the number of infections due to pneumococcal serotypes not included in the vaccine, as well as an increase in the proportion of nontypable *H. influenzae* and *M. catarrhalis.* Two second-generation pneumococcal conjugated vaccines are in development that will include additional serotypes not currently included in the PCV7. The 2013 AAP guideline on AOM recommends that clinicians recommend the pneumococcal conjugate vaccine and the influenza vaccine to all children according to the schedule of the Advisory Committee on Immunization Practices, AAP, and the American Academy of Family Practice. Antibiotic resistance is increasing among the bacteria causing AOM, with at least one-third of *S. pneumoniae* being penicillin- and amoxicillin-resistant. Macrolide resistance is also an increasing problem. In AOM, at least 20% of *H. influenzae* produces b-lactamase. If signs and symptoms of AOM persist after 48 to 72 hours of antibiotic treatment, it is likely the pathogen is resistant.

■ Diagnosis

In recent years, efforts have been made to standardize the diagnosis and treatment of OM. According to the 2013 AAP guideline on AOM a diagnosis of AOM should be made in children who present with moderate to severe bulging of the tympanic membrane (TM), or new onset of otorrhea not due to acute otitis externa. In addition a diagnosis of AOM can be made if there is mild bulging of the TM *and* recent onset of ear pain (holding, tugging, rubbing of the ear in a nonverbal child) or intense erythema of the TM. Clinicians should not diagnose AOM in children who do not have a middle ear effusion (MEE) based on pneumatic otoscopy and/or tympanometry. Otitis media with effusion (OME) is defined as fluid in the middle ear without signs or symptoms of acute ear infection. The key distinguishing feature between AOM and OME is that only AOM has acute signs and symptoms.

■ Management

Acute Otitis Media

Antibiotic therapy plays a major role in the selection of increasingly resistant bacteria, so the observation option (watchful waiting) has been increasingly advocated over the past several years. Prophylactic antibiotics should *not* be prescribed to reduce the frequency of episodes of AOM in children with recurrent AOM. Antibiotic treatment has not been shown to speed up resolution of middle ear fluid or to prevent the development of asymptomatic MEEs. The AAP's 2013 AOM guidelines recommend an assessment of pain; if pain is present the clinician should recommend treatment to reduce pain. Recommendations for antimicrobial therapy depend on the severity of the symptoms and the age of the patient. For the child with unilateral or bilateral severe AOM (i.e., moderate or severe otalgia or otalgia for at least 48 hours, or temperature 39°C [102.2°F]), who is 6 months of age and older, the clinician should prescribe antibiotic therapy. For nonsevere (mild otalgia for < 48 hours, temperature < 39°C) bilateral AOM in

children younger than 24 months of age, antibiotics should also be prescribed. If the infection is in a child age 6 to 23 months and is unilateral and mild, the clinician can either prescribe antibiotic therapy *or* offer observation with close follow-up based on joint decision making with a parent/caregiver. When observation is recommended, there should be a mechanism in place to ensure follow-up and begin antibiotic therapy if the child worsens or fails to improve within 48 to 72 hours. In the older child (≥ 24 months) with nonsevere AOM the clinician can either prescribe antibiotic therapy *or* offer observation with close follow-up. Children less than 6 months of age should be treated with antibiotics, regardless of whether the diagnosis is certain. Approximately 7 to 10 children must be treated with antibiotics for just one to derive benefit from the treatment.

Should antibiotic treatment be required, current guidelines recommend amoxicillin as the first-line drug of choice in the patient who has not received amoxicillin in the past 30 days and who does not have concurrent purulent conjunctivitis and is not allergic to penicillin. Amoxicillin is generally effective against susceptible and intermediately resistant *S. pneumoniae.* The drug is also safe, inexpensive, tastes good, and has a relatively narrow microbiological spectrum. The recommended dosage is 40 to 90 mg/kg/d, divided into two daily doses. The prescribed dose within this range should be determined based on the incidence of antibiotic resistance in the geographic area. Children who have received amoxicillin in the past 30 days *or* who have concurrent purulent conjunctivitis *or* have a history of recurrent AOM unresponsive to amoxicillin should be prescribed an antibiotic with additional b-lactamase coverage (high-dose amoxicillin–clavulanate). If the initial antibiotic treatment fails the child should be treated with amoxicillin–clavulanate or ceftriaxone.

Symptoms of a type I immunoglobulin (Ig) E-mediated hypersensitivity reaction include urticarial rash, pruritus, flushing, angioedema, wheezing, and/or anaphylaxis. If the patient is allergic to amoxicillin and the allergic reaction was not a type I IgE-mediated hypersensitivity reaction, cefdinir (14 mg/kg/d in one or two doses), cefpodoxime (10 mg/kg/d once daily) or cefuroxime axetil (30 mg/kg/d in two divided doses) can be used. If a type I IgE-mediated hypersensitivity reaction occurred, then azithromycin (10 mg/kg/d on day 1, followed by 5 mg/kg/d for 4 days as a single dose) or clarithromycin (15 mg/kg/d in two divided doses) can be prescribed.

Immediate versus delayed treatment (if symptoms do not resolve within 48–72 hours) with amoxicillin has a modest benefit compared with placebo regarding symptom resolution, but antibiotic use may also be associated with diarrhea and rash. Of 100 average-risk children with AOM, ~ 80 would likely get better within ~ 3 days without antibiotics. If all were treated immediately with amoxicillin, an additional 12 would likely improve, but 3 to 10 children would develop a rash and 5 to 10 diarrhea. No antibiotic has been found to have a higher rate of success than amoxicillin.

Historically, the standard duration of antibiotic therapy for AOM has been 10 days. However, around the world the duration of treatment varies widely, with treatment regimens of 3 to 7 days often being recommended. Treatment with a 5-day course of short-acting antibiotics has been shown to slightly increase the risk of a child's developing signs or symptoms ~ 2 weeks after treatment, although the side effects of the antibiotics are lessened (decreased diarrhea). The trend worldwide is clearly away from the standard North American regimen of 10 days and toward a shorter antibiotic course. Currently, the 2013 AAP guideline recommends a 10 day course in children younger than 2 years, a 7 day course in children 2 to 5 years with mild or moderate AOM, and a 5 to 7 day course for children 6 years and older with mild to moderate symptoms.

Recurrent AOM (defined as three episodes in 6 months or four episodes in a year) continues to be a controversial indication for ventilation tube insertion. The 2013 American Academy of Otolaryngology–Head and Neck Surgery (AAO-HNS) Clinical Practice Guideline on Tympanostomy Tubes in Children recommends that clinicians *not* perform tympanostomy tube insertion in children with recurrent AOM who do not have middle ear effusion in either ear at the time of assessment for tube candidacy. If a unilateral or bilateral MEE is present at the time of assessment then clinicians should offer bilateral tympanostomy tube insertion to children with recurrent AOM. In prospective studies, adenoidectomy has not been found to reduce the number of episodes of AOM.

Chronic Otitis Media with Effusion

Treatment for chronic OME (OME that is present for at least 3 months) has changed considerably over the last decade. Well-designed prospective studies have demonstrated that oral antibiotics, mucolytics, antihistamines, oral decongestants, and topical nasal steroids are not effective. Oral steroids, especially when combined with antibiotic treatment, speed resolution of OME in the short term but have not been shown to have longer-term benefit, and there is no evidence they improve hearing loss. The term *autoinflation* refers to the opening of the eustachian tube by blowing air into it. Autoinflation can be accomplished by forced exhalation with a closed mouth and nose (Valsalva), blowing up a balloon with the nose, or using an anesthetic mask or a Politzer device. Although the data are not extensive,

autoinflation has been shown to hasten resolution of OME compared with a placebo.

When documented bilateral OME has been present for 3 months the chance of spontaneous resolution is ~ 20% within an additional 3 months, 25% after 6 months, and 30% after 1 additional year of observation. According to the 2013 Guideline on Tympanostomy Tubes once OME has been present for 3 months a hearing evaluation is recommended to determine the degree of hearing loss. The average hearing loss in a child with OME is 28 dB, although it can vary from 0 dB to 55 dB. An average hearing level between 0 and 20 dB is considered normal. If hearing loss is identified, and OME has been present for 3 months, tympanostomy tubes should be offered to the patient and family. Tympanostomy tubes should *not* be offered to the children with a single episode of OME of less than 3 months duration. The alternative to tympanostomy tube placement is surveillance at 3 to 6 month intervals, with audiological follow-up as indicated. When considering tympanostomy tubes it is important to identify children at risk for developmental or speech delay who may be more affected by the conductive hearing loss that results from a middle ear effusion. The primary benefits of tympanostomy tube placement are reduced prevalence of middle ear effusion resulting in improved hearing and improved patient and caregiver quality of life. Tubes have been shown to temporarily improve hearing by ~ 12 dB at 3 months and 4 dB at 6 to 9 months, but no improvement has been found at 12 to 18 months following surgery. This is not surprising, given that short-term grommet-style tubes were used in most studies. The expected longevity and risks of tympanostomy tubes should be discussed with the patient's caregivers prior to surgery. If OME has been present for 3 months but the child does not have documented hearing loss tympanostomy tubes may be considered if other symptoms are likely attributable to the OME such as vestibular dysfunction, poor school performance, behavioral problems, or ear pain. Similarly if OME has been present for 3 months in a developmentally at-risk child, and the effusion is unlikely to resolve quickly (i.e., child with Down syndrome or cleft palate), tympanostomy tubes can be considered. Children who do *not* have documented hearing loss or any of the preceding findings likely attributable to OME can safely be observed for 6 to 12 months without developmental sequelae or reduced quality of life. If a child is scheduled to undergo tympanostomy tube placement the caregivers should be educated regarding the expected duration of tube function, recommended follow-up schedule, and detection of complications. Clinicians should *not* encourage routine, prophylactic water precautions for children with tympanostomy tubes.

■ Controversial Issues

Recommendations for the treatment of AOM and OME have changed considerably over the past decade but have become clearer since the publication of the 2013 AAP Clinical Practice Guideline on Acute Otitis Media and the 2013 AAO-HNS Clinical Practice Guideline on tympanostomy tubes in children. There are stringent guidelines for the diagnosis of AOM and clear trends toward less antibiotic use and more watchful waiting. Recommendations for tympanostomy tube placement have been clarified for the first time with recommendations for fewer tube placements in children with recurrent AOM without middle ear effusions, and the increased use of hearing screening to help in the decision making regarding tube placement in children with OME.

■ Practice Guidelines, Consensus Statements, and Measures

Lieberthal AS, Carroll AE, Chonmaitree T, et al. The diagnosis and management of acute otitis media [published correction in Pediatrics 2014;133(2):346. Dosage error in article text]. Pediatrics 2013;131(3):e964–e999 doi; 10.1542/peds.2012-3488

Rosenfeld RM, Culpepper L, Doyle KJ, et al; American Academy of Pediatrics Subcommittee on Otitis Media with Effusion; American Academy of Family Physicians; American Academy of Otolaryngology--Head and Neck Surgery. Clinical practice guideline: Otitis media with effusion. Otolaryngol Head Neck Surg 2004;130(5, Suppl): S95–S118

Rosenfeld RM, Schwartz SR, Pynnonen MA, et al. Clinical practice guideline: Tympanostomy tubes in children. Otolaryngol Head Neck Surg 2013;149(1, Suppl):S1–S35 doi: 10.1177/0194599813487302

■ Suggested Reading

Azarpazhooh A, Limeback H, Lawrence HP, Shah PS. Xylitol for preventing acute otitis media in children up to 12 years of age. Cochrane Database Syst Rev 2011;(11):CD007095

Browning GG, Rovers MM, Williamson I, Lous J, Burton MJ. Grommets (ventilation tubes) for hearing loss associated with otitis media with effusion in children. Cochrane Database Syst Rev 2010; (10):CD001801

Burton MJ, Derkay CS, Rosenfeld RM. Extracts from the Cochrane Library: "Grommets (ventilation tubes) for hearing loss associated with otitis media with effusion in children". Otolaryngol Head Neck Surg 2011;144(5):657–661

Coker TR, Chan LS, Newberry SJ, et al. Diagnosis, microbial epidemiology, and antibiotic treatment of acute otitis media in children: a systematic review. JAMA 2010;304(19):2161–2169

Damoiseaux RA, Rovers MM. AOM in children. Clin Evid (Online) 2011;2011

Griffin G, Flynn CA. Antihistamines and/or decongestants for otitis media with effusion (OME) in children. Cochrane Database Syst Rev 2011;(9):CD003423

Hellström S, Groth A, Jörgensen F, et al. Ventilation tube treatment: a systematic review of the literature. Otolaryngol Head Neck Surg 2011;145(3):383–395

Kozyrskyj A, Klassen TP, Moffatt M, Harvey K. Short-course antibiotics for acute otitis media. Cochrane Database Syst Rev 2010;(9):CD001095

Leibovitz E, Broides A, Greenberg D, Newman N. Current management of pediatric acute otitis media. Expert Rev Anti Infect Ther 2010;8(2):151–161

Lous J, Ryborg CT, Thomsen JL. A systematic review of the effect of tympanostomy tubes in children with recurrent acute otitis media. Int J Pediatr Otorhinolaryngol 2011;75(9):1058–1061

Pelton SI, Leibovitz E. Recent advances in otitis media. Pediatr Infect Dis J 2009;28(10, Suppl):S133–S137

Perera R, Haynes J, Glasziou P, Heneghan CJ. Autoinflation for hearing loss associated with otitis media with effusion. Cochrane Database Syst Rev 2006;(4):CD006285

Rosenfeld RM, Jang DW, Tarashansky K. Tympanostomy tube outcomes in children at-risk and not at-risk for developmental delays. Int J Pediatr Otorhinolaryngol 2011;75(2):190–195

Simpson SA, Lewis R, van der Voort J, Butler CC. Oral or topical nasal steroids for hearing loss associated with otitis media with effusion in children. Cochrane Database Syst Rev 2011;(5):CD001935

Smith DF, Boss EF. Racial/ethnic and socioeconomic disparities in the prevalence and treatment of otitis media in children in the United States. Laryngoscope 2010;120(11):2306–2312

van den Aardweg MT, Schilder AG, Herkert E, Boonacker CW, Rovers MM. Adenoidectomy for otitis media in children. Cochrane Database Syst Rev 2010;(1):CD007810

Vergison A, Dagan R, Arguedas A, et al. Otitis media and its consequences: beyond the earache. Lancet Infect Dis 2010;10(3): 195–203

72 Pediatric Congenital Sensorineural Hearing Loss

◼ Introduction

This chapter provides the practicing otolaryngologist with an algorithm for the evaluation and management of children with congenital sensorineural hearing loss (SNHL). Within the team of hearing loss specialists—including audiologists, geneticists, speech-language pathologists, social workers, and educators—the otolaryngologist has the role of performing a comprehensive history and complete head and neck examination, coordinating diagnostic testing to determine the etiology of the hearing loss, and directing appropriate medical or surgical interventions. This chapter discusses the rationale and background information for a diagnostic algorithm that will enable the otolaryngologist to provide optimal care for children with congenital SNHL.

Early identification and intervention of congenital SNHL are critical to avoid serious detrimental consequences on a child's speech, language, academic, emotional, and social development. In the early 1990s, both the Joint Committee on Infant Hearing (JCIH) and the National Institutes of Health's National Institute of Deafness and Communication Disorders (NIH-NIDCD) issued recommendations for universal newborn hearing screening (UNHS). The most recent JCIH statement in 2007 outlines the goals for screening, evaluation, intervention, and surveillance for hearing loss. In an effort to optimize outcomes for children with hearing loss, JCIH recommends UNHS by 1 month of age, comprehensive audiological evaluation for "referred" infants by 3 months of age, and appropriate intervention for those with confirmed hearing loss by 6 months of age. The 2007 JCIH update also includes recommendations for the surveillance of children with delayed-onset hearing loss and auditory neuropathy or auditory dyssynchrony (AN/AD). The American Academy of Audiology has also recently published guidelines for hearing screening of children from 6 months of age through the teenage years. Both the

NIH-NIDCD and the Centers for Disease Control and Prevention (CDC) have established data tracking systems to verify progress of universal screening and intervention services.

With the advent of UNHS, most children with congenital hearing loss are detected soon after birth. With an incidence of nearly 3 per 1,000 children born in the United States, hearing loss is the most common birth defect, with the vast majority of these losses being SNHL. According to the CDC Early Hearing Detection and Intervention data from 2009, more than 97% of the births in the United States underwent newborn hearing screening, and 1.4 of 1,000 newborns screened were diagnosed with hearing impairment; however, many children will present later in childhood, either because they were not screened at birth (e.g., home births), or as a result of progressive or delayed expression of a congenital etiology. At 4 years of age, the incidence of SNHL increases significantly, from 186 per 100,000 live births to 270 per 100,000. This fact underscores the importance of continued surveillance, especially for children at risk for hearing loss.

Genetic Hearing Loss

Roughly 30 to 50% of childhood SNHL is due to genetic factors, with the remainder due to acquired factors or factors that are not currently recognized as inheritable. These proportions will vary with the population, depending on access to immunization programs and perinatal care. As our understanding of the interaction between genetic etiologies and environmental factors advances, some causes thought to be acquired may be found to have a significant genetic basis or predisposition, such as the mitochondrial MTRNR1 gene, which predisposes the individual to aminoglycoside ototoxicity.

Approximately 30% of children diagnosed with genetic SNHL have other abnormalities and are designated as having syndromic SNHL. The concept of syndromic versus nonsyndromic SNHL is evolving. Advances in diagnostic genetic testing have made these traditional classifications less meaningful. Should a child's SNHL with an identified genetic cause and an associated enlarged vestibular aqueduct (EVA) on imaging or a specific auditory phenotype (e.g., AN/AD) be considered syndromic or nonsyndromic? To complicate matters further, we now recognize that one syndrome may be the result of mutations in several different genes (genetic heterogeneity) or that one gene may cause more than one phenotype (genetic pleiotropy).

The majority of SNHL syndromes have autosomal-recessive (AR) inheritance, compared with roughly 20% having autosomal-dominant (AD) inheritance, and only a small fraction have X-linked or mitochondrial inheritance. For nonsyndromic SNHL cases, current genetic research has identified more than 40 genes with AR inheritance (designated deafness B or DFNB), 25 genes with AD inheritance (designated DFNA), and 3 genes with X-linked inheritance (designated DFNX). Some genes may have both AD and AR inheritance patterns, such as the connexin gene GJB2 (DFNA3A and DFNB1A). In addition, SNHL may be caused by mutations in two complementary genes, such as GJB2 and GJB6. Finally, a single gene may cause both syndromic and nonsyndromic SNHL (e.g., the SLC2A4 gene causing Pendred syndrome or DFNB4). **Table 72.1** presents details of gene products and inheritance patterns for common syndromic and nonsyndromic SNHL.

Pathophysiology and Embryology

It is important for the clinician to have an understanding of the pathophysiology and embryology that lead to congenital SNHL. A dysfunction anywhere within the complex auditory system may result in SNHL. Much of our current understanding of the molecular pathophysiology of SNHL stems from the study of gene expression in the cochlea. An important example of this is the recognition that the connexin genes (e.g., GJB2 and GJB6) code for gap junction proteins that we now know are responsible for the recycling of potassium and maintenance of the endocochlear potential.

A failure of any step in the development of the cochlea will result in the anatomical characteristics of that developmental stage. An otocyst forms at the 4th week of gestation with invagination of the otic placode, and progresses to the fully formed cochlea at 22 to 24 weeks. Complete labyrinthine aplasia (Michel aplasia) stems from arrest in development prior to the 4th week and the formation of the otocyst. If inner ear development stops at the 4th week, a common cavity deformity (essentially an otocyst)

may form. Arrested development at the 5th week may result in a pear-shaped structure (cochlear agenesis). If development ceases at the 6th week, the patient will have cochlear hypoplasia with some rudimentary differentiation of cochlear structures, but without the spiral turns of the cochlea. If development is halted between the 6th and 11th weeks, the cochlear turns will not be completed and the interscalar septum will be absent, resulting in Mondini deformity. A cochlea with complete turns but failed membranous labyrinthine development (Scheibe cochleosaccular dysplasia) occurs after the 12th week. The final stage of cochlear development involves sequential ossification of the otic capsule from the 14th to the 22nd week. The last portion of the otic capsule to ossify is the bone overlying the superior and posterior semicircular canals, the failure of which may result in semicircular canal dehiscence. Because the inner ear is fully mature by 22 to 24 weeks of gestation, the otolaryngologist should pay particular attention to any potentially teratogenic events during the first half of pregnancy.

■ Evaluation: Diagnostic Algorithm

Fig. 72.1 presents a stepwise approach to the diagnosis of congenital SNHL, based on the child's individual history and clinical findings, including physical examination, audiometry, and laboratory and imaging studies. By using this algorithm, the otolaryngologist can avoid unnecessary and costly tests. The otolaryngologist may ask a series of questions listed in this section that will ultimately lead to a diagnosis specific to the child. The order of these questions may vary slightly, depending on the age of the child, severity of the SNHL, and family concerns.

Is There Any History of Perinatal Risk Factors?

The otolaryngologist should first determine if the child has a history of any known risk factors. History should include an inquiry about toxic exposure during early pregnancy, intrauterine infections, Apgar scores, postnatal infections, respiratory distress, jaundice, medications, postnatal meningitis, or other neonatal complications. The otolaryngologist should also ask about other medical problems, such as eye or renal disease. Finally, a detailed inquiry should be made about any family members with hearing loss prior to the age of 40 years or with history of sudden death. In 2007, the JCIH revised the list of risk indicators associated with hearing loss in children

Table 72.1 Genetic causes of hearing loss

Syndrome	Gene(s)	Inheritance	Clinical features	Cochlear expression
Usher type I	MYO7A USH1Cª CDH23ª PCDH15 USH1G (SANS)	AR	Retinitis pigmentosaª in 1st decade Vestibular dysfunction Congenital profound SNHL	Stereocilia
Usher type II	USH2A GPR98/VLGR1 DFNB31/WHRN	AR	Retinitis pigmentosa in 1st–2nd decade Normal vestibular function Congenital sloping SNHL	Stereocilia
Usher type III	CLRN1(USH3A)	AR	Variable onset of retinitis pigmentosa Variable vestibular function Progressive SNHL	Stereocilia
Waardenburg type I	PAX3	AR	Dystopia canthorum Pigmentary abnormalities SNHL	Melanocytes
Waardenburg type II	MITF SNAI2	AR	No dystopia canthorum Pigmentary abnormalities Variable SNHL	Melanocytes
Jervell Lange-Nielsen	KCNQ1 KCNE1	AR	Prolonged QT Interval on EKG Syncope/sudden death Profound SNHL	Potassium channels
Branchio-oto-renal (BOR)	EYA1 SIX1 SIX5	AD	Branchial cysts/fistulae Urinary collecting system dysplasia Cataracts (variable) Conductive hearing loss or SNHL	N/A
Pendred	SLC26A4	AR	Goiter (failure of iodine organification) Enlarged vestibular aqueduct SNHL (goiter may be absent— nonsyndromic)	Endolymphatic sac/ duct Saccule/utricle
Alport	COLA3 COLA4 COL4A5	AD AR X-Linked	Variable onset glomerulonephritis Variable anterior lenticonus/ cataracts Progressive/variable SNHL	Basilar membrane Spiral ligament Stria vascularis
Nonsyndromic				
DFNB1A DFNA3A DFNB1B	GJB2 GJB2 GJB6	AR AD AR	Severe to profound SNHL	Connexin gap function proteins in spiral ligament
DFNB9	OTOF	AR	Auditory neuropathy/dyssynchrony	Hair cell synapses
Mitochondrial	MTRNR1	Mitochondrial	Aminoglycoside induced/worsened SNHL	N/A

Abbreviations: AD, autosomal dominant; AR, autosomal recessive; EKG, electrocardiogram; N/A, not applicable; SNHL, sensorineural hearing loss.

ª May also be nonsyndromic.

to include acquired, genetic, delayed-onset, and progressive hearing loss as shown in **Table 72.2**. In recent studies of neonatal intensive care unit (NICU) graduates, only intrauterine TORCH (toxoplasmosis, other [syphilis], rubella, cytomegalovirus, herpes simplex virus) infections, craniofacial abnormalities, known SNHL syndromes, bacterial meningitis, or asphyxiation were identified as significant independent risk factors for SNHL. Some risk factors that deserve special consideration are highlighted next.

In Utero TORCH Infections

Cytomegalovirus (CMV)

The most important of the TORCH intrauterine infections, cytomegalovirus (CMV) infections occur in 0.4 to 2.3% of all newborns, 85 to 90% of which are asymptomatic. CMV-associated SNHL can vary in severity, laterality, onset, and progression and is the most common cause of late-onset, prelinguistic

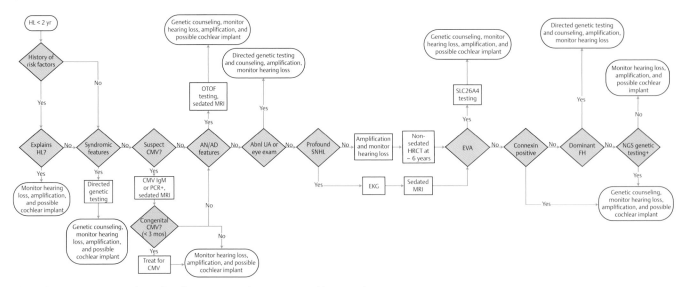

Fig. 72.1 Diagnostic algorithm for congenital sensorineural hearing loss.

SNHL, and unilateral SNHL in infancy. SNHL is identified in roughly 7% of asymptomatic CMV-infected babies and may present as progressive (50%), delayed (18%), or fluctuating (22%). Overall, CMV is believed to account for approximately 20% of nonsyndromic congenital SNHL cases and treatment for CMV in young infants has been shown to improve hearing loss outcomes. Therefore, diligent screening and frequent surveillance are critical when CMV-related SNHL hearing loss is suspected.

Since CMV is ubiquitous and seropositivity may be due to acquired infection in children > 3 weeks of age, the diagnosis of intrauterine CMV infection can be difficult. Roughly, 25% of infants will be seropositive for CMV by 7 months of age. The presence of CMV infection may be confirmed by elevated serum immunoglobulin M (IgM), or the virus itself may be identified in urine or saliva using polymerase chain reaction (PCR) or in culture. Positive CMV IgM or PCR samples obtained within the first 3 weeks of life are diagnostic, and positive samples taken within the first 3 months in the context of SNHL are highly suggestive for congenital CMV infection. Characteristic MRI findings (e.g., cerebellar hypoplasia and abnormal myelination) may also be helpful in confirming the diagnosis of congenital CMV in an older child. One creative approach to confirm the diagnosis is to retroactively test the dried blood spot (DBS) samples from birth if these are available. Antiviral treatment (ganciclovir) should be initiated in confirmed cases if they are identified within the first few months of life.

NICU Stay > 5 Days or Hypoxia Requiring Extracorporeal Membrane Oxygenation or Assisted Ventilation

In these cases, the inner ear is highly metabolically active. Even brief periods of hypoxia may result in permanent SNHL. Neonatal respiratory distress most commonly from prematurity, as evidenced by low Apgar scores or prolonged ventilatory support, has been shown to be an independent risk factor for hearing loss.

Hyperbilirubinemia

Infants with hyperbilirubinemia with neurological sequelae (kernicterus) or requiring exchange transfusions are certainly at high risk for hearing loss. These patients are also at risk for AN/AD. In one study of neonates requiring exchange transfusion for hyperbilirubinemia, 46% developed AN/AD.

Neonatal Meningitis

Meningitis is a significant risk for hearing loss in children of any age, with the highest prevalence in those less than 4 years of age. In addition to *Streptococcus pneumoniae*, meningitis within the first month of life is commonly caused by group B *Streptococcus*, *Escherichia coli*, or *Listeria monocytogenes*. Steroid administration reduces the incidence of SNHL. Children under 2 years old and those with pneumococ-

Table 72.2 High-risk indicators and associated frequency of hearing loss

High-risk indicator	Frequency of SNHL in children with risk indicator (%)
Caregiver concerns (re: hearing, speech, language, or developmental delay)	< 10
Family history of permanent childhood hearing loss	> 15
Neonatal intensive care unit (NICU) stay for more than 5 days	< 15
ECMO	> 20
Assisted ventilation or severe asphyxia	> 15
Ototoxic medications (aminoglycosides or loop diuretics)	< 10
Hyperbilirubinemia requiring exchange transfusion	< 20
In utero (TORCH) infections	> 15
Craniofacial anomalies	> 50
Physical findings or known syndromes associated with hearing loss	< 10
Postnatal infections associated with SNHL (e.g., meningitis)	> 10
Head trauma, especially temporal bone trauma requiring hospitalization	< 10
Chemotherapy	< 10

Abbreviations: ECMO, extracorporeal membrane oxygenation; SNHL, sensorineural hearing loss; TORCH, toxoplasmosis, other (syphilis), rubella, cytomegalovirus, herpes simplex virus.

cal infections are at the highest risk for SNHL. One important feature of bacterial meningitis is the possibility of cochlear osteoneogenesis (labyrinthitis ossificans). Intracochlear fibrosis and bone growth may begin to form within weeks of infection and may eventually prevent the placement of a cochlear implant. Therefore, it is imperative that children with meningitis are evaluated promptly for the possibility of SNHL and that the option of early cochlear implantation is discussed with the family in cases of profound hearing loss.

Do These Risk Factors Adequately Explain the Hearing Loss?

The answer to this question will depend on the risk factor exposure and the severity of the hearing loss. If the hearing loss is adequately explained by the exposure, additional diagnostic workup may not be necessary. As can be seen in **Table 72.2**, the actual frequency of SNHL in children with risk factors may be relatively low. A pneumococcal meningitis infection that temporally correlates with the onset of the SNHL does not need further evaluation, whereas further testing is recommended for severe hearing loss in a case with mild jaundice or uncomplicated prematurity. In general, the otolaryngologist should be somewhat skeptical of presumed explanations for SNHL and should pursue additional studies if suspicion for other etiologies arises.

Is there Evidence of Syndromic Features on Physical Exam?

A complete, age-appropriate head and neck examination should be performed, with particular attention to clinical features of syndromic hearing loss. **Table 72.3** presents a list of physical exam findings associated with some known hearing loss syndromes. If syndromic features are present, a directed genetic evaluation for those syndromes should be considered, along with genetic counseling.

Usher Syndrome

Usher syndrome is characterized by retinitis pigmentosa and SNHL. The three types of Usher syndrome vary in onset and severity of the SNHL, onset of the retinitis pigmentosa, and presence of vestibular symptoms (see **Table 72.1**). The potential development of blindness in Usher syndrome may make visually based communication (sign language) difficult. Retinal findings are generally not present until later in childhood or adolescence, but preclinical signs can be seen with electroretinography. The use of this test for the diagnosis of Usher syndrome has been largely supplanted by genetic testing.

Table 72.3 Physical findings associated with hearing loss

Areas examined	Physical signs	Associated syndromes
Ears	Preauricular pits	—
	Auricular malformations	Branchiootorenal
Eyes	Retinitis pigmentosa	Usher
	Dystopia canthorum	Waardenburg
	Heterochromia irides	Waardenburg
	Coloboma	CHARGE
	Cataracts	Rubella
	Keratitis	Cogan
	Severe myopia	Stickler
Neck	Goiter	Pendred
	Branchial cysts/fistulas	BOR
Musculoskeletal	Fusion of vertebrae	Klippel–Feil
	Dwarfism	Achondroplasia
Integumentary	White forelock	Waardenburg
	Hypopigmentation	Albinism
	Ectodermal dysplasia	Ichthyosis
Neurological	Ataxia	—
	Mental retardation	—

Abbreviation: CHARGE, coloboma of the eye, heart anomaly, choanal atresia, retardation, genital and ear anomalies.

Waardenburg Syndrome

Waardenburg syndrome is characterized by a variable penetrance and phenotype with four classifications. Type I is the most common, with the clinical features of dystopia canthorum and pigmentation abnormalities (heterochromia irides and white forelock). Type II is differentiated by the absence of dystopia canthorum. SNHL occurs in 2 to 50% of Waardenburg cases.

Jervell and Lange-Nielsen Syndrome

This syndrome is characterized by severe-to-profound SNHL and a prolonged QT interval on electrocardiogram (EKG), with potential for syncope and even sudden death. Otolaryngologists should obtain an EKG on all infants having severe-to-profound SNHL or those with a family history of sudden infant death.

Branchiootorenal (BOR) Syndrome

Branchiootorenal (BOR) syndrome is associated with a variety of abnormalities of branchial development, the external ear, and the urinary collecting system. The hearing loss may be conductive, mixed, or sensorineural. Clinical examination may reveal branchial cleft sinus, cyst, or fistula or preauricular sinus or auricular deformity. The urinary anomalies can be detected by renal ultrasonography and may present with recurrent urinary tract infections or urinalysis abnormalities.

Pendred Syndrome

Pendred syndrome is associated with EVA and thyroid goiter (abnormal perchlorate discharge test). Most patients are euthyroid, but they may be hypothyroid or hyperthyroid. Patients with mutations of the same gene (SLC26A4) may also present with nonsyndromic SNHL and EVA without goiter.

Are There Audiometric Features of Auditory Neuropathy/Dyssynchrony?

AN/AD is characterized by an auditory brainstem response (ABR) that is absent, except for the cochlear microphonic and present otoacoustic emissions. An AN/AD pattern may be seen in an immature auditory system, especially in premature neonates; therefore, the ABR should be repeated after 1 year of age. AN/AD may be due to genetic (i.e., otoferlin or OTOF gene) or acquired (e.g., kernicterus) causes. Children with AN/AD should be evaluated with an OTOF genetic test, and cochlear implantation may be considered.

Are There Abnormalities on the Urinalysis or on an Ophthalmology Consult?

Routine diagnostic testing of all children with congenital SNHL has been shown to have a low yield; however, directed laboratory testing and specialized (ophthalmology, cardiology, nephrology) consultations may supplement the clinical examination. A urinalysis is inexpensive and may provide evidence of latent renal disease that would not be apparent on physical examination. Findings of hematuria or proteinuria may prompt a renal ultrasound, nephrology consult, and genetic testing for BOR or Alport syndrome. Likewise, findings from an ophthalmological exam may reveal retinitis pigmentosa, cataracts, or myopia and may prompt genetic testing for Usher, Alport, or Stickler syndrome.

Is the SNHL Severe or Profound?

Individuals with early onset of severe-to-profound SNHL should have an EKG to evaluate for prolonged QT to rule out Jervell and Lange-Nielsen syndrome. Although this diagnosis is relatively rare, a missed diagnosis may result in sudden infant death. If the child has severe or profound SNHL, the otolaryngologist should discuss communication strategies and possible cochlear implantation with the family. If cochlear implantation is under consideration, imaging of the cochlea is required. For children who are not cochlear implant candidates, a computed tomographic (CT) scan can be delayed until 5 to 6 years of age, so that it can be performed without sedation. If imaging is required, magnetic resonance imaging (MRI) scan with high-resolution T2-weighted fast imaging employing steady-state acquisition (FIESTA) images outlining fluid in the labyrinth, vestibular aqueduct, and internal auditory canal is the study of choice in preparation for cochlear implantation, especially if there is a history of meningitis or a concern for other central nervous system (CNS) pathology. Fibrosis of the labyrinth in early labyrinthitis ossificans can be seen on an MRI scan before calcification is seen on a CT scan. Likewise, cochlear nerve hypoplasia may be present even if the bony internal auditory canal (IAC) is normal and can only be seen on an MRI scan.

Are There Abnormalities, Such as Mondini Deformity or EVA, on Imaging?

Imaging of the ear can determine an underlying etiology for hearing loss in roughly 10 to 20% of cases. Imaging is required in preparation for cochlear implantation as already mentioned, and may provide prognostic information. The optimal timing and imaging modality (MRI vs. CT scan) must be weighed against the risk of radiation exposure (CT) and need for anesthesia for sedation (MRI). A high-resolution temporal bone CT scan without contrast demonstrates the bony anatomy of the labyrinth and temporal bone. CT may be performed without sedation in older children and is the study of choice for mixed hearing loss or when semicircular canal dehiscence is suspected. An MRI scan has some advantages, as already discussed, and has no radiation exposure, but, as mentioned, is more likely to require sedation.

EVA is the most common imaging abnormality found in children with congenital SNHL. An EVA is considered if the diameter of the vestibular aqueduct is > 1 mm in its midportion. SNHL associated with EVA is often progressive and may be aggravated by relatively minor head injuries. Therefore, children with EVA are generally advised to avoid participation in contact sports. Approximately 40% of EVA cases will have a mutation in the Pendred syndrome gene SLC26A4, with no evidence of goiter. If EVA is diagnosed, an SLC26A4 gene test should be requested. The finding of cochlear dysplasia or Mondini deformity on imaging also influences the diagnostic inquiry. Imaging abnormalities are uncommon in GJB2-related SNHL. If there is no evidence of EVA or other abnormalities on imaging, or if the family wishes to defer imaging until the child is older, a genetic test for GJB2 and GJB6 should be considered.

Is the Genetic Testing Positive for GJB2 or GJB6 Mutation?

Genetic testing can provide the etiologic diagnosis of hearing loss and can supply the medical providers, patients, and families with data to aid in management and intervention of children with SNHL. For example, patients with GJB2/GJB6 SNHL have statistically better outcomes after cochlear implantation. Because mutations in the GJB2 genes account for 30 to 40% of nonsyndromic SNHL in developed countries, genetic testing generally begins with an analysis of these genes. The most common GJB2 mutation in Caucasians is the 35delG mutation, but the prevalence of specific GJB2 mutations varies with ethnicity. Therefore, mutation-specific testing is rarely adequate. Other connexin genes (GJB6, GJB3) are also significant contributors to congenital SNHL, and biallelic (GJB2 and GJB6) mutations may present with variable degrees of SNHL. Nearly 20% of GJB2-related SNHL is progressive. If pathogenic mutations are discovered on GJB2 or GJB6 genetic testing, the family should be referred for genetic counseling, and the hearing loss should be managed appropriately. If the connexin tests are negative, more comprehensive genetic testing by next generation sequencing that includes other nonsyndromic, mitochondrial, and syndromic genetic causes of SNHL should be considered.

Are There Pathogenic Mutations Identified on Next-Generation Sequencing-Based Gene Panels?

With more than 110 loci and more than 65 genes identified that cause nonsyndromic SNHL, the decision of which genes to test and the interpretation of these results can be challenging. Physicians may use the results of diagnostic tests and imaging to choose the appropriate genetic tests. Parallel next-generation sequencing (NGS) analysis of most of the SNHL genes is now available. One example of this technology is the OtoGenome, which tests for 70 SNHL genes simultaneously. Because the test for a single gene can have higher sensitivity and lower cost than parallel sequencing tests, most centers recommend a tiered approach, with testing for GJB2 and GJB6 mutations first.

Genetic counseling should be recommended in cases with positive genetic test results. Additional consultations may be requested if other organ systems are implicated. For example, a child with a genetic test for Usher, Alport, or Stickler syndrome should be referred to an ophthalmologist for evaluation and monitoring. Similarly, aminoglycosides should be avoided at all costs in children with mitochondrial hearing loss related to the MTRNR1 gene.

■ Practice Guidelines, Consensus Statements, and Measures

American Academy of Audiology. Childhood Hearing Screening Guidelines. September 2011. http://www.cdc.gov/ncbddd/hearing loss/documents/AAA_Childhood%20Hearing%20Guidelines_ 2011.pdf

Joint Committee on Infant Hearing. Year 2007 Position Statement: Principles and Guidelines for Early Hearing Detection and Intervention Programs. http://www.cdc.gov/ncbddd/hearingloss/ documents/JCIH_2007.pdf and http://pediatrics.aappublications .org/content/120/4/898.full.pdf+html

U.S. Preventive Services Task Force. Universal Screening for Hearing Loss in Newborns, Recommendation Statement. http://www .uspreventiveservicestaskforce.org/uspstf08/newbornhear/ newbhearrs.htm

■ Management

After diagnosis of the etiology of SNHL, management focuses on routine monitoring of hearing loss and aural habilitation. Surgical management is limited to tympanostomy tube placement for SNHL children with recurrent acute otitis media or otitis media with effusion, and cochlear implantation in selected children.

Aural Habilitation

Infants have a critical period for speech and language development, so it is important that auditory stimulation begin as soon after birth as possible. For those children with hearing loss, aural habilitation with a hearing aid trial and speech therapy should begin immediately (preferably prior to 6 months of age) and should never be delayed while searching for a specific diagnosis. A hearing aid trial is indicated regardless of the severity of the SNHL, but it should be approached cautiously in children with AN/AD. Aggressive amplification in these children may result in noise-induced hair cell loss. Families of children with profound SNHL should be counseled regarding long-term communications options, including sign language education or cochlear implantation. Although somewhat controversial, there appears to be no contraindication to a family's augmenting aural communication with sign language, especially in the face of profound SNHL. Details of pediatric aural habilitation and communication options can be found elsewhere.

■ Suggested Reading

Albert S, Blons H, Jonard L, et al. SLC26A4 gene is frequently involved in nonsyndromic hearing impairment with enlarged vestibular aqueduct in Caucasian populations. Eur J Hum Genet 2006;14(6):773–779

American Academy of Audiology. Childhood Hearing Screening Guidelines. http://www.cdc.gov/ncbddd/hearingloss/documents/AAA_Childhood%20Hearing%20Guidelines_2011.pdf. Accessed July 2012

American Academy of Pediatrics. Joint Committee on Infant Hearing 1994 position statement. Pediatrics 1995;95(1):152–156

American Academy of Pediatrics. Joint Committee on Infant Hearing. Year 2007 position statement: Principles and guidelines for early hearing detection and intervention programs. Pediatrics 2007;120(4):898–921

Centers for Disease Control and Prevention. Hearing Loss in Children. http://www.cdc.gov/ncbddd/hearingloss/index.html

Centers for Disease Control and Prevention. Summary of 2009 National CDC EDHI Data. http://www.cdc.gov/ncbddd/hearingloss/2009-Data/2009_EHDI_HSFS_Summary_508_OK.pdf. Accessed July 2012

Cincinnati Children's Hospital Medical Center, Molecular Genetics Laboratory and the Ear and Hearing Center. Genetic Testing for Hearing Loss. http://www.cincinnatichildrens.org/service/g/genetic-hearing-loss/tests/. Accessed July 2011

Cone-Wesson B, Vohr BR, Sininger YS, et al. Identification of neonatal hearing impairment: infants with hearing loss. Ear Hear 2000;21(5):488–507

Demmler GJ. Infectious Diseases Society of America and Centers for Disease Control. Summary of a workshop on surveillance for congenital cytomegalovirus disease. Rev Infect Dis 1991;13(2):315–329

Denoyelle F, Weil D, Maw MA, et al. Prelingual deafness: high prevalence of a 30delG mutation in the connexin 26 gene. Hum Mol Genet 1997;6(12):2173–2177

Fowler KB, McCollister FP, Dahle AJ, Boppana S, Britt WJ, Pass RF. Progressive and fluctuating sensorineural hearing loss in children with asymptomatic congenital cytomegalovirus infection. J Pediatr 1997;130(4):624–630

Green GE, Scott DA, McDonald JM, Woodworth GG, Sheffield VC, Smith RJ. Carrier rates in the midwestern United States for GJB2 mutations causing inherited deafness. JAMA 1999;281(23):2211–2216

Hille ET, van Straaten HI, Verkerk PH; Dutch NICU Neonatal Hearing Screening Working Group. Prevalence and independent risk factors for hearing loss in NICU infants. Acta Paediatr 2007;96(8):1155–1158

Jackler RK. Congenital malformations of the inner ear. In: Flint PW, ed. Cummings Otolaryngology–Head and Neck Surgery. 5th ed. Philadelphia, PA: Mosby Elsevier; 2010

Lee KH, Larson DA, Shott G, et al. Audiologic and temporal bone imaging findings in patients with sensorineural hearing loss and GJB2 mutations. Laryngoscope 2009;119(3):554–558

Meyer C, Witte J, Hildmann A, et al. Neonatal screening for hearing disorders in infants at risk: incidence, risk factors, and follow-up. Pediatrics 1999;104(4 Pt 1):900–904

Morton CC, Nance WE. Newborn hearing screening—a silent revolution. N Engl J Med 2006;354(20):2151–2164

National Institute on Deafness and Other Communications Disorders. Quick Statistics. http://www.nidcd.nih.gov/health/statistics/Pages/quick.aspx. Accessed July 2012

National Institutes of Health. Early Identification of Hearing Impairment in Infants and Young Children: NIH Consensus Development Conference Statement. Vol 11. Bethesda, MD: National Institutes of Health; 1993:1–24. http://consensus.nih.gov/1993/1993HearingInfantsChildren092html.htm

Partners HealthCare Center for Personalized Genetic Medicine, Laboratory for Molecular Medicine. Hearing Loss Gene Tests. http://pcpgm.partners.org/lmm/tests/hearing-loss. Accessed July 2011

Rao A, Schimmenti LA, Vestal E, et al. Genetic testing in childhood hearing loss: review and case studies. Audiology Online 2011. http://www.audiologyonline.com/articles/article_detail.asp?article_id=2376

Saluja S, Agarwal A, Kler N, Amin S. Auditory neuropathy spectrum disorder in late preterm and term infants with severe jaundice. Int J Pediatr Otorhinolaryngol 2010;74(11):1292–1297

Shearer AE, DeLuca AP, Hildebrand MS, et al. Comprehensive genetic testing for hereditary hearing loss using massively parallel sequencing. Proc Natl Acad Sci U S A 2010;107(49):21104–21109

Smith RJH, Bale JF Jr, White KR. Sensorineural hearing loss in children. Lancet 2005;365(9462):879–890

Smith RJH, Shearer AE, Hildebrand MS, et al. Deafness and hereditary hearing loss overview. (Feb 14, 1999. Updated Jan 5, 2012.) In: Pagon RA, Bird TD, Dolan CR, et al., eds. GeneReviews™. Seattle, WA: University of Washington; 2012. http://www.ncbi.nlm.nih.gov/books/NBK1434/July

Speleman K, Kneepkens K, Vandendriessche K, Debruyne F, Desloovere C. Prevalence of risk factors for sensorineural hearing loss in NICU newborns. B-ENT 2012;8(1):1–6

Van Camp G, Smith RJH. The Hereditary Hearing Loss Homepage. 2010. http://www.hereditaryhearingloss.org. Accessed July 2011

Van Riper LA, Kileny PR. ABR hearing screening for high-risk infants. Am J Otol 1999;20(4):516–521

Wangemann P. Supporting sensory transduction: cochlear fluid homeostasis and the endocochlear potential. J Physiol 2006;576(Pt 1):11–21

Withrow KA, Tracy KA, Burton SK, et al. Impact of genetic advances and testing for hearing loss: results from a national consumer survey. Am J Med Genet A 2009;149A(6):1159–1168

Yoshinaga-Itano C, Baca RL, Sedey AL. Describing the trajectory of language development in the presence of severe-to-profound hearing loss: a closer look at children with cochlear implants versus hearing aids. Otol Neurotol 2010;31(8):1268–1274

73 Congenital Auricular Deformities

■ Introduction

There is no consensus in the classification of congenital auricular malformations. There have been at least five classification schemes in the past century. The most quoted was proposed by Weerda in 1988 (**Table 73.1**). Acceptance of Weerda's classification likely may be due to the schema allowing all congenital deformities to be grouped under an umbrella of three increasing degrees of dysplasia. Because microtia (anotia) is the most studied and researched malformation, most of the information referenced in this chapter deals with microtia.

Relevant Basic Science

Advances in microtia research are based on a variety of genetic approaches, including linkage analysis, direct sequencing from affected individuals, the study of single-gene disorder, identification of cytogenetic rearrangements, and animal models.

Relevant Anatomy

The auricle is formed from several protuberances in the first and second branchial arches called hillocks of His. The hillocks grow, fuse, and undergo morphogenesis that begins at the sixth week of embryogenesis. The hillock of the first arch forms the tragus, and the hillocks of the second arch form the lobule, the antihelix, and the dorsocaudal part of the helix.

Etiology

The etiology of microtia rests on genetic and environmental factors and the interplay between the two. It can occur in isolation or as a part of a spectrum of anomalies or a syndrome. Approximately 20 to 60% of children with microtia have associated anoma-

Table 73.1 Weerda's classification of congenital auricular deformities

A. First degree dysplasia—Most structures of a normal auricle are recognizable

- Macrotia
- Protruding ears
- Cryptotia
- Absence of upper helix
- Small deformities
- Colobomata
- Lobule deformities
- Cup ear deformities

B. Second degree dysplasia—Some structures of a normal auricle are recognizable

- Cup ear deformity type III
- Mini ear

C. Third degree dysplasia—None of the structures of a normal auricle are recognizable

- Unilateral
- Bilateral
- Anotia

Adapted with permission from Weerda H. Classification of congenital deformities of the auricle. Facial Plast Surg 1988; 5(5): 385–388.

lies or an identifiable syndrome. The more common syndromes familiar to otolaryngologists include Klippel–Feil, Nager, Treacher Collins, and branchiootorenal syndromes. The most notable known risk factors through case-control and cross-sectional studies include male gender, low birth weight, higher maternal parity, maternal acute illness, advanced maternal age, low maternal education, use of medications (retinoids, thalidomide, immunosuppressants, and mycophenolate mofetil), maternal diabetes mellitus, high altitude (above 2,500 m), and Hispanic ethnicity.

Incidence/Epidemiology

Prevalence rates of microtia range from 0.83 to 4.34 per 10,000 births. The variance may be due to inclusion criteria and case ascertainment because less severe forms of microtia may be under- or overreported. Population-based studies in the United States showed increased prevalence in certain ethnic groups (higher in Asian, Pacific Islanders, and Hispanic populations).

Pathogenesis

Microtia is both etiologically and pathogenetically heterogeneous. Although single gene mutations are seen in syndromic and familial cases, the cause is likely multifactorial (genetic and environmental) or polygenic in sporadic cases. The several existing hypotheses include neural crest cell disturbance, vascular disruption, and altitude. Defects or insults (both genetic and environmental) affecting neural crest cell delamination, proliferation, apoptosis, or migration, or their reciprocal interaction with mesoderm, endoderm, or overlying ectoderm, can explain the various forms of microtia. Vascular disruption as a hypothesis is based on ischemia and necrosis secondary to vessel occlusion, vasoconstriction, and underdevelopment of the arterial system. Altitude has been shown to have an increased prevalence of microtia in high-altitude as compared with low-altitude cities in South America.

Pathology

Using the Weerda classification, it becomes apparent that congenital auricular deformity can be classified as a continuum, but the schema helps the clinician to group the deformities of increasing anatomical derangement into three stages of dysplasias. In the first degree of dysplasia, most of the auricular structures are recognizable (e.g., protruding ears and cryptotia). In the second degree, some of the structures are recognizable (e.g., cup ear deformity type III). And in the third degree, none of the structures is visible (e.g., microtia/anotia).

■ Evaluation

Clinical Findings

Because certain types of congenital auricular malformation, in particular microtia, have familial, genetic, and syndromic association, a family history could be very helpful.

A thorough head and neck examination is mandatory. In particular, associated maxillary and mandibular dysplasia needs to be considered because auricular embryology encompasses the first two branchial arches. The association with branchiootorenal syndrome necessitates the search for branchial sinuses, fistulas, and cysts. When dealing with the less severe forms of auricular dysplasias, the clinician needs to pay special attention to the specific deformities because all surgical repairs are customized. Special attention needs to be paid to the size (cupped ear) and depth (prominent ear) of the conchal bowl, the degree of antihelical fold deformity (prominent ear), the helical root (cryptotia), and the presence of a third crux (Stahl ear). As other dysmorphic features are identified, it may be beneficial to refer the patient to a medical geneticist.

It is also important during the initial appointment to set surgical goals and contain the patient's and family's expectations, as with all aesthetic procedures. Complications unique to repair of auricular deformities need to be addressed as well. Clearly, there are psychosocial issues to consider in making a decision for the timing of surgical intervention beyond clinical factors.

Imaging

Routine imaging is not required in the management of congenital auricular deformities. Even in the case of microtia, computed tomography only plays a role in determining surgical candidacy in bilateral microtia patients because few otolaryngologists would pursue repair of unilateral canal atresia. A cervical spine series may aid in the diagnosis of Klippel–Feil syndrome by characterizing fusion of the cervical vertebrae.

Audiology

Behavioral audiometry to establish the presence or absence of sensorineural or conductive hearing loss is mandatory as part of the evaluation of a child with congenital auricular malformation.

■ Management

Nonsurgical Options

The basis for intervention of the cartilages of the nose and ear with congenital deformity during the neonatal period is purportedly due to high-circulating estrogens in newborns within the privileged period.

Since the 1980s, the Japanese have been avid proponents of nonsurgical correction of various congenital auricular malformations. Early papers reported the correction of lop ears and cryptotias using a variety of methods of splinting materials and even a butterfly venipuncture needle, primarily in neonates and up to 1 year of age. The current method of correcting a variety of congenital auricular deformities that include cryptotias, lop ears, Stahl ear, and prominent ears with varying rates of success relies on using dental wax and Steri-Strips (3M, St. Paul, MN) to secure the mold in newborns as proposed by Brown et al in 1986. The molding/splinting procedure lasts a total of 4 to 6 weeks. The author has no experience of molding or splinting older children. A customized molding system is available commercially, but the cost is prohibitive.

Surgical Options

Microtia Repair Approaches

The classic Brent total reconstruction of the microtic ear using autogenous rib graft is a four-stage procedure.

Brent Stage 1 Repair

The first stage consists of obtaining en bloc rib cartilages from the side contralateral to the ear being reconstructed. A template using unexposed X-ray films to trace out the opposite normal ear is made. This template is used to determine both the height of the ear being constructed in the preoperative phase and the extent of rib resection intraoperatively. The cartilage framework is made up of a main block from the synchondrosis of ribs 6 and 7 and a helical rim from the floating rib cartilage. Meticulous carving, shaping, and suturing are performed to complete the framework. This is followed by the removal of the microtic cartilage and insertion of the framework. Suction drains are placed to improve coaptation of the skin flap to the framework.

Brent Stage 2–4 Repair

The second stage consists of rotation of the vertically oriented lobule to a more normal-looking horizontal orientation using a Z-plasty approach. The third stage achieves tragal construction and defines the conchal bowl. A composite graft from the normal ear's anterolateral conchal surface is harvested. A j-shaped incision is made in the conchal region, whereby underlying extraneous soft tissues are removed and the composite graft is inserted. The last stage is for the elevation of the posterior auricular skin and covering the defect with a split skin graft.

Repair with Alloplastic Materials

Alloplastic materials, including Silastic, stainless steel, and other materials, have been used for microtia repair. The most frequently used alloplastic material for the traditional autogenous rib graft method currently is prefabricated porous polyethylene (Medpor, Stryker, Kalamazoo, MI). Another alternative is the implantation of bone-anchored implant screws (Vistafix, Cochlear Americas, Centennial, CO), affixing them using magnets to a silicone ear prosthesis sculpted by an anaplastologist. Frequently, the Vistafix screws are implanted at the same time when the bone-anchored hearing device (Baha System, Cochlear Americas, Centennial, CO) is implanted. In children, both Vistafix and Baha screws are placed as a two-stage procedure. separated by 4 to 6 months to enhance osseointegration.

Otoplasty

Otoplastic surgery is tailored to correcting specific auricular deformities, which are grouped under three primary areas: depth of the concha, prominence of the antihelix fold, and a combination of the two. The goal is to attain smooth, regular lines without sharp edges. From an anterior view, the helix needs to rest beyond the antihelical fold, and the auricle has to have an auriculomastoid angle of ~ 23 degrees. In reality, one or more surgical techniques may be employed to achieve the desired aesthetic goals.

The depth of the concha can be altered by conchal setback described by Furnas. Mattress sutures are placed that penetrate the full thickness of cartilage of the conchal wall and the thick layer of mastoid fascia. The depth of the concha can also be altered by resection of a piece of full-thickness crescent of conchal cartilage through an anterior incision. This method is seldom used, most likely due to the need for an anterior skin incision. Alternatively, the "Gibson principle" has also been described to decrease the depth of the conchal bowl by scoring and thereby weakening the appropriate portion of the bowl.

Methods to alter the antihelical fold include suturing of the cartilage on either side of the desired height of the antihelical fold, or the so-called Mustardé sutures. Generally two to three sutures would be sufficient to achieve the desired results. A modification of the traditional Mustardé suture method for the correction of the "lop" ear was introduced by Fritsch in 1995. It is termed incisionless otoplasty and is used alone or in conjunction with other methods. The Gibson principle has also been described in this instance by weakening the anterior surface of the antihelix using a subcutaneous tunnel and rasping the desired region in conjunction with Mustardé stitches.

Other useful minor surgical methods have been described. The prominent upper auricular pole can be altered by placing full-thickness mattress sutures from the triangular fossa or scaphoid fossa or both to the temporal scalp periosteum. Undesirable lobule orientation can be corrected by placing a suture in the adipose tissue of the lobule and anchoring it to the concha or the fascia of the sternocleidomastoid muscle. Excision of the postauricular muscle or soft tissue is used to further decrease the conchomastoid angle.

Prevention and Management of Surgical Complications

A hemostatic dressing of sufficient pressure is placed when major cartilage work has taken place. In the first-stage microtia repair using autogenous rib graft, suction drains are also placed. Excessive pain or surgical wound bleeding may signal the formation of hematoma that requires timely evacuation. Postoperative cellulitis can occur, and broad-spectrum antibiotic therapy is required to prevent progression to chondritis. Suture extrusion and granuloma can occur. The use of monofilament sutures can decrease occurrence.

■ Controversial Issues

The timing of canal atresia surgery as it relates to microtia surgery has been controversial. It is well accepted today that microtia surgery should precede canal atresia surgery.

■ Suggested Reading

Brent B. Microtia repair with rib cartilage grafts: a review of personal experience with 1000 cases. Clin Plast Surg 2002;29(2): 257–271, vii

Brown FE, Colen LB, Addante RR, Graham JM Jr. Correction of congenital auricular deformities by splinting in the neonatal period. Pediatrics 1986;78(3):406–411

Fritsch MH. Incisionless otoplasty. Laryngoscope 1995;105(5 Pt 3, Suppl 70):1–11

Furnas DW. Otoplasty for prominent ears. Clin Plast Surg 2002;29(2):273–288, viii

Gibson T, Davis WB. The distortion of autogenous cartilage grafts: its cause and prevention. Br J Plast Surg 1958;10:257–274

Luquetti DV, Heike CL, Hing AV, Cunningham ML, Cox TC. Microtia: epidemiology and genetics. Am J Med Genet A 2012;158A(1): 124–139

Weerda H. Classification of congenital deformities of the auricle. Facial Plast Surg 1988;5(5):385–388

74 Pediatric Laryngotracheal Stenosis

■ Introduction

The management of pediatric laryngotracheal stenosis (PLTS) in children poses multiple challenges for treating clinicians. Children presenting with PLTS have complex medical issues, and their appropriate care requires a high level of integration of multiple medical services, led by an otolaryngologist. In general, multidisciplinary expertise in anesthesia, surgery, pulmonology, gastroenterology, intensive care management, and general medicine is requisite to adequately manage these patients. Furthermore, expertise in nursing, speech therapy, and social service is required for patient/parent teaching, counseling, rehabilitation, social assessment, tracheotomy care instruction, and home care assessment.

Definition and Classification

With the improved survival of premature neonates, the use of prolonged intubation and ventilatory support has increased. Although a heightened awareness of the potential damage to the subglottis related to intubation has led to a decrease in acquired subglottic stenosis (SGS), the incidence remains 1 to 2% of neonates. SGS is present when the subglottic airway measures < 4 mm (or 3 mm in a preterm infant). In general, PLTS is characterized by etiology, area involved, and the nature and degree of the stenosis.

PLTS is considered congenital when there is no history of other potential causes, including intubation. SGS of congenital origin is less common than acquired SGS and can only be diagnosed with certainty in a child before a first intubation. It is not known what proportion of those intubated neonates who develop PLTS have a smaller than normal larynx prior to the intubation. The posterior glottis and/or subglottis is almost universally involved in children with acquired PLTS, which occurs most commonly secondary to prolonged intubation, but may be due to other factors as well (**Table 74.1**).

The grading scale most universally employed to categorize SGS was proposed by Myer and Cotton in 1994. The scale describes grade 1 SGS as 0 to 50% narrowing, grade 2 SGS as 50 to 75% narrowing, grade 3 SGS as 75 to 99% narrowing, and grade 4 SGS as no detectable lumen (**Fig. 74.1**). This grading scheme is important in outcomes assessment, for planning therapy, and in discussing objective disease severity among parents and colleagues. The nature of the stenosis can be further qualified as soft, firm, or a combination of the two.

■ Evaluation

The evaluation of children with suspicion of PLTS should include a careful history and physical assessment. Most infants with acquired SGS will have had a history of neonatal intubation. For neonates presenting with inflammatory SGS and multiple failures

Table 74.1 Etiology of pediatric laryngotracheal stenosis

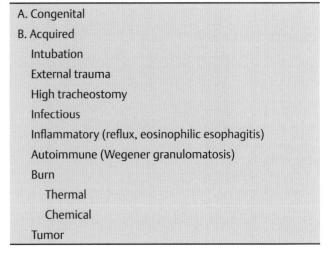

A. Congenital

B. Acquired

Intubation

External trauma

High tracheostomy

Infectious

Inflammatory (reflux, eosinophilic esophagitis)

Autoimmune (Wegener granulomatosis)

Burn

Thermal

Chemical

Tumor

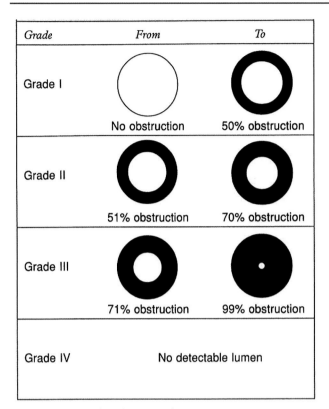

Grade	From	To
Grade I	No obstruction	50% obstruction
Grade II	51% obstruction	70% obstruction
Grade III	71% obstruction	99% obstruction
Grade IV	No detectable lumen	

Fig. 74.1 SGS Classification Scheme.

to extubate, the neonatology and otolaryngology teams must be in close cooperation. Close attention should be paid to the patient's medical condition, with emphasis on cardiopulmonary status, ventilation status, oxygen requirements, and the details of previous extubation failures.

Assuming that steroids and racemic epinephrine have been used appropriately, the duration of extubation prior to reintubation is an important determinant for the need for consideration of tracheotomy; the shorter the interval, measured in hours, the more likely a tracheotomy is necessary. Possible concomitant presence of gastroesophageal reflux disease (GERD) should be investigated and treated; many have reported a correlation between the presence of GERD and SGS and that GERD may affect surgical healing after laryngotracheoplasty (LTP). Patients with dysphagia, or severe laryngeal and hypopharyngeal inflammation, should be considered for eosinophilic esophagitis because this emerging disorder has also recently been shown to be associated with SGS and influences negative healing and outcomes after LTP.

Preoperative radiographic imaging plays little to no role in surgical planning, except to help characterize and determine the length of a stenotic airway segment. Undoubtedly, the gold standard in the

preoperative airway evaluation and SGS characterization is a rigid direct microlaryngoscopy and bronchoscopy (DLB) procedure under general anesthesia. Almost universally, the anesthetic management for this evaluation can be accomplished in children with spontaneous ventilation with oxygen insufflation using a combination of inhalational agents and propofol for induction. This approach allows for a dynamic assessment of the laryngotracheobronchial tree, while manipulating the airway without needing intubation or ventilation through a rigid bronchoscope. The surgeon is able to simply use narrow rigid fiberoptic "naked" telescopes for diagnostic purposes, minimizing airway trauma associated with the larger-diameter ventilating bronchoscope. Use of the ventilating bronchoscope is then reserved for cases where therapeutic or interventional maneuvers have to be performed in the trachea and mainstem bronchi.

After DLB is performed, to objectively determine the severity of the stenosis, the lumen of the stenotic airway is typically sized with endotracheal tubes (ETTs). DLB is supplemented in all patients by flexible nasopharyngolaryngoscopy, which is important in nonintubated patients, where one should carefully assess the nasopharynx, oropharynx, and particularly the vocal cord level. Abnormalities of glottic mobility due to neurological problems, scarring of the glottis, or involvement of the cricoarytenoid joints complicate surgical therapy.

In selected patients, flexible laryngobronchoscopy under anesthesia is also complementary to rigid DLB. It is particularly useful in patients with severe micrognathia to assess the degree of possible obstruction at the tongue base, and in patients with chronic lower airway disease to reach and examine the distal aspects of the bronchial tree. Flexible laryngobronchoscopy under anesthesia is also best accomplished without intubation, under spontaneous ventilation with oxygen insufflation through the side port of the flexible scope. With this approach the endoscopist is not limited to performing flexible endoscopy through the lumen of an ETT, which in infants is often too small to allow for passage of a flexible scope with suction capability.

For patients with PLTS without an existing tracheotomy tube, further and definitive reconstructive management is based on the clinical picture and the severity of the stenotic segment. The presence of chronic pulmonary disease, often represented by baseline oxygen requirement in the setting of bronchopulmonary dysplasia and poor pulmonary functional reserve, disallows for single-stage LTP, necessitating placement of a tracheotomy prior to or during the LTP. This is because reconstructive laryngotracheal surgery requires lung function adequate to withstand not only the surgery but also the post-operative course in the neonatal intensive care unit (NICU) and subsequent extubation. Indeed, those children with significant pulmonary disease should undergo consultation by a pediatric pulmonologist. In general, it is inadvisable to perform LTP in children with anything more than a mild nighttime oxygen requirement; in selected cases, continued oxygen administration may be possible by nasal prongs after decannulation.

■ Management

Endoscopic Treatment

In general, endoscopic treatment is limited to acquired (and not congenital) airway stenoses. Classically, endoscopic treatment has taken the form of laser ablation of narrowing lesions, but is only useful for nonmature, noncircumferential, short, soft lesions that constitute mild grade 1 or 2 stenoses. Recent small case series have also described the use of balloon-dilating catheters as potential tools that may successfully treat some patients with SGS, even if severe, but larger confirmatory studies are necessary to validate this approach. In any circumstance, dilation may certainly help temporize obstructive symptoms. Multiple, serial repeated dilations may eventually weaken the airway lateral walls, effectively worsening the pathology.

Anterior Cricoid Split (ACS)

The anterior cricoid split (ACS) procedure was introduced by Cotton and Seid in 1980 as an alternative approach to tracheotomy, as a result of failing to extubate premature neonates with healthy lungs but laryngeal obstruction due to edema and early stenosis. To qualify for this procedure, the only reason for extubation failure must be laryngeal obstruction, and the neonate should have grown to 3.3 lb, have no assisted ventilatory support for 10 days, have no supplemental oxygen need greater than an FiO_2 of 35%, and have no evidence of congestive heart failure.

The procedure consists of making an anterior vertical split through the first tracheal ring, cricoid cartilage, and lower thyroid cartilage, followed by nasotracheal intubation for 10 to 14 days in the NICU. If criteria are strictly and carefully followed, case series have demonstrated ACS to be successful in avoiding tracheotomy in a majority of neonates. During ACS, placement of a small piece of thyroid ala cartilage into the vertical split has also been described, and some have shown it can improve the success of the surgery.

Laryngotracheoplasty with Cartilage Grafting

LTP with interposition of cartilage graft was introduced by Fearon and Cotton in 1972 as a means to expand an otherwise narrowed subglottic airway segment. The principle of the procedure is to distract the cricoid cartilage anteriorly and/or posteriorly by suturing cartilaginous grafts in place over a luminal, appropriately sized stent.

In single-stage LTP procedures, the stent used is an endotracheal tube, which is left in place while the child is nasotracheally intubated and sedated in the pediatric intensive care unit (PICU) for a period of 5 to 14 days. Large outcome studies demonstrate success (defined by avoidance of tracheotomy need) of single-stage LTP surgery in more than 80% of children. The only factor associated with surgical failure was found to be the presence of tracheomalacia. Management of the child in the postoperative period while intubated in the PICU is often difficult and continually evolving. Reports suggest that older children (> 3 y) tolerate the intubation period better and often require minimal sedation or ventilatory assistance.

In double-stage procedures, a tracheotomy tube is either placed temporarily or left in place after the surgery. A sutured indwelling suprastomal stent is left in place postoperatively while the grafts heal. Usually the stents are left in place for a period of 2 to 6 weeks. Double-stage approaches are necessary when the child has a need for prolonged stenting, more complex airway lesions, or a concomitant airway pathology (such as tracheomalacia, impaired vocal cord mobility, or tongue base obstruction), or in revision surgical cases. In cases when the reconstructed tracheal walls are flaccid, resulting in poor graft stability, or if the anatomy is highly distorted due to previous multiple failed reconstruction attempts, stenting periods longer than 6 weeks are warranted. Traditionally, in adults the most commonly used long-term laryngotracheal stent has been the Montgomery T-tube. Recently, it has also been demonstrated to be an effective, reliable stent in children, allowing for long-term stenting (> 2 mon). T-tubes provide for stable, long-term laryngeal stenting, with the possibility of vocalization. However, due to possible increased problems with obstruction and aspiration, they are restricted to children older than 4 years.

Cricotracheal Resection (CTR)

Resection of a narrowed laryngotracheal airway segment was first introduced in adults by Conley in 1953 and was later popularized in children by Monnier in the 1990s. Multiple reports have since demonstrated that this procedure is more likely to achieve decannulation or avoid a tracheotomy tube in children with severe grade 3 or grade 4 stenosis, where success rates of > 90% have been reported.

The concept of this procedure is to resect the narrowed subglottic airway, including the anterolateral cricoid cartilage ring, sparing the posterior cricoid cartilaginous plate, maintaining functional cricoarytenoid joints. As with LTP procedures, cricotracheal resection (CTR) can be done in a single- or double-stage fashion. Added postoperative considerations include the use of chin-to-chest sutures for 7 to 10 days postoperatively to prevent neck extension and anastomotic dehiscence.

Postoperative Considerations

The postoperative considerations for patients undergoing laryngotracheal reconstructive procedures depend on the nature of the surgery. For patients undergoing single-stage procedures, the use of sedation protocols for PICU management is likely to be helpful in minimizing complications. Children who require high doses of sedation, paralytic agents, and controlled, assisted ventilation are at higher risk of pneumonia, narcotic withdrawal, and need for reintubation. These morbidities are especially salient in the young neonates and infants less than 3 years of age. Older children are less likely to require high levels of ventilatory and anesthetic support.

For double-stage patients, meticulous care of the tracheotomy tube is mandatory. This is especially the case considering the presence of a suprastomal stent above the tracheotomy tube—a fact that further confers the child completely dependent on the tracheotomy tube for an airway. In this setting, accidental decannulation and tracheotomy mucous plugging are potentially lethal events without the appropriate level of nursing and monitoring. Given that children with suprastomal stents, and certainly those with Montgomery T-tubes, are likely to aspirate to a varying degree, there is also a small risk of pneumonia. Careful cooperation with a speech and language pathologist to gauge the child's ability to swallow or the aspiration risk is critical in postoperative double-stage patients with indwelling stents.

◼ Controversial Issues

Timing of Reconstruction

The ideal timing of LTR surgery remains somewhat ill defined. Although some studies have demonstrated that children younger than 24 months have higher rates of reconstruction failure despite lesser degrees of stenotic pathology when compared with older children, more recent larger series have shown that (1) although younger children have a higher rate of reintubation after single-stage procedures, eventually they are able to extubate, and (2) age alone is not a predictor for reconstructive failure (defined as failure to decannulate or avoid tracheotomy). In children with existing tracheotomies, any LTR timing decisions must consider the fact that severe SGS managed with tracheotomy, where formal LTR is deferred, is potentially life threatening because yearly tracheotomy-specific mortality in children due to tracheotomy tube obstruction is 1 to 3.4%. Associated tracheotomy tube morbidity also includes the need for comprehensive nursing care and monitoring, delayed speech and language development, feeding difficulties, and infection. Therefore, now many authors propose reconstruction as early as possible so as to avoid tracheotomy.

Decannulation

The decannulation process begins once DLB indicates an adequate airway, including adequate vocal cord movement. The first step is typically a reduction in size of the tracheotomy tube in a controlled environment using a speaking valve, followed by plugging the tracheotomy tube in a monitored setting. The tube is plugged initially while the patient is awake. The tracheotomy tube remains plugged as long as the child shows no clinical evidence of respiratory distress or oxygen desaturation. If the child tolerates plugging while awake, then nighttime plugging of the tracheotomy tube is appropriate in a monitored setting, including pulse oximetry. Decannulation itself is performed in a monitored setting (for at least 48 h) to evaluate for any significant oxygen desaturations.

If a child fails plugging at some point during this process, several possibilities should be considered, including supraglottic collapse, inadequate vocal cord movement, residual laryngeal stenosis, suprastomal collapse, and tracheobronchomalacia. If there is any question about the adequacy of the airway or the ability of the child to clear secretions, then plugging the tracheotomy tube for a period of 3 months is advisable, during which time the child should be able to tolerate an upper respiratory infection without unplugging.

One month following decannulation the child should be evaluated, either endoscopically or with imaging, for intratracheal granulation tissue at the previous stomal site.

■ Suggested Reading

Bagwell CE. CO2 laser excision of pediatric airway lesions. J Pediatr Surg 1990;25(11):1152–1156

Bailey M, Hoeve H, Monnier P. Paediatric laryngotracheal stenosis: a consensus paper from three European centres. Eur Arch Otorhinolaryngol 2003;260(3):118–123

Carr MM, Poje CP, Kingston L, Kielma D, Heard C. Complications in pediatric tracheostomies. Laryngoscope 2001;111(11 Pt 1): 1925–1928

Carron JD, Derkay CS, Strope GL, Nosonchuk JE, Darrow DH. Pediatric tracheotomies: changing indications and outcomes. Laryngoscope 2000;110(7):1099–1104

Choi SS, Zalzal GH. Changing trends in neonatal subglottic stenosis. Otolaryngol Head Neck Surg 2000;122(1):61–63

Conley JJ. Reconstruction of the subglottic air passage. Ann Otol Rhinol Laryngol 1953;62(2):477–495

Cotton RT, Seid AB. Management of the extubation problem in the premature child: anterior cricoid split as an alternative to tracheotomy. Ann Otol Rhinol Laryngol 1980;89(6 Pt 1):508–511

Dauer EH, Ponikau JU, Smyrk TC, Murray JA, Thompson DM. Airway manifestations of pediatric eosinophilic esophagitis: a clinical and histopathologic report of an emerging association. Ann Otol Rhinol Laryngol 2006;115(7):507–517

Durden F, Sobol SE. Balloon laryngoplasty as a primary treatment for subglottic stenosis. Arch Otolaryngol Head Neck Surg 2007;133(8):772–775

Dutton JM, Palmer PM, McCulloch TM, Smith RJ. Mortality in the pediatric patient with tracheotomy. Head Neck 1995;17(5): 403–408

Eze NN, Wyatt ME, Hartley BE. The role of the anterior cricoid split in facilitating extubation in infants. Int J Pediatr Otorhinolaryngol 2005;69(6):843–846

Fearon B, Cotton R. Surgical correction of subglottic stenosis of the larynx: preliminary report of an experimental surgical technique. Ann Otol Rhinol Laryngol 1972;81(4):508–513

Forte V, Chang MB, Papsin BC. Thyroid ala cartilage reconstruction in neonatal subglottic stenosis as a replacement for the anterior cricoid split. Int J Pediatr Otorhinolaryngol 2001;59(3):181–186

George M, Ikonomidis C, Jaquet Y, Monnier P. Partial cricotracheal resection in children: potential pitfalls and avoidance of complications. Otolaryngol Head Neck Surg 2009;141(2):225–231

Gustafson LM, Hartley BE, Liu JH, et al. Single-stage laryngotracheal reconstruction in children: a review of 200 cases. Otolaryngol Head Neck Surg 2000;123(4):430–434

Halstead LA. Gastroesophageal reflux: a critical factor in pediatric subglottic stenosis. Otolaryngol Head Neck Surg 1999;120(5): 683–688

Hartley BE, Rutter MJ, Cotton RT. Cricotracheal resection as a primary procedure for laryngotracheal stenosis in children. Int J Pediatr Otorhinolaryngol 2000;54(2-3):133–136

Hartnick CJ, Hartley BE, Lacy PD, et al. Surgery for pediatric subglottic stenosis: disease-specific outcomes. Ann Otol Rhinol Laryngol 2001;110(12):1109–1113

Jacobs BR, Salman BA, Cotton RT, Lyons K, Brilli RJ. Postoperative management of children after single-stage laryngotracheal reconstruction. Crit Care Med 2001;29(1):164–168

Lee KH, Rutter MJ. Role of balloon dilation in the management of adult idiopathic subglottic stenosis. Ann Otol Rhinol Laryngol 2008;117(2):81–84

Maddalozzo J, Holinger LD. Laryngotracheal reconstruction for subglottic stenosis in children. Ann Otol Rhinol Laryngol 1987;96(6):665–669

Maronian NC, Azadeh H, Waugh P, Hillel A. Association of laryngopharyngeal reflux disease and subglottic stenosis. Ann Otol Rhinol Laryngol 2001;110(7 Pt 1):606–612

Monnier P, Savary M, Chapuis G. Partial cricoid resection with primary tracheal anastomosis for subglottic stenosis in infants and children. Laryngoscope 1993;103(11 Pt 1):1273–1283

Myer CM III, O'Connor DM, Cotton RT. Proposed grading system for subglottic stenosis based on endotracheal tube sizes. Ann Otol Rhinol Laryngol 1994;103(4 Pt 1):319–323

Preciado D, Zalzal G. Laryngeal and tracheal stents in children. Curr Opin Otolaryngol Head Neck Surg 2008;16(1):83–85

Rutter MJ, Hartley BE, Cotton RT. Cricotracheal resection in children. Arch Otolaryngol Head Neck Surg 2001;127(3):289–292

Schroeder JW Jr, Holinger LD. Congenital laryngeal stenosis. Otolaryngol Clin North Am 2008;41(5):865–875, viii

Smith LP, Chewaproug L, Spergel JM, Zur KB. Otolaryngologists may not be doing enough to diagnose pediatric eosinophilic esophagitis. Int J Pediatr Otorhinolaryngol 2009;73(11): 1554–1557

Smith LP, Zur KB, Jacobs IN. Single- vs double-stage laryngotracheal reconstruction. Arch Otolaryngol Head Neck Surg 2010;136(1):60–65

Stenson K, Berkowitz R, McDonald T, Gruber B. Experience with one-stage laryngotracheal reconstruction. Int J Pediatr Otorhinolaryngol 1993;27(1):55–64

Stern Y, Willging JP, Cotton RT. Use of Montgomery T-tube in laryngotracheal reconstruction in children: is it safe? Ann Otol Rhinol Laryngol 1998;107(12):1006–1009

Walner DL, Stern Y, Gerber ME, Rudolph C, Baldwin CY, Cotton RT. Gastroesophageal reflux in patients with subglottic stenosis. Arch Otolaryngol Head Neck Surg 1998;124(5):551–555

Werkhaven JA, Weed DT, Ossoff RH. Carbon dioxide laser serial microtrapdoor flap excision of subglottic stenosis. Arch Otolaryngol Head Neck Surg 1993;119(6):676–679

White DR, Bravo M, Vijayasekaran S, Rutter MJ, Cotton RT, Elluru RG. Laryngotracheoplasty as an alternative to tracheotomy in infants younger than 6 months. Arch Otolaryngol Head Neck Surg 2009;135(5):445–447

White DR, Cotton RT, Bean JA, Rutter MJ. Pediatric cricotracheal resection: surgical outcomes and risk factor analysis. Arch Otolaryngol Head Neck Surg 2005;131(10):896–899

Willis R, Myer C, Miller R, Cotton RT. Tracheotomy decannulation in the pediatric patient. Laryngoscope 1987;97(6):764–765

Yellon RF, Parameswaran M, Brandom BW. Decreasing morbidity following laryngotracheal reconstruction in children. Int J Pediatr Otorhinolaryngol 1997;41(2):145–154

Younis RT, Lazar RH, Astor F. Posterior cartilage graft in single-stage laryngotracheal reconstruction. Otolaryngol Head Neck Surg 2003;129(3):168–175

Zalzal GH, Choi SS, Patel KM. Ideal timing of pediatric laryngotracheal reconstruction. Arch Otolaryngol Head Neck Surg 1997;123(2):206–208

75 Pediatric Vascular Anomalies

■ Introduction

There has been a long history of misleading nomenclature for the various vascular anomalies. The source of the current classification is the 1996 International Society for the Study of Vascular Anomalies, which is based on natural history, cellular turnover, and histology. The new classification calls for replacing improper terms with new terms (**Table 75.1**).

Pediatric vascular anomalies are divided into two broad categories: vascular tumors and vascular malformations. Vascular tumors include infantile hemangiomas, congenital hemangiomas (noninvoluting and rapidly involuting types), kaposiform hemangioendotheliomas, and tufted angiomas. Vascular malformations include low-flow lesions (capillary, lymphatic, and venous malformations) and high-flow lesions (arteriovenous [AV] malformations and AV fistulas). Mixed lesions are common.

Vascular Tumors

Infantile hemangiomas are the most common tumor of infancy (10% of Caucasian infants by 1 year of age). Risk factors include low birth weight, prematurity, female, Caucasian ethnicity, multiple gestation pregnancy, advanced maternal age, and placental abnormalities. There is a triphasic growth pattern: proliferation (first 2 months of life), plateau (3–5 months of age), and involution (3 years of age). Segmental infantile hemangioma is clinically important in PHACES syndrome (*p*osterior fossa malformation, *h*emangioma, *a*rterial anomaly, *c*oarctation of the aorta, *e*ye abnormality, *s*ternal cleft/raphe). Intracranial vascular anomalies resulting in neurological sequelae are most devastating in this syndrome.

Congenital hemangiomas are rare compared with infantile hemangiomas and are subdivided into noninvoluting and rapidly involuting types. Both types are fully formed at birth and have no postnatal growth phase. The rapidly involuting type involutes by 12 months of age, whereas the noninvoluting type does not and requires surgical excision. Both types are differentiated by their natural history.

Kaposiform hemangioendotheliomas and tufted angiomas are rare in the head and neck. However, they are significant for the otolaryngologist in an event called Kasabach–Merritt syndrome, which is characterized by severe coagulopathy due to platelet trapping within the tumor, and is the most common life-threatening complication.

Vascular Malformations

It is postulated that growth hormone receptors may play a role in the natural history of the various types of vascular malformation. A recent report found overexpression of growth hormone receptor in venous malformations, lymphatic malformations, and AV malformations, but failed to find overexpression in androgen, estrogen, and progesterone receptors.

The most common low-flow vascular malformations are venous malformations. They are generally sporadic, but autosomal-dominant inheritance pattern has been reported. In the head and neck presentation, deep structures (muscle, orbit, and underlying bones) are frequently involved, resulting in an assortment of long-term sequelae, including pain, facial deformity, malocclusion, feeding issues, and obstructive sleep apnea.

Capillary malformations (formerly called portwine stains) involve the superficial layers of skin that progress over years to become nodular lesions. Of importance to the otolaryngologist is Sturge–Weber syndrome, which is characterized by facial capillary malformation and ipsilateral ocular and leptomeningeal anomalies. Ocular lesions include glaucoma and choroidal vascular malformation. Neurological involvements include seizures, hemiparesis/hemiplegia, migraines, developmental delay, and behavioral disorders.

Table 75.1 Misleading and appropriate terms for vascular anomalies

Misleading terms	Appropriate terms
Vascular tumors	
Strawberry hemangioma	Infantile hemangioma
Capillary hemangioma	Infantile hemangioma
Cavernous hemangioma	Venous malformation, deep/missed hemangioma
Vascular malformations	
Port-wine stain	Capillary malformation
Lymphangioma	Microcystic lymphatic malformation
Cystic hygroma	Macrocystic lymphatic malformation

Used with permission from Adams MT, Saltzman B, Perkins JA. Head and neck lymphatic malformation treatment: a systematic review. Otolaryngol Head Neck Surg 2012 147(4):627–639.

Lymphatic malformations are most frequently found in the head and neck (75% of all cases). Fifty percent are detectable at birth and 90% by age 2. The incidence is estimated to be between 1 in 6,000 to 16,000 live births. The subtypes of lymphatic malformations (macrocystic and microcystic) are determined by their radiographic appearance, although both subtypes can coexist in the same lesion. Lymphatic malformations have a greater risk of progression in adolescence than in childhood, which is suggestive of the role of pubertal hormones. Spontaneous regression, primarily in the macrocystic subtype, has been reported. Furthermore, mixed lesions are common among vascular malformations, with combinations of capillary, lymphatic, and venous components.

AVMs of the head and neck are infrequently encountered within the broad classification of vascular anomalies, which include a direct communication from arteries to veins (AV shunting) and a lack of a normal capillary network. Typically during puberty or adolescence, the initial congenital quiescent lesion progresses to an expansive mass with cosmetic and functional disturbance, resulting in disfigurement, uncontrollable bleeding, ulceration, pain, and even output failure. This lesion has a notorious track record for recurrence.

■ Evaluation

History

The presence or absence of hemangiomas at birth would be useful to differentiate between congenital and infantile hemangiomas. Knowledge of the triphasic growth pattern of an infantile hemangioma is helpful in determining the life-cycle phase of a lesion, and it is also useful in providing family counseling.

Fever and irritability in the presence of a lymphatic malformation would suggest an infectious process.

Physical Examination

The common finding of all pediatric vascular anomalies, with the exception of a capillary malformation, is that of a mass. The size and discoloration of the mass vary according to the type of lesion and the state of growth and depth of the lesion. Generally, these lesions are not tender, except in an infected lymphatic malformation. Venous malformations could engorge with a Valsalva maneuver or placing the head and neck in a dependent position. A bruit may be heard in an AVM.

Clinical Laboratory Studies

Laboratory testing is generally not required to establish the diagnosis of vascular anomalies. However, platelet count would be diagnostic for Kasabach–Merritt syndrome when thrombocytopenia will be encountered.

Imaging

Imaging tools that have proven useful in the diagnosis of vascular anomalies include ultrasound with Doppler, magnetic resonance imaging (MRI), computed tomography (CT), and arteriography. Ultrasound with Doppler has become the first-line imaging tool, due to its availability, lack of ionizing radiation, and limited need for sedation. It is unique in its ability to assess depth of lesion and flow characteristics. MRI is useful in its superior soft tissue contrast. In particular, magnetic resonance angiography is used to assess vascular supply and to evaluate arterial feeders and venous drainage. CT is playing a decreasing role, except in evaluating osseous involvement. Angiography is used primarily in the diagnosis and treatment of AVM.

Patients suspected to have PHACES or Sturge–Weber syndrome should undergo brain MRI to rule out intracranial anomalies and vascular malformations.

Diagnosis

The diagnosis of pediatric vascular anomalies is generally straightforward, once imaging studies have been performed. The only exception is that the noninvoluting and rapidly involuting subtypes of congenital hemangioma can be distinguished from each other only in retrospect.

■ Management

Nonsurgical Management

When lymphatic malformation becomes infected, directed antimicrobial therapy alone is sometimes adequate. Aspiration of the infected fluid is followed by coverage from a broad-spectrum antibiotic (e.g., amoxicillin-clavulanate).

Microcystic lymphatic malformation is not amenable to medical therapy. Current alternative medical therapy for macrocystic lymphatic malformation is sclerotherapy. Agents that have shown promise include OK-432, doxycycline, ethanol, bleomycin, and Ethibloc (Ethicon, Somerville, NJ). At this writing, OK-432 is not available as an investigational agent, but it was previously made available through a trial sponsored by the National Institutes of Health based at the University of Iowa. Interventional radiologists at Children's Hospital Colorado prefer doxycycline, and occasionally use ethanol.

Past medical treatments for infantile hemangiomas have included corticosteroids, interferon alpha, and vincristine. All of these have significant side effects. In 2008, Léauté-Labrèze et al serendipitously treated two hemangioma patients accompanied by cardiac complications with propranolol. Their work has revolutionized the medical treatment of infantile hemangiomas. Obviously, this is an off-label use of propranolol, and no standards are established.

Menezes et al recently summarized the status of using propranolol for the treatment of infantile hemangioma, basing their findings on six published studies that had treated more than 10 patients. Propranolol therapy was initiated during infancy in 92.9% of patients with a mean age of 4.5 months. About two-thirds of the patients received a dose of 2 mg/kg/d dose. Five out of six studies admitted their patients for treatment at least part of a day. Treatment was ongoing for 46% of the patients at the time of the study's publication. Average treatment duration in the remaining patients was 5.1 months. Rebound hemangioma growth occurred in 21% of the patients. Adverse events occurred in 18.1% of the patients, including hypotension, somnolence, insomnia/agitation/nightmares, cool hands/night sweats, wheezing, gastroesophageal reflux disease, and rash. The authors reported a favorable outcome, but efficacy was not standardized.

The use of propranolol for the treatment of subglottic hemangioma has also been reported, but the response rate has not been as universal as that for infantile cutaneous hemangiomas. Javia et al reported that 8 of 12 patients responded to propranolol therapy alone, whereas Roal et al reported that 2 of 3 patients responded to propranolol therapy. Both institutions discussed their changing treatment paradigm of using propranolol and the continued role of surgical intervention.

Surgical Management

Surgical management of both lymphatic malformation and infantile hemangioma will change in response to advances in medical management. The surgical management of lymphatic malformation should be reserved for cosmesis, repeated infections in microcystic lymphatic malformation, and failure to respond to sclerotherapy in macrocystic lesions. The philosophy of surgical management has varied from complete excision to temporizing surgery to save vital structures and maintain function. Generally, it is felt by most clinicians that normal anatomy and, most important, bodily functions should not be sacrificed to accomplish complete resection of these benign lesions.

Although the long-term impact of propranolol on surgical management of cutaneous hemangioma is unknown, the need to revise hemangioma sites for cosmetic reasons will remain. The partial response to propranolol for subglottic hemangioma keeps open the options of endoscopic laser procedures and open excisions.

■ Controversial Issues

In 2009, the University of Iowa Collaborative Study Group published its safety and efficacy data on the treatment of lymphatic malformation using OK-432. The group concluded that OK-432 is an effective, safe, and simple treatment option for managing macrocystic cervicofacial lymphatic malformation. However, recent publications suggest that the efficacy of OK-432 may not be different from that of other treatment modalities, including bleomycin or alcohol. Furthermore, the superiority of sclerotherapy versus surgical excision is not settled, due to a lack of well-designed trials.

■ Suggested Reading

Adams MT, Saltzman B, Perkins JA. Head and neck lymphatic malformation treatment: a systematic review. Otolaryngol Head Neck Surg 2012;147(4):627–639

Churchill P, Otal D, Pemberton J, Ali A, Flageole H, Walton JM. Sclerotherapy for lymphatic malformations in children: a scoping review. J Pediatr Surg 2011;46(5):912–922

Javia LR, Zur KB, Jacobs IN. Evolving treatments in the management of laryngotracheal hemangiomas: will propranolol supplant steroids and surgery? Int J Pediatr Otorhinolaryngol 2011; 75(11):1450–1454

Kulungowski AM, Hassanein AH, Nosé V, et al. Expression of androgen, estrogen, progesterone, and growth hormone receptors in vascular malformations. Plast Reconstr Surg 2012;129(6): 919e–924e

Léauté-Labrèze C, Dumas de la Roque E, Hubiche T, Boralevi F, Thambo JB, Taïeb A. Propranolol for severe hemangiomas of infancy. N Engl J Med 2008;358(24):2649–2651

Menezes MD, McCarter R, Greene EA, Bauman NM. Status of propranolol for treatment of infantile hemangioma and description of a randomized clinical trial. Ann Otol Rhinol Laryngol 2011;120(10):686–695

Puttgen KB, Pearl M, Tekes A, Mitchell SE. Update on pediatric extracranial vascular anomalies of the head and neck. Childs Nerv Syst 2010;26(10):1417–1433

Raol N, Metry D, Edmonds J, Chandy B, Sulek M, Larrier D. Propranolol for the treatment of subglottic hemangiomas. Int J Pediatr Otorhinolaryngol 2011;75(12):1510–1514

Smith MC, Zimmerman MB, Burke DK, Bauman NM, Sato Y, Smith RJ; OK-432 Collaborative Study Group. Efficacy and safety of OK-432 immunotherapy of lymphatic malformations. Laryngoscope 2009;119(1):107–115

Wiegand S, Eivazi B, Zimmermann AP, Sesterhenn AM, Werner JA. Sclerotherapy of lymphangiomas of the head and neck. Head Neck 2011;33(11):1649–1655

76 Pediatric Head and Neck Masses

■ Introduction

Pediatric head and neck masses, cysts, and lesions encompass a heterogeneous group of entities that taken together have a tremendous variety of clinical presentations. Individual entities, however, have more characteristic presentations that are helpful for making a proper diagnosis. A thorough understanding of the embryology, anatomy, typical presentation, and expected clinical course and consequences of these lesions is essential when selecting an effective evaluation and management plan. This chapter is organized by categorizing these lesions into five groups: congenital lesions, infectious lesions, salivary gland lesions, thyroid lesions, and soft tissue masses.

■ Congenital Lesions

Thyroglossal Duct Cyst

Thyroglossal duct cyst (TGDC) is the most common congenital anomaly that presents as a pediatric neck mass. Up to 7% of the population at autopsy has evidence of a TGDC. It occurs due to persistence of the thyroglossal duct, often with thyroid tissue elements, along the path of thyroid gland descent during embryological development.

The thyroglossal duct course is from the foramen cecum at the base of the tongue to the final thyroid gland location in the lower anterior neck. During the fourth week of fetal development, epithelium located in the floor of the pharynx that later forms the foramen cecum of the tongue evaginates to form the thyroglossal duct. The duct descends to the lower midline neck, where its distal end becomes bilobed and differentiates into the thyroid gland. Thyroid development is completed at the 8th week of gestation. Between the 8th and 10th weeks, the duct normally involutes.

TGDCs most commonly present as a midline cervical lump, often in close association with the hyoid bone. More rarely, they present in the base of the tongue (lingual TGDC), suprasternal, or intrathyroid. Untreated TGDCs have a propensity for infection, and the treatment of choice is surgical removal. A malignant TGDC is very rare and typically has well-differentiated thyroid carcinoma histology.

Evaluation

Neck examination will often show a soft or hard lump in the perihyoid area in the midline of the neck. The association with the hyoid bone leads to movement of the lump with protrusion of the tongue. If infected, overlying skin may be erythematous or may have a draining fistula. Neck ultrasonography can help differentiate a TGDC from other pathology, such as a dermoid cyst, lymph node, or ectopic thyroid tissue. Computed tomography (CT) or magnetic resonance imaging (MRI) is typically not needed but may be useful in recurrent or complicated cases. Some surgeons recommend thyroid functions tests (TFTs), but this may not be necessary in a symptomatically euthyroid patient with normal thyroid tissue in the expected location on neck ultrasound.

Management

The recommended treatment for a TGDC is surgical extirpation by the Sistrunk procedure. This involves removal of the cyst and remnant thyroglossal duct tract in continuity with the middle third of the hyoid bone and involved tongue musculature. Recurrence rates after the Sistrunk procedure are ~ 2 to 6%, but have been shown to be higher (up to 20%) if there is a history of infection of the cyst. Recurrence may be lower if the middle third of the hyoid bone and involved perihyoid tissue are thoroughly removed. Simple cystectomy alone has an unacceptably high recurrence rate.

Key anatomical landmarks in the surgery are the midline strap muscles, thyrohyoid membrane, hyoid bone, and tongue musculature. Broad-spectrum antibiotics with or without incision and drainage are used for an infected TGDC. It is preferable to delay definitive surgery until the infection is resolved. Other complications with the Sistrunk procedure are typically minor and wound related, but can be more serious and include violation of the airway, neurovascular injury, or hematoma with airway obstruction.

Branchial Cleft Anomalies

Branchial cleft anomalies are the second most common congenital lesion that can present as a mass in the pediatric neck, representing 30% of such masses. The etiology is failure of the clefts and pouches of the pharyngeal apparatus to obliterate during embryogenesis. The pharyngeal arches (also known as branchial arches), of which four are dominant and two are much smaller, are evident by the fourth to fifth week of gestation. Each arch is composed of mesoderm, along with a primary blood vessel, nerve, and cartilage bar, and is separated from the next arch by an external cleft lined by ectoderm and an internal pouch lined by endoderm. This pharyngeal apparatus gives rise to the primary structures of the head and neck.

Branchial anomalies can present as solitary cysts, sinuses (tract either to pharynx or skin), vestigial remnants, or complete pharyngocutaneous fistulas. A complete fistula results from a connection between a persistent pouch and cleft forming a tract from the pharynx to the skin of the neck. The lining of the cyst or tract is typically squamous or respiratory epithelium. Branchial cleft anomalies are named by the arch/cleft/pouch of origin. Embryology ensures a predictable relationship to the surrounding anatomy, particularly neurovascular structures. A thorough understanding of these relationships is the foundation of safe surgical planning.

Branchial cleft anomalies can cause recurrent infection, abscess formation, and drainage from fistulas. When large, they can have problematic mass effects that impact the airway or swallowing. Malignancies in these lesions are extremely rare.

First Branchial Cleft Anomalies

The first pharyngeal arch, with maxillary and mandibular processes, differentiates to form many structures of the midface, mandible, middle ear, and muscles innervated by the motor root of the mandibular nerve of the third vertebra (V3). The first cleft and pouch form much of the eustachian tube, middle ear and mastoid cavities, and external auditory canal.

First branchial cleft anomalies represent up to 8% of all branchial cleft anomalies. They can present as a cutaneous pit in the neck, parotid area, external auditory meatus, or periauricular area, or with swelling and infectious complications at any of these sites.

Two types of first branchial cleft anomalies are commonly described. Type I is an ectoderm-derived duplication of the membranous external auditory canal and travels lateral to the facial nerve. Type II is ectoderm and mesoderm derived, can have a tract medial to the facial nerve, and often presents with swelling or pits around the auricle or as far inferior as the angle of the mandible and submandibular area.

Evaluation

Neck examination will often show a hard or soft swelling or pit in the periauricular area, parotid area, or upper neck. There may be infectious symptoms. Occasionally, involvement of the external auditory canal or tympanic membrane can be seen. Although ultrasound can help identify an underlying cyst, CT or MRI provides more anatomical detail and can better define any parotid gland involvement, which allows for better preoperative planning and assessment of facial nerve risk prior to surgical intervention. Laboratory studies are typically not useful. Some surgeons advocate fistulogram studies.

Management

The recommended treatment of first branchial cleft anomalies is surgical excision of the lesion. This often involves superficial (rarely total) parotidectomy and facial nerve dissection. Involvement of the external auditory canal or middle ear may require reconstruction. Complications typically involve wound issues, recurrence, or facial nerve weakness. The risk of recurrence can range from 3% for primary resections to 20% for revision cases. Facial nerve weakness is rare and typically temporary.

Second Branchial Cleft Anomalies

The second pharyngeal arch differentiates to form part of the hyoid bone and the muscles innervated by the facial nerve (cranial nerve [CN] VII). The second pouch forms the palatine tonsils. The second cleft normally obliterates by the seventh week of gestation.

Second branchial cleft anomalies account for 70 to 90% of all brachial cleft anomalies. They can present as a solitary cyst, but they may have a cutaneous pit at the anterior border of the sternocleidomastoid (SCM) muscle in the lower third of the neck. Solitary cysts present at an older age and are more likely to have a history of recurrent infection. Complete fistulas represent a minority of all second cleft anomalies but are not uncommon.

A complete fistula has a described course. Traveling from the cutaneous pit anterior to the SCM muscle, it pierces the platysma and investing layer of the deep cervical fascia; ascends superficial to the strap muscles; and travels between the carotid artery bifurcation, over the hypoglossal nerve, and around the glossopharyngeal nerve to reach the tonsillar fossa.

Evaluation

When evaluating a fistula, cervical ultrasound can help screen for an underlying cyst or cartilage component. Ultrasound is also useful for differentiating a cyst from a soft tissue mass or lymph node, when this is not clear on physical examination. When a cyst is evident on physical examination, CT or MRI may be more useful to better define the anatomy for surgical planning. Some clinicians find CT and MRI useful in identifying a tract, whereas others find them less useful. Some clinicians advocate fistulography, whereas others do not find this necessary. Laboratory studies are typically not useful. Complete fistulas are more common on the right, and bilateral anomalies have a higher association with branchiootorenal syndrome (BORS).

Management

The recommended treatment for second branchial cleft anomalies is surgical excision of the lesion. Pits are typically excised by an elliptical skin incision, in continuity with the underlying tract. Tracts are followed from inferior to superior, taking care to protect adjacent structures, such as the internal jugular vein, carotid artery, and nerves. For long tracts, a "step ladder" incision has been described, but this is often unnecessary. Described methods to assist in identifying the tract are cannulation with lacrimal probes and injection with liquid such as saline or methylene blue. Following the tract superior to the hyoid bone is a useful landmark to help facilitate complete removal of a complete fistula. Solitary cysts are removed by traditional open neck surgery.

Third and Fourth Branchial Cleft Anomalies

Third and fourth branchial cleft anomalies present similarly and are difficult to differentiate from each other. The third arch gives rise to part of the internal carotid artery, hyoid bone, epiglottis, thymus, and stylopharyngeus muscle controlled by the glossopharyngeal nerve (CN IX), and the third pouch gives rise to the inferior parathyroid glands and pyriform fossa. The fourth arch gives rise to the arch of the aorta; cartilages, including thyroid, cuneiform, and part of the epiglottic cartilage; and muscles controlled by the superior laryngeal nerve (branch of CN X). The fourth pouch forms the superior parathyroid glands.

The theoretical course of third and fourth branchial cleft anomaly tracts has been extensively described based on anatomical principles. Of significance, the tracts pass posterior to the carotid artery, have a variable association with the thyroid gland, and enter the pharynx in the pyriform fossa. The presentation of these lesions is most often recurrent neck abscesses (40%) and suppurative thyroiditis (30–45%).

Evaluation

Neck examination will less commonly show a pit in the cervical skin. A cyst with or without an internal opening in the pyriform sinus is more common. Evidence of previous incision and drainage of neck abscess or tenderness due to thyroiditis may be present. Barium swallow, direct laryngoscopy, and MRI are the most useful diagnostic studies. Barium esophagram has a 50 to 80% sensitivity for identifying the internal opening of a third or fourth branchial fistula. Thyroid ultrasound may be helpful in cases of recurrent thyroiditis. These lesions are more common on the left.

Management

The recommended treatment is surgical removal of the lesion. Direct laryngoscopy, with particular attention to the pyriform sinus, is important to identify the tract opening in this location. Pyriform sinus openings can be closed by such techniques as monopolar or chemical cautery, chemical sealants, or suture. Hemithyroidectomy may be necessary in cases of recurrent thyroiditis. Recurrence rates have been shown to depend on the method of treatment: incision and drainage (90%), endoscopic cauterization of the opening in the pyriform sinus (15%), open neck surgery with excision of the lesion and tract (15%), and open neck surgery with hemithyroidectomy (8–15%).

Cervical and Nasal Dermoid Cysts

Dermoid cysts result from trapped epithelial elements (ectoderm and endoderm) along embryological lines of fusion. They often present in a midline or paramedian location in the neck, or as a midline nasal dorsum cyst. Other head, face, or neck locations are possible. Dermoid cysts are lined by epithelium and can contain skin elements, such as hair and sebaceous glands. They enlarge over time due to accumulation of sebaceous material. The contents have a characteristic "cheeselike" quality.

Midline cervical dermoid cysts need to be differentiated from TGDCs and lymph nodes. Imaging can help, but definitive identification can often be made only during surgery and final histopathology. Midline cervical dermoid cysts present commonly as a soft or hard, midline, nontender lump anywhere from the sternal notch to the submentum and floor of the mouth, with intact overlying skin or mucosa. Some of these cysts have a history of infection, although this is rare. Cervical dermoid cysts represent 20% of head and neck dermoids and are usually diagnosed before 3 years of age.

Nasal dermoid cysts represent 4 to 13% of head and neck dermoids, can present as a swelling on the nasal dorsum anywhere from the glabella to the nasal tip, and are sometimes associated with a cutaneous pit. A pit and tract can be present without an associated swelling or defined cyst. An estimated 5 to 45% of nasal dermoid cysts can have intracranial extension. The etiology is thought to be failure of a normal dura mater diverticulum to involute during embryogenesis. This dural diverticulum forms around 8 weeks of gestation, travels from the anterior cranial base through the foramen cecum to the prenasal space and nasal skin, and involutes after closure of the frontal and nasal bones. Imaging prior to surgical removal is critical to evaluate for intracranial extension and to help differentiate the cyst from an encephalocele or glioma.

Evaluation

Midline cervical dermoid cysts are typically superficial to the strap muscles and well encapsulated. They can be subcutaneous and move with the skin or deep to the investing cervical fascia. Cervical ultrasound can help define the extent and depth of the lesion and, sometimes, differentiate it from TGDCs and lymph nodes. CT or MRI is usually not needed but may be helpful for large or atypical lesions.

Nasal dermoid cysts require CT, MRI, or both preoperatively to assess for possible intracranial extension and to rule out other pathology, particularly encephalocele. A bifid crista galli or enlarged foramen cecum on CT scan is suggestive of intracranial involvement. MRI, with better soft tissue definition, can more directly visualize intracranial involvement as a high-intensity T1 signal. Physical exam is important because an encephalocele can have a bluish color, can swell with Valsalva maneuvers or crying (Furstenberg sign), and is not associated with a pit.

Management

The recommended treatment for a dermoid cyst is excision. Midline cervical dermoid cysts can usually be removed by simple excision from a horizontal incision in the skin crease. The surgeon should be prepared to convert to a Sistrunk procedure if the intraoperative appearance is characteristic of a TGDC. Some surgeons recommend Sistrunk procedure for a dermoid cyst that is attached to the hyoid bone, to ensure complete removal and account for a possible atypical TGDC. Recurrence is rare if the cyst is completely excised, and complications are typically minor and wound related.

Nasal dermoid cysts can be removed through a horizontal or vertical incision that includes an ellipse around a cutaneous pit, if present. The entire tract and cyst need to be removed to avoid recurrence. The tract can proceed superficial to, deep to, or through the nasal bones. If no skin pit is present, an open rhinoplasty approach can avoid an incision on the nasal dorsum. When intracranial extension is present, a neurosurgeon assists in surgery. Large lesions may require additional incisions or a bicoronal incision. More recently, endoscopic or endoscopically assisted removal has been described. Complications are typically minor and wound related, unless intracranial involvement introduces location-specific risk, such as meningitis, cerebrospinal fluid leakage, or brain injury.

Midline Cervical Cleft

Congenital midline cervical cleft is very rare, with fewer than 100 cases reported as of 2009. The leading etiology is thought to be failure of midline fusion of the first or second branchial arches during embryogenesis. The appearance is a midline skin defect with an erythematous, vertical line of variable thickness and length, anywhere from the mandible to the sternal notch, associated with a skin protuberance at the superior end and sinus tract at the inferior end. The cleft is lined with stratified squamous epithelium. The tract has respiratory or columnar epithelial lining and the protuberance may contain muscle or cartilage. The lesion has a tendency to tether the neck and restrict cervical extension. It can be associated with more severe midline clefting extending superiorly into the mandible, lower lip, and tongue.

Evaluation

The physical exam is characteristic and diagnostic if the examiner is familiar with the anomaly. Palpation will often show a firm, subcutaneous fibrous cord along the length of the lesion. The lesion is superficial (surface and subcutaneous), and imaging is typically not needed.

Management

The recommended treatment is early surgical removal, to avoid infection and reduce the restriction on cervical extension. After excision, repair by Z-plasty (single or multiple adjacent) is recommended, serving both to reorient the closure in a relaxed skin tension line horizontally and to lengthen the closure, thereby relieving the restriction on cervical motion.

Preauricular Cyst

Preauricular skin pits with associated sinus tract and cyst are common congenital lesions. The reported incidence range is 1 to 10% of the population, with the highest rate occurring in parts of Africa. Preauricular cysts have a squamous lining and are theorized to form along the fusion points of the six auricular hillocks during external ear formation near the sixth week of embryogenesis.

Evaluation

The physical exam for preauricular cysts is characteristic and diagnostic, with attention given for signs of infection or drainage. Imaging is typically not needed. If cysts are seen in conjunction with branchial anomalies, hearing loss, external ear malformations, or family history of hearing loss, renal ultrasonography and further workup for possible BORS should be considered.

Management

Preauricular cysts are often asymptomatic and can be observed. However, frequent drainage or a history of infection is an indication for surgical removal. The entire pit, tract, and associated cyst, if present, need to be removed to avoid recurrence. An ellipse around the pit, oriented so closure will align in the preauricular crease, is incised, and the tract is followed to the cyst. Extension of the incision, inferiorly in the preauricular crease, or superiorly curving posteriorly under the superior pinna, is helpful for exposure, especially for recurrent lesions. The cyst is superficial to the temporalis fascia. The small cuff of tragal cartilage is often removed due to a close association of the cartilage/perichondrium with the tract or cyst. Some clinicians advocate injection of the tract with saline or dye preoperatively.

■ Infectious Lesions

Nontuberculous Mycobacterial Infections

Nontuberculous (atypical) mycobacteria (NTM) cervical lymphadenitis can present as a mass in the pediatric neck, typically in ages 1 to 5 years. The infection is indolent and is often not associated with systemic illness signs, such as fever or chills. Early infections may present as a soft or hard, mobile or fixed mass along the cervical lymph node regions with intact skin. This mass must be differentiated from other inflammatory, congenital, or neoplastic lesions, including *Mycobacterium tuberculosis* cervical adenitis (scrofula). The broad differential diagnosis at this point can lead to a delay in diagnosis.

The causative bacteria of NTM infections are endemic to the soil in many regions, particularly the midwestern and southwestern United States. Organisms may include *Mycobacterium avium-intracellulare*, *Mycobacterium scrofulaceum*, and *Mycobacterium kansasii*. Organisms may be introduced through a defect in the skin or oral mucosa, leading to lymphadenitis. Over time, the overlying skin develops a characteristic erythematous or violaceous color that can aid in diagnosis. Untreated, this skin will eventually break down, leading to fistula formation and thick drainage.

Evaluation

The history of NTM infections often reveals a child with frequent outdoor activity in areas with exposed soil, such as a yard or farm. Physical examination will demonstrate the mass, possibly with the characteristic violaceous overlying skin. The color change is less obvious in pigmented skin. In many cases, the history and physical exam can be highly suggestive of NTM infections. In other cases, the lack of skin color change or suggestive history makes diagnosis more difficult. Purified protein derivative (PPD) testing is appropriate, and a positive result in active NTM infections ranges in studies from 4 to 67%. A positive PPD demands consideration of a *Mycobacterium tuberculosis* infection. Imaging is helpful to define the disease burden. Cervical ultrasonography is useful with mild disease, whereas MRI or CT scan is useful with more bulky disease or a large mass. CT characteristically shows asymmetric cervical lymphadenopathy with low-density, necrotic, ring-enhancing masses. Acid-fast staining may show the mycobacteria. Culture of the offending organism through fine-needle aspiration (FNA) or open incision is diagnostic. Open surgery can be highly suggestive of the diagnosis because the infected lymph nodes have a characteristic "cheesy" quality.

Management

Treatment of NTM adenitis is by antibiotics, surgery, or both. Complete surgical excision when possible is the treatment of choice. The nature of these bacteria makes antibiotics alone less effective, especially with bulky disease. Clarithromycin and rifabutin have been shown to be efficacious alone or in combination with surgery. Prolonged antibiotic courses of 6 months or more may be required. Decreasing the disease burden by incision and curettage or, preferably, complete excision of the lesion is often required. Consideration for appropriate isolation of the operative suite is reasonable if typical tuberculosis is in the differential diagnosis. If NTM lymphadenitis is completely excised, antibiotic therapy may not be needed, and the cure rate approaches 100%. When complete excision is not possible, revision surgery and/or antibiotics may be necessary. Involving infectious disease specialists in the care of these patients can be helpful. Human-to-human transmission has not been described, and isolation of patients is not necessary.

Reactive Lymphadenitis

Lymphadenopathy is a common cause of cervical masses in the pediatric population. Nodes larger than 10 mm are considered abnormal. Most commonly in children, adenopathy is a response to inflammatory conditions, such as infections, and is termed reactive lymphadenitis. Nodal enlargement occurs as a result of cellular hyperplasia, leukocyte infiltration, and tissue edema. The masses present in typical lymph node locations, such as periauricular, submental, submandibular, along the jugular vein, supraclavicular, or in the posterior cervical triangle. More rarely, neoplastic lesions cause pediatric lymphadenopathy.

Evaluation

The history may reveal a recent infection of the head or neck, such as otitis media, sinusitis, upper respiratory infection, or skin infection. Physical exam shows a hard or rubbery mobile mass that may be tender. Bacterial infections may show suppuration of the involved nodes, leading to a fluctuant mass with overlying skin erythema. The primary care physician typically orders laboratory tests early for evidence of microorganisms and evaluates for adenopathy outside of the head and neck. The many infectious possibilities are described in the literature. Otolaryngologists typically become involved with chronic head or neck lymphadenopathy.

Cervical ultrasonography can establish the nodal morphology and size and differentiate a solid lesion from one with fluid density, as in a congenital cyst or suppuration. Serial ultrasonography is helpful to follow for nodal growth or changes over time. CT or MRI may be more helpful with a large mass or bulky disease. Persistent adenopathy raises more concerns. Nodes that are painless, firm, or immobile, or single-dominant nodes that persist for more than 6 weeks, increase concern for neoplastic lesions.

Management

Treatment of reactive lymphadenitis depends on the cause of lymphadenopathy. Reactive cervical lymphadenitis with an appropriate history suggestive of this diagnosis can be followed conservatively for a period of time. Some clinicians advocate a trial of broad-spectrum antibiotics, especially with strong evidence of bacterial infection (skin erythema, purulent drainage). Often the initial management is by the primary care physician. With an atypical history, large masses, or evidence of consistent mass growth, referral to a surgeon should be considered for needle or open biopsy to evaluate for other pathology, such as neoplasia or congenital cyst. Failure to respond to routine antibiotics can also occur with nontuberculous mycobacterial lymphadenitis.

■ Salivary Gland Lesions

Pediatric salivary gland masses are rare. Parotid gland masses are most common and include inflammatory lesions, first branchial cleft cysts, venolymphatic malformations, or neoplastic lesions. Inflammatory lesions include infections of intraparotid lymph nodes, or chronic inflammation from infection or autoimmune disease. Less than 5% of all salivary gland neoplasms occur in children. In the parotid gland, the most common benign nonepithelial neoplastic lesion is hemangioma, and the most common benign epithelial lesion is pleomorphic adenoma. The most common malignant pediatric parotid gland tumor is mucoepidermoid carcinoma. Other rarer lesions include acinic cell carcinoma and adenoid cystic carcinoma. Similar epithelial tumors even more rarely can present in the submandibular, lingual, or minor salivary glands.

Evaluation

History and physical exam help differentiate infectious, congenital, or neoplastic lesions. The parotid gland, including intraparotid lymph nodes, submandibular gland, sublingual gland, or minor salivary glands, can be involved. Imaging by ultrasonography, CT, or MRI is often useful to demonstrate the extent of disease. Imaging can be diagnostic, with a high degree of accuracy for some lesions, particularly hemangioma and venolymphatic malformations. Lesions that do not respond to medical management, especially if there is concern for neoplasia (solid lesions), require biopsy by needle aspiration or excisional biopsy. Incisional biopsy is not recommended for parotid lesions because facial nerve injury may occur.

Management

Management depends on identifying the etiology. Infectious or inflammatory lesions may respond to appropriate medical therapy. Hemangioma has unique treatment. Other congenital and neoplastic lesions often require excision. For malignant lesions, appropriate surgical, medical, and radiation therapy is directed, based on oncological principles.

■ Thyroid Lesions

Thyroid nodules are less common in pediatric patients than adults, with an estimated incidence of less than 1.8%. However, pediatric solitary thyroid nodules have an estimated 20% likelihood of malignancy. The most common pediatric thyroid malignancy is papillary thyroid carcinoma (80–85% of cases), followed by medullary thyroid carcinoma. Unlike incidence in adults, follicular thyroid carcinoma is less common in children. Radiation exposure, either therapeutic (Hodgkin lymphoma treatment most commonly) or accidental (environmental accidents), results in increased risk for thyroid carcinoma. Children are more susceptible to the effect of radiation exposure, especially when younger than 10 years. Development of thyroid malignancy is associated with certain syndromes, such as Cowden and Gardner syndromes. Germline point mutations in the RET proto-oncogene result in multiple endocrine neoplasia syndromes (MEN2A or MEN2B) and increased risk for medullary thyroid carcinoma and other endocrine malignancies.

Evaluation

A full history, including family history of thyroid carcinoma and personal history of radiation exposure, and physical examination are critical. Ultrasonography is useful to establish the size and echogenicity of a nodule. It can also identify bilateral or multiple lesions and cervical lymph node enlargement. FNA biopsy is highly sensitive and specific (up to 100% and 95%, respectively) for identifying papillary, medullary, or anaplastic thyroid malignancies. When FNA is unable to identify a concerning nodule, open biopsy through hemi- or total thyroidectomy is warranted. TFT and thyroid autoimmune antibodies can be helpful for identifying nodules caused by Graves disease or Hashimoto thyroiditis. Radionuclide imaging with technetium-99m pertechnetate can show a hyper- or hypofunctioning nodule but cannot establish whether a nodule is malignant.

Management

Benign nodules can be followed by serial examination, ultrasonography, and fine-needle biopsy. Suspected or biopsy-confirmed thyroid carcinoma is treated by thyroidectomy when possible. Small (< 1 cm) solitary, well-differentiated papillary or follicular carcinomas can be treated by hemithyroidectomy. Total thyroidectomy is indicated for larger, multifocal, or bilateral well-differentiated lesions. Neck dissection is indicated to remove involved lymph node basins. Pediatric papillary or follicular carcinoma has a survival rate higher than 90%. Medullary thyroid carcinoma is treated with total thyroidectomy and removal of involved lymph nodes. Total thyroidectomy is recommended by age 6 years in patients with MEN2A and by age 1 year in patients with MEN2B. Radioiodine (131I) is administered postoperatively for some forms of metastatic thyroid cancer. Surveillance by whole-body scanning, thyroglobulin levels, imaging, and examination is important.

■ Soft Tissue Neck Masses

Fibromatosis Colli

Fibromatosis colli (also known as SCM tumor of infancy) presents as a hard, minimally mobile mass in the neonatal neck intimately associated with the SCM muscle. The incidence is 0.4% of live births. The etiology is presumed to be a fibrotic reaction to SCM trauma during the birth process.

Evaluation

Physical examination shows a mass in the mid to lower lateral neck, associated with the SCM muscle. This lesion must be differentiated from other congenital, inflammatory, or neoplastic lesions. The involved muscle is often shortened from the fibrosis, resulting in muscular torticollis, with the head turned to the opposite side. Cervical ultrasonography, when combined with history and physical exam, is often diagnostic. Ultrasound typically shows a hyperechoic mass or diffuse SCM enlargement with mixed echogenicity. MRI, CT scan, or biopsy is rarely needed. When necessary, FNA biopsy can be diagnostic and shows benign fibroblasts and atrophic skeletal muscle.

Management

Physical therapy and time result in resolution of the fibrotic mass and torticollis in 90% or more cases. Surgical excision is not indicated.

Neoplastic Lesions

Pediatric neoplastic neck lesions are relatively rare. Benign or malignant lesions have cells of origin from varied tissues, including epithelial, mesenchymal, neural, thyroid, salivary, and lymphoid. They can be congenital or acquired later in infancy or childhood. These lesions include a diverse group of pathologies, and the individual incidence, evaluation, and management are equally diverse. The role of the head and neck surgeon is varied. Biopsy is often required to guide medical therapy (e.g., rhabdomyosarcoma and lymphoma), or surgical excision may be required to best treat the lesion (e.g., nonrhabdomyosarcoma and many benign lesions). A full discussion of all such lesions is beyond the scope of this chapter. Nevertheless, it is critical for the pediatric otolaryngologist to be familiar with these lesions when patients present with a cervical mass.

■ Suggested Reading

Acierno SP, Waldhausen JH. Congenital cervical cysts, sinuses and fistulae. Otolaryngol Clin North Am 2007;40(1):161–176, vii–viii

Al-Dajani N, Wootton SH. Cervical lymphadenitis, suppurative parotitis, thyroiditis, and infected cysts. Infect Dis Clin North Am 2007;21(2):523–541, viii

Bajaj Y, Dunaway D, Hartley BE. Surgical approach for congenital midline cervical cleft. J Laryngol Otol 2004;118(7):566–569

Bentley AA, Gillespie C, Malis D. Evaluation and management of a solitary thyroid nodule in a child. Otolaryngol Clin North Am 2003;36(1):117–128

Black CJ, O'Hara JT, Berry J, Robson AK. Magnetic resonance imaging of branchial cleft abnormalities: illustrated cases and literature review. J Laryngol Otol 2010;124(2):213–215

Enzinger FM, Weiss SW. Fibrous tumors of infancy and childhood. In: Weiss SW, Goldblum JR, eds. Enzinger and Weiss's Soft Tissue Tumors. 4th ed. St. Louis, MO: Mosby; 2001:347–408

Hirshoren N, Neuman T, Udassin R, Elidan J, Weinberger JM. The imperative of the Sistrunk operation: review of 160 thyroglossal tract remnant operations. Otolaryngol Head Neck Surg 2009;140(3):338–342

Maddalozzo J, Rastatter JC, Dreyfuss HF, Jaffar R, Bhushan B. The second branchial cleft fistula. Int J Pediatr Otorhinolaryngol 2012;76(7):1042–1045

Manning SC, Bloom DC, Perkins JA, Gruss JS, Inglis A. Diagnostic and surgical challenges in the pediatric skull base. Otolaryngol Clin North Am 2005;38(4):773–794

Mirilas P. Lateral congenital anomalies of the pharyngeal apparatus: part I. Normal developmental anatomy (embryogenesis) for the surgeon. Am Surg 2011;77(9):1230–1242

Mirilas P. Lateral congenital anomalies of the pharyngeal apparatus: part III. Cadaveric representation of the course of second and third cleft and pouch fistulas. Am Surg 2011;77(9):1257–1263

Munck K, Mandpe AH. Mycobacterial infections of the head and neck. Otolaryngol Clin North Am 2003;36(4):569–576

Nicoucar K, Giger R, Jaecklin T, Pope HG Jr, Dulguerov P. Management of congenital third branchial arch anomalies: a systematic review. Otolaryngol Head Neck Surg 2010;142(1):21–28, e2

Nicoucar K, Giger R, Pope HG Jr, Jaecklin T, Dulguerov P. Management of congenital fourth branchial arch anomalies: a review and analysis of published cases. J Pediatr Surg 2009;44(7):1432–1439

Orvidas LJ, Kasperbauer JL, Lewis JE, Olsen KD, Lesnick TG. Pediatric parotid masses. Arch Otolaryngol Head Neck Surg 2000;126(2):177–184

Tracy TF Jr, Muratore CS. Management of common head and neck masses. Semin Pediatr Surg 2007;16(1):3–13

Zapata S, Kearns DB. Nasal dermoids. Curr Opin Otolaryngol Head Neck Surg 2006;14(6):406–411

77 Pediatric Rhinosinusitis

■ Introduction

Paranasal Sinus Anatomy

The paranasal sinuses are air-filled cavities within the skull. They include four paired sinuses: maxillary, ethmoid, sphenoid, and frontal. Each sinus is lined with respiratory mucosa and is in communication with the nasal cavity through an ostium.

Maxillary Sinus

The maxillary sinus is the first to develop, is present in the neonate, and continues to grow until early adulthood. The maxillary sinus ostium is located along the medial wall of the maxillary sinus and drains into the middle meatus.

Ethmoid Sinus

The ethmoid sinus is divided into anterior and posterior ethmoid air cells, separated by the basal lamella, which is the bony attachment of the middle turbinate. The ethmoid sinuses are also present at birth and have nearly completed development by 12 years of age. Anterior ethmoid cells drain into the middle meatus, whereas the posterior sinuses drain into the superior meatus.

Sphenoid Sinus

The sphenoid sinus does not pneumatize until 5 years of age and has typically completed its development by age 12 to 15 years. The sphenoid ostium is situated on the anterior face of the sphenoid and drains into the superior meatus.

Frontal Sinus

The frontal sinus is the last to develop, with pneumatization beginning between ages 4 to 8 years. Development is not complete until the late teenage years. The frontal recess drains into the middle meatus. The significance of the paranasal sinuses is largely unknown. An accepted function is that the cilia within the sinuses beat toward the natural ostium and allow clearance of mucous and prevention of infection.

Incidence

Pediatric rhinosinusitis (RS) is a commonly encountered problem. Children develop on average six to eight upper respiratory infections each year, in contrast to adults, who develop only two to three. In this population, 90% of children would be expected to have an associated viral sinusitis and 0.5 to 2% would develop a bacterial superinfection. Symptoms can include cough, purulent nasal discharge, headache, facial pain, and fever.

Sinusitis typically involves an inciting event or process, followed by inflammation and obstruction of a sinus ostium. Sinus ventilation is impaired, which results in negative pressure formation; nasal and nasopharyngeal contents are trapped in the sinus.

Categories of Bacterial Rhinosinusitis

Bacterial RS in children is subdivided into five categories, as described in the clinical practice guidelines published by the American Academy of Pediatrics: acute, subacute, recurrent acute, acute on chronic, and chronic. Acute rhinosinusitis (ARS) usually begins as an upper respiratory infection, which then persists beyond the expected 7 to 10 days. It will last fewer than 30 days in total duration. Subacute sinusitis lasts 30 to 90 days, followed by complete resolution. Recurrent acute sinusitis involves episodes of acute infection lasting fewer than 30 days, separated by a minimum of 10-day intervals during which the patient is asymptomatic. Acute or chronic infections have underlying chronic symptoms and intermittent development of new symptoms. Chronic rhinosinusitis (CRS) occurs for longer than 90 days. Patients often have persistent residual symptoms, including cough, rhinorrhea, or nasal obstruction.

■ Etiologies

Causative factors of ARS and CRS are vital to review because they will determine the appropriate management scheme. These causes have been described in prior literature, and the more common factors are summarized here. Viral upper respiratory infection is the most common precursor to pediatric ARS. Bacterial pathogens causing ARS parallel those causing acute otitis media and include *Streptococcus pneumoniae, Haemophilus influenzae*, and *Moraxella catarrhalis*. CRS has a different spectrum of bacterial infection, with the most common organisms including viridans streptococci, *Streptococcus pneumoniae, Staphylococcus aureus*, and anaerobes. Allergy is an important causative factor of CRS; ~ 80% of children with RS have a family history of allergy, as opposed to a frequency of 15 to 20% in the general population. The adenoid pad can act as a reservoir for bacterial organisms, and removal of the adenoid will improve RS for 70 to 80% of children. Gastroesophageal reflux disease (GERD) has been implicated in CRS in children. A prospective analysis of children with CRS found that 63% of patients had GERD, and 79% had improvement after treatment for GERD. Less common factors include immunodeficiency, ciliary dyskinesia, anatomical abnormalities of the nasal cavity and/or sinuses, and nonallergic rhinitis. Finally, cystic fibrosis (CF) is an important causative factor in pediatric chronic RS and will be discussed in detail.

CRS has a severe physical impact on the health of children. A child presenting with CRS should be fully evaluated for the previously described causative factors. Medical factors should be controlled if possible prior to consideration of surgical management. Allergy should be considered in children with a history of signs or symptoms consistent with seasonal, environmental, or food allergy; allergic rhinitis; asthma; or eczema. If these signs and symptoms are present, treatment by a pediatric allergist is warranted. Environmental exposures, including secondhand smoke and day care, should be eliminated.

Cystic Fibrosis

CRS is a consistent feature of the autosomal recessive disorder of CF. Its prevalence is ~ 1 in 3,500 live births. CF is caused by a mutation in the CF transmembrane regulator (CFTR) gene. The pathophysiology within the airway is thought to occur by the inability to secrete salt, and secondarily water, resulting in inadequate water on the airway surface to hydrate the secretions. As a result, secretions become viscous and difficult to remove via mucociliary clearance. The secretions are then retained in the airway and can cause obstruction and chronic inflammation. Respiratory symptoms include bronchiectasis, pneumonia, nasal polyposis, sinusitis, and reactive airway disease. Patients with CF have an increased prevalence of infection with *Pseudomonas aeruginosa*, and the presence of the mucoid phenotype of *pseudomonas* is highly suggestive of CF. Testing for CF has historically involved obtaining sweat sodium chloride levels. More recently, genetic testing has been used as a more accurate method of obtaining this diagnosis.

There are also data to suggest that there is increased incidence of CRS in carriers of the CFTR gene who do not meet criteria for CF. Specifically, adult literature has shown an association between the development of CRS and the presence of the CFTR gene. A study of 58 children with CRS who did not satisfy criteria for CF were found to have an increased prevalence of the CFTR mutation (12%), as compared with the expected rate of 3 to 4% without CRS. Therefore, it has been suggested that the presence of the CFTR gene, even in the absence of a CF diagnosis, results in increased predisposition to CRS. CFTR dysfunction and resultant lower expression levels may compromise the function of the CFTR in uptake and removal of bacterial pathogens, such as *Pseudomonas aeruginosa*, leading to persistent inflammation. A conclusion from these data is that children with CRS and an absence of frank CF may have heterozygosity of the CFTR gene and therefore may be more susceptible to infection by such pathogens as *Pseudomonas*, which are more commonly associated with classic CF. This may have implications for disease severity, the need for longer-term medical regimens, and the need for endoscopic sinus surgery.

■ Evaluation

An acute viral respiratory illness typically resolves within 10 days. Clinical findings to indicate development of ARS include fever, purulent nasal discharge, cough, and halitosis. Findings in CRS differ from those in acute sinusitis and can include headache, facial pain, and irritability in addition to nasal congestion, cough, and halitosis. Differentiating a viral upper respiratory infection from sinusitis can be difficult and is often based primarily on clinical presentation. A finding of purulent drainage from the middle meatus is highly suggestive of sinusitis but can be challenging to assess in younger children. However, anterior rhinoscopy can reveal purulent nasal drainage, leading to the diagnosis of sinusitis. Radiographic imaging in the form of computed tomography (CT) is typically reserved for refractory cases of sinusitis that do not respond to medical management or for complications of sinusitis. This is discussed in detail later in this chapter.

In children with a history suggestive of GERD, it may be reasonable to initiate a trial of antireflux medication; the literature has shown that this may decrease the need for surgical intervention. Immune testing should be considered in cases of refractory sinusitis and should include testing of humoral immune function with serum levels of immunoglobulin A (IgA), total IgG, and IgG subclasses. Immunoglobulin replacement may be a helpful adjuvant therapy. Primary ciliary dyskinesia can be evaluated by obtaining a nasal or tracheal brushing and examining the ciliary structure; however, no specific treatment is available for this condition. Finally, CF evaluation should be considered, especially in children with chronic or recurrent acute sinusitis in conjunction with other upper and lower respiratory infections. Sinonasal anatomy should be evaluated, and the mainstay of imaging is CT. Magnetic resonance imaging (MRI) can also be performed.

■ Management

The treatment of CRS in children is often a multistep process. The goal is to achieve maximal medical therapy in the hope of avoiding a surgical procedure. The exception to this is when there are acute complications of sinusitis, in which case surgical intervention is typically warranted. As previously discussed, causative factors, including allergens, environmental smoke exposure, GERD, and day care exposure, should be eliminated. It is recommended to treat patients with antibiotics for 3 to 6 weeks, although there are no randomized clinical trials to support this longer course of treatment. Adjunctive measures, including saline nasal sprays, mucolytic agents, and antihistamines, aid in the clearance of secretions. When nasal polyposis is present, nasal steroids can be considered, as well as oral steroids in the setting of severe polyposis.

There is no consensus approach for determining when a child with RS needs surgery. One described approach states that surgery is indicated in children with CRS who have failed maximal medical therapy,

do not have untreated allergy or GERD, and do not have an untreated systemic disease, including CF. First-line surgical treatment consists of adenoidectomy to eliminate the bacterial reservoir that can exist in the adenoid pad. A significant correlation has been shown with sinonasal symptom scores and colony-forming units of adenoid core pathogens. Following adenoidectomy, the expected rate of improvement is 70 to 80%. An alternate therapy for children with refractory CRS after oral antibiotics consists of maxillary sinus aspiration and irrigation with or without adenoidectomy, followed by culture-directed intravenous (IV) antibiotics and oral prophylaxis. In a study of this treatment, 89% of patients had resolution of symptoms, and 11% went on to require endoscopic sinus surgery (ESS). Similar results were seen in the stepwise protocol described by Don et al, in which children with CRS were treated with maxillary sinus aspiration and irrigation with selective adenoidectomy, followed by 1 to 4 weeks of culture-directed IV antibiotic therapy. Of the 70 patients studied, 89% had complete resolution of symptoms, and 11% required ESS.

In patients who have failed medical and conservative surgical measures, ESS should be considered. Although generally considered a safe surgery, reluctance to operate exists secondary to concerns regarding the effects on facial growth. A prospective study of 23 patients with CF, 14 of whom underwent ESS and 9 of whom served as controls, found no statistically significant difference on cephalometric measurements between the two groups after a minimum follow-up time of 10 years. This finding is in agreement with those of other studies that used CT volumetrics and quantitative anthropomorphic analysis of human midfacial growth following ESS and found no significant differences in development.

Preoperative CT imaging is necessary to evaluate the extent of sinonasal disease, as well as to determine whether anatomical abnormalities exist to cause a structural obstruction. In this era, it is important to note that health care workers as well as the general public are becoming increasingly aware of the potential long-term risk of cumulative radiation exposure in children to cause future malignancies. A recent study evaluated the cumulative radiation dose for 77 children with CF attending a tertiary CF center. This study found that the average cumulative radiation dose was 6.2 milliSieverts per CF patient, and these patients had undergone an average of 57 CT scans, 51 of which were thoracic. The authors' recommendation was to avoid unnecessary radiation exposure in this population.

The majority of imaging in CF patients comes in the form of thoracic CT. It has been recently suggested that MRI be used in place of CT for thoracic imaging to reduce overall radiation exposure. In adults, sinonasal imaging using MRI has been compared with imaging using CT. The findings were relevant for Lund–Mackay staging of sinus disease by MRI to be closely correlated to staging based on CT. MRI was found not to significantly overstage or overclassify patients with sinus disease. Imaging is essential for preoperative planning for ESS; however, it is important for the clinician to remain cognizant of the risk of radiation to the child and to minimize the cumulative radiation dose by reducing the radiation dosage per CT scan when possible; replacing CT with other modalities, such as MRI; and reducing the overall number of CT scans obtained.

The goal of ESS is to enlarge the natural ostia of the affected sinuses while preserving sinus mucosa. A meta-analysis of outcomes of ESS in the pediatric population found the rate of positive outcome to be 88.4% and the incidence of major complications to be 0.6%, thereby concluding that ESS is a safe and effective treatment for medically refractory pediatric CRS. CF comprises a special patient population. Chronic sinusitis is extremely common in this population, and the most common presenting symptoms include nasal obstruction and headache. It is estimated that many patients with CF will ultimately fail medical management of CRS, and 10 to 20% of these patients will undergo ESS. Surgery was found to provide a marked and lasting improvement in these patients. Unfortunately, this population frequently requires revision procedures.

A study by Becker et al of 81 patients (50 pediatric, 31 adult) found that patients with high Lund–Mackay scores at the time of initial surgery were more likely to undergo several revision surgeries. There was no significant correlation between increased number of surgeries and patient age, gender, ethnicity, CF genotype, presence of asthma or aspirin triad, exposure to smoking, pulmonary function test results, months to recurrence, or presence of nasal polyps. This study concluded that patients with high Lund–Mackay scores at the time of initial surgery should be considered for alternative and possibly more aggressive management of their sinus disease at presentation.

■ Controversial Issues

Balloon Sinuplasty

Balloon sinuplasty is a newer technique that has been used in other organ systems and now has been introduced for the treatment of CRS. Initially investigated in 10 adults, this technique was found to effectively dilate 18 sinus ostia in 10 patients without any observed complications. The advantages of balloon sinuplasty are the relative preservation of mucosa and the minimized destruction of tissue or circumferential scarring of the sinus ostia.

A multicenter study of 115 adults who underwent balloon sinuplasty and were prospectively evaluated at 24 week follow-up found that 80.5% had patent sinuses; patency could not be determined in 17.9%. No serious adverse events occurred. Overall symptom improvement in the study group was reported to be 84% at 24 weeks. Revision surgery was required in less than 1% of patients.

This technique has been more recently investigated in children who have failed medical therapy with oral antibiotics for at least 3 weeks, systemic and topical steroids, and allergy management for at least 6 months. Those children with CT evidence of CRS underwent balloon sinuplasty with sinus wash and adenoidectomy if the adenoids were not previously removed. This treatment was found to be successful in 91% of the sinuses and was primarily ineffective when a hypoplastic maxillary sinus was present.

A study of the outcome of this balloon sinuplasty in children found that 50% of children had significant improvement in quality of life (QOL), 29% had moderate improvement, 4% remained the same, and 8% had worsening QOL scores. The disadvantage to the technique used in the previously described studies was the use of fluoroscopic guidance, thereby subjecting patients as well as the surgeon to small quantities of radiation. More recently, balloon sinuplasty technology has been changed from fluoroscopic guidance to the use of an illuminated guidewire. This technology has been shown to be as safe and effective as fluoroscopic methods, except for the sphenoid sinus, which cannot be transilluminated. The safety and efficacy of illuminated guidewire have not yet been shown in children. It is also important to note that these early studies have excluded patients with CF. Further research will be required to determine whether balloon sinuplasty is as effective in this population.

■ Conclusion

In conclusion, many factors, both genetic and environmental, contribute to the development of acute and chronic sinusitis in children. Treatment consists of controlling contributing factors (such as daycare, smoking exposure, allergy, and GERD) and medical treatment with sinus rinse, nasal topical steroid sprays, and antibiotics. Should these measures fail, surgical treatment proceeds in a stepwise fashion to include adenoidectomy with or without maxillary sinus lavage, and finally endoscopic sinus surgery for refractory cases. Areas of controversy include the safety and efficacy of balloon sinuplasty in children, as well as the frequency and type of imaging modality used to monitor disease extent.

■ Practice Guidelines, Consensus Statements, and Measures

American Academy of Otolaryngology–Head and Neck Surgery. Clinical Practice Guideline: Adult Sinusitis. Alexandria, VA: AAO–HNS; 2007

American Academy of Otolaryngology–Head and Neck Surgery. Clinical Practice Guideline: Clinical Consensus statement: CT

Imaging Indications for Paranasal Sinus Disease. Alexandria, VA: AAO–HNS. Under development.

American Academy of Pediatrics. Subcommittee on Management of Sinusitis and Committee on Quality Improvement. Clinical practice guideline: management of sinusitis. Pediatrics 2001;108(3):798–808

■ Suggested Reading

Becker SS, de Alarcon A, Bomeli SR, Han JK, Gross CW. Risk factors for recurrent sinus surgery in cystic fibrosis: review of a decade of experience. Am J Rhinol 2007;21(4):478–482

Bolger WE, Brown CL, Church CA, et al. Safety and outcomes of balloon catheter sinusotomy: a multicenter 24-week analysis in 115 patients. Otolaryngol Head Neck Surg 2007;137(1):10–20

Bothwell MR, Parsons DS, Talbot A, Barbero GJ, Wilder B. Outcome of reflux therapy on pediatric chronic sinusitis. Otolaryngol Head Neck Surg 1999;121(3):255–262

Bothwell MR, Piccirillo JF, Lusk RP, Ridenour BD. Long-term outcome of facial growth after functional endoscopic sinus surgery. Otolaryngol Head Neck Surg 2002;126(6):628–634

Brown CL, Bolger WE. Safety and feasibility of balloon catheter dilation of paranasal sinus ostia: a preliminary investigation. Ann Otol Rhinol Laryngol 2006;115(4):293–299, discussion 300–301

Buchman CA, Yellon RF, Bluestone CD. Alternative to endoscopic sinus surgery in the management of pediatric chronic rhinosinusitis refractory to oral antimicrobial therapy. Otolaryngol Head Neck Surg 1999;120(2):219–224

Chan KH, Winslow CP, Levin MJ, et al. Clinical practice guidelines for the management of chronic sinusitis in children. Otolaryngol Head Neck Surg 1999;120(3):328–334

Cunningham MJ, Chiu EJ, Landgraf JM, Gliklich RE. The health impact of chronic recurrent rhinosinusitis in children [published correction available in Arch Otolaryngol Head Neck Surg. 2014 Apr;140(4):356. Cunningham, JM corrected to Cunningham, MJ]. Arch Otolaryngol Head Neck Surg 2000;126(11):1363–1368

Don DM, Yellon RF, Casselbrant ML, Bluestone CD. Efficacy of a stepwise protocol that includes intravenous antibiotic therapy for the management of chronic sinusitis in children and adolescents. Arch Otolaryngol Head Neck Surg 2001;127(9):1093–1098

Friedman M, Wilson M. Illumination guided balloon sinuplasty. Laryngoscope 2009;119(7):1399–1402

Gentile VG, Isaacson G. Patterns of sinusitis in cystic fibrosis. Laryngoscope 1996;106(8):1005–1009

Goldsmith AJ, Rosenfeld RM. Treatment of pediatric sinusitis. Pediatr Clin North Am 2003;50(2):413–426

Gwaltney JM Jr. Acute community-acquired sinusitis. Clin Infect Dis 1996;23(6):1209–1223, quiz 1224–1225

Hebert RL II, Bent JP III. Meta-analysis of outcomes of pediatric functional endoscopic sinus surgery. Laryngoscope 1998;108(6): 796–799

Kliegman RM, Behrman RE, Jensen HB, Stanton BF. Nelson Textbook of Pediatrics. 18th ed. Philadelphia, PA: Saunders Elsevier; 2007:Chapter 400

Lee D, Rosenfeld RM. Adenoid bacteriology and sinonasal symptoms in children. Otolaryngol Head Neck Surg 1997;116(3): 301–307

Lieser JD, Derkay CS. Pediatric sinusitis: when do we operate? Curr Opin Otolaryngol Head Neck Surg 2005;13(1):60–66

Lin HW, Bhattacharyya N. Diagnostic and staging accuracy of magnetic resonance imaging for the assessment of sinonasal disease. Am J Rhinol Allergy 2009;23(1):36–39

O'Reilly R, Ryan S, Donoghue V, Saidlear C, Twomey E, Slattery DM. Cumulative radiation exposure in children with cystic fibrosis. Ir Med J 2010;103(2):43–46

Phipps CD, Wood WE, Gibson WS, Cochran WJ. Gastroesophageal reflux contributing to chronic sinus disease in children: a prospective analysis. Arch Otolaryngol Head Neck Surg 2000;126(7):831–836

Puderbach M, Eichinger M. The role of advanced imaging techniques in cystic fibrosis follow-up: is there a place for MRI? Pediatr Radiol 2010;40(6):844–849

Ramadan HH. Safety and feasibility of balloon sinuplasty for treatment of chronic rhinosinusitis in children. Ann Otol Rhinol Laryngol 2009;118(3):161–165

Ramadan HH, McLaughlin K, Josephson G, Rimell F, Bent J, Parikh SR. Balloon catheter sinuplasty in young children. Am J Rhinol Allergy 2010;24(1):e54–e56

Raman V, Clary R, Siegrist KL, Zehnbauer B, Chatila TA. Increased prevalence of mutations in the cystic fibrosis transmembrane conductance regulator in children with chronic rhinosinusitis. Pediatrics 2002;109(1):E13

Ramesh S, Brodsky L, Afshani E, et al. Open trial of intravenous immune serum globulin for chronic sinusitis in children. Ann Allergy Asthma Immunol 1997;79(2):119–124

Ramsey B, Richardson MA. Impact of sinusitis in cystic fibrosis. J Allergy Clin Immunol 1992;90(3 Pt 2):547–552

Rosenstein BJ, Cutting GR; Cystic Fibrosis Foundation Consensus Panel. The diagnosis of cystic fibrosis: a consensus statement. J Pediatr 1998;132(4):589–595

Senior B, Wirtschafter A, Mai C, Becker C, Belenky W. Quantitative impact of pediatric sinus surgery on facial growth. Laryngoscope 2000;110(11):1866–1870

Shin KS, Cho SH, Kim KR, et al. The role of adenoids in pediatric rhinosinusitis. Int J Pediatr Otorhinolaryngol 2008;72(11): 1643–1650

Steele RW. Rhinosinusitis in children. Curr Allergy Asthma Rep 2006;6(6):508–512

Vandenberg SJ, Heatley DG. Efficacy of adenoidectomy in relieving symptoms of chronic sinusitis in children. Arch Otolaryngol Head Neck Surg 1997;123(7):675–678

Vanlerberghe L, Joniau S, Jorissen M. The prevalence of humoral immunodeficiency in refractory rhinosinusitis: a retrospective analysis. B-ENT 2006;2(4):161–166

Van Peteghem A, Clement PA. Influence of extensive functional endoscopic sinus surgery (FESS) on facial growth in children with cystic fibrosis. Comparison of 10 cephalometric parameters of the midface for three study groups. Int J Pediatr Otorhinolaryngol 2006;70(8):1407–1413

Wang X, Moylan B, Leopold DA, et al. Mutation in the gene responsible for cystic fibrosis and predisposition to chronic rhinosinusitis in the general population. JAMA 2000;284(14):1814–1819

78 The Management of Drooling

■ Introduction

Most children will develop salivary "continence" by the age of 18 months, although it is common to drool up to the age of 3 years. After age 4, sialorrhea, or excessive drooling, during waking hours is abnormal. This condition primarily affects people with neurological disorders, particularly cerebral palsy and Parkinson disease, although it can affect patients with anatomical abnormalities of the lips, mandible, or oral cavity.

Drooling is a social and physical detriment to patients. Medically, it can lead to the development of skin irritation, dehydration, unpleasant odor, and impairment of speech. The drooling individual often has problems avoiding damage to books, communication aids, and/or computers. Socially, sialorrhea can lead to reduced self-confidence and poor interpersonal relationships, ultimately resulting in social isolation.

Healthy, neurologically intact people typically produce between 1,000 and 1,500 mL of saliva daily. Children prior to puberty produce significantly less—750 to 900 mL/d. Many families will complain that the patient produces too much saliva, when in fact the drooling is actually due to an impaired swallowing mechanism or an inadequate rate of swallowing or both.

The submandibular glands produce the bulk of saliva in the unstimulated state (70%), which is semiviscous. The paired sublingual glands produce a more viscous saliva that makes up ~ 3 to 4% of the unstimulated daily production. The saliva produced by the parotid glands is watery and ~ 25% of the total. The minor salivary glands produce only a trace of the total saliva. When the salivary glands are stimulated by smell, taste, or chewing, the proportion of saliva produced by the submandibular and parotid glands is reversed.

Parasympathetic stimulation is the principal impetus for salivary gland secretion, which is of large volume and low protein content. The salivary glands are also innervated by the sympathetic nervous system, leading to production of low volumes of saliva with a high protein content (the saliva is more viscous). Pharmacological interventions for drooling are principally aimed at blocking the parasympathetic system.

■ Evaluation of the Drooling Patient

At some medical centers, a "drooling team" made up of various professionals, such as a dentist, otolaryngologist, neurologist, speech and/or occupational (swallowing) therapist, pediatrician, psychologist, and rehabilitation specialist, is available and can be consulted. In many areas, no such team is available, and the otolaryngologist is responsible for primary evaluation of the patient.

In obtaining the patient's history, the practitioner should focus on aspects of oral motor control (e.g., does the patient eat orally); history of aspiration; and aspects that may increase the problem of the drooling, such as posture, medications, dental health, and neurological status. The family should be questioned regarding the number of bibs or shirt changes that are required in an average day, and the Thomas-Stonell and Greenberg drooling rating scale (**Table 78.1**) may be used. The scale is particularly useful when quantifying the problem before and after treatment.

On physical examination, particular attention should be paid to dental health (poor dentition can cause an increase in drooling), head position, salivary flow from the mouth, bib status, and the ability of patients to wipe their mouth and swallow.

■ Management of Drooling

Various approaches are used to manage drooling.

Table 78.1   Drooling rating scale: Thomas-Stonell and Greenberg

Drooling severity
1. Dry—never drools
2. Mild—wet lips only
3. Moderate—wet lips and chin
4. Severe—damp clothing
5. Profuse—damp clothing, hands, and surrounding objects
Drooling frequency
1. Never—no drooling
2. Occasionally
3. Frequently
4. Constantly

Data from Thomas Stonell N, Greenberg SJ. Three treatment approaches and clinical factors in the reduction of drooling. Dysphagia 1988;3:73–78

Behavior Management

Behavior management assists patients with managing their own saliva independently (e.g., by wiping their mouth).

Oromotor or Swallowing Therapy

Oromotor or swallowing therapy aims to establish or restore oral coordination for the patient's eating or swallowing capabilities.

Pharmacological Treatment

If behavior management and oromotor therapy are not successful in controlling the drooling, pharmacological therapy is often considered. For many years, anticholinergic agents have been the mainstay of drug therapy. These medications reduce the volume of saliva produced by reversibly blocking the cholinergic muscarinic receptors, specifically the muscarinic receptor subtype 3 (M3), which is thought to be responsible for salivation. Due to the lack of selectivity of these agents for the salivary glands, undesirable adverse effects can occur, such as dry mouth, constipation, urinary retention, restlessness, irritability, drowsiness, and flushing.

Glycopyrrolate, benztropine, and scopolamine have all been used off-label for treatment of drooling. Glycopyrrolate comes in tablet form as well as an intravenous preparation that has been used for patients who need a liquid formulation. In 2010, an oral solution of glycopyrrolate (1 mg/5 mL) was approved by the U.S. Food and Drug Administration (FDA) for children ages 3 to 18 years with neurological disorders and chronic severe drooling. The manufacturer recommends an initial dose of 0.02 mg/kg/dose administered orally (or by feeding tube) three times a day. Doses may be increased by 0.02 mg/kg every 5 to 7 days to a maximum of 0.1 mg/kg/dose three times a day or 0.2 to 3 mg/kg/dose three times a day.

Prospective studies have shown that anticholinergic medications are effective in reducing the quantity of saliva and thus the drooling. However, a significant proportion of patients experience side effects. The benefits of using glycopyrrolate over the other agents include its long duration of action and its inability to cross the blood–brain barrier, thus minimizing central nervous system adverse effects, such as sedation dysphoria and restlessness. Both benztropine and scopolamine cross the blood–brain barrier, thereby reducing their usefulness in patients sensitive to such effects.

Botulinum Toxin

Botulinum toxin A (BoNT-A) is frequently used off-label to control drooling. The medication is injected directly into the submandibular and/or parotid glands and works by blocking the release of acetylcholine. No official recommendations have been made regarding dosing or the time interval between each treatment, but most clinicians consider the minimum interval to be 3 months.

To avoid serious side effects, BoNT-A should be injected using ultrasound guidance. Possible complications of the injection include hematoma in the periglandular region, thickening of the saliva, and dysphagia and/or dysarthria due to diffusion of the BoNT-A into the surrounding muscular tissue. When injecting the parotid gland, diffusion of BoNT-A into the masseter muscle is possible, causing weakness in chewing. Several prospective trials have demonstrated the BoNT-A to be effective in decreasing the drooling in a significant percentage of patients injected, but there are few randomized, prospective trials.

Intraoral Appliances

Intraoral appliances aim to improve motor function and consequently oral control of saliva. However, their efficacy has not been proven.

Acupuncture

Tongue acupuncture has been reported.

Surgical Therapy

Many surgical options have been described to control drooling; this suggests that no single option is perfect in its efficacy or lack of side effects. Surgical therapy is not recommended until the patient is 6 years old, to ensure the child has had a chance to mature and learn to control the saliva. The goal of surgery is to reduce the amount of drooling but maintain a moist mouth. Dry mouth is a severe complication because it can lead to increased difficulty with dental caries and swallowing.

Most surgical procedures aim to reduce the amount of saliva produced, including submandibular gland excision, sublingual gland excision, parotid and/or submandibular duct ligation, and transtympanic neurectomy. Submandibular duct relocation aims to move the saliva from the front of the mouth to the rear so that the patient may swallow it more easily; this surgery should not be performed in patients with a history of aspiration. The most common procedures performed include submandibular gland excision with or without parotid duct ligation or submandibular duct relocation. If submandibular duct relocation is performed, it is recommended that the sublingual glands also be removed to prevent ranula formation.

■ Controversial Issues

In recent years, there has been a marked increase in the number of drooling patients who are treated with BoNT-A therapy. There is no consensus regarding treatment algorithms for the type of drooling treatment or, in the case of BoNT-A, the quantity and frequency of treatment. Surgery provides a more permanent solution, but it is not fully effective in all patients.

■ Suggested Reading

Chanu NP, Sahni JK, Aneja S, Naglot S. Four-duct ligation in children with drooling. Am J Otolaryngol 2012;33(5):604–607

Eiland LS. Glycopyrrolate for chronic drooling in children. Clin Ther 2012;34(4):735–742

Fairhurst CBR, Cockerill H. Management of drooling in children. Arch Dis Child Educ Pract Ed 2011;96(1):25–30

Khan WU, Campisi P, Nadarajah S, et al. Botulinum toxin A for treatment of sialorrhea in children: an effective, minimally invasive approach. Arch Otolaryngol Head Neck Surg 2011;137(4): 339–344

Reddihough D, Erasmus CE, Johnson H, McKellar GMW, Jongerius PH; Cereral Palsy Institute. Botulinum toxin assessment, intervention and aftercare for paediatric and adult drooling: international consensus statement. Eur J Neurol 2010;17(Suppl 2):109–121

Scheffer AR, Erasmus C, van Hulst K, et al. Botulinum toxin versus submandibular duct relocation for severe drooling. Dev Med Child Neurol 2010;52(11):1038–1042

Scheffer AR, Erasmus C, van Hulst K, van Limbeek J, Jongerius PH, van den Hoogen FJ. Efficacy and duration of botulinum toxin treatment for drooling in 131 children. Arch Otolaryngol Head Neck Surg 2010;136(9):873–877

Walshe M, Smith M, Pennington L. Interventions for drooling in children with cerebral palsy. Cochrane Database Syst Rev 2012;2:CD008624

79 Cleft Lip and Cleft Palate

■ Introduction

Anatomy

Classifications of cleft lip and palate are based on the embryological distinction between the primary and secondary palate. The primary palate consists of the lip and the alveolar ridge bearing the incisor teeth, with a triangular portion of the hard palate extending back to the incisive foramen—that is, the premaxilla. The remainder of the hard palate and the soft palate is the secondary palate.

Clefts may be unilateral or bilateral, complete or incomplete. Complete clefts extend into the nose, whereas incomplete clefts have varying amounts of soft tissue and/or bone separating the lip or palate from the nasal cavity. Submucous cleft palate is an intact palate with a bifid uvula and absence of muscle continuity in the midline of the palate, often resulting in a bluish streak (zona pellucida) and a palpable notch in the posterior edge of the hard palate. On oral examination, the palate of a patient with an occult cleft palate appears normal with a single uvula, but it is not completely functional, resulting in velopharyngeal incompetence.

Palatal musculature includes the tensor veli palatini muscle whose aponeuroses form the anterior third of the soft palate, the levator veli palatini, palatopharyngeus, palatoglossus, and musculus uvulae muscles. The most important muscle for palatal elevation is the levator veli palatini muscle. The levator, palatopharyngeus, and palatoglossus muscles form the so-called levator sling in the middle third of the soft palate.

Etiology

The etiology of clefting is probably a combination of factors, including genetic aberrations, environmental influences, and chance. Approximately 70% of clefts occur as isolated malformations, whereas 30% occur with other malformations, chromosomal aberrations, or syndromes. Children with Robin sequence (micrognathia, glossoptosis, and usually cleft palate) have an associated syndrome, such as Stickler syndrome or velocardiofacial syndrome, ~ 30% of the time. The incidence of associated anomalies is almost five times higher in isolated cleft palate than in cleft lip and palate. Drugs associated with clefting include phenytoin, retinoic acid (vitamin A derivatives), and folic acid antagonists. Smoking and ethanol in the first trimester of pregnancy have been associated with an increased risk of clefting. Multivitamins started before pregnancy are associated with a reduced risk of clefting.

Incidence

Unilateral clefts occur 80% and bilateral clefts occur 20% of the time. Cleft lip and palate is more common in males and isolated cleft palate is more common in females. In addition, males tend to have more severe clefts. There is a racial variability in clefting, with ~ 3.6 per 1,000 live births occurring in Native Americans, 1 per 1,000 live births in Caucasians, and 0.3 per 1,000 live births in African Americans.

■ Evaluation of the Cleft Patient

The foundation of cleft management is the multidisciplinary approach based on the recognition that no single discipline has the expertise for the variety of cleft problems, and that the best approach is patient oriented rather than specialty oriented. Basic team members consist of a surgeon, dentist, and speech-language pathologist and an audiologist. A full team also includes an otolaryngologist/otologist, a pedodontist, a prosthodontist, an orthodontist, an oral surgeon, a geneticist, a social worker, a psychiatrist or psychologist, a nutritionist, and a pediatric specialty nurse.

Ideally, patients are evaluated as soon as possible after birth for a general examination and genetic assessment, and nutrition and feeding information and support are provided. Infants with Robin sequence and upper airway obstruction may require emergency airway management (prone positioning, intubation, mandibular advancement, lip–tongue adhesion, or tracheotomy). Infants with only a cleft lip may be able to successfully breast-feed. More severe clefts generally require a special feeder, such as a Mead Johnson squeeze bottle feeder (Mead Johnson and Company, LLC, Evansville, IN) or a Haberman feeder. The parents of older children with a cleft should be queried regarding snoring at night and other symptoms of obstructive sleep apnea, as well as a history of ear disease. A polysomnogram should be considered for any cleft child with snoring. Children with a previously repaired, submucous, or occult cleft palate who are identified with hypernasal speech should undergo nasopharyngoscopy and/or speech videofluoroscopy to evaluate the closure pattern of the velopharyngeal inlet.

■ Management: Surgical Options

Surgery is required to repair oral clefts. The age at cleft repair and type of surgery both affect future facial form. More extensive undermining of soft tissue, especially periosteum, closure of clefts under tension, and repair at a very young age tend to have the greatest adverse affect on facial growth.

Lip Adhesion

The lip adhesion is a tension-relieving procedure for use in extremely wide cleft lips. The basic procedure is a side-to-side closure of the lip, with minimal undermining of soft tissues and no attempt to align landmarks. The chief advantage of this procedure is it allows a definitive cleft lip repair under the more favorable condition of decreased tension. Its disadvantages are an additional operation, the risk of breakdown due to excessive tension, and some increased risk of scar tissue in the lip.

Definitive Cleft Lip Repair

The two most commonly performed types of unilateral cleft lip repair are the rotation advancement technique described by Millard, and the single or double triangular flap repairs. In both techniques, the lip landmarks are carefully measured and marked. In the Millard repair, the elevated cupid's bow peak on the medial side of the cleft is dropped into a normal position by means of the curving rotation incision. This leaves a gap below the nose that is filled by the advancement flap from the lateral lip. Its advantages include a lip scar that simulates the position of the philtral column and accurate placement of the alar base. Its disadvantages include the need for extensive undermining of soft tissue from the maxilla in wide clefts without a lip adhesion and a tendency to overadvance the nose, which results in stenosis. Considerable surgical experience and judgment are required to obtain optimal results.

The triangular flap techniques produce precisely measured geometrical single or double triangular flaps, which interdigitate to create a symmetrical lip. On the medial side of the cleft, the elevated cupid's bow peak is lowered by an oblique incision extending into the philtrum. The resulting defect is filled by the triangular flap from the lateral lip. The advantage is greater ease of closure in wide clefts. Disadvantages include the zigzag lip scar and difficulty in adjusting the repair once the flaps have been created.

Bilateral Cleft Lip Repair

The bilateral cleft lip is challenging due to the greater severity of the deformity, the often protrusive premaxilla, and the frequently deficient prolabium, which becomes the philtrum of the reconstructed lip. Definitive repair may be a one- or two-stage procedure. If the two-stage procedure is the preferred method, a unilateral cleft lip repair technique (rotation advancement or triangular flap) is performed on one side. After 2 to 3 months for healing, the opposite cleft is closed by the same technique. Because many of these deformities are symmetrical or nearly so, there are advantages to repairing both sides in one stage. This method has numerous advantages, including the creation of a symmetrical lip and nose with orbicularis oris muscle continuity anterior to the premaxilla, with the cupid's bow and midline lip tubercle reconstructed from lateral lip vermilion flaps, a deep labial sulcus, and the ability to save tissue for later columella lengthening.

Cleft Palate Repair—Palatoplasty

Normal speech requires an intact functional palate. Therefore, the primary goal of palatoplasty is to reconstruct a valve or sphincteric mechanism to achieve normal nasal resonance and articulation. Optimal timing of palate repair is still controversial. The trend since the early 1980s has been for earlier surgery—that is, by 12 months of age. Very early and extensive palatal surgery may increase facial growth disturbances, with maxillary hypoplasia and malocclusion. Although delayed closure of the hard palate for several years (Schweckendiek procedure) is beneficial for facial growth, it has been shown to result in significantly poorer speech. Current techniques emphasize lengthening of the soft palate when possible, reconstructing the levator muscle sling, and minimally elevating the periosteum from the hard palate.

In the von Langenbeck palatoplasty, bipedicle mucoperiosteal flaps are elevated from the hard and soft palates and advanced medially to close narrow palatal defects. There is relatively little exposed palatal bone and minimal dissection, and the procedure is rapid. Its disadvantages include lack of palatal lengthening and usefulness in the narrow clefts only.

The V to Y pushback method creates three or four unipedicle flaps, depending upon the extent of the cleft. The larger posterior flaps consist of the velum and a portion of hard palatal mucoperiosteum based on the neurovascular bundle (descending palatine artery). Closure is in a V to Y fashion, with at least theoretical lengthening of the velum. The V to Y pushback method is applicable in wider clefts, where it produces better speech results than the von Langenbeck method. Disadvantages in the complete cleft lip and palate are difficulty in handling the small anterior flaps and greater likelihood of fistula formation at the distal aspects of the approximated flaps, where the mucoperiosteum is thinnest and under greatest tension.

The two-flap palatoplasty (Bardach) produces a large mucoperiosteum flap from the entire palatal shelf on either side and includes the velum as well. This technique is useful in complete clefts of the lip and palate. Its advantages are that wide clefts may also be repaired by this technique, and there is a very low incidence of fistula formation at or near the hard–soft palate junction. As with the pushback procedure, levator muscles are readily dissected and approximated. Alveolar clefts are not closed unless done previously at lip repair.

The Furlow double-reversing Z-plasty operation (1986) is an extremely useful procedure in narrow or submucous cleft palates. Four triangular flaps are created with the two muscle-bearing flaps from the oronasal side of the palate transposed posteriorly to reconstruct the anterior soft palate. Its main disadvantage is the difficulty or impossibility of closing wider clefts.

Postoperatively, palatoplasty patients are monitored closely for airway obstruction and bleeding. The principal long-term complication of palatoplasty is hypernasal speech.

Velopharyngeal Insufficiency (VPI) and Speech Disorders

After palatoplasty, failure to achieve normal palatal function may result in a hypernasal resonant quality to the voice, audible nasal emission of air through the nose, nasal turbulence, and the inability to produce sounds requiring increasing oral pressure (plosives). Articulation abnormalities, which include the omission, substitution, and abnormal production of speech sounds (phonemes), may result. Evaluation of the cleft patient with a speech problem may include some or all of the following: speech pathology evaluation with standard articulation tests and clinical examination, including fiberoptic nasoendoscopy, multiview videofluoroscopy, and quantitative measures of differential nasal and oral resonance (nasometer).

Treatment of Velopharyngeal Insufficiency

Speech therapy alone may be sufficient to correct very mild or inconsistent VPI. Other patients, more severely affected, require intervention. Treatment may consist of nonsurgical modalities, such as palatal obturators and lifts. These devices are constructed by a prosthodontist to attach to the teeth and extend posteriorly, either to raise the velum closer to the posterior nasopharyngeal wall or to fill the space behind the soft palate. The usefulness of these devices in young children is limited by factors of cooperation and motivation.

Surgical correction of VPI includes the following procedures: palatal elongation–pushback, posterior pharyngeal wall implants, sphincter pharyngoplasty, and pharyngeal flap. Small gaps in velar elevation as determined radiographically or endoscopically may be corrected by a palatal pushback procedure, as described for primary palatoplasty. This procedure is rarely performed alone, however, and is usually combined with another secondary procedure, such as a pharyngeal flap. A posterior pharyngeal wall implant may be indicated with defects of a few millimeters or less and a mobile soft palate.

A sphincter pharyngoplasty may be considered when diagnostic studies have shown good velar elevation and poor mobility of the lateral pharyngeal walls. The operation creates a single smaller midline opening that is valved by the soft palate. The procedure consists of elevating bilateral mucosal and muscular superiorly based flaps from the lateral pharyngeal walls, rotating them 90 degrees into a horizontal incision placed across the posterior pharyngeal wall, and suturing them end-to-end or overlapping to create an even smaller midline opening.

A superiorly based posterior pharyngeal flap is still considered by many surgeons to be the gold standard for correction of secondary velopharyngeal insufficiency. Classically, it is indicated when diagnostic studies show poor velar elevation and good medial mobility of the lateral pharyngeal walls. Lateral wall mobility allows valving of the lateral ports for speech. The operation consists of elevating a superiorly based flap consisting of mucosa, submucosa, and superior constrictor muscle down to the prevertebral fascia. It is attached to the soft palate by either creating a pocket into the palate (sandwich technique) or dividing the palate in the midline and suturing it into the apex of the divided velum. Wider flaps are more obstructive to the airway, and obstructive sleep apnea is a complication of very wide flaps. Persistent obstructive sleep apnea that is documented by polysomnography may require revision of the flap ports or even complete release of the flap. Fortunately, recurrence of VPI following a superiorly based posterior pharyngeal flap is extremely uncommon.

Dental Management

Children with cleft lip and palate have frequent dental problems, including congenitally missing teeth, supernumerary teeth, and abnormally formed or positioned teeth. For children in the mixed dentition state, orthodontic expansion for anterior and/or posterior crossbite may be indicated. Secondary bone grafting or the alveolar graft is performed prior to eruption of the permanent cuspid tooth, usually between 8 and 11 years of age. Patients with maxillary hypoplasia and class III occlusion (underbite) may require orthognathic surgery with Le Fort advancement of the maxilla and/or mandibular recession.

Ear Disease

The incidence of eustachian tube dysfunction and middle ear disease is extremely high in the cleft palate population. This is because of the abnormal insertion of the tensor veli palatini muscle, which is a dilator of the eustachian tube. Repair of the cleft palate probably has little or no effect on the incidence of middle ear disease, although almost all children needing repair have significant middle ear problems by the time their palate is repaired. At least half of these children require more than one ventilation tube insertion. Indications for ventilating tube insertion are the same as for non-cleft patients. Patients should be followed at 3 to 6 month intervals until their middle ear problems are resolved.

■ Controversial Issues

There is no consensus among cleft surgeons regarding the best surgical procedure for cleft lip repair, cleft palate repair, and surgical correction of velopharyngeal insufficiency. Surgical decisions are typically made on the basis of scant surgical literature comparing techniques and, more important, surgeon experience.

■ Suggested Reading

Chen YW, Chen KT, Chang PH, Su JL, Huang CC, Lee TJ. Is otitis media with effusion almost always accompanying cleft palate in children?: the experience of 319 Asian patients. Laryngoscope 2012;122(1):220–224

Fisher DM, Sommerlad BC. Cleft lip, cleft palate, and velopharyngeal insufficiency. Plast Reconstr Surg 2011;128(4):342e–360e

Furlow LT Jr. Cleft palate repair by double opposing Z-plasty. Plast Reconstr Surg 1986;78(6):724–738

Johnson CY, Little J. Folate intake, markers of folate status and oral clefts: is the evidence converging? Int J Epidemiol 2008; 37(5):1041–1058

Kummer AW. Perceptual assessment of resonance and velopharyngeal function. Semin Speech Lang 2011;32(2):159–167

Mackay DR. Controversies in the diagnosis and management of the Robin sequence. J Craniofac Surg 2011;22(2):415–420

MacLean JE, Hayward P, Fitzgerald DA, Waters K. Cleft lip and/or palate and breathing during sleep. Sleep Med Rev 2009;13(5): 345–354

Williams WN, Seagle MB, Pegoraro-Krook MI, et al. Prospective clinical trial comparing outcome measures between Furlow and von Langenbeck palatoplasties for UCLP. Ann Plast Surg 2011;66(2):154–163

80 Nasopharyngeal Stenosis and Velopharyngeal Insufficiency

■ Introduction

Anatomy of the Velopharyngeal Sphincter

The nasopharynx is fundamentally a cuboidal space bounded superiorly by the base of the skull and anterior wall of the sphenoid sinus, anteriorly by the choanae and posterior aspect of the vomer, posteriorly by the superior extension of the posterior pharyngeal wall, and laterally by the tori tubariae and fossae of Rosenmüller. Inferiorly, the nasal surface of the soft palate (velum) and the uvula constitute its dynamic floor. Six muscles make up the velopharyngeal sphincter. The levator veli palatini is the major elevator of the soft palate. Its fibers fan out in the soft palate and blend with the contralateral levator. The tensor veli palatini arises from the scaphoid fossa, the spine of the sphenoid, and the cartilaginous portion of the eustachian tube. It inserts into a tendon winding around the hamular process. Innervated by the mandibular branch of cranial nerve V, it tenses the soft palate and opens the eustachian tube during swallowing.

The musculus uvulae arises from the palatal aponeurosis posterior to the hard palate and inserts into the uvula mucosa. It functions to add bulk to the dorsal aspect of the uvula. The palatoglossus muscle forms the anterior tonsillar pillar, simultaneously lowers the velum and elevates the tongue upward and backward, and depresses the palate for nasal speech. The superior pharyngeal constrictor produces medial movement of the pharyngeal walls, narrowing the pharynx from side to side. The inferior portion of this muscle forms the Passavant ridge. Disruption of the coordinated function of this velopharyngeal sphincter produces two conditions that represent extremes on the spectrum of palatal positioning: (1) complete or near-complete closure, or *nasopharyngeal stenosis*, and (2) persistent or near-persistent lack of closure, or *velopharyngeal insufficiency*.

■ Nasopharyngeal Stenosis

Nasopharyngeal Stenosis Incidence

Historically, most cases of nasopharyngeal stenosis (NPS) were of syphilitic origin. The advent of penicillin therapy has shifted the etiology of this condition to one occurring iatrogenically after adenotonsillectomy (T&A), uvulopalatopharyngoplasty (UPPP), or radiation therapy. The exact incidence of NPS is unknown but appears to be exceedingly low. No recent reports of overall NPS incidence after T&A exist, but in 1944 Imperatori reported it to be three cases for every 100,000 procedures performed. Although the incidence of NPS following UPPP is not known, it is undoubtedly low; only 46 cases were reported during a 9 year period following introduction of the operation in the United States. Rhinoscleroma, lupus, diphtheria, tuberculosis, acid burn, scarlet fever, and aggressive velopharyngeal insufficiency repair can also rarely cause NPS.

After T&A, NPS may occur due to approximation of raw mucosal surfaces during the healing process. The mucosal trauma may have occurred intraoperatively as a result of denuding the nasal surface of the palate, imprecise exuberant use of electrocautery, or use of the potassium titanyl phosphate laser for adenoidectomy. It may also develop postoperatively from local infection. Use of meticulous surgical technique is the key to minimizing this complication after T&A. After UPPP, NPS may occur due to technical errors, including excessive excision and cauterization of the posterior tonsillar pillars or undermining the posterior and lateral pharyngeal walls. In addition, adenoidectomy in conjunction with UPPP carries an increased risk of nasopharyngeal stenosis.

Nasopharyngeal Stenosis Classification

A classification system of NPS has been proposed by Krespi and Kacker. In type I stenosis, the mildest form, the lateral aspects of the palate are adherent to

521

the posterior pharynx wall. There is circumferential scarring in type II stenosis, with a central opening of 1 to 2 cm. The most severe grade, type III, features a residual opening of < 1 cm. Treatment of type I stenosis has been amenable to office-based surgery, but most cases of types II and III have required operating room facilities.

Nasopharyngeal Stenosis Evaluation

Rigid nasal endoscopic examination and/or flexible nasopharyngolaryngoscopy should be performed to assess the thickness, nature, and extent of the stenosis and the deformity of the posterolateral aspect of the nasal cavity and to further delineate anatomical deformities at the level of the vomer and the posterior nasal cavity. Computed tomographic (CT) imaging (without contrast) may help characterize the nature and extent of the scar as well.

Nasopharyngeal Stenosis Management

Careful operative technique should help prevent NPS. However, if this complication does develop, repair should not be planned until inflammation, erythema, and infection have resolved. Excellent reviews are available describing numerous techniques of historical interest, including simple finger dilation, suturing, and various types of flaps or grafts. Variation in thickness and extent of stenoses makes a choice of operations desirable.

Recently, there have been reports of the successful use of balloon-dilating catheters in cats and dogs and, more recently, in selected human cases. Although there is limited outcome evidence in the literature, the balloon technique appears to be useful in less severe forms of NPS. In adults, it can be employed in an office-based setting. For more severe forms of NPS, for patency to be maintained long term, the raw edges of the stenosis must be mucosally lined—an objective in general requiring either the use of regional flaps or long-term stenting. An approach using a carbon dioxide laser to excise the major components of the scar, followed by a 6 month stenting period with nasal obturators and the topical application of mitomycin-C, was reported with success in three patients. Madgy et al treated three cases of severe NPS with plasma radiofrequency-based coblation "plasma hook," followed by prolonged stenting.

When employing local rotational flaps, because of the extent of the contracture, these will not often retain their outlined size and will tend to return to their original positions, leaving denuded areas uncovered. To circumvent this problem, Cotton described a versatile lateral-based posterior pharyngeal advancement flap that is elevated as a mucomuscular flap at the plane of the prevertebral fascia. The inferior limit of the flap is dissected as far back as possible, and the pharyngeal mucomuscular flap is mobilized and sewn into position, covering the denuded area of the lateral walls of the nasopharynx and oropharynx. Smaller posterior pharyngeal Z-plasties may also be adequate. Techniques based on palatal flaps include McDonald et al's use of a unilateral mucoperiosteal flap that includes the hard palate, and the bivalved palatal transposition flap described by Toh et al in 2000.

Postoperative complications include the potential for airway obstruction and bleeding, but these have not been reported to date. More likely, postoperative contracture can be expected and will cause some degree of retraction and restenosis. The exact need for revision surgery is unclear. Velopharyngeal insufficiency after NPS repair has been reported but, due to restenosis, may gradually resolve.

■ Velopharyngeal Insufficiency

Velopharyngeal insufficiency (VPI) results from inadequate closure of the velopharyngeal sphincter during speech, which gives an abnormally hypernasal resonance to the voice. Occasionally, in severe cases, there may be nasal escape of swallowed foods as well. The ability to communicate through well-articulated speech is integral to being human and can have a large impact on the quality of life.

Velopharyngeal Insufficiency Incidence

In general, VPI can be classified into two groups: anatomical (overt or submucous cleft palate) or functional (neuromuscular disorders, cerebral palsy, postcerebral infarction). A history of cleft palate either before or after repair is the most common cause of VPI, where it has been reported in as many as 30 to 50% of patients following palate repair. Submucous cleft palate occurs when there is a deficiency of the musculus uvulae and diastasis of the levator veli palatini in the midline raphe of the soft palate, with or without the presence of an overt bifid uvula. Because of this abnormal musculature, these patients may be predisposed to VPI at baseline or after adenoidectomy. Transient VPI with hypernasal resonance following adenoidectomy, with or without tonsillectomy, is not uncommon, especially in patients with submucous cleft palate. This condition may persist for several days to weeks and usually resolves spontaneously. Incidence of persistent VPI after adenoidectomy has been reported to be ~ 1 per 1,500 patients. Children at particular risk of developing persistent VPI after adenoidectomy include those with a repaired cleft palate, a submucous cleft palate, 22q11 deletion syndrome, or neuromuscular problems.

VPI may be the presenting manifestation of velo-cardiofacial (VCF) syndrome. VCF syndrome was first described in 1978 in a case series of patients with the repeated physical findings of conotruncal cardiac anomalies, dysmorphic facial features, VPI, and learning disabilities. In 1992, an associated genetic deletion on the long arm of chromosome 22 was discovered in patients with VCF syndrome, providing a means to diagnose the disorder via fluorescence in situ hybridization chromosomal testing for the deletion. VPI has been reported to be present in ~ 75% of patients with 22q11 deletions, but only 10% of those patients showed actual submucous clefts. An isolated autosomal-dominant genetic inheritance pattern to VPI has also been reported without an identifiable genetic or chromosomal locus cause.

Velopharyngeal Insufficiency Evaluation

Prevention of VPI in a patient at risk undergoing adenoidectomy is of paramount importance. An examination of the uvula, the depth of the nasopharynx, and the contour of the edge of the hard palate should be routine during anesthesia prior to T&A. If a submucous cleft is suspected upon visual inspection, a diastasis in the musculi uvulae can be confirmed by nasal endoscopy or by transillumination through the nasal floor, where the characteristic midline thinness of the soft palate may be visible. If an overt submucous cleft palate is found, it is probably preferable to avoid adenoidectomy completely. However, if absolutely necessary, a superior half adenoidectomy can be performed.

Once VPI is suspected, the evaluation consists of a thorough history, physical examination, velopharyngeal assessment, and speech resonance analysis. Clearly, a multidisciplinary approach consisting of an initial assessment conducted by an otolaryngologist and a speech pathologist probably works best as the primary tool in determining the severity of VPI by the trained ear. Although subjective, it offers the most insight into the overall assessment of speech intelligibility, consistency, and articulation.

As an initial step, the examining clinical team should focus on the voiceless consonants, such as *p, t, k, s, f,* and *sh,* which require maximal pulmonary pressures and thus can be used as a brief screening measure for integrity of plosive sounds. Phonemes that require velopharyngeal closure, such as *sk, six, sp,* or *pt,* should also be elicited. Finally, overall intelligibility in running, spontaneous, connected speech should also be ascertained. This assessment of perceptual speech has been shown to be useful in predicting relative velopharyngeal gap size. The Pittsburgh Weighted Speech Scale is a useful tool to assist in quantifying the perceived severity of VPI.

Objective tools for assessment of hypernasality also exist. Nasalance, a measure of hypernasality, can be determined by a nasometer, a tool that can evaluate the ratio of nasal-to-oral sound emission during speech. Although results from nasometry are compared with normalized values for standard speech passages, they do not correlate well with the size of the velopharyngeal gap and do not necessarily correlate well with treatment outcomes for VPI. Aerodynamic measurements of absolute nasal airflow in mL/s can provide a useful adjunct in the objective assessment of VPI but have not been as universally used in most treatment centers.

Physical assessment of velopharyngeal sphincter closure and function is performed by nasoendoscopy, by radiographic multiview videofluoroscopy (MVF), or by both. The use of these studies certainly assists in the surgical planning of corrective procedures for VPI, allowing for direct "tailoring" of the surgical procedure to the defect. Without adequate evaluation of the VP sphincter area during phonation, optimal surgical planning is difficult.

For MVF, barium instilled through the nose coats the surface of the velum and posterior pharyngeal wall, allowing visualization of these structures. Lateral, anterior/posterior, and base views are required to obtain true measurements of the velopharyngeal sphincter. However, difficulties with overlapping shadows, positioning, and asymmetry can make the interpretation of MVF difficult. Concerns with radiation dosages have tempered the enthusiasm for MVF in many centers, especially considering the existence of useful alternative velopharyngeal assessment methods, such as nasoendoscopy. Nasoendoscopy provides a two-dimensional "bird's-eye" view of the velopharyngeal sphincter, shedding light on the location and size of the velopharyngeal gap during active speech production. Studies have demonstrated fairly good interrater reliability with the use of nasoendoscopy to assess VPI, and nasoendoscopy has been shown to correlate better with VPI severity than MVF.

Velopharyngeal Insufficiency Management

The treatment of VPI begins with directed speech therapy to correct compensatory misarticulations. Early speech therapy results in increased speech accuracy and can help improve long-term outcomes. In cases where speech therapy has not resolved VPI, surgery is indicated. Increasingly, an approach tailoring the choice of surgical procedure to the specific defect noted in the patient has been proposed. In general, surgical procedures employed to treat VPI can be classified as palatal, palatopharyngeal, or pharyngeal.

Palatal Surgical Procedures

Palatal procedures most often include the Furlow palatoplasty, which involves a double Z-plasty lengthening of the palate. This technique appears to work best when the orientation of the palatal levator musculature is sagittal or when a small preoperative velopharyngeal gap size is noted.

Palatopharyngeal Surgical Procedures

A common palatopharyngeal technique employed is the superiorly based pharyngeal flap. This procedure involves creation of a superiorly based myomucosal flap from the pharyngeal wall that is inserted into the nasal surface of the soft palate, creating two lateral pharyngeal ports. It is best used when there is severe hypernasality in the setting of a large central velopharyngeal gap and good lateral wall movement. A drawback to this surgery is the potential for prolonged postoperative obstructive sleep apnea development in up to 50% of patients.

Pharyngeal Surgical Procedures

Pharyngeal procedures for VPI treatment include augmentation of the posterior pharyngeal wall and sphincter pharyngoplasty. Augmentation pharyngoplasty is contemplated when VPI is mild and characterized by a small coronal gap. However, results of rolled muscle flaps to augment the coronal gap and pharynx have not been encouraging. The sphincter pharyngoplasty consists of raising two myomucosal flaps of the posterior lateral pharynx and approximating these to form a sphincter along the posterior pharyngeal wall just superior to the level of the velum.

■ Controversial Issues

Some clinicians claim that successful outcomes in fact depend on matching the functional capability of the patient with the surgical procedure. However, undoubtedly, the greatest predictor for postoperative final speech outcomes from VPI surgery is the preoperative condition of the patient. Children with syndromes, such as VCF, as compared with those with anatomical, nonsyndromic causes of VPI, are more likely to have suboptimal outcomes after VPI surgery. The type of surgical procedure employed does not seem to be as important as the experience of the surgeon. A large, prospective, randomized study from Spain found no difference in outcomes when comparing sphincter pharyngoplasty to pharyngeal flaps, regardless of the preoperative velopharyngeal sphincter characteristics. In summary, outcomes after VPI surgery are probably dependent on a multitude of factors, including severity of preoperative VPI, gap size, presence or absence of comorbidities or syndromes, and surgeon comfort.

■ Conclusion

NPS and VPI are rare conditions that may arise as complications of adenoidectomy/adenotonsillectomy and UPPP, which can usually be prevented with careful operative technique. If postoperative stenosis does develop, correction requires resurfacing of the stenotic area with mucosal flaps and using stents if needed. To avoid postadenoidectomy/adenotonsillectomy VPI, a meticulous preoperative examination is essential. If VPI does occur, speech therapy is necessary, and in many cases, a surgical procedure will be required. Posterior pharyngeal flaps or sphincter pharyngoplasties are the preferred techniques.

■ Suggested Reading

Collins J, Cheung K, Farrokhyar F, Strumas N. Pharyngeal flap versus sphincter pharyngoplasty for the treatment of velopharyngeal insufficiency: a meta-analysis. J Plast Reconstr Aesthet Surg 2012;65(7):864–868

Cotton RT. Nasopharyngeal stenosis. Arch Otolaryngol 1985; 111(3):146–148

Dailey SA, Karnell MP, Karnell LH, Canady JW. Comparison of resonance outcomes after pharyngeal flap and furlow double-opposing z-plasty for surgical management of velopharyngeal incompetence. Cleft Palate Craniofac J 2006;43(1):38–43

Dudas JR, Deleyiannis FW, Ford MD, Jiang S, Losee JE. Diagnosis and treatment of velopharyngeal insufficiency: clinical utility of speech evaluation and videofluoroscopy. Ann Plast Surg 2006; 56(5):511–517, discussion 517

Friedman M, Duggal P, Joseph NJ. Revision uvulopalatoplasty by Z-palatoplasty. Otolaryngol Head Neck Surg 2007;136(4): 638–643

Lam DJ, Starr JR, Perkins JA, et al. A comparison of nasendoscopy and multiview videofluoroscopy in assessing velopharyngeal insufficiency. Otolaryngol Head Neck Surg 2006;134(3):394–402

Lee SC, Tang IP, Singh A, Kumar SS, Singh S. Velopharyngeal stenosis, a late complication of radiotherapy. Auris Nasus Larynx 2009;36(6):709–711

Losken A, Williams JK, Burstein FD, Malick DN, Riski JE. Surgical correction of velopharyngeal insufficiency in children with velocardiofacial syndrome. Plast Reconstr Surg 2006;117(5): 1493–1498

Ruda JM, Krakovitz P, Rose AS. A review of the evaluation and management of velopharyngeal insufficiency in children. Otolaryngol Clin North Am 2012;45(3):653–669, viii

Rudnick EF, Sie KC. Velopharyngeal insufficiency: current concepts in diagnosis and management. Curr Opin Otolaryngol Head Neck Surg 2008;16(6):530–535

Scherer NJ, D'Antonio LL, McGahey H. Early intervention for speech impairment in children with cleft palate. Cleft Palate Craniofac J 2008;45(1):18–31

Wan DC, Kumar A, Head CS, Katchikian H, Bradley JP. Amelioration of acquired nasopharyngeal stenosis, with bilateral Z-pharyngoplasty. Ann Plast Surg 2010;64(6):747–750

Wang QY, Chai L, Wang SQ, Zhou SH, Lu YY. Repair of acquired posterior choanal stenosis and atresia by temperature-controlled radio frequency with the aid of an endoscope. Arch Otolaryngol Head Neck Surg 2009;135(5):462–466

Ysunza A, Pamplona C, Ramírez E, Molina F, Mendoza M, Silva A. Velopharyngeal surgery: a prospective randomized study of pharyngeal flaps and sphincter pharyngoplasties. Plast Reconstr Surg 2002;110(6):1401–1407

81 Current Concepts in Medical and Surgical Therapy for Tonsil and Adenoid Disorders

■ Introduction

Anatomy

The faucial tonsils are paired collections of lymphoid tissue bounded by the palatoglossus muscles anteriorly (anterior tonsillar pillars) and the palatopharyngeus muscles posteriorly (posterior tonsillar pillars). The superior pharyngeal constrictor creates the deep bed of the tonsillar fossa. The vascular supply is from the external carotid system. The tonsillar branches of the ascending pharyngeal and lesser palatine arteries enter the superior tonsil pole, whereas the tonsillar branches of the facial, dorsal lingual, and ascending palatine arteries enter the inferior pole. The facial artery contribution is the greatest. The venous outflow from the tonsil is through a venous plexus around the tonsillar capsule, draining into the lingual vein and pharyngeal plexus.

The lymphatics drain predominantly into the upper deep cervical nodes, with other communications with the submandibular and superficial cervical lymph node chains. There are no afferent lymphatics to the tonsils. The nerve supply to the tonsil is the glossopharyngeal nerve inferiorly, and descending branches from the lesser palatine nerves superiorly. The pharyngeal tonsil (adenoid) resides in the nasopharynx. The blood supply to the adenoid is via the pharyngeal, facial, and internal maxillary branches of the external carotid system. Sensory innervation is from the glossopharyngeal and vagus nerves.

Physiology

The function of both tonsil and adenoid tissue is to process antigens and present them to the germinal centers of the lymphoid follicle. This modulates both B and T cell populations within the tonsils and affects circulating immunoglobulin levels and classes dur-ing early childhood. Clinical studies have failed to show any change in the incidence of systemic infections following removal of tonsil and adenoid tissue.

Epidemiology

An estimated 90% of acute pharyngotonsillar infections are attributable to group A b-hemolytic *Streptococcus*, *Mycoplasma*, or viruses (including adenovirus, parainfluenza, influenza, and Epstein-Barr virus). Meanwhile, the majority of nasopharyngitis infections are secondary to viral infections with adenovirus, influenza, parainfluenza, and enterovirus.

Group A b-hemolytic streptococci are the predominant pathogenic bacteria that infect the tonsils. Their significance is due to their association with acute rheumatic fever and acute glomerulonephritis. Group A b-hemolytic streptococci are subdivided into more than 80 serotypes based on distinct M-protein antigens located on the cell wall of the bacterium. The M-serotype has predictive value with respect to the incidence of systemic complications; it also affects the virulence of the strain by resisting phagocytosis. Other aerobic bacterial isolates from the tonsils include B, C, and G streptococci, *Streptococcus pneumoniae*, *Haemophilus influenzae*, viridans streptococci, *Neisseria* spp., and *Haemophilus parainfluenzae*. Anaerobic isolates are rare. The lack of systemic complications makes the treatment of infection from these organisms less imperative, but significant pain and feeding difficulties may develop that may warrant antibiotic treatment.

Viral infection also frequently affects the tonsils and adenoids, with adenovirus, influenza A and B, parainfluenza, and herpes simplex viruses routinely cultured from inflamed tonsils and the pharynx. Epstein-Barr virus is the causative agent of mononucleosis. It is associated with mononuclear lymphocytosis and a positive heterophile antibody "mono" test in 90% of cases. The mono test may be negative early, and diagnosis is suggested by an elevated white blood cell count and atypical lymphocyte percentage.

◼ Acute Tonsillitis

Acute tonsillitis is a self-limiting disease of one or both tonsils. It is diagnosed by clinical examination. The onset of fever is sudden, with throat pain developing over several days. The symptoms usually persist for less than 1 week without treatment, and it is generally a self-limiting disease. The tonsils show enlargement and a patchy exudate that frequently coalesces over the tonsil surface during the acute infection. Complications may develop from acute tonsillitis, including pharyngeal inflammation leading to airway obstruction, peritonsillar abscess, deep neck infection, and septicemia.

Management

Classic treatment of acute tonsillitis has been limited to those infections caused by group A b-hemolytic streptococci. Other pathogens, however, cause tonsillar disease and require intervention when symptomatic complaints develop. The goal of antibiotic treatment is fourfold: (1) to hasten clinical recovery, (2) to render the patient noninfectious to contacts, (3) to avoid suppurative complications of acute infection, and (4) to prevent rheumatic fever. Identification of group A b-hemolytic streptococci requires either a throat culture or an antigen detection test (rapid strep test). The throat culture requires 24 to 48 hours to obtain a result. In contrast, the antigen detection tests require only a few minutes, and their specificity is > 90%. If the antigen test is negative, however, a culture should be used as the definitive study to rule out group A b-hemolytic streptococci. Appropriate antibiotic therapy can be initiated from a rapid antigen detection test when positive.

Penicillin V remains the drug of choice for the treatment of group A b-hemolytic streptococci but requires frequent dosing. Amoxicillin is frequently substituted because of its once daily dosing schedule. In penicillin-allergic patients, macrolides (azithromycin, clarithromycin, or erythromycin) are the drugs of choice. To prevent rheumatic fever, the antibiotic should be given for at least 10 days, regardless of the speed of clinical recovery. In cases of suspected poor compliance, intramuscular benzathine penicillin G (600,000 units for children under 60 pounds and 1.2 million units for older children) ensures adequate blood levels and avoids compliance issues.

Sulfonamides were previously used for continuous prophylaxis, but they fail to eradicate group A b-hemolytic streptococci from the pharynx. Continuous prophylaxis is no longer recommended. For children, tetracyclines should be avoided because of the permanent staining of the enamel of unerupted teeth.

Beta-lactamase-producing upper respiratory tract flora may inactivate penicillin class antibiotics and thus shield group A β-hemolytic streptococci. In treatment failures, β-lactamase-stable antibiotics (amoxicillin-clavulanate, clindamycin, dicloxacillin) are useful. With the increasing prevalence of penicillin-resistant *Streptococcus* (which is generally multidrug resistant), sensitivity testing is required to ensure correct treatment and eradication of the organism. Consultation with infectious disease specialists may be appropriate for multiple-resistant organisms if surgery is not indicated.

◼ Chronic Tonsillitis

Chronic tonsillitis usually represents persistent inflammatory changes within the tonsils for at least 3 months. Throat pain and cervical adenopathy may continue despite antibiotic therapy. Throat cultures are usually negative in these children. The tonsillar tissue may become hyperplastic in response to the chronic stimulation, or it may become small and fibrotic. The chronically inflamed tonsils may become a persistent nidus of upper respiratory infections, exacerbating chronic and reactive lung disease.

Management

Antibiotic therapy and improved oral hygiene may be effective in alleviating chronic adenotonsillitis. Alternatively, surgical therapy may be indicated, although the 2011 tonsillectomy guidelines from the American Academy of Otolaryngology–Head and Neck Surgery (AAO–HNS) did not include recommendations specific to chronic tonsillitis.

◼ Adenotonsillar Hypertrophy

Tonsillar hypertrophy results from an increase in the size of existing tonsillar tissue. It begins in early childhood and continues for the first 2 to 5 years. At puberty, atrophy occurs. Tonsillar hypertrophy is normal growth of the tonsil and adenoid tissue. On the other hand, hyperplasia causes enlargement of the tonsil and adenoid tissue, because of increases in the number of cells and cellular activity in the germinal centers in response to an acute inflammatory response, chronic antigen stimulation, or chronic irritation. Therefore, the actual cellular content of the tissue increases. Tonsillar size becomes clinically significant when mechanical obstruction of the oropharynx or nasopharynx interferes with respiration or deglutition. These patients frequently present with loud snoring, irregular breathing, restless sleep patterns, and frequent awakenings. Adults often complain of daytime somnolence, and children may develop chronic open-mouth posturing, drooling, and dysphagia for solid food materials.

Both the AAO–HNS and the American Academy of Sleep Medicine (AASM) published guidance on the use of polysomnography (PSG) in children in 2011. The AAO–HNS guidelines recommend that children with "obesity, Down syndrome, craniofacial abnormalities, neuromuscular disorders, sickle cell disease or mucopolysaccharidoses" undergo PSG prior to tonsillectomy. In addition, they note that a PSG should be advocated in children with a discrepancy between tonsil size and sleep-disordered breathing severity. The AASM practice parameter goes further in recommending PSG in all children with suggested obstructive sleep apnea and in all children for whom adenotonsillectomy is being considered. The expense, inconvenience, and lack of widely available pediatric PSG are also acknowledged in the AAO–HNS guidelines, which note that home-administered PSG may be considered if in-laboratory PSG is not available, but that its routine use is not recommended because there are very few data validating home study use in children.

■ Indications for Surgery

After it has been determined that medical therapy has been unsuccessful at resolving the adenotonsillar problems, surgical intervention may be considered. These indicators are generally broken into three broad categories: infection, obstruction, and neoplasia.

Infection

Recurrent infections of the tonsils and adenoids are a burden to the patient and family. AAO–HNS guidelines recommend that adenotonsillectomy should be considered if a patient has experienced seven episodes of adenotonsillitis in a year, five episodes of adenotonsillitis in each of 2 preceding years, or three episodes in each of the preceding 3 years, along with documentation of sore throat and at least one of the following: positive group A b-hemolytic streptococci test, temperature over 38.3°C, exudative tonsillitis, or cervical lymphadenopathy. The documentation of group A b-hemolytic streptococcal infection is not necessary for the recommendation of surgical intervention.

The effect of the infections on daily activities must also be considered when contemplating surgery.

Days missed from work or school numbering at least 2 weeks, or hospitalizations resulting from severe infection, or the development of complications of adenotonsillitis should sway the decision toward a surgical approach to the management of recurrent adenotonsillar infection. Coexisting morbidity must also be evaluated when making a decision to recommend surgical intervention. The AAO–HNS tonsillectomy guidelines also suggest looking at "modifying factors," such as antibiotic intolerance/allergy, history of recurrent peritonsillar abscess, and *p*eriodic *f*ever, *a*phthous stomatitis, *p*haryngitis, and *a*denitis (PFAPA).

Upper Airway Obstruction

Adenotonsillar hypertrophy with upper airway obstruction requires surgical intervention to alleviate the acute obstruction and to prevent long-term sequelae that might develop if left untreated. The classic long-term complications of obstructive sleep apnea (OSA) in adults are cor pulmonale, right ventricular hypertrophy, congestive heart failure, cardiomegaly, hypoventilation syndrome, pulmonary hypertension, neurological damage, failure to thrive, and death. Although there is some evidence of early cardiovascular changes in children with OSA, much of the short-term concern has focused on neurocognitive outcomes, such as lowered school performance, short-term memory, intelligence quotient (IQ), and executive functions skills. These complications can often be reversed by adenotonsillectomy.

The criteria for the diagnosis of significant OSA in the pediatric age group are not as clearly defined as they are for adults, although it is clear that adult criteria are not directly applicable to children. The basis of the diagnosis is taken from the history. Manifestations of OSA include respiratory pauses, snoring, noisy breathing, chronic mouth breathing, frequent arousals, restless sleep patterns, repositioning throughout the night, hyperextension of the neck while sleeping, and paradoxical chest wall motion. Some children may develop behavioral abnormalities, enuresis, decreased school performance, learning disabilities, and daytime somnolence. In children, prolonged partial airway obstruction during sleep may result in significant hypoxemia and hypercarbia without frank apneic events. Adenotonsillar hypertrophy with sleep-disordered breathing is an indication for adenoidectomy, tonsillectomy, or adenotonsillectomy, even in the absence of actual apneic episodes. This is reinforced by recent studies citing decreased neurocognitive function in children who snore despite a lack of scorable events on a sleep study.

Malignancy

Asymmetric tonsils raise the question of malignancy. In patients with a malignancy, there is often an area of ulceration or the mucosa overlying the affected tonsil is friable. Palpation of the affected tonsil may demonstrate a hard mass, in contrast to the typical rubbery consistency of the tonsillar tissue. Lymphoma is the most common malignancy to be identified in pediatric tonsils, whereas squamous cell carcinoma is most common in adult tonsils. Biopsy is warranted in all cases of suspected malignancy, and the biopsy procedure should be a complete tonsillectomy. The tonsils should be sent immediately in a fresh condition for pathological evaluation, so that special tumor markers can be performed if indicated.

Peritonsillar Abscess

Peritonsillar abscesses may develop as a complication of acute tonsillitis. They may be managed in the older child and adult with needle aspiration with or without incision and drainage. In the uncooperative or young child, general anesthesia is typically required for this procedure.

A tonsillectomy could also be performed as the procedure to drain the abscess and prevent recurrent infections in the future. The "quinsy" tonsillectomy is more technically difficult to perform than the standard tonsillectomy because acute inflammatory changes are present. Frequently, the tissues are edematous and the electrocautery technique of tissue dissection is tedious. However, final hemostasis is generally not difficult, and the posttonsillectomy hemorrhage rates do not appear higher than in the standard tonsillectomy.

There is potential for recurrence of a peritonsillar abscess after the first event. Elective tonsillectomy, at least 4 weeks after treatment of the first peritonsillar abscess to allow resolution of the inflammatory process, is another reasonable alternative. The AAO–HNS tonsillectomy guidelines note that tonsillectomy in this setting is controversial because the need for tonsillectomy after a single episode of peritonsillar abscess is only 10 to 20%. Peritonsillar abscess, however, does not appear as common in children without a long history of tonsillitis.

Otitis Media

The proximity of the adenoids to the eustachian tube orifice raises the possibility that bacteria residing within or in biofilms over the surface of the adenoids contribute to the development of otitis media. The physical size of the adenoids may interfere with proper eustachian tube function. Removal of the adenoids may lessen the incidence of otitis media. Tonsillectomy has not been shown to have an affect on the incidence of otitis media.

Other Indications

Tonsillar hypertrophy can narrow the oropharyngeal inlet to the extent that dysphagia results, even in the absence of signs of respiratory difficulties. In severe cases, failure to thrive is the result of combined respiratory compromise and feeding difficulties. Hemorrhage from superficial tonsillar vessels that are difficult to control or recurrent in nature require removal of the tonsil. Hypertrophic tonsils have been noted on occasion to project superiorly into the nasopharynx, causing velopharyngeal insufficiency. Adenoid hypertrophy may obstruct the nasopharynx and posterior choanae, leading to hyponasal speech and difficulties with speech intelligibility. Adenoid obstruction of the nasal passages can produce chronic rhinorrhea and can contribute to the development of sinusitis. Malocclusion (anterior open bite) may develop from a chronic open-mouth posture, resulting from chronic nasal obstruction. PFAPA is an indication for tonsillectomy according to the latest guidelines; however, *p*ediatric *a*utoimmune *n*europsychiatric *d*isorders *a*ssociated with *s*treptococcal infections (PANDAS) is not.

■ Preoperative Management

Evaluation

Unless underlying medical conditions dictate, preoperative laboratory studies are of questionable value, but there is no consensus of opinion. In general, no laboratory studies are required prior to adenotonsillectomy. A baseline complete blood count rarely identifies any abnormality. Screening for coagulopathies should generally be limited to a history of problems in the patient or in the patient's family history, and detailed coagulation and bleeding studies should be performed only if risk factors are identified.

Contraindications to Adenotonsillectomy

Velopharyngeal insufficiency occurs postoperatively in 1 in 1,500 adenoidectomy procedures. Many patients in whom this complication develops have underlying abnormalities of the soft palate. A thorough preoperative evaluation of the palate is essential in all patients being considered for adenoidectomy. A history of cleft palate in the patient or family, a submucous cleft of the palate, and a history of feeding difficulties as a young child all raise the risk of velopharyngeal insufficiency developing following adenoidectomy. Neurological abnormalities associated with poor oral motor skills may also be associated with poor velar function. If the obstructive symptoms are severe, an adenoidectomy may be required, despite the risk of velopharyngeal insufficiency. In this situation, superior half-adenoidectomy should be performed to alleviate the obstruction of the posterior choana, while maintaining the adenoid pad inferiorly to assist with closure of the velopharyngeal sphincter.

Hematologic contraindications to adenotonsillectomy involve disorders of hemostasis. If the patient has a known disorder of coagulation, or a positive family history of bleeding disorders is obtained, the coagulation cascade must be evaluated with a bleeding time, prothrombin time, partial thrombin time, and platelet count. Hematologic correction of all deficiencies must be obtained, as well as assurances that the correction can be maintained for at least 10 days postoperatively, before the adenotonsillectomy can be performed. Life-threatening hemorrhage is always a possibility following adenotonsillectomy, despite normal preoperative laboratory studies.

Surgical Technique

The specific technique used for removal of tonsil and adenoid tissue is a matter of individual surgeon preference. Conventional sharp dissection, electrocautery, radiofrequency ablation, harmonic scalpel, argon beam coagulator, and lasers have all been described and can be used safely in skilled hands. The benefits of reduced time of operation, blood loss, and postoperative pain must all be balanced with the increased cost of highly complex equipment.

The AAO–HNS guidelines strongly recommend that a single dose of dexamethasone be given intravenously during the adenotonsillectomy to reduce emesis and fever, and to increase oral intake at 24 hours postoperatively. In addition, it is strongly recommended that perioperative antibiotics not be given; a 2010 Cochrane review also found that there was no evidence that they reduce "the main morbid outcomes after tonsillectomy."

◼ Postoperative Management and Controversies

Postoperatively, patients experience throat pain, referred otalgia, odynophagia, and neck stiffness. Dehydration and weight loss occurring over the 2 week recovery period are common. Oral intake must be encouraged to minimize the risk of dehydration. Generally, in an attempt to maximize oral intake, no restrictions are placed on the patient with respect to the types of food to be consumed after the operation. The majority of patients prefer liquid and soft diets for the first postoperative week.

Although it was previously thought that all non-steroidal anti-inflammatory drugs (NSAIDs) should be avoided after adenotonsillectomy, recent pooled analysis shows that NSAIDs, with the exception of ketorolac, do not have a significant impact on acute or delayed bleeding rates. Ketorolac has been shown to increase bleeding rates after surgery and is not recommended. The AAO–HNS guidelines also address the use of pain medication after surgery and recommend that pain management be emphasized in communications with caregivers. In addition, they recommend avoiding the use of acetaminophen with codeine because issues with codeine metabolism render it ineffective for some and dangerous for other children. There is debate about allowed activity levels after surgery, with some otolaryngologists recommending no restriction and others recommending limitation of strenuous activity for the first 2 weeks postoperatively.

Although disposition following adenotonsillectomy has generated much controversy in the literature, there has been a clear migration to outpatient adenotonsillectomy. A period of observation is required for all patients postoperatively to ensure that there is no bleeding from the operative site, to ensure minimal emesis, and to ensure that the patient is tolerating oral fluids well. This time varies from 2 to 4 hours for most outpatient procedures. The patients who should be observed overnight for signs of developing airway compromise or disordered breathing include those with underlying craniofacial abnormalities, Down syndrome, neurological impairments, cor pulmonale, morbid obesity, upper airway obstruction, chronic medical problems, severe OSA, and age younger than 3 years.

Complications

Hemorrhage

Hemorrhage within the first 24 hours of adenotonsillectomy is a technical problem related to the surgery, with a rate ranging from 0.2 to 2.2%. Hemorrhage beyond the first 24 hours (delayed hemorrhage) occurs in 0.1 to 3% of patients and generally has no identifiable causes. Delayed hemorrhage tends to occur between postoperative days 5 and 10, which is the period of eschar separation from the tonsillar fossa. If bleeding is encountered postoperatively, patients must be evaluated for signs of continued hemorrhage or clot formation in the tonsillar fossa.

Treatment may range from observation at home to hospital admission to evaluation in the operating room, with possible control of bleeding. The need for evaluation of an underlying coagulation disorder is not well defined after a single episode of delayed bleeding, but it is definitely warranted in children with recurrent postoperative hemorrhage. A blood count is best obtained after fluid equilibration to determine the extent of the bleeding.

Postoperative Dehydration

Postoperative dehydration occurs in nearly all patients after adenotonsillectomy, with ~ 3% of patients requiring hospital admission. Ineffective postoperative pain control is frequently the basis for significant dehydration.

Airway Obstruction

Airway obstruction is most likely to occur in children 3 years of age or younger. Edema of the uvula, posterior soft palate, or lateral tongue encroaches on and obstructs the airway. Intravenous steroids (dexamethasone) may decrease the extent of edema development. Rarely, nasal trumpets or endotracheal intubation are required to secure the airway until the edema resolves. Airway obstruction is also more common in patients with craniofacial anomalies, obesity, and neurological disorders.

Significant OSA can disrupt the normal respiratory control centers. The normal elevation of carbon dioxide that should trigger respiration has been replaced by a system that is driven by low blood oxygen levels. This altered physiology persists for a period postoperatively and may impair normal respiration and require respiratory support.

Obstructive Sleep Apnea

Severe cases of OSA may be associated with pulmonary edema that develops immediately upon relief of the upper airway obstruction and leads to hypoxia and tachypnea. Postobstructive pulmonary edema generally requires admission to the intensive care unit for close observation and treatment. Diuretics and positive airway pressure—either continuous positive airway pressure or endotracheal intubation—are the mainstays of treatment for severe cases.

Transient Velopharyngeal Insufficiency

Transient velopharyngeal insufficiency frequently occurs after removal of a large adenoid pad. Generally, if the musculature of the palate is normal, the palate may be retrained to extend further posteriorly to close the velopharyngeal port. If there is any abnormality in the structure or neural control of the palate, velopharyngeal insufficiency will persist until surgical intervention corrects the problem.

Nasopharyngeal and Oropharyngeal Stenosis

Though uncommon, nasopharyngeal and oropharyngeal stenoses are devastating complications of adenotonsillectomy. The technique of adenotonsillectomy does not seem to be related to the development of stenosis. However, if the surgical defect results in the apposition of two de-epithelialized surfaces, stenosis may develop. The use of a nasopharyngeal or nasotracheal tube also increases the risk of this complication. Additionally, concurrent lingual tonsillectomy or partial midline glossectomy has been shown to increase the rate of oropharyngeal stenosis.

■ Practice Guidelines, Consensus Statements, and Measures

Baugh RF, Archer SM, Mitchell RB, et al; American Academy of Otolaryngology-Head and Neck Surgery Foundation. Clinical practice guideline: tonsillectomy in children. Otolaryngol Head Neck Surg 2011;144(1, Suppl):S1–S30

Roland PS, Rosenfeld RM, Brooks LJ, et al; American Academy of Otolaryngology–Head and Neck Surgery Foundation. Clinical practice guideline: polysomnography for sleep-disordered breathing prior to tonsillectomy in children. Otolaryngol Head Neck Surg 2011;145(1, Suppl):S1–S15

■ Suggested Reading

Academy of Otolaryngology–Head and Neck Surgery. Clinical Indicators Compendium. Alexandria, VA: American Academy of Otolaryngology–Head and Neck Surgery; 1999. http://www.entnet.org/Practice/clinicalIndicators.cfm. Accessed August 10, 2012

Aurora RN, Zak RS, Karippot A, et al; American Academy of Sleep Medicine. Practice parameters for the respiratory indications for polysomnography in children. Sleep 2011;34(3):379–388

Baltimore RS. Re-evaluation of antibiotic treatment of streptococcal pharyngitis. Curr Opin Pediatr 2010;22(1):77–82

Baugh RF, Archer SM, Mitchell RB, et al; American Academy of Otolaryngology-Head and Neck Surgery Foundation. Clinical practice guideline: tonsillectomy in children. Otolaryngol Head Neck Surg 2011;144(1, Suppl):S1–S30

Brodsky L, Moore L, Stanievich JF, Ogra PL. The immunology of tonsils in children: the effect of bacterial load on the presence of B- and T-cell subsets. Laryngoscope 1988;98(1):93–98

Cherry JD. Pharyngitis. In: Feigin RD, Cherry JD, eds. Textbook of Pediatric Infectious Diseases. 4th ed. Philadelphia, PA: WB Saunders; 1998:148–156

Cardwell M, Siviter G, Smith A. Non-steroidal anti-inflammatory drugs and perioperative bleeding in paediatric tonsillectomy. Cochrane Database Syst Rev 2005;2(2):CD003591

Darrow DH, Kludt NA. Adenotonsillar disease. In: Mitchell RD, Pereira KD, eds. Pediatric Otolaryngology for the Clinician. New York, NY: Humana Press; 2009:187–195

Dhiwakar M, Clement WA, Supriya M, McKerrow W. Antibiotics to reduce post-tonsillectomy morbidity. Cochrane Database Syst Rev 2010;7(7):CD005607

Gates GA, Avery CA, Prihoda TJ, Cooper JC Jr. Effectiveness of adenoidectomy and tympanostomy tubes in the treatment of chronic otitis media with effusion. N Engl J Med 1987;317(23):1444–1451

Halbower AC, Degaonkar M, Barker PB, et al. Childhood obstructive sleep apnea associates with neuropsychological deficits and neuronal brain injury. PLoS Med 2006;3(8):e301

Hollinshead WH. The pharynx and larynx. In: Anatomy for Surgeons. Vol 1. Philadelphia, PA: Lippincott-Raven; 1982:389–403

Kaplan EL. The rapid identification of group A beta-hemolytic streptococci in the upper respiratory tract. Current status. Pediatr Clin North Am 1988;35(3):535–542

Prager JD, Hopkins BS, Propst EJ, Shott SR, Cotton RT. Oropharyngeal stenosis: a complication of multilevel, single-stage upper airway surgery in children. Arch Otolaryngol Head Neck Surg 2010;136(11):1111–1115

Roland PS, Rosenfeld RM, Brooks LJ, et al; American Academy of Otolaryngology–Head and Neck Surgery Foundation. Clinical practice guideline: polysomnography for sleep-disordered breathing prior to tonsillectomy in children. Otolaryngol Head Neck Surg 2011;145(1, Suppl):S1–S15

Steward DL, Welge JA, Myer CM. Steroids for improving recovery following tonsillectomy in children. Cochrane Database Syst Rev 2003;1(1):CD003997

Taylan I, Özcan I, Mumcuoğlu I, et al. Comparison of the surface and core bacteria in tonsillar and adenoid tissue with Beta-lactamase production. Indian J Otolaryngol Head Neck Surg 2011;63(3):223–228

VIII

Rhinology and Allergy

82 Allergy and Immunotherapy

Introduction

Allergy describes a hypersensitive response to a foreign protein called an allergen through ingestion, contact, or inhalation exposure. An estimated 50 million, or 1 in 5, Americans suffer from some form of allergy, and its prevalence has been noticeably increasing since the 1990s. This makes allergy the fifth most common of chronic diseases suffered by Americans, ranking as the second most common reason patients seek out a health care professional (behind dental care).

A widely used classification of hypersensitivity immune responses, the Gell and Coombs classification, categorizes hypersensitive immune responses into four types (**Table 82.1**). This review focuses primarily on immunoglobulin E (IgE)-mediated allergic responses, and specifically allergic rhinitis. Other causes of rhinitis include adverse responses to certain food and chemical stimuli.

Allergic rhinitis is a condition consisting of nasal congestion with obstruction of airflow, mucous production, and drainage, resulting from adverse reaction to an environmental or ingested stimulus. Allergic rhinitis affects 20 to 30 million people, accounting for an estimated 3% of all physician office visits. More than 10% of the world's population is believed to have symptoms of allergic rhinitis.

The development of allergic rhinitis in an atopic patient requires, first, sensitization, followed by reexposure to a given allergen. During sensitization, a low-dose exposure of the antigen is taken up by an antigen-presenting cell (dendritic cell, macrophage, Langerhans cell). The antigen-presenting cell processes the antigen and expresses antigenic proteins on its cell surface via the major histocompatibility complex class II receptor. These processed allergens are then recognized by T-helper cells, resulting in the production of T-helper 2 (Th2) cytokines, such as interleukin (IL)-4, IL-5, and IL-13. IL-4 and IL-13 are the two cytokines that primarily activate B cells to produce antigen-specific IgE and incite mucus

production. IL-5 is the primary cytokine involved in recruitment and maintenance of eosinophils important in the allergy response. The IgE molecules are then recognized by high-affinity receptors located on mast cells.

Upon reexposure, the fixated IgE molecules recognize the allergens, leading to the activation of mast cells and the release of several preformed proinflammatory mediators, including histamine. These mediators stimulate blood vessels, nerves, and mucus glands, which leads to the classic acute symptoms associated with allergic rhinitis (rhinorrhea, nasal congestion, nasal irritation, and sneezing). These acute symptoms are followed by a late-phase response that is predominated by nasal congestion. This late-phase response, which follows several hours after the initial antigen exposure, is characterized by an influx of inflammatory cells, including eosinophils, mast cells, basophils, and lymphocytes.

Evaluation

Clinical Findings

The diagnosis of allergic rhinitis is highly dependent on obtaining a good history and physical examination. One of the goals of the history is to differentiate allergic rhinitis from other causes of rhinitis. In addition, a good history will allow classification of allergic rhinitis severity based on recent Allergic Rhinitis and Its Impact on Asthma (ARIA) guidelines into mild or moderate/severe and intermittent and persistent symptoms. Features consistent with allergic rhinitis include the seasonality of symptoms, symptoms associated with a specific exposure or environment, symptoms improved with air-conditioned environments, and symptoms predominated by itchiness, ocular irritation, nasal congestion, sneezing, and rhinorrhea. The physical exam may reveal dark circles around the eyes ("allergic shiners"). Other physical

Table 82.1 Classification of hypersensitivity

Type	Clinical manifestations	Major mediator	Major effectors	Sensitization	Mechanisms of injury
I (Anaphylactic)	Local anaphylaxis (atopic allergies); systemic anaphylaxis	IgE	Histamine; slow-reacting substance of anaphylaxis (SRS-A)	Inhalation (respiratory mucosa); ingestion (gastrointestinal mucosa); parenteral	IgE attached to mast cells causes releases of histamine and SRS-A on reacting with specific antigen
II (Cytotoxic)	Hemolytic disease of the newborn, drug-induced hemolytic hypersensitivity, transfusion reactions, graft rejection, autoimmune diseases	IgG	Complement; K cell	Parenteral, ingestion, transplantation	Activation of complement to give lysis and opsonization; K cell cytotoxicity for antibody-coated target cells
III (Immune complex)	Local: Arthus reaction; systemic: serum sickness	IgG	Antigen-antibody complexes; complement; polymorphonuclear leukocytes	Parenteral (inoculation of antigen or antiserum), inhalation (rare)	Activation of complement by antigen-antibody complexes chemotactic for polymorphonuclear leukocytes, which leads to vasculitis
IV (Cell-mediated immunity [CMI])	Delayed-type hypersensitivity (DH), contact hypersensitivity, cytotoxicity (graft and tumor rejection), autoimmune disease	CMI: T cells	Lymphokines (DH type), cytotoxic T cells	Parenteral, contact, transplantation	Lymphokines: migration inhibition factor (MIF), chemotactic factor, etc., lead to vascular necrotic injury; cell membrane injury by direct cytotoxicity of the cytotoxic cells leads to invasive-destructive injury

Abbreviations: IgE, immunoglobulin E; IgG, immunoglobulin G.

findings typical of rhinitis include boggy inferior turbinates, nasal congestion, and cobblestoning of the nasopharynx as a result of persistent postnasal drainage.

Diagnostic Evaluation

The goal of specific antigen testing is to determine which, if any, antigenic substance may be causing a patient's symptoms. One should not forget this basic goal. Testing techniques can determine only whether the patient has IgE antibodies to the antigen and, in some cases, can estimate the quantity of antibody available. Cross-reactivity exists between antigens and may lead to misdiagnosis if allergy results are not viewed in a context of history. Various forms of testing exist to assess the patient's sensitivity to a test antigen. These tests are performed either on the patient's skin (called in vivo testing or, more simply, skin testing) or on the patient's serum in a laboratory (termed in vitro testing, or blood tests). Testing is discussed here in the context of these categories.

Skin Testing

Skin Prick Testing (SPT)

Skin prick testing (SPT) identifies allergic sensitivity by eliciting a skin reaction to the specific antigen. A drop of antigen is introduced with a lancet-type (solid point) needle just below the epidermis. Antigens are identified as positive based on the extent of skin response, including wheal and flare. Although the response is qualitative, the extent of reaction is used by some practitioners to categorize positive test results into low- and high-sensitivity responses. This modality should be distinguished from the scratch testing technique. Although the prick test does not reach the depth of intradermal testing, the type of skin opening is deeper and more standardized than the obsolescent scratch test.

The benefits of SPT include identification of the allergic response directly from the patient's skin with a simple needle stick. Also, because the antigen is introduced into a relatively superficial layer, SPT has a low risk of systemic reaction.

Disadvantages of SPT include the fact that this test does not determine the precise level of sensitivity for specific antigens. Additionally, there is no opportunity to detect allergic disease at sensitivities below the concentration of the antigen injected. However, this drawback may not be serious. It can be argued that low-sensitivity antigens, while potentially important from an environmental standpoint, are not likely to be used in immunotherapy; therefore, the lack of ability to detect them is of minor consequence.

At the conclusion of SPT, the practitioner knows which antigens are positive and which are historically important and has only a rough sense of the level of the patient's sensitivity to each antigen.

Intradermal Dilution Testing (IDT) (or Skin Endpoint Titration)

Intradermal dilution testing (IDT) is a form of skin testing conducted by intradermal injection of a specific antigen. By sequential injection of increasing antigen concentration, the physician may identify a patient's level of sensitivity to the specific antigen. The dilution of antigens used may vary with physician training and preference, but the 1:5 dilution is the technique taught in otolaryngic allergy courses as a safe, standard protocol. The mathematics of 1:5 dilutions result in dilution ratios of 1:2,500, 1:12,500, 1:62,500, and so on. To simplify charting and avoid error, each dilution is assigned a number. In this system, diluting a 1:20 concentrate by fivefold obtains a 1:100 concentration, termed the number 1 dilution. Sequential fivefold dilutions are numbered as shown in **Table 82.2**.

The no. 6 dilution is sufficiently dilute that anaphylaxis is extremely unlikely. This dilution is injected into the skin as a 4 mm wheal and is observed for 10 minutes. Following this, a sequence of stronger intradermal injections is administered into the skin at 10 minute intervals, each creating a 4 mm wheal. The endpoint is defined as follows, noted on the series of skin wheals:

1. The *endpoint* is the dilution in which the wheal size increases by at least 2 mm from the wheal size created by the preceding less concentrated dilution within 10 minutes, and is followed by a more concentrated dilution that creates a larger wheal by at least 2 mm or more within 10 minutes, called the *confirmatory wheal.*

2. If two or more dilutions match the 2 mm size increase, the true *endpoint* is the dilution immediately before the confirmatory wheal. This endpoint identifies the patient's level of sensitivity to the antigen and provides a safe point for the initiation of immunotherapy.

In summary, IDT permits a semiquantitative determination of antigen sensitivity. The technique allows differentiation of idiosyncratic responses from true sensitivities. Each antigen may now be started independently at the strongest safe concentration. Of equal importance, each antigen's relative sensitivity is preserved with respect to the other antigens. This avoids having a very sensitive antigen cause a skin reaction and delay advancement of therapy.

The disadvantage of IDT is that testing involves several needle sticks for each antigen. This requires both an increased time requirement and increased cost. As a consequence of these disadvantages, a modified quantitative testing (MQT) method was proposed.

Modified Quantitative Testing

MQT combines skin testing with IDT to identify an endpoint from which to start immunotherapy. The technique starts with an SPT using a multiunit application device. The wheal size from the SPT determines the dilution from which to perform the IDT. The size of the consequent wheal from the IDT then dictates the endpoint dilution. This fused technique serves to minimize the time and cost of the conventional IDT, while providing the quantitative data that an SPT lacks.

In vitro Testing

In vitro, literally meaning "in glass," refers to testing performed outside the patient's body. It is a generic term, not one that specifies any particular testing technique. The in vitro tests that allow therapeutic decisions and the initiation of immunotherapy are variations of the "sandwich" type immunoassay. In these studies, specific IgE antibody is identified by allowing it to bind with a known antigen. The specific IgE antibody attached to the antigen is itself immunologically identified by an "antihuman" IgE molecule tagged with a tracer material. Tracers may use a variety of techniques, including fluorescence, radioactivity, and chemiluminescence.

Table 82.2 1:5 Dilution and corresponding concentration

Dilution	**1**	**2**	**3**	**4**	**5**	**6**
Concentration 1:20 weight/volume (w/v)	1:100 w/v	1:500 w/v	1:2500 w/v	1:12,500 w/v	1:62,5000 w/v	1:312,500 w/v

Antibody assays using radioactive labels are termed radioallergosorbent tests (RASTs). The RAST, particularly the modified RAST, has been considered a standard against which other immunoassays are judged. The modified RAST yields a reading of 0 (nonallergic), 0/1 (equivocal), or allergy class 1 through 6, with larger numbers indicating higher concentrations of specific IgE and therefore greater sensitivity to a given antigen. A modified RAST result of a class 4 allergy to June grass is designed to correlate to an endpoint of 4 using IDT techniques. As a consequence, in vitro technology can reproduce quantitative information about antigen sensitivity without risking systemic reactions, flash responses, or a patient's ability to cooperate with the repeated pricks or injections associated with skin testing.

A valuable safety technique when using in vitro testing is to move the in vitro endpoints to one dilution less concentrated before preparing immunotherapy vials. This shift of endpoints across the spectrum of an individual patient's in vitro results is called "treating at RAST $n - 1$."

This approach provides a margin of safety when initiating immunotherapy. Note that the minus sign does not indicate an arithmetic minus, but is an indication that a more dilute mixture has been selected. The name may be confusing, but it is deeply rooted in the literature at this point.

With particularly brittle patients, such as asthmatics, patients who have had severe reactions in the past, or at times when therapy has begun coseasonally, alteration of the endpoint to RAST $n - 2$, or less concentrated by two endpoints, provides an additional margin of safety. More important, the relative levels of sensitivity between antigens are preserved. In vitro testing results must still be confirmed by skin testing before initiating immunotherapy.

◼ Management

The management of allergic rhinitis is categorized into environmental control, pharmacotherapy, and immunotherapy.

Allergen Avoidance and Environmental Control

For patients with a limited allergen profile, avoidance of the allergens causing patients' symptoms may be a very effective management technique, such as patients with an isolated cat or dog allergy. Although completely avoiding outdoor allergens, such as pollen, may be impractical, minimizing outdoor exposure on dry, sunny, windy days during pollen season would reduce symptoms. Environmental control measures are also recommended to patients with allergies to indoor allergens, such as dust mites or molds. These measures can include minimizing carpeting and indoor humidity, using filters, and frequently washing bed linens in hot water. Although the effectiveness of these measures as standalone treatments is limited, they are recommended as part of an overall defense strategy.

Pharmacotherapy

H₁ Blockers

H_1 blockers, or antihistamines, have both oral and intranasal preparations. This is one of the possible first-line treatments, particularly if the patient does not have a complaint of nasal obstruction or has mild-to-moderate allergic rhinitis. For intermittent symptoms or mild persistent symptoms, use of oral or intranasal H_1 blockers is recommended with or without a decongestant. Antihistamines are recommended in patients with moderate-to-severe persistent symptoms, together with intranasal steroids.

The second-generation H_1 blockers have significantly less sedating side effects as compared with their first-generation counterparts. They serve as competitive inhibitors to the histamine 1 receptor. Examples of antihistamines available in the United States include cetirizine, levocetirizine, fexofenadine, and loratadine.

Leukotriene Receptor Antagonists (LTRAs)

Leukotriene receptor antagonists (LTRAs) prevent the action of leukotrienes that are released by mast cells and eosinophils to drive the pathophysiology of allergic rhinitis. Montelukast has the approval of the U.S. Food and Drug Administration (FDA) for the treatment of seasonal and perennial allergic rhinitis. LTRAs are a treatment option for intermittent symptoms and mild persistent symptoms and a second-line option for moderate-to-severe persistent symptoms.

Intranasal Steroids

Several intranasal steroids are available in the United States. As a treatment option, intranasal steroids are highly efficacious, primarily with controlling nasal congestion, sneezing, itching, and rhinorrhea. Intranasal steroids should be considered as a first-line treatment option in patients with allergic rhinitis, particularly with moderate-to-severe intermittent symptoms and in all patients with persistent disease. Several different formulations are available, but basically all are geared to reduce inflammation within the nasal mucosa.

Intranasal Cromolyns

Intranasal cromolyns are mast cell stabilizers that can be considered in patients with moderate-to-severe intermittent symptoms and patients with persistent symptoms. Their effect is modest compared with that of intranasal steroids. However, they have an excellent safety profile and are considered safe to be used in children and pregnant women.

Intranasal Antihistamines

Currently two intranasal antihistamines are FDA approved for the treatment of allergic rhinitis. Azelastine and olopatadine are both second generation H1-receptor antagonists. Compared to oral antihistamines, the intranasal preparations offer the advantage of rapid onset of action within 15 minutes, higher concentration of drug in the targeted area and fewer adverse effects. Side effects of antihistamine nasal sprays may include a bitter taste, drowsiness or fatigue.

Immunotherapy

Immunotherapy involves exposing patients over an extending period of time to allergen(s) in an attempt to modulate the immune response away from an IgE-mediated hypersensitive response. The two available delivery methods are subcutaneous immunotherapy (SCIT) and sublingual immunotherapy (SLIT). SCIT introduces antigens through subcutaneous shots, whereas SLIT administers antigens under the tongue. In 2014, the FDA approved SLIT tablets for ragweed, Timothy, and grass mix. SLIT drops are still not approved, making them an "off-label" route of administration. SLIT seems to have some advantages over SCIT, such as an improved safety profile and ability to deliver therapy at home and not in a clinical office.

Although the mechanism of immunotherapy for allergies has not been completely elucidating, it appears to decrease IgE production and increase IgG produc-

tion, which may serve as an IgE-blocking antibody. Other possible effects include increased IL-10 production, which can suppress Th2 lymphocyte and mast cell activity. In addition, there is evidence of increased T regulatory cells and reduced Th2 cells with immunotherapy. These effects of immunotherapy serve to suppress the IgE-mediated hypersensitivity response.

Subcutaneous Immunotherapy

SCIT is typically initiated at a given safe, low-dose concentration of antigen. As already discussed, IDT, MQT, and modified RAST serve to identify the endpoint from which to initiate therapy. The patient undergoes (1) a buildup phase in which an increasing amount of antigen is introduced, and (2) a maintenance phase in which the most effective dose of antigen is provided over a regular interval for an extended period of time. During the buildup phase, patients typically require injections 1 to 2 weeks. Once a maintenance dose is reached, the time between injections is extended to 2 to 4 weeks.

Preparation of Antigen Treatment Vials

Not all positive antigen responses require inclusion in immunotherapy. Antigens should be considered based on patient history to ensure that they are significant contributors to a patient's overall care plan. The practitioner must be aware of antigen cross-reactivity. Antigens within a family relationship may have similar epitopes. Cross-reactivity explains the multiple responses within a given family of antigens. For example, a patient may have a class 5 response to June grass, with lesser levels of positive reactions to other grasses, such as timothy, which may not exist in the patient's environment. Recognition of cross-reactivity is important to successful allergy therapy, because cross-reacting antigens do not represent a true environmental allergy, and adding them to an immunotherapy regimen provides an unintended increase in the antigen presented during immunotherapy.

Mixing and Dosage Advancement

There has been little-to-no recent change in the methods used for vial preparation. An endpoint, identified by IDT, MQT, or in vitro determinations, defines the safe starting concentration for therapy.

Methods of dose advancement depend more upon patient factors than the format of testing used. So-called conventional schedules for inhalant allergens begin with an IDT dose of 0.05 to 0.1 mL. Following this, otolaryngic allergy dosage schedules often proceed on a weekly basis, with an increase of 0.05 to 1 mL each week. After reaching 0.5 mL, the concentration injected is now equivalent to 0.1 mL of the next-higher dilution (again using 1:5 as an example), and dosage escalation continues to the point of symptom relief, which becomes the maintenance dose.

Rush Immunotherapy

The biggest drawback to immunotherapy from a practical standpoint is the length of time required to complete a safe dose escalation. Faster advancement, called rush therapy, has been attempted at various times through the years. These protocols have been associated with an increased incidence of reactions. The tradeoff between slow advancement and increased side effects has been the subject of continued study. Rush immunotherapy studies the ability to provide therapy in a considerably decreased time period, such as 2 to 5 days.

Premedication before rush injection protocols decreased the incidence of severe reaction to less than 16%, with a per-injection reaction rate of 3 to 7%. It appears that rush therapy methods, even with aggressive premedication, will not achieve a safety profile acceptable to physicians and patients for generalized use with current antigen preparations.

Practical Use of Immunotherapy

Immunotherapy should be considered in the following scenarios:

1. Pharmacotherapy insufficiently controls symptoms or produces undesirable side effects.
2. Appropriate avoidance measures of indoor allergens fail to control symptoms.
3. There is a history of allergic rhinitis for at least two seasons (seasonal) or 6 months (perennial).
4. There are positive skin tests or serum-specific IgE that correlates with rhinitis symptoms.

The following conditions are considered relative contraindications and must be specifically evaluated before considering immunotherapy:

1. Concomitant therapy with a β-blocker
2. Contraindication to the administration of adrenaline (epinephrine)
3. Noncompliance by patient
4. Autoimmune disease
5. Induction but not maintenance therapy during pregnancy
6. Uncontrolled asthma
7. Human immunodeficiency virus status

When SCIT is indicated, the potential dangers, as well as the optimal duration of therapy, should be thoroughly discussed with the patient prior to initiation of therapy. SCIT should be prescribed by a specially trained physician practitioner and administered under the supervision of a physician trained to manage anaphylaxis. Adrenaline (epinephrine), corticosteroids, and equipment for respiratory resuscitation must be readily available.

Administration of Immunotherapy

Debate remains active (and definitive data are lacking) on the topic of where immunotherapy can be safely administered. In particular, the removal of a patient from an allergy specialist's office to the primary care provider raises issues of managed care, responsibility for outcomes, and overall safety. It is generally considered safe to transfer shot therapy to a primary care physician's office after the maintenance dosage shot level is reached, although some patients have been sent to well-trained primary care physicians after the first buildup vial is complete. Though home therapy is still under evaluation, it may be safe once antigen doses have reached stable maintenance levels under certain circumstances (i.e., an adult nonasthmatic patient).

Safety Concerns

To minimize risk and improve efficacy, it has been recommended that immunotherapy be prescribed by specially trained physician practitioners and administered under the supervision of physicians trained to manage systemic reactions, with the immediate availability of adrenaline (epinephrine) should anaphylaxis occur. In the United States, controversy continues on various topics. Administration of shots outside the medical office environment has provoked debate. Can immunotherapy be given at home during buildup, during maintenance, or not at all? Another concern relates to how long a patient must remain in the office for observation following an allergy injection. Twenty minutes has been suggested as an appropriate interval. Definitive data are lacking. Asthmatic patients also create a clinical dilemma. Although patients with allergic disease contributing to bronchospasm can benefit from immunotherapy by decreased asthmatic response to antigenic challenge, they have been noted to suffer a disproportionately greater number of severe reactions to the injection therapy.

Cessation of Therapy

It is unclear how long patients require immunotherapy to achieve maximum benefit, or if the positive immunomodulatory effects are conferred for life. Particular questions relate to whether immunotherapy should be modified or stopped at 1 year if no improvement is seen, and whether 5 years is a reasonable length of time to attain a maximal effect. With patients who attain substantial system relief with immunotherapy, it is reasonable to stop the therapy in the 3 to 5 year range to ascertain whether immunotherapy has conferred a long-lasting allergy tolerance, or whether at least shots must be continued indefinitely.

Sublingual Immunotherapy

Although commonly offered in Europe, SLIT is less commonly used in the United States as compared with SCIT, primarily because it is not covered by insurance companies. Typically, the liquid or tablet antigen(s) are applied to the underside of the tongue three or more times a week. The main difference between SCIT and SLIT is that the safety profile seems to be better with SLIT, and as a consequence it can be offered as a home treatment, although anaphylaxis has been reported in patients receiving SLIT. The most common side effect reported from patients is irritation at the site of allergen application.

■ Practice Guidelines, Consensus Statements, and Measures

There have been several practice guidelines that have been published on the management of allergic rhinitis, including one supported by the Standards of Care Committee of the British Society for Allergy and Clinical Immunology, the American Academy of Allergy, Asthma and Immunology, and the Global Allergy and Asthma European Network. The AAO-HNS Allergic Rhinitis Clinical Practice Guideline will be released in 2015.

■ Suggested Reading

Akdis CA, Blesken T, Akdis M, Wüthrich B, Blaser K. Role of interleukin 10 in specific immunotherapy. J Clin Invest 1998;102(1):98–106

ARIA (Allergic Rhinitis and Its Impact on Asthma). ARIA Guidelines. http://www.whiar.org/Documents&Resources.php

Benninger M, Farrar JR, Blaiss M, et al. Evaluating approved medications to treat allergic rhinitis in the United States: an evidence-based review of efficacy for nasal symptoms by class. Ann Allergy Asthma Immunol 2010;104(1):13–29

Blaiss M, Maloney J, Nolte H, Gawchik S, Yao R, Skoner DP. Efficacy and safety of timothy grass allergy immunotherapy tablets in North American children and adolescents. J Allergy Clin Immunol 2011;127(1):64–71, e1–e4

Brozek JL, Bousquet J, Baena-Cagnani CE, et al; Global Allergy and Asthma European Network; Grading of Recommendations Assessment, Development and Evaluation Working Group. Allergic Rhinitis and its Impact on Asthma (ARIA) guidelines: 2010 revision. J Allergy Clin Immunol 2010;126(3):466–476

Calderón M, Brandt T. Treatment of grass pollen allergy: focus on a standardized grass allergen extract—Grazax®. Ther Clin Risk Manag 2008;4(6):1255–1260

Cingi C, Gunhan K, Gage-White L, Unlu H. Efficacy of leukotriene antagonists as concomitant therapy in allergic rhinitis. Laryngoscope 2010;120(9):1718–1723

Durham SR; GT-08 investigators. Sustained effects of grass pollen AIT. Allergy 2011;66(Suppl 95):50–52

Esteitie R, deTineo M, Naclerio RM, Baroody FM. Effect of the addition of montelukast to fluticasone propionate for the treatment of perennial allergic rhinitis. Ann Allergy Asthma Immunol 2010;105(2):155–161

Frati F, Incorvaia C, Lombardi C, Senna G. Allergen immunotherapy: 100 years, but it does not look like. Eur Ann Allergy Clin Immunol 2012;44(3):99–106

Hirata H, Arima M, Yukawa T. Effect of rush immunotherapy (RIT) on cytokine production in hymenoptera allergy. Dokkyo J Med Sci. 2000;27(1):27–40

James LK, Shamji MH, Walker SM, et al. Long-term tolerance after allergen immunotherapy is accompanied by selective persistence of blocking antibodies. J Allergy Clin Immunol 2011;127(2):509–516, e1–e5

Kesavanathan J, Swift DL, Fitzgerald TK, Permutt T, Bascom R. Evaluation of acoustic rhinometry and posterior rhinomanometry as tools for inhalation challenge studies. J Toxicol Environ Health 1996;48(3):295–307

King HC. An Otolaryngologist's Guide to Allergy. New York, NY: Thieme; 1990:27:145

Krouse HJ. Diagnostic testing for inhalant allergies. ORL Head Neck Nurs 2007;25(2):9–14

Nelson HS, Nolte H, Creticos P, Maloney J, Wu J, Bernstein DI. Efficacy and safety of timothy grass allergy immunotherapy tablet treatment in North American adults. J Allergy Clin Immunol 2011;127(1):72–80, e1–e2

Ratner PH, Hampel F, Van Bavel J, et al. Combination therapy with azelastine hydrochloride nasal spray and fluticasone propionate nasal spray in the treatment of patients with seasonal allergic rhinitis. Ann Allergy Asthma Immunol 2008;100(1):74–81

Scadding GK, Durham SR, Mirakian R, et al; British Society for Allergy and Clinical Immunology. BSACI guidelines for the management of allergic and non-allergic rhinitis. Clin Exp Allergy 2008; 38(1):19–42

Wallace DV, Dykewicz MS, Bernstein DI, et al; Joint Task Force on Practice; American Academy of Allergy; Asthma & Immunology; American College of Allergy; Asthma and Immunology; Joint Council of Allergy, Asthma and Immunology. The diagnosis and management of rhinitis: an updated practice parameter. J Allergy Clin Immunol 2008;122(2, Suppl):S1–S84

83 Lateral Nasal Wall and Sinus Surgical Anatomy: Contemporary Understanding

■ Introduction

Sinus surgery evolved into the modern era due to the pioneering work of Messerklinger, who described paranasal sinus anatomy and physiology in his seminal publication in 1978. This work highlighted the role of the ostiomeatal complex in the pathophysiology of chronic sinusitis. New focus was directed to the study of sinonasal anatomy after 1985, when Kennedy introduced the technique of functional endoscopic sinus surgery (ESS) to the United States.

The endoscope affords visualization of the nasal and sinus anatomy in great detail and magnification. Identification of sinonasal anatomical landmarks and recognition of variations are imperative in conducting safe and efficient ESS, and limiting complications. This chapter offers a concise review of the relevant anatomy of the lateral nasal wall and the paranasal sinuses. Standardized nomenclature based on the recommendations of the Anatomic Terminology Group at the International Conference on Sinus Disease is used in this chapter. Older terms will be discussed for the sake of clarity. Uniform and accurate use of anatomical terms is important in communicating clinical problems, surgical procedures, outcomes, and new ideas.

■ Basic Embryology

The adult nose has three or four turbinates: inferior, middle, superior, and occasionally supreme. Each has an attachment to the lateral nasal wall. Lateral to each of the turbinates is an associated space or "meatus" named after it. The frontal, maxillary, and anterior ethmoid sinuses drain into the middle meatus; the posterior ethmoids drain into the superior meatus; and the sphenoid sinus drains into the sphenoethmoid recess. The nasolacrimal duct opens into the inferior meatus.

The inferior turbinate is derived from the maxilloturbinal, whereas the middle, superior, and supreme turbinates develop from the ethmoturbinals. The ethmoturbinals develop from the ethmoid bone and therefore have a vertical attachment to the ethmoid skull base. Each ethmoturbinal has an ascending part (pars ascendens), which is more anterior and vertical, and a descending part (pars descendens), which is more horizontal and posterior. There are as many as five to seven of these ethmoturbinals and intervening grooves or furrows on the embryological lateral nasal wall (**Fig. 83.1**).

The ascending portion of the first ethmoturbinal (AP 1st ET) becomes the agger nasi region. The descending portion (DP 1st ET) becomes the uncinate process. The first furrow or groove becomes the ethmoid infundibulum. The AP 2nd ET, when it persists, becomes the ethmoid bulla lamella attached to the skull base at the location of the anterior ethmoid artery. The DP 2nd ET becomes the ethmoid bulla itself. When the bulla lamella is absent or does not attach to the skull base, a space is present over the ethmoid bulla, named the suprabullar recess. The frontal recess then communicates with the suprabullar recess.

The second furrow or groove, when it persists, becomes the retrobullar recess (RBR). The ethmoid bulla is then separated from the middle turbinate basal lamella (**Figs. 83.2** and **83.3**). This space was previously known as the sinus lateralis. The two-dimensional opening into this space is the semilunar hiatus posteriores, which sometimes communicates with the ethmoid infundibulum over the top of the bulla. If the bulla lamella does not persist, the retrobullar recess communicates over the bulla via the suprabullar recess with the ethmoid infundibulum.

The third ET becomes the middle turbinate. The AP 3rd ET contributes the vertical attachment to the skull base and the vertical portion of the basal lamella. The DP 3rd ET becomes the body of the middle turbinate and the horizontal basal lamella attachment to the lamina papyracea.

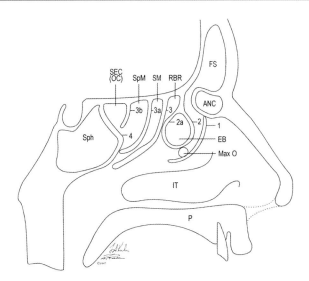

Fig. 83.1 Left lateral nasal wall with middle, superior, and supreme turbinates removed; uncinate process removed; and ethmoid bulla and agger nasi cell uncapped. 1, uncinate process attachment (1st embryological ethmoturbinal [EET]); 2, face of ethmoid bulla (2nd EET); 2a, posterior wall, ethmoid bulla (2nd EET); 3, middle turbinate basal lamella (3rd EET); 3a, superior turbinate basal lamella (4th EET); 3b, supreme turbinate basal lamella (5th EET); 4, sphenoid face; FS, frontal sinus (2nd embryological frontal furrow); ANC, agger nasi cell (1st embryologic frontal furrow); EB, ethmoid bulla; Max O, maxillary sinus ostium; IT, inferior turbinate; P, palate; RBR, retrobullar recess; SM, superior meatus; SpM, supreme meatus; SEC (OC), sphenoethmoid cell (Onodi cell); Sph, sphenoid sinus.

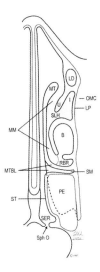

Fig. 83.3 Half axial view of the sinuses above the level of the maxillary sinus ostium. LD, Nasolacrimal duct; OMC, Ostiomeatal complex (*shaded area*); LP, Lamina papyracea; I, ethmoid infundibulum; U, uncinate process; MT, middle turbinate; SLH, semilunar hiatus; MM, middle meatus; B, ethmoid bulla; RBR, retrobullar recess; SM, superior meatus; MTBL, middle turbinate basal lamella; PE, posterior ethmoids; ST, superior turbinate; SER, sphenoethmoidal recess; Sph O, sphenoid ostium.

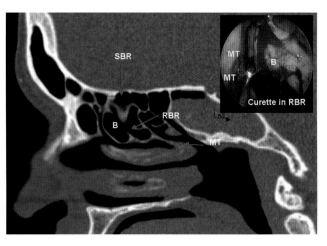

Fig. 83.2 Parasagittal computed tomography demonstrating the suprabullar recess (SBR), a space between the ethmoid bulla (B) and the skull base when the bulla or bulla lamella does not reach the skull base. The retrobullar recess (RBR) is the space behind the bulla separating it from the oblique basal lamella of the middle turbinate (MT). Inset: Endoscopic view of the left middle meatus with a curette in the left RBR.

The fourth ET becomes the superior turbinate and the fifth ET the supreme turbinate, when present.

These lamella can be used to establish landmarks (constant and variable; **Table 83.1**) during ESS to execute surgery safely (**Table 83.2**).

■ Key Anatomical Structures and Concepts

Ostiomeatal Complex (OMC)

The ostiomeatal complex (OMC) is a functional concept, rather than an anatomical structure with defined boundaries. It represents the final common pathway for drainage and ventilation of the ethmoid, maxillary, and frontal sinuses. Though the OMC's exact boundaries are not defined, it is bound by the medial orbital wall and the middle turbinate. The OMC comprises the uncinate process, ethmoid infundibulum, semilunar hiatus, and anterior ethmoid cells, and the ostia of the anterior ethmoid, maxillary, and frontal sinuses (**Figs. 83.3, 83.4, 83.5**). The goal of naming this area was to call attention to the concept that inflammation in the OMC can lead to anatomical and functional obstruction of the anterior sinuses. Medical and surgical strategies are devised to eliminate OMC obstruction and restore function.

Table 83.1   Lamella identification for endoscopic sinus surgery: constant and variable parallel landmarks

A. Four constant parallel landmarks

   1. Uncinate process

   2. Face of ethmoid bulla

   3. Middle turbinate basal lamella

   4. Sphenoid face

B. Three variable parallel landmarks

   1. Posterior bulla wall

   2. Superior turbinate basal lamella

   3. Supreme turbinate basal lamella

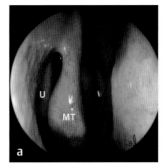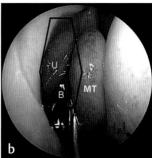

Right Nasal Cavity

Fig. 83.4   The ostiomeatal complex (OMC) is a functional concept, and its anatomical boundaries are not strictly defined but lie in the middle meatus. (**a**) View of the right nasal cavity with the middle turbinate (MT) and the uncinated process (U); the OMC lies in relation to these structures. (**b**) A close-up view of the same area with the MT pushed medially shows the bulla (B) in addition. The OMC is bound by the medial orbital wall and the middle turbinate (enclosed space). It contains the uncinate process (U), bulla (B), ethmoid infundibulum, semilunar hiatus, and ostia of the anterior ethmoid, maxillary, and frontal sinuses.

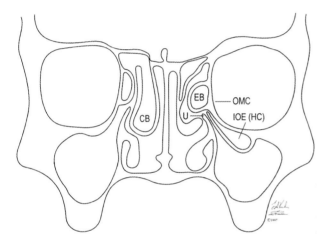

Fig. 83.5   Coronal view of the sinuses and orbits. CB, concha bullosa, right middle turbinate; U, uncinate process; EB, ethmoid bulla; IOE (HC), infraorbital ethmoid cell (Haller cell); OMC, ostiomeatal complex (shaded area).

Table 83.2   The steps in endoscopic ethmoidectomy

Step 1: Remove uncinate process (1st parallel lamella). This step is almost always incomplete, because the inferior-posterior uncinate remnant usually persists, lying over the maxillary sinus ostium, and requires special attention.

Step 2: Remove inferior uncinate remnant, visually identify and clear maxillary sinus ostium. This step requires the use of 30-, 45-, or 70-degree scopes.

Step 3: Remove ethmoid bulla face (second constant parallel lamella) and posterior wall (see **Fig. 83.1**, anatomical reference 2) if separate from middle turbinate basal lamella.

Step 4: Identify posteroinferior horizontal part of the middle turbinate basal lamella (third constant parallel lamella), come up 1.5 to 2 cm, and penetrate into the posterior ethmoid sinus.

Step 5: *Stay low.* Penetrate the superior and supreme turbinate basal lamellae (**Fig. 83.1**, anatomical references 3a and 3b), and clear until reaching the lamina papyracea.

Step 6: Identify the sphenoid face (fourth constant parallel lamella).

Step 7: Identify the posterior skull base; follow the sphenoid face up to the skull base, identifying the sphenoethmoid/Onodi cell if present (the most superoposterior ethmoid cell).

Step 8: Clean the skull base from posterior to anterior.

Step 9: (Optional) Perform sphenoidotomy through the medial inferior triangle of the posterior ethmoid box (**Fig. 83.24**).

Step 10: (Optional) Identify the frontal recesses, perform frontal sinusotomy.

Step 11: (Optional) Scarify the medial middle turbinate surface and septum, pack or suture the middle turbinate to the septum for floppy, unstable middle turbinate (Bolger maneuver).

Step 12: (Optional) Place a middle meatal spacer.

Middle Turbinate (MT)

The middle turbinate (MT) is a boomerang-shaped structure (**Figs. 83.6** and **83.7**) that can be conveniently thought of in four parts (**Fig. 83.8**): (1) the anterior turbinate buttress, where it attaches to the agger nasi region; (2) the vertical attachment to the skull base and cribriform (**Fig. 83.9**), lying in the sagittal plane; (3) an oblique orientation in the coronal/ frontal plane that attaches to the medial orbital wall (**Fig. 83.10**); and (4) the posterior buttress, lying in an axial plane (**Fig. 83.11**). This most posterior part attaches to the lateral nasal wall at the lamina papyracea, maxilla, and perpendicular process of the palatine bone. The MT basal lamella is the entire MT attachment to the lateral nasal wall (**Figs. 83.7, 83.8, 83.9, 83.10, 83.11**). It extends from the posterior MT attachment all the way up to the skull base.

The basal lamella is the only part of the MT that can be sacrificed without compromising the integrity of the turbinate. If the anterior buttress and vertical attachment are fractured, the MT will lateralize and scar down the middle meatus. If too much horizontal basal lamella is removed and the posterior buttress is damaged, the posterior MT will lateralize and make access to the posterior ethmoids impossible.

Ethmoid Roof

The ethmoid roof consists of two bones: laterally, the thicker orbital plate of the frontal bone, which covers most of the ethmoid sinus; and medially, the thin lateral cribriform plate lamella (LCPL) (**Fig. 83.12**). The orbital plate's inferior surface has pits or depressions

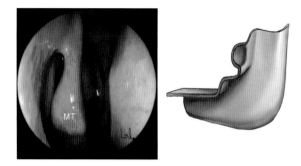

Endoscopic view from anterior aspect　　Schematic view from lateral aspect

Fig. 83.6 Middle turbinate: endoscopic view of right middle turbinate (image panel on left) and a schematic representation (image panel on right).

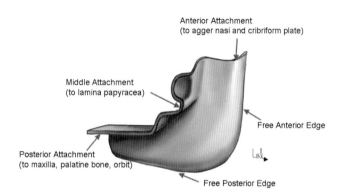

Fig. 83.7 Schematic view of the right middle turbinate as viewed from the lateral aspect. The three areas of attachments of the middle turbinate are depicted. The anterior attachment to the agger nasi and cribriform lies in a vertical, parasagittal plane; the middle attachment to the lamina papyracea lies in an oblique, coronal plane, and the posterior attachment to the maxilla, palatine bone, and orbit lies in a horizontal, axial plane. The free anterior and posterior edges of the middle turbinate can be easily visualized on nasal endoscopy.

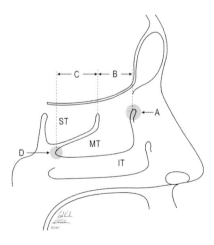

Fig. 83.8 Middle turbinate divisions. A, anterior middle turbinate attachment or buttress; B, vertical middle turbinate attachment to skull base; C, middle turbinate basal lamella; D, posterior middle turbinate buttress; ST, superior turbinate; MT, middle turbinate; IT, inferior turbinate.

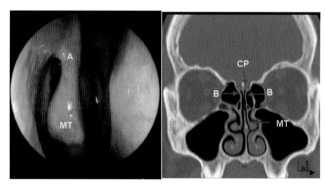

Fig. 83.9 The anterior attachment (B) of the middle turbinate (MT) is first at the agger nasi (A) and then at the junction of the lateral lamella and medial part of the cribriform plate (CP). These attachments are oriented in the sagittal plane. These figures show the endoscopic view (left panel) and radiographic correlate on computed tomographic scan (panel on right).

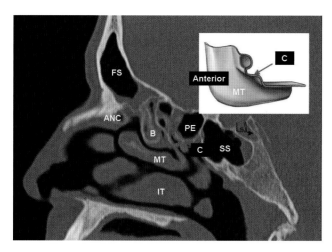

Fig. 83.10 Middle turbinate (MT) basal lamella. The midpart of the middle turbinate (C) attaches to the lamina papyracea via the basal lamella. The inset, schematic panel of the middle turbinate is now being correlated with the magnified computed tomographic (CT) scan correlate. The CT image selected is in the parasagittal plane to show the middle attachment of the middle turbinate (C, as also seen in the schematic inset). This middle part of the basal lamella (C) is oriented obliquely in the coronal plane. This basal lamella separates the anterior ethmoid (B) from the posterior ethmoid (PE) cells. FS, frontal sinus; ANC, agger nasi cell; SS, sphenoid sinus; IT, inferior turbinate. Inset: schematic view of the left middle turbinate from the lateral aspect.

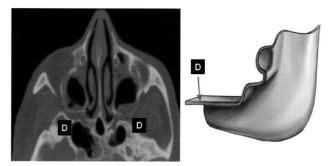

Fig. 83.11 The posterior attachment of the middle turbinate (D) is horizontal, oriented in the axial plane. The computed tomographic (CT) scan (left image panel) and the schematic view of the middle turbinate (image panel on the right) are being correlated. The CT image selected is in the axial plane to show the horizontal, posterior attachment of the middle turbinate, which attaches (anterior to posterior) to the lamina papyracea, medial wall of the maxilla, and perpendicular process of the palatine bone. In these figures, D shows the most posterior attachment of the basal lamella to the medial maxilla and the palatine bone. It is important not to destabilize this attachment to prevent lateralization and synechia formation in the posterior ethmoids.

caused by pneumatization from the ethmoid cells it covers. Each of these pits or depressions is a fovea ethmoidalis, so there are many foveae. Hence, the term *fovea ethmoidalis* is a misnomer for the ethmoid roof; it should simply be called the ethmoid roof, recognizing that two different bones contribute to it.

The LCPL extends vertically from the MT attachment to the cribriform plate forming the medial ethmoid roof, and may be only 0.1 to 0.2 mm thick. It forms the lateral wall of the olfactory groove, which has been classified into three configurations by Keros: shallow (**Fig. 83.13a**), medium (**Fig. 83.13b**), and deep (**Fig. 83.13c**). A patient with a Keros type III olfactory groove (**Fig. 83.13c**) is at higher risk for penetration of the medial ethmoid roof. If the orbital plate is thin and the LCPL is more horizontal (**Fig. 83.13d**), the thin ethmoid roof may appear to be another ethmoid cell and may provide very little resistance to penetration. The cribriform area can also be asymmetric.

A recent study uses the ratio of posterior ethmoid cell height compared with the maxillary sinus height for assessing the posterior ethmoid skull base. If the maxillary sinus is high, the posterior ethmoid is lower and suggests a lower-lying skull base. During an endoscopic ethmoidectomy, one should dissect low through the ethmoids until the sphenoid face

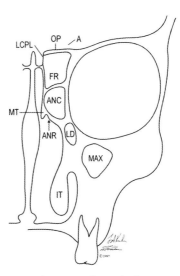

Fig. 83.12 Coronal section through the anterior portion of the maxillary sinus and frontal recess. A, area of ethmoid roof; OP, orbital plate of frontal bone; LCPL, lateral cribriform plate lamella; FR, frontal recess; ANC, agger nasi cell; ANR, agger nasi region; MT, most anterior portion of the middle turbinate; LD, lacrimal duct; MAX, maxillary sinus; IT, inferior turbinate.

is identified, then follow it up to identify the skull base posteriorly. The ethmoid partitions are then removed from the skull base in a posterior to anterior direction. This allows bony lamella removal by pulling forward away from the skull base, rather than pushing back into it. Particular attention should be paid to the position of the anterior and posterior eth-

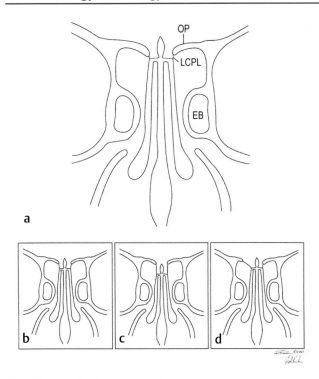

Fig. 83.13 Configurations of the ethmoid roof and the lateral cribriform plate lamella. (**a**) Keros type I olfactory groove/lateral cribriform plate lamella. (**b**) Keros type II. (**c**) Keros type III. (**d**) Asymmetrical ethmoid roof with right lateral cribriform plate lamella, very thin and long at an oblique angle, including much of the right ethmoid roof. OP, orbital plate, frontal bone; LCPL, lateral cribriform plate lamella; EB, ethmoid bulla.

moid arteries, because they traverse the skull base from the orbit toward the nasal septum. Sometimes these arteries may be exposed or may lie pedicled in a partition within the ethmoid space (**Fig. 83.14**); their injury could result in bleeding in the orbit or intracranially.

Uncinate Process, Ethmoid Infundibulum, and Semilunar Hiatus

The uncinate process is the first structure encountered in the middle meatus when the MT is medialized. It is a sickle-shaped bone with fibrous and bony attachments along the lateral nasal wall. It lies in the sagittal plane forming the medial wall of the ethmoid infundibulum. The ethmoid infundibulum is a funnel-shaped three-dimensional space between the uncinate process and the lamina papyracea (**Fig. 83.15**). The maxillary sinus opens into the inferior aspect of the ethmoid infundibulum at a 45 degree angle (**Fig. 83.16**). The semilunar hiatus is a two-dimensional slit that lies between the free edge of the uncinate process and the ethmoid bulla. It is a cleft that connects the middle meatus into the infundibulum laterally (**Figs. 83.3** and **83.15**).

Depending on the anterosuperior attachment of the uncinate process, the frontal sinus may open into the superior part of the infundibulum. When the uncinate attaches to the skull base or MT, the frontal sinus drains into the infundibulum (**Fig. 83.17**, see labels B and C). However, more commonly, the uncinate process attaches laterally to the orbit below the internal frontal ostium (**Fig. 83.17**, see label A), forming a terminal recess (recessus terminalis). In this case, the frontal sinus drains medial to the uncinate into the middle meatus, and not into the infundibulum. The uncinate process must be removed to gain access to the anterior ethmoid sinuses, the maxillary sinus, and the frontal recess. Its posteroinferior portion overlies the maxillary sinus ostium and must be removed to identify the natural maxillary ostium.

Fontanelles and Accessory Ostia

The lateral nasal wall has two areas where bone is absent underneath the mucosa, called fontanelles. One fontanelle is anterior to the uncinate bone, and

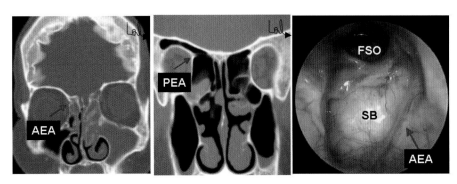

Fig. 83.14 The location of the ethmoid arteries must be determined prior to skull base (SB) dissection. On a computed tomographic (CT) scan, these arteries appear as conical projections from the orbit. The arteries may sometimes lie within the ethmoid space, pedicled (outside the skull base). The anterior ethmoid artery (AEA) is located in the skull base posterior to the frontal sinus ostium (FSO) in the ethmoid SB, and is labeled in the first CT image panel. The posterior ethmoid artery (PEA) is located just anterior to the sphenoid, in the larger-appearing posterior ethmoid cells, and is labeled in the second CT image panel. The endoscopic image panel shows a 70-degree endoscope view of the AEA in the ethmoid SB.

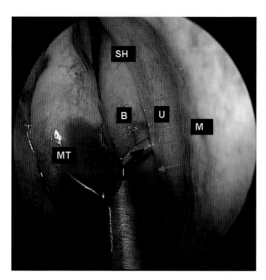

Fig. 83.15 The uncinate process (U) is a crescent-shaped bone attaching anteriorly to the maxillary bone (M) adjacent to the nasolacrimal duct. It runs in the sagittal plane, and its posterior free margin parallels the ethmoid bulla (B). The semilunar hiatus (SH, *red arrows*) is a two-dimensional cleft between the free edge of the uncinate process and the ethmoid bulla. It is the gap through which the nasal cavity communicates with the ethmoid infundibulum (I). The infundibulum (I, *solid black arrow*) is a three-dimensional space between the uncinate process and the lamina papyracea. This endoscopic figure shows the maxillary ball probe being passed through the cleft of the SH into the infundibulum, with the probe tip within that three-dimensional space.

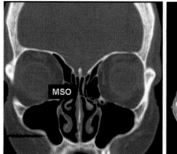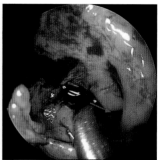

Fig. 83.16 Maxillary sinus ostium (*red arrows*) is located posteroinferiorly in the infundibulum. This is visualized on a coronal computed tomographic (CT) image (image panel on left) as opening at a 45-degree angle into the ethmoid infundibulum. Therefore, for best visualization endoscopically, the uncinate process must be resected, and an angled endoscope (30 or 45 degree) looking at 5 o'clock (for the left maxillary sinus ostium) and 7 o'clock for the right maxillary sinus should be used. The endoscopic image panel on the right shows the left maxillary sinus ostium being identified (*arrow*) in the posteroinferior part of the infundibulum after uncinectomy; a 30-degree endoscope looking sideways at about the 5 o'clock position is being used.

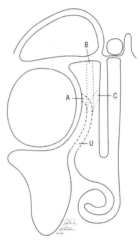

Fig. 83.17 The three possible attachments of the uncinate process (U). A, to the medial orbital wall; B, to the anterior skull base; C, to the middle turbinate. In the case of A, the frontal recess drains into the middle meatus. In the case of B, the frontal sinus generally drains to the middle meatus. In the case of C, the frontal sinus drains into the ethmoid infundibulum.

the other is posterior. Any accessory ostia that may be present in these fontanelles (**Fig. 83.18**) must be distinguished from the natural maxillary sinus ostium on computed tomography (CT) and on endoscopy. Since the maxillary sinus mucus flow is always toward the natural maxillary ostium, a posterior fontanelle accessory ostium or antrostomy is not functional. If the natural ostium has some patency, mucus flows out of it and may drop back into the maxillary sinus through the posterior ostium/antrostomy, creating recirculation. A maxillary antrostomy that has incorporated the natural ostium has a pearlike appearance (**Fig. 83.19**).

Anterior and Posterior Ethmoids

The MT basal lamella is the boundary between the anterior and posterior ethmoid cells. Any cell opening into the middle meatus is considered an anterior ethmoid cell. Any cell opening into the superior meatus is a posterior ethmoid cell. *There are no middle ethmoid cells.*

Previously called the Haller cell, the infraorbital ethmoid cell is an anterior ethmoid cell that pneuma-

tizes into the orbital floor above the maxillary sinus ostium (**Figs. 83.5** and **83.20**) and may compromise its patency. When this cell's common wall with the maxillary sinus ostium is not adequately resected, edema may develop, obstructing the maxillary sinus ostium. The lateral wall of the infraorbital ethmoid cell may be attached to the infraorbital nerve canal.

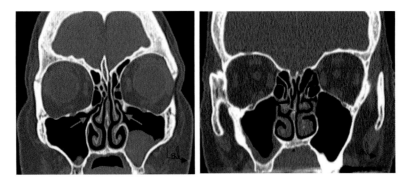

Fig. 83.18 The accessory maxillary ostium is located in the posterior fontanelle, as opposed to the natural ostium located in the posteroinferior part of the infundibulum. The computed tomographic (CT) image panel on the left shows the natural maxillary sinus ostium (*red arrows*) to be located between the orbit laterally and the uncinated process medially in the inferior part of the infundibulum. The CT image panel on the right shows an accessory ostium of the left maxillary sinus (*arrow*) to be located in the posterior fontanelle. We do not see the uncinate process in this coronal view; instead, the posterior ethmoid complex and the superior turbinate start coming into view in this more posterior location.

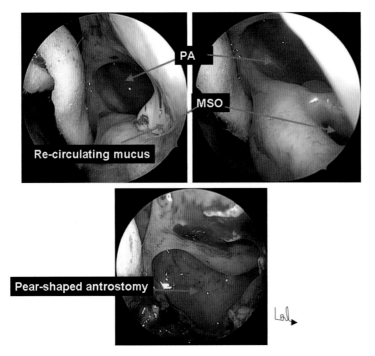

Fig. 83.19 An antrostomy in the posterior fontanelle (PA) is not helpful, as the maxillary sinus mucociliary clearance continues toward the natural maxillary sinus ostium (MSO). Mucus recirculates back into the maxillary sinus via the posteriorly placed surgical antrostomy as shown in the top, left, and right images. Once the tissue between the two openings is removed to prevent recirculation and incorporate the natural ostium, the desired pear shape of the maxillary antrostomy can be verified with a 45-degree endoscope (bottom image).

Superior Turbinate, Superior Meatus

The superior turbinate is separated from the MT by the superior meatus, into which the posterior ethmoid cells drain (**Fig. 83.21**). The basal lamella of the superior turbinate lies *behind* and *not above* the basal lamella of the MT. This is an important concept, because confusion is caused by parasagittal sections of the lateral nasal wall, where the *attachment* of the superior turbinate is seen above the MT attachment. The space lateral to the superior turbinate is the superior meatus and drains the posterior ethmoids. The superior turbinate serves as an important medial landmark for completion of posterior ethmoidectomy (**Fig. 83.22**).

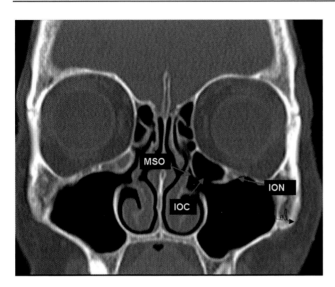

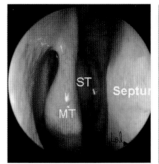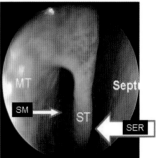

Fig. 83.20   An infraorbital ethmoid cell (IOE), or Haller cell, narrows the ethmoid infundibulum and maxillary sinus ostium (MSO). It may attach laterally to the infraorbital canal (ION).

Fig. 83.21   Endoscopic views of the right superior turbinate (ST) and superior meatus (SM). The panel on the right shows a close-up view of the panel on the left, by showing a more magnified view of the area between the right middle turbinate and the nasal septum. Anteriorly, the ST shares the skull base attachment with the middle turbinate (MT). The ST runs in a sagittal plane like the MT. Inferiorly, the ST forms the lateral wall of the sphenoethmoidal recess (SER, *blue arrow*). The SM (*orange arrow*) is therefore posterior and medial to the medial half of the middle portion of the basal lamella of the MT.

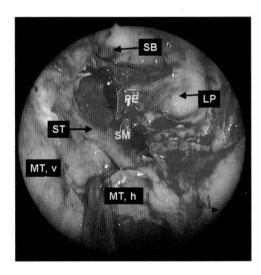

Fig. 83.22   The left superior meatus (SM) has been exposed by dissecting through the oblique basal lamella of the middle turbinate (suction tip). The boundaries of the posterior ethmoidectomy are the superior turbinate medially, lamina papyracea laterally, skull base superiorly, and horizontal attachment of the middle turbinate inferiorly. MT, v, middle turbinate, vertical part; MT, h, middle turbinate horizontal part; ST, superior turbinate; SB, skull base; LP, lamina papyracea; PE, posterior ethmoid cells.

Sphenoethmoid Recess

As the superior turbinate attaches to the sphenoid face, it bends laterally. This creates a narrow vertical space between the superior turbinate and septum, called the sphenoethmoidal recess. The sphenoid ostium (**Figs. 83.3** and **83.23**) opens into the sphenoethmoidal recess.

Posterior Ethmoid and Sphenoid: The Parallelogram Box

The medial orbital wall is roughly parallel to the superior turbinate, which attaches to the sphenoid face. The posterior ethmoid roof is parallel to the posterior ethmoid floor (the superior turbinate basal lamella). These four structures form a parallelogram-shaped box bounded posteriorly by the sphenoid face (**Fig. 83.24**). If a diagonal is drawn from the superior medial corner down to the lateral inferior corner, it delineates the triangular-shaped medial inferior portion of the sphenoid face. This is the safe area on the sphenoid face to penetrate from the posterior ethmoid into the sphenoid, because the optic nerve and internal carotid artery are normally located behind the superior-lateral triangle of the sphenoid face. **Table 83.3** summarizes the basic steps in ethmoidectomy.

Sphenoid Sinus: Septa, Internal Carotid, Optic Nerve

The sphenoid sinus lies medial and inferior to the last posterior ethmoid cell. The optic nerve and internal carotid artery are related to the lateral sphenoid wall, with the optic nerve above and internal carotid artery below. The sphenoid sinuses are separated by one or more intersinus septations. These septa may commonly insert on the bony canal of the internal carotid artery, which also sometimes may be dehiscent. When removing these septa, care should be exercised to bite the bone and not twist it (**Fig. 83.25**).

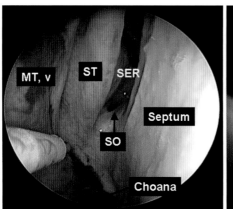
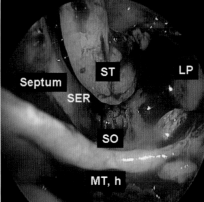

Right Sphenoid ostium, transnasal view   **Left Sphenoid ostium, transethmoid view**

Fig. 83.23   The sphenoid ostium (SO) drains into the sphenoethmoid recess (SER), medial to inferior third of the superior turbinate. The image panel on the left side shows a transnasal view of the right SO and SER, which has been obtained by looking medial to the middle and superior turbinates. The image panel on the right shows a transethmoid view of the left ST, SO, and SER, which has been obtained after removing the oblique part of the middle turbinate; note that the horizontal attachment of the middle turbinate (MTh) has been left intact. The SO is usually located at the junction of the upper third and lower two-thirds on the sphenoid face, ~ 1.5 cm superior to the choana. MT, v, middle turbinate, vertical part; MT, h, middle turbinate, horizontal part; ST, superior turbinate; LP, lamina papyracea.

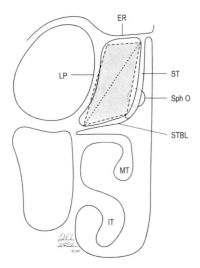

Fig. 83.24   Right posterior coronal section demonstrating the posterior ethmoids and the "box" of Bolger. ER, ethmoid roof; LP, lamina papyracea; ST, superior turbinate; Sph O, sphenoid ostium; STBL, superior turbinate basal lamella; MT, middle turbinate; IT, inferior turbinate. The shaded area is the parallelogram roughly approximating the shape of the posterior ethmoids with the diagonal extending from superior medial to lateral inferior indicating the safe zone of penetration through the medial inferior triangle into the sphenoid sinus.

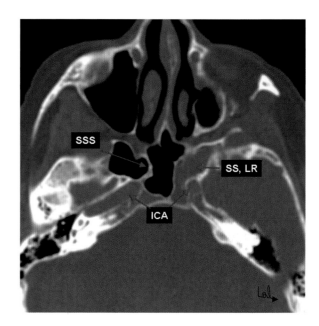

Fig. 83.25   The sphenoid sinus (SS) has variable pneumatization and septations (SSS). Extensive lateral pneumatization creates a lateral recess (LR). The intersinus septae (SSS) divide the SS asymmetrically and commonly attach to the bony canal of the internal carotid artery (ICA).

Table 83.3 Some known frontal recess cells

Agger nasi cell
Frontal cells
Frontoethmoid cells: types I, II, III, and IV
Supraorbital ethmoid cell
Interfrontal sinus septal cell
Frontal bulla cell
Suprabullar cell

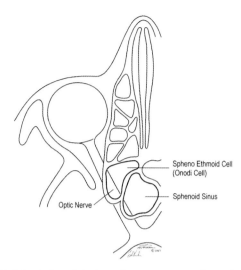

Fig. 83.26 Left axial view demonstrating the sphenoethmoid cell's impingement on the optic nerve and the optic nerve's potential path through both the sphenoethmoid cell and the sphenoid sinus.

Sphenoethmoid Cell

The last most posterosuperior ethmoid cell can sometimes pneumatize above, lateral, and posterior to the sphenoid face (**Figs. 83.26** and **83.27**). Previously known as an Onodi cell, this is currently called the sphenoethmoid cell. In this instance, the sphenoid sinus lies in a more inferior and medial relation to the posterior ethmoid. The optic nerve may lie in relation to or in the sphenoethmoid cell (**Fig. 83.26**). This relation of the optic nerve to the sphenoethmoid cell is reported to occur in as many as 50% of Asian specimens.

Frontal Sinus/Frontal Recess

Knowledge of frontal sinus embryology is helpful in understanding its adult anatomy. Schaffer and Kasper described four embryological frontal pits or furrows on the lateral frontal recess wall above the developing uncinate and bulla. The first frontal pit or furrow develops into the agger nasi cell, the second pneumatizes into the frontal bone to become the frontal sinus, the third often becomes the supraorbital ethmoid cell, and the fourth often becomes other anterior ethmoid cells. The frontal sinus is originally an anterior ethmoid cell. The connection between the frontal sinus and anterior ethmoids is not a tube or duct, but an inverted funnel-shaped space or recess whose narrow upper opening is the internal frontal ostium (**Figs. 83.28** and **83.29**).

The posterior frontal recess wall is the skull base. The anterior wall extends from the internal frontal ostium down to the MT's anterior attachment (**Fig. 83.28**). This recess is frequently filled with various anterior ethmoid cells called frontal recess cells, which consequently narrow the frontal sinus drainage pathway. Many times, the frontal recess is only a potential space. The narrow, convoluted drainage pathway out of the frontal sinus may easily be subject to obstruction by relatively minor swelling.

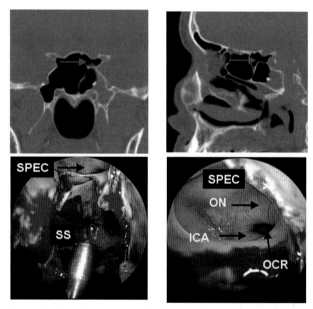

Fig. 83.27 The sphenoethmoid cell or Onodi cell (SPEC/OC) is a posterior ethmoid cell that is lateral and superior to the sphenoid sinus (SS). In this situation, the sphenoid sinus is usually smaller, pushed medially and inferiorly. It is important to recognize the SPEC to avoid optic nerve (ON) or internal carotid artery (ICA) injury. These four figure panels show how the SEC appears on coronal and sagittal views on the computed tomographic (CT) scan (top two figures, respectively). The figures show red arrows pointing to a left SPEC on coronal and sagittal CT cuts. Endoscopic views of the SEC are shown in the endoscopic images (bottom two). The endoscopic image on the left demonstrates the relationship of the SPEC to the SS. The endoscopic view on the right is a closeup of the SPEC showing the ON, ICA, and opticocarotid recess (OCR) on the lateral wall.

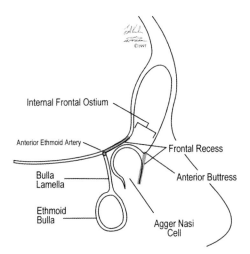

Fig. 83.28 Left lateral nasal wall demonstrating frontal recess and internal frontal ostium. The frontal recess begins at the internal frontal ostium, extending posteriorly along the skull base to the region of the anterior ethmoid artery and down the anterior wall to the most anterior attachment of the middle turbinate. The frontal recess in this case is occupied by an agger nasi cell impinging on the ethmoid bulla lamella.

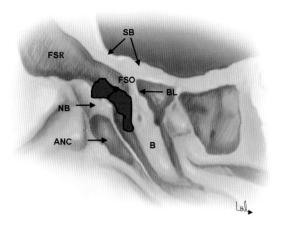

Fig. 83.29 The frontal sinus recess (FSR) is an hourglass-shaped space (purple shaded area) with the waist at the frontal sinus ostium (FSO), which is its narrowest part. In the simplest configuration, the boundaries of the frontal recess are limited by the agger nasi cell (ANC) and nasal beak (NB) anteriorly, the bulla ethmoidalis (B) and the bulla lamella (BL) posteriorly, the anterior skull base (SB) posterosuperiorly, the cribriform plate and middle turbinate medially, and the lamina papyracea laterally.

Table 83.3 presents a partial listing of the known frontal recess cells. The three most important are the agger nasi cell, the four types of frontal cells, and the supraorbital ethmoid cell (**Fig. 83.30**). These cells, the interfrontal sinus septal cell, and the uncinate attachments cause most of the different frontal sinus problems. The frontal recess anatomy must be studied in axial, coronal, and parasagittal views to construct a mental three-dimensional impression of the frontal sinus drainage pathway.

Messerklinger described frontal sinus muco-ciliary flow in 1955. Mucus flows up the intersinus septum across the frontal sinus roof laterally, then medially along the floor to the frontal sinus ostium, and down into the frontal recess. An estimated 40 to 60% of this mucus flows back up the medial frontal recess wall to the intersinus septum and then recirculates up the intersinus septum to the roof.

Agger Nasi Cell

The agger nasi cell is the most anterior of all ethmoid cells and the most constant, occurring in 98.5% of CT scans. The agger nasi cell is key in frontal sinus surgery. It may pneumatize so far superiorly into the frontal sinus as to be mistaken for the sinus itself when viewed endoscopically from below. A common

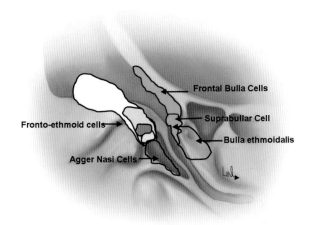

Fig. 83.30 The Kuhn classification divides frontal recess cells into an anterior group (the agger nasi cell [ANC] and fronto-ethmoidal cells), and posterior group (suprabullar, frontal bulla cell, and supraorbital cells) and interfrontal sinus septal cells. Frontoethmoidal cells are anterior ethmoidal cells associated with the frontal process of the maxilla (the "nasal beak"). These cells are distinct from those associated with the bulla ethmoidalis, the suprabulla cells. If a suprabulla cell migrates along the skull base into the frontal sinus, it is termed a frontal bulla cell. Finally, the cell associated with the intersinus septum of the frontal sinus is termed the intersinus septal cell.

mistake is to remove the floor and posterior cell wall, leaving the cap or dome of the cell lying against the posterior frontal recess wall, or a partially resected ethmoid bulla lamella leading to iatrogenic frontal sinus obstruction.

Frontal Cells

Frontal cells occur above the agger nasi cell and pneumatize into the frontal sinus (**Fig. 83.31**). As classically described by Kuhn, there are four types: type I is a single cell occurring above an agger nasi cell, type II is a tier of two or more cells occurring above an agger nasi cell, type III is a single massive cell pneumatizing into the frontal sinus from the middle meatus, and type IV is a single isolated cell within the frontal sinus, appearing as an air bubble with no apparent connection to the frontal recess. With modern imaging techniques affording parasagittal sections, most type IV cells are found to drain into the frontal recess area. PJ Wormald has therefore suggested a modification of the Kuhn classification, defining a type IV cell as one that extends into the frontal sinus for > 50% of the frontal sinus height. Although most of these cells can be reached endoscopically, some may require the addition of anterior frontal sinus trephination.

Supraorbital Ethmoid Cells

The supraorbital ethmoid (SOE) cell derives its name by pneumatizing into the orbital plate of the frontal bone, sometimes all the way over the orbit (**Fig. 83.32**). On a coronal CT, the frontal sinus appears to be septated. Axial, coronal, and parasagittal CT views confirm that the lateral "frontal sinus cell" actually lies posterior to the frontal sinus (**Fig. 83.32a–c, e**). It drains via a separate opening into the frontal recess (**Fig. 83.32d, e**). Three major problems with the SOE cell are (1) mistaking it for the frontal sinus, (2) missing it altogether, or (3) not resecting the partition (commonly the bulla lamella) separating the SOE from the frontal sinus high enough into the frontal recess to make a common antechamber into which the frontal sinus and the SOE may empty. The SOE cell lies anterior to the bulla lamella. The anterior ethmoid artery (AEA) commonly is at the skull base attachment of the bulla lamella, usually behind the SOE cell (**Fig. 83.32d**). The internal frontal ostium lies anteromedial to the SOE (**Fig. 83.32d, e**).

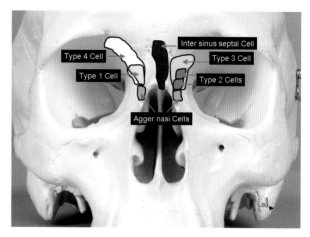

Fig. 83.31 The type 1 frontoethmoid cell is a single cell occurring above an agger nasi cell; type 2 is a tier of two or more cells occurring above an agger nasi cell; type 3 is a single massive cell pneumatizing into the frontal sinus above the frontal sinus ostium level, and a type 4 cell is one that extends into the frontal sinus for greater than 50% of the frontal sinus height.

Interfrontal Sinus Septal Cell

This cell occurs in the septum between the two frontal sinuses and usually opens into one frontal recess medial to the internal frontal ostium. This cell may pneumatize only the lower intersinus septum or extend all the way to the top of the frontal sinus.

Pneumatized Structures: Middle Turbinate, Uncinate, and Superior Turbinate

MT pneumatization, called a concha bullosa (**Fig. 83.5**), may be in just the vertical portion attached to the skull base or all the way down into the body of the MT. When the vertical portion only is pneumatized, it is difficult to resect. When the concha bullosa pneumatizes the entire MT, it may compromise the middle meatus. When resecting a large concha bullosa, the lateral half to two-thirds should be removed, leaving the middle third. Any residual lateral lamella going up to the skull base should be carefully removed to prevent disruption of mucociliary clearance (**Fig. 83.33**).

A pneumatized uncinate is rare but can contribute to OMC obstruction. A superior turbinate concha bullosa is also rare, and its clinical significance is variable.

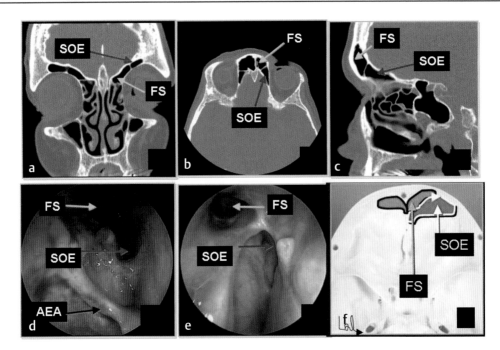

Fig. 83.32 The supraorbital ethmoid cell (SOE) pneumatizes into the orbital plate of the frontal bone, sometimes all of the way out over the orbit to the lateral skull wall. When seen in this extreme pneumatization on coronal computed tomography (CT), the frontal sinus appears to be septated. Axial sections with coronal and sagittal reconstructions will demonstrate that the SOE lines up posterior to the frontal sinus (FS) and drains via a separate opening into the frontal recess. (**a–c**) How a left SOE cell appears on coronal, axial, and parasagittal CT sections, respectively. (**a**) The classic "septate" appearance of the FS on the coronal CT view, which should prompt suspicion of an SOE being present. (**b**) Axial view; note that the SOE lies posterior to the FS. (**c**) Parasagittal CT view shows pneumatization of the SOE into the orbital roof, behind the FS. (**d, e**) Endoscopic view using a 45-degree endoscope after complete left frontoethmoidectomy has been performed. (**d**) Relationship of the anterior ethmoid artery (AEA) to the SOE and the FS; note that the AEA is posterior to the SOE, and not in the partition between the FS and SOE. (**e**) Close-up view, showing that the SOE cells drain posterior and lateral to the FS, (i.e., the FS ostium lies anterior and medial to the SOE opening). (**f**) Schematic showing that the SOE cell is formed by pneumatization of an anterior ethmoidal call into the orbital roof, behind the frontal sinus.

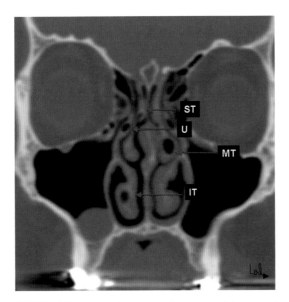

Fig. 83.33 The coronal computed tomographic scan shows an unusually extensive pneumatization of bilateral uncinate processes (U), left middle turbinate (MT concha bullosa), right inferior turbinate (IT), and right superior turbinate (ST).

■ Suggested Reading

Bent JP, Cuilty-Siller C, Kuhn FA. The frontal cell in frontal sinus obstruction. Am J Rhinol 1994;2:31–37

Bolger WE, Keyes AS, Lanza DC. Use of the superior meatus and superior turbinate in the endoscopic approach to the sphenoid sinus. Otolaryngol Head Neck Surg 1999;120(3):308–313

Casiano R. Endoscopic Sinonasal Dissection Guide. New York, NY: Thieme; 2011

Kasper KA. Nasofrontal connections: a study based on one hundred consecutive dissections. Arch Otolaryngol 1936;23:322–343

Kennedy DW, Hwang PH, eds. Rhinology: Diseases of the Nose, Sinuses, and Skull Base. New York, NY: Thieme; 2012

Kennedy DW, Zinreich SJ, Hassab MH. The internal carotid artery as it relates to endonasal sphenoethmoidectomy. Am J Rhinol 1990;4:7–12

Kuhn FA. Chronic frontal sinusitis: the endoscopic frontal recess approach. Oper Tech Otolaryngol--Head Neck Surg 1996;7:222–729

Messerklinger W. Endoscopy of the Nose. Baltimore, MD: Urban & Schwarzenberg; 1978

Messerklinger W. On the drainage of the normal frontal sinus of man. Acta Otolaryngol 1967;63(2):176–181

Meyers RM, Valvassori G. Interpretation of anatomic variations of computed tomography scans of the sinuses: a surgeon's perspective. Laryngoscope 1998;108(3):422–425

Orlandi RR, Smith B, Shah L, Wiggins RH III. Endoscopic verification of the sphenoid sinus. Int Forum Allergy Rhinol 2012;2(1):16–19

Ramakrishnan VR, Suh JD, Kennedy DW. Ethmoid skull-base height: a clinically relevant method of evaluation. Int Forum Allergy Rhinol 2011;1(5):396–400

Schaeffer JP. The genesis, development and adult anatomy of the nasofrontal region in man. Am J Anat 1916;20:125–146

Stamm AC, Draf W. Micro-Endoscopic Surgery of the Paranasal Sinuses and the Skull Base. New York, NY: Springer; 2000

Stammberger H. Functional Endoscopic Sinus Surgery. St. Louis, MO: Mosby; 1991

Stammberger HR, Kennedy DW; Anatomic Terminology Group. Paranasal sinuses: anatomic terminology and nomenclature. Ann Otol Rhinol Laryngol Suppl 1995;167:7–16

Stankiewicz JA, Lal D, Connor M, Welch K. Complications in endoscopic sinus surgery for chronic rhinosinusitis: a 25-year experience. Laryngoscope 2011;121(12):2684–2701 doi: 10.1002/lary.21446

VanAlyea O. Ethmoid labyrinth: anatomic study with consideration of the clinical significance of its structural characteristics. Arch Otolaryngol 1939;29:881–901

Wormald PJ. Endoscopic Sinus Surgery: Anatomy, Three Dimensional Reconstruction and Surgical Technique. Stuttgart, Germany: Thieme; 2008

Wormald PJ. Surgery of the frontal recess and frontal sinus. Rhinology 2005;43(2):82–85

84 Assessing Olfactory Disorders

■ Introduction

Symptoms of Olfactory Disorders

Olfaction is deeply rooted to human emotions, both anatomically and behaviorally, and dysfunction of this special sense is often a major emotional stress for patients. The most important service a physician can offer patients with an olfactory complaint is an accurate diagnosis and concern for their plight. Even though some patients may not complain of distortions in olfactory perception, the distortions do bother them and should be addressed to allay their concerns. Making an accurate diagnosis may allow these patients to regain their olfactory ability or, at the very least, understand why it cannot be treated and learn ways to safely enjoy living.

Normal Anatomy and Physiology

Anatomy

The neurons that perceive inhaled chemicals (odorants) are almost all associated with the olfactory nerve, but the trigeminal nerve has receptors for pungent smells throughout the nasal and pharyngeal cavities, and the glossopharyngeal and vagus nerves provide a minor chemosensory function to the pharyngeal area. The ciliated olfactory receptors are located in a 2 cm^2 patch of specialized mucosa centered beneath the cribriform plate of each nasal cavity. This patch straddles the upper septum, the superior turbinate, and the upper middle turbinate. Within this specialized mucosa are ~ 10 to 20 million primary olfactory neurons.

Primary olfactory neurons are bipolar cells with a single dendrite that has a thickened ending called the olfactory knob. The olfactory knob of each neuron extends into the nasal mucosa and contains non-mobile sensory cilia, where odor molecules bind to their receptors. The cell bodies of primary olfactory neurons are in the *nasal* mucosa too. Each primary olfactory neuron also has an axon, and the axons from primary olfactory neurons come together to form nerve bundles called *fila olfactoria*. The latter go *up* through the cribriform plate to synapse in the olfactory bulb. Although most of the neural processing is ipsilateral, there is some left–right interaction at the level of the bulb and some of the more central olfactory circuits.

Compared with other special sensory neurons, such as vision or hearing, olfactory neurons have the unique ability to regenerate. As has been demonstrated in other mammals, human olfactory neurons are assumed to regenerate every 3 to 6 months. The mechanism whereby each neuron can send its axon to the "correct" part of the olfactory bulb is suspected to be by following the axon sheath of the dying axon that is being replaced. As long as the basal cells of the olfactory epithelium remain healthy, this regeneration can take place. However, inhaled toxins or pathogens that come in with the inspired airflow have access to these olfactory neurons and can destroy the primary neurons. In addition, toxins and pathogens can access the central nervous system (CNS) through the foramina where the fila olfactoria cross the cribriform plate. If the concentration of toxins or pathogens is too high for too long a time, the basal cells can be destroyed, thus eliminating any chance for neural regeneration.

The Process of Smelling

As air flows through the nasal cavity, ~ 10 to 20% moves through the olfactory cleft. Like most nasal passageways, this cleft is ~ 1 to 2 mm wide, and ~ 7 cm from the nostrils. Very little olfactory perception occurs without airflow, as laryngectomized patients can demonstrate. Once the odorant chemical reaches the wall of the olfactory mucosa, it must stick to and become dissolved in the mucus overlying that mucosa; therefore, more soluble chemicals are smelled faster and better than less soluble ones. In air-breathing vertebrates, including humans, soluble binding proteins in the olfactory mucus, called odorant-binding proteins (OBPs), enhance the access of the odorants to the receptors by increasing their concentration there. These OBP molecules may also act to remove odorant molecules from the region of the receptors after transduction. Odorants can also be detected when they rise from the nasopharynx and pass through the nose posteriorly to the olfactory epithelium. This is known as retronasal olfaction and is believed to play a role in the sensation of flavor.

The actual transformation of chemical information into an electrical action potential occurs as a result of specific interactions between the odorant molecules and receptor proteins on the surface of the olfactory cilia. Genes specific for these proteins have been identified, and the inability to perceive particular odorants (anosmia) or an abnormally exaggerated sense of smell (hyperosmia) has been associated with the loss of specific genes or downstream signaling pathways. Several second messenger systems then assist in depolarizing the cell and initiating the action potential. The main second messengers are cyclic adenosine monophosphate (AMP) and inositol phosphate, although other systems involving nitric oxide/guanylyl cyclase have also been identified.

Once the peripheral olfactory receptor cells are depolarized, a convergence of electrical information toward the olfactory bulb begins. Both genetic and spatial (location on the olfactory mucosa, number of neurons stimulated) information seems to at least preliminarily code the differences among the different odorants. The coding is completed with some processing at the olfactory bulb and central olfactory neurons. Currently, the exact coding mechanism is unknown. This entire process, from the odorant flowing into the nose to the identified odor perception, takes several hundred milliseconds, with up to 400 ms separating "slow" odorants from "fast" ones.

Once the odor has been identified, there is the opportunity for multiple associations to be made with it (baking bread smell and Mother). Much of olfactory memory, along with association areas, is in the medial anterior temporal lobes of the brain. Although some studies have suggested that humans have a better side for olfactory ability, this conclusion seems to depend on the testing paradigm. Odor memory seems to be better using birhinal presentation of odorants.

Pathophysiology of Olfaction

Although the exact mechanism(s) of how odorants are perceived is not completely clear, it is well known that patients who lose significant olfactory ability often have difficulty in distinguishing among differ-

ent odorants or have an altered perception of odorants. When obtaining the history from a patient with a chemosensory complaint, it is important to clearly define the symptoms. Patients with concerns about their chemosensory ability will frequently state that they "cannot taste or smell." Although this is sometimes true, it is more likely that they have *only* a smell problem. This can be explained by the brain's routine combination of taste (salt, sweet, sour, and bitter) and smell into "flavor." Up to 80% of the flavor of a meal is due to olfactory input.

Another important consideration is whether the patient's compliant is related to decreased intensity (hyposmia or anosmia), changed perception of the quality of inhaled odorants (parosmia or troposmia), an abnormally exaggerated/acute sense of smell (hyperosmia), or a persisting smell in the absence of an odorant stimulus (phantosmia or hallucination). All of these can occur together, and usually at least some hyposmia is associated with either a distorted or a persisting smell. Damage to or loss of some of the neurons seems to result in abnormal sensory perception.

Although dysfunction in trigeminal chemosensory ability (common chemical sense) is extremely rare, changes in olfactory ability are quite common and fall into two main categories: conductive and neural losses. Conductive losses occur because odorant molecules cannot reach the nasal olfactory receptors due to some type of obstruction. Neural losses are related either to destruction, malfunction, or absence of the primary olfactory neurons in the nasal mucosa, or to abnormal function of the olfactory bulb or more central olfactory neurons.

It is common for patients to have more than one likely cause for an olfactory loss, and often it is difficult to separate the etiologies. For example, patients with chronic rhinosinusitis (CRS) have evidence of inflammatory changes in the olfactory epithelium that can range from squamous metaplasia with the presence of abnormal olfactory neurons to erosion of both supporting respiratory epithelial cells and primary olfactory neurons coupled with the infiltration of immune and inflammatory cells. Furthermore, the histopathological changes have been correlated with the degree of olfactory disturbance. These observations support both conductive and neural processes associated with the olfactory deficits observed in patients with CRS.

◼ Etiology

Obstructive Nasal and Sinus Disease

Any process in the nasal or sinus cavities that causes total cessation of airflow to the olfactory receptors along the nasal cavity roof can block olfaction. This blockage must be essentially total, because even a little airflow will allow olfactory transduction. CRS is among one of the most common conditions obstructing the sinonasal airway, with ~ 61 to 83% of CRS patients experiencing some degree of olfactory impairment. In fact, hyposmia is considered one of four signs and symptoms in CRS diagnostic criteria in the 2007 Adult Sinusitis Guidelines from the American Academy of Otolaryngology–Head and Neck Surgery. Patients with ethmoid disease primarily can have inflammation spread through the middle turbinate to cause membrane edema that blocks the olfactory cleft. Other causes, in descending order of likelihood, include nasal edema from the common cold or allergies, nasal polyps, scarring after intranasal surgery, and intranasal neoplasms. Intranasal deformities due to nasal septal deviation or trauma are essentially never complete enough to block airflow to the olfactory cleft. Patients with obstructive nasal and sinus disease usually have fluctuating losses, with intermittent return of normal olfactory ability. A 1- or 2-week trial of oral steroid therapy will often resolve this blockage and allow a return of olfactory ability while the patient is taking the medication, with occasional long-term results.

Result of an Upper Respiratory Infection

The typical history for this etiology is a middle-aged woman (70 to 80% are female) who had a good sense of smell, caught an upper respiratory infection (URI), and noted a marked decrease in olfactory ability several days after the URI resolved. This loss is thought to be due to a virus that invades and destroys primary olfactory neurons in the nasal epithelium; however, this has not been proven. This loss is often permanent, with the possibility of a small return of function.

Head Trauma

A small percentage of individuals who receive head trauma (probably < 5%) will have a loss of olfactory ability. This is especially likely if the trauma is either occipital or frontal. The theoretical cause of this loss is a stretching or tearing of the fila olfactoria fibers as they leave the top of the cribriform plate when the brain and olfactory bulbs are displaced inside the cranium during even minor trauma. Some individuals, especially those younger than 30 years of age and those with minor losses, may regain some olfactory ability within weeks of the injury. Although the exact numbers are unknown, it is likely that the majority of patients who lose their olfactory ability after head trauma will have little or no olfactory function return. Human olfactory biopsy studies after head trauma have suggested that the regrowing olfactory

neurons cannot find the olfactory bulbs or the holes in the cribriform plate, and therefore the olfactory ability does not return.

Aging

Aging is thought to have the most significant impact on olfactory decline in the general population. After age 60 or 70, even healthy individuals have a natural loss in olfactory ability. The cause of this loss is unknown, but it parallels losses in balance, vision, and hearing. There are also losses of olfactory ability noted in individuals with some dementias and dementia-related diseases, such as Alzheimer and Parkinson diseases. These losses tend to occur early in the disease process but are not diagnostic of the disease. Neurohistochemical alterations can be found all along the olfactory pathways into the brain in these patients, and the etiological agent or process is unknown.

Toxin Exposure

Some patients have olfactory losses after exposures to toxic chemicals. Common chemicals noted to cause olfactory loss include formalin compounds, cyanoacrylates, cigarette smoke, herbicides, and pesticides. The length of exposure required to cause a loss obviously relates to the toxicity of the chemical, and can range from hours to decades. These losses are usually permanent.

Congenital Dysfunction

Some individuals have never had an olfactory ability. This is usually discovered near the end of their first decade of life. The diagnosis is difficult to make, because other causes, such as head trauma and post-URI, must be ruled out. Although there are usually no other congenital problems associated with this condition, Kallmann syndrome (hypogonadotropic hypogonadism) can be present. Failure to develop secondary sexual characteristics in an anosmic male should prompt a referral to an endocrinologist. Specialized magnetic resonance imaging (MRI) scanning may be able to demonstrate the lack of olfactory bulbs.

Postsurgical Loss

Sometimes, there is a loss of olfactory ability after septal or sinus surgery. If the airways are patent, this loss is likely related to a direct trauma and destruction of the olfactory neurons. Decreased olfactory function is especially noticeable if there had already been a loss of many of the neurons prior to surgery and the last few neurons are destroyed intraoperatively. Surgery in the frontal recess region also has a higher risk of subsequent olfactory disturbance. Obviously, anterior craniofacial resection will result in anosmia. Alternatively, there may be scarring postoperatively that makes the olfactory neurons nonfunctional. Patients who have tracheotomies have a major diversion of airflow away from the olfactory receptors and thus have a decreased olfactory ability.

Miscellaneous Etiologies

In addition to the foregoing etiologies that account for the majority of losses, numerous conditions are associated with decreased or absent olfactory ability. In most of these instances, the exact pathophysiology causing the olfactory problem is unknown. This list includes human immunodeficiency virus infection, epilepsy, brain tumors, depression, autoimmune diseases, Down syndrome, conditions associated with endocrine changes (pregnancy), schizophrenia, and some vitamin deficiencies. In addition, certain medications, such as antibiotics, opiates, sympathomimetics, and chemotherapy agents, can affect olfactory function as well. Currently, the exact mechanisms creating these olfactory disturbances are also unknown. Finally, there is a group of ~ 30 to 40% of patients with olfactory dysfunction for whom an etiology cannot be determined other than to say that it is a neural loss. There is no proven therapy for this group.

■ Evaluation

Subjective Testing

Until recently, olfactory testing was done either poorly or not at all, or it was so complicated that few patients were tested. As in any sensory system, tests of threshold, discrimination, and identification can be performed. Because the identification tests are performed at a suprathreshold level, they are easier to perform and can give reliable results in shorter times. Commonly described olfactory tests probably all measure the same function. The Smell Identification Test uses scratch-and-sniff technology and assesses the response of a patient to 40 odorants. This test is portable and reliable and has a version that is available for many cultures. Notably, it can be used to assess a patient's olfactory ability on multiple occasions, such as before and after therapeutic interventions.

Objective Testing

Tests that do not require patient cooperation have been developed, but only a handful of places are conducting them because of their expense and the technical needs of presenting warmed and humidified air and odorants in an unobtrusive manner. Nevertheless, the use of these tests is increasing, and more patients are being referred for evaluation, increasing the possibility that the tests will continue to evolve so that they can become more readily available in the future.

The electro-olfactogram is the most peripheral of the objective tests. It measures the response of the olfactory primary neurons to odorant stimulation with a catheter placed through the nose touching the neurons. This test is difficult to perform and causes some discomfort to the patient. Another more commonly used test measures the brain-evoked potentials after an odorant is introduced into the nose. This test can identify differences between trigeminal and olfactory odorants.

Imaging

When evaluating a patient for olfactory dysfunction, the most important determinant for deciding whether therapy can be provided is whether the upper nasal airways are patent. A coronal computed tomographic (CT) scan of the nasal cavity can easily give this information and is sometimes more helpful than the endoscopic nasal examination. Plain films of the nasal and sinus regions have no place in this evaluation. Magnetic resonance imaging (MRI) does not image bones and tends to magnify the nasal and sinus mucosa, thus limiting its value for analysis of airway patency. However, MRI is useful for imaging the olfactory bulbs and for assessing for possible brain tumors.

■ Treatment

General

All patients who have an olfactory loss need to protect themselves against fire and dangerous gases with smoke detectors and by eliminating the possibility of exposure to methane, propane, and other harmful agents. If it is impossible to live in an all-electric or wood- or oil-heated residence, then an electrical sensor for these gases should be installed. To add quality to an otherwise drab eating experience, pungent foods, such as mustards or hot peppers can be added, since the trigeminal system is likely still functioning. Tastants, such as sour and bitter, can also be added with few health consequences.

Medical Therapy

Nasal airway obstruction is the only type of olfactory dysfunction that can be successfully treated. There is currently no proven therapy for patients with neural losses. The usual nasal/sinus treatments of antibiotics, decongestants, antihistamines (in proven allergic patients), oral and topical steroids, and saline irrigations have been helpful. Especially helpful for patients with olfactory cleft blockage is the application of an aqueous topical nasal steroid with the head inverted into the head down-and-forward position. Many publications have suggested that various vitamins, minerals, and pharmaceuticals will help olfactory disorders (e.g., zinc, B vitamins, vitamin A, theophylline, antiseizure medications). There have been no good studies that have demonstrated effectiveness for any of these preparations.

Surgical Therapy

Surgical therapy for patients with decreased olfactory ability due to inflammatory or infectious disease may be helpful if medical therapy has been ineffective. The surgical therapy (endoscopic sinus surgery) should be directed to open the sinuses and allow ventilation. Because of the proximity of the olfactory cleft to the ethmoid sinus, if the latter can be restored to an air-containing space lined by pink, thin mucosa, the olfactory cleft will open and also become healthy. Direct instrumentation of the olfactory cleft carries a high risk of obstructive scarring. A small number of individuals with phantosmia have been helped by surgery to excise the olfactory mucosa from the bottom of the cribriform plate. This difficult and risky endoscopic operation should be performed by an experienced surgeon.

Future Directions

Due to the olfactory epithelium's capability to regenerate new sensory neurons, there has been interest in using olfactory epithelial grafts to restore olfactory function in patients with anosmia. Grafts of olfactory epithelium have already been successfully transplanted to different parts of the brain in animal models and have retained their olfactory characteristics. However, before any procedures can be applied to humans, several technical problems have to be worked out, including testing the functional capacity of these grafts. Nevertheless, preliminary data appear promising.

■ Summary

Although the basic mechanisms of olfaction are still being discovered, a firm foundation has been laid for effective clinical evaluation of olfactory disorders. A thorough and empathetic evaluation that includes standardized and repeatable olfactory testing, and possibly imaging, is important. With such an assessment, the patient can be maximally helped.

■ Suggested Reading

Bromley SM, Doty RL. Odor recognition memory is better under bilateral than unilateral test conditions. Cortex 1995;31(1):25–40

Costanzo RM, Yagi S. Olfactory epithelial transplantation: possible mechanism for restoration of smell. Curr Opin Otolaryngol Head Neck Surg 2011;19(1):54–57

Corwin J, Loury M, Gilbert AN. Workplace, age, and sex as mediators of olfactory function: data from the National Geographic Smell Survey. J Gerontol B Psychol Sci Soc Sci 1995;50(4):179–186

Cowart BJ, Flynn-Rodden K, McGeady SJ, Lowry LD. Hyposmia in allergic rhinitis. J Allergy Clin Immunol 1993;91(3):747–751

Davidson TM, Murphy C, Jalowayski AA. Smell impairment. Can it be reversed? Postgrad Med 1995;98(1):107–109, 112–118

Doty RL, Marcus A, Lee WW. Development of the 12-item Cross-Cultural Smell Identification Test (CC-SIT). Laryngoscope 1996;106(3 Pt 1):353–356

Downey LL, Jacobs JB, Lebowitz RA. Anosmia and chronic sinus disease. Otolaryngol Head Neck Surg 1996;115(1):24–28

Duncan HJ, Seiden AM. Long-term follow-up of olfactory loss secondary to head trauma and upper respiratory tract infection. Arch Otolaryngol Head Neck Surg 1995;121(10):1183–1187

Furukawa M, Kamide M, Ohkado T, Umeda R. Electro-olfactogram (EOG) in olfactometry. Auris Nasus Larynx 1989;16(1):33–38

Golding-Wood DG, Holmstrom M, Darby Y, Scadding GK, Lund VJ. The treatment of hyposmia with intranasal steroids. J Laryngol Otol 1996;110(2):132–135

Hahn I, Scherer PW, Mozell MM. Velocity profiles measured for airflow through a large-scale model of the human nasal cavity. J Appl Physiol (1985) 1993;75(5):2273–2287

Herz RS, Cupchik GC. The emotional distinctiveness of odor-evoked memories. Chem Senses 1995;20(5):517–528

Hummel T. Retronasal perception of odors. Chem Biodivers 2008;5(6):853–861

Ikeda K, Sakurada T, Suzaki Y, Takasaka T. Efficacy of systemic corticosteroid treatment for anosmia with nasal and paranasal sinus disease. Rhinology 1995;33(3):162–165

Jafek BW, Eller PM, Esses BA, Moran DT. Post-traumatic anosmia. Ultrastructural correlates. Arch Neurol 1989;46(3):300–304

Kern RC. Chronic sinusitis and anosmia: pathologic changes in the olfactory mucosa. Laryngoscope 2000;110(7):1071–1077

Kimmelman CP. The risk to olfaction from nasal surgery. Laryngoscope 1994;104(8 Pt 1):981–988

Leopold DA, Hornung DE, Youngentob SL. Olfactory loss after upper respiratory infection. In: Getchell, Bartoshuk LM, Doty RL, Snow J, eds. Smell and Taste in Health and Disease. New York, NY: Raven; 1991

Leopold DA, Schwob JE, Youngentob SL, Hornung DE, Wright HN, Mozell MM. Successful treatment of phantosmia with preservation of olfaction. Arch Otolaryngol Head Neck Surg 1991; 117(12):1402–1406

Li C, Yousem DM, Doty RL, Kennedy DW. Neuroimaging in patients with olfactory dysfunction. AJR Am J Roentgenol 1994;162(2): 411–418

Litvack JR, Mace JC, Smith TL. Olfactory function and disease severity in chronic rhinosinusitis. Am J Rhinol Allergy 2009;23(2): 139–144

Menashe I, Abaffy T, Hasin Y, et al. Genetic elucidation of human hyperosmia to isovaleric acid. PLoS Biol 2007;5(11):e284

Miller G. 2004 Nobel Prizes. Axel, Buck share award for deciphering how the nose knows. Science 2004;306(5694):207

Mozell MM, Hornung DE, Leopold DA, Youngentob SL. Initial mechanisms basic to olfactory perception. Am J Otolaryngol 1983; 4(4):238–245

Nordin S, Murphy C, Davidson TM, Quiñonez C, Jalowayski AA, Ellison DW. Prevalence and assessment of qualitative olfactory dysfunction in different age groups. Laryngoscope 1996; 106(6):739–744

Pinto JM. Olfaction. Proc Am Thorac Soc 2011;8(1):46–52

Rawson NE. Olfactory loss in aging. Sci SAGE KE 2006;2006(5): pe6

Rawson N, Huang L. Symposium overview: Impact of oronasal inflammation on taste and smell. Ann N Y Acad Sci 2009;1170: 581–584

Reed RR. The molecular basis of sensitivity and specificity in olfaction. Semin Cell Biol 1994;5(1):33–38

Rosenfeld RM, Andes D, Bhattacharyya N, et al. Clinical practice guideline: adult sinusitis. Otolaryngol Head Neck Surg 2007; 137(3, Suppl):S1–S31

Ship JA, Pearson JD, Cruise LJ, Brant LJ, Metter EJ. Longitudinal changes in smell identification. J Gerontol A Biol Sci Med Sci 1996; 51(2):M86–M91

Tcatchoff L, Nespoulous C, Pernollet JC, Briand L. A single lysyl residue defines the binding specificity of a human odorant-binding protein for aldehydes. FEBS Lett 2006;580(8):2102–2108

Yamagishi M, Fujiwara M, Nakamura H. Olfactory mucosal findings and clinical course in patients with olfactory disorders following upper respiratory viral infection. Rhinology 1994;32(3):113–118

Zucco GM, Negrin NS. Olfactory deficits in Down subjects: a link with Alzheimer disease. Percept Mot Skills 1994;78(2):627–631

85 Imaging of the Nasal Cavity and Paranasal Sinuses

Introduction

With the advent of innovative techniques to treat sinus pathology, particularly functional endoscopic sinus surgery (FESS) and balloon sinus dilation, clinicians and surgeons who treat these problems must have extensive knowledge of the anatomy of the nasal cavity and paranasal sinuses. However, knowledge of the anatomy is not enough. Clinicians should be familiar with the essentials of imaging to more effectively understand and treat sinus pathology. This chapter provides an overview of the anatomy of the nasal cavity and paranasal sinuses, with an emphasis on indications for specific imaging studies, and the role of imaging in the treatment and follow-up of sinus disease. The reader is encouraged to have diagrams and photographs available (provided in many current texts) when reading this chapter.

Anatomy

Mucociliary Clearance

For a clear understanding of the regional anatomy and the importance of the anterior ethmoid sinus structures, it is critical that one understand the flow pattern of the mucous blanket coating the major sinuses (mucociliary clearance). Further, one must be acquainted with the concept that inflammatory sinus disease is largely the result of compromise of the drainage portals (ostiomeatal channels) of the individual sinus cavities.

The mucosal lining of the paranasal sinuses is made up of a ciliated cuboidal epithelium. In turn, a mucous blanket is found on the surface. The cilia are in constant motion and act in concert to propel the mucus in a specific direction. The pattern of flow is specific for each sinus, and will persist even if alternative openings are surgically created in the sinus. Therefore, FESS and the more recent balloon sinus technology have gained widespread accep-

tance, because their goal is to restore drainage of the sinuses via their natural pathways.

There are two main ostiomeatal channels, both of which are at risk for blockage by a small amount of mucosal thickening. The anterior ostiomeatal unit includes the frontal sinus ostium, frontal recess, maxillary sinus ostium, infundibulum, and middle meatus. These channels provide communication between the ipsilateral frontal, anterior ethmoid, and maxillary sinuses. The posterior ostiomeatal unit consists of the sphenoid sinus ostium, sphenoethmoidal recess, and superior meatus. The radiological representation of the anatomy should emphasize display of these ostiomeatal channels.

An understanding of the normal anatomy of the lateral nasal wall and its relationship to adjacent structures is essential and is well demonstrated by imaging. The paranasal sinuses are close to the anterior cranial fossa cribriform plate, the internal carotid arteries, the cavernous sinuses, the orbits and their contents, and the optic nerves as they exit the orbits.

Anatomical Variations

Even though the nasal anatomy varies significantly from patient to patient, certain anatomical variations are observed commonly in the general population and are often seen more frequently in patients with chronic inflammatory disease. The significance of a particular anatomical variant is determined by its relationship to the ostiomeatal channels and nasal air passages. The ability of the variation to obstruct the air passages implies a role in the recurrence of sinusitis. The most common variations are discussed in this section.

Concha Bullosa

A concha bullosa is defined as an aeration in a middle turbinate. It may be unilateral or bilateral. Less frequently, aeration of the superior turbinate may occur, whereas aeration of the inferior turbinate is infrequent. A concha bullosa in the middle turbinate may enlarge to obstruct the middle meatus or the infundibulum. The air cavity in a concha bullosa is lined with the same epithelium as the rest of the nasal cavity, so these cells can undergo the same inflammatory disorders experienced in the paranasal sinuses. Obstruction of the drainage of a concha can lead to mucocele formation.

Nasal Septal Deviation

This deviation is an asymmetric bowing of the nasal septum that may compress the middle turbinate laterally, narrowing the middle meatus. Bony spurs, which are often associated with septal deviation, may further compromise the ostiomeatal unit. Nasal septal deviation is usually congenital, though it may be a posttraumatic finding in some patients.

Paradoxic Middle Turbinate

The middle turbinate usually curves medially toward the nasal septum. However, its major curvature can project laterally, and thus narrow the middle meatus and infundibulum. Such a variant is called a paradoxic middle turbinate. The inferior edge of the middle turbinate may assume various shapes with excessive curvature, which in turn may obstruct the nasal cavity, infundibulum, and middle meatus.

Variations in the Uncinate Process

The course of the "free edge" of the uncinate process has several variations. In most cases, it either extends slightly obliquely toward the nasal septum, with the free edge surrounding the inferior-anterior surface of the ethmoid bulla, or extends more medially to the medial surface of the ethmoid bulla. Sometimes, the free edge of the uncinate is noted to adhere to the orbital floor/inferior aspect of the lamina papyracea. This is referred to as an atelectatic uncinate process. This variant is usually associated with a hypoplastic, and often opacified, ipsilateral maxillary sinus due to closure of the infundibulum. It is important to note this variant for surgical planning, because the ipsilateral orbital floor will be low-lying due to the hypoplastic maxillary sinus. This increases the risk of inadvertent penetration of the orbit during surgery. An additional variation of the uncinate is its extension superiorly to the roof of the anterior ethmoid sinus, thus causing the superior infundibulum to end as a "blind pouch," referred to as the lamina terminalis. Here, the infundibulum drains via the posterior aspect of the middle meatus.

If the free edge of the uncinate deviates laterally, there can be obstruction of the infundibulum. Less frequently, "medial curling" of the uncinate is encountered, which will encroach upon the middle meatus.

Aeration of the Uncinate

This infrequently occurring anomaly expands the width of the uncinate, thus potentially compromising the infundibulum. Functionally, it acts like a concha bullosa or an enlarged ethmoid bulla.

Infraorbital Ethmoid Cells (Haller Cells)

These ethmoid air cells extend along the medial roof of the maxillary sinus. They can have a variable appearance and size and may cause narrowing of the infundibulum when they are large. Haller cells may exist as discrete cells or may open into the maxillary sinus or infundibulum.

Onodi Cells

These rare "cells" are lateral and posterior extensions of the posterior ethmoid air cells. They extend the paranasal sinus cavity close to the optic nerves as they exit the orbits. Onodi cells may surround the optic nerve tract and put the nerve at risk during surgery.

Giant Ethmoid Bulla

The largest of the ethmoid air cells, the ethmoid bulla may enlarge to narrow or obstruct the middle meatus and infundibulum.

Extensive Pneumatization of the Sphenoid Sinus

Pneumatization of the sphenoid sinus can extend into the anterior clinoids and clivus, surrounding the optic nerves. When this occurs, the optic nerves are at increased risk of being damaged during surgical exploration.

Medial Deviation and/or Dehiscence of the Lamina Papyracea

This anatomical variation may be a congenital finding or the result of prior facial trauma. In either case, the intraorbital contents are at risk during surgery due to the common dehiscences in the area, as well as the ease of confusing this "medial bulge" with the ethmoid bulla. Both excessive medial deviation and bony dehiscence tend to occur most often at the site of the insertion of the basal lamella into the lamina papyracea, thus rendering this portion of the lamina papyracea fragile.

Aerated Crista Galli

Aeration of this normally bony structure can occur. When aerated, these cells may communicate with the frontal recess. Obstruction of this ostium can lead to chronic sinusitis and mucocele formation. It is important to recognize this entity preoperatively and to differentiate it from an ethmoid air cell to avoid extension of surgery into the cranial vault.

Cephalocele

Preoperative computed tomographic (CT) scanning is useful in assessing for congenital abnormalities, such as cephaloceles. These abnormalities may be spontaneously present or may occur as a result of previous ethmoid/sphenoid sinus surgery. Their presence needs to be considered when dealing with an isolated soft tissue mass adjacent to the ethmoid or sphenoid roof, especially if associated bony erosion is present. The differential diagnosis includes mucocele, neoplasm, cephalocele, and, less likely, a polyp associated with an adjacent bony dehiscence. Coronal CT scanning best displays the extent of bony erosion, and sagittal and coronal magnetic resonance imaging (MRI) is very helpful in narrowing the differential diagnosis.

Posterior Nasal Septal Air Cells

Air cells are commonly found within the posterior-superior portion of the nasal septum. When they are present, the communication is with the sphenoid sinus. Like any other air cell within the paranasal sinuses, posterior nasal septal air cells may also be affected with mucosal inflammation, which may obliterate them. In such cases, these cells may resemble a cephalocele. CT scanning and MRI may be beneficial in defining the involved pathology.

Asymmetry in Ethmoid Roof Height

It is important to make note of any asymmetry in height of the ethmoid roof. Measurement of the height in millimeters of the cribriform to the roof of the ethmoids, first described by Keros in 1965, will allow classification of this height as type I (1–3 mm),

II (4–7 mm), or III (> 8 mm). There is a higher incidence of intracranial penetration during FESS when this anatomical variation occurs. The intracranial penetration is more likely to occur on the side where the position of the roof is lower.

■ Techniques of Radiological Evaluation of the Nose and Paranasal Sinuses

Standard Radiographs

Despite their frequency of use, standard radiographs offer only limited information due to the problem of structural superimposition. The anterior-posterior and Waters views best demonstrate the frontal and maxillary sinuses. The lateral view best displays the sphenoid sinus. However, the fine bony detail of the ethmoid sinuses is poorly displayed on all views because of overlapping structures. Although of limited value in the evaluation of patients with chronic inflammatory disease, standard radiographs may be of value in the assessment of patients with acute inflammatory disease. Here, a single Caldwell or Waters view may be very informative.

Computed Tomography

CT is currently the modality of choice in the evaluation of the paranasal sinuses and the nasal cavity. Its ability to optimally display bone and air facilitates accurate definition of regional anatomy and extent of disease. In patients with inflammatory disease, imaging in the coronal plane is preferred as the initial screening technique. The cross-sectional plane that most closely correlates with the surgical approach is the coronal plane.

The coronal plane optimally displays the ostiomeatal unit and the relationship of the brain and ethmoid roof, and it depicts the relationship of the orbits to the paranasal sinuses. Coronal images correlate with the endoscopic surgical approach; therefore, they should always be obtained for patients with inflammatory sinus disease who are surgical candidates. Axial imaging is important in the evaluation of trauma and neoplasms in this region.

To evaluate the sinuses, a patient is placed in a prone position with the chin hyperextended on the bed of the CT scanner. The scanner gantry is angled so that it is as perpendicular to the hard palate as possible. Scanning is performed from the anterior frontal sinus and nasal tip posteriorly through the sphenoid sinus. Contiguous 3 mm images are obtained. Scans should overlap if thicker slices are used, so that multiplanar reconstructions can still be performed. The field of view is adjusted to include only the areas of interest. This helps reduce artifact from the teeth and associated metallic restorations and magnifies the small structures of the nasal cavity and adjacent paranasal sinuses.

Windows are chosen to accentuate the air passages, the bony detail, and the soft tissues. Experience shows that a window width of + 2,000 with a level of – 200 is the best starting point. The potentiometers can then be manually manipulated to optimally display the anatomical detail of the uncinate process and ethmoid bulla. This same setting is then used to film the entire study.

With CT, sagittal reconstructions can be obtained for a morphological orientation. Various distances and angles can be measured to aid in the passage of instruments during surgery on these views. In displaying the position of the internal carotid arteries with respect to the bony margins of the sphenoid sinus, axial reconstructions can be helpful.

Modern multidetector CT scanners use very thin slices, such that the length and width of a pixel are the same as the slice width. This yields a voxel (pixel in three dimensions) with equal length, width, and height. The axial images can be reformatted into coronal or sagittal images that have almost exactly the same resolution as the direct slice. Reformatting with specific protocols and skin surface markers also forms the basis for image guidance technology. This essentially allows for navigation of the sinuses in the manner of a global positioning system, using a detection array or mask worn by the patient that correlates with the formatted navigation system protocol utilized.

Magnetic Resonance Imaging

MRI provides better visualization of soft tissue than CT, but it is not well suited to routine evaluation of the paranasal sinuses. Cortical bone and air yield no MRI signal and thus are not depicted on the images. Furthermore, the signal intensity of the mucosal lining during the edematous phase of the nasal cycle is similar to the appearance of mucosal inflammation. The nasal cycle is a physiological phenomenon in which the nasal mucosa undergoes alternating cycles of left- and right-sided mucosal swelling. The cycle varies from 20 minutes to 6 hours. Although inflammation of the mucosa gives very bright signal intensity on T2-weighted images, neoplastic processes are usually of intermediate increased signal intensity on T2-weighted images. Fungal concretions have a very low signal intensity on T2-weighted images.

Radiographic Evaluation following Functional Endoscopic Sinus Surgery

The emphasis of the postoperative evaluation of patients is similar to that of the preoperative evaluation. Ideally, patients should be followed with coronal CT. Given the fact that a surgical procedure has been performed, one must first establish the type and extent of surgery. The emphasis should be on understanding the underlying anatomy as it appears following surgery. Areas that merit close scrutiny follow.

Frontal Recess

The frontal recesses should be identified to determine their patency. Postoperatively, recurrence of disease is often due to persistent obstruction in this area. It should be noted that persistence of the agger nasi cell (if it remains) may continue to narrow the frontal recess.

Ostiomeatal Unit

The extent of the uncinectomy and removal of the ethmoid bulla should be noted. The outline of the middle turbinate should be examined to determine whether a middle turbinectomy has been performed. If so, then careful attention should be paid to both the vertical attachment of the middle turbinate to the cribriform plate, as well as the attachment of the basal lamella to the lamina papyracea. Traction applied during middle turbinectomy can inflict damage at these sites.

Lamina Papyracea

The entire course of the lamina papyracea should be inspected to evaluate its integrity. Postoperative dehiscences are not uncommonly found just posterior to the nasolacrimal duct at the level of the ethmoid bulla and basal lamella attachment.

Sphenoid Sinus Area

The margins of the sphenoid sinus should be evaluated for bony dehiscence or cephalocele.

Imaging to Identify Operative Complications following Functional Endoscopic Sinus Surgery

In general, complications can be divided into minor and major. Minor complications include periorbital emphysema, epistaxis, postoperative nasal synechiae, and tooth pain and do not require postoperative radiological evaluation. Major complications are rarer but can be severely devastating or fatal. Loss of integrity of the lamina papyracea can permit intra-orbital fat to herniate into the ethmoid sinuses. Pre-existing dehiscence of the lamina papyracea may be due to prior trauma or erosion from chronic sinus disease. Intraoperative disruption of the lamina papyracea can occur during resection of the middle turbinate if the ground lamella is resected back to its attachment to the lamina papyracea. Another major complication is direct damage to the medial rectus muscle, superior oblique muscle, or other orbital contents, which can occur if there is preexisting or intraoperative disruption of the lamina papyracea.

If intraorbital and intraocular pressure builds up due to an expanding hematoma or to air being forced into the orbit from the nasal cavity (via a dehiscent lamina papyracea), then visual impairment or blind-ness secondary to ischemia can result. Blindness due to injury of the optic nerve can occur during poste-rior ethmoidectomy if the bony limit of the sinus is violated. Trauma to the vascular supply of the optic nerve can also result in visual loss. Thin-section axial and coronal CT can be of benefit in evaluation of such cases.

Massive hemorrhage from direct injury to major vessels can also occur. Laceration of the internal carotid artery has been reported and is often a fatal complication. Emergent angiography with balloon occlusion of the lacerated artery can be performed. Patients who report severe postoperative headache or photophobia, or who have signs that suggest sub-arachnoid hemorrhage, should have a noncontrast head CT. If subarachnoid blood is found, cerebral angiography is recommended to detect vascular injury. Postoperative cerebrospinal fluid (CSF) leak-age is another major complication of FESS. These leaks occur following inadvertent penetration of the dura. Extension of the injury to involve the cribri-form plate, ovea ethmoidalis, anterior cranial fossa, and skull base have all been reported. Secondary nasal encephalocele or deep penetration of the cere-brum can be seen following violation of the cranial vault. CSF leaks may not become clinically apparent for up to 2 years after surgery. Although they will often close spontaneously with conservative mea-sures (i.e., lumbar drain), if they persist, radionuclide CSF study is indicated. If the radionuclide test is posi-tive (directly or indirectly) then a contrast CT cister-nography is performed to define the anatomy and pinpoint the site of leakage.

CT for Staging of Sinus Pathology

CT is the imaging modality of choice for evaluation of sinus disease. Recently, the value of CT in stag-ing of sinus pathology has been explored. Kennedy reported that, particularly with regard to outcome, CT scanning preoperatively is indicative of disease severity and is related to outcome. Gliklich and Met-son compared four proposed sinus CT staging sys-tems with regard to their value in outcomes research. They emphasized that the statistical attributes of a staging system directly affect its usefulness in clini-cal trials and concluded that a staging system based on anatomical disease site would be most beneficial with regard to outcomes research.

In another study, Friedman and Katsantonis pro-posed a four-stage system. Stage I disease included single-focus disease radiographically, either unilat-erally or bilaterally. Stage II was defined as discon-tiguous or patchy areas of disease radiographically with symptomatic response to medication. Stage III included contiguous disease throughout the eth-moid labyrinth, with or without other major sinus opacity, with symptomatic response to medication. Stage IV included contiguous hyperplastic disease involving all sinuses with minimal or no symptom-atic response to medication. Stage I disease indi-cated primarily medical treatment, whereas stages II through IV indicated surgical treatment. Friedman and Katsantonis concluded that this four-stage sys-tem is most indicative of clinical course and eventual outcome.

It is clear that careful radiographic evaluation, particularly the use of CT for staging of sinus pathol-ogy, is a critical component—if not the prime deter-minant—for staging and clinical outcome.

Finally, the Lund–Mackay staging system uses numerical scoring of six anatomical sites, includ-ing maxillary sinus, anterior and posterior ethmoid sinus, sphenoid sinus, frontal sinus, and the ostiome-atal unit, assigning a score of 0 for no mucosal thick-ening, 1 for partial, and 2 for complete opacification of each site, for a total possible score of 24. A study by Hopkins et al, in the October 2007 issue of *Otolar-yngology–Head and Neck Surgery* concluded that the Lund–Mackay staging system was useful when com-bined with validated symptom questionnaires such as the Sino-Nasal Outcome Test (SNOT-22) in pre-dicting whether surgery is going to provide symp-tomatic relief to patients, and demonstrates positive predictive value in counseling patients about risk of complications from surgery.

■ Suggested Reading

Aaløkken TM, Hagtvedt T, Dalen I, Kolbenstvedt A. Conventional sinus radiography compared with CT in the diagnosis of acute sinusitis. Dentomaxillofac Radiol 2003;32(1):60–62

Benson ML, Oliverio PJ, Zinreich SJ. Techniques of imaging of the nose and paranasal sinuses. In: Advances in Otolaryngology–Head and Neck Surgery. Vol 10. St. Louis, MO: Mosby–Year Book; 1996

Bhattacharyya N, Fried MP. The accuracy of computed tomography in the diagnosis of chronic rhinosinusitis. Laryngoscope 2003;113(1):125–129

Dessi P, Moulin G, Triglia JM, Zanaret M, Cannoni M. Difference in the height of the right and left ethmoidal roofs: a possible risk factor for ethmoidal surgery. Prospective study of 150 CT scans. J Laryngol Otol 1994;108(3):261–262

Fatterpekar GM, Delman BN, Som PM. Imaging the paranasal sinuses: where we are and where we are going. Anat Rec (Hoboken) 2008;291(11):1564–1572

Friedman WH, Katsantonis GP. Staging systems for chronic sinus disease. Ear Nose Throat J 1994;73(7):480–484

Gliklich RE, Metson R. A comparison of sinus computed tomography (CT) staging systems for outcomes research. Am J Rhinol 1994;8:291–297

Hopkins C, Browne JP, Slack R, Lund V, Brown P. The Lund-Mackay staging system for chronic rhinosinusitis: how is it used and what does it predict? Otolaryngol Head Neck Surg 2007;137(4): 555–561

Kennedy DW. Prognostic factors, outcomes and staging in ethmoid sinus surgery. Laryngoscope 1992;102(12 Pt 2, Suppl 57):1–18

Laine FJ, Smoker WR. The ostiomeatal unit and endoscopic surgery: anatomy, variations, and imaging findings in inflammatory diseases. AJR Am J Roentgenol 1992;159(4):849–857

Mafee MF. Imaging of paranasal sinuses and rhinosinusitis. Clin Allergy Immunol 2007;20:185–226

Mafee MF. Preoperative imaging anatomy of nasal-ethmoid complex for functional endoscopic sinus surgery. Radiol Clin North Am 1993;31(1):1–20

Sargi ZB, Casiano RR. Surgical anatomy of the paranasal sinuses. In: Kountakis SE, Onerci M, eds. Rhinologic and Sleep Apnea Surgical Techniques. Berlin, Germany: Springer; 2007:17–26

Shah RK, Dhingra JK, Carter BL, Rebeiz EE. Paranasal sinus development: a radiographic study. Laryngoscope 2003;113(2): 205–209

Shanker L, Evans K. Atlas of Imaging of the Paranasal Sinuses. 2nd ed. London, England: Informa Healthcare; 2006

Wippold FJ II. Head and neck imaging: the role of CT and MRI. J Magn Reson Imaging 2007;25(3):453–465

Yousem DM. Imaging of sinonasal inflammatory disease. Radiology 1993;188(2):303–314

Yousem DM, Kennedy DW, Rosenberg S. Ostiomeatal complex risk factors for sinusitis: CT evaluation. J Otolaryngol 1991;20(6): 419–424

Zinreich SJ. Imaging of chronic sinusitis in adults: X-ray, computed tomography, and magnetic resonance imaging. J Allergy Clin Immunol 1992;90(3 Pt 2):445–451

Zinreich SJ. Progress in sinonasal imaging. Ann Otol Rhinol Laryngol Suppl 2006;196:61–65

86 Functional Endoscopic Sinus Surgery: Contemporary Instrumentation and Prevention of Complications

■ Introduction

The initial instrumentation that was available for endoscopic sinus surgery (ESS) consisted primarily of instruments without suction, such as the Blakesley forceps and cupped forceps, which tended to strip mucosa from the underlying bone. It soon became evident that this lack of control of mucosal removal and poor intraoperative visualization as a result of bleeding were frequently limiting factors in the surgical procedure and a common cause of intraoperative complications. The introduction of suction forceps was an advance in this regard, but not a satisfactory solution, because early versions tended to be bulky, and suction was not available for all instruments.

■ Contemporary Instrumentation

Nonpower Instrumentation

Recognition of the importance of mucosal preservation has led to modification in nonpower instrumentation. Experience has shown that when mucosa is stripped, healing is slowed, and more intensive postoperative care is required, which can result in formidable scarring. Also, areas of stripped mucosa may result in new bone growth and provide a nidus for chronic infection. This complication becomes even more critical in the important area of the frontal recess, where mucosal scarring and new bone growth can lead to complete stenosis and persistent infection.

Through-Cutting Instrumentation

With this in mind, the most significant nonpower development has been through-cutting instrumentation. Low-profile heads and ergonomic designs have added to the usefulness of nonpower instruments. Furthermore, convenient shapes for accessing the frontal recess, where the use of through-cutting instrumentation is critically important, have been a significant advance. The aim of functional endoscopic sinus surgery (FESS) should be to open diseased sinuses at the natural ostium and, wherever possible, to completely remove the underlying bony partitions in areas adjacent to chronic disease. At the same time, an intact mucosa-lined cavity should be achieved. This approach leads to more rapid healing with less crusting, reduced incidence of persistent disease, and a more favorable postoperative course.

Powered Instrumentation

Microdebrider Technology

Powered instrumentation using soft tissue shavers offers a significant advance to the endoscopic sinus surgeon. These instruments achieved widespread use in orthopedic surgery before their potential application in sinus surgery was recognized. In 1994, Setliff and Parsons were the first to report the use of soft tissue shavers for ESS. The shavers have since become widely accepted for the removal of polyps and soft tissue masses.

All currently available instruments work along a similar principle, with an electrically powered disposable cutting blade open only through a small window on the side and/or tip. Oscillation of the blade is accompanied by continuous suction through a hollow shaft to remove debris and blood from the operative field. The sharp oscillating blade allows for precise cutting of polyps and mucosa, while leaving adjacent tissue intact. However, perhaps the most significant advantage of the soft tissue shaver is its ability to maintain a bloodless field with continuous suction. It improves visualization and safety during a procedure, particularly in the setting of massive nasal polyposis, where the use of these instruments dramatically advances surgeons' ability to reduce bleeding and maximizes their ability to identify the anatomy.

Angled microdebrider blades allow improved access to different parts of the nasal cavity and paranasal sinuses. Variations on microdebrider technology include a bipolar microdebrider, which delivers bipolar energy to the end of the blade, permitting the added ability to control bleeding, not merely suction it clear.

Endoscopic Drills

When bone is thicker than microdebrider blades can handle, endoscopic drills can be used. Endoscopic drills have built-in suction, allowing for removal of blood and debris from the surgical field. They may also offer a sheath to protect tissue from the posterior aspect of the drill bit, helpful in drilling in the frontal recess. Both cutting and diamond drill bits are available, allowing for efficient removal of damaged tissue while minimizing risks to surrounding healthy tissue.

Coblation Technology

Coblation uses radiofrequency to energize electrolytes within a conductive medium, typically saline. This creates a plasma field that disrupts molecular bonds within the surrounding tissue at a relatively low temperature, leading to less thermal damage to surrounding structures. Coblation technology has been proposed for the removal of nasal polyps and nasal tumors because its hemostatic properties allow for a clear operating field. However, coblation lacks the ability to remove bone, limiting its utility in ESS within the ethmoid sinus. The removal of soft tissue seems to be the most appropriate use of coblation technology, but further studies are necessary to determine its exact role in ESS.

Balloon Catheter Technology

Balloon catheter technology has been presented as a potentially less invasive alternative for patients undergoing sinus surgery. An adaptation of cardiac-like devices, the technology received U.S. Food and Drug Administration approval in 2005 for use in the sinuses. Balloon dilatation employs a noncompliant balloon with the ability to displace bone and tissue to enlarge the sinus ostia.

Several studies have sought to clarify the role of balloon dilation. The 2007 CLEAR study was a prospective, multicenter trial of 109 patients with chronic rhinosinusitis without nasal polyps, unresponsive to medical management, undergoing balloon dilatation with or without concurrent ethmoidectomy. Follow-up evaluations were performed

at 1, 12, and 24 weeks after surgery. The authors report ostial patency rates of 80.5%, as well as consistent improvement in quality-of-life measures over baseline. However, 52% of these patients underwent FESS as well as balloon sinus dilation, leading to a "hybrid" group of patients. For those patients undergoing balloon-only procedures, their burden of disease was limited, with a Lund–Mackay score of 6.1. This radiological score seeks to quantify disease burden on computed tomography (CT) and should be compared with an incidental Lund–Mackay score of 4.26 in the general population. Also, the study does not define explicitly the medical or surgical therapy used in these patients. Finally, the measurement of ostial patency was not blinded, leading to a likely optimistic view on actual patency. This uncontrolled, observational study does not provide adequate data to determine the role for balloon dilatation.

In 2008, a balloon registry reported on 1,036 patients across 27 practices. This study found a 95.2% improvement rate in symptoms, with 3.8% unchanged and 1% worse. Eight complications were reported, including two cerebrospinal fluid leaks and six episodes of minor epistaxis. Although this study seems to demonstrate the relative safety of balloon dilatation, definitive conclusions regarding patient improvement cannot be drawn, because the disease burden and surgery indications were not defined, and no validated symptom measurement tools were used.

Based on the data to date, it is clear that balloon catheter technology likely has a role in the management of chronic rhinosinusitis, but that role has not yet been fully defined. Further controlled studies comparing balloon dilatation to FESS are needed to better understand its applications.

Surgical Navigation

Surgical navigation represents another technological advancement used during ESS. Navigation systems help identify anatomical landmarks by locating surgical instruments in space, calculating the location of the instrument tip in relation to the patient and projecting the instrument location onto a previously obtained imaging study, usually CT. Magnetic resonance imaging data can also be loaded into an image guidance system and used for intraoperative navigation. This is especially useful for intracranial procedures, sinonasal neoplasms, and encephaloceles.

The American Academy of Otolaryngology–Head and Neck Surgery has published indications for surgical navigation. These are (1) revision sinus surgery; (2) distorted sinus anatomy of development, postoperative, or traumatic origin; (3) extensive sinonasal polyposis; (4) pathology involving the frontal, posterior ethmoid, and sphenoid sinuses; (5) disease abutting the skull base, orbit, optic nerve, or carotid artery; (6) cerebrospinal fluid rhinorrhea or conditions where there is a skull base defect; and (7) benign and malignant sinonasal neoplasms. Most ESS, however, can be performed safely and effectively without the use of surgical navigation. Therefore, the use of image guidance is not the standard of care.

A recent survey found that more than 80% of respondents believe surgical navigation provides safer ESS than surgery without the use of navigation. Although complication rates have been shown to increase in revision ESS without the use of surgical navigation, these data are from 1988 to 1998, and there are likely to have been other improvements in ESS since that first review. More recent studies have found no significant difference in complication rates between ESS performed with and without surgical navigation.

Surgical navigation systems are accurate between 1 and 2 mm. However, the systems can provide misleading information. When the information provided by the image guidance system conflicts with clinical judgment, surgeons should trust their clinical judgment.

■ Prevention of Complications

General Principles and Bleeding

When considering the avoidance of complications in functional ESS, the wise surgeon should keep a few critical principles foremost in mind: (1) a detailed knowledge of general sinus anatomy and the patient's specific anatomy is primary in the avoidance of complications; (2) a recent CT scan should be available in the operating room for frequent referral; and (3) the field should be kept as clear as possible.

Prior to initiation of surgery, many surgeons apply topical oxymetazoline, either via spray in the preoperative holding area or on pledgets once the patient is under anesthesia. Injection of local anesthesia with epinephrine also allows for some degree of vasoconstriction. Typical injection sites include the posterior attachment of the middle turbinate, near the site of the sphenopalatine artery, as well as the anterior attachment of the middle turbinate. Care should be taken to aspirate the needle prior to injection to avoid direct injection of air into blood vessels. During surgery, pledgets soaked with topical vasoconstrictors, such as oxymetazoline or 1:1,000 epinephrine, are helpful to maintain a clean operative field. If the surgeon uses 1:1,000 epinephrine, this can easily be confused with other clear liquids on the field if not properly marked. Coloring one liquid with fluorescein or the end of a surgical marker will help to sufficiently distinguish clear liquids.

The anesthesiologist plays a significant role in surgical safety. Experienced anesthesiologists can provide total intravenous anesthesia, which can noticeably decrease the intraoperative bleeding. If circumstances in the course of surgery compromise an acceptable margin of safety and visualization, *the surgeon should stop operating*. It is far better to return another day to complete an operation than to proceed in an unsafe situation and experience a complication.

Experience and knowledge of the surgical anatomy are paramount in the prevention of complications. Although improvements in instrumentation may assist the surgeon and help to decrease the incidence of complications, there is no substitute for a detailed knowledge of the surgical anatomy. Frequent cadaveric dissection practice with the use of endoscopes, especially for the less experienced surgeon, is very helpful.

A detailed history and physical examination play an important role in avoidance of complications. Bleeding disorders and medications, such as aspirin, should be recognized and addressed. A history of prior sinus surgery alerts the surgeon that the landmarks may be obscured. Endoscopic examination in the office can be correlated with the CT scan for appropriate presurgical planning.

Major Complications

Major complications in FESS include intracranial injury, visual disturbances, and hemorrhage. Other significant complications include periorbital hematoma, periorbital cellulitis, subcutaneous orbital emphysema, epiphora, synechia, and scarring with obstruction.

Intraorbital or intracranial injury can occur by violating important anatomical boundaries. By identifying and operating lateral to the middle turbinate, the lateral lamella of the cribriform plate may be avoided. The superior limit of the ethmoid cavity and skull base may be delineated by using the planum sphenoidale as a landmark. The medial orbital wall should be identified early in the surgery to determine the lateral extent of dissection. The ethmoid roof, sphenoid rostrum, frontal recess, and medial orbital wall demarcate the operative field.

The importance of preoperative and intraoperative review of the patient's CT scan cannot be overemphasized. In cases of severe nasal polyposis or revision surgery, more frequent referral to the CT scan is generally required. Although image guidance technology may be used to provide anatomical confirmation during the surgery, it is no substitute for definitive anatomical knowledge.

Entrance into the orbital cavity or violation of the skull base requires immediate attention. Visual changes require emergent evaluation and consultation by an ophthalmologist. Visual changes may be due to orbital hematoma or direct injury to the optic nerve in its course throughout the sphenoid or orbit. Immediate diagnosis and early intervention may prevent permanent visual damage.

Prior to surgery, the eyes should be palpated to determine the firmness of the orbital contents. If the eye becomes hard and proptotic, and intraorbital bleeding (as in the case of an injured ethmoid artery that has retracted into the orbit) is the suspected cause of visual loss, an emergent lateral canthotomy/cantholysis with or without medial orbital decompression may prevent or ameliorate permanent visual damage. If visual loss is secondary to direct optic nerve injury, then there is little hope of recovery.

Cerebrospinal fluid leak, if noted at the time of surgery, can usually be satisfactorily repaired intraoperatively. Neurosurgical consultation may be necessary, depending on the severity of the injury. A capable otolaryngologist should never hesitate to obtain consultation in the face of complication.

Some bleeding after sinus surgery is to be expected. However, significant bleeding can come from injury to arterial structures during the surgery. This may present at the time of surgery, or it may occur postoperatively. Possible sources of significant bleeding include the anterior ethmoid artery, posterior ethmoid artery, or sphenopalatine artery. The posterior septal branch of the sphenopalatine artery can be encountered when opening the natural sphenoid ostium inferiorly. If arterial bleeding is noted during the surgery, bipolar cautery should be used for control. If the vessel reopens postoperatively, a return to the operating room is often required for control.

Other Complications

Synechia, the most common complication, can generally be diminished by meticulous surgical technique with minimal abrasion of adjacent tissue and meticulous postoperative cleaning. Adhesions and synechiae that do form can generally be lysed in the office under direct endoscopic guidance. Natural ostia closure and severe synechiae may occasionally require revision surgery.

Epiphora due to damage to the nasolacrimal duct can be avoided by paying special attention to anatomical detail during maxillary antrostomy. Generally, epiphora resolves without treatment. If not, a dacrocystorhinostomy may be required for repair. Periorbital hematoma, cellulitis, and subcutaneous orbital emphysema are complications from violation of the medial orbital wall. Local care with the avoidance of nose blowing, the use of cool compresses, and observation will usually be sufficient management. However, progression of symptoms and visual disturbance require further evaluation and treatment.

Postoperative care deserves special mention with regard to prevention of complications. Patients must understand the need for frequent postoperative office visits for examination and cleaning. This reduces the incidence of postoperative scarring, synechiae, and recurrence of surgical disease. Topical nasal decongestion and anesthesia in the office allow for thorough endoscopic evaluation and cleaning. Continued follow-up is a mainstay of successful treatment of chronic sinusitis.

◼ Suggested Reading

American Academy of Otolaryngology–Head and Neck Surgery. Intra-Operative Use of Computer Aided Surgery. http://www.entnet.org/Practice/policyIntraOperativeSurgery.cfm. Accessed November 27, 2012

Bolger WE, Brown CL, Church CA, et al. Safety and outcomes of balloon catheter sinusotomy: a multicenter 24-week analysis in 115 patients. Otolaryngol Head Neck Surg 2007;137(1):10–20

Bruggers S, Sindwani R. Evolving trends in powered endoscopic sinus surgery. Otolaryngol Clin North Am 2009;42(5):789–798, viii

Hepworth EJ, Bucknor M, Patel A, Vaughan WC. Nationwide survey on the use of image-guided functional endoscopic sinus surgery. Otolaryngol Head Neck Surg 2006;135(1):68–73

Levine HL, Sertich AP II, Hoisington DR, Weiss RL, Pritikin J; PatiENT Registry Study Group. Multicenter registry of balloon catheter sinusotomy outcomes for 1,036 patients. Ann Otol Rhinol Laryngol 2008;117(4):263–270

Setliff RC III, Parsons D. The "human" new instrumentation for functional endoscopic sinus surgery. Am J Rhinol 1994;8:275–278

Tewfik MA, Wormald PJ. Ten pearls for safe endoscopic sinus surgery. Otolaryngol Clin North Am 2010;43(4):933–944

87 Diagnosis and Therapy of Rhinologic Causes of Headache and Facial Pain

■ Introduction

Headache and facial pain, which are among the most frequent patient complaints, often accompany nasal pathology. With the recent refinements in both endoscopic instruments and imaging protocols, the diagnosis of these conditions has improved dramatically. However, there are still controversies with respect to the management of these patients.

Anatomy

The vast majority of the general sensory nerve fibers to the sinonasal tract are provided by the ophthalmic (V1) and maxillary (V2) divisions of the trigeminal nerve, with a very small contribution from the greater petrosal branch of the facial nerve. V1 traverses the cavernous sinus lateral to the sphenoid sinus and enters the posterior aspect of the orbit through the superior orbital fissure. Within the orbit, V1 gives rise to the nasociliary nerve. The nasociliary nerve branches into the anterior ethmoid (AE) and posterior ethmoid (PE) nerves. These two branches leave the orbit medially, course along the ethmoid roof/skull base, and enter the lateral lamella of the cribriform plate. Before entering the cribriform plate, AE and PE nerve branches supply sensory input to the superior and middle turbinates and the upper portion of the septum.

V2 exits the cranium via the foramen rotundum into the pterygopalatine (or sphenopalatine) fossa, and then courses along the roof of the maxillary sinus as the infraorbital nerve. The nasopalatine nerve, a major branch of V2, originates in the pterygopalatine fossa and exits the sphenopalatine foramen into the nasal cavity. The nasopalatine nerve then branches to supply the nasal septum via the posterosuperior medial nasal nerve, and the lateral nasal wall via the posterosuperior and posteroinferior lateral nasal nerves.

The parasympathetic supply of the nasal mucosa is derived from the greater superficial petrosal nerve (GSPN), which originates from the geniculate ganglion of the facial nerve and carries preganglionic parasympathetic fibers from the superior salivary nucleus. The GSPN joins the deep petrosal nerve, which carries sympathetic fibers from the sympathetic plexus on the internal carotid artery to form the vidian nerve. The latter then travels through the pterygopalatine ganglion, where the preganglionic parasympathetic nerves of the GSPN synapse. From the pterygopalatine ganglion, the postsynaptic parasympathetic fibers of the GSPN travel to innervate the nose, palate, and lacrimal glands.

Basic Science

Peripheral sensory nerve terminals can be found throughout the nasal mucosa on a microscopic level. Their greatest concentration is found in the subepithelial mucosa. Some of these sensory neurons respond to painful stimuli and are known as nociceptors. Normally, hypersensitivity to pain after injury is an adaptive response and aids in the healing process. However, nociceptors can become more sensitive to stimuli and sensory inputs following tissue injury, producing an exaggerated and prolonged pain. Hyperalgesia, or hypersensitivity to pain, is thought to involve both peripheral and central mechanisms.

Peripheral sensitization refers to a reduction in threshold and an increase in responsiveness of the peripheral ends of nociceptors transferring input from target organs to the central nervous system (CNS). Direct mechanical trauma appears to be one trigger for peripheral sensitization. In skin, nociceptors become sensitized following tissue injury, accounting for hyperalgesia to sustained pressure or static mechanical hyperalgesia at the site of the injury. Focal injuries to a peripheral nerve that leave it in continuity are frequently associated with pronounced hyperalgesia. This phenomenon is likely similar in nature to what takes place in areas of mucosal contact within the nasal cavity.

The effects of chemical agents or mediators released around the site of tissue damage or inflammation are also suspected of precipitating peripheral sensitization. Some agents can directly activate the ends of the peripheral nociceptors, signaling the presence of inflamed tissue and producing pain. Other agents, such as the inflammatory mediators bradykinin, histamine, and prostaglandin E_2 (PGE_2), are produced by activated cells at the site of injury or inflammation. Bradykinin acts on endothelial cells, causing them to increase vascular permeability and vasodilation, which generates the erythema, edema, and pain associated with acute inflammation. Histamine increases paracellular permeability through tight junctions and facilitates the interaction between antigens and T cells.

PGE_2 is produced by inflammatory cells via the cyclooxygenase (COX) pathway and also contributes to development of inflammatory pain. Enhanced extracellular levels of serotonin produced by mast cells and basophils have been detected during inflammatory states. Serotonin has also been implicated in the modulation of cytokine production by monocytes.

Central sensitization, the other mechanism thought to cause or exacerbate hyperalgesia, creates increased CNS neuron excitability to the point where normal inputs begin to produce abnormal responses. When synaptic connections between the nociceptor and the neurons of the spinal cord are altered after an insult, low-threshold sensory fibers begin to activate neurons in the CN that normally only respond to noxious stimuli. As a result, an input that would normally evoke an innocuous sensation now produces pain. Neurotransmitters and modulators such as excitatory synaptic transmitter glutamate and neuropeptides, including substance P (SP) and calcitonin gene-related peptide (CGRP), are released by the nociceptor central terminals and act on specific CNS receptors that increase the excitability of these neurons. In addition, the modification of CNS endogenous opioids contributes to central sensitization. Dynorphin is one such endogenous opioid that increases neuronal excitability, and COX-2, the enzyme that produces PGE_2.

The concentration of SP has been found to vary with the presence and type of sinus disease. Stammberger and Wolf measured SP concentrations in sinonasal mucosa of control patients and compared it to that of the sinonasal mucosa from chronic sinusitis patients. The control samples averaged ~ 2 ng SP/g of mucosa, and the diseases cohort averaged ~ 0.75 ng SP/g of mucosa. No SP was detected in nasal polyp tissues. These findings correlate well with the variability in pain severity seen in the clinical spectrum of sinus disease. Typically, acute sinusitis is associated with more severe pain than chronic sinus disease or nasal polyposis.

The presence of higher SP concentrations in normal mucosa can also explain how mucosal contact may give rise to pain of greater intensity than that associated with chronic sinusitis. Furthermore, airway epithelium elaborates enzymes, such as neural endopeptidase (NEP), which degrade the excitatory neuropeptides SP and CGRP. Should the sinonasal epithelium be denuded, not only are nerve terminals in the submucosa more exposed to stimulation, but the inhibiting effects of NEP are also lost. Sensitization is likely the result.

Following tissue damage, primary hyperalgesia occurs in the region of injury. Secondary hyperalgesia is located in the surrounding undamaged area or, in the case of referred pain, in a distant region. The trigeminal nucleus caudalis receives input from most of the ethmoidal afferent nerve fibers, as well as the nerves supplying other cephalic structures, providing a neuroanatomical mechanism for referred pain of rhinologic origin. Local anesthesia prevents the development of primary or secondary hyperalgesia, suggesting that both types of hyperalgesia depend on activity established in nerve fibers supplying the damaged area. The distribution of referred pain and secondary hyperalgesia depends on the intensity and duration of the noxious stimuli. The influence of the duration of stimulus on the spread of pain was shown experimentally by McAuliffe and Wolff, who noted that brief stimulation of the maxillary sinus ostium resulted in localized intranasal pain, whereas prolonged stimulation of the same area caused the spread of pain over the ipsilateral head and face.

In their classic experiments on human volunteers, McAuliffe, Goodell, and Wolff determined the intensity and patterns of referred pain resulting from stimulation of various intranasal structures. Their findings can be summarized as follows: (1) the mucosa covering the sinus ostia was the most pain sensitive in the sinonasal tract, followed by turbinate and septal mucosa, and the mucosa lining the sinus cavities was found to be least sensitive; (2) stimulation of structures within the sinonasal cavities produced referred pain rather than pain at the site of stimulation; and (3) inflammation and engorgement of turbinate mucosa, rather than the sinus mucosa itself, were responsible for the referred headache accompanying sinusitis.

Clerico and Grabo report in an unpublished communication that they repeated the experiments performed by McAuliffe et al with the aid of rigid nasal telescopes for precise placement of the stimuli. In contrast to McAuliffe's findings, they found that the posterosuperior aspect of the nasal cavity, in the region of the superior turbinate, is the most pain-sensitive area of the entire sinonasal tract. This corresponds anatomically to the area of greatest nerve trunk density. The sinus ostia were the next most sensitive, and the inferior turbinate and anterior septum were the least sensitive.

■ Pathology

The two broad categories of sinonasal pathology that can cause headache are sinus inflammatory disease (acute or chronic) and mucosal contact. In some patients, both exist simultaneously.

Sinus Inflammatory Disease

Headache/facial pain may accompany acute or chronic sinusitis. The pain associated with acute sinusitis is usually localized to the involved sinus(es), acute in onset, worse with bending and physical activity, worse in the morning on awakening, and accompanied by obvious nasal symptoms like congestion, obstruction, and purulent discharge. Less frequently, pain may radiate to neighboring structures, such as the temple, ear, and over the teeth and gums. Acute sinusitis typically follows a viral upper respiratory infection, and fever is more common in children than adults. Occasionally, the spread of an acute infection to the periorbital, ocular, and intracranial structures may necessitate urgent or emergent surgery. Acute sphenoidal sinusitis represents an exception to the foregoing patterns in that the location of pain can be the vertex, the occiput, retroorbital, or diffuse and poorly localized. Palpation over the sinus is impossible.

Headache pain from chronic sinusitis may exist in the absence of nasal symptoms such as congestion, rhinorrhea, and postnasal drip, making it more of a diagnostic challenge. The location of pain may be over the involved sinus, or it may be referred. The severity of pain in chronic sinus disease bears little relation to the extent of inflammatory disease, suggesting that other factors play a role in pain causation. Patients most frequently describe the pain as a pressure sensation, but it can take on almost any quality.

Sinogenic pain may be constant or intermittent and is often most intense in the morning. Headaches may increase in frequency or intensity with viral upper respiratory infections and changes in barometric pressure, such as often accompany weather changes.

Several authors have reported typical primary headache syndromes resulting from occult sinonasal pathology like migraine, cluster, and tension-type headaches. This suggests that the distinction between primary headaches and sinus-related headaches is not as clear as previously thought.

Mucosal Contact

Mucosal contact is becoming increasingly recognized as a source of referred headache. As early as 1888, septal-turbinate contact was described as a cause of referred headache in the absence of nasal symptoms. Numerous clinical studies have left little doubt that septal-turbinate compression can cause chronic headaches. Although mucosal contact can serve as the mechanical stimulus that compresses nerve terminals/axons in nasal mucosa, not all subjects demonstrating mucosal contact on nasal endoscopy or computed tomography (CT) have complaints of headaches.

The location, extent, and duration of mucosal contacts are three important factors that likely influence whether a patient has pain associated with a mucosal contact. Since the anterior-inferior aspects of the nasal cavity are generally less pain sensitive than the posterior-superior regions, mucosal contacts that are located posteriorly or superiorly tend to be more symptomatic. Mucosal contacts with long-standing large areas of contact would also be more likely to cause pain because larger areas of contact involve a greater number of stimulated nerve endings. In addition, central pain-modulating mechanisms like the release of endogenous opioids and the integrity of the mucosal neuropeptide-degrading enzymes, such NEP, may be compromised in clinical pain states and therefore impact the degree of facial pain or headache experienced by patients. Finally, hormonal, autonomic, and psychological factors can also influence the perception of pain in general.

■ Evaluation

History

In addition to the chief complaint and history of present illness, a thorough history of the facial pain or headache should include specific questions regarding the quality, duration, and associated symptoms and triggers of the patient's pain. The answers to these questions will yield invaluable clues regarding the patient's diagnosis and sometimes may help detect an impending cerebrovascular accident in an elderly patient that presents with an acute and severe headache. Patients with throbbing and pulsing pain often have vascular headaches, whereas those with a tight and drawing sensation commonly have a tension-type headache. The pain lasts for hours or days in migraine and tension headaches. Migraine is almost always accompanied by one or more associated symptoms, which include nausea, vomiting, photophobia, phonophobia, and dizziness. Migraines are frequently triggered by cigarette smoke, perfume, menses, chocolate, and wine.

Sharp, burning and boring pain is most often seen with cluster headaches. Cluster headache pain is usually very intense, but typically patients are pain-free for many weeks or even months between cluster attacks. Cluster headaches are characterized by lacrimation, rhinorrhea, and Horner syndrome ipsilateral to the side of the pain. Trigeminal neuralgia pain is usually described as a brief, sharp, and lancing pain that recurs. Headache and facial pain can manifest with any combination of these qualities. Similarly, although headache pain of sinogenic origin often presents with a pressure sensation, it can also be associated with any combination of the qualities already delineated.

■ Physical Exam

Nasal symptoms, such as obstruction, congestion, and postnasal drip, are an unreliable indicator of underlying nasal pathology, so the absence of nasal symptoms does not preclude a rhinologic origin of the headache. Conversely, the presence of nasal symptoms in a headache patient does not guarantee that the pain is of rhinologic origin. The clinician must bear in mind that comorbid conditions may exist in individual patients and should systematically and thoroughly evaluate each patient. Physical examination of the headache patient should consist of a complete head and neck exam, including palpation of the temporomandibular joints and cranial nerve evaluation. Although anterior rhinoscopy may be of some value in diagnosing acute sinusitis, it often fails to identify foci of disease in chronic ethmoid labyrinth disease or mucosal contacts. Therefore, diagnostic nasal endoscopy should be performed on most, if not all, of these patients. Rigid telescopes are preferred because of superior optical quality and the ability to use the other hand for instrumentation.

Although visualization of the ostiomeatal complex (OMC) is paramount in the sinusitis patient, the most important region in the chronic headache sufferer is the posterosuperior aspect of the nasal cavity. In particular, septal–turbinate mucosal contact at the level of the middle and superior turbinates should be noted. Such contact may result from septal abnormalities, such as deviations and spurs, or from turbinate anomalies, such as bony hypertrophy, pneumatization, paradoxical curvature, or other abnormalities. The otorhinolaryngologist should make every attempt to determine the significance of mucosal contact by seeing the patient during a headache attack, and applying a diagnostic block to the area of mucosal contact. If headache pain improves or resolves with anesthetizing the area of mucosal contact, then this contact is presumed to be the source of headache.

■ Imaging

Plain sinus radiographs have some value in the evaluation of a patient with acute sinusitis, unlike those with chronic sinusitis. Diagnostic nasal endoscopy and coronal CT of the paranasal sinuses should be used adjunctively in the workup of chronic sinus patients. Coronal sinus CT scans can help identify mucosal contact areas that are not readily apparent on direct nasal endoscopy. CT may therefore provide a roadmap for performing a diagnostic block. In this way, the role of CT scanning differs in the headache patient compared with the chronic sinus patient, where CT is generally obtained only after an adequate course of medical therapy. Both nasal endoscopy and CT should be employed in the workup of the headache patient.

■ Management

Medical

Treatment should start with conservative therapy and should proceed to endoscopic surgery only in refractory cases. Topical and systemic decongestants and topical and systemic glucocorticosteroids are first-line agents when mucosal contact alone is present. Patients with infrequent headaches may require no more than over-the-counter medications for occasional relief of pain. Inflammatory sinus disease should be treated with broad-spectrum antibiotics according to established protocols. Many times, a trial of medical therapy consisting of broad-spectrum oral antibiotics, nasal corticosteroid spray, decongestants, and/or oral steroids may provide clues as to the etiology of headache. If a patient responds with decreasing headache to the foregoing regimen, underlying sinonasal disease is likely present. However, failure to respond to such a regimen does not rule out headache of sinonasal origin. Topical anesthetics sprayed intranasally may be of both diagnostic and therapeutic value if mucosal contact is the etiology of the headache pain. Narcotic analgesics should be used sparingly.

Surgical

The endoscopic procedure of choice will differ for each patient, depending on the anatomy, presence of absence of sinusitis, and area(s) of mucosal contact.

Headache relief may be achieved by simply resecting a septal spur, or may require extensive pansinus surgery. In cases where septal–turbinate contact is the only finding, Clerico favors preserving the turbinate structures and resecting the lateral bony supports, such as the lateral lamella of a concha bullosa, or performing an ethmoidectomy if necessary. In rare cases, a pneumatized superior turbinate contacting the septum can be approached transnasally without ethmoidectomy. Great care must be taken when manipulating the superior turbinate due to its proximity to the cribriform plate. In some cases, the turbinate can simply be outfractured laterally with an elevator, avoiding the need for resection. Standard endoscopic approaches that do not specifically address mucosal contact areas are unlikely to provide long-term headache relief. Turbinate lateralization and/or partial resection should follow ethmoidectomy only in appropriate cases.

■ Controversies

Although a few anecdotal reports have shown that underlying sinonasal abnormalities or disease can masquerade as primary headache syndromes, the prevalence of mucosal contact points in the sinonasal tract is somewhat controversial. Moreover, it is still unclear whether these mucosal contact points are responsible for migraine, cluster, tension-type, and other primary headache syndromes. Only one study exists in which a systematic evaluation of the sinonasal cavity was performed in a group of migraine sufferers. In that study, a high prevalence of septal–turbinate contact in migraine patients was found by diagnostic nasal endoscopy and sinus CT. The CT prevalence of contact was significantly greater than that of the nonmigraine control group. Endoscopic sinonasal surgery, with particular intent to eliminate areas of mucosal contact, was highly successful at providing long-term headache relief, suggesting a cause-and-effect relationship between migraine and mucosal contact. Additional studies are needed to confirm these findings.

■ Suggested Reading

Chow JM. Rhinologic headaches. Otolaryngol Head Neck Surg 1994;111(3 Pt 1):211–218

Clerico DM. Pneumatized superior turbinate as a cause of referred migraine headache. Laryngoscope 1996;106(7):874–879

Clerico DM. Rhinopathic headaches. In: Gershwin ME, Incaudo GA, eds. Diseases of the Sinuses. Totowa, NJ: Humana Press; 1996:403–423

Clerico DM. Sinus headaches reconsidered: referred cephalgia of rhinologic origin masquerading as refractory primary headaches. Headache 1995;35(4):185–192

Clerico DM, Evan K, Montgomery L, Lanza DC, Grabo D. Endoscopic sinonasal surgery in the management of primary headaches. Rhinology 1997;35(3):98–102

Clerico DM, Grabo DJ. An experimental study of pain referred from the sinonasal cavity. Unpublished data

Dürk T, Panther E, Müller T, et al. 5-Hydroxytryptamine modulates cytokine and chemokine production in LPS-primed human monocytes via stimulation of different 5-HTR subtypes. Int Immunol 2005;17(5):599–606

Faleck H, Rothner AD, Erenberg G, Cruse RP. Headache and subacute sinusitis in children and adolescents. Headache 1988;28(2):96–98

Goldsmith AJ, Zahtz GD, Stegnjajic A, Shikowitz M. Middle turbinate headache syndrome. Am J Rhinol 1993;7:17–23

Hardy JD, Wolff HG, Goodell H. Pain sensations and reactions. Baltimore, MD: Williams and Wilkins; 1952

Hoover S. The nasal patho-physiology of headaches and migraines: diagnosis and treatment of the allergy, infection and nasal septal spurs that cause them. Rhinol Suppl 1987;2:1–23

Hucho T, Levine JD. Signaling pathways in sensitization: toward a nociceptor cell biology. Neuron 2007;55(3):365–376

Janković BD. Neuroimmunomodulation: facts and dilemmas. Immunol Lett 1989;21(2):101–118

Kawabata A. Prostaglandin E2 and pain—an update. Biol Pharm Bull 2011;34(8):1170–1173

Latremoliere A, Woolf CJ. Central sensitization: a generator of pain hypersensitivity by central neural plasticity. J Pain 2009;10(9):895–926

Lee M, Silverman SM, Hansen H, Patel VB, Manchikanti L. A comprehensive review of opioid-induced hyperalgesia. Pain Physician 2011;14(2):145–161

Lucier GE, Egizii R. Characterization of cat nasal afferents and brain stem neurones receiving ethmoidal input. Exp Neurol 1989;103(1):83–89

Maurer M, Bader M, Bas M, et al. New topics in bradykinin research. Allergy 2011;66(11):1397–1406

McAuliffe GW, Goodell H, Wolff HG. Experimental studies on headache: pain from the nasal and paranasal structures. Res Publ Assoc Res Nervous Ment Dis 1943;23:185–206

Okano M. Mechanisms and clinical implications of glucocorticosteroids in the treatment of allergic rhinitis. Clin Exp Immunol 2009;158(2):164–173

Pearce JMS. Chronic headache: the role of deformity of the nasal septum. [letter to the editor] Br Med J (Clin Res Ed) 1984; 288(6422):1005–1006

Roe JO. The frequent dependence of persistent and so-called congestive headaches upon abnormal conditions of the nasal passages. Med Record 1888;34:200–204

Ryan RE Sr, Ryan RE Jr. Headache of nasal origin. Headache 1979;19(3):173–179

Schønsted-Madsen U, Stoksted P, Christensen PH, Koch-Henriksen N. Chronic headache related to nasal obstruction. J Laryngol Otol 1986;100(2):165–170

Silverman SM. Opioid induced hyperalgesia: clinical implications for the pain practitioner. Pain Physician 2009;12(3):679–684

Stammberger H, Wolf G. Headaches and sinus disease: the endoscopic approach. Ann Otol Rhinol Laryngol Suppl 1988; 134(Suppl 134):3–23

Takano K, Kojima T, Go M, et al. HLA-DR- and CD11c-positive dendritic cells penetrate beyond well-developed epithelial tight junctions in human nasal mucosa of allergic rhinitis. J Histochem Cytochem 2005;53(5):611–619

Takeshima T, Nishikawa S, Takahashi K. Cluster headache like symptoms due to sinusitis: evidence for neuronal pathogenesis of cluster headache syndrome. Headache 1988;28(3):207–208

Willis WD Jr. Hyperalgesia and allodynia, summary and overview. In: Willis WD Jr, ed. Hyperalgesia and Allodynia. New York, NY: Raven; 1992:1–11

Woolf CJ. Central sensitization: implications for the diagnosis and treatment of pain. Pain 2011;152(3, Suppl):S2–S15

88 New Approaches to the Management of Epistaxis

Introduction

Epistaxis is a relatively common condition that is usually benign and self-limited, and only infrequently comes to the attention of health care providers. Even then, it is usually straightforward and successfully managed in a primary care setting. Paradoxically, epistaxis may present as a life-threatening condition that can challenge the skill and judgment of the most experienced otolaryngologist. Successful management requires knowledge of current treatment options and individualized decision making for each patient.

Epidemiology

The etiology of epistaxis is multifactorial and in 80% of patients remains idiopathic after thorough evaluation. In spite of this, there is an estimated global lifetime incidence of 60%. From an otolaryngological standpoint, epistaxis may account for up to 33% of emergency admissions with a median age of 70 years. The overall age of onset describes a bimodal distribution, with an increased incidence in childhood followed by a peak incidence in the sixth decade. Bleeding may also be classified as primary epistaxis (or idiopathic), which accounts for the majority of cases, or secondary epistaxis, which results from known local or systemic factors (**Table 88.1**).

There are many local causes of epistaxis, including sinonasal tumors, granulomatous disease, and septal perforation. However, the majority of these causes are iatrogenic or posttraumatic. In adolescent males with unilateral epistaxis and nasal obstruction, the presence of a juvenile nasopharyngeal angiofibroma should be ruled out. Systemic causes may include hypertension. In patients with multiple cutaneous, lip, oral, and intranasal telangiectasias, the diagnosis of hereditary hemorrhagic telangiectasia must be considered. Bleeding diatheses—the most common of which are hemophilia A followed by von Willebrand disease—are significant causes, with recent studies showing that disorders of primary hemostasis may play an even more significant role.

McGarry et al reported that 46% of patients with severe epistaxis exhibited a prolonged bleeding time. Also in their study they found a significant association between alcohol consumption and prolongation of the bleeding time. Alcohol inhibits platelet aggregation by reducing the activity of platelet cyclic adenosine monophosphate and decreasing thromboxane synthesis. These same antithrombotic effects are thought to be responsible for the reduced risk of coronary artery disease associated with moderate alcohol consumption (the French paradox). The antiplatelet effects of alcohol are dose related and are present at low levels of consumption. Alcohol consumption has also been associated with hemodynamic changes, such as hypertension and vasodilation, which may intensify its hemostatic effects.

There exists a correlation between epistaxis and the use of aspirin and other nonsteroidal anti-inflammatory drugs (NSAIDs). NSAIDs interfere with platelet function by altering the cyclooxygenase pathway of arachidonic acid metabolism. Epistaxis should be considered a potential complication of NSAID treatment, along with the more commonly recognized problems with gastrointestinal bleeding. This possibility is particularly important, given the increased NSAID use in the United States, with widespread over-the-counter availability and marketing to an aging population. Some studies have also suggested a seasonal variation in the incidence of epistaxis with episodes being more common in the fall and winter. Although this may reflect an overall decrease in the ambient humidity during the colder months, these findings have not been universally accepted.

Vascular Anatomy of the Nose

The nasal mucosa is supplied by blood vessels derived from both the internal and the external carotid arterial systems. These arborizations travel within the mucoperiosteal/perichondrial layers, except for

Table 88.1 Local and systemic factors for secondary epistaxis

Local	Systemic
Trauma (blunt, digital, devices)	Drugs (warfarin, NSAID, ASA)
Surgery (sinus, endoscopic skull base)	Bleeding diatheses
Anatomical deformities (septal deviation, spurs)	Hematologic malignancy
Sinonasal tumors (benign, vascular, malignant)	Hypertension
Foreign bodies	Hepatobiliary disease
Inflammation, granulomatous disease	Alcoholism
Topical medications	Vascular/connective tissue disorders
Low humidity	Malnutrition

Abbreviations: ASA, acetylsalicylic acid; NSAID, nonsteroidal anti-inflammatory drug.

small branches, which traverse bony canals within the inferior and middle turbinates.

Internal Carotid Arterial System

The internal carotid artery (ICA) supplies the nose via the ophthalmic artery, which gives off the anterior and posterior ethmoidal arteries. These arteries penetrate the anterior and posterior ethmoidal foramina within the frontoethmoid suture line to travel in bony canals within the ethmoid roof, finally entering the anterior cranial fossa through the lateral lamella of the cribriform plate. Intracranially, both arteries give rise to terminal branches that supply the anterior fossa dura and superior nasal cavity.

External Carotid Arterial System

The external carotid system provides contributions to the nasal mucosa via the facial artery and internal maxillary artery (IMA). The facial artery branches give rise to the superior labial artery, which projects a septal branch onto the anterior septum. Posteriorly, the IMA traverses the pterygopalatine fossa and enters the posterolateral nasal cavity as the sphenopalatine artery (SPA) via the sphenopalatine foramen. This branch carries the greatest volume of blood to the nose and is the source of most posteriorly based bleeds.

The crista ethmoidalis represents an important landmark for the position of the SPA and is located anteromedial to the sphenopalatine foramen in almost all cases. Although the number of SPA branches varies according to the reports, in one study, 73 of 75 cadaveric specimens demonstrated two or more branches of the SPA medial to the crista ethmoidalis. Consequently, when performing an SPA ligation, it is essential to explore the lateral wall of the nose, a maneuver that often requires resection of the crista ethmoidalis to enhance exposure. Once

the SPA exits the sphenopalatine foramen, its more distal posterolateral contributions may continue to exhibit significant variability. The posterior nasal branch of the SPA passes below the sphenoid ostium and travels anteriorly to anastomose in the Kiesselbach plexus.

■ Evaluation and Management of Anterior Epistaxis

When considering the management and prognosis of patients with epistaxis, it is useful to classify the bleeding site into anterior or posterior. Although there is no precise anatomical distinction between the two, anterior bleeds are more common and tend to originate on the septum, whereas posterior bleeds are generally higher volume and arise laterally from branches of the SPA. Anterior epistaxis usually arises from the septal vasculature. Within the literature, this area has been referred to as both the Little area, after James Little (an American physician who described four patients with a bleeding ulcer at this site) and the Kiesselbach plexus, after Wilhelm Kiesselbach (a German physician who subsequently described three patients with bleeding from distended vessels from this site). Control of bleeding from this area is usually not problematic when suction, lighting, and local anesthesia are adequate. The bleeding site may be cauterized with silver nitrate, electrocautery, or laser. Commonly used lasers include potassium-titanyl-phosphate and argon lasers. It is generally taught that cautery must not be applied bilaterally to the anterior nasal septum simultaneously, to avoid the potential risk of septal perforation. Although this is largely anecdotal and highly unlikely, the resultant perforation can be quite difficult to manage; thus bilateral cauterization is not recommended.

Anterior packing is used when the site cannot be visualized. This approach is less desirable than cautery because treatment is not focused. Although various products exist, globally they may be divided into absorbable and nonabsorbable materials. The development of biodegradable topical hemostatic agents has enabled a shift away from the exclusive use of nonabsorbable packing. These materials include oxidized cellulose, microfibrillar collagen, porcine or bovine gelatin, and human thrombin solutions, all of which serve to provide a platform for fibrin and platelet aggregation. In one randomized, nonblinded trial sponsored by Baxter Biosurgery that compared the gelatin-based agent Floseal (Baxter Healthcare Corp., Deerfield, IL) to nonabsorbable nasal packing, Floseal was found to significantly reduce the rate of rebleeding at 1 week. Although patient satisfaction and comfort were also improved with the absorbable agent, it should be noted that these agents tend to be more expensive than traditional packing.

An alternative mechanism for hemostasis has been exploited by a new class of aminopolysaccharide known as chitosan. Chitosan is strongly cationic and is able to attract red blood cells at the site of a vascular injury, thereby promoting hemostasis independent of the innate clotting cascade. A chitosan/dextran gel studied by Valentine et al was found to be both hemostatic and capable of inhibiting adhesion formation following sinus surgery.

If absorbable packing is ineffective, larger nonabsorbable packs may be considered. Modern expandable polyvinyl acetate (PVA) polymer sponges have largely replaced the traditional use of layered Vaseline petrolatum gauze strips. No statistically significant difference has been demonstrated between the use of ribbon gauze and a PVA sponge, but the latter is much easier to insert and more comfortable for the patient. Nasal packing containing lipid materials, such as petroleum, should be used with caution because they have been shown to be associated with myospherulosis.

Toxic shock syndrome (TSS) is a rare possibility associated with packing. TSS has not been shown to be associated with any particular type of packing, and it can neither be predicted nor prevented by prophylactic antibiotics. Given that most packs are removed after 1 to 7 days, the need for antibiotics is controversial, although they are still commonly used.

Intranasal balloon catheters are a popular option for control of epistaxis in the emergency room setting. They are less traumatic to the patient and more convenient for the physician to insert than gauze packs. Balloon catheters with a central airway have the added advantage of impacting less on arterial blood gases than conventional nasal packs. McGarry and Aitken performed anatomical studies to determine the mechanism of action of these devices in the human nose. They found that, contrary to manufacturers' descriptions, these devices do not conform to the internal contours of the nose. They tend to inflate along lines of least resistance, displacing the

septum and ala and expanding to fill the nasopharynx. Pressure necrosis of the nasal mucosa with a resultant septal perforation or intranasal adhesions is the most common local complication of intranasal balloon catheters. The incidence of complications is increased when the balloon is overinflated, when bilateral tamponade is required, or when the duration of inflation is > 24 hours.

■ Evaluation and Management of Posterior Epistaxis

Posterior epistaxis is active hemorrhage into the posterior pharynx, without identifiable anterior bleeding or severe nasal hemorrhage refractory to anterior packing. Intractable posterior epistaxis, estimated at 5% of all cases of epistaxis seen in primary care settings, is the most common ear, nose, and throat emergency requiring admission to a hospital. Both the condition and its various treatment options carry risks of serious complication and death, making it an important clinical entity.

Posterior epistaxis arises from large-bore arborizations of the internal maxillary and SPA and thus produces typically high-volume bleeds. Although initial management is similar to that of anterior epistaxis, tamponade must be directed toward the posterior nasal cavity and nasopharynx. Balloon packing with both anterior and posterior balloons has been developed for this purpose and provides excellent tamponade. If balloon packing is unavailable, the Foley catheter has also been used as a posterior nasal pack for several decades. Hartley and Axon investigated various methods of inflation and recommended a size 12 catheter with a 30 mL balloon.

Although considered conservative treatment, posterior nasal packing is far from benign. Bilateral posterior packs can theoretically induce the nasopulmonary reflex, leading to hypercarbia, hypoxia, and decreased lung volume. Thus hospital admission with telemetry monitoring is recommended. Posterior packing is poorly tolerated in some individuals because of extreme discomfort or adverse impact on cardiopulmonary dynamics; in these cases, early surgical intervention is warranted.

Although the question of when conservative measures should be abandoned and surgery or embolization should be considered remains unanswered, a trial of conservative management is usually recommended as first-line treatment. The success rate is dependent on the skill and care used in placing the pack and managing the patient while it is in place. Surgical management of epistaxis is typically reserved for patients whose bleeding is refractory to more conservative therapies, who have chronic or recurrent episodes, or who have had a single life-threatening bleed. The choice of procedure depends on a variety of preoperative factors, including, most important, the suspected site of bleeding.

Sphenopalatine Artery Ligation

The SPA can be exposed endoscopically by raising a posterolateral mucosal flap over the orbital process of the palatine bone. As the flap is elevated, the crista ethmoidalis and accessory posterolateral neurovascular bundles will be encountered. The SPA can then be identified and dissected from the surrounding tissue using a ball-tipped probe. The artery may be occluded using clips, bipolar cautery, or some combination thereof. If bipolar cautery is to be used, it should precede clip application, because tissue desiccation may shrink the tissue away from a previously applied clip.

Dissection should be continued posteriorly toward the choanal arch to rule out the possibility of an additional posterior nasal branch that may enter the nose through a separate foramen posterior to the SPA. Alternatively, the artery may be traced laterally into the pterygopalatine fossa to ligate it prior to its terminal bifurcation. The mucosal flap may then be replaced, which hastens remucosalization and can often avoid the need for nasal packing.

Ethmoidal Artery Ligation

The ethmoidal vessels may be accessed within the orbit using a limited medial canthal (Lynch) incision. This incision is often broken into a seagull shape to prevent linear contracture postoperatively. The anterior ethmoidal artery is identified running from the periorbita into its foramen at the frontoethmoidal suture. This suture line is typically located immediately superior to the medial canthus, so care should be taken not to disrupt the canthal tendons during the periorbital dissection. The posterior ethmoidal artery may be found ~ 12 mm posterior to the anterior ethmoidal artery. Once exposed, the arteries can be clipped or divided following diathermy or suture ligature. Some authors have also described endoscopic identification and cauterization of the anterior ethmoid artery, either within the ethmoid roof or intraorbitally, following removal of the lamina papyracea.

■ Embolization

Selective angiography with embolization of the distal IMA (with or without embolization of the facial artery) was introduced in 1974 as an alternative to vessel ligation in intractable epistaxis. Over the following decades, several series have confirmed the efficacy of angiographic embolization in treating intractable epistaxis. This technique requires an experienced neuroradiologist and sophisticated equipment, which are not available at all medical centers. Angiographic embolization is indicated as a primary treatment if arterial ligation has been unsuccessful and for epistaxis secondary to vascular anomalies, bleeding disorders, trauma, or tumor. Unlike arterial ligation, angiographic embolization can be performed under local anesthesia, making it a useful modality in the medically compromised patient with high anesthetic risk.

The most common complications of angiographic embolization are temporofacial pain, paresthesias, trismus, and skin necrosis due to local tissue ischemia. Inadvertent reflux of embolic material into the ICA with resultant blindness or stroke is a rare but potentially serious complication. Angiographic embolization is contraindicated in patients with middle meningeal artery–ophthalmic artery anastomoses; retrograde supply to the IMA by the artery of the foramen rotundum; middle meningeal artery as the primary supply to the ipsilateral cerebral cortex; or other ICA–external carotid artery anastomoses. Angiographic embolization is also contraindicated when bleeding is from the anterior ethmoid artery.

The most frequently reported major complication of angiographic embolization is facial paralysis. Aberrant embolization of the petrosal branch of the middle meningeal artery, which originates from the IMA, may compromise blood flow to the geniculate ganglion and facial nerve. In the facial canal, the nerve is supplied by anastomoses between the petrosal branch of the middle meningeal artery, the caroticotympanic branch of the ICA, and the stylomastoid branch, which originates from either the occipital or the retroauricular artery. Recent technical refinements, including the use of a superselective coaxial catheter system, may decrease the risks of aberrant embolization of IMA branches that do not contribute to nasal blood supply.

■ Summary

Epistaxis is a common problem and requires intervention in the minority of cases. Nasal endoscopy is recommended as an important diagnostic technique in the evaluation of the site and etiology of epistaxis, which is critical when determining treatment options. Conservative measures should be used as a first-line intervention, although in refractory, recurrent, or life-threatening bleeding, surgical management should be considered.

Angiographic embolization is typically reserved for patients who fail to respond to or are not candidates for surgical management. Controversy regarding which of these two options constitutes optimal treatment exists in the literature. The lack of uniform reporting criteria defining success and complication rates makes it difficult to state which of the available treatment options is the procedure of choice. Optimal treatment of posterior epistaxis must be highly individualized. It must be based on the needs of the patient, on the experience and training of the physician, and on the availability of resources.

■ Suggested Reading

Bleier BS, Kennedy DW, Palmer JN, Chiu AG, Bloom JD, O'Malley BW Jr. Current management of juvenile nasopharyngeal angiofibroma: a tertiary center experience 1999-2007. Am J Rhinol Allergy 2009;23(3):328–330

Bleier BS, Schlosser RJ. Endoscopic anatomy of the postganglionic pterygopalatine innervation of the posterolateral nasal mucosa. Int Forum Allergy Rhinol 2011;1(2):113–117 doi: 10.1002/alr.20011

Bray D, Giddings CE, Monnery P, Eze N, Lo S, Toma AG. Epistaxis: are temperature and seasonal variations true factors in incidence? J Laryngol Otol 2005;119(9):724–726

Corbridge RJ, Djazaeri B, Hellier WPL, Hadley J. A prospective randomized controlled trial comparing the use of Merocel nasal tampons and BIPP in the control of acute epistaxis. Clin Otolaryngol Allied Sci 1995;20(4):305–307

Faughnan ME, Palda VA, Garcia-Tsao G, et al; HHT Foundation International - Guidelines Working Group. International guidelines for the diagnosis and management of hereditary haemorrhagic telangiectasia. J Med Genet 2011;48(2):73–87

Hartley C, Axon PR. The Foley catheter in epistaxis management—a scientific appraisal. J Laryngol Otol 1994;108(5):399–402

Livesey JR, Watson MG, Kelly PJ, Kesteven PJ. Do patients with epistaxis have drug-induced platelet dysfunction? Clin Otolaryngol Allied Sci 1995;20(5):407–410

Mathiasen RA, Cruz RM. Prospective, randomized, controlled clinical trial of a novel matrix hemostatic sealant in patients with acute anterior epistaxis. Laryngoscope 2005;115(5):899–902

McGarry GW, Aitken D. Intranasal balloon catheters: how do they work? Clin Otolaryngol Allied Sci 1991;16(4):388–392

McGarry GW, Gatehouse S, Vernham G. Idiopathic epistaxis, haemostasis and alcohol. Clin Otolaryngol Allied Sci 1995;20(2):174–177

Metson R, Lane R. Internal maxillary artery ligation for epistaxis: an analysis of failures. Laryngoscope 1988;98(7):760–764

Pletcher SD, Metson R. Endoscopic ligation of the anterior ethmoid artery. Laryngoscope 2007;117(2):378–381

Rotenberg B, Tam S. Respiratory complications from nasal packing: systematic review. J Otolaryngol Head Neck Surg 2010;39(5):606–614

Shires CB, Boughter JD, Sebelik ME. Sphenopalatine artery ligation: a cadaver anatomic study. Otolaryngol Head Neck Surg 2011;145(3):494–497

Simmen DB, Raghavan U, Briner HR, Manestar M, Groscurth P, Jones NS. The anatomy of the sphenopalatine artery for the endoscopic sinus surgeon. Am J Rhinol 2006;20(5):502–505

Sindwani R, Cohen JT, Pilch BZ, Metson RB. Myospherulosis following sinus surgery: pathological curiosity or important clinical entity? Laryngoscope 2003;113(7):1123–1127

Snyderman CH, Goldman SA, Carrau RL, Ferguson BJ, Grandis JR. Endoscopic sphenopalatine artery ligation is an effective method of treatment for posterior epistaxis. Am J Rhinol 1999;13(2):137–140

Strong EB, Bell DA, Johnson LP, Jacobs JM. Intractable epistaxis: transantral ligation vs. embolization: efficacy review and cost analysis. Otolaryngol Head Neck Surg 1995;113(6):674–678

Valentine R, Athanasiadis T, Moratti S, Hanton L, Robinson S, Wormald PJ. The efficacy of a novel chitosan gel on hemostasis and wound healing after endoscopic sinus surgery. Am J Rhinol Allergy 2010;24(1):70–75

Viehweg TL, Roberson JB, Hudson JW. Epistaxis: diagnosis and treatment. J Oral Maxillofac Surg 2006;64(3):511–518

Walker TWM, Macfarlane TV, McGarry GW. The epidemiology and chronobiology of epistaxis: an investigation of Scottish hospital admissions 1995-2004. Clin Otolaryngol 2007;32(5):361–365

Weber R, Keerl R, Hochapfel F, Draf W, Toffel PH. Packing in endonasal surgery. Am J Otolaryngol 2001;22(5):306–320

Winstead W. Sphenopalatine artery ligation: an alternative to internal maxillary artery ligation for intractable posterior epistaxis. Laryngoscope 1996;106(5 Pt 1):667–669

89 Endoscopic Management of Cerebrospinal Fluid Rhinorrhea

■ Introduction

Anatomy

Cerebrospinal fluid (CSF) is predominantly produced (50–80%) in the choroid plexus. Other sites of CSF production include the ependymal surface layer and capillary ultrafiltration. CSF is produced at a rate of 20 mL/h or ~ 500 mL/d. At any given time, ~ 90 to 150 mL of CSF is circulating throughout the central nervous system. CSF produced at the choroid plexus typically circulates from the lateral ventricles to the third ventricle via the aqueduct of Sylvius. From the third ventricle, the fluid circulates into the fourth ventricle and exits the fourth ventricle into the subarachnoid space via the foramina of Magendie and Luschka. After circulating through the subarachnoid space, CSF is reabsorbed via the arachnoid villi.

CSF is composed of water, electrolytes, glucose, amino acids, and various proteins, including b-2-transferrin, a protein found only in CSF, aqueous humor, and perilymph. It is not found in saliva, tears, sputum, serum, or routine nasal secretions.

With its presence within the subarachnoid space, CSF is separated from the nasal cavity via multiple layers. The arachnoid surrounds the brain and spinal cord and is attached to the inside of the dura mater. The bone of the skull base also separates CSF from the nasal cavity. No matter the cause, disruption in the arachnoid and dura mater, coupled with an osseous defect and a CSF pressure gradient that is continuously or intermittently greater than the tensile strength of the disrupted tissue, is the underlying defect in CSF rhinorrhea.

■ Etiology and Epidemiology

The causes of CSF rhinorrhea may be categorized as congenital, traumatic, or spontaneous.

Congenital CSF Rhinorrhea

Congenital CSF rhinorrhea results from failed closure of the anterior neuropore, with herniation of central nervous tissue through the skull base. Although these defects may be diagnosed in childhood, many patients present as adults with long-standing histories of CSF rhinorrhea.

Traumatic CSF Rhinorrhea

The cause of CSF rhinorrhea is most often traumatic. Traumatic CSF rhinorrhea may be related to blunt force or penetrating injury. It may further be subdivided into iatrogenic and tumor-related trauma. Blunt or penetrating trauma may lead to CSF rhinorrhea from disruption of the bony skull base and dura, with the bony disruption usually identified on computed tomography (CT). The leak may present immediately or may be delayed. If delayed, the leak usually presents within 3 months. Iatrogenic CSF rhinorrhea is typically caused during functional endoscopic sinus surgery (FESS) or neurosurgical procedures. However, in terms of the total number of FESS cases, CSF leaks are relatively uncommon, occurring in < 1% of cases. Many iatrogenic injuries occur at the lateral lamella of the cribriform plate, highlighting the importance of evaluating the height of the olfactory fossa on preoperative imaging. Other sites include the posterior fovea ethmoidalis and the posterior aspect of the frontal recess. Neurosurgical procedures that lead to CSF rhinorrhea include transsphenoidal hypophysectomy and other endoscopic resection of sellar and suprasellar lesions. Aggressive nasal tumors can cause the erosion of bone and disruption of dura, leading to CSF rhinorrhea.

Spontaneous CSF Rhinorrhea

Spontaneous CSF leaks occur in the absence of congenital or traumatic causes. However, in many cases, spontaneous CSF leaks may actually represent a variant of benign intracranial hypertension, also known as idiopathic intracranial hypertension, or pseudotumor cerebri. Increased intracranial pressure (ICP) leads to a thinning of the bone of the skull base, typically along the cribriform plate or lateral recess of the sphenoid sinus. Eventually, a skull base defect develops with herniation of meninges, or meninges and brain parenchyma. In some cases, multiple defect sites form. Dural injury can then lead to CSF rhinorrhea. Patients affected are typically middle-aged, obese females.

Not all spontaneous CSF leaks exhibit elevated ICP. Patients with normal ICP, but no other cause for a CSF leak, may develop rhinorrhea from focal atrophy, rupture of arachnoid projections that accompany the fibers of the olfactory nerve, and persistence of an embryonic olfactory lumen.

■ Evaluation

Patients with CSF rhinorrhea usually complain of unilateral, or sometimes bilateral, nasal discharge. This may be worsened with changes in head position. In the absence of a significant surgical or trauma history, patients are often treated for extended periods of time for rhinitis without any significant improvement. In addition to rhinorrhea, patients may complain of headaches, pulsatile tinnitus, or visual disturbances, which may be indications of ICP. Headaches may be improved with an increase in rhinorrhea, which leads to a decrease of the ICP. Patients should also be questioned about a history of meningitis.

In patients with a question of CSF rhinorrhea, a complete head and neck exam should be performed, including nasal endoscopy. Nasal endoscopy may reveal a meningocele or encephalocele, and can show the state of the sinuses after sinus surgery. Drainage of CSF may be elicited by having the patient perform a Valsalva maneuver. In patients without obvious rhinorrhea, evidence of a CSF leak can be elicited by placing them in the "provocative position," with their head immediately above their knees while sitting in a chair. If rhinorrhea is noted, the fluid can be collected for analysis. The simplest form of analysis is to place several drops of the CSF on filter paper or a paper tissue. CSF is relatively devoid of the protein present in blood and mucus, and should leave a clear, homogeneous ring as the fluid spreads on the paper. When CSF is mixed with blood, a series of concentric rings appears as the fluid is absorbed by the paper. However, this "halo sign" is problematic, because mucus and other body fluids mixed with blood can give a false-positive sign.

A more specific analysis is a CSF test for the presence of b-2-transferrin. Beta-2-transferrin is a protein found in CSF, perilymph, and aqueous humor.

Its detection confirms the presence of a CSF leak. In patients with a confirmed CSF leak based on b-2-transferrin, a high-resolution CT scan of the paranasal sinuses may specify the location of the leak. CT scan may reveal specific disruption of the bony skull base or the presence of opacification in the paranasal sinuses, indicating possible encephalocele or meningoencephalocele. Magnetic resonance imaging can specifically show continuity of these lesions with the intracranial cavity. Imaging findings suggestive of elevated intracranial pressures such as empty sella or increased tortuosity of the optic nerves may also add to the suggestion of CSF leak. In all cases of confirmed leakage, it is recommended that brain imaging be accomplished to rule out other pathology, such as tumors, that may be contributing.

In some cases, patients are unable to elicit fluid for laboratory evaluation, and high-resolution CT scanning does not reveal any evidence of the leak site. In such cases, where the presence of a CSF leak remains in question, isotope cisternography may be performed. This procedure involves the placement of a radioisotope-labeled agent within the subarachnoid space, followed by scanning of the head for evidence of CSF draining into the nose. Neurosurgical cottonoids or pledgets of cotton are also placed within the nasal cavity to attempt to isolate the site of leakage of CSF into the nose. Specifically, cottonoids are placed in the nasopharynx, beneath the middle turbinate, and between the middle turbinate and septum.

Detection of elevated radioactivity relative to plasma radioactivity on cottonoids placed within the nasopharynx suggests the site of the fistula may be in the ear, with fluid emerging via the eustachian tube, or from an injury to the middle fossa or sphenoid sinus. Radioactivity of the middle meatus cottonoid suggests an injury to the roof of the ethmoid sinus. The presence of the radioactive agent on cottonoids placed in the olfactory cleft is consistent with a communication from the subarachnoid space via the cribriform plate or at its articulation with the septum or middle turbinates. This study may help confirm the presence and narrow the focus for location of a CSF leak in the absence of clear laboratory and other radiological findings. However, it should be noted that this study is associated with a significant false-positive rate.

■ Management

Once the presence of a CSF leak has been established, the goals of treatment are to establish a watertight closure and prevent ascending meningitis. If a CSF leak occurs during a surgery and is noticed immediately, repair should be performed at the time of surgery, provided the operating surgeon feels comfortable with the repair of skull base injuries.

In traumatic CSF leaks, it is reasonable to attempt conservative measures, including stool softeners, bed rest, and lumbar drainage for a period of time to assist with spontaneous closure of the traumatic defect. However, long-term postinjury follow-up has demonstrated up to a 29% incidence of subsequent meningitis in these patients, leading to the question of whether more of these leaks should be repaired.

In traumatic CSF leaks that fail to respond to conservative measures, and in all other instances of CSF rhinorrhea, surgical management is indicated. An endoscopic approach to closure of the CSF fistula has shown initial success rates of over 90% in multiple series, making it the approach of choice in most cases of CSF rhinorrhea. The procedure begins with identification of the specific leak site. If preoperative imaging does not provide information regarding the site of the defect, the use of intrathecal fluorescein can greatly assist identification of the CSF leak site. A solution of 0.1 mL of 10% fluorescein mixed with 10 mL of the patient's own CSF or nonbacteriostatic saline is injected intrathecally through a lumbar puncture. Because intrathecal fluorescein is not approved by the U.S. Food and Drug Administration for intrathecal injection, its use should be accompanied by fully informed consent. Complications of intrathecal fluorescein include seizures, headaches, and cranial nerve deficits. However, the safety of low-dose intrathecal fluorescein (as described here) infused slowly has been established in many series.

Once the leak site has been identified, the mucous membrane and fragments of bone and arachnoid must be debrided from around and within the fistula site. Less than meticulous preparation of the defect site will result in failure of closure. Furthermore, failure to remove the nasal mucosa, if then covered by the repair materials, may lead to mucocele formation in the future. Meningoceles or encephaloceles should be reduced with bipolar cautery or coblation.

Multiple studies have shown that the type of tissue used for leak closure does not significantly affect success rates. Materials used include fat, fascia, acellular dermis, and pericranium, to name a few. Free grafts are shown to have good success in closure of CSF fistula. Some surgeons use tissue glues to provide additional sealant of the graft. Also, some studies indicate improved success in the closure of large defects with pedicled septal flaps based on the sphenopalatine artery. No matter what graft material is used, it needs to be kept in place with some combination of absorbable or nonabsorbable packing. The specific type of packing used varies from series to series, and one type has not been established as the material of choice. Examples include Gelfoam, Surgicel, and Merocel packing.

Postoperatively, patients should be placed on stool softeners to avoid straining, which increases intracranial pressure. Nose blowing is discouraged, and opening of the mouth is recommended on sneezing, to avoid pneumocephalus. Some authors advocate bed rest for a period of time after surgery, whereas others do not believe such restrictions are necessary.

In patients with spontaneous CSF leaks, further evaluation of ICP may be required to ensure successful treatment. Elevated ICP does not become evident until after closure of the CSF fistula, so evaluation should occur after successful closure of the fistula. Patients with elevated ICP may benefit from treatment with acetazolamide, a carbonic anhydrase inhibitor diuretic that decreases CSF production, thereby decreasing ICP. Ventriculoperitoneal shunts are occasionally needed in patients with spontaneous leaks that recur postclosure, in patients with very high intracranial pressures, or for patients who fail to respond to acetazolamide.

◼ Controversial Issues

The use of lumbar drains postoperatively is controversial. Although some surgeons routinely use lumbar drains postoperatively, others do not use them as standard practice. These drains are often used diagnostically, in conjunction with intrathecal fluorescein. However, their role postoperatively is not clearly elucidated. The concept of using a lumbar drain after CSF leak repair, to lower intracranial pressure and allow the graft to heal, does make intuitive sense. However, many series have shown good closure success without the use of postoperative lumbar drainage.

The use of prophylactic antibiotics in traumatic CSF leaks is another area of controversy. In an attempt to decrease the incidence of meningitis, prophylactic antibiotics are often used to prevent contamination of the intracranial space from the nasal cavity. However, other surgeons believe the use of prophylactic antibiotics leads to the selection of resistant organisms. A recent Cochrane review concluded that the evidence does not support the use of prophylactic antibiotics to reduce the risk of meningitis in patients with skull base fractures or skull base fractures with active CSF leak. The evidence failed to identify a benefit of prophylactic antibiotic use. Therefore, routine use of prophylactic antibiotics in CSF leaks is not supported by current literature.

◼ Conclusion

Overall, the endoscopic repair of patients with congenital, traumatic, or spontaneous CSF rhinorrhea has resulted in a successful permanent closure rate of over 90%.

■ Suggested Reading

Banks CA, Palmer JN, Chiu AG, O'Malley BW Jr, Woodworth BA, Kennedy DW. Endoscopic closure of CSF rhinorrhea: 193 cases over 21 years. Otolaryngol Head Neck Surg 2009;140(6):826–833

Bernal-Sprekelsen M, Bleda-Vázquez C, Carrau RL. Ascending meningitis secondary to traumatic cerebrospinal fluid leaks. Am J Rhinol 2000;14(4):257–259

Hadad G, Bassagasteguy L, Carrau RL, et al. A novel reconstructive technique after endoscopic expanded endonasal approaches: vascular pedicle nasoseptal flap. Laryngoscope 2006;116(10):1882–1886

Placantonakis DG, Tabaee A, Anand VK, Hiltzik D, Schwartz TH. Safety of low-dose intrathecal fluorescein in endoscopic cranial base surgery. Neurosurgery 2007;61(3, Suppl):161–165, discussion 165–166

Prosser JD, Vender JR, Solares CA. Traumatic cerebrospinal fluid leaks. Otolaryngol Clin North Am 2011;44(4):857–873, vii

Psaltis AJ, Schlosser RJ, Banks CA, Yawn J, Soler ZM. A systematic review of the endoscopic repair of cerebrospinal fluid leaks. Otolaryngol Head Neck Surg 2012;147(2):196–203

Ratilal B, Costa J, Sampaio C. Antibiotic prophylaxis for preventing meningitis in patients with basilar skull fractures. Cochrane Database Syst Rev 2006;(1):CD004884

Stankiewicz JA. Cerebrospinal fluid fistula and endoscopic sinus surgery. Laryngoscope 1991;101(3):250–256

Wang EW, Vandergrift WA III, Schlosser RJ. Spontaneous CSF Leaks. Otolaryngol Clin North Am 2011;44(4):845–856, vii

90 Optic Canal Decompression and Dacryocystorhinostomy

■ Optic Canal Decompression

Introduction

Compression of the optic nerve can be attributable to a wide variety of etiologies, including trauma, hyperostosis, neoplastic lesions, vascular malformations, and sinus disease, which can all produce a compartment syndrome. Left untreated, the optic nerve can undergo ischemia, resulting in optic neuropathy and, ultimately, irreversible vision loss.

The optic nerve consists of ~ 1 to 1.2 million ganglion cell axons. It initially traverses the sclera through the lamina cribrosa, at which point it acquires both a myelin coating and a dural sheath. Although the intraorbital segment of the optic nerve spans ~ 28 mm to the optic canal, the distance from the posterior aspect of the globe to the orbital apex is only 18 mm. This extra length allows the globe to rotate freely and also accommodates axial shifts within the orbit. The vast majority of blood supply for the optic nerve is derived from branches of the ophthalmic artery.

The optic canal is located within the lesser wing of the sphenoid bone, running in a superior (15 degree) and medial (45 degree) direction for ~ 8 to 10 mm. The orientation and course of the optic canal allow for the visualization of its medial wall using an anterior surgical approach through the sphenoid sinus. The optic nerve, ophthalmic artery, and sympathetic nerves all pass through the optic canal. As the nerve enters the canal, its dural sheath fuses with the periorbita, leaving the intracanalicular segment particularly susceptible to traumatic injury. Upon its exit from the canal, the nerve passes under the falciform ligament, where it subsequently runs for 8 to 12 mm prior to termination at the optic chiasm.

Evaluation

The clinical evaluation of patients with suspected optic nerve dysfunction is directed toward the detection, quantification, and localization of the cul-prit lesion. The examination focuses on assessment of best-corrected visual acuity, color vision testing, pupillary testing, funduscopy, and visual field testing, which all serve as markers of optic nerve function.

Appropriate imaging in this setting is largely dependent on the suspected etiology. Computed tomography (CT) is ideal for traumatic injuries, because it allows for the detection of bony fractures and hemorrhages. However, it is important to note that traumatic optic neuropathy can also occur in the absence of fractures. CT is also useful in the detection of fibro-osseous tumors within the orbit because these lesions often exhibit characteristic patterns on imaging. For instance, fibrous dysplasia often exhibits a poorly defined ground-glass appearance, stemming from the lucency and sclerosis of bone. In contrast, magnetic resonance imaging (MRI) is preferred over CT in cases of suspected neoplastic, inflammatory, and cystic lesions.

Management

Decompression of the optic canal can be considered in cases of progressive constriction that impairs or threatens optic nerve function. The goal of surgical intervention is predicated on relieving pressure within the canal caused by optic nerve edema. However, there is a complex interplay between ischemia, demyelination, and axonal degeneration that makes the potential functional benefit of surgery difficult to predict.

Adequate decompression of the optic canal involves removal of half the circumference of the osseous canal, removal of bone in a longitudinal dimension that spans the extent of the canal, and total longitudinal incision of the dural sheath that includes the annulus of Zinn. Multiple surgical approaches have been described in the literature, including extracranial, transcranial, and endoscopic transnasal techniques. The appropriate surgical approach is dependent on a wide range of clinical considerations, such as the location of the lesion, and often entails a thorough multidisciplinary assessment. For instance, the transcranial approach provides optimal access to the roof of the optic canal and can also be used to address concurrent intracranial pathology. On the other hand, the endoscopic approach provides infero-medial access to the canal, whereas the extracranial transethmoidal approach tends to be preferred for pathology that is limited to the intracanalicular portion of the optic nerve.

Controversial Issues

In general, data favoring optic canal decompression are strongest in the setting of compression by extrinsic tumors and secondary mass lesions, as seen in fibrous dysplasia. In contrast, decompression for intracanalicular meningiomas and traumatic optic nerve sheath hematomas is supported only by anecdotal reports. Appropriate management for traumatic optic neuropathy is even less clear and remains a controversial topic. Although some groups favor treatment with high-dose corticosteroids, others support surgical intervention, particularly if bone fragments are seen on imaging. Close observation also appears to be a reasonable strategy. The International Optic Nerve Trauma Study, a prospective observational study published in 1999, did not show any clear functional benefit in patients treated with high-dose steroids or surgical canal decompression, compared with those who were simply observed. Of note, 57% of the observation group exhibited an improvement in visual acuity of three lines or greater, reflecting the potential for spontaneous improvement following trauma.

Summary

Ultimately, the efficacy of optic canal decompression remains unproven and carries many inherent risks related to the technical difficulty of the procedure. As a result, its use is relatively rare in common practice and is typically reserved for only a select subset of patients.

◼ Dacryocystorhinostomy

Introduction

The lacrimal drainage system originates at the puncta, which are located on the medial aspect of the upper and lower eyelids. Each punctum leads to a canaliculus, which extends inferiorly for 2 mm into an ampulla, turns 90 degrees, and then runs an additional 8 to 10 mm medially prior to drainage into the lacrimal sac. The upper and lower canaliculi com-

bine to form a common canaliculus in nearly 100% of patients. Reflux within the drainage system is prevented by a combination of the acute angle taken by the common canaliculus into the lacrimal sac as well as the valve of Rosenmüller, a fold of mucous membrane with multiple anatomical variants that is present at this junction.

The lacrimal sac is situated within a bony fossa, where it subsequently leads into the nasolacrimal duct (NLD). The NLD measures ~ 12 mm and ultimately opens into the nasal cavity through an ostium located underneath the inferior turbinate. This ostium is covered by a mucosal fold known as the valve of Hasner.

Obstruction can occur at any point within the lacrimal drainage system, leading to conditions such as epiphora and dacryocystitis. Acquired nasolacrimal duct obstruction (NLDO) can be associated with a wide variety of etiologies, including involutional stenosis, dacryoliths, sinus disease, inflammation, trauma, and neoplasia.

Evaluation

Because patients with NLDO most commonly present with excess tearing, the clinical examination revolves around distinguishing hypersecretion of tears (lacrimation) from impaired drainage (epiphora). This can be accomplished through careful assessment of the tear meniscus and tear film breakup time, as well as Schirmer testing. It is important to note that both lacrimation and epiphora may be present concurrently.

Further evaluation is warranted in patients determined to have restricted outflow. In the dye disappearance test, fluorescein dye is placed into the conjunctival fornices and assessed for any persistence or discrepancy in the rate of drainage at 5 minutes. Similarly, the Jones I test involves checking for fluorescein at the ostium following its instillation into the fornices. If unsuccessful, the clinician can then perform the Jones II test by irrigating the drainage system with saline. The composition of the irrigated fluid, in conjunction with the reflux pattern, is used to characterize and localize the underlying obstruction.

Irrigation can also be implemented as a stand-alone measure to assess the patency of the lacrimal drainage system. This procedure is performed by advancing an irrigating cannula into the horizontal canaliculus, followed by saline injection. Again, the location and degree of reflux from the system is used to identify the site of obstruction. Probing can confirm obstructions of the punctum, canaliculus, or lacrimal sac.

The primary imaging modalities used in the setting of NLDO include endoscopy, which provides direct visualization of the nasal passages and lacrimal drainage system, as well as contrast dacryocystography and dacryoscintigraphy. CT and MRI are typically used only as adjunctive modalities in the evaluation of patients with concurrent sinus or nasal disease.

Management

Dacryocystorhinostomy (DCR) is the treatment of choice for patients with acquired NLDO. Because NLDO can often lead to dacryocystitis, surgery must be deferred until any active infection has been adequately treated.

DCR involves the creation of a rhinostomy between the lacrimal sac fossa and the nasal cavity, and can be performed using either an external or an internal (endoscopic) approach. Classically, external DCR has been associated with a higher efficacy rate, although recent reports have estimated success rates of internal DCR to be ~ 90%, which is at least comparable to the rates reported using the external technique.

External DCR involves the creation of a skin incision to gain adequate access for the creation of an osteotomy. Anterior mucosal flaps, and occasionally posterior flaps, are then created between the lacrimal sac and the nasal mucosa. Once the flaps have been secured, Crawford tubes are passed through the canaliculi into the ostium and tied together in the nose. After the system has been intubated, the flaps and skin incision are closed.

In the internal approach, an osteotomy is performed to remove the frontal process of the maxilla and the lacrimal bone overlying the lacrimal sac. After appropriate access has been obtained, the lacrimal sac is then opened and marsupialized into the nose. In contrast to the external technique, flaps are usually not created during endoscopic DCR. Following creation of the fistula, bicanalicular intubation is then performed. Many variations of the internal approach have been described in the literature, such as the implementation of balloon catheters and laser.

Summary

Choosing between the external and internal DCR approaches is dependent on multiple factors, including the context and severity of symptoms, various anatomical considerations, and prior surgical history, as well as patient and surgeon preference. A report released by the American Academy of Ophthalmology in 2001 did not offer any definitive guidelines due to the lack of data directly comparing the two techniques. Nevertheless, the endoscopic DCR technique has grown in popularity in recent times, because it offers some inherent advantages over the external approach, including the avoidance of cutaneous scarring, less intraoperative bleeding, a shorter postoperative recovery course, and the ability to concurrently treat intranasal pathology.

■ Suggested Reading

Acheson JF. Optic nerve disorders: role of canal and nerve sheath decompression surgery. Eye (Lond) 2004;18(11):1169–1174

Bartley GB, Fatourechi V, Kadrmas EF, et al. Clinical features of Graves' ophthalmopathy in an incidence cohort. Am J Ophthalmol 1996;121(3):284–290

Ben Simon GJ, Joseph J, Lee S, Schwarcz RM, McCann JD, Goldberg RA. External versus endoscopic dacryocystorhinostomy for acquired nasolacrimal duct obstruction in a tertiary referral center. Ophthalmology 2005;112(8):1463–1468

Daffner RH, Kirks DR, Gehweiler JA Jr, Heaston DK. Computed tomography of fibrous dysplasia. AJR Am J Roentgenol 1982;139(5):943–948

Forbes G, Gorman CA, Brennan MD, Gehring DG, Ilstrup DM, Earnest F IV. Ophthalmopathy of Graves' disease: computerized volume measurements of the orbital fat and muscle. AJNR Am J Neuroradiol 1986;7(4):651–656

Goldberg RA, Steinsapir KD. Extracranial optic canal decompression: indications and technique. Ophthal Plast Reconstr Surg 1996;12(3):163–170

Gupta AK, Bansal S. Primary endoscopic dacryocystorhinostomy in children – analysis of 18 patients. Int J Pediatr Otorhinolaryngol 2006;70(7):1213–1217

Joseph MP, Lessell S, Rizzo J, Momose KJ. Extracranial optic nerve decompression for traumatic optic neuropathy. Arch Ophthalmol 1990;108(8):1091–1093

Kacker A, Kazim M, Murphy M, Trokel S, Close LG. "Balanced" orbital decompression for severe Graves' orbitopathy: technique with treatment algorithm. Otolaryngol Head Neck Surg 2003;128(2):228–235

Kazim M, Goldberg RA, Smith TJ. Insights into the pathogenesis of thyroid-associated orbitopathy: evolving rationale for therapy. Arch Ophthalmol 2002;120(3):380–386

Kountakis SE, Maillard AA, Urso R, Stiernberg CM. Endoscopic approach to traumatic visual loss. Otolaryngol Head Neck Surg 1997;116(6 Pt 1):652–655

Lehmann GM, Feldon SE, Smith TJ, Phipps RP. Immune mechanisms in thyroid eye disease. Thyroid 2008;18(9):959–965

Levin LA, Beck RW, Joseph MP, Seiff S, Kraker R. The treatment of traumatic optic neuropathy: the International Optic Nerve Trauma Study. Ophthalmology 1999;106(7):1268–1277

Mourits MP, Koornneef L, Wiersinga WM, Prummel MF, Berghout A, van der Gaag R. Orbital decompression for Graves' ophthalmopathy by inferomedial, by inferomedial plus lateral, and by coronal approach. Ophthalmology 1990;97(5):636–641

Muellner K, Bodner E, Mannor GE, Wolf G, Hofmann T, Luxenberger W. Endolacrimal laser assisted lacrimal surgery. Br J Ophthalmol 2000;84(1):16–18

Papay FA, Morales L Jr, Flaharty P, et al. Optic nerve decompression in cranial base fibrous dysplasia. J Craniofac Surg 1995;6(1):5–10, discussion 11–14

Reifler DM. Results of endoscopic KTP laser-assisted dacryocystorhinostomy. Ophthal Plast Reconstr Surg 1993;9(4):231–236

Ressiniotis T, Voros GM, Kostakis VT, Carrie S, Neoh C. Clinical outcome of endonasal KTP laser assisted dacryocystorhinostomy. BMC Ophthalmol 2005;5:2

Sellari-Franceschini S, Berrettini S, Santoro A, et al. Orbital decompression in Graves' ophthalmopathy by medial and lateral wall removal. Otolaryngol Head Neck Surg 2005;133(2):185–189

Silbert DI, Matta NS. Outcomes of 9 mm balloon-assisted endoscopic dacryocystorhinostomy: retrospective review of 97 cases. Orbit 2010;29(3):131–134

Sofferman RA. An extracranial microsurgical approach to the optic nerve. J Microsurg 1979;1(3):195–202

Thornton J, Kelly SP, Harrison RA, Edwards R. Cigarette smoking and thyroid eye disease: a systematic review. Eye (Lond) 2007;21(9):1135–1145

Tsirbas A, Davis G, Wormald PJ. Mechanical endonasal dacryocystorhinostomy versus external dacryocystorhinostomy. Ophthal Plast Reconstr Surg 2004;20(1):50–56

Woog JJ, Kennedy RH, Custer PL, Kaltreider SA, Meyer DR, Camara JG. Endonasal dacryocystorhinostomy: a report by the American Academy of Ophthalmology. Ophthalmology 2001;108(12):2369–2377

Zoumalan CI, Joseph JM, Lelli GJ Jr, et al. Evaluation of the canalicular entrance into the lacrimal sac: an anatomical study. Ophthal Plast Reconstr Surg 2011;27(4):298–303

91 Tumors of the Nasal Cavity and Paranasal Sinuses

Introduction

Tumors of the sinonasal tract are rare. They arise from the bony cartilaginous skeleton and the lining skin and respiratory mucosa. They are of epithelial, neural, fibro-osseous, hamartomatous, vascular, and odontogenic origin (**Tables 91.1** and **91.2**). Tumors of the nasal cavity have equal benign and malignant pathology, but most tumors of the paranasal sinuses are malignant. The most common tumors are osteomas, followed by inverted papillomas. Malignant sinonasal tumors are rare, occurring in fewer than 1 in 100,000 people per year in the United States.

Clinical Findings

Most tumors present with the same symptoms as inflammatory pathology (obstruction, congestion, loss of smell, and drainage) and may be misdiagnosed as rhinitis or sinusitis. Symptoms are usually unilateral. Vascular and large tumors present with epistaxis. Symptoms reflect the location of the tumor and extension into adjacent structures. Benign tumors remodel bone, whereas rapidly growing malignant tumors invade bone. Nasolacrimal duct obstruction leads to epiphora. Sinus obstruction causes recurrent or chronic sinusitis. Facial deformity, proptosis, diplopia, and loss of vision occur very late. Pain, paresthesia, and numbness should alert one to a malignant process. Neurological involvement can include single or multiple cranial nerves (CNs), orbital apex (CN II, III, IV, VI), cavernous sinus (CN II–VI), and brain (headache, mental status changes, confusion, lethargy). Involvement of the maxillary nerve and its branches, olfactory nerve, and vidian nerve is not infrequent. Palatal involvement can present with pain, loose teeth, nonhealing extraction, ill-fitting dentures, or mass. Nasopharyngeal involvement can cause hearing loss, middle ear effusion, pain, and bilateral nasal obstruction. Infra-temporal fossa involvement can cause trismus and metastatic neck nodes.

Delayed diagnosis is a major problem with sinonasal malignancies. The time from initial symptoms to diagnosis may exceed 6 months. Patients may remain asymptomatic and even present very late with metastases. On initial presentation, cervical metastasis is present in 1 to 26% and distant metastasis in less than 7%; these patients have poor prognoses. Regional spread via lymphatic drainage is to the primarily echelon pretubal plexus and lateral retropharyngeal nodes, followed by secondary echelon drainage to the deep jugular nodes. The anterior nasal cavity and skin drain to the submandibular nodes.

Evaluation

A complete head and neck examination followed by nasal endoscopy should be performed. Tumors are often more white and fleshy than inflammatory polyps, but they can be difficult to distinguish from polyps. Malignant tumors are more solid with areas of hemorrhage and necrosis. The oral cavity should be inspected for palatal erosion or loosening of teeth. Orbital, eye, and cranial nerve examination should be performed.

Imaging

Computed tomography (CT) and magnetic resonance imaging (MRI) are complementary and used to characterize the tumor and determine its location, extent, and possible site of origin. CT is usually used for initial evaluation. It is superior to MRI in demonstrating bony architecture, bony remodeling, and erosion of the orbit and skull base. It may be used for intraoperative image guidance. CT with contrast or CT angiography (CTA) demonstrates tumor vascular-

Table 91.1 Benign tumors of the sinonasal cavity, World Health Organization classification

Origin of tumor	Tumor
Epithelial	Sinonasal papilloma (inverted, exophytic, oncocytic); salivary adenomas (pleomorphic, oncocytoma, myoepithelioma)
Vascular	Hemangioma, juvenile nasopharyngeal angiofibroma, pyogenic granuloma, hemangiopericytoma
Fibro-osseous	Osteoma, fibrous dysplasia, ossifying fibroma, chondroma
Neural	Schwannoma, neurofibroma, meningioma
Soft tissue	Respiratory epithelial adenoid hamartoma (REAH)
Neuroectodermal	Ameloblastoma, craniopharyngioma

Used with permission from Lund VJ, Stammberger H, Nicolai P, et al. European position paper on endoscopic management of tumors of the nose, paranasal sinuses and skull base. Rhinol Suppl 2010;(22):1–143.

Table 91.2 Malignant tumors of the sinonasal cavity, World Health Organization classification

Origin of tumor	Tumor
Epithelial	Squamous cell carcinoma, undifferentiated carcinoma, adenocarcinoma, adenoid cystic carcinoma, mucoepidermoid carcinoma, lymphoepithelial carcinoma
Neuroendocrine	Olfactory neuroblastoma, small-cell neuroendocrine carcinoma, mucosal melanoma, ameloblastoma
Fibro-osseous	Osteosarcoma, chondrosarcoma
Neural	Meningioma, malignant schwannoma
Hematolymphoid	NK-T cell lymphoma, extranodal B cell lymphoma, plasmacytoma
Soft tissue	Fibrosarcoma, angiosarcoma, rhabdomyosarcoma, leiomyosarcoma
Skull base tumors	Meningioma, craniopharyngioma, chordoma

Used with permission from Lund VJ, Stammberger H, Nicolai P, et al. European position paper on endoscopic management of tumors of the nose, paranasal sinuses and skull base. Rhinol Suppl 2010;(22):1–143.

ity and its relationship to the internal carotid artery. However, CT scans cannot differentiate tumor from secretions and soft tissue.

MRI is superior to CT in distinguishing tumor from inflammatory mucosa and secretions (**Fig. 91.1**). An MRI scan of the sinonasal cavity, orbit, and brain with gadolinium enhancement should be obtained. Tumor enhances to an intermediate degree on T1 sequences with gadolinium, whereas the lining of inflamed mucosa enhances more intensely. Secretions are bright on T2 images. MRI is also useful for detecting perineural invasion and invasion of the dura, orbit, or brain. It may also be "merged" with a CT scan for intraoperative image guidance.

Other diagnostic tests include positron-emission tomography CT, chest X-ray, and lactate dehydrogenase levels to study distant metastases. Angiography (with embolization) is helpful in vascular tumors and may be used to study internal carotid involvement.

Biopsy

An office biopsy for histopathology is usually possible for accessible tumors, unless contraindicated. Radiographic imaging may suffice for diagnosing osteoma or fibrous dysplasia. For vascular tumors, such as angiofibroma, office biopsy is contraindicated due to the risk of major hemorrhage. If there is

skull base erosion, the risk of causing cerebrospinal fluid (CSF) leakage should be considered.

■ Management

It is important to recognize the biological behavior of each tumor type because this determines both management and prognosis. Benign tumors are treated surgically or observed. Malignant tumors can be treated with surgery, radiation, chemotherapy, or a combination thereof. In general, early malignant tumors (T1, T2) may be treated with either surgery or radiation. For T3 tumors, treatment is surgery followed by radiation; for T4 tumors, treatment is surgery with radiation or chemoradiation. Long-term follow-up with clinical examination and imaging (CT, MRI) is necessary for oncological surveillance.

Surgery

Surgery is the cornerstone of treatment for most sinonasal benign tumors and malignancies. Tumors may be removed via the traditional open approach

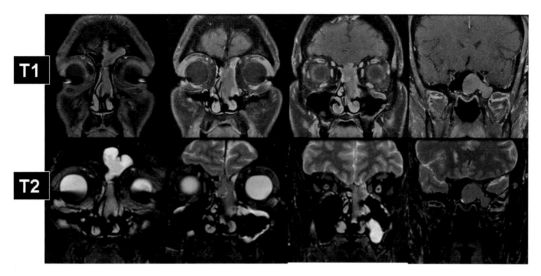

Fig. 91.1 Magnetic resonance imaging of a left high-grade adenocarcinoma extending from the sinonasal cavity intracranially. Figures show T1 (with gadolinium contrast) and T2 sequences. The T1-weighted sequence shows an intermediate enhancing tumor in the nose, ethmoid, sphenoid, and intracranially. The T2-weighted sequence shows the presence of fluid (bright) in the frontal sinus. Mucosa in the left maxillary enhances brightly. Tumor attachment is likely in the medial ethmoid skull base.

or through newly described endoscopic or combined techniques. Traditionally, resection was performed en bloc via open approaches, such as alotomy, lateral rhinotomy, midfacial degloving, the Weber–Ferguson approach, and external craniofacial resection. Advanced malignancies may require orbital exenteration, maxillectomy, or anterior cranial base resection.

Recent advances have made endoscopic resection of sinonasal tumors a viable alternative to the traditional techniques. Endoscopic techniques can be designed to mimic the resection from many open approaches, including endoscopic skull base and dural resection from the crista galli to the planum sphenoidale. The development of vascularized pedicled flap, such as the nasoseptal flap, has revolutionized skull base reconstruction and reduced complications. Advantages of the endoscopic technique include absence of an external facial incision; shorter inpatient stay; and reduced postoperative pain, infraorbital numbness, and trismus. However, the biggest advantage is improved visualization and magnification that can help discriminate tumor from normal tissue. The duration of endoscopic surgery is a relative disadvantage. Complications of the endoscopic approach are similar to total sphenoethmoidectomy. Resection starts with tumor debulking to identify the attachments of the tumor, which are carefully identified and widely resected with adequate margins with frozen section control. A "minimal access" corridor, which is needed for both tumor resection and surveillance, is used. However, the resection itself is not "minimal"; a customized procedure can be designed for aggressive tumor resection.

Radiation

Radiation as the sole modality is recommended for lymphoreticular tumors (lymphoma, plasmacytoma), unresectable cases, and poor surgical candidates. Conventional photon therapy or particles (neutron) can be used. Intensity-modulated radiation therapy has replaced conventional external beam and can minimize the dose delivered to vital structures adjacent to the tumor (cornea, lens, brain, spine). Surgery and adjuvant radiotherapy with or without chemotherapy are used in advanced tumors (T3 and T4), positive surgical margins, perineural spread, perivascular invasion, cervical lymphatic metastasis, and recurrent tumors.

Chemotherapy

Chemotherapy is used as a radiosensitizer, for palliation, and as an adjuvant for high-risk patients. Platinum-based agents are most commonly used.

Complications

Surgical complications include bleeding, wound infection, reconstructive flap necrosis, visual loss, CSF leaks, pneumocephalus, and intracranial infection. Late sequelae include globe malposition, diplopia, epiphora, blepharitis/conjunctivitis, eyelid malposition, and facial disfigurement. Radiation therapy is associated with significant ocular complications, such as dry eye, cataracts, and keratitis.

▪ Factors in Outcome and Prognosis of Malignant Tumors

Advanced disease, dural, and brain invasion have poor prognosis. Obtaining clean, tumor-free margins intraoperatively has prognostic value independent of tumor type and extent.

Tumor histopathology is an independent prognostic factor. Overall 5 year survival is best for low-grade neoplasms, such as esthesioneuroblastoma (78%), low-grade sarcomas (69%), intermediate- to high-grade sarcomas (57%), adenocarcinoma (52%), salivary malignancies (46%), and squamous cell carcinoma (44%). Prognosis is worst for undifferentiated/anaplastic carcinoma (37%) and mucosal melanoma (18%).

Although an extensive discussion on individual tumors is beyond the scope of this chapter, brief summaries highlighting salient features of common sinonasal tumors follow.

Benign Tumors

Fibro-osseous Tumors

Osteoma

Osteoma is the most common sinonasal tumor, seen in 3% of routine CT sinus scans. These slow-growing tumors (0.44–6 mm per year) are most frequently located in the frontal sinus (57%) (**Fig. 91.2**). There are three types: ivory/compact (composed of dense cortical bone), mature (composed of cancellous bone), and mixed (**Fig. 91.2**). Most patients remain asymptomatic, with incidental diagnosis on imaging. The most common presenting symptom is frontal headache or facial pain. Malignant transformation has not been reported. Management depends on symptoms, location, and rate of growth.

Fibrous Dysplasia

Fibrous dysplasia usually presents in the first 2 decades of life. The two classic forms are polyostotic (15–30%), involving more than one bone, and monostotic (70–85%), involving only one bone. McCune–Albright syndrome is a rare syndrome with polyostotic fibrous dysplasia, precocious puberty, and cutaneous pigmentation. Asymptomatic fibrous dysplasia is incidentally found on imaging, with the sphenoid and central skull base being frequently involved. Growth slows after puberty. A low rate of malignant transformation has been reported, occurring in 0.5% of polyostotic forms and in 4% of lesions in McCune–Albright syndrome. Histologically, the medullary bone is replaced by abnormal fibrous tissue and bone metaplasia. CT scan with a homogeneous ground-glass appearance on the bone window is almost diagnostic (**Figs. 91.3** and **91.4**). Clinical presentation includes facial asymmetry, facial pain, and ocular and neurological changes. Surgery is indicated based on symptoms, age, and extent of the tumor.

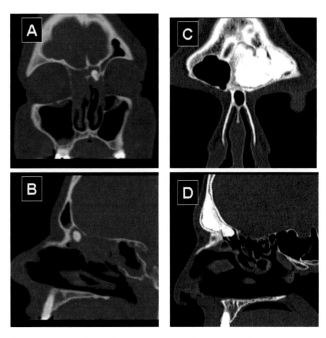

Fig. 91.2 Osteomas are often discovered incidentally on computed tomographic scans. They are most commonly located in the frontal sinus recess. (**a, b**) Small, incidentally noted osteoma in the left frontal recess. (**c, d**) Large osteomas can present with symptoms, such as frontal headaches and pain, as in this patient.

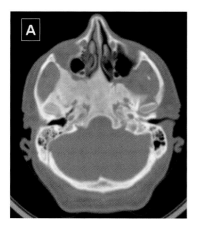

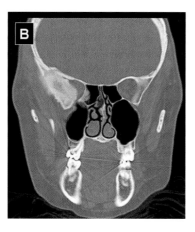

Fig. 91.3 (**a**) Fibrous dysplasia has a relatively homogeneous, ground-glass appearance on the bone window and commonly affects the central skull base. (**b**) Right zygomatic bone. Ossifying fibroma shows a characteristic sharply demarcated, expansile mass covered by a thick shell of bone; the tumor mass appears to be multiloculated and is of varying density.

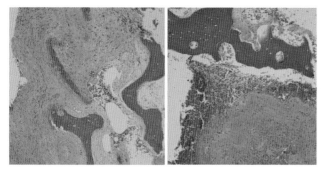

Fig. 91.4 Fibrous dysplasia hematoxylin and eosin (H&E) stained section. The medullary bone is replaced by abnormal fibrous tissue and bone metaplasia (low- and high-power views).

Ossifying Fibroma

Ossifying fibroma is more commonly found in females, usually affecting the mandible (75%) or maxilla (10–20%). Trauma has been implicated in its etiology. Histologically, distinct regions of fibrous tissue with varying amounts of mineralized or calcified psammomatoid bodies are seen. CT shows a characteristic sharply demarcated, expansile, multiloculated mass of varying density covered by a thick shell of bone (**Fig. 91.3**). Tumors invading the midface and sinonasal tract behave more aggressively and may need wide surgical resection.

Inverted Papilloma

Papilloma is the most common sinonasal tumor for which surgery is performed. It is found in 0.5 to 4% of surgically resected nasal tumor specimens. These specimens are subdivided into inverted papilloma (IP), fungiform papilloma, and cylindrical cell papilloma.

IPs have a locally aggressive behavior. They can be associated with malignancy, and they tend to recur after surgery. IPs affect all ages (highest in fifth to sixth decades of life) and are two to five times more common in males than in females (2–5:1). IPs tend to be fleshy and vascular (**Fig. 91.5**). Calcification within the tumor may be occasionally seen. Most IPs arise from the lateral nasal wall and extend into the adjacent sinuses and nasopharynx. The ethmoid sinuses are the next most frequent site of origin (48%), followed by the maxillary (28%), sphenoid, and frontal sinuses. The role of human papilloma virus (HPV) in pathogenesis is controversial. Hyperostosis on CT adjacent to the tumor has been proposed to be the site of tumor attachment.

On histopathology, the epithelial lining of the IP inverts into the underlying stroma, but the basement membrane remains intact (**Fig. 91.6**). Atypia and dysplasia are seen in 1 to 2%. Carcinoma (squamous cell, transitional cell, adenocarcinoma, mucoepidermoid, verrucous) within IP is seen in ~ 7% of resected specimens (0–53%). Therefore, most of the tumor should be sent for histopathology. Squamous cell carcinomas arising in IP have an aggressive course and may have poor survival. Metachronous carcinomas occur in 3.6% of IP. The incidence of metachronous carcinomas is higher in association with recurrent IP (11%). These metachronous carcinomas arise after a mean interval duration of 52 months (range 6–180 months).

The most common and newest staging systems for IP are summarized in **Table 91.3**. Historically, the surgical gold standard was an external approach constituting a medial maxillectomy. Vrabec reported a recurrence rate of only 2% using a lateral rhinotomy on mean follow-up of 8.9 years. Endoscopic techniques for resection have been gaining favor and show promising early results.

The principal cause of recurrence is incomplete resection at the site of origin. A recent systematic review of 63 case series found recurrence to be 12.8%

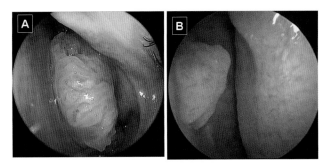

Fig. 91.5 Schneiderian papilloma. (**a**) Large inverted papilloma arising from the left lateral nasal wall. (**b**) Fungiform (everted) papilloma on the left nasal septum; it has a frondlike appearance, and the anterior septum is a common location.

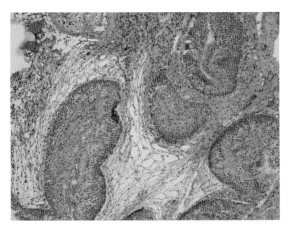

Fig. 91.6 Inverted papilloma histopathology section (hematoxylin and eosin stain) shows the lining ciliated respiratory columnar epithelium to invert toward the stroma. The basement membrane remains intact.

Table 91.3 Staging systems for inverted papilloma

Krouse	
Type 1	Tumor totally confined to nasal cavity; must not extend into sinuses or any extranasal structure; no concurrent malignancy
Type 2	Tumor involving ostiomeatal complex, ethmoid sinus, and/or medial part of maxillary sinus, with/without nasal cavity; no concurrent malignancy
Type 3	Tumor involving lateral, inferior, superior, anterior, or posterior walls of maxillary sinus; sphenoid sinus, and/or frontal sinus, with/without involvement of medial maxillary sinus, ethmoid sinus, or nasal cavity; no concurrent malignancy
Type 4	All tumors with extranasal/extrasinus extension (orbit, intracranial, or pterygomaxillary space); all tumors with concurrent malignancy
Han	
Group 1	Tumor limited to nasal cavity, lateral nasal wall, medial maxillary sinus, ethmoid sinus, and sphenoid sinus
Group 2	Group 1 plus tumor extends lateral to the medial maxillary wall
Group 3	Tumor extends to involve frontal sinus
Group 4	Tumor extends outside sinonasal cavity (orbital or intracranial extension)
Oikawa	
T1	Tumor limited to nasal cavity
T2	Tumor limited to ethmoid sinus and/or medial and superior maxillary sinus
T3	Tumor involves lateral, inferior, anterior, or posterior walls of maxillary sinus, sphenoid sinus, or frontal sinus. T3-A: without extension to frontal sinus or supraorbital recess. T3-B: involving frontal sinus or supraorbital recess
T4	Tumor extends outside sinonasal cavity (orbit/intracranial) or is associated with malignancy
Cannady	
Group A	Inverted papilloma confined to the nasal cavity, ethmoid sinuses, or medial maxillary wall
Group B	Inverted papilloma with involvement of any maxillary wall (other than the medial wall), or frontal sinus, or sphenoid sinus
Group C	Inverted papilloma with extension beyond the paranasal sinuses

Used with permission from Lund VJ, Stammberger H, Nicolai P, et al. European position paper on endoscopic management of tumors of the nose, paranasal sinuses and skull base. Rhinol Suppl 2010;(22):1–143.

for endoscopic procedures (n = 484), 17% for lateral rhinotomy with medial maxillectomy (n = 1,025), and 34.2% for limited resections, such as nasal polypectomy (n = 600). However, the follow-up duration of the endoscopic cohort was shorter (3.1 years) than the open series (5.2 years). Complete resection of the involved mucosa and mucoperiosteum is advocated, with some surgeons drilling the bone at the site of attachment. Recurrence is higher in revision cases. Most IPs recur within the first 10 to 20 months (range 30–56 months).

Juvenile Angiofibroma

Juvenile angiofibroma is a benign vascular tumor accounting for 0.5% of all head and neck tumors. The median age at diagnosis is 18.5 years (range 18–35 years), and all patients are males. Patients complain of increasing unilateral nasal obstruction (80–90%), drainage, and recurrent epistaxis (45–60%). A hormonal etiology has been proposed, because androgen and/or estrogen receptors have been found in tumor tissue, and recent studies have found partial or total loss of the Y chromosome and gains in the X chromosome in tumor tissue. Some clinicians believe juvenile angiofibroma to be a vascular malformation

from a nonresorbed first brachial arch artery. Histologically, these tumors are composed of large and small ectatic vessels with variable amounts of fibrous tissue (**Fig. 91.7**). Office biopsy is not recommended for risk of major hemorrhage.

Angiofibromas have a characteristic growth pattern on CT and MRI (**Fig. 91.7**). They originate around the pterygopalatine fossa, starting from the basisphenoid and the sphenopalatine foramen. They can be locally aggressive, growing into the nose, nasopharynx, paranasal sinuses, orbit, skull base, and intracranially (**Fig. 91.7**). Dumb-belling of the tumor around the sphenopalatine foramen and basisphenoid may be noted. Bowing of the posterior maxillary wall is noted with infratemporal fossa extension. MRI shows several signal voids within the tumor on T1 and T2 images, reflecting its vascularity. Angiography should be performed preoperatively for studying the vascular supply and embolization. Embolization should be performed within 24 to 48 hours of the planned resection and may reduce bleeding by 60 to 70%. The major vascular supply is usually from the internal maxillary artery, the ascending pharyngeal artery, and the vidian artery. Major vascularization from the internal carotid artery is problematic, because branches from the internal carotid arteries cannot be embolized due to risk of stroke.

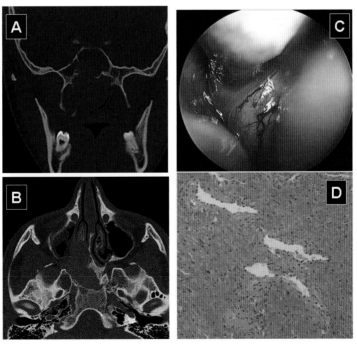

Fig. 91.7 Right sinonasal angiofibroma. (**a, b**) The plain computed tomographic scans show erosion of the right basisphenoid and vidian canal, as well as the subtle expansion of the right pterygopalatine fossa; a large part of the tumor dumb-bells into the nasopharynx. (**c**) Endoscopy shows a smooth vascular mass. (**d**) Histopathology shows tumors to be vascular with large ectatic vessels that branch into progressively smaller capillary-sized vessels. The cells are bland, evenly spaced, and stellate in a variable component of fibrous stroma.

Table 91.4 highlights some classic, commonly used, and new staging systems. Surgery has conventionally been performed by open approaches. However, the endoscopic approach is being increasingly used for selected angiofibromas. Key to preventing recurrences is subperiosteal dissection of the tumor attachment at the basisphenoid, with drilling of the denuded bone to remove any residual disease. Extensive tumors remain a challenge. Nonsurgical treatment options include external beam therapy and stereotactic radiation for unresectable tumors, residual and recurrent tumors, and extensive intracranial extension. Chemotherapy has a limited role.

Lobular Capillary Hemangioma (Pyogenic Granuloma)

Lobular capillary hemangioma (pyogenic granuloma) is relatively common, located in the anterior parts of the nasal septum and turbinates, and presents as a polypoid vascular submucosal mass with intact surface mucosa. It is usually found in females. Nasal trauma and hormonal etiology have been proposed. These are surgically resected and rarely recur.

Table 91.4 Select staging systems for angiofibroma

Stage	Session (1981)	Fisch (1983)	Radkowski (1996)	Snyderman (2010)
I	IA: limited to posterior nasal cavity and choana IB: IA plus involvement of at least one paranasal sinus	Limited to nasal cavity and nasopharynx; without any bony destruction	IA: limited to posterior nasal cavity and choana IB: IA plus involvement of at least one paranasal sinus	No significant extension beyond site of origin; tumor remains medial to the midpoint of the pterygopalatine space
II	IIA: Minimal lateral extension to the pterygopalatine fossa IIB: Extension into entire pterygopalatine fossa with or without orbital bone erosion	Invading the pterygopalatine fossa and the maxillary, ethmoid, and sphenoid sinus with bone destruction	IIA: Minimal lateral extension to the pterygopalatine fossa IIB: Extension into entire pterygopalatine fossa with or without orbital bone erosion IIC: Extension posterior to pterygoid plates	Extension to the paranasal sinuses and lateral to the midpoint of the pterygopalatine space
III	IIIA: Skull base erosion (e.g., middle fossa, pterygoid plates) with minimal intracranial invasion IIIB: Extensive intracranial extension with or without cavernous sinus invasion	Invasion of infratemporal fossa, orbit, and parasellar region remaining lateral to the cavernous sinus	IIIA: Erosion of the skull base with minimal intracranial extension IIIB: Extensive intracranial extension with or without cavernous sinus invasion	Locally advanced with skull base erosion or extension to additional extracranial spaces, including orbit and infratemporal fossa; no residual vascularity following embolization
IV		Massive invasion of cavernous sinus, the optic chiasmal region or pituitary fossa		IV: Skull base erosion or extension to additional extracranial spaces, including orbit and infratemporal fossa; residual vascularity following embolization
V				V: Intracranial extension, residual vascularity M: medial extension L: lateral extension

Used with permission from Lund VJ, Stammberger H, Nicolai P, et al. European position paper on endoscopic management of tumors of the nose, paranasal sinuses and skull base. Rhinol Suppl 2010;(22):1–143.

Glomangiopericytoma

Glomangiopericytomas are rare tumors of the nose and paranasal sinuses. They have borderline, low potential for malignancy and tend to recur in 7 to 40% of the population.

Other Benign Tumors

Hamartomas

Hamartomas are tumors composed of cell rests from the embryological period. These are categorized into epithelial, mesenchymal, and mixed epithelial/mesenchymal types. Respiratory epithelial adenomatoid hamartoma (REAH), the most common type, presents as a polypoid mass in adult males. It has prominent glandular proliferations lined by ciliated respiratory epithelium that can be confused grossly and microscopically with IP and squamous cell carcinoma (SCC). Seromucinous hamartoma can be misdiagnosed as low-grade adenocarcinoma.

Pleomorphic Adenoma

Pleomorphic adenoma, arising from the minor salivary glands, is the third most common benign tumor of the sinonasal tract. The nasal septum is most frequently affected.

Malignant Sinonasal Tumors

Malignant sinonasal tumors represent 1% of all malignancies and 3 to 5% of all head and neck malignancies. They are more common in males than in females (1.2–2.7:1). Epithelial tumors usually present in the fifth and sixth decades of life. The nose is the primary site in 25% of cases and the sinuses in 75%. Of these cases, 75 to 80% are SCC or its variants (anaplastic, undifferentiated, transitional). Salivary gland cancers (adenocarcinoma, adenoid cystic, colonic type, mucoepidermoid) represent ~ 10% of sinonasal malignancies, and sarcomas (chondrosarcoma, osteogenic, malignant fibrous histiocytoma) represent ~ 6%. Rare tumors, such as melanoma, lymphoma, esthesioneuroblastoma (olfactory neuroblastoma), represent 4%.

Occupational exposure has strong association with malignant tumors. Nickel exposure is associated with squamous and anaplastic cancer. Increased risk of SCC is seen with exposure to leather tanning, mineral oils, isopropyl oils, lacquer paint, metal, textile, mining, agriculture, soldering, and welding. Adenocarcinoma is associated with wood dust exposure; hardwoods and formaldehyde inhalation increase risk. Thorium dioxide (Thorotrast) increases the risk for squamous and mucoepidermoid carcinomas. Chronic infection, tobacco, alcohol, previous radiation, and HPV do not appear to increase risk.

Squamous Cell Carcinoma

SCC commonly originates in the maxillary sinus (60–73%) in males in the fifth and sixth decades of life. Occupational exposure is a risk factor. Treatment of SCC depends on the stage of the disease (**Tables 91.5A** and **91.5B**). Early lesions (T1–T2) are usually treated by surgery or radiation therapy. Advanced disease (T3–T4) is treated with combination therapy (surgery followed by radiation or chemoradiation). Elective treatment of the neck is not indicated for necks with no regional lymph node metastases unless there is soft tissue invasion. Local recurrences occur in 30 to 40%, and systemic metastasis in 10% of patients. The 3- and 5-year survival rates are 86% and 69%, respectively.

Adenoid Cystic Carcinoma (ACC)

Adenoid cystic carcinoma (ACC) accounts for < 1% of all head and neck malignancies. Sinonasal ACC represents 10 to 25% of head and neck ACC. Most patients are Caucasians, nonsmokers, and nondrinkers. The maxillary sinus (47%) and the nasal cavity (30%) are the most commonly affected. ACC shows a propensity for perineural and bony invasion, leading to significant skull base and intracranial extension. Negative margins are frequently difficult to obtain.

There are three subtypes: cribriform, tubular, and solid. The cribriform pattern is most common, having the classic "Swiss cheese" appearance. The tubular subtype has the best prognosis, and solid has the worst. These tumors can also be classified into grades I through III based on the percentage of each histological subtype, with grade I having the best prognosis.

Surgery followed by radiotherapy is the treatment of choice. Radiotherapy is strongly recommended for positive margins and for advanced and high-grade tumors. Neutron beam radiation may have advantages over photons in ACC. Five-year survival rates range from 50 to 86%, with a recurrence rate of 51 to 65%. Distant hematogenous metastases to the lung, liver, and bones may occur in 26 to 40% of cases in spite of control at the primary site. Of note, more than 20% of patients with distant metastasis can survive 5 years or longer. Long-term follow-up is needed because tumors may recur 10 to 20 years after the initial treatment. The survival rate of patients with ACC continues to decrease after 5 years.

Table 91.5a T staging for sinonasal carcinoma

T1	Tumor is limited to maxillary sinus mucosa with no erosion or destruction of bone
T2	Tumor is causing bone erosion or destruction, including extension into the hard palate and/or the middle of the nasal meatus, except extension to the posterior wall of maxillary sinus and pterygoid plates
T3	Tumor invades any of the following: bone of the posterior wall of maxillary sinus, subcutaneous tissues, floor or medial wall of orbit, pterygoid fossa, ethmoid sinuses
T4a	Moderately advanced local disease: tumor invades anterior orbital contents, skin of cheek, pterygoid plates, infratemporal fossa, cribriform plate, sphenoid or frontal sinuses
T4b	Very advanced local disease: tumor invades any of the following: orbital apex, dura, brain, middle cranial fossa, cranial nerves other than V2, nasopharynx, or clivus

Used with the permission of the American Joint Committee on Cancer (AJCC), Chicago, Illinois. The original source for this material is the AJCC Cancer Staging Manual, Seventh Edition (2010) published by Springer Science and Business Media LLC, www.springer.com.

Table 91.5b Staging for nasal cavity and ethmoid sinus

T1	Tumor is restricted to any one subsite, with or without bony invasion
T2	Tumor invades 2 subsites in a single region or extending to involve an adjacent region within the nasoethmoidal complex, with or without bony invasion
T3	Tumor extends to invade the medial wall or floor of the orbit, maxillary sinus, palate, or cribriform plate
T4a	Moderately advanced local disease: Tumor invades any of the following: anterior orbital contents, skin of nose or cheek, minimal extension to anterior cranial fossa, pterygoid plates, sphenoid or frontal sinuses
T4b	Very advanced local disease: Tumor invades any of the following: orbital apex, dura, brain, middle cranial fossa, cranial nerves other than V2, nasopharynx, or clivus

Used with the permission of the American Joint Committee on Cancer (AJCC), Chicago, Illinois. The original source for this material is the AJCC Cancer Staging Manual, Seventh Edition (2010) published by Springer Science and Business Media LLC, www.springer.com.

Adenocarcinoma

Adenocarcinoma is the third most common sinonasal epithelial malignancy (8–15% of all sinonasal cancers). Mean age of presentation is 60 to 65 years. Men are at fourfold greater risk compared with women, due to occupational risks. Adenocarcinoma is located most frequently (85%) in the ethmoid sinuses and upper part of the nasal cavity. Sinonasal adenocarcinomas are divided into intestinal and nonintestinal types. Nonintestinal-type adenocarcinomas represent over 90% of sinonasal adenocarcinoma and are further divided into low- and high-grade subtypes. Low-grade tumors are well differentiated, with low mitotic activity, usually recurring only locally. High-grade tumors are poorly differentiated, with high mitotic activity, and they have a higher propensity for distant metastasis (30% of these patients have distant metastases at initial presentation). Low-grade adenocarcinoma has excellent 5-year survival (85%), whereas high-grade has poor 3-year survival (20%). Intestinal adenocarcinomas are similar to those in the in the colon and are rare in the sinonasal tract. They are classified into papillary, sessile, and alveolar mucoid types. Papillary tumors are associated with the best prognosis, and alveolar mucoid type with the worst.

Surgery is the treatment of choice for adenocarcinoma. Postoperative radiotherapy is recommended for patients with positive margins, and for high-grade or advanced-stage tumors. The use of topical 5-fluorouracil postoperatively has been reported but needs further validation.

Round Cell Tumors

These rare tumors of the sinonasal cavity include esthesioneuroblastoma, sinonasal undifferentiated carcinoma (SNUC), small-cell undifferentiated carcinoma, extrapulmonary neuroendocrine carcinoma, lymphoma, melanoma, and sarcoma. Round cell tumors appear similar on standard stains. Routine hematoxylin and eosin (H&E) sections are insufficient in diagnosis and differentiating types. Immunohistochemistry is invaluable for differentiation of these tumors (**Table 91.6**).

Esthesioneuroblastoma (Olfactory Neuroblastoma)

These tumors are reported rarely, with an incidence of 0.4 cases/million, but they likely represent more than 5% of all nasal malignancies. They occur over a wide age range (3–90 years) and have bimodal peaks in the second and sixth decades of life. Esthesioneuroblastoma has no known etiology. Microscopically, round cells arranged into rosettes, pseudorosettes, or sheets and clusters are seen. Neuron-specific enolase, chromogranin, and synaptophysin are positive. Hyams described four grades of differentiation

Table 91.6 Immunohistochemistry stains to differentiate round cell sinonasal malignancies

Carcinoma	Keratin stain
Melanoma	S-100, HMB-45
Lymphoma	Leukocyte common antigen
Neuroendocrine carcinoma or esthesioneuroblastoma	Synaptophysin, neuron-specific enolase
Rhabdomyosarcoma	Actin, desmin, myoglobin

Table 91.7a Kadish staging for esthesioneuroblastoma

Stage A	The tumor is limited to the nasal fossa.
Stage B	The tumor extends to the paranasal sinuses.
Stage C	The tumor extends beyond the paranasal sinuses.

Table 91.7b University of California–Los Angeles staging for esthesioneuroblastoma

T1	The tumors involve the nasal cavity, paranasal sinuses, or both (excluding sphenoid), sparing the most superior ethmoidal air cells.
T2	The tumors involve the nasal cavity, paranasal sinuses, or both (including the sphenoid), with extension to or erosion of the cribriform plate.
T3	The tumors extend into the orbit or protrude into the anterior cranial fossa.
T4	The tumors involve the brain.

Note: Orbital and extradural invasions are considered separately from intracranial intradural invasion.

that correlate with prognosis. Surgical resection is the treatment of choice for esthesioneuroblastoma. Anterior skull base resection is considered the gold standard. Endoscopic resection is replacing craniofacial resection with good results in a multicenter study. Postoperative radiation improves results. The 5-year disease-free survival for all stages is 65% after combined surgery with radiotherapy but is worse with advanced disease. The Kadish and University of California–Los Angeles (UCLA) staging systems (**Tables 91.7A** and **91.7B**) are the most commonly used. In the University of Virginia study, the disease-free survival was 86.5% and 82.6% at 5 and 15 years, respectively. Long-term follow-up is recommended because mean time to recurrence was 6 years.

Sinonasal Undifferentiated

These are rare tumors, occurring more commonly in males than in females (2–3:1) in a wide age range (median in sixth decade). There are no known etiologic agents. SNUC is negative for Epstein-Barr virus (EBV) (differentiating it from undifferentiated nasopharyngeal carcinoma). These tumors are very aggressive, growing frequently and rapidly into the orbit and intracranial cavity (**Fig. 91.8**). They stain positive for cytokeratin and neuron-specific enolase. The prognosis for SNUC is poor, in spite of aggressive therapy with combined surgery, radiation, and chemotherapy. Median survival is 18 months. Chemoradiation or radiation alone is used for palliation. Locoregional recurrence is 20 to 30%, and distant metastasis occurs in 25 to 30% of patients.

Sinonasal Lymphomas

These lymphomas are the second most common malignant tumor of the sinonasal tract, following carcinomas. Most are non-Hodgkin lymphomas (B and T-NK subtypes) occurring in the elderly. In Asia, EBV-positive T cell lymphomas are more common. The 5-year overall survival for all subtypes is 52%. Younger age, early stage, and use of combination chemoradiation correlate with a better prognosis.

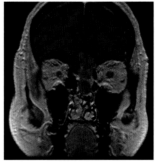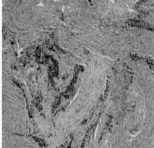

Fig. 91.8 Tumors with intracranial extension: Magnetic resonance imaging (MRI) shows a sinonasal undifferentiated carcinoma extending from the left sinonasal cavity intracranially. The hematoxylin and eosin stained section of the resected tumor shows sheets of undifferentiated round cells around the olfactory fibers. In the hands of experienced surgeons, this type of tumor can be removed by external or endoscopic approaches.

Sinonasal Mucosal Melanomas

Sinonasal melanoma represents 4% of all sinonasal neoplasms. These tumors are rare, making up 0.3 to 2% of all melanomas and 4% of head and neck melanomas. They commonly occur equally in men and women and are more prevalent in African Americans and older patients. S-100 and HMB-45 stains confirm diagnosis. Mucosal melanomas are considered to be advanced disease (**Table 91.8**). Although most mucosal melanomas present with disease localized to the primary site, regional or distant metastases must be evaluated in all cases. One-third of all patients have neck metastases. More than 50% of mucosal melanomas recur locally and then show distant metastases. Overall prognosis and survival rates are poor, with median survival of 19 to 21 months, and overall 5-year survival of 22% of patients. Most patients succumb within 3 years. Surgery is the treatment of choice. Radiotherapy is used to improve locoregional control. Adjuvant therapies, such as interferon and vaccines, are being evaluated.

Metastatic Tumors

Most malignant tumors of sinonasal regions are primary. The most common sites for metastatic tumors are the maxillary sinus (50%), followed by the ethmoid sinus (18%) and nasal cavity (15%). More than 50% of sinonasal metastases originate from a renal carcinoma. Other sources are lung, urogenital ridge, breast, and the gastrointestinal tract.

■ Controversies and Contemporary Issues

What Makes a Tumor Inoperable?

Absolute contraindications to surgery include major medical morbidities. The presence of distant metastases, invasion of prevertebral fascia, and invasion of the cavernous sinus or internal carotid artery in bilateral invasion of the optic nerves or optic chiasm may be contraindications too. Relative contraindications include extensive invasion of brain and neural structures, leading to poor prognosis.

When Should Orbital Exenteration Be Performed?

The extent of orbital invasion for which exenteration should be performed is controversial. Studies show little difference in local recurrence and survival between orbital preservation and exenteration. A detailed discussion is beyond the scope of this chapter, but invasion of the orbital apex, retrobulbar fat, extraocular eye muscles, and bulbar conjunctiva or sclera may be indications for orbital exenteration.

Table 91.8 Staging system for mucosal melanoma of the head and neck

Primary tumor
T3: Mucosal disease
T4a: Moderately advanced disease; tumor involving deep soft tissue, cartilage, bone or overlying skin
T4b: Very advanced disease; tumor involving brain, dura, skull base, lower cranial nerves (IX, X, XI, XII), masticator space, carotid artery, prevertebral space, or mediastinal structures
Regional lymph nodes
NX: Regional lymph nodes cannot be assessed
N0: No regional lymph node metastases
N1: Regional lymph node metastases present
Distant metastasis
M0: No distant metastasis
M1: Distant metastasis present
Clinical stage
Stage III: T3 N0 M0
Stage IVA: T4a N0 M0
T3–T4a N1 M0
Stage IVB: T4b Any N M0
Stage IVC: Any T Any N M1

Used with the permission of the American Joint Committee on Cancer (AJCC), Chicago, Illinois. The original source for this material is the AJCC Cancer Staging Manual, Seventh Edition (2010) published by Springer Science and Business Media LLC, www.springer.com.

What Are the Major Concerns about Endoscopic Approaches?

The primary concern with endoscopic approaches is adherence to oncological principles of "en-bloc resection." Experience with transoral resection of laryngopharyngeal cancers has shown that en bloc excision is not always necessary. Early oncological outcomes with the endoscopic technique show promising results, but long-term follow-up and larger cohorts of patients are needed to validate these. Contraindications to a completely endoscopic approach include invasion of superficial soft tissues and bony skeleton, as well as extension far lateral over the orbital roof.

■ Conclusion

A thorough knowledge of the diverse tumor biology and treatment modalities is essential for optimum management of sinonasal tumors.

Acknowledgments

The author acknowledges the Department of Pathology, Mayo Clinic, Arizona, for histopathology images and Dr. Michael H. Hinni for pictures of external medial maxillectomy.

■ Suggested Reading

Edge SB, Byrd DR, Compton CC, Fritz AG, Greene FL, Trotti A, eds. AJCC Cancer Staging Manual. 7th ed. New York, NY: Springer Science + Business Media; 2010

Bell D, Hanna EY. Sinonasal undifferentiated carcinoma: morphological heterogeneity, diagnosis, management and biological markers. Expert Rev Anticancer Ther 2013;13(3):285–296

Carrau RL, Ong YK, Solares CA, et al. Malignant tumors of the sinonasal cavity. Emedicine. August 24, 2011. http://emedicine.medscape.com/article/846995-overview

Douglas R, Wormald PJ. Endoscopic surgery for juvenile nasopharyngeal angiofibroma: where are the limits? Curr Opin Otolaryngol Head Neck Surg 2006;14(1):1–5

Fitzhugh VA, Mirani N. Respiratory epithelial adenomatoid hamartoma: a review. Head Neck Pathol 2008;2(3):203–208

Folbe A, Herzallah I, Duvvuri U, et al. Endoscopic endonasal resection of esthesioneuroblastoma: a multicenter study [published correction appears in Am J Rhinol Allergy 2009;23(2):238. Kassam, Amin Bardai added; Morcos, Jacques J added]. Am J Rhinol Allergy 2009;23(1):91–94

Howard DJ, Lloyd G, Lund V. Recurrence and its avoidance in juvenile angiofibroma. Laryngoscope 2001;111(9):1509–1511

Husain Q, Kanumuri VV, Svider PF, et al. Sinonasal adenoid cystic carcinoma: systematic review of survival and treatment strategies. Otolaryngol Head Neck Surg 2013;148(1):29–39

Lawson W, Patel ZM. The evolution of management for inverted papilloma: an analysis of 200 cases. Otolaryngol Head Neck Surg 2009;140(3):330–335

Loy AH, Reibel JF, Read PW, et al. Esthesioneuroblastoma: continued follow-up of a single institution's experience. Arch Otolaryngol Head Neck Surg 2006;132(2):134–138

Lund VJ, Chisholm EJ, Takes RP, et al. Evidence for treatment strategies in sinonasal adenocarcinoma. Head Neck 2012;34(8):1168–1178

Lund VJ, Chisholm EJ, Howard DJ, Wei WI. Sinonasal malignant melanoma: an analysis of 115 cases assessing outcomes of surgery, postoperative radiotherapy and endoscopic resection. Rhinology 2012;50(2):203–210

Lund VJ, Stammberger H, Nicolai P, et al; European Rhinologic Society Advisory Board on Endoscopic Techniques in the Management of Nose, Paranasal Sinus and Skull Base Tumours. European position paper on endoscopic management of tumours of the nose, paranasal sinuses and skull base. Rhinol Suppl 2010; (22):1–143

Mirghani H, Mortuaire G, Armas GL, et al. Sinonasal cancer: Analysis of oncological failures in 156 consecutive cases. Head Neck 2014;36(5):667–674

Mirza S, Bradley PJ, Acharya A, Stacey M, Jones NS. Sinonasal inverted papillomas: recurrence, and synchronous and metachronous malignancy. J Laryngol Otol 2007;121(9):857–864

National Comprehensive Cancer Network. NCCN Guidelines for Head and Neck Cancers. http://www.nccn.org/professionals/physician_gls/f_guidelines.asp#head-and-neck

Nicolai P, Castelnuovo P. Benign tumors of the sinonasal tract. In: Cummings CW, Flint PW, Haughey BH, et al., eds. Cummings Otolaryngology: Head and Neck Surgery, 5th ed. Philadelphia, PA: Elsevier Mosby; 2010:

Rawal RB, Gore MR, Harvey RJ, Zanation AM. Evidence-based practice: endoscopic skull base resection for malignancy. Otolaryngol Clin North Am 2012;45(5):1127–1142

Suárez C, Ferlito A, Lund VJ, et al. Management of the orbit in malignant sinonasal tumors. Head Neck 2008;30(2):242–250

Zimmer LA, Carrau RL. Neoplasms of the nose and paranasal sinuses. In: Bailey BJ, Johnson JT, Newland SD, eds. Head & Neck Surgery–Otolaryngology. 4th ed. Philadelphia, PA: Lippincott, Williams & Wilkins; 2006

IX

Facial Plastic and Reconstructive Surgery

92 Rhytidectomy

■ Introduction

Rhytidectomy as a cosmetic procedure has evolved from simple undermining and advancement of skin to a measured relocation of facial structures. Technical advances and anatomical knowledge have improved the efficacy and safety of the procedure, and social factors have caused an explosion in cosmetic surgery in general.

In 1974, Skoog described elevating the platysma muscle with the cutaneous flap. This method helped define the neck and jawline, but it did little to improve the midface and nasolabial folds. Mitz and Peyronie published their report in 1976 describing the superficial musculoaponeurotic system (SMAS) in the parotid and cheek area. This paper promulgated several facelift procedures that involved either elevation or imbrication of the SMAS to rejuvenate the face. Because the SMAS is a distinct fascial layer of the skin superficial to the parotideomasseteric fascia that spreads into the face and envelops the flat facial muscles, elevation and advancement of the SMAS should also advance the platysma and other facial muscles. The facial nerve is beneath the parotideomasseteric fascia and should be safe if the elevation is in the correct plane. The SMAS rhytidectomy produced excellent results in the jawline and neck but still poorly rejuvenated the midface and nasolabial fold area.

The deep-plane rhytidectomy was described by Hamra in 1990. This technique is designed to reposition the ptotic malar fat pad after separation from the underlying zygomatic musculature. Elevation of the midface soft tissue by raising a subplatysmal musculocutaneous flap above the jawline should help flatten the nasolabial fold and rejuvenate the midface. The midface elevation is superficial to the parotideomasseteric fascia, the facial nerve lying deep to this fascia, and the zygomaticus muscles. Hamra later described the composite rhytidectomy, which included elevation of the orbicularis oculi muscle with the midface flap, stating that this helps to reju-venate the periorbital area in conjunction with the other facial structures being elevated.

Not all authors support the theory and safety of the deep-plane rhytidectomy. Baker warned of the dangers of deep-plane dissection to the facial nerve and cited a lack of evidence that the aesthetic results were superior to the traditional techniques. As surgeons gained more experience with these more aggressive procedures, many concluded that for the majority of patients, the results were no better, and the morbidity and complications were greater. A trend back to more traditional SMAS rhytidectomies and trials of even more conservative approaches resulted that minimized the risk of complications. A notable contribution to this trend was the minimal access cranial suspension (MACS) lift introduced by Tonnard in 2002. This procedure, which uses SMAS suspension and a short scar, is useful in well-selected patients. However, its long-term results are still being evaluated.

Despite this trend toward more conservative approaches, several authors have found support for the deep-plane and composite rhytidectomy techniques. Kamer reported on a series of 100 consecutive deep-plane dissections and found no facial nerve injuries. Complications were about the same as expected for traditional SMAS rhytidectomy techniques. It appears that in experienced hands, the deep-plane rhytidectomy may provide a safe facelift alternative that has increased surgeons' ability to rejuvenate the midface in addition to the neck and jawline. Kamer also found that the thicker SMAS-skin flap developed in a deep-plane lift is hardier and less prone to marginal necrosis—an advantage especially important in patients who smoke.

The subperiosteal facelift, described by Ramirez, involves a subperiosteal elevation of the midface and periorbital area from both sublabial and forehead approaches. Both direct and endoscopic techniques are used to free the midfacial soft tissues for elevation. This procedure has been particularly helpful in the forehead and brow region, but further long-term results are necessary in the midface to judge its efficacy.

Rhytidectomy continues to be a surgical procedure in development, with innovations introduced with increasing frequency. Technological and anatomical advancements will further innovation in the next few years. Meaningful prospective evaluation of results is needed. A recent systematic review comparing efficacy and complication rates among rhytidectomy techniques revealed that there are no quality data on which to rely to choose one technique over another.

■ Patient Evaluation and Selection

Patient selection may be the most important factor in a successful rhytidectomy procedure. The surgeon must develop a sense of both the physical and the psychological factors that influence the final outcome. Patients must be screened for unrealistic expectations, depression, and manipulative or abrasive behavior. It is always an advantage to recognize these personalities prior to surgery.

Surgeon preference and experience are probably the major factors in choosing the technique of rhytidectomy. With respect to choosing deep-plane techniques versus more conservative SMAS techniques, including plication, it is the opinion of some authors that older patients may require a more aggressive technique to achieve outcomes similar to those of younger patients undergoing more conservative techniques.

Many patients arrive for a surgical consultation well prepared to describe their goals. They frequently can describe particular perceived defects, and they ask directly about improving these areas. The patient who has difficulty describing these desires, or who cannot focus on specific anatomical areas, may be psychologically unfit for surgery. There is no specific or reliable preoperative test of a patient's personality to screen for potential psychiatric problems after surgery.

Medical History

A medical history is essential before deciding upon rhytidectomy. The general health of the patient must be assessed with regard to anesthesia concerns and the ability to heal well. Systemic problems, such as diabetes, hypothyroidism, cardiovascular disease, and pulmonary reserve, are important factors in patient assessment. This evaluation may be performed by an independent physician, such as the patient's family physician or internist. Because of the microvascular effects of nicotine and the danger of flap necrosis in the postoperative period, smoking history is vital and must be specifically sought. Active smoking is considered a relative contraindication to rhytidectomy. The risk of marginal flap necrosis in active smokers is 12.6 times the rate of necrosis in nonsmokers after superficial-plane rhytidectomy. This rate decreases with smoking cessation beginning 4 to 6 weeks preoperatively and continuing 2 to 4 weeks postoperatively.

Skin Disorders

Several genetic skin disorders will affect the decision to proceed with rhytidectomy—most notably, Ehlers–Danlos syndrome, cutis laxa, and pseudoxanthoma elasticum, characterized by an abnormality in collagen maturation, a decrease in the size and number of elastic fibers in the dermis, and degeneration of elastic fibers in the skin, respectively. All of these disorders cause premature skin laxity. Rhytidectomy in patients with Ehlers–Danlos syndrome should be avoided due to poor wound healing. However, cutis laxa and pseudoxanthoma patients are good candidates for rhytidectomy because they have no significant problems with wound healing. Other conditions with strong relative contraindications to rhytidectomy include systemic autoimmune conditions that may affect the face, such as scleroderma, systemic lupus erythematosus, and sarcoidosis.

Preoperative Precautions

Any use of aspirin and anti-inflammatory drugs must be discontinued at least 2 weeks prior to the planned surgical date. The need for preoperative laboratory studies, electrocardiogram, and chest X-rays will vary according to medical conditions and local community standards.

Age

There is no ideal age for facelift surgery. Patients show signs of facial aging as early as in their 30s. We are seeing more patients present in their 40s with the goal of preserving, rather than obtaining a youthful appearance. At this age, the skin is still relatively elastic and able to adapt to the operative repositioning and edema. Patients in their 50s through 80s are still good candidates for rhytidectomy, with excellent results obtainable for properly selected individuals.

Physical Evaluation

The physical evaluation should note not only anatomical signs of facial aging but also the condition of the skin and facial skeleton. In assessing patients for rhytidectomy, the surgeon should document signs of aging, such as brow position, jowls, platysma and skin laxity, and the nasolabial folds. The temporal and occipital hairline must be noted, especially if previous surgery has been performed. The presence of excessive submental and facial fat is evaluated and incorporated into the proposed technique. Skeletal factors, such as midface hypoplasia and retrognathia, are noted and are addressed as the patient desires with appropriate ancillary procedures. The cranial nerves should be evaluated and documented on the chart prior to surgery.

In assessing the condition of the skin, elasticity, actinic damage, and rhytids are observed and discussed with the patient. A well-designed skin care program started several weeks preoperatively can enhance surgical results and make patients active participants in their own care. The surgeon must emphasize that rhytidectomy surgery will do little to erase fine rhytids, and ancillary procedures, such as chemical peel or laser resurfacing, may be indicated.

Patient Education

After sharing the evaluation and surgical recommendations with the patient, the surgeon answers questions as thoroughly as possible. It is important to make sure that the patient understands not only the technical procedure planned, but also the expected morbidity and recovery period. The surgeon then lists and describes complications prior to obtaining an informed consent from the patient.

The display of previous patients' pre- and postoperative photographs is of some value in teaching patients about the benefits and limitations of facelift surgery. It is helpful to find an example of a patient of about the same age and face structure for best comparison. Computer imaging is also of some value but must be used with caution to avoid expectations that are not easily obtainable. Preoperative photographs are then taken in a standardized and consistent fashion. In general, the views obtained include frontal, submental, profile, and three-quarter views. These are reviewed prior to surgery and very often help in surgical planning. Often the photographs will reveal characteristics not initially appreciated on physical examination. The photographs are also an essential part of medical documentation.

Financial Arrangements

Financial arrangements and scheduling are then discussed, with the patient encouraged to consider all of the session's information prior to scheduling a procedure. Printed informational brochures and preoperative instructions are also given to the patient for review.

■ Management

Gender Considerations

Male patients are seeking cosmetic facial surgery in increasing numbers. In some areas, men may constitute 25% of rhytidectomy patients. For men and women in the workplace, the benefits of appearing youthful and energetic are increasing. The concept of women adorning themselves with makeup, jewelry, or cosmetic surgery is easy for our society to accept, but male adornment has been much slower to develop and is still not readily accepted in Western societies.

The major anatomical differences between male and female facelift patients involve the hairline, beard pattern, and skin characteristics. It is important to maintain male characteristics, such as the hairless area anterior to the ear, and the temporal hairline. The natural progression of male pattern baldness must be considered when planning rhytidectomy in male patients. The presence of a beard in men leads to thicker, less elastic, and rougher skin than in female patients. A richer subdermal plexus to enrich the beard is also present and has been cited as a source of increased hematoma complications in men. For this reason, some authors have recommended a deep-plane dissection to minimize the actual subcutaneous dissection. The deep-plane technique creates a myocutaneous flap with less chance of injuring the subdermal plexus.

Men seem more concerned with laxity in the cheek and neck, whereas women focus on the upper face and eyes. Most male facelift patients are middle-aged professionals with busy lifestyles. Because men have few peers who have undergone facial cosmetic surgery, they may have unrealistic expectations about results and recovery periods. The surgeon must spend considerable time explaining both the limitations of surgery and the expected period of recuperation. Men must be informed that shaving may now involve an area behind the ear, and that temporary hypesthesia may make shaving with a sharp blade difficult for several months.

In the immediate postoperative period men are less likely than women to complain of pain or ask for medications. On the other hand, men are noted to be less patient with regard to the resolution of normal postoperative ecchymosis and edema. After healing, male patients are generally quite pleased and ask for minor revisions less often than women.

The operative technique is modified in men to protect the sideburn and temporal hair. A hairless strip of skin is preserved in front of the ear, and vascular complications are minimized by a deep dissection. To preserve the sideburn and temporal hair, the incision is made 1 cm anterior to the tragus and just inferior to the temporal tuft. An endoscopic treatment of the brow area is recommended to avoid large incisions in a potentially balding scalp. Ancillary procedures, such as blepharoplasty, mentoplasty, and brow lift, are common.

Anesthesia

Rhytidectomy can be safely performed under general or local anesthesia. This decision is made jointly by the surgeon and the patient in consultation with the anesthesiologist.

Increasingly, surgeons are using general anesthesia for the comfort of the patient and better control of the airway during a lengthy surgery. The endotracheal tube can be stabilized to the teeth using dental floss, leaving the chin and submental areas free for surgery. With the deep-plane techniques, it is also more difficult to obtain local comfort in the anterior midface region without injecting around the facial nerve branches. Improved anesthetic agents with reduced toxicity and faster half-lives have improved the overall safety of anesthesia for cosmetic surgery.

Complications

Patients undergoing aesthetic surgery are usually not prepared to expect complications, even minor problems. Therefore, the surgeon must inform and educate patients that rhytidectomy is a major operation and has definable risks like any other medical intervention. The possibility of unforeseen secondary procedures should be addressed prior to surgery. The unhappy patient is usually the result of a less than perfect outcome in combination with not enough preoperative discussion about possible complications. In this early postoperative period, unforeseen psychological traits may emerge, causing great anxiety for both patient and surgeon. Many patients suffer postoperative depression of variable degree and may benefit from the surgeon's recognition of this state.

Hematoma Formation

The most commonly reported complication of rhytidectomy is hematoma formation. The reported incidence of significant hematoma is 1 to 8%. It is generally noted that hematoma is more prevalent in male patients, attributed to the rich subdermal plexus beneath the bearded skin. Prevention is best obtained by meticulous intraoperative hemostasis and careful screening for bleeding disorders, aspirin ingestion, and recent anti-inflammatory medications. Appropriate pressure dressings and ice compresses in the immediate postoperative period may also reduce the risk of hematoma. Careful blood pressure control in the perioperative period may also prevent hematomas.

Grover found a 4.2% hematoma rate in a series of 1,078 consecutive rhytidectomies. Significant factors included platysmaplasty, systolic blood pressure, male sex, use of aspirin, and smoking. Rhytidectomy technique—whether primary or secondary, surgeon, and the use of Tisseel (Baxter Healthcare Corp., Deerfield, IL) were not associated with an increased risk of hematoma. Once a hematoma is recognized, it must be treated immediately with evacuation and hemostasis. Irrigation of the wound will also prevent secondary infection. Failure to recognize and correct the problem may lead to decreased blood flow to the skin flaps and necrosis.

Late hematoma formation can occur up to 2 weeks following rhytidectomy. In some cases, this has been found to be due to an unrecognized injury to the superficial temporal artery and is set off by strenuous activity or a rise in blood pressure. This formation can be prevented by ligation of vessels if injury is suspected during surgery. Treatment will require exploration and appropriate ligation of the offending vessels.

Infection

Infection after rhytidectomy is rare. It is more common in areas of untreated hematoma, even in small isolated pockets. Prophylactic antibiotics to cover for *Staphylococcus aureus* are routinely used by many surgeons. Any infection should be treated aggressively with drainage of abscesses, debridement of necrotic tissues, and appropriate cultures to guide antibiotic selection.

Tissue Loss

Tissue loss following rhytidectomy may be minor or catastrophic. The most common area of loss is in the postauricular area. Preauricular skin loss is also seen, most often in conjunction with a hematoma or failure to stop smoking. Technical problems in elevating the flaps may also be associated with flap loss. Aggressive cautery on the underside of the flaps, or even hot operating room lights, has been associated with skin flap necrosis. Strangulating postoperative dressings may also contribute to decreased blood flow and complications.

Local wound care and appropriate debridement of necrotic eschar will accelerate healing and minimize obvious scarring. Frequent follow-up and reassurance are essential for these patients.

Nerve Injury

The greater auricular nerve is the most frequent nerve injury site in rhytidectomy.

Many patients have temporary hypesthesia of the lateral face and earlobe following surgery. If the greater auricular nerve continuity has been preserved, sensation should return within 2 to 6 months. If the greater auricular nerve is severed or severely damaged, this anesthetic area may be permanent and bothersome to the patient. A simple act, such as inserting earrings, may become extremely difficult. If there is a persistent painful neuralgia, treatment may involve such interventions as surgery for the management of a neuroma and the use of such medicines as gabapentin.

Facial nerve injuries are relatively uncommon in rhytidectomy. It is important that the surgeon understand the anatomy of the facial nerve. The frontal branch is vulnerable as it crosses the zygomatic arch, especially from traction applied during a coronal flap for brow lift. The marginal mandibular branch arches below the mandible lateral to the facial notch and may be injured if a subplatysmal dissection is attempted in this area. Weakness of the cervical branch due to platysma modification or direct nerve injury may result in a pseudomarginal mandibular nerve injury appearance, which resolves over time. The buccal branch passes deep to the zygomatic muscles in the midface and may be injured during deep-plane dissections if the elevation does not proceed superficial to the musculature. Unilateral nerve injuries can sometimes be camouflaged by causing temporary paralysis on the opposite side with selective injections of botulinum toxin.

Hypertrophic Scarring or Keloid Formation

Hypertrophic scarring or keloid formation can occur in several places after rhytidectomy. The most common area is the postauricular incision, especially in non-Caucasian or young patients. Preventive actions include avoiding excessive tension at the closure site and the timely removal of sutures or staples. Postoperative intralesional steroid injections at the first sign of hypertrophy are thought to be helpful. This can be repeated every 3 to 4 weeks until the wound has stabilized. Scar revision may be necessary later if the response to observation and steroids is not satisfactory.

Hair Loss

Hair loss after rhytidectomy in the temporal or postauricular regions may be very light or obvious. This is more common in elderly patients, smokers, and those with very sparse hair density. Preventive measures include placing the incisions inferior to the hairline, avoiding excessive cautery or tension, and ensuring the patient's cessation of smoking at least 1 month prior to surgery. The flap dissection should be deep to the hair follicles, preventing direct sharp injury.

Most areas of postoperative alopecia are temporary and will resolve spontaneously in 3 to 4 months. If the loss is permanent, the use of hair micrografts will restore hair density and create a natural hair density. Hundreds of grafts may be necessary.

Earlobe Deformity

Earlobe deformity is one of the most obvious facelift complications. The pulled down "devil's ear" or "pixie ear" deformity is usually recognized by surgeon and layperson alike. The usual cause is overaggressive skin flap excision anterior and inferior to the earlobe. Scar contracture during healing may make this complication even more obvious. Careful trimming of the skin flap to ensure a tension-free closure in this area will usually prevent this complication. If the defect is recognized immediately, surgical repair is recommended early in the postoperative period.

The hairline may be moved upward by one or more facelift procedures. The sideburn and temporal tuft of hair will move above the anterior ear into the scalp unless steps are taken to prevent this movement. If the hairline is high preoperatively, the surgeon may wish to select an incision along the anterior edge of the temporal tuft before curving into the scalp area. This will prevent further upward migration. The same practice can be used to prevent elevation of the postauricular hairline.

Pain

Pain after facelift surgery is usually limited and not severe. The compressive dressing applied the first night is often referred to as "very uncomfortable but not painful." Extreme pain and edema may signal the formation of hematoma or other complication, so the dressing should be removed and the area closely inspected at the earliest opportunity. Rapid diagnosis and treatment of complications will minimize damage and prevent further sequelae.

Summary

The rhytidectomy is a collection of procedures that must be individualized for each patient. The diversity of patient characteristics, surgeon preferences, and patient motivation make selection of an ideal procedure an art form. Patient education and preparation are essential to minimize postoperative dissatisfaction. Meticulous surgical technique and close clinical follow-up are necessary to minimize complications.

■ Suggested Reading

Becker FF, Bassichis BA. Deep-plane face-lift vs superficial musculoaponeurotic system plication face-lift: a comparative study. Arch Facial Plast Surg 2004;6(1):8–13

Beighton P, Bull JC. Plastic surgery in the Ehlers-Danlos syndrome. Case report. Plast Reconstr Surg 1970;45(6):606–609

Beighton P, Bull JC, Edgerton MT. Plastic surgery in cutis laxa. Br J Plast Surg 1970;23(3):285–290

Chang S, Pusic A, Rohrich RJ. A systematic review of comparison of efficacy and complication rates among face-lift techniques. Plast Reconstr Surg 2011;127(1):423–433

Goin J, Goin M. Changing the Body: The Psychological Effects of Plastic Surgery. Baltimore, MD: Williams & Wilkins; 1981

Goldwyn RM. Late bleeding after rhytidectomy from injury to the superficial temporal vessels. Plast Reconstr Surg 1991;88(3):443–445

Griffin JE, Jo C. Complications after superficial plane cervicofacial rhytidectomy: a retrospective analysis of 178 consecutive facelifts and review of the literature. J Oral Maxillofac Surg 2007;65(11):2227–2234

Grover R, Jones BM, Waterhouse N. The prevention of haematoma following rhytidectomy: a review of 1078 consecutive facelifts. Br J Plast Surg 2001;54(6):481–486

Hamra ST. Composite Rhytidectomy. St. Louis, MO: Quality Medical Publishing; 1993

Hamra ST. The deep-plane rhytidectomy. Plast Reconstr Surg 1990;86(1):53–61, discussion 62–63

McCollough EG. Facelifting in the male patient. Facial Plast Surg Clin North Am 1993;1(2):217–229

Mitz V, Peyronie M. The superficial musculo-aponeurotic system (SMAS) in the parotid and cheek area. Plast Reconstr Surg 1976;58(1):80–88

Nahai F. The Art of Aesthetic Surgery: Principles and Techniques. St. Louis, MO.: Quality Medical Publishing; 2005

Ng AB, O'Sullivan ST, Sharpe DT. Plastic surgery and pseudoxanthoma elasticum. Br J Plast Surg 1999;52(7):594–596

Papel ID, Lee E. The male facelift: considerations and techniques. Facial Plast Surg 1996;12(3):257–263

Perkins S, Naderi S. Rhytidectomy. In: Patel I, ed. Facial Plastic and Reconstructive Surgery. New York, NY: Thieme; 2008:207–225

Ramirez OM. Endoscopic techniques in facial rejuvenation: an overview. Part I. Aesthetic Plast Surg 1994;18(2):141–147

Rees TD, Liverett DM, Guy CL. The effect of cigarette smoking on skin-flap survival in the face lift patient. Plast Reconstr Surg 1984;73(6):911–915

Schuster RH, Gamble WB, Hamra ST, Manson PN. A comparison of flap vascular anatomy in three rhytidectomy techniques. Plast Reconstr Surg 1995;95(4):683–690

Thomas JR. Thomas Procedures in Facial Plastic Surgery: Facelift. Shelton, CT: People's Medical Publishing House–USA; 2011

Tonnard P, Verpaele A, Monstrey S, et al. Minimal access cranial suspension lift: a modified S-lift. Plast Reconstr Surg 2002;109(6):2074–2086

93 Endoscopic Aesthetic Facial Surgery

■ Introduction

Endoscopy is an important area of clinical practice developed by otolaryngologists. As smaller endoscopes and endoscopic instruments were perfected for nasal cavity and paranasal sinus disease, some surgeons became interested in using these techniques for aesthetic surgery of the face and neck. In 1993, Keller et al published the first paper using endoscopic techniques for removal of forehead rhytids and furrows. Since then, endoscopic aesthetic surgery has advanced rapidly. Despite the experience and standardization associated with the endoscopic forehead lift, a recent systematic literature review found no prospective randomized trials. Based on a series of retrospective reviews, endoscopic approaches have similar complication rates compared with open approaches. The choice of appropriate technique (endoscopic vs. open) should be based on careful patient selection criteria.

The endoscopic forehead lift is commonly performed nearly exclusively with visualization through endoscopes. Other facial cosmetic procedures, including facelifting, may be conducted with the aid of an endoscope to limit the length of incisions in conspicuous areas or to minimize skin vascular compromise. These endoscopically assisted procedures are less well described, and there are only a few reports regarding long-term results. Endoscopically assisted rhytidectomies are generally performed to limit visible scarring in male patients, in smokers at risk for flap necrosis, and in secondary facelifting cases, when only limited tissue movement or skin excision is needed. Nevertheless, it is a full facelifting technique subject to complications similar to those associated with classic facelifting. Only the forehead lift has evolved sufficiently to become relatively standardized. The endoscopic forehead lift is designed to treat the muscles causing undesired rhytids and to reposition the eyebrows to a more aesthetic position. As other treatments are readily available to treat forehead rhytids, such as botulinum toxin (Botox,

Allergan, Irvine, CA), the endoscopic forehead lift is primarily used for reshaping and elevating the brows.

The youthful forehead is usually smooth and without significant wrinkling, except in animation. As described by Ellis, habitual patterns of forehead movement develop at an early age and lead to consistent patterns of forehead wrinkling. Individuals who chronically lift their brows develop strong horizontal lines from the action of the frontalis muscle. Those who consistently frown develop the vertical lines from the action of the procerus muscle. Individuals who consistently squint develop lateral brow ptosis. These various muscle use patterns have been addressed with endoscopic surgical techniques, Botox, and selected nerve sections.

The youthful brow is positioned above the orbital rim and is slightly higher laterally than medially. The male brow is usually more horizontal and positioned more inferiorly than is the female brow. The female brow is usually more arched, with the peak of the eyebrow located between the lateral limbus and the lateral canthal angle.

Relevant Anatomy

Overactivity of several muscles results in forehead and glabellar wrinkling, whereas skin aging and gravitational effects cause forehead ptosis. Muscles involved in wrinkle formation include the frontalis, procerus, and corrugators. The frontalis muscle is an extension of the galea aponeurotica. It inserts into the dermis of the upper brow, and contraction produces transverse forehead wrinkling. Procerus and corrugator muscles are primarily medial brow depressors. The procerus originates from the upper nasal bones and inserts into the glabellar dermis. Procerus muscular contraction depresses the medial brow, causing transverse wrinkling of the nasal radix. The corrugator muscles work to depress the medial brow, taking their origin from the superomedial orbital rim and inserting into the medial brow skin. Corrugator contraction results in vertical and oblique glabellar wrinkle formation. The corrugator muscles are the primary focus of forehead lifting procedures and must be adequately addressed for satisfactory results.

The endoscopic forehead lift is the most standardized of the face and neck endoscopic procedures. It is designed to replace the coronal and trichophytic forehead lifts in patients who are suitable candidates. The surgical goal of the forehead lift is to aesthetically reposition the eyebrows and remove or improve forehead rhytids, creases, and glabellar furrows caused by the action of various periorbital muscles. Brow aesthetics as well as the musculature responsible for forehead rhytids, creases, and furrows have been well described.

The central forehead and scalp consist of five characteristic layers. The skin is thick and is densely adherent to the abundant underlying subcutaneous tissue. The galea aponeurotica, or epicranial aponeurosis, is a thin, tendinous sheet of connective tissue that envelops the entire skull. It is a mobile structure located just superficial to the loose areolar tissue. The galea aponeurotica splits anteriorly to surround the frontalis muscle and posteriorly to encircle the occipitalis muscle. Below the superior temporal line, the galea becomes confluent with the temporoparietal fascia. The superficial temporal vessels and the temporal branch of the facial nerve lie within and just deep to the temporoparietal fascia. This layer is also continuous with the superficial musculoaponeurotic system (SMAS), below the zygomatic arch.

The temporal fossa, also an area of concern in endoscopic forehead lifts, is bounded by the superior temporal line (superiorly), the frontal process of the zygomatic bone (anteriorly), and the zygomatic arch (inferiorly). It contains the temporalis muscle and its overlying fascia, the superficial and deep temporal vessels, the temporal branch of the facial nerve, and the auriculotemporal nerve.

The temporoparietal fascia of the temporal fossa is continuous with the epicranial aponeurosis of the forehead and scalp. This layer also contains the temporal branch of the facial nerve, which arises from the upper division of the facial nerve and crosses the midportion of the zygomatic arch on its superficial surface. The temporal branch ramifies into three to five branches, all of which ascend into the forehead no higher than 2 cm above the lateral aspect of the eyebrow. These nerves supply the frontalis, corrugator, procerus, and orbicularis oculi muscles. The subaponeurotic plane (loose areolar tissue) of the temporal fossa is located deep to the temporoparietal fascia and superficial to the deep temporal fascia.

The deep temporal fascia covers the temporalis muscle. It contains the deep temporal vessels, which supply the underlying muscle. The deep temporal fascia splits ~ 2 cm above the zygomatic arch to envelop the temporal fat pad and also invests the zygomatic arch

on both its superficial and its deep surfaces. Branches of the superficial temporal artery and vein can be seen in the temporal parietal fascia more superficially. The middle temporal artery arises from the superficial temporal artery at the level of the zygomatic arch, or 1 to 2 cm below it. The middle temporal artery always courses superficial to the arch, and it enters the superficial layer of the deep temporalis fascia just above the arch. The middle temporal artery supplies the fascia and sends a few branches to the temporalis muscle. A branch of the middle temporal vein traverses the surface of the temporalis muscle, inferior to the line of fusion of the temporalis fascias; becomes superficial at about the frontozygomatic suture line; and pierces the fascial layers. This may represent the "sentinel vein" described in some clinical literature.

The zygomaticotemporal nerve provides sensation to the anterior portion of the temporal fossa and is encountered as one dissects inferiorly and anteriorly toward the arch and lateral orbital rim. Just above the zygomatic arch lies the temporal parietal fat pad. The temporal branch of the facial nerve runs just superficial to this fat on the undersurface of the temporal parietal fascia. At the lateral orbital rim beginning at the zygomaticofrontal suture line is the area of fascial blending.

Descending from the midline of the forehead in the subaponeurotic or subperiosteal planes, one encounters the supraorbital and supratrochlear vessels and nerves. They can originate from either a notch (60%) or two foramina (40%). The supraorbital vessels generally travel with the nerves. The supratrochlear vessels are intimately associated with the supratrochlear nerves. There is considerable variation in the relative size and initial branching pattern of these nerves. They pierce the frontalis muscle at various levels, with the more medial branches becoming superficial before the lateral branches. The corrugator, procerus, and medial branches of the orbicularis oris (depressor supercilii) muscles are seen clearly from this plane but may blend with each other.

Extending over the orbital rim, the arcus marginalis is encountered. After releasing the attachments of the enveloping fascia of the frontalis muscle (SMAS) from the periosteum, the retro-orbicularis oculi fat (ROOF), or eyebrow fat pad, is expressed. Medially, the ROOF is adherent to the periosteum and extends as a more filamentary layer inferiorly between the orbicularis oculi and the orbital septum.

■ Evaluation

Patient Selection

Selection criteria for the endoscopic forehead lift are the same as for open forehead lifts. However, because no skin excision is performed, elevation of the brows also raises the hairline. Therefore, a high hairline is a relative contraindication to this procedure (as it is with the coronal lift). In a patient with a high forehead (> 5 cm), an anterior hairline incision should be performed to avoid elevating the hairline further. This should be discussed during the consultation and documented on the consent form. In addition, in patients who on profile have a prominent frontal bone angle (scalp to forehead) at the hairline, it may be difficult to pass the rigid endoscope over the supraorbital region. This situation is more common in patients with high hairlines. The trichophytic forehead lift may be more suitable in these situations.

Preoperative Evaluation

In a well-illuminated room, the characteristics of the forehead should be assessed, including the degree of wrinkling in the forehead and glabella. Forehead height, hairline position, and hair density are also important elements in the initial examination. Brow position should be noted with respect to the underlying bony orbital rim and how its position affects upper eyelid fullness. Brow position may have a profound effect on upper eyelid fullness, and raising the brow could obviate the need for blepharoplasty. The ideal brow position has been described by Ellenbogen as follows:

- It starts medially at a vertical line perpendicular to the alar base.
- The lateral brow ends at an oblique line through the nasal ala and lateral canthus.
- The medial and lateral ends lie approximately at the same horizontal level.
- The apex of the brow intersects the vertical line through the lateral limbus.
- The brow arches above the supraorbital rim in females and following the supraorbital rim in males.

■ Management

Surgical Technique

An endoscopic forehead lift is generally performed under a general anesthesia, although limited endoscopic lifts focusing on, for example, the lateral brow can easily be performed under local anesthesia. Incision sites and the entire supraorbital rim are infiltrated using lidocaine 1% with epinephrine to assist in anesthesia and to enhance hemostasis. The forehead may be infiltrated using lidocaine 0.5% with epinephrine or with a tumescent solution into the subperiosteal plane as an aid in dissection.

Although traditional coronal brow lifts most often involve dissection in the subgaleal layer, endoscopic approaches are most often performed in the subperiosteal layer, because the focus is entirely on lifting with limited skin movement. Scarring of the periosteum to the underlying frontal bone adds to the permanency of the lift. Theoretically, the disadvantage to this approach is that some bone resorption may occur, because the frontal bone has been separated from the periosteum that provides its blood supply.

The basic instrumentation for performing endoscopic brow elevation includes a 5 mm rigid scope with a 30-degree angle and a standard light source, angled endoscopic periosteal elevators, graspers, scissors, and cautery. The procedure begins with preoperative markings at the planned incision sites. There are three to five sites through which the endoscope and instruments will gain access. Each incision is 2 cm long and placed 3 to 5 mm posterior to the anterior hairline: There are several patterns described for the placement of the incisions. The general location of the supraorbital and supratrochlear nerves as a reference is marked prior to the dissection.

The dissection begins in the temporal scalp after the incisions are made. The dissection proceeds through the temporoparietal fascia in a subgaleal plane over the temporal fascia through the lateral incisions and up to the lateral orbital rims to the anterior two-thirds of the zygomatic arch. To prevent injury to the superficial temporal vessels, dissection in the region of the posterior zygomatic arch should be avoided. After the temporal dissections are completed, the central dissection begins.

The central dissection is carried toward the supraorbital rims in the subperiosteal plane. The supratrochlear and supraorbital nerves should be identified near the orbital rims. The lateral dissection joins the temporal dissection. The surgical goal at this point is to release the temporal line and identify the "sentinel vein" described by de la Plaza. This vein is a constant landmark and lies ~ 5 mm lateral to the frontozygomatic suture line. The frontal branch of the facial nerve lies in proximity to the sentinel vein. The nerve is generally within a 10 mm radius cephalad to the vein, lying on the deep surface of the temporoparietal fascia. The temporoparietal fascia from the endoscopic vantage point is the undersurface of the flap being elevated, which is commonly covered (deep surface) by a thin layer of fat. Just anterior to the sentinel vein along the temporal line is a ligament-like confluence of fascia, referred to by some surgeons as the "conjoint tendon" and by others as the "orbital ligament." This ligament spans from the frontozygomatic suture area along the temporal line to the superficial temporal fascia, which in turn is tightly adherent to the overlying skin. If elevation of the lateral brow is an important goal, this periosteal-cutaneous ligament requires release. The sentinel vein will usually need to be divided for access to this ligament. Cauterization and transection of this vein must be performed on the deep side to prevent risk of frontal nerve branch injury. Once this ligament is released, the posterior border of the lateral bony orbit will be visualized. Subperiosteal elevation along the lateral orbital rim to the lateral canthus completes the dissection.

Upon completion of the entire dissection, the superior aspect of the arcus marginalis of both orbits from lateral canthus to lateral canthus is incised using an elevator, endoscopic scissors, or laser fiber. Dissection is continued until the ROOF is reached. Release of the arcus marginalis results in a 1 to 3 mm elevation of the eyebrows by itself.

The corrugators and procerus muscles are exposed, cut, and partially resected. For glabellar vertical and horizontal lines, corrugator and procerus myotomies are performed with endoscopic scissors or laser. Myotomies of the depressor supercilii and orbital portion of the orbicularis can also be performed if desired. Free fat grafting may be necessary to avoid a glabellar depression after muscle resection. Incision of the frontalis muscle to improve horizontal dynamic and static rhytids and creases of the forehead is not usually necessary. These rhytids and creases are greatly ameliorated or disappear without frontalis muscle work after release of the arcus marginalis.

Positioning the eyebrows and fixing the flap to maintain that position are the final steps. The amount of overcorrection recommended by various surgeons for elevation of the flap varies from 1 to 2 mm to near maximal overcorrection laterally. Similarly, the method of flap fixation, as well as the duration of flap fixation, remains quite variable among surgeons.

The forehead periosteum is supported and fixed to the frontal bone using titanium screws, bone tunnels, or absorbable retention devices. If screws are used, they are usually ~ 1.5 mm in diameter and 12 to 16 mm long. They are placed 4 mm into the bone through two or three of the central incisions. The screws are removed 10 to 14 days postoperatively

after the flap has sufficiently scarred into place. The temporoparietal fascia is plicated to the deep temporal fascia using 3–0 polydioxanone suture (PDS) to suspend the tissues in the temporal regions. Generally, the incisions are closed in two layers, the second layer being staples. A drain may be used and is removed on postoperative day 3. The staples and fixation screws may be removed 10 to 14 days postoperatively.

Alternatively, bioabsorbable screws may be used as a semipermanent fixation method. This method provides longer-term support for the periosteum and forehead tissue layers. Semipermanent fixation with bioabsorbable screws has at least a theoretical advantage over titanium screws, which must be removed before the periosteum is fully adhered to the underlying skull, which takes at least 6 weeks.

Adjuvant procedures, such as chemical peels or laser skin resurfacing of the forehead, can be performed concomitantly with the endoscopic forehead lift, because the flap is full thickness, and the principal axial blood supply is not interrupted. Upper blepharoplasties can be performed at the same time but are usually delayed 3 to 6 months to allow more precise judgment of skin removal.

Complications

Complications, similar to those seen in open approaches, include hematoma, alopecia, paralysis of the frontalis muscle, loss of sensation, scar pain and itching, and skin necrosis. Hematomas should be promptly evacuated to avoid flap necrosis and alopecia. Excessive tension on the flap may result in alopecia. Frontalis muscle paralysis is rare but may occur due to injury to the frontal branch of the facial nerve. Disadvantages specific to the endoscopic forehead lift include the cost of equipment and training, extended operative time, and increased risk to nerve or vessel injury due to poor visualization.

■ Suggested Reading

Aiache AE. Endoscopic facelift. Aesthetic Plast Surg 1994;18(3):275–278

Citarella ER, Sterodimas A, Condé-Green A. Endoscopically assisted limited-incision rhytidectomy: a 10-year prospective study. J Plast Reconstr Aesthet Surg 2010;63(11):1842–1848

Codner MA, Kikkawa DO, Korn BS, Pacella SJ. Blepharoplasty and brow lift. Plast Reconstr Surg 2010;126(1):1e–17e

Daniel RK, Tirkanits B. Endoscopic forehead lift: aesthetics and analysis. Clin Plast Surg 1995;22(4):605–618

Ellenbogen R. Transcoronal eyebrow lift with concomitant upper blepharoplasty. Plast Reconstr Surg 1983;71(4):490–499

de la Paza R, de la Cruz L. Can some facial rejuvenation techniques cause iatrogenia? Aesthetic Plast Surg 1994;18(2):205–209

De La Plaza R, Valiente E, Arroyo JM. Supraperiosteal lifting of the upper two-thirds of the face. Br J Plast Surg 1991;44(5):325–332

Ellis DA, Masri H. The effect of facial animation on the aging upper half of the face. Arch Otolaryngol Head Neck Surg 1989;115(6):710–713

Graham DW, Heller J, Kurkjian TJ, Schaub TS, Rohrich RJ. Brow lift in facial rejuvenation: a systematic literature review of open versus endoscopic techniques [published correction in Plast Reconstr Surg. 2011;128(5):1151. Note: Kirkjian, T Jonathan corrected to Kurkjian, T Jonathan]. Plast Reconstr Surg 2011;128(4):335e–341e

Hönig JF. The fiber endoscope with guidable and flexible working instruments for endofacelift: a new instrument in facial surgery. Aesthetic Plast Surg 1994;18(4):373–375

Iro H, Hosemann W. Minimally invasive surgery in otorhinolaryngology. Eur Arch Otorhinolaryngol 1993;250(1):1–10

Isse NG. Endoscopic facial rejuvenation: endoforehead, the functional lift. Case reports. Aesthetic Plast Surg 1994;18(1):21–29

Keller GS. Endoscopic Facial Plastic Surgery. St. Louis, MO: Mosby–Year Book; 1997

Keller GS, Razum NJ, Elliott S, Parks J. Small incision laser lift for forehead creases and glabellar furrows. Arch Otolaryngol Head Neck Surg 1993;119(6):632–635, discussion 636

Knize DM. An anatomically based study of the mechanism of eyebrow ptosis. Plast Reconstr Surg 1996;97(7):1321–1333

Knize DM. Muscles that act on glabellar skin: a closer look. Plast Reconstr Surg 2000;105(1):350–361

Larrabee WF Jr, Nishioka GJ. Laser blepharoplasty and laser assisted endoforehead lift. In: Krespi Y, ed. Office-Based Surgery of the Head and Neck. Philadelphia, PA: Raven-Lippincott; 1998

McKinney P, Mossie RD, Zukowski ML. Criteria for the forehead lift. Aesthetic Plast Surg 1991;15(2):141–147

Naini FB. Facial Aesthetics: Concepts and Clinical Diagnosis. Chichester, West Sussex, UK: Wiley-Blackwell; 2011:xix

Paul MD, Calvert JW, Evans GR. The evolution of the midface lift in aesthetic plastic surgery. Plast Reconstr Surg 2006;117(6):1809–1827

Ramirez OM. Endoscopic subperiosteal browlift and facelift. Clin Plast Surg 1995;22(4):639–660

Romo T III, Sclafani AP, Yung RT, McCormick SA, Cocker R, McCormick SU. Endoscopic foreheadplasty: a histologic comparison of periosteal refixation after endoscopic versus bicoronal lift. Plast Reconstr Surg 2000;105(3):1111–1117, discussion 1118–1119

Sclafani AP. Thomas Procedures in Facial Plastic Surgery: Aesthetic Surgery of the Forehead and Upper Third of the Face. Shelton, CT: People's Medical Publishing House–USA; 2010

Toledo LS. Video-endoscopic facelift. Aesthetic Plast Surg 1994;18(2):149–152

Vasconez LO, Core GB, Gamboa-Bobadilla M, Guzman G, Askren C, Yamamoto Y. Endoscopic techniques in coronal brow lifting. Plast Reconstr Surg 1994;94(6):788–793

94 Blepharoplasty

■ Introduction

Blepharoplasty is an aesthetic procedure of the upper and lower eyelids. Although occasionally a functional upper lid blepharoplasty is performed to correct a visual field deficit, aesthetic blepharoplasty is the focus of this discussion.

The purpose of aesthetic blepharoplasty is to rejuvenate the eyelids. The physical findings that patients would like corrected are not pathological elements; to a patient, findings of excess lid skin, excess or swagging of the orbicularis muscle, pseudoherniation of orbital fat, and creping of lid skin are aesthetic problems. The otolaryngologist/facial plastic surgeon who undertakes the treatment of aesthetic facial plastic problems must be sympathetic—not judgmental—about a patient's self-image.

■ Evaluation

Ideal Patients

Ideal patients seek blepharoplasty after thoughtful consideration. They reasonably recognize their aesthetic issues, but they do not overly dramatize them. They already have a good self-image and wish to make some improvement but are not expecting some fantasy secondary gain. They reasonably comprehend the surgical procedure and have a realistic understanding of the outcomes. It is helpful for patients to have the support of a significant other, but they should not be coerced by someone to have the procedure performed. Physically, such patients appear appropriate in their mode of dress, manner, and expressions; that is, ideal patients do not display any extreme in dress (extremely fastidious or sloppy) or behavior.

Questionable Patients

Questionable patients make a sudden decision about aesthetic surgery. They behave inappropriately during examination, have a general physical appearance that would not be helped by the procedure, or have a significant psychiatric history.

History

Medical History

Any medical history that would contraindicate any other elective surgical procedure would be a contraindication to blepharoplasty. Especially important is any history of a coagulopathy, diabetes, or untreated hypothyroidism. Because local anesthesia containing epinephrine is imperative to the procedure, any medical condition that would be worsened by the use of epinephrine or elevation of blood pressure would be a contraindication to the procedure.

Ophthalmologic History

An ophthalmologic history should address vision, previous eyelid surgery, eyelid trauma, eyelid skin allergy, glasses and/or contact lenses, tearing, burning, conjunctivitis, herpes infection, chalazion, recurrent eyelid edema, or use of any ophthalmic medications or treatments. If there is any indication of dry-eye syndrome, an ophthalmologic consultation may be requested to determine the advisability of blepharoplasty. Conservative blepharoplasty may be tolerated in the patient with mild dry eye syndrome. Blepharoplasty is contraindicated in the patient with moderate to severe dry-eye syndrome, because it will always worsen the condition.

Surgical Anatomy

The orbicularis muscle is intimately attached to lid skin. It is divided by location into a ring superficial to the tarsus (pretarsal orbicularis), a ring over the orbital septum (preseptal orbicularis), and an outer ring that extends under the brow and over the inferior orbital rim (orbitalis). The orbital septum is separated from the overlying orbicularis muscle by areolar tissue. It is contiguous with the tarsal plates. The orbital septum attaches peripherally to the orbital rim and with the tarsal plates to form a diaphragm protecting the intraorbital structures.

The orbital fat compartments, which pseudoherniate in some individuals on a hereditary basis, occupy two spaces in the upper lid and three spaces in the lower lid. In the upper lid, the central and medial compartments are divided by the superior oblique muscle. The lacrimal gland sits in the lateral compartment. In the lower lid, the central and medial compartments are separated by the inferior oblique muscles. The central and lateral compartments are separated by the arcuate expanse of the capsulopalpebral fascia. The floor of the fat compartments in the upper lid is formed by the levator aponeurosis. The levator aponeurosis attaches to the superior tarsal plate to elevate the lid. In the lower lid the lower lid refractors attach to the inferior tarsal plate. The lateral canthal ligament inserts behind the lateral orbital rim at the orbital (Whitnall) tubercle. The inferior and superior preseptal muscles blend together laterally over the orbital tubercle as the lateral palpebral raphe.

Physical Examination

Palpation indicates the position of the eyebrow in relationship to the orbital rim. The medial brow should be at the orbital rim, the central brow should be just slightly above the rim, and the lateral brow should be definitely above the lateral orbital rim. If the central or lateral brow is below the orbital rim, a brow lift procedure may be indicated and should be considered. A blepharoplasty performed on a brow that is below the orbital rim may draw the brow farther downward.

In the patient with a normally positioned brow, the amount of excess skin is estimated by gathering the redundant skin gently in a forceps without elevating the lid margin. The natural tarsal crease is identified. The amount of medial and central fat pseudoherniation is estimated by digitally raising the brow maximally to look for bulging of the fat. The lateral compartment of the upper lid is normally absent of fat. The space just beneath the orbital rim in the lateral compartment is occupied by the lacrimal gland. If the lacrimal gland is noted to be below the orbital rim, a plan is made to secure it to the inner orbital rim with a single permanent suture once an X-ray study has shown the enlargement does not represent a tumor.

In the lower lid, the orbital rim is also palpated to rule out a prominent orbital rim mimicking orbital fat pseudoherniation. The lower lid is gently pulled away from the globe and released to measure its elastic integrity. It should snap back to contact the globe quickly. If the lid fails to snap back until the patient blinks, then a standard blepharoplasty is contraindicated. A lid lacking elasticity will most likely droop following standard blepharoplasty, to cause at least a scleral show and, possibly, at worst, an ectropion. Eyelid closure strength is tested to ensure seventh nerve function. At the same time, the lids are gently separated while the patient is attempting to close them, to determine presence or absence of a Bell phenomenon.

The amount of lower skin excess is noted by gently gathering the skin using a blunt forceps. The amount of lower lid fat pseudoherniation is estimated by having the patient look upward, then laterally. This test projects the fat outward in the medial, central, and lateral compartments and makes the excess very obvious.

Any skin crepe (fine wrinkling), skin pigmentation, or skin lesions (i.e., hypertrophic sebaceous glands, syringoma, or trichoepithelioma) are noted, so that the patient can be told that removal of these lesions is not ordinarily part of blepharoplasty.

Any inequality of the palpebral fissure is noted. If this has been present for an extended period of time and is < 2 mm, then the patient is shown the inequality and told that it will not change with blepharoplasty. If the inequality is > 2 mm, then ptosis repair on the dependent lids should be considered. This can be done by a surgeon familiar with this very specific surgery, or a referral can be made to an oculoplastic surgeon.

The patient is shown in a mirror the approximate appearance of the blepharoplasty result by rolling the upper lid skin upward with the wooden end of a cotton tip applicator or by elevating the brow to a position that will mimic the blepharoplasty result. If the surgeon is artistic and comfortable with computer imaging, the patient is shown the anticipated result by this medium. It is not imperative that computer imaging be done, but if it is, no promises should be made about the computer image representing a postoperative result.

Once agreement about the goal of surgery is achieved, the patient is informed about preparation and techniques of surgery.

■ Management

Surgery

Preparing the Patient

For ~ 2 weeks prior to surgery and for 1 week following surgery, the patient should avoid any medication that might interfere with coagulation (i.e., aspirin, nonsteroidal anti-inflammatory drugs, and vitamin E). Alcohol should be avoided immediately preoperatively and 1 week postoperatively. Caffeine, because it is a vasodilator, should be avoided postoperatively. The patient should be told what to expect at the time of surgery (e.g., the type of anesthesia the surgeon prefers, the length of the procedure, and the anticipated postoperative course). The patient should also be informed about any complications and their frequency. Finally, the choice of place for the procedure (office procedure or outpatient hospital) should be discussed.

Photographs

As with all aesthetic procedures, photodocumentation is required. This may be done personally by the surgeon, or it may be delegated either to another person in the office or to an outside professional. It is the surgeon's responsibility, however, to be sure that the photographs are taken and are adequate. Acceptable views for blepharoplasty include full face frontal, close-up frontal with eyes open, close-up frontal with upward gaze, close-up frontal with eyes closed, close-up oblique left and right, and close-up lateral left and right.

Anesthesia

Blepharoplasty can be performed under local anesthesia, local with intravenous analgesia, or general anesthesia. All procedures are conducted with local infiltrative anesthesia with epinephrine, whether using local, intravenous, or general anesthesia. The local anesthesia is usually Xylocaine (AstraZeneca Pharmaceuticals LP, Wilmington, DE) 2% with epinephrine 1:100,000. Lesser concentrations do not provide enough time for the average surgeon to complete the procedure before return of sensation and loss of vasoconstriction. Approximately 1 to 1.5 mL of subcutaneous local anesthesia is required per eyelid for the upper lid and skin muscle flap lower lid blepharoplasty. Transconjunctival lower lid anesthesia requires the use of topical tetracaine into the lower lid conjunctival cul-de-sac prior to instillation of Xylocaine 2% with epinephrine into the subconjunctival space. The anesthesia is infiltrated with a 27- to 30-gauge needle.

Procedures

Upper Lid Blepharoplasty

Prior to infiltration of anesthesia, the skin is marked with a thin surgical marking pen. The patient should be positioned upright. The initial line is drawn at the natural tarsal crease if the crease is 8 to 10 mm above the lid margin. If the natural crease is > 10 mm or < 8 mm above the lid margin, or if no discernible crease exits, then the line is drawn 8 to 10 mm above the margin. The brow is gently depressed to mimic its natural position when the patient is standing. The upper boundary of the lid skin excision is determined by grasping the lid skin with a blunt forceps in an amount that incorporates all of the redundant skin but without elevating the lid margin. By removing just this amount of skin, no lagophthalmos will be produced. The lateral portion of the upper lid skin marking beyond the orbital rim should swing gently upward, so that the lateral hooding is eliminated. The medial and lateral ends of the excision should end in a 30-degree angle to prevent any standing cone deformity.

If all four lids are being operated on, usually the two upper lids are anesthetized at the same time. The lower lids are then anesthetized following completion of the upper lids. In this manner, anesthesia will be optimal as the skin incisions are made.

The skin is stretched taught as the initial incision is made with a no. 15 blade or a no. 67 Beaver blade along the inferior lid marking. The superior lid marking is then incised. The 30-degree angle must be precise and sharp. The skin is then removed using a Brown–Adson forceps and a curved Stevens tenotomy scissors down to, but not including, the orbicularis muscle. Care is taken not to remove too much skin at the medial end of the excision if there is a large amount of medial fat. A large amount of fat resection will leave a defect over which the skin must be closed. If the skin is closed under tension, a scar will result. A small amount of orbicularis muscle is then removed along a central trough equally distant from the superior and inferior skin edges in most cases. This muscle excision, which creates an increased definition of the natural upper lid cleft, is not performed in the eyelid that has exceedingly thin skin and scant muscle. The muscle is removed down to the level of the orbital septum. The fat pseudohernias are then removed as necessary from the central and medial compartments. This is done by incising the orbital septum and then teasing the fat into the operative field. No more fat than that which flows outward should be removed. The fat is removed by fine hemostat clamping excision and cautery of the fat stump. If the patient is being operated on under local anesthesia, each fat removal is preceded by a small local anesthesia injection. The initial subcutaneous anesthesia injection does not penetrate the orbital septum. The lateral compartment contains fat only rarely. This can be anticipated in patients with extraordinarily heavy upper lids. Occasionally, the lacrimal gland is ptotic and protrudes into the lateral compartment. This ptosis may be repaired with a single permanent suture between the gland capsule and the superior periorbita.

The most tension in the wound closure exists at the most lateral aspect of the eyelid, where the wound is the widest. This lateral area is closed with multiple interrupted permanent sutures. The remaining central and medial portions of the wound are closed with a single subcuticular suture that is taped to the skin at each end. Monofilament non-absorbable suture is better than braided suture or absorbable suture. Braided suture tends to develop scars and suture tunnels, whereas absorbable suture can be reactive when used in the skin.

Lower Lid: Skin–Muscle Flap Approach

A skin–muscle flap is used in the older patient who demonstrates fat pseudoherniation and some degree of skin redundancy and possibly orbicularis hypertrophy or swag. The ideal patient for skin muscle lower lid blepharoplasty requires some skin and muscle excision and usually some overall lid tightening.

The lower lid incision is made at 2.5 mm below the eyelash line. This places the incision in a natural skin crease, below the lash follicles, and high enough to avoid any obvious scar. An initial skin-only flap of 3 mm preserves the pretarsal orbicularis muscle. A skin–muscle flap is then elevated over the orbital septum down to the orbital rim, thus exposing the entire orbital septum. The lateral compartment, which lies at the 8 o'clock position in the patient's right eye and 4 o'clock in the left eye, is opened by creating a fenestration through the septum. The globe is gently palpated to encourage herniation of fat through the fenestration. The amount of fat that can be easily drawn into the wound is clamped with a fine hemostat and divided with cautery after a small amount of local anesthesia has been infiltrated into the fat. Fat management for the central and medial compartments varies according to surgical philosophy. Traditionally, central and medial fat is excised. The remaining fat in all three compartments should lie 1 mm below the orbital rim. This ensures that the fat will no longer register as a pseudohernia protrusion, and the bony, orbital rim will not be prominent enough to create a hollow.

Alternatively, instead of fat resection, fat from the central and medial pockets can be repositioned over the inferior orbital rim. This transfers fat volume away from an area of volume excess (pseudoherniation behind the orbital septum) to an area of relative volume loss (over the orbital rim, which underlies

the nasojugal fold). In this case, the orbital septum is opened widely from the medial canthus to the lateral canthus at the inferior orbital rim to liberate the retroseptal fat. Care is taken not to injure the inferior oblique muscle, which separates the medial and central fat pads. The fat is then positioned in either a supraperiosteal pocket or a subperiosteal pocket over the inferior orbital rim. A suture is used to maintain the positioning of the fat during the initial healing period. This suture is passed transcutaneously inferomedial to the nasojugal fold into the sub/supraperiosteal pocket, through the repositioned fat, then back out transcutaneously. This is then tied over a bolster, which is later removed 5 to 7 days postoperatively.

At this point, the skin muscle flap is draped upward. With the patient's eyes closed, it will most likely appear that there is a large amount of redundant skin to be removed. The amount of skin that can be safely removed, however, is determined by having the patient look upward and open the mouth slightly. This safe amount is then removed. If the lid skin and muscle demonstrated considerable swag preoperatively, then a small additional amount of skin and muscle is removed and a suspension suture is used.

The suspension suture is placed between the preseptal orbicularis muscle and the lateral orbital periosteum at the position of the orbital tubercle. The suture is placed so that pull is vertically upward. The major purpose of the suspension suture is to maintain a lateral tightness to the lower lid to (1) overcome a mild to moderate loss of lid tone and prevent scleral show, (2) eliminate muscle swag, and (3) correct some skin wrinkling by gently stretching the skin. Once hemostasis is established, the incision is closed with a running monofilament nonabsorbable suture.

Lower Lid: Transconjunctival Approach

The transconjunctival approach to lower lid blepharoplasty is used in younger patients, where the pseudoherniation of fat is the cardinal feature. Skin redundancy and skin wrinkling should be minimal. There should be little or minimal muscle hypertrophy. Skin wrinkling and, to some extent skin looseness, can be overcome by simultaneous carbon dioxide (CO_2) laser skin resurfacing. These features, if combined with muscle laxity or hypertrophy, cannot be properly diminished by laser if they are a major factor in the examination of the eyelid. In the properly selected case, the transconjunctival approach is efficient and effective.

The procedure is begun by using a retractor to expose the inferior cul-de-sac. Some protection of the cornea is indicated. A corneal shield can be used or the proximal portion of the transconjunctival incision can be brought across the cornea as a protective mechanism. Following the retraction of the lower lid to expose the inferior edge of the tarsal plate, an incision is made just below the tarsal plate margin with a very fine electrodissection needle guarded to expose only the tip. The arcuate vessels immediately below the conjunctival surface can bleed briskly if not incised with the electrodissection needle.

The inferior lid refractors are then incised with a small scissors. The proximal conjunctival flap can be retracted over the cornea with one or two retraction sutures draped vertically over the patient's head. The orbicularis muscle is bluntly dissected from the orbital septum down to the orbital rim. Management of the orbital fat can be through methods similarly described as with the skin muscle flap. To check for aesthetic contour following fat management, the lid is released, draped into its normal position, and examined. Gentle pressure is placed on the globe to note any pulsation in the three positions of usual fat herniation. Additional fat is removed as needed. If a laser resurfacing procedure has been planned, it is done prior to releasing the retraction sutures to continue the corneal protection. The retraction sutures are released, and the lid is lifted vertically as far superiorly as possible and released. The transconjunctival incision falls into place without the need for sutures. The procedure is essentially complete.

Postoperative Care

The patient should remain at rest for the remainder of the postoperative day. Cold compresses are applied to the eyes to help prevent edema and ecchymosis. An ophthalmic ointment is applied to the incisions to prevent crusting. In the case of transconjunctival blepharoplasty, the ointment is applied along the lash margin. Any blood coming from the conjunctival incision will otherwise fuse the eyelashes together. The patient is advised to look down only if necessary. This is especially true when the patient is lying down. In this position, downward gaze could theoretically allow the skin to slide downward over the deeper structures, causing an ectropion or scleral show. Other postoperative care is scheduled as follows:

- *First day:* The patient may ambulate without exertion. Cold compresses are used each hour for ~ 20 minutes.
- *Second day:* The maximal postoperative edema occurs on the second day when the patient begins to ambulate. The patient should be told that the increased edema is expected so that a complication is not suspected.
- *Third day:* The patient may go out with sunglasses.
- *Fourth day:* Sutures are removed.
- *Sixth day:* Makeup may be applied directly to the incisions.

- *Two weeks:* Moderate exercise begins. Prior to this time, exercise may produce edema in the operative area.
- *One month:* Full athletic activity is possible. The specialized pre- and postoperative care for CO_2 laser skin resurfacing is not within the scope of this chapter.

Complications

Problems Shortly after Surgery

The following problems occurring shortly after surgery will resolve in 1 or 2 weeks:

- Chemosis of the lower lid conjunctiva
- Subconjunctival hemorrhage
- Mild scleral show
- Tearing
- Burning sensation
- Visual blurring secondary to ointment
- Edema of the lids
- Pain
- Numbness of the upper lids

Problems after Two Weeks

These problems can be expected to resolve after the second postoperative week:

- *Eyelid ecchymosis*, especially in dark-skinned people
- *Tearing*, secondary to minor separation of the lids during sleep
- *Contact lens prescription no longer corrective*—change may be required in some patients because eyelid shape is altered.
- Recurrence of *dormant chalazion*
- *Wound problems*, secondary to overlapping skin edges
- *Persistent sensation of tightness*, usually self-limited
- *Contact dermatitis*, secondary to ophthalmic ointments

Aesthetic Problems

The following aesthetic problems are associated with blepharoplasty:

- *Persistence of fat pseudohernias*, most common in the lateral compartment of the lower lid. and the medial compartment of the upper lid. Recurrent or persistent fat of the lower lid is removed via the transconjunctival approach. Upper lid redundant fat is removed via the original incision.
- *Persistent skin of lower lid*, most common medially.

- *Persistent skin of the upper lid*, most common laterally.
- *Prominent ridge* just below the lower lid incision, secondary to redundant hypertrophic orbicularis, removed using a minor skin flap.
- *Asymmetric upper lid scar*, secondary to not placing the incisions in identical locations above the upper lid margin.
- *Webbed scar* at the medial end of the upper lid incision, usually the result of placing the incision onto the nasal skin.
- *Suture marks*, usually due to excess tension and leaving sutures beyond the fourth day.
- *Suture tunnels*, usually secondary to use of braided rather than monofilament suture.

Problems of Lower Lid Position

The following problems are associated with the lower lid position:

- *Scleral show* can occur even when little or no skin is removed. May not be seen as a problem by the patient. Squinting exercises reduce the problem.
- *Ectropion*, usually secondary to excess removal of skin or blepharoplasty on a patient with lax lids. These cases may require a horizontal lid-shortening procedure.

Problems of Upper Lid Position

The following problems are associated with the upper lid position:

- *Blepharoptosis* can occur if the levator aponeurosis is injured during upper lid blepharoplasty. The levator is the floor of the upper lid fat compartment. It is especially vulnerable in the central compartment.
- *Lagophthalmos*, most common following secondary or tertiary upper lid blepharoplasty when the patient complains of skin redundancy with the eyes open but in fact there is little or no redundant skin when the eyes are closed.

Hematoma

Hematoma of the upper lid is rare. Usually subcutaneous, it may require reopening of the wound. Hematoma of the lower lid is significant if expansion is documented and it is differentiated from ecchymosis and edema. Ecchymosis and edema are soft, whereas a hematoma is firm. An expanding hematoma requires opening of the surgical wound and hemostasis.

Overcorrection of the Fat Pockets

Only the amount of fat that flows easily into the surgical area should be removed from the central compartment of the upper lid. If fat is pulled from the intraorbital space, a retraction will occur in the central upper lid sulcus. In the lower lid, a sulcus will occur just above the orbital rim if the fat removal extends lower than 1 mm below the rim. Correction may require fat grafts.

Functional Problems

The following functional problems are associated with blepharoplasty:

- *Dry-eye syndrome* following blepharoplasty is almost always a result of worsening of an occult dry-eye syndrome present preoperatively. Very specific questioning preoperatively is essential.
- *Epiphora* beyond the first week or two may be caused by external rotation of the lacrimal puncta secondary to extending the lower lid incision too far medially.
- *Orbital hematoma* is a rare complication. Sudden intense pain associated with lid edema and proptosis is an emergency. To prevent damage to the orbital nerve, the wounds are opened, clots are expressed, and the bleeding is controlled. If the intraocular pressure approaches 80 mm hemoglobin, a lateral canthotomy should be performed. This will relieve the pressure on the central retinal artery.
- *Blindness* is a rare complication. No specific causal relationship may exist between blindness and blepharoplasty. The suspected causes—toxic amblyopia, idiopathic optic nerve atrophy, retrobulbar optic neuritis, or optic nerve changes secondary to systemic diseases—are beyond preventability. Such causes have all followed lower lid blepharoplasty and have been unilateral.
- *Diplopia.* The muscle at most risk during blepharoplasty is the inferior oblique between the central and medial fat compartments. Most diplopia is transient, but blind clamping or cautery can cause permanent damage to this muscle and also to the superior oblique and lateral rectus.

■ Suggested Reading

Collar RM, Lyford-Pike S, Byrne P. Algorithmic approach to lower lid blepharoplasty. Facial Plast Surg 2013;29(1):32–39 doi: 10.1055/s-0033-1333836

Fagien S. Advanced rejuvenative upper blepharoplasty: enhancing aesthetics of the upper periorbita. Plast Reconstr Surg 2002; 110(1):278–291, discussion 292

Honrado CP, Pastorek NJ. Long-term results of lower-lid suspension blepharoplasty: a 30-year experience. Arch Facial Plast Surg 2004;6(3):150–154

Hamra ST. The role of the septal reset in creating a youthful eyelid-cheek complex in facial rejuvenation. Plast Reconstr Surg 2004;113(7):2124–2141, discussion 2142–2144

Jacobs SW. Prophylactic lateral canthopexy in lower blepharoplasties. Arch Facial Plast Surg 2003;5(3):267–271

Leatherbarrow B, Saha K. Complications of blepharoplasty. Facial Plast Surg 2013;29(4):281–288 doi: 10.1055/s-0033-1349362

McCann JD, Pariseau B. Lower eyelid and midface rejuvenation. Facial Plast Surg 2013;29(4):273–280 doi: 10.1055/s-0033-1349361

McCord CD, Boswell CB, Hester TR. Lateral canthal anchoring. Plast Reconstr Surg 2003;112(1):222–237, discussion 238–239

Muzaffar AR, Mendelson BC, Adams WP Jr. Surgical anatomy of the ligamentous attachments of the lower lid and lateral canthus. Plast Reconstr Surg 2002;110(3):873–884, discussion 897–911

Nassif PS. Lower blepharoplasty: transconjunctival fat repositioning. Otolaryngol Clin North Am 2007;40(2):381–390

Perkins SW, Batniji RK. Rejuvenation of the lower eyelid complex. Facial Plast Surg 2005;21(4):279–285

Rohrich RJ, Coberly DM, Fagien S, Stuzin JM. Current concepts in aesthetic upper blepharoplasty. Plast Reconstr Surg 2004; 113(3):32e–42e

Terella AM, Wang TD, Kim MM. Complications in periorbital surgery. Facial Plast Surg 2013;29(1):64–70 doi: 10.1055/s-0033-1333838

Weissman JD, Most SP. Upper lid blepharoplasty. Facial Plast Surg 2013;29(1):16–21 doi: 10.1055/s-0033-1333833

95 Current Concepts of Chemical Peeling and Dermabrasion

Introduction

Skin aging results from both intrinsic (hereditary) and extrinsic factors. Photodamage produces rough textural change, pigmentary dyschromia, and loss of elasticity. Reductions in dermal volume produce fine and coarse rhytids. Histological correlates include a thickened stratum corneum; thinner, atrophic epidermis; epidermal atypia; and irregular melanin deposition. Dermal elastic fiber breakdown produces amorphous elastotic masses and increases in reticulin fibers.

Type I collagen appears irregularly arranged and smudged. Therefore, skin rejuvenation strategies strive to create a thinner, more compact stratum corneum; an increase in new, compact, orderly type I and type III dermal collagen; an increase in dermal glycosaminoglycans; and more uniform arrays of melanin. Treatment modalities currently available to realize these goals include chemical peels, mechanical dermabrasion, and laser ablation. Tailoring these options to accomplish resurfacing objectives centers on the control of treatment depth. Combining the use of different resurfacing modalities represents a major advance in customizing individual treatment strategies.

Evaluation

Evaluating a patient for resurfacing begins with a complete medical history. Some dermatologic conditions, such as rosacea, atopic dermatitis, and psoriasis, may increase the risk for complications, including disease exacerbation, prolonged erythema, or delayed healing. A history of herpes simplex virus (HSV) merits pretreatment with antiviral prophylaxis (e.g., acyclovir). Prophylaxis in patients without a history of herpetic infection remains controversial. Previous studies have shown a 6.6% HSV infection rate in patients who underwent chemical peels who had no history of infection.

Current medications should be known. It is generally recommended waiting at least 6 to 12 months after discontinuing oral isotretinoin therapy before resurfacing. Photosensitizing agents and anticoagulants should be discontinued 2 weeks before dermabrasion, if medically possible. The details of prior resurfacing procedures should be sought. A personal or family history of hypopigmentation or hyperpigmentation, keloid scars, or hypertrophic scars should be examined. The surgical history is relevant, because patients who have undergone extensive undermining of the area to be resurfaced have vascular compromise. Surgeons must determine any history of radiation therapy, cardiac disease, hepatic or renal insufficiency, and collagen vascular disease. Finally, it is important to have patients clearly explain their treatment goals.

Patients' facial skin types are classified during the examination. Three schemes have been used in this regard.

- Fitzpatrick types I through VI range from the inability to tan and only burn, to the high propensity to darkly tan and never burn. Fitzpatrick skin types III and IV, although at higher risk, are still appropriate candidates for chemical peeling. Skin types V and VI should be limited to superficial chemical peels.
- Glogau types I through IV qualify the level of photodamage from mild to severe, respectively. Clinically, wrinkling with acne scarring and actinic keratoses are included within this classification.
- Rubin established the level of photodamage based on the depth of visible signs. Level I photodamage is confined to the epidermis. Level II photodamage extends into the papillary dermis, and level III pathology exhibits changes in the reticular dermis.

Chemical Peeling

Chemical peeling is an accelerated form of chemexfoliation induced by the topical application of one or more chemical cauterant or escharotic agents. This results in the destruction and subsequent regeneration of the epidermis and/or dermis. Two mechanisms have been proposed to account for the beneficial effects of chemical peels: a quantitative increase in dermal glycosaminoglycans and a qualitative change in dermal collagen.

McKee, a British dermatologist, began chemical peeling for acne in 1903, but it wasn't until the 1960s, when plastic surgeons (e.g., Brown, Litton, and Baker) developed phenol formulations, that chemical peeling became widely used for rejuvenation. Unfortunately, most of these treatments produced deep-depth injury, so their widespread implementation was limited. In the 1980s, however, Brody and others began using more superficial wounding agents to vary the depth of treatment.

Types of Chemical Peels

Peels of very superficial depth exfoliate the stratum granulosum, whereas superficial-depth peels produce full-thickness epidermal injury (**Table 95.1**). These peels can be accomplished with varying concentrations of glycolic acid, salicylic acid, malic acid, lactic acid, citric acid, tartaric acid, malic acid, resorcinol, 5-fluorouracil (5-FU), 10 to 20% trichloroacetic acid (TCA), and Jessner solution. These peels are most useful for mild conditions, such as postinflammatory erythema, mild photoaging, or comedonal acne.

Medium-depth peels extend into the papillary dermis and upper reticular dermis (**Table 95.1**) and can be achieved with agents such as 30 to 35% TCA alone, 35% TCA with Jessner solution, 35% TCA with 70% glycolic acid, 35% TCA with carbon dioxide (CO_2) laser treatment, or phenol 88%. Of these preparations, 35% TCA has been the gold standard medium-depth peel. Use of solid CO_2, Jessner solution, or 70% glycolic acid prior to 35% TCA disrupts the epidermal barrier, permitting a more even and complete penetration of TCA. Medium-depth peels are most useful for the removal of superficial/epidermal lesions and the improvement of skin texture in moderate photodamaged skin.

Deep-depth peels are characteristic of phenol-based preparations, with or without occlusion. Although 45 to 50% TCA has been used historically, its use is limited due to a higher risk of untoward scarring. Phenol (carbolic acid, C_6H_5OH) is an aromatic hydrocarbon derived organically from coal tar. Full-strength 88% phenol without dilution can create an upper reticular dermal chemical peel (**Table 95.1**). The Baker–Gordon peel is generally considered the classic deep-depth peeling agent. The solution consists of 3 mL (mL) 88% phenol, 8 drops Septisol (Steris Corp., Mentor, OH), 3 drops croton oil, and 2 mL distilled water. Croton oil is an extract of the seed of the plant *Croton tiglium*. These treatments affect the midreticular dermis. In contrast to the keratocoagulation seen with pure phenol peels, the Baker–Gordon peel denatures keratin via disruption of intermolecular sulfur bridges; this permits even deeper peel penetration. The peel depth is further augmented with croton oil, which acts as an irritant, and Septisol, which lowers skin surface tension. Reducing the number of drops of croton oil, in turn, reduces the depth of the peel.

Multiple factors govern the ultimate depth of a chemical peel. As already noted, the type of agent chosen is the best way to control peel depth. However, increasing the concentration of an agent can increase the depth of penetration (such as increasing glycolic acid from 40 to 70% or increasing TCA from 10 to 50%). Phenol-based peels constitute an exception to this rule; the stronger the concentration of phenol, the less deep the peel. The phenol creates such an intense surface protein keratocoagulation that it limits the extent of its own penetration.

The number of times a peeling agent is applied during a single treatment may also increase the depth of wounding. This is particularly true of TCA and not true of phenol. The pre-peel preparation of the skin may directly affect the penetration of the peeling solution. Applying retinoic acid (Retin-A, DRAXIS Specialty Pharmaceuticals, Inc., Kirkland, QC, Canada) or alphahydroxy acids for several weeks prior to the peel removes keratin and allows more rapid and even penetration of the peeling solution.

Table 95.1   Classification of chemical peels by depth of cutaneous injury and key histological correlates

Type of peel	Depth of peel	Key histology
Light superficial peel	Stratum corneum	Stimulation of epidermal growth via exfoliation of stratum corneum
Full superficial peel	Full-thickness epidermis	Destruction of epidermis with induction of epidermal regeneration
Medium	Papillary dermis	Epidermal destruction with induction of inflammation in papillary dermis
Deep	Superficial–midreticular dermis	Inflammatory response in midreticular dermis induces collagenesis and production of ground substance

Degreasing the skin at the time of a chemical peel will also optimize the effects of the peeling agent. Epi-abrading the facial skin with gauze soaked in acetone, for instance, will prepare the skin in a manner akin to 6 weeks of an exfoliant.

Inherent patient skin types affect peel penetration as well. Thick, oily skin with advanced photoaging will not be affected nearly as readily by the wounding agent as thin, dry skin. This holds true across individuals and across facial subunits within an individual. For example, one might choose a deeper peeling agent for advanced perioral photoaging and wrinkling and select a medium-depth peel for the remainder of the face.

Chief Indications for Chemical Peels

The chief indications for chemical peeling are as follows:

- Photodamage, with dyschromia
- Actinic preneoplasia and other epidermal processes, such as freckles, lentigenes, and seborrheic keratoses
- Fine and coarse rhytid
- Pigmentary dyschromias
- Superficial scarring
- Acne
- Blending photoaged skin with laser resurfacing

In general, peels improve skin texture, improve the uniformity of pigmentation, and reduce rhytids. Medium-depth peels are indicated for signs of moderate photoaging: fine rhytids, cross-hatched lines, crinkly skin, and sallow dyschromia. The more advanced changes seen with deeper grooves and rhytids, pebbly appearance of the skin, and more pronounced gravitational change of Glogau III and IV photoaging skin require deep peels and laser resurfacing. Peels can accompany the medical treatment of acne because they are useful against both comedonal and inflammatory acneiform lesions. Although chemical peels may also be used for melasma, the irregular patches of darkened skin resulting from excess melanin may prove refractory to treatment.

Dermabrasion

Dermabrasion is a procedure relied on and trusted over the years to improve facial skin contour. Dermabrasion was conceived by Dr. Kromayer, a German dermatologist, in 1905. Dermabrasion became a useful procedure when the equipment was refined in the 1950s by Noel Robbins. The current state of the art in dermabrasion equipment uses a variable-speed electrically driven hand unit with a variety of diamond fraises or wire brushes. Dermabrasion is

generally considered a deep reticular dermal–depth treatment indicated for the following conditions:

- Post-acne scarring
- Traumatic scarring
- Postoperative scars
- Traumatic tattoos
- Acne rosacea
- Rhinophyma
- Telangiectasias refractory to laser
- Angiofibromas of tuberous sclerosis
- Photoaging skin conditions, such as solar elastosis, actinic keratoses, and seborrheic keratoses
- Cosmetic removal of rhytids, especially perioral regions

Major Indications for Dermabrasion

A major indication for dermabrasion is to improve the appearance of acne scars. Shallow craterlike scars are more amenable to improvement than "ice-pick" scars or deeper depressions from post-acne atrophy. Punched-out scars, ice-pick scars, and other scars too deep for improvement from a single dermabrasion procedure can be treated with punch excision of scars with primary closure, punch elevation of the base of scars, and/or punch excision with composite grafted skin. Leveling the scars with these modalities allows for subsequent improvement with dermabrasion. These predermabrasion procedures need to be performed at least 6 weeks prior to the dermabrasion procedure.

Yarborough has shown that dermabrading posttraumatic and postsurgical scars at 4 to 6 weeks following injury is optimal for scar effacement in many situations. This also holds true for postscar revision with Z-plasty, W-plasty, and geometric broken-line techniques. Scars from flap reconstruction after skin cancer ablation are improved significantly with dermabrasion.

Dermabrasion may be the best technique for effacement of deep (grade III–IV) perioral rhytids. Compared with chemical peels for rhytid removal, dermabrasion is more consistent in removing deep-depth rhytids. Improvement continues for up to 4 to 6 months following the procedure, as collagen reorganization in the papillary and upper reticular dermis matures. Dermabrasion may be relied upon for touch-up procedures for residual rhytids after chemical peels and laser resurfacing. Finally, dermabrasion combined with dermaplaning remains an excellent cost-efficient treatment for rhinophyma.

Relative Contraindications to Dermabrasion

Dermabrasion is sometimes contraindicated for patients with Fitzpatrick types III through V skin types. These light-skinned African Americans,

Asians, Hispanics, and patients of Mediterranean origin have a high propensity for unpredictable hyper- and hypopigmentation. Pretreatment with bleaching agents, such as topical 4% hydroquinone or Tri-Luma (Galderma Laboratories, LP, Fort Worth, TX), can reduce this propensity for pigmentary dyscrasias.

Absolute Contraindications to Dermabrasion

Dermabrasion is absolutely contraindicated for the following:

- Patients without skin appendages, such as those with postradiation changes and loss of vellus hairs
- Patients recently treated with isotretinoin for acne. There is disagreement about how long one needs to wait after stopping isotretinoin before performing a resurfacing procedure. Depending on the author, the waiting period ranges from at least 6 months to 2 years.
- Patients with autoimmune cutaneous or vascular conditions, such as scleroderma

Infection Prophylaxis for Dermabrasion

Because dermabrasion aerosolizes skin particles, preoperative human immunodeficiency virus (HIV) and hepatitis evaluations are appropriate. Blood and tissue are aerosolized during dermabrasion; thus protective facemasks with eyeshields should be worn. There have been no known cases of transmission of the HIV virus with dermabrasion. Patients with a history of atopy or impetigo may be prescribed antibiotic prophylaxis. Finally, retinoic acid 0.05% cream applied once daily 2 weeks before dermabrasion has been shown to expedite reepithelialization.

■ Management

Chemical Peeling

Prepeel Procedures

Preparing for resurfacing 2 to 12 weeks in advance of the procedure can enhance the ultimate outcome. Topical retinoids (e.g., tretinoin 0.05%) exfoliate keratinocytes, thin the stratum corneum, and activate fibroblasts. A smoother stratum corneum results, permitting more even penetration of the peel. Topical retinoids may also speed healing. A bleaching agent (e.g., hydroquinone 4–8%) may reduce the likelihood of postinflammatory hyperpigmentation in dark-skinned patients. Sunscreen and exfoliants, such as 5 to 10% glycolic acid lotion, are also used to opti-

mally prepare the facial skin for the peel. Finally, on the day of the peel, vigorous cleaning and degreasing with acetone are necessary for even penetration of the solution.

Technique of Chemical Face Peeling

Very superficial peels and superficial peels can be routinely performed by an aesthetician, because they do not require anesthesia and limit injury to the epidermis. Level I frosting occurs with erythema and a stingy appearance. Superficial peels may be safely used in patients with dark complexions. They are tolerated with mild discomfort, such as transient burning, irritation, and erythema.

Most full-face medium- and deep-depth chemical peels will require sedation anesthesia and local anesthesia for regional anesthetic blocks. By contrast, very superficial- and superficial-depth peels do not require any type of anesthesia. Regional peeling, even with a deep-chemical-peeling agent such as phenol, can be done without anesthesia, but it does create an intense sting lasting for several seconds. The sting and burn will subside for ~ 20 or 30 minutes and then will begin to burn increasingly over the next 4 to 6 hours. Regional-block anesthesia will generally result in a higher level of patient satisfaction in the postoperative period. To effectively administer a regional block anesthesia, it can be helpful to premedicate the patient with analgesics and anxiolytics, such as diazepam.

Level II frosting is defined as white-coated frosting with erythema showing through. A level III frosting, which is associated with penetration through the papillary dermis, is a solid white enamel frosting with little or no background of erythema. The level II to level III white frost from 35% TCA indicates keratocoagulation or keratin denaturation and matures within 30 seconds to 2 minutes. Even application should eliminate the need to go over treated areas a second or third time. However, if the frosting is incomplete or uneven, the solution should be reapplied. The surgeon should wait at least 3 to 4 minutes after the application of TCA to ensure that the frosting has peaked. Careful feathering of the solution into the hairline and around the mandible conceals the line of demarcation between peeled and non-peeled skin.

Prior to a phenol-based deep-depth peel, patients should be considered to have an electrocardiogram and complete blood count. Patients with known heart disease should be considered for clearance from their cardiologist. Before applying the peel solution, the skin is meticulously degreased with acetone-soaked gauze and locally anesthetized. Because phenol is directly toxic to the myocardium, full-face deep-depth peels are usually performed in the operating suite under sedation anesthesia with continuous cardiopulmonary monitoring and intravenous hydration (1,500 to 2,000 mL). Application of the peel must be separated into five regions, staged 15 to 20 minutes apart. If the peel is performed in less than 30 minutes, the risk of arrhythmia increases. Hydration and diuresis promote metabolism and excretion of phenol, thus reducing the risk of arrhythmia. Antiarrhythmia medications, such as lidocaine or propranolol, are needed if arrhythmias occur. The peel should be feathered into the hairline and across the mandibular line into the shadow area of the submandibular neck. This will minimize sharp lines of demarcation from treated areas of relative hypopigmentation to sun-damaged, untreated skin. The usual end point of a deep peel occurs when the skin appears ivory-white to gray-white. Monitoring is discontinued 60 to 90 minutes after the procedure if there are no adverse events.

Certain areas and skin lesions require special attention. Thicker keratoses do not absorb peel solutions well; additional applications rubbed vigorously into the lesion may be needed for sufficient solution penetration. Wrinkled skin should be stretched to allow an even coating of solution into the folds. Oral rhytids require the peel solution to be applied with the wood portion of the cotton-tipped applicator and extended into the vermilion of the lip. Deeper furrows, such as expression lines, will not be eradicated with the peel and thus should not be treated too aggressively.

Postpeel Procedures

Postoperative care following a chemical peel centers on maintaining a moist, well-lubricated healing environment. This can be accomplished with a variety of occlusive agents, such as waterproof zinc oxide nonpermeable tape, occlusive moisturizers, antibiotic ointments, and biosynthetic occlusive dressings. If occlusion is not desired, the patient is left without an emollient for the first 12 to 24 hours postpeel. After this period elapses, the patient is instructed to apply a thick lubricating agent, such as Aquaphor (Beiersdorf, Inc., Wilton, CT), an antibiotic ointment, or petroleum jelly. The patient is instructed to keep the wound bed well lubricated, and to apply compresses to the treated skin with dilute acetic acid rinses up to six times a day. After 24 hours, patients may shower and use a mild nondetergent cleanser. Erythema intensifies as desquamation becomes complete within 4 to 5 days; lubrication and massage during this period allow separation of the epidermal and upper dermal layers. Continuing this lubrication regimen over the ensuing 5 to 7 days permits epithelial regeneration without surface drying. It is critical that patients follow instructions carefully to maintain a

clean healing environment without infection. It is also imperative that the surgeon monitor patients every 2 to 3 days to ensure that instructions are followed and wound healing progresses as expected.

Usually by the day 7 to 10 after a medium-depth peel, reepithelialization has occurred; this regenerative process requires 10 to 14 days for deep-depth peels. Intense erythema is most likely present and can often be mitigated with a mild hydrocortisone cream when epithelialization is complete. Makeup camouflage and sun-protection strategies can be discussed at this time.

Follow-up care continues with the patient at appropriate intervals, such as at 6 weeks, 3 months, and 6 months. This allows the surgeon to watch for postinflammatory hyperpigmentation and assess the final results of the chemical peel. It takes 3 to 6 months for the collagen and elastin layers to reorganize before a patient can appreciate the full clinical results of deeper medium-depth and deep-depth chemical peeling procedures.

Even after healing has concluded, postpeel regimens that include cleansing, toning, exfoliation, sunscreen, and moisturization are recommended to maintain the skin in a rejuvenated state.

Complications of Chemical Peels

Conditions that are considered normal sequelae after chemical face peeling include pain, swelling, erythema, and occasional milia. Complications are often related to the depth of the treatment and include pigmentary changes, infections, allergic reactions, hypersensitivity, disease exacerbation, improper healing/scarring, and events due to operator error.

Acneiform eruptions after chemical peels may occur immediately after reepithelialization. The etiology is related either to exacerbation of previous acne or to overgreasing newly formed skin. Short-term systemic antibiotics, together with discontinuation of topical oily preparations, will usually resolve the condition.

It is not unusual to have some degree of hypopigmentation and, rarely, areas of depigmentation. Occluded Baker solution phenol peels will commonly produce hypopigmentation, whereas unoccluded Baker peels rarely produce significant hypopigmentation. Although decreasing pigmentation through chemical peels is part of the normal treatment of pigmentary dyschromias, excess hypopigmentation is usually not seen for 6 to 12 months postpeel. Delayed hypopigmentation after phenol peels is proportional to peel depth, amount of peel solution used, and inherent skin color.

In the first several weeks of the healing period, reactive hyperpigmentation is common, particularly for medium-depth peels. TCA peels often stimulate transient hyperpigmentation 3 to 6 weeks postpeel. Accentuation of the pigment in previously existing intradermal nevi is common and should be recognized when it occurs to avoid any unnecessary alarm of a changing mole. Pretreatment with bleaching agents, such as kojic acid or 4 to 5% hydroquinone (which inhibits the enzyme tyrosinase), can limit this hyperpigmentation. Alternatively, bleaching agents may be introduced 2 to 3 weeks postpeel until the hyperpigmentation subsides. A mixture of 0.1% retinoic acid (Retin-A) with 4 to 5% hydroquinone and 1% hydrocortisone cream can also be used at night. The routine use of sunscreen is imperative to prevent further hyperpigmentation postpeel.

Scarring remains the most dreadful complication of chemical peels. Scarring is caused by uncontrolled penetration of the peeling agent into the deeper layers of the skin. Special precautions should be taken while peeling the lower and lateral face following rhytidectomy, even years postoperatively. This is because vascular compromise following the undermining of the skin interferes with healing. Additionally, neck skin, which is a bad candidate for deep peels, is elevated to the face with facelift surgery. Delayed healing and persistent redness 3 months or more following a deep peel herald impending scarring. Potent steroid preparations should be promptly introduced in this scenario.

Infections can occur with any open wound resulting from chemical peels or dermabrasion. Proper cleansing with diluted acetic acid soaks will prevent most infections. It is nonetheless customary to treat patients prophylactically with a broad-spectrum antistaphylococcal antibiotic. Occasionally, however, a superficial infiltrative infection with *Pseudomonas aeruginosa* occurs. If an adherent, yellowish-green crust forms 2 to 4 days postpeel, it must be treated with 0.25% acidic acid soaks and an antibiotic appropriate for covering *Pseudomonas*.

The most common outbreak in the perioral region is from HSV type 1. Fever blisters or cold sores may erupt in the perioral area and then spread over the entire peeled area if the patient has any previous history of herpetic outbreaks and has not received the herpes zoster immunization. Herpes zoster infections can be adequately prevented by prophylactic treatment with ~ 2000 mg per day of acyclovir or ~ 1,000 mg/d of valacyclovir. If herpetic outbreaks occur, the dosage should increase to 4,000 mg/d of acyclovir or 2,000 mg/d of valacyclovir.

Candida albicans is a more unusual infection that may occur in the postpeel patient who has been given a broad-spectrum antibiotic or topical steroid treatment. It is appropriately treated with antifungal agents and by stopping the antibiotic prophylaxis.

The most common long-term complication of chemical peels is disappointment in the result because of residual rhytids. The surgeon and the patient, however, having chosen an appropriate, safe chemical peel, must accept some remaining photoaging and residual rhytids. The alternative is to peel too deeply and incur more severe complications, such as permanent depigmentation and scarring. Hypertrophic scarring from chemical peeling is rare but possible, most commonly in the upper lip, chin, and eyelids. It is more common with 50% TCA than with Baker solution chemical peeling

Dermabrasion

Technique of Facial Dermabrasion

Dermabrasion requires proper skin tumescence to maintain a uniform depth of dermabrasion and maximize the control of the dermabrader. Several methods can be used to accomplish this, including skin refrigerants, infiltration with local anesthetic, and mechanically stretching the skin surface to create skin tension. The skin surface may be prepared with gentian violet or the ink from a marking pen to stain the epidermis. Therefore, once the epidermis has been removed the surgeon no longer sees the stain.

Regional facial segments are sequentially treated when a full-face procedure is performed. Slowly and evenly moving the dermabrading fraise perpendicular to the direction of rotation will yield good control of the abrasion depth and minimize the risk of skin gouging. Extreme care must be taken to ensure the diamond fraise tip is rotating away from the vermilion border and eyelids. In contrast to fraises, wire brushes create microscopic lacerations oriented at right angles to one another, thereby creating micro-Z-plasty effects. Fraises are more forgiving, and they are less dependent on skin turgor than wire brushes. Regardless, dermabrasion should never extend onto eyelid skin.

Dividing the face into small regions and freezing each region sequentially will allow the surgeon to proceed in an orderly fashion. Diffuse pinpoint bleeding heralds entry into the papillary dermis. A yellow chamois color characterizes the reticular dermis, with the superficial reticular dermis characterized by parallel-oriented strands, and the deeper reticular dermis by frayed white strands. The procedure must be terminated at this point to permit proper healing and avoid untoward scar formation.

Postoperative Dermabrasion Care

Similar to chemical peels, postdermabrasion care centers on the commitment to maintain a moist wound healing environment. However, because there is already a loss of the epidermis, papillary dermis, and upper reticular dermis, the wound needs to have some kind of sealant dressing for the first 24 hours. Xeroform gauze may be applied over the dermabraded area the first night. The following morning, emollients, such as Aquaphor ointment or bacitracin, are applied. Over the ensuing 5 to 7 days, emollients need to be rinsed off with mild, nondetergent soap and water. Emollients are then reapplied six times a day after the wounds are cleaned with a dilute acetic acid solution. Complete reepithelialization generally occurs in 7 to 14 days.

Once reepithelialization has occurred, topical hydrocortisone cream can be applied to avoid prolonged erythema. Sun avoidance and sunscreen precautions are recommended, especially during the first year following the procedure. Camouflage makeup may also be applied after reepithelialization has occurred. In 2 to 3 weeks postdermabrasion, postinflammatory hyperpigmentation may be observed. When this phenomenon is recognized, the "splotchy" pigmentary dyscrasias are treated until resolved with retinoic acid (Retin-A), combined with hydroquinone or alphahydroxy acids (such as kojic acid), or combined with hydroquinone.

Complications of Dermabrasion

Commonly observed and expected side effects of dermabrasion are edema, erythema, crust formation, pain, pruritus, milia, and dermatitis. When these effects occur, patients are instructed to have patience, because these conditions resolve either spontaneously or with minimal treatment. Pruritus can be treated with antihistamines. The incidence of postdermabrasion milia can be lowered by pretreating the skin with 0.05% retinoic acid (Retin-A), applied once daily 1 week before the procedure. Milia can be treated with retinoic acid (Retin-A), facials, or direct unroofing. Dermatitis can occur in up to 10% of patients and can be treated with topical, intralesional, or systemic steroids.

Pigmentary changes represent the most common complication. Erythema is expected, commonly lasts for weeks to months, and generally resolves with time. However, similar to the case with chemical peels, patients susceptible to reactive hyperpigmentation may be pretreated with bleaching agents, such as 4 to 5% topical hydroquinone. Hyperpigmentation can also be exacerbated by estrogen use and sun exposure.

Hypopigmentation can occur within an area of deeper treatment, as is also the case with deep chemical peels. Although uncommon, patients nonetheless need to be informed of possible hypopig-

mentation, particularly in conjunction with efforts to efface deeper scars with deeper dermabrasion treatments. Hypopigmentation may be associated with zones of demarcation, depending on the extent to which the treatment is feathered or tapered into adjoining untreated facial subunits. Hypopigmentation will not be evident for 6 months or longer following a dermabrasion procedure. Unfortunately, no medical treatment exists for hypopigmentation; makeup may be the only remedy.

Infections seen with chemical peels can also occur with dermabrasion. They are treated similarly. Hypertrophic scarring with dermabrasion is more common in the upper lip, lip–chin regions, mandibular borders, and over bony prominences. Dermabrasion is very technique-dependent, with a difficult learning curve. The most common factors associated with postdermabrasion scarring are hereditary predisposition, wound depth, postoperative infection, and isotretinoin use. Dermabrasion has limited ability to treat periocular rhytids and scars, due to the thin skin of the eyelids.

■ Summary

Because surgeons have a variety of choices and methods for rejuvenating facial skin, resurfacing has become a highly honed surgical art. The addition of laser resurfacing has further increased the scope and variability of treatment for photoaging. Combined with proper patient selection and knowledge of the spectrum of resurfacing agents, a surgeon can treat superficial-, medium-, and deep-depth photoaging problems. Different methods of resurfacing can be used in different facial subunits to achieve the desired results for each patient. The results generally achieved with dermabrasion and a Baker–Gordon peel remain a benchmark standard of care for single-session patient treatment. This is especially true for severe photoaging and deep rhytidoses, such as are commonly encountered in the perioral region.

Finally, understanding the physiology of wound healing and proper postoperative wound care following facial skin resurfacing permits surgeons to minimize the morbidity of resurfacing procedures. By mastering the management of the normal nuances of healing and the potentially avoidable complications of chemical peels and dermabrasion, a surgeon will develop the confidence to perform these procedures for even early photoaging in patients who increasingly seek these modalities of rejuvenation.

■ Suggested Reading

Baker TJ, Gordon HL. Chemical face peeling and dermabrasion. Surg Clin North Am 1971;51(2):387–401

Branham GH, Thomas JR. Rejuvenation of the skin surface: chemical peel and dermabrasion. Facial Plast Surg 1996;12(2):125–133

Brody HJ. Complications of chemical peeling. J Dermatol Surg Oncol 1989;15(9):1010–1019

Brody HJ. The art of chemical peeling. J Dermatol Surg Oncol 1989;15(9):918–921

Fitzpatrick TB. The validity and practicality of sun-reactive skin types I through VI. Arch Dermatol 1988;124(6):869–871

Monheit GD. Medium-depth chemical peels. Dermatol Clin 2001;19(3):413–425, vii

Perkins SW, Balikian R. Treatment of perioral rhytids. Facial Plast Surg Clin North Am 2007;15(4):409–414, v

Perkins SW, Sandel HD. Management of aging skin. In: Flint PW, Haughey BH, Lund VJ, Niparko JK, Richardson MA, Robbins KT, Thomas JR, eds. Cummings Otolaryngology–Head and Neck Surgery. 5th ed. Philadelphia, PA. Mosby Elsevier; 2010:390–404

Perkins SW, Sklarew EC. Prevention of facial herpetic infections after chemical peel and dermabrasion: new treatment strategies in the prophylaxis of patients undergoing procedures of the perioral area. Plast Reconstr Surg 1996;98(3):427–433, discussion 434–435

Surowitz JB, Shockley WW. Enhancement of facial scars with dermabrasion. Facial Plast Surg Clin North Am 2011;19(3):517–525

Yarborough JM. Scar revision by dermabrasion. In: Roenigk RK, Roenigk HH, eds. Dermatologic Surgery. 2nd ed. New York, NY. Marcel Dekker; 1996:911–922

96 Hair Restoration

■ Introduction

Hair loss is a common affliction, with androgenic alopecia affecting up to 40% of the adult population. The inheritability pattern of male pattern baldness remains debatable. Early studies were consistent with an autosomal-dominant inheritance pattern in men and autosomal-recessive in women. However, more recent work indicates male pattern baldness is likely a multifactorial inheritance pattern, with twin studies showing that up to 80% of androgenic alopecia is attributable to an inherited form. Furthermore, it is important to note that androgenic alopecia has been associated with other health conditions, including benign prostatic hypertrophy, coronary artery disease, and even prostate cancer.

Hair growth is not uniform throughout the body or even on the head. Hair growth involves four separate phases (**Table 96.1**). The growth phase is known as anagen. The catagen phase is the transition that takes place from the anagen phase to the dormant, or telogen phase. The shedding of hairs is known as the exogen phase. Scalp hairs remain in the anagen phase anywhere from 2 to 8 years, which explains why continued growth can take place when compared with the rest of the body. The telogen phase lasts ~ 3 months, and then anagen begins again, with most people losing around 50 to 150 scalp hairs every day.

At the histological level, hairs are derived from invaginations of the epidermal epithelium, forming elongated keratinized structures that extend from the skin's surface. At the base of each hair follicle is a hair bulb with an associated dermal papilla, which contains the vasculature for the follicle. Extending up from the dermal papilla are epithelial cells, which form the root and shaft. The shaft includes the medulla (present in thicker hair cells) made of vacuolated, moderately keratinized cells and a cortex, which is heavily keratinized. This is then surrounded by the hair cuticle, which covers the cortex. Surrounding the shaft is the internal root sheath followed by the external root sheath. The glassy membrane is a noncellular layer composed of hyaline, which separates the follicle from the surrounding dermis. Within the surrounding dermis are smooth muscle cells known as erector pili, which are responsible for erection of the hair shaft. The basic unit of the scalp is the follicular unit, which consists of up to four terminal hairs and its surrounding sebaceous glands, erector muscles, and neurovascular plexus. On the scalp, hair follicle density varies between races, with Caucasians having the highest density at 3.1 hair follicles per square millimeter (mm^2), and Koreans having the lowest density at 1.2 hair follicles/mm^2.

Biologically, male pattern baldness has been associated with increased levels of dihydrotestosterone (DHT) in hair follicles and increased expression of androgen receptors. DHT is more potent than its precursor molecule, testosterone, from which it is converted by the action of 5a-reductase. Variations in the androgen receptor as well as a gene locus on chromosome 20 have been associated with heritable, male pattern baldness. The pathognomonic finding in male pattern baldness is miniaturization of hair follicles, which occurs in the presence of androgens. The terminal follicles decrease in size until they become more like vellus hair cells, although they continue to have residual connective tissue and nerves as well as atrophied erector pili muscles (**Fig. 96.1**).

Notice the decrease in caliber and overall size of the hair cells in comparison to the normal size hair cell featured most prominently to the left of the picture.

Table 96.1 Hair growth cycle

Phase	Characteristic
Anagen	Growth
Catagen	Transition from growth to rest
Telogen	Rest
Exogen	Shedding

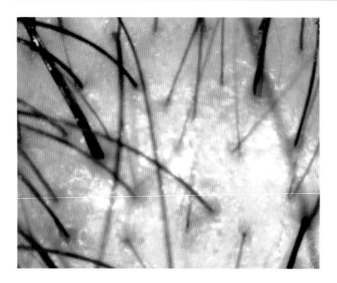

Fig. 96.1   Hair cell miniaturization.

■ Evaluation

Although androgenic alopecia is the most common cause of alopecia, the differential diagnosis is extensive when the presentation is not straightforward. After considering both androgenic alopecia and female pattern hair loss, other categories include endocrine disorders, dermatological conditions that include both scarring and nonscarring alopecia, nutritional deficiencies, infectious diseases, systemic illnesses and stress, and, finally, traumatic hair loss.

Endocrinopathies causing alopecia include disorders of thyroid function, as well as hypoparathyroidism, diabetes mellitus, growth hormone deficiency, hyperprolactinemia, polycystic ovary syndrome, Cushing syndrome, and androgen-producing tumors. Dermatological conditions include alopecia areata, a type of nonscarring alopecia with episodic patches of hair loss that may progress to complete hair loss, as well as cicatricial alopecia or scarring alopecia. Infectious etiologies, such as syphilis, alopecia from tick bites, and tinea capitis, exist. Systemic illnesses can also lead to alopecia. Autoimmune diseases, such as systemic lupus erythematosus (SLE), fall into this category, as does toxic alopecia, which is related to systemic toxicities, commonly from chemotherapeutic agents, but it also can be seen with heavy metal poisoning. Telogen effluvium is the result of hair follicles prematurely entering into the telogen phase. This can be seen following stresses on the body, including childbirth, initiation of oral contraceptive pills, surgery, anemia, and malnutrition. Chronic diseases, including renal and liver failure, can also be associated with a diffuse telogen hair loss pattern. Patient activities can lead to traumatic alopecia. Both trichotillomania and traction alopecia are

in this category. Trichotillomania is an impulse control disorder, as classified under the *Diagnostic and Statistical Manual of Mental Disorders*, fourth edition (*DSM-IV*), where patients compulsively pull out their hair; traction alopecia is associated with prolonged or repetitive tension on the hair. Pressure alopecia is caused by prolonged pressure on the skin, leading to hair loss, frequently occurring on the occiput.

A thorough examination of the scalp in addition to the patient history may provide the etiology of the alopecia. With the most common type, androgenic alopecia, men tend to have frontal hairline recession and vertex balding, whereas women tend to have a diffuse balding pattern with preservation of the frontal hairline, but there are exceptions. The degree of hair loss is most commonly quantified using the Hamilton-Norwood Baldness scale in men and the Ludwig classification in women. Originally described in 1951 by Hamilton and in 1975 by Dr. O'Tar Norwood, the scale ranges from I to VII (**Table 96.2; Fig. 96.2**). The Ludwig classification has only three stages and was developed in 1977 to more appropriately address the female pattern of hair loss (**Table 96.3; Fig. 96.3**).

If the diagnosis is not apparent, based on the patient history and physical exam, ancillary tests may be ordered. Because thyroid disorders can be associated with alopecia, thyroid-stimulating hormone (TSH) as well as levels of T3 and T4 should be obtained. Given the association of various autoimmune diseases with alopecia, including SLE, antinuclear antibody titers may be ordered. A complete blood count (CBC) may be considered because anemia has been associated with alopecia. Secondary syphilis produces a moth-eaten pattern of hair loss, and syphilis serology may be indicated in select patients with risk factors. Loss of iron stores has been implicated, with women being more susceptible than men, given menstruation. Although studies have indicated that women with depleted serum ferritin levels are more likely to have alopecia than healthy women, other studies have failed to validate this finding. Therefore, judgment should be used as to whether to order iron studies (**Table 96.4**).

Various tests exist for evaluating and quantifying hair loss that is suspected to be caused by other issues than androgenic alopecia. These tests are not commonly performed and are ordered when the history of physical examination warrants further investigation. These include the wash test, which is mainly a historical test designed to differentiate telogen effluvium from androgenic alopecia. A larger number of hairs are lost with telogen effluvium. The hair pull test is an in-office test performed on a patient who has not washed his hair in 24 hours. Approximately 60 hairs are grasped between the index and middle fingers and the thumb. Gentle pressure is applied as the fingers are pulled away from the hair. If six or more hairs are pulled out, this is considered abnor-

Table 96.2 Hamilton–Norwood classification

Type	Description
I	Minimal hair loss
II	Frontotemporal hairline recession, does not extend to within 2 cm of the external auditory canal
IIA	Entire frontal hairline recession, does not extend to within 2 cm of the external auditory canal
III	Frontotemporal recession to within 2 cm of a coronal plane bisecting the external auditory canal
III vertex	Hair loss in the crown
IIIA	Entire frontal hairline recession to within 2 cm of a coronal plane bisecting the external auditory canal
IV	Frontotemporal recession greater than type III, combined with crown hair loss, but a generous amount of hair remains between the crown and frontal hairlines
IVA	Recession of the entire frontal hairline posterior to the midcoronal line
V	More extensive hair loss than IV, with only a narrow band of hair separating the frontotemporal hair line from the crown hair loss
VA	Recession of the hairline into the vertex
VI	Frontotemporal hair loss extending to the crown and extending both laterally and posteriorly
VII	Hair loss with only a narrow horseshoe pattern of hair remaining

Data from Norwood, OT. Male pattern baldness: classification and incidence. South Med J 1975;68(11): 1359–1365.

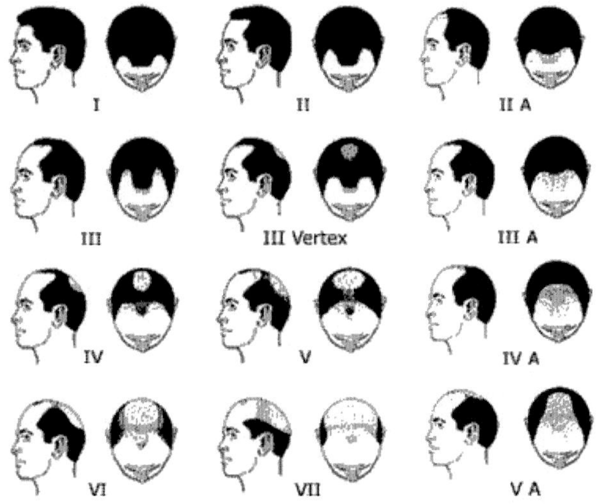

Fig. 96.2 Hamilton–Norwood classification. Used with permission from Norwood, OT. Male pattern baldness: classification and incidence. South Med J 1975;68(11): 1359–1365.

mal. The extracted hairs are those in the telogen phase and can be seen in telogen effluvium. However, the test lacks specificity and sensitivity, because the amount of pressure applied to remove the hairs varies between evaluators and from test to test.

The unit area trichogram involves plucking hairs from a defined area to evaluate the hair follicle density, anagen-to-telogen ratio, and hair shaft diameter. This test is also limited by sampling error, because no skin is resected to determine the exact size of the sampled area. The trichogram uses a rubber-armed forceps to extract ~ 100 hairs with a single pluck in two separate regions. The first location is 2 cm posterior to the frontal hairline and then 3 cm lateral to the midline. The second site is 2 cm lateral from the occipital protuberance. The hair roots can be evaluated via microscopy to determine the phase of growth. Like many other tests, it is most useful in evaluating for the presence of telogen effluvium because a greater percentage of hairs will be in the telogen phase.

A phototrichogram uses photography to evaluate for hair growth. A macro lens is used to evaluate up to three areas of the scalp. These three areas are shaved, a photo is taken, and then another photo is taken 3 days later. Hairs in the anagen phase will have shown growth, but hairs in the telogen phase will not.

The TrichoScan is similar but automated. Trichoscopy uses high magnification of the scalp to evaluate the hairs. Particular attention is paid in distinguishing terminal hairs from vellus hairs, as well as to evaluate the hair follicle. This method may be useful in evaluating androgenic alopecia and alopecia areata.

Light microscopy can be used to evaluate the hair shaft for thickness and the presence of other anomalies, but its overall usefulness is limited. The use of polarized light with specialized microscopes can add further utility to evaluate for anomalies.

The gold standard for evaluating the etiology of alopecia is the punch biopsy. This allows for complete evaluation of the hair follicle as in other tests, as well as evaluation of the ratio of anagen to telogen. What separates the punch biopsy from other tests is its ability to evaluate the surrounding skin for abnormalities (**Table 96.5**).

Table 96.3 Ludwig classification

Stage	Description
I	Minimal hair loss
II	Widening of the midline part, with thinning anterior to the crown
III	Complete alopecia of the crown, with preservation of the hairline

Data from Ludwig E. Classification of the types of androgenetic alopecia (common baldness) occurring in the female sex. Br J Dermatol 1977;97:247–254.

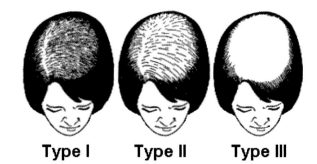

Type I   **Type II**   **Type III**

Fig. 96.3 Ludwig classification. Used with permission from Ludwig E. Classification of the types of androgenetic alopecia (common baldness) occurring in the female sex. Br J Dermatol 1977;97:247–254.

Table 96.4 Ancillary laboratory tests

Medical disorder	Diagnostic test
Endocrinopathies	Thyroid-stimulating hormone, T3, T4, testosterone, prolactin, dehydroepiandrosterone sulfate, estrogen
Autoimmune disease	Antinuclear antibody, systemic lupus erythematosus tests, including double-stranded DNA and anti-Smith antibodies
Infections	Complete blood count, syphilis serology
Iron depletion	Ferritin level, total iron-binding capacity
Nutritional	Vitamin D levels

Table 96.5 Hair examination techniques

Test	Summary	Limitation
Wash test	Hair is washed and number of hairs that came out evaluated	Only useful for differentiating telogen effluvium from androgenic alopecia
Hair pull test	60 hairs grasped and pulled	Only useful for differentiating telogen effluvium from androgenic alopecia
Unit area trichogram	Plucking hairs to evaluate follicular density, anagen-to-telogen ratio, shaft diameter	Sampling error
Trichogram	Plucking of 100 hairs from defined locations	Only useful for differentiating telogen effluvium from androgenic alopecia
Phototrichogram	Macroscopic view, hairs shaved, 3 days later area reevaluated	Only evaluates anagen to telogen ratio
TrichoScan	Camera evaluates numbers of hairs automatically, hairs shaved, 3 days later area reevaluated	Only evaluates anagen to telogen ratio
Trichoscopy	High magnification of scalp hairs	Limited to evaluating for androgenic alopecia and alopecia areata
Polarized light microscopy	Hairs removed and evaluated under a polarized light and microscope	Only evaluates hair thickness and presence of other hair anomalies
Punch biopsy	Punch biopsy of skin and hair taken	Gold standard for complete evaluation

◼ Medical Management

Once the etiology of the alopecia has been determined, management can be initiated. The abnormalities should be corrected for the reversible causes, such as endocrinopathies and nutritional deficiencies. For the remaining patients, there are both medical and surgical options. Medical options include the use of topical minoxidil (Rogaine, McNeil-Ppc., Inc., Fort Washington, PA), oral finasteride (Propecia, Merck and Company, Whitehouse Station, NJ), and various laser and light technologies such as the HairMax LaserComb (Lexington International, LLC, Boca Raton, FL).

Minoxidil was developed as an antihypertensive medication but was found to induce hair regrowth. The exact mechanism of regrowth remains elusive, but its mechanism of action involves potassium channel opening. Studies have shown that 5% minoxidil solution applied topically causes a significant increase in hair regrowth when compared with both placebo and a 2% minoxidil solution. It should be noted that there was increased pruritus and local irritation in the higher-concentration group. This irritation can be improved by using the minoxidil 5% foam, which lacks propylene glycol. Patients should be cautioned that discontinuation of minoxidil in those who are responders will lead to recurrent alopecia.

Finasteride works by inhibiting the 5a-reductase enzyme responsible for the conversion of testosterone to the more active DHT. Studies have shown that finasteride decreases the levels of DHT in the scalp. A randomized clinical trial evaluating the efficacy of 1 mg a day of oral finasteride compared with placebo showed hair regrowth ranging from 37% in patients with frontal balding to 61% in patients with vertex balding. It also demonstrated that 80% of patients with vertex baldness and 70% of patients with frontal baldness had the hair loss arrested with 2 years of follow-up. Finasteride (1 mg/d) has also been shown to significantly increase the anagen to telogen ratio at 1 year.

In a head-to-head comparison of 1 mg/d finasteride with 5% topical minoxidil solution over a 12 month period, there was a greater improvement in the alopecia in the finasteride group. However, there were more side effects in finasteride patients, with loss of libido being the most common effect.

The HairMax LaserComb has recently received clearance from the U.S. Food and Drug Administration (FDA) for both female and male pattern hair loss. The exact mechanism of action remains unknown, but a 26-week randomized, controlled trial showed that 86.1% of patients using the LaserComb had an increase in hair density, compared with 5% of placebo patients. Mild paresthesia and mild urticaria were the only reported side effects. Treatment involved using the LaserComb three times a week for 15 minutes each on nonconsecutive days.

Surgical Evaluation

For patients who fail to respond to medical therapy, surgical corrective methods should be discussed. The goal of any of the surgical hair restoration procedures is to decrease the areas of non-hair-bearing skin. This can be accomplished by donating hair from other portions of the scalp, with either rotational flaps or hair transplants or by scalp reduction surgeries.

When deciding on operating, selecting the appropriate candidate is the most important aspect of the evaluation. Experiences by Rousso and Brandy have shown that younger patients are less likely to be satisfied with the results. Reasons provided for the poorer satisfaction include unrealistic expectations, as well as the likelihood of continued hair loss with aging. Brandy has gone on to develop 20 criteria that each patient is scored on, which are then normalized to determine whether a patient is a good surgical candidate. Several of these criteria that portend a worse prognosis following surgery include a younger age, larger area of baldness, decreased donor hair shaft diameter and density, minimal scalp laxity, straight hair, contrasting hair and skin color, and keloid formers. With this in mind, it is important to plan for the future and not just the patient's current hair pattern. Evaluation of the patient's family's hair loss pattern may shed light on the likely, although not guaranteed, pattern of hair loss. As the hair loss progresses, the donor hair site will decrease, and poorly planned grafts that were previously placed will appear unnatural with few options for correction.

When deciding on donor sites, it is important to properly analyze the scalp. The midoccipital area has the highest density of hair follicles, which makes it the most appropriate area for the donor site. When designing the recipient site, the most important areas to consider are the frontal hair line and the vertex transition point. The frontal line in an adult should recede toward the temples. Failure to properly transition this zone will create an unnatural hair pattern. The vertex transition point occurs where the hairs transition from pointing forward to being in a more radial distribution.

The number of transplant sessions should be minimized to decrease trauma to the donor site, which can decrease vascularity and lead to alopecia. The frontal hairline with extension to the vertex point should be performed at the first session. Future sessions can be used to increase the density of the intervening hair. The total number of follicular units needed for a complete restoration is dependent on the Norwood classification, with 900 to 1,500 units indicated for a Norwood III, but as many as 4,000 to 6,600 needed for a Norwood VII. The goal follicular unit density is > 25 units/cm², but achieving this density in one session can impede hair growth and graft survival.

Surgical Management

Scalp reduction surgery employs the concept of resecting nonhair-bearing scalp. Although this can create a more "hairy" head, it is unlikely to create a natural hair pattern. As a result, most of these techniques are relegated to reconstruction and are included for historical purposes only. A variety of incisions have been developed to help minimize the scars, including crescents, triangles, and Mercedes-shaped incisions. The more common complications included the production of a midline slot where divergent hair from the temporal areas was brought to the midline, creating a noticeable deficit, the formation of visible scars on the scalp, the loss of potential donor hair sites, and finally the continued progression of alopecia leaving a "doughnut" of bald scalp around a central hair-bearing donor site.

Another surgical approach involved scalp lifting. This was described by Brandy and involved lifting the bilateral occipitoparietal skin after elevating down to the neck. However, it also involved ligation of the occipital artery, which could lead to further alopecia. This was further aided by the use of tissue extenders, which are designed to help stretch the donor site using mechanical creep and allow for further excision of the hairless scalp, as well as tissue expanders, which use biological creep prior to scalp reduction surgery.

Other methods of transferring hair-bearing tissue included axial-based flaps described by Juri. Similar to the scalp reduction surgeries, these axial flaps are rarely performed because they created an abrupt hair line and with continued alopecia would often have bald areas posterior to the flap.

The current state of the art for hair transplantation is the follicular unit transfer (FUT). This represents the continued refinement of the mini- and micrograft techniques, which involved removing ever smaller donor hair units. FUT involves excision of a 1 to 2 cm wide donor strip and then dissecting the strip into follicular unit grafts. This method allows for harvesting of a large number of follicular units. The donor site of harvest is then closed with a one- or two-layer fine-suture closure. Beveling the edge—the upper or lower edge or both edges—of the donor site wound before closure, as described by Juri and Kabaker for axial flaps, allows for hair to grow through the scar, breaking it up and making it less noticeable. The follicular units can then be carefully dissected into varying sizes to help create appropriate transition zones and allow for a natural hair pattern.

The follicular unit extraction (FUE) is similar to FUT but involves the use of 1 mm punches to make small circular incisions around the upper part of a follicular unit followed by blunt dissection. This is the most recent advancement in hair restoration surgery. Accordingly, there are no published data on long-term results, as well as hair follicle survival rates. The proposed benefit is that by avoiding long incisions as with FUT, there is no continuous linear scar. This can be very important in patients who have had scarring from previous transplantation, as well as those who want to keep their hair short. FUE procedures are generally more time consuming. Another limitation to FUE harvesting techniques is that most surgeons experience a higher transection rate of the hair shafts, as high as 10% of donor hairs, compared with 2% with FUT. This may prove to be an important hindrance for widespread acceptance because higher Norwood classification patients have fewer donor sites available. While obtaining the grafts, it is important to keep in mind that FUE leaves very small 0.5 mm scars that can become noticeable if the area is overharvested.

The follicular units are implanted into the bald recipient area by placing the grafts into sites created by using various gauge needles to create holes or specialized knives to create slits; the units are then secured in place by friction. These sites can be created prior to the initiation of transplantation to allow for a designed hair distribution density and hair growth direction. The benefit of this style is that once the follicular units are harvested, the surgeon can focus purely on insertion of the grafts instead of having to concentrate on both the design of the hair lines and the insertion. Another technique is creation of the implantation sites at the time when each individual graft is set. The latter stick-and-place method also allows the needle to facilitate insertion of the graft atraumatically. Also, no recipient holes or slits are created that are not used, and there is no doubling up of grafts, which can happen when multiple grafts are placed in the same recipient site.

Postoperative Care

The hair should be cleansed with a nonabrasive shampoo on posttransplant day 1 and should be cleaned daily to minimize crusting. Patients should be advised not to pick at any crusts, because this can dislodge the transplanted hair. Avoiding sun exposure with sunscreen for 3 months is advised. A restriction to only light physical activity for up to 6 weeks postoperatively is recommended to prevent stretching of the donor site and breakdown of the donor wound. If nonabsorbable sutures are used, they should be removed in 7 to 10 days.

It is important to note that smoking adversely affects flap viability, as well as the density of follicular units that can be transplanted at a single session. Therefore, patients should be counseled on smoking cessation.

■ Practice Guidelines, Consensus Statements, and Measures

The International Society of Hair Restoration Surgery has set forth core competencies for a surgeon to be able to perform both safe and aesthetically pleasing hair restoration surgery. A summary of these recommendations includes appropriate counseling, recommendations for nonandrogenetic hair loss, formulation of an appropriate combination of medical and surgical methods, operating room setup, hair harvest techniques, follicular unit preparation for both donor and recipient sites, appropriate anesthetic administration, recommendations for revision surgery, management for complications, and the appropriate way to train the hair restoration team.

■ Suggested Reading

Arca E, Açikgöz G, Taştan HB, Köse O, Kurumlu Z. An open, randomized, comparative study of oral finasteride and 5% topical minoxidil in male androgenetic alopecia. Dermatology 2004; 209(2):117–125

Bernstein RM, Rassman WR. Follicular unit transplantation: 2005. Dermatol Clin 2005;23(3):393–414, v

Brandy DA. An evaluation system to enhance patient selection for alopecia-reducing surgery. Dermatol Surg 2002;28(9):808–816

Ellis JA, Stebbing M, Harrap SB. Polymorphism of the androgen receptor gene is associated with male pattern baldness. J Invest Dermatol 2001;116(3):452–455

Epstein JS. Evolution of techniques in hair transplantation: a 12-year perspective. Facial Plast Surg 2007;23(1):51–59, discussion 60

Finner AM. Alopecia areata: Clinical presentation, diagnosis, and unusual cases. Dermatol Ther 2011;24(3):348–354

Frechet P. Scalp extension. J Dermatol Surg Oncol 1993;19(7): 616–622

Junqueira L, Carneiro J. Basic Histology Text and Atlas. 11th ed. New York, NY: McGraw-Hill; 2005:368–370

Juri J. Use of parieto-occipital flaps in the surgical treatment of baldness. Plast Reconstr Surg 1975;55(4):456–460

Kaufman KD, Olsen EA, Whiting D, et al; Finasteride Male Pattern Hair Loss Study Group. Finasteride in the treatment of men with androgenetic alopecia. J Am Acad Dermatol 1998;39(4 Pt 1): 578–589

Leavitt M, Charles G, Heyman E, Michaels D. HairMax LaserComb laser phototherapy device in the treatment of male androgenetic alopecia: A randomized, double-blind, sham device-controlled, multicentre trial. Clin Drug Investig 2009;29(5):283–292

Lotufo PA, Chae CU, Ajani UA, Hennekens CH, Manson JE. Male pattern baldness and coronary heart disease: the Physicians' Health Study. Arch Intern Med 2000;160(2):165–171

Ludwig E. Classification of the types of androgenetic alopecia (common baldness) occurring in the female sex. Br J Dermatol 1977;97(3):247–254

McElwee KJ, Shapiro JS. Promising therapies for treating and/or preventing androgenic alopecia. Skin Therapy Lett 2012;17(6): 1–4

Norwood OT. Male pattern baldness: classification and incidence. South Med J 1975;68(11):1359–1365

Nyholt DR, Gillespie NA, Heath AC, Martin NG. Genetic basis of male pattern baldness. J Invest Dermatol 2003;121(6):1561–1564

Olsen EA, Whiting D, Bergfeld W, et al. A multicenter, randomized, placebo-controlled, double-blind clinical trial of a novel formulation of 5% minoxidil topical foam versus placebo in the treatment of androgenetic alopecia in men. J Am Acad Dermatol 2007; 57(5):767–774

Paus R, Cotsarelis G. The biology of hair follicles. N Engl J Med 1999;341(7):491–497

Puig CJ. Incorporating hair replacement into your practice. Facial Plast Surg 2008;24(4):462–466

Puig CJ, Beehner ML, Cotterill PC, et al. Core competencies for hair restoration surgeons recommended by the International Society of Hair Restoration Surgery. Dermatol Surg 2009;35(3):425–427, discussion 427–428

Richards JB, Yuan X, Geller F, et al. Male-pattern baldness susceptibility locus at 20p11. Nat Genet 2008;40(11):1282–1284

Rousso DE, Presti PM. Follicular unit transplantation. Facial Plast Surg 2008;24(4):381–388

Seager D. The one-pass hair transplant: a six-year perspective. Hair Transplant Forum International. 2003;12:176–178

Unger MG. The Y-shaped pattern of alopecia reduction and its variations. J Dermatol Surg Oncol 1984;10(12):980–986

Van Neste D, Fuh V, Sanchez-Pedreno P, et al. Finasteride increases anagen hair in men with androgenetic alopecia. Br J Dermatol 2000;143(4):804–810

97 Laser Resurfacing

■ Introduction

Lasers are commonly used in otolaryngology–head and neck surgery. However, over the past 22 years, a new role has evolved: rejuvenation of the skin in lieu of dermabrasion or chemical peeling. Key to this application is control of thermal damage to achieve clinical improvement without unusual or adverse healing. The laser is capable of producing highly specific vaporization of photodamaged epidermis and epidermal lesions, including seborrheic keratoses, solar lentigenes, and actinic keratosis. Penetration into the dermis will result in contraction of dermal collagen by its thermal effects, with reduction in static wrinkles and, to some degree, active wrinkles of the face. Additionally, lasers can treat scars from trauma or acne.

The significant advantages of the pulsed laser cutaneous resurfacing are precise control of tissue vaporization, minimization of residual thermal damage, dermal heating, and excellent hemostasis. Different laser wavelengths interact with chromophores in the tissue, such as water, melanin, or hemoglobin, for a desired effect. As most of the epidermis is water, resurfacing lasers frequently target water for tissue heating or vaporization. Lasers used for resurfacing can be ablative or nonablative, determined by their ability to destroy skin epithelium. Both types of laser can produce rejuvenation from dermal heating.

The carbon dioxide (CO_2) laser wavelength (10,600 nuclear magnitude [nm]) is efficiently absorbed by water with penetration to 30 μm. Upon absorption, heat transfer results in instantaneous heating to > 100°C with vaporization and cellular ablation. The erbium:yttrium-aluminum-garnet (Er:YAG) laser (2,940 nm) is 10 times more efficiently absorbed by water, resulting in more precise and superficial ablation. Nonablative lasers, such as the neodymium:yttrium-aluminum-garnet (Nd:YAG) (1,320 nm) and diode (1,450 nm), penetrate the dermis and cause thermal damage and induce neocollagenesis, while leaving the epidermis intact. The degree of dermal penetration is generally directly correlated with the wavelength of the laser. Induction of dermal remodeling without epidermal ablation can be appealing because the recovery time is reduced, but this also means the rejuvenation result is less dramatic.

Although tissue damage is necessary for clinical improvement, excess tissue damage can lead to complications or delayed healing. Recently developed fractionated lasers attempt to maximize rejuvenation while further minimizing undesired effects, by creating patterned pillars of tissue damage surrounded by undamaged skin. This pattern of untreated skin surface being interspersed with treated skin causes patients to experience quicker healing and recovery times. The risk of hyperpigmentation and hypopigmentation is also decreased.

■ Patient Evaluation and Education

Careful preoperative evaluation and counseling of the laser resurfacing patient will simplify postoperative care. The first concern is whether the patient is an appropriate candidate for laser resurfacing.

Patient History

A careful history is helpful and should include the following specific points:

- Smoking history
- Alcohol intake history
- History of keloid or hypertrophic scar formation. Patients with a former keloid/hypertrophic scar are not good candidates for laser resurfacing
- History of prior aesthetic procedures (e.g., dermabrasion, chemical peel)

- History of use of topical facial medications, including a-hydroxy acid, Retin-A (DRAXIS Specialty Pharmaceuticals, Inc., Kirkland, QC, Canada), among others
- History of isotretinoin use
- History of prior and current infections, specifically the following:
  - Herpes simplex infections
  - Yeast infections
  - *Staphylococcus* infections and acne
  - Current nasal infections or prior nasal vestibulitis
- History of cutaneous cancers or changing lesions of the face

Patient Skin Type

The patient should be classified according to skin type on the Fitzpatrick Classification Scale:

I. Always burns, never tans
II. Always burns, sometimes tans
III. Sometimes burns, tans easily
IV. Never burns, always tans
V. Moderately pigmented skin
VI. Deeply pigmented skin

Note that patients with type I through III skin are more likely to develop freckling, solar lentigenes, and actinic keratosis. Patients with type III skin or higher will be more likely to have temporary or permanent hyperpigmentation. Patients with type III through VI skin will all require treatment with some bleaching preparation, such as 4% hydroquinone or kojic acid in the preoperative period.

Wrinkles

Wrinkles may be classified as I through IV, with I being the most superficial etching of the skin with just an epidermal component, and IV extending all the way through the dermis. Wrinkles are also classified as static or active. Laser resurfacing will treat effectively types I through III, but it will not adequately treat type IV wrinkles. Static wrinkles can be effectively treated, whereas active wrinkles, caused primarily by underlying musculofascial attachments as opposed to skin changes, are usually resistant to this therapy. It is important to discuss with the patient preoperatively these findings and realistic expectations. The Glogau photoaging scale is a well-recognized method of categorizing wrinkles and other photodamage characteristics of the skin.

Acne Scarring

Shell- or disc-shaped acne scars are most amenable to resurfacing, whereas the deeper ice-pick scars extending through the dermis are more resistant

to laser resurfacing. White fibrotic scars and stellate acne scars are not amenable to this treatment, although the surrounding irregularities will be less prominent. The greater the surface area treated, the greater the tightening effect and reduction in surface irregularity seen postoperatively. Texture improvement with laser resurfacing in the acne patient is significant. The patient should never be promised complete erasure, but rather a degree of improvement. Pre- and postoperative photographs of patients who have had this procedure are frequently helpful in the discussion with patients considering laser resurfacing.

Treatment of Scars

Laser technology has also proven effective in the treatment of atrophic, hypertrophic, and keloid scars. Proper assessment of scar characteristics guides the choice of laser to be used. Depressed scars respond quite well to laser resurfacing with both CO_2 and erbium lasers. In addition, the nonablative 1,064 nm Nd:YAG laser has been shown to be effective and safe for treatment of these mature scars, even in patients with Fitzpatrick skin types III through VI. Hypertrophic scars and keloids have been treated with fully ablative CO_2 lasers, but this method has high rates of recurrence and is not generally recommended. Red hypertrophic scars can be treated effectively with the pulsed-dye laser (PDL); the results have been reliable and comparable to the use of intralesional steroid injections. The 585 nm wavelength PDL is thought to target vasculature and to modulate cytokines and collagen production as well as alignment.

■ Management

Preprocedure Preparation

Patients are often advised to avoid sunlight for weeks prior to treatment to minimize pigmentation of skin. Some surgeons advocate preparing the skin with retinoic acid cream for 3 weeks to accelerate posttreatment reepithelialization. Similarly, hydroquinone can be initiated 3 weeks prior to minimize potential postprocedural inflammatory hyperpigmentation, especially in darker skin types. If the patient has pigmentation in prior scars or has irregular pigmentation, a bleaching cream, such as hydroquinone or kojic acid, should be used twice a day for up to 6 weeks prior to the surgical procedure to condition the skin to have a more uniform melanocytic activity. Antibiotics are generally started 1 to 2 days prior to treatment. When treating the perioral region, antivirals can also be initiated 2 days preoperatively and continued for over 1 week postoperatively. In general, these medications are continued until reepithelialization is complete.

Anesthesia

Anesthesia for laser resurfacing can be accomplished with topical anesthesia with or without regional nerve blocks (e.g., the great auricular, meatal, infraorbital, and supraorbital nerves), together with field blocks as appropriate. Sedation or general anesthesia may also be used on occasion. The skin can also be chilled prior to the procedure.

Technique

On the day of the procedure, patients are instructed to cleanse their skin and not apply any skin products, such as makeup or moisturizer. The skin can be washed again using mild soap immediately prior to the procedure, but it should completely dry before starting laser treatment. Strict safety precautions must be taken to avoid disastrous events. Any outlets for light escape from the room should be covered. A sign warning of laser use should be placed outside the room. Everyone in the room should wear the eye protection appropriate for the laser wavelength being used. Fire extinguishers or a water source should be readily available.

The surgeon then confirms the desired settings for power, density, and duration of pulse. Segmental versus a full-face laser resurfacing procedure should be discussed in detail with the patient. A full-face procedure, with feathering of the treated area into the hairline and the neck, is the easiest of the procedures to manage aesthetically in the postoperative period, from the patient's perspective. If a segmental (e.g., perioral or periorbital) area is treated, the contrast with the remaining skin requires makeup until the redness has dissipated. Pilosebaceous glands are necessary for normal healing after laser resurfacing. These are numerous in the face, but there are few in the neck; therefore, the neck is not an optimal site for full ablative laser resurfacing. However, the neck may be cautiously treated using fractionated technologies.

The differences in the thickness of the epidermis and dermis in the individual zones of the face are important. The eyelids may have as thin an epidermal/dermis structuring as 350 μm or may be as thick as 800 or 900 μm. The thickest epidermis lies in the forehead and anterior mental area. It is important to outline with a surgical marker the areas needing treatment, with the patient in an upright position. As a guide, a line may be drawn 2 cm below the lower border of the horizontal ramus of the mandible. The area between this line and the inferior border of the mandible is the zone where superficial removal of the epidermis will permit a transition of color. Other techniques may be used to further diminish the appearance of this transition.

Depth of Resurfacing

During full ablative CO_2 laser resurfacing, if the laser eschar is removed after the first application of the laser, then variations of the underlying skin will be apparent. These variations change with each subsequent pass with the laser, denoting the depth of penetration of the skin. For example, residual epidermal appendages create a pink look, removal of the papillary reticular dermis creates a gray look, and removal of the deep reticular dermis and/or subcutaneous tissue creates a yellow appearance. The objective is to limit the laser penetration to a maximum depth of the superficial reticular dermis in order to preserve the pilosebaceous glands, which are essential for healing. With use of a fractionated laser, an eschar, as already described, is usually not actively removed as is typical with full ablative resurfacing. The depth of resurfacing is instead established depending on the laser settings and knowledge of the patient's skin characteristics.

Postoperative Care

The myriad of methods for postprocedural skin care all attempt to keep the skin clean and protected. The cleansing effect can be achieved with mild soap and water, diluted peroxide, or a mixture of water and vinegar. Reepithelialization will be facilitated with the use of moist occlusive dressings. Appropriate occlusive dressings include a layer of petroleum-based ointment, vegetable oil, Aquaphor (Beiersdorf, Inc., Wilton, CT), or even Preparation H (Pfizer, New York, NY). Crusts and eschars can be gently removed in this way without producing scarring. This process is continued until the skin is completely epithelialized, which may take up to a week or more. The patient is also advised to avoid sunlight and to wear sunscreen after reepithelialization. The patient should avoid scratching the affected skin because this may cause hypertrophic scarring.

Complications

Complications of laser resurfacing are fortunately few. Fractionated CO_2 lasers carry an even further reduced risk of complications. Hypertrophic scarring can be treated with silicone sheeting, topical or injected steroids, and, on occasion, further laser treatment. Dyschromia (light or dark changes in the skin) is the most common complication seen with laser resurfacing procedures. Hyperpigmentation is generally self-limited, but hypopigmentation may be permanent. Prolonged erythema can last months after treatment, but it can be ameliorated by topical ascorbic acid or steroid creams. Acne or milia can result from the occlusive post-procedural dressing.

■ Conclusion

Laser resurfacing is an effective and evolving skin resurfacing technique. The benefits obtained from tissue damage are counterbalanced by the duration of recovery. Different lasers, including ablative, nonablative, and fractionated laser technologies, combined with varying laser settings, allow the surgeon to produce diverse results. Complications, although rare, must be recognized and treated or prevented.

■ Suggested Reading

Alster T. Laser scar revision: comparison study of 585-nm pulsed dye laser with and without intralesional corticosteroids. Dermatol Surg 2003;29(1):25–29

Alster TS, Apfelberg DD. Cosmetic Laser Surgery. New York, NY: Wiley-Liss; 1998

Alster TS, Tanzi EL. Complications in laser and light surgery. In: Goldberg DJ, ed. Lasers and Lights. Vol 2. Philadelphia, PA: Saunders Elsevier; 2008:99–112

Alster T, Zaulyanov L. Laser scar revision: a review [published correction in Dermatol Surg 2007;33(6):770. Note: Zaulyanov-Scanlon, Larissa corrected to Zaulyanov, Larissa]. Dermatol Surg 2007;33(2):131–140

Apfelberg DB, Maser MR, White DN, Lash H. Failure of carbon dioxide laser excision of keloids. Lasers Surg Med 1989;9(4):382–388

Avram MM, Tope WD, Yu T, Szachowicz E, Nelson JS. Hypertrophic scarring of the neck following ablative fractional carbon dioxide laser resurfacing. Lasers Surg Med 2009;41(3):185–188

Badawi A, Tome MA, Atteya A, Sami N, Morsy IA. Retrospective analysis of non-ablative scar treatment in dark skin types using the sub-millisecond Nd:YAG 1,064 nm laser. Lasers Surg Med 2011;43(2):130–136

Chernoff WG, Cramer H. Rejuvenation of the skin surface: laser exfoliation. Facial Plast Surg 1996;12(2):135–145

Doshi SN, Alster TS. 1,450 nm long-pulsed diode laser for nonablative skin rejuvenation. Dermatol Surg 2005;31(9 Pt 2):1223–1226, discussion 1226

Fitzpatrick TB. Ultraviolet-induced pigmentary changes: benefits and hazards. Curr Probl Dermatol 1986;15:25–38

Fitzpatrick RE, Goldman MP, Satur NM, Tope WD. Pulsed carbon dioxide laser resurfacing of photo-aged facial skin. Arch Dermatol 1996;132(4):395–402

Riggs K, Keller M, Humphreys TR. Ablative laser resurfacing: high-energy pulsed carbon dioxide and erbium:yttrium-aluminum-garnet. Clin Dermatol 2007;25(5):462–473

Tanzi EL, Alster TS. Comparison of a 1450-nm diode laser and a 1320-nm Nd:YAG laser in the treatment of atrophic facial scars: a prospective clinical and histologic study. Dermatol Surg 2004;30(2 Pt 1):152–157

98 Biomaterials and Facial Contouring

■ Introduction

The role of augmentation procedures has been expanded not only to include increasing skeletal dimension but also to perform facial rejuvenation and contour correction. The present trend is a customized approach to problems in contour restoration. Even for the most experienced surgeon, facial contouring poses a major challenge in the application of both methodology and implant design to achieve both the surgeon's and the patient's vision of the result. Facial contouring now comprises the art and science of patient evaluation, clinical indications, selection of implant materials, and implant shape.

■ Biomaterials

Knowledge of the safe and effective use of biomaterials requires an understanding of the histopathology of the implant–tissue interface and the host response to all implant materials. Adverse reactions are a consequence of an unresolved inflammatory response to implant materials. The behavior is also a function of not only the material, but also the configuration characteristics of the site of implantation—for example, the thickness of the skin overlying the implant, the scarring of the tissue bed, and the underlying bone architecture, all of which facilitate stabilization of the implant.

The method used to stabilize the implant is also important for predictable clinical outcome as well as for the longevity of the clinical result. Implants that are mobile cause reaction between the tissue and the implant at their interface, which increases and compromises implant longevity.

■ The Ideal Implant

The ideal implant material is cost-effective, nontoxic, nonantigenic, and noncarcinogenic. The material should be inert, easily shaped, able to maintain the desired form, and permanently accepted. There must be host acceptability with high resistance to infection. Biocompatibility is also influenced by the physical characteristics of the implant, such as firmness and surface characteristics.

Surgical technique, size of the device, and preparation also play a role in the success of the implant procedure. Ideally, the implant's posterior anatomical configuration should conform to the bony surface of the facial skeleton, and the anterior surface shape should imitate the desired natural anatomical configuration. The implants should be readily implantable, and the margins must be tapered to blend onto the bony surface so that they will be nonpalpable. The implants should also be malleable, conformable, and readily exchangeable. Permanent fixation or fabrics to immobilize them from the surrounding tissue are often undesirable, particularly if the patient desires to change augmentation characteristics in later years. The natural encapsulation process of silicone ensures immobility, yet provides exchangeability without damage to surrounding soft tissue. The implants should be easily modifiable by the surgeon before and during the procedure.

Implant Biomaterials

Polymeric Materials/Solid Polymers

Silicone Polymers

Silicone has a long history of clinical use with a reasonable safety-efficacy profile. The chemical name for silicone is polysiloxane. This material has been categorized into two forms of elastomers: heat-temperature vulcanized (HTV) polysiloxane elastomer, and room-temperature vulcanized (RTV) polysiloxane elastomer. RTV applies only to the elastomer that is supplied in a prefabricated form, whereby the surgeon or technician mixes components in an exothermic chemical reaction to produce a custom implant. Currently, this material is

646

not approved by the U.S. Food and Drug Administration's (FDA's) Good Manufacturing Practice guidelines. However, the FDA has approved other commercial custom implant processes, such as three-dimensional AccuScan, developed by Implantech Associates, Inc., Ventura, California. Even with commercially manufactured, FDA-approved HTV implants, differences in manufacture have significance for the purity and stability of the product. For example, the harder the implant, the more stable it is. An implant that is less than a hardness (durometer) of 10 will approach characteristics of a gel and over time will potentially leach or leak some of its internal molecular substances. However, the most recent studies on breast implant gel silicone have shown no objective cause and effect for silicone in producing scleroderma, lupus erythematosus, or other collagen vascular diseases.

Tissue reaction to solid silicone implants is characterized by a fibrous tissue capsule without tissue ingrowth. When unstable or placed without adequate soft tissue coverage, the implants are subject to moderate ongoing inflammation and possible seroma formation.

Polymethacrylate (Acrylic) Polymers

These polymers are supplied as a powdered mixture and catalyzed to produce a very hard material. The rigidity and hardness of the acrylic implants cause difficulty in many of the applications for using large implants inserted through small openings. In the preformed state, there is difficulty in conforming the implant to the underlying bony contour.

Polyethylene

This material can be produced in a variety of consistencies, now most commonly a porous form. Porous polyethylene, also known as Medpor (Stryker, Kalamazoo, MI), suggests stability with minimal inflammatory cell reaction. Porous polyethylene is harder and more friable than silicone and is somewhat more difficult to sculpt. Porous polyethylene allows satisfactory fibrous tissue ingrowth, which provides an advantage for enhanced implant stability.

Polytetrafluoroethylene (PTFE)

Polytetrafluoroethylene (PTFE) comprises a group of materials that have had a defined history of clinical application. The brand name PTFE is Proplast, which is no longer made in the United States because of the complications related to its use in temporomandibular joints. Under excessive mechanical stress, this implant material was subject to breakdown, intense inflammation, thick capsule formation, infection, and ultimate extrusion or explantation.

Expanded Polytetrafluoroethylene (ePTFE) (Gore-Tex)

This material was originally produced for cardiovascular applications. Animal studies showed ePTFE (Gore-Tex, W.L. Gore and Associates, Inc., Newark, DE) to elicit limited fibrous tissue ingrowth without capsule formation and minimum inflammatory cell reaction. The reaction seen over time compared favorably with many of the materials in use for facial augmentation. ePTFE has found acceptable results in subcutaneous tissue augmentation.

Mesh Polymers

Mesh polymers have the advantage of increased fibrous tissue ingrowth. However, their shortcomings have outweighed their ability to be used on a wide scale. For example, polyamide mesh has been shown to cause inflammatory cell reaction with numerous multinucleated giant cells. However, like other mesh materials, polyamide mesh can be folded, sutured, and shaped with relative ease. Other meshes include Marlex (Marlex Pharmaceuticals, Inc., New Castle, DE), Dacron, and Mersilene (Ethicon, Somerville, NJ).

■ Facial Contouring

Facial contouring means changing the shape of the face. Modern hallmarks of beauty are distinguished by bold facial contours that are accentuated by youthful malar-midface configurations and a sharp, well-defined jawline. The most important component of beauty is determined by the major architectural promontories of the facial skeleton. The configurations of the nose, malar-midface area, and mandible (jawline) create the fundamental proportions and contours. Any of these promontories that are too small or too large affect the aesthetic importance of the others. Reduction of the nasal prominence causes both the malar-midface and the mandibular-jawline volume and projection to appear relatively more distinct. Accentuating the malar-midface or enhancing the mandibular or malar-midface volumes makes the nose appear smaller and less imposing. By altering the volumetric relationships of the skeletal structures, the surgeon can create or restore facial harmony, balance, and beauty. Secondary promontories, such as the superior or inferior orbital ridge, the temporal mound, and the premaxilla, are all subtleties in contour that must also be considered.

The term *profileplasty* was traditionally applied to nose–chin relationships. However, because traditional chin implants were small, centrally placed, and poorly designed, excessive reduction in the nasal bridge was frequently performed in an attempt to improve contour. This type of chin augmentation often resulted in a protuberant, buttonlike, abnormally bulging central chin mound. Newer implants permit extended premandible augmentation across the entire lower third facial segment, thereby facilitating a natural-looking jawline contour. These implants are placed on the deepest or fourth skeletal plane. The other three planes are the skin, the subcutaneous fat, and the superficial musculoaponeurotic system (SMAS). Despite the most radical or extensive deep-plane SMAS techniques, enhancement in facial contour with rhytidectomy does not significantly change in most instances. Only judicious alterations of mass and volume in different anatomical regions produce contour changes. This balance of three major regions of volume and mass creates the classic balance of facial beauty. Technically, this is accomplished through selecting implants with the proper shape and design, and controlling their position on the facial skeleton.

Pathophysiological Considerations of Aging

Involutional soft tissue changes brought on by age, weight loss, or even excessive exercise may bring about facial flaws that appear progressively more obvious and pronounced with age. Recognizing these various defects and configurations caused by aging is also a part of the subject of facial contouring. During the aging process, depending on the underlying skeletal structure, different but definable configurations of the face are formed. These include the development of a generalized flattening of the midface, thinning of the vermilion border of the lips, the formation of jowls, and areas of deep cavitary depressions of the cheek. Other soft tissue configurations include the prominence of the nasolabial folds, as well as flattening of the soft tissue button of the chin and formation of the prejowl sulcus, in part by the relaxation of the soft tissue surrounding an area of bone resorption along the body of the mandible.

In the midface, most soft tissue deficiencies are found within the anatomical recess described as the submalar triangle. This inverted triangular area of midfacial depression is bordered above by the prominence of the zygoma, medially by the nasolabial fold, and laterally by the body of the masseter muscle. In cases of degenerative changes of the skin, the combination of soft tissue and/or loss of fat with deficient underlying bone structure exaggerates the gravitational effects of aging and may prevent rhytidectomy from completely rejuvenating the face. In contrast, exceptionally prominent cheekbone structure, if combined with thin skin lacking in subcutaneous or deep supporting fat, further emphasizes facial depressions. This type of pattern causes a gaunt or haggard appearance in an otherwise healthy person.

Preoperative Analysis for Facial Contouring

Augmentation of the facial skeleton with alloplastic implants changes the deepest skeletal plane of the face with a three-dimensional modality. The three elements necessary to alter facial form are shape, size, and positioning. However, correct analysis and identification of distinctive and recognizable configurations of facial deficiency are essential to choosing the optimal implant shape and size to obtain the best overall result in facial contour.

Zonal Principles of Skeletal Anatomy: The Premandibular Jawline Region

The premandibular space is the anatomical region that, when augmented, creates significant change in the shape and volume contour of the jawline and lower third of the face. Delineation of zonal principles of the anatomy within this space allows the surgeon to create specific chin and jawline contours. Traditional chin implants have essentially been placed between the mental foramina. This familiar location (zone 1) constitutes only one segment or zone of the mandible that can be successfully altered. Implants placed in the central segment alone and without extension often produce abnormal round protuberances that are unattractive.

A midlateral zone (zone 2) within the premandibular space can be defined as the region extending from the mental foramen posteriorly to the oblique line of the horizontal body of the mandible. When this zone is augmented, in addition to the central mentum, the anterior jawline contour widens. This is the basis for the development of the extended and prejowl chin implant. The posterior lateral zone is a third zone of the premandibular space, which encompasses the posterior half of the horizontal body, including the angle of the mandible and the first 2 to 4 cm of the ascending ramus. This zone can be modified with a mandibular angle implant, which can augment the area in a lateral or posterior direction. This will either widen or elongate the posterior mandibular angle to produce a strong posterior jawline contour.

Zonal Principles of Skeletal Anatomy: The Midface

Zonal principles of skeletal anatomy are useful for conceptualizing the malar-midfacial region into distinct anatomical zones.

- *Zone 1*, the largest area, includes the major portion of the malar bone and the first third of the zygomatic arch. Augmentation within this zone maximizes the projection of the malar eminence and produces a high, sharp, angular appearance.

- *Zone 2* overlies the middle third of the zygomatic arch. Enhancement of this zone along with zone 1 accentuates the cheekbone laterally, producing a broader dimension to the upper third of the face.
- *Zone 3*, the paranasal area, lies midway between the infraorbital foramen and the nasal bone. A vertical line drawn from the intraorbital foramen marks the lateral border of zone 3, which is the medial extent of the dissection usually done for malar augmentation. Augmentation of zone 3 gives medial fullness to the infraorbital region.
- *Zone 4* overlies the posterior third of the zygomatic arch. Augmentation in this area produces an unnatural appearance and in most cases is not indicated. The tissues overlying this zone are quite adherent to the bone. Therefore, dissection must be performed cautiously because the zygomaticotemporal division of the facial nerve passes superficially within the temporoparietal fascia over the zygomatic arch and would be prone to injury.
- *Zone 5* is the submalar triangle.

Classifying Midfacial Contour Defects

A topographical classification has recently proven to be more useful as a basic reference guideline to correlate distinctive anatomical patterns of deformity with specific implants.

Type I Deformity

This deformity occurs in a patient with good midfacial fullness but insufficient malar skeletal development. In this case, a malar implant would be desirable to augment the zygoma and create a higher arch to the cheekbone. Terino prefers the malar shell implant to augment this type of area. The shell concept provides a larger surface area to impart greater implant stability, which helps to reduce rotation or displacement.

Type II Deformity

The second type of deformity occurs in the patient who has atrophy or ptosis of the midfacial soft tissues in the submalar area and adequate malar development. In this case, submalar implants are used to augment or fill these depressions and/or to provide anterior projection to a relatively wide, flat face.

Type III Deformity

This deformity occurs in patients who have thin skin and very prominent malar eminences. These characteristics combine to cause an abrupt transition from the cheekbone superiorly to an extreme area of hollowness found within the submalar region, producing an exceptionally gaunt or skeletonized facial appearance. In this group of patients, a second-generation submalar implant is used to fill the abrupt midfacial hollow that in some cases may actually be exaggerated by rhytidectomy alone.

Type IV Deformity

This deformity is the result of malar hypoplasia and submalar soft tissue deficiency, which is described as the volume-deficient face. In this situation, a single combined malar-submalar implant must serve two purposes: to proportionally augment a deficient skeletal structure and to fill the void created by absent midfacial soft tissue.

"Tear-Trough" (Type V) Deformity

This deformity is specifically limited to a deep groove that commonly occurs at the junction of the thin eyelid and the thicker cheek skin. In this deformity, a pronounced nasal fold extends downward and laterally from the inner canthus of the eye across the infraorbital rim and the suborbital component of the malar bone. Flowers uses a tear-trough silicone elastomer implant, and Schoenrock and Chernoff use a Gore-Tex implant to augment this region.

■ Procedure

Considering the infinite variations of facial form, most analytical measurements used in determining aesthetic guidelines have been unreliable. By following the principles of skeletal zonal anatomy and by identifying the specific type of topographical anatomy or deformity, the surgeon will be able to determine the optimal course for correct implant selection and placement.

The safest level of dissection in the face is on bone where all anatomical landmarks, such as foramina and the exiting nerves, are familiar to the surgeon. In this subperiosteal plane, implants become firmly secured and attached to the skeleton by fibrosis and are usually stable within several days. Dissection is facilitated by adequate infiltration of dilute local anesthetic agents. The dissected compartments should be larger than the implant to accommodate it comfortably.

Surgical Technique for Mandibular Augmentation

Elevation of the soft tissues from the anterior and inferior borders of the mandible should be safe and simple. The basic principles for augmenting the malar-midface and premandibular spaces are identical. Controlling the shape, size, and positioning of the implants determines the overall final facial contour. Five basic technical rules for safe and accurate augmentation are as follows:

1. Stay on bone. Placement of implants on bone in the subperiosteal plane creates a firm and secure attachment of the implant to the bony skeleton. There is a strong adherence of the periosteum along the inferior border of the mandible and surrounding the mental foramina. This area contains the origins of the anterior mandibular ligament, which defines the prejowl sulcus at the inferior aspect of the aging marionette crease.
2. Gently elevate the soft tissues in a nonbony area.
3. Adequately expand the dissection space to accommodate the prosthesis comfortably. A sharp dissecting instrument may be used on the central bone, but only blunt instruments should be used around the nerves and adjacent to soft tissues.
4. Avoid the mental nerve by directing the elevator along the inferior border of the mandible and gently sweeping it below the mental foramen. The course of the mental nerve is directed superiorly into the lower lip, which helps to protect it from dissection trauma. Temporary hypesthesia of the mental nerve is not uncommon for several days to several weeks after surgery. Permanent nerve damage is extremely rare and represents less than half of 1% of statistically large numbers of cases.
5. Maintain a dry operative field, which is essential for accurate visualization, precise dissection, and proper implant placement.

Choice of Incisions

Access to the premandibular space can be accomplished by either an intraoral or an external route. The advantages of the external route are that it does not involve intraoral bacterial floral contamination; it has direct access to the inferior mandibular border, where cortical bone is present; it does not require significant retraction of the mental nerves; and it allows the implant to be secured to the periosteum along the inferior mandibular border, providing a method of fixation and preventing either side-to-side or vertical malposition. The intraoral route provides the obvious advantage of leaving no external scars.

The entry wound for the intraoral route is a transverse incision made through the mucosa and then through the mentalis muscle, which is divided vertically in the midline raphe to avoid transection of the muscle belly or total detachment from the bony origins. This midline aperture provides adequate access inferiorly onto the bone of the central mentum and eliminates potential muscle weakness that may occur if transected. The external route uses a v-shaped 1.5 cm incision that immediately accesses the inferior border of the mandible. First a narrow Joseph periosteal elevator or a 4-mm-wide blunt spatula elevator is used to perform the dissection along the inferior mandibular border. Care is taken to stay inferiorly to avoid injury to the mental nerve. One side of the implant is inserted into the lateral portion of the pocket on one side and then, if one is using a silicone implant, it is folded upon itself and the contralateral portion of the implant is inserted into the other side of the pocket. The implant is then adjusted in position.

Mandibular Angle Implants

The angle of the mandible is accessed through a 2 cm mucosal incision at the retromolar trigone placed ~ 8 mm lateral to the angle. Once again, dissection is performed on bone and beneath the masseter muscle to elevate the periosteum around the posterior angle of the mandible up along the ramus and then anteriorly along the body of the mandible. This permits accurate placement of the angle implants that are specifically designed to fit the posterior bony border of the adjacent ascending ramus and enhance angle definition. These implants are secured with a titanium screw.

Choosing Premandibular Implants

Implants extending into the midlateral (parasymphyseal) zone accomplish anterior widening of the lower third of the facial segment. The average central and midlateral projection necessary is 6 to 9 mm for men and 4 to 7 mm for women. Occasionally in a patient with severe microgenia, implants of up to 10 to 12 mm in projection may be necessary to create a more normal profile and a broader jawline.

Surgical Techniques for Malar and Midface Contouring

As in mandibular augmentation the safest level of dissection is on bone, in the subperiosteal plane, where all anatomical landmarks are identified. The various routes for entering the malar-midfacial area are as follows:

- Intraoral
- Subciliary (lower blepharoplasty)
- Rhytidectomy
- Zygomatic or temporal
- Transcoronal
- Transconjunctival

Intraoral Route

The intraoral route is the most common approach used for malar-midface augmentation and currently is the preferred route for most midfacial implants, with the exception of the tear-trough implant. After infiltration of the anesthetic solution, a 1 cm incision is made through the mucosa in a vertical oblique direction above the buccal-gingival line over the canine tooth and carried down to the bone. A large, broad-based Tessier-type elevator (~ 10 mm wide) is directed through the zygomaticus muscle onto the bone in the same orientation as the incision. While keeping the elevator directly on bone, the soft tissues are elevated obliquely upward off the maxillary buttress and the maxillary eminence. The elevator is kept on the bone margin along the inferior border of the malar eminence and the zygomatic arch.

For routine malar-submalar augmentation procedures, no attempt is made to visualize or dissect within the vicinity of the infraorbital nerve unless an implant is intended for this area. The submalar space is created by elevating the soft tissues inferiorly over the tendinous attachments of the masseter muscle below the zygoma. The surgeon can discern the correct plane of dissection of the glistening white fibers of the masseter tendons by direct vision. It is important to note that these masseteric attachments should not be cut. They are left completely intact to provide a supporting framework upon which the implant may rest. As the dissection moves posteriorly along the zygomatic arch, the space becomes tighter and is not as easily enlarged as the medial segment. However, this part of the space can be opened by gently advancing and elevating the tissues with a heavy, blunt periosteal elevator. It is of utmost importance that the dissection be extended sufficiently so that the implant fits passively within the pocket. A pocket that is too small will force the implant toward the opposite direction, causing implant displacement or extrusion. Implant selection is aided by observing the actual topographical changes produced by placement of the different implant "sizers" into the pocket.

Final implant placement must correspond to the external topographical defects outlined on the face preoperatively. In submalar augmentation, the implant may reside below the zygoma and zygomatic arch, over the masseter tendon, or it may overlap both bone and tendon. The larger shell-type malar implants reside primarily on bone in a more superior, lateral position and may extend partly into the submalar space. The combined implant will occupy both areas. Any implant placed in patients with noticeable facial asymmetry, thin skin, or an extremely prominent bone structure may require modification to reduce its thickness or length and avoid potential ridging or abnormal projections.

Once the implant position has been established, it is often necessary to secure it. This can be accomplished by several methods. Internal suture fixation relies on the presence of an adjacent stable segment of periosteum or tendinous structure upon which to anchor the implant. Stainless steel or titanium screws can also be used. Two methods of external fixation are used to stabilize midfacial implants:

1. The *indirect lateral suspension technique* uses 2–0 Ethilon sutures (Ethicon, Somerville, NJ) wedged on large Keith needles and placed through the implant tail. These needles are then inserted through the pocket and directed superiorly and posteriorly to exit percutaneously posterior to the temporal hairline. The sutures are then tied over a bolster, exerting traction on the tail of the implant. This technique is more suitable for a malar implant that treats a type I deformity.

2. The *direct method of external fixation* is often used on patients either with gross asymmetry or in whom the implants are placed in the midfacial or submalar area of the face. In these situations, the direct external method of fixation will prevent slippage in the immediate postoperative period. In this method, the implants are positioned directly to correspond with marks on the skin that correspond with the two most medial fenestrations of the implant. A double-armed suture is made with 1 in straight needles, which are then passed through the two medial fenestrations of the implant from a posterior to anterior direction. The needles are advanced through the pocket, passed perpendicularly through the skin, and exited at the respective external markings. The implant, following the needles, is guided into the pocket, and is then secured in place by tying the sutures over bolsters comprising two dental rolls.

Subciliary (Lower Blepharoplasty) Approach

Since the introduction of the newer, larger-surface-area implants, the subciliary approach is seldom used. However, this is the preferred approach for the insertion of the tear-trough implant. In malar augmentation, if only zones 1 or 2 require volumetric filling to achieve high-arch cheekbones, the blepharoplasty approach may be adequate. The advantages of the subciliary approach over the intraoral approach are the lack of oral contamination and the soft tissue support inferiorly, which reduces the chances for implant rotation or descent. However, this technique can also precipitate an ectropion in the presence of a weak tarsus.

Rhytidectomy Approach

The malar space may be safely entered through zone 1 of the malar region. Penetration of the SMAS is made medial to the zygomatic eminence and then bluntly carried down to bone. There are no significant facial nerve branches in this area. The malar pocket is then created primarily by retrograde dissection. This approach affords direct access to the area being augmented. However, insertion of an implant via this approach can introduce technical difficulties during SMAS dissection and elevation during rhytidectomy.

Zygomatic Temporal and Coronal Approaches

The cranial facial techniques used in subperiosteal face lifts have provided ready access to the malar zygomatic region. However, for the inexperienced surgeon, these techniques present an unwarranted risk of frontalis nerve damage.

Transconjunctival Approach

The transconjunctival approach has been used for insertion of midfacial implants, but it may also require disinsertion of the lateral canthal tendon. This necessitates secondary resuspension canthoplasty, with the attendant risk of lower eyelid asymmetry, distortion, and change in shape of the eye aperture.

■ Complications

Complications of implants in facial augmentation include bleeding, hematoma, infection, exposure, extrusion, malposition, displacement, fistula, seroma, persistent edema, abnormal prominence, pain and inflammatory action, and nerve damage. However, in most of the complications listed, very few are due solely to the implant material itself. In assessing complications, it is extremely difficult to distinguish among the surgical technique, the surrounding circumstances of the individual operation, and the individual patient factors as to problems associated with the implant material itself.

Extrusion should never occur if the technical rules already outlined have been observed. A secure, two-layer closure of both muscle and mucosa for both the chin and the midfacial implants assists in preventing movement and wound dehiscence. The anatomical contouring of the larger or extended implants that fit along the midface and mandibular contours minimizes malposition and malrotation. Dissection of the subperiosteal space to create midlateral and posterolateral tunnels in the mandible and the desired pockets in the midface will maintain the implant in proper position.

In mandibular augmentation, the mandibular branch of the facial nerve passes just anterior to the midportion of the mandible in the midlateral (parasymphyseal) zone. It is important not to traumatize the tissues that overlie this area. Similarly, the temporal branch of the facial nerve passes posterior to the middle aspect of the zygomatic arch, so care must be exercised when dissecting in this area. In mandibular augmentation, the mental nerve is directed in an upward path into the lower lip. Dissection that remains inferior to the foramen along the lower border of the mandible will minimize danger to the nerve. Permanent anesthesia of the mental nerve is rare. Temporary anesthesia or paresthesia for several weeks after surgery is not uncommon.

If encroachment on the nerve is detected by misplacement or malposition of the implant, then the implant should be repositioned below the nerve as early as possible. Infection in facial implants, particularly in silicone elastomer implants, is also uncommon. Irrigation with bacitracin, 50,000 units per liter of sterile saline, is used to fully irrigate the wounds and to soak the implant during the procedure. Drainage techniques are not ordinarily necessary in mandibular augmentation but may be used in midfacial augmentation, particularly if there is more than the normal amount of bleeding.

In mandibular augmentation, bone resorption is more common than not for most alloplastic implants. Findings of bone erosion after chin implants were reported in the 1960s but have not proved to be clinically significant since. Almost no clinical evidence has appeared in the literature, nor has any been revealed by surveying large audiences of plastic surgeons to substantiate any significant number of serious dental or mandibular problems associated with bone resorption. The condition appears to stabilize at a certain level of ingrowth without the loss of cosmetic gain.

◼ Conclusion

Facial contouring provides patients with significant changes in their facial appearance. The adjustment process for a patient, particularly one who has undergone a large degree of augmentation, is sometimes difficult. For this reason, the patient must be well counseled preoperatively to properly anticipate the postoperative course of swelling and to be able to cope with the change. At the same time, there are very few procedures that can provide the major rewards that facial contour procedures are able to offer.

◼ Suggested Reading

Badie B. Cosmetic reconstruction of temporal defect following pterional [corrected] craniotomy. Surg Neurol 1996;45(4):383–384

Beekhuis GJ. Use of silicone-rubber in nasal reconstructive surgery. Arch Otolaryngol 1967;86(1):88–91

Binder W. A comprehensive approach for aesthetic contouring of the midface in rhytidectomy. Facial Plast Surg Clin North Am 1993;1:231–255

Binder WJ. Submalar augmentation: an alternative to face-lift surgery. Arch Otolaryngol Head Neck Surg 1989;115(7):797–801

Binder WJ. Submalar augmentation: a procedure to enhance rhytidectomy. Ann Plast Surg 1990;24(3):200–212

Binder W, Schoenrock L, eds. Facial Plastic Surgery Clinics of North America: Facial Contouring and Alloplastic Implants. Philadelphia, PA: WB Saunders; 1994

Braley S. Symposium on synthetics in maxillofacial surgery, I: The silicones in maxillofacial surgery. Laryngoscope 1968;78(4):549–557

Braley S. Use of silicones in plastic surgery. Arch Otolaryngol 1963;78:669–675

Conrad K, Chapnik JS, Reifen E. E-PTFE (Gore-Tex) suspension cervical facial rhytidectomy. Arch Otolaryngol Head Neck Surg 1993;119(6):694–698

Flowers RS. Periorbital aesthetic surgery for men. Eyelids and related structures. Clin Plast Surg 1991;18(4):689–729

Flowers RS. Tear trough implants for correction of tear trough deformity. Clin Plast Surg 1993;20(2):403–415

WL Gore and Associates, Inc. Technical Considerations in Plastic and Reconstructive Surgery. Gore-Tex, SAM facial implant information pamphlet. Flagstaff, AZ: WL Gore and Associates, Inc.

Hollinger JO. Biomedical Application of Synthetic Biodegradable Polymers. Boca Raton, FL: CRC Press; 1995

Lagrotteria L, Scapino R, Granston AS, Felgenhauer D. Patient with lymphadenopathy following temporomandibular joint arthroplasty with Proplast. Cranio 1986;4(2):172–178

Lykins CL, Friedman CD, Ousterhout DK. Polymeric implants in craniomaxillofacial reconstruction. Otolaryngol Clin North Am 1994;27(5):1015–1035

Millard DR Jr. Chin implants. Plast Reconstr Surg (1946) 1954;13(1):70–74

Mittelman H. The anatomy of the aging mandible and its importance to facelift surgery. Facial Plast Surg Clin North Am 1994;2:301–311

Neel HB III. Implants of Gore-Tex. Arch Otolaryngol 1983;109(7):427–433

Peled IJ, Wexler MR, Ticher S, Lax EE. Mandibular resorption from silicone chin implants in children. J Oral Maxillofac Surg 1986;44(5):346–348

Romm S. Art, love, and facial beauty. Clin Plast Surg 1987;14(4):579–583

Schoenrock LD, Chernoff WG. Subcutaneous implantation of Gore-Tex for facial reconstruction. Otolaryngol Clin North Am 1995;28(2):325–340

Schultz RC. Reconstruction of facial deformities with alloplastic material. Ann Plast Surg 1981;7(6):434–446

Shemen LJ. Expanded polytef for reconstructing postparotidectomy defects and preventing Frey's syndrome. Arch Otolaryngol Head Neck Surg 1995;121(11):1307–1309

Silver FH, Maas CS. Biology of synthetic facial implant materials. Facial Plast Surg Clin North Am 1994;2:241–253

Staffel G, Shockley W. Nasal implants. Otolaryngol Clin North Am 1995;28(2):295–308

Terino EO. Alloplastic facial contouring by zonal principles of skeletal anatomy. Clin Plast Surg 1992;19(2):487–510

Terino EO. Implants for male aesthetic surgery. Clin Plast Surg 1991;18(4):731–749

Tobias GW, Binder WJ. The submalar triangle: its anatomy and clinical significance. Facial Plast Surg Clin North Am 1994;2:255–264

Watanabe K, Miyagi H, Tsurukiri K. Augmentation of temporal area by insertion of silicone plate under the temporal fascia. Ann Plast Surg 1984;13(4):309–319

Wellisz T. Clinical experience with the Medpor porous polyethylene implant. Aesthetic Plast Surg 1993;17(4):339–344

Wellisz T. Reconstruction of the burned external ear using a Medpor porous polyethylene pivoting helix framework. Plast Reconstr Surg 1993;91(5):811–818

Wellisz T, Dougherty W. The role of alloplastic skeletal modification in the reconstruction of facial burns. Ann Plast Surg 1993;30(6):531–536

Wellisz T, Dougherty W, Gross J. Craniofacial applications for the Medpor porous polyethylene flexblock implant. J Craniofac Surg 1992;3(2):101–107

Yih WY, Zysset M, Merrill RG. Histologic study of the fate of autogenous auricular cartilage grafts in the human temporomandibular joint. J Oral Maxillofac Surg 1992;50(9):964–967, discussion 968

99 Rehabilitation of the Paralyzed Face

■ Introduction

Rehabilitation of the paralyzed face continues to be a challenge, despite the advent of numerous advances in treatment in the last decades. Individualization of the treatment plan is obviously necessary, because the needs of a young patient with idiopathic facial paralysis are vastly different from those of an elderly person with facial paralysis after a resection for malignancy that included the facial nerve. Developmental facial nerve paralysis is uncommon and requires a unique approach. Therefore, the appropriate rehabilitative options and patient expectations will likewise be different. An important function of the physician is to educate the patient as to the possible rehabilitative options and their potential outcomes.

Anatomy and Physiology

The facial nerve (cranial nerve [CN] VII) is the nerve of facial expression. It allows humans to communicate many thoughts and emotions nonverbally. Accordingly, CN VII plays a major role in our interactions with others. The loss of this ability is obviously devastating and disabling.

The facial nerve is composed of ~ 7,000 fibers. It is primarily thought of as a motor nerve, but it has a large somatosensory and secretomotor component. The nerve arises in the pons and then traverses the cerebellopontine angle and enters the internal auditory meatus along with the eighth nerve. After passing through the internal auditory canal, the facial nerve fibers synapse at the geniculate ganglion and then pass into the fallopian canal, through the middle ear, and into the mastoid after the second genu. The nerve continues in the bony canal (the entire length of which is the longest bony canal of any nerve in the body), until it exits the skull base at the stylomastoid foramen, deep to the mastoid tip and lateral to the styloid process. It then turns anteriorly, where it is enveloped by the parotid gland.

The facial nerve divides into an upper and lower division at the pes anserinus, shortly after entering the parotid gland. These two main divisions then give rise to five main branches with extensive and variable arborization and communicating branches. These five main branches are (in order from superior to inferior): the temporal (frontal), zygomatic, buccal, marginal mandibular, and cervical. The zygomatic and buccal branches typically have the most extensive arborization and anastomotic branches. The distal nerve fibers generally enter the muscles of facial expression along the deep surface of the muscle.

■ Evaluation of the Patient

Initial evaluation should attempt to elucidate as completely as possible the cause and duration of the paralysis. The status of the integrity of the proximal and distal portions of the facial nerve is of prime importance. If the nerve is known to be transected, favorable factors for regeneration include clean transection, distal injury, immediate repair, and younger age. The nerve distal to the injury is the conduit for regeneration to the facial musculature; therefore, the integrity and continuity of the nerve to the muscles must be precisely determined. In injuries less than 72 hours old, distal stimulation is possible. After this, only visual surgical identification is possible.

The Sunderland Classification

The Sunderland classification of nerve injury ranges from type 1, which is no architectural disruption of the nerve with only temporary disruption of sodium ion channels, to type 5, with total anatomical disruption.

Electroneurography

Electroneurography can only distinguish between Sunderland type 1 injury and all other types, but serial Electroneurography comparing the normal to the injured side will reveal either continued near-normal responses in the case of incomplete injury, or progressive decline in the case of more severe injury.

Electromyography

Electromyography (EMG) is the most helpful method for assessing facial muscle innervation in the presence of paralysis of ~ 12 months or longer. Nascent, polyphasic, or normal voluntary action potentials indicate that innervation is present but inadequate to produce movement. Fibrillation or denervation potentials reflect viable but denervated muscle. Electrical silence reflects denervation atrophy of the muscles of facial expression.

Patient factors, such as advancing age, diabetes, poor nutrition, surgical or traumatic scarring, and history of radiation therapy, all have negative implications for rehabilitation and neural regeneration. The facial nerve deficit should be documented precisely from the physical examination.

House–Brackmann Scale

The most commonly used scale for description of facial paralysis is the House–Brackmann scale, where a score of 1 designates normal movement and a score of 6 is no movement at all. Several other scales, notably the Sunnybrook and Sidney scales, have been developed but are not as commonly used. Central and peripheral lesions should be differentiated, and other associated cranial nerve deficits should be identified. In particular, the status of the trigeminal nerve (corneal sensation, muscles of mastication) and hypoglossal nerve should be noted because these nerves have important implications for therapy and future rehabilitation. Surgical or traumatic scars should be noted because they may have an impact on future access or design of flaps.

◼ Management

Medical Protection of the Eye

After the initial assessment of the extent of nerve injury, evaluation of the eye and eyelids is most important. Numerous factors must be considered in deciding what is the most appropriate treatment for the patient. Young patients with good skin tone and

Bell phenomenon (outward and upward rolling of the eye on the attempt to close the affected side, thus providing lubrication and protection of the cornea) may need only reassurance and close observation. The older patient with poorer muscle tone will likely suffer more with both ectropion and brow ptosis.

Many patients in both groups will require liberal use of lubricant artificial tears during the day and ophthalmic ointment at night. Many excellent ocular moisturizing agents are available over the counter today. Ointment tends to blur vision and is not as well tolerated by patients during the day. Additional protection can be obtained with the use of careful taping or cellophane wrap occlusal dressings sealed in place on the skin with ointment. This can be held in place with a standard eyepatch.

Patients with increasing degrees of lower lid laxity can be helped by temporary repositioning of the lower eyelid with tape. It is applied along the lateral portion of the lower eyelid with tension exerted in a superolateral direction, thus elevating and tightening the lower lid. Corneal protection from debris, wind, and sunlight can be enhanced with the use of glasses during the time that the blink reflex is diminished or absent. This is particularly important in patients who have an associated trigeminal lesion with diminished or absent corneal sensation.

Surgical Protection of the Eye

If adequate ocular protection is not achieved with the maneuvers described, surgical intervention may be necessary. Temporary suture tarsorrhaphies (without denuding of the eyelid margins) are useful, simple short-term solutions. These are reserved for patients who are unable to administer supportive care or to buy time until a definitive procedure can be performed. Permanent lid-adhering tarsorrhaphies are functionally and cosmetically inferior to more contemporary procedures but may play a role in the older patient with extreme lower lid laxity and in whom cosmesis may be less of an issue. The Bick type of tarsorrhaphy is reversible and can provide excellent protection for a procedure that can be performed under local anesthesia in an office setting in a short period of time.

Paralysis of the orbicularis oculi muscle results in corneal exposure due to retraction of the upper lid, with failure of closure and blink and lower eyelid ectropion. This exacerbates dryness of the cornea by interfering with the lacrimal lake and proper tear film distribution, but it may also lead to excessive tearing, since eversion of the lower punctum causes overflow of tears (epiphora) because they are unable to drain into the lacrimal system.

Probably the most commonly performed procedure for facial paralysis at this time is upper eyelid loading with gold or platinum weights, which come in a variety of shapes and sizes. Eyelid closure is obtained by a combination of mass effect and reflex inhibition of CN III input during attempted closure. The weight is implanted in the pretarsal space of the mid–upper eyelid and sutured directly onto the tarsal plate. This procedure has a very high success rate and is easily reversible. It thus can be used very early in the course of the paralysis, even if it is expected to be temporary. In young people who do not have lower eyelid paralytic ectropion, it is often the only procedure necessary and may even obviate the need to use artificial tears. Its major drawback is that it is gravity dependent and, therefore, not dynamic in all positions, particularly when the patient is supine. Complications include extrusion of the implant, infection, malposition, failure to completely close the lid, visual changes due to deformity of the cornea from the weight of the implant, and visibility of the implant.

Surgical repositioning of the lower eyelid is performed with a variety of procedures, including, most commonly, lateral canthoplasty (canthotomy, inferior cantholysis, and superior resuspension), and tightening by excising a lateral tarsal strip. These maneuvers functionally and cosmetically reappose the lower eyelid to the globe, bring the tear film into closer approximation with the cornea, and improve the lacrimal pump system. Conchal cartilage support grafts, palpebral springs, and Silastic slings are not as commonly used due to extrusion and need for frequent revisions.

Other procedures to correct the symptoms of dry eye include placement of temporary punctal plugs and permanent punctual occlusion. However, these procedures are usually outside of the practice realm of the otolaryngologist. It is imperative that all patients with facial paralysis have a complete baseline ophthalmologic exam and appropriate interim follow-up.

Surgical Rehabilitation

Neurorrhaphy

The best chance for return of function after surgical or traumatic disruption of the facial nerve occurs if the nerve is repaired immediately. In the event a delay is required (medical instability, etc.) careful tagging of the nerve stumps and an operative diagram should be used. The distal branches will not respond to stimulation after 3 days and, therefore, become much more difficult to identify. The decision to operate becomes more difficult when a patient is evaluated between the first and approximately fourth month after injury, because this is beyond the ideal time for primary nerve repair and around the time when spontaneous recovery may begin to occur. In this situation, surgical exploration is indicated in the presence of total paralysis, lack of response to electrical stimulation, or absence of polyphasic or volitional potentials on EMG.

Direct repair of the exposed facial nerve and epineurium is performed with 8-0 to 10-0 monofilament permanent suture material in an interrupted fashion. A single suture may suffice to reapproximate the nerve lying in the facial canal or near the brain stem. More distally, as few sutures as possible are used to achieve a tension-free coaptation of the nerve ends. If the injury is beyond the point where the nerve has arborized to enter the facial muscles (lateral orbital rim, nasolabial crease area), soft tissue approximation is all that is necessary and technically possible.

In recent years there have been no major technical advances with wide clinical application in the repair of severed or damaged peripheral nerves. Intense investigation and use of regeneration chambers, lasers, tissue adhesives, and growth factors in the basic science realm will hopefully yield clinical applications in the near future.

Interposition Nerve Grafts

When neural tissue is deficient, a conduit for regeneration is reestablished by grafting. The two most commonly used donor nerves are the greater auricular and the sural nerves. The greater auricular nerve is found overlying the sternocleidomastoid muscle, bisecting a line connecting the mastoid tip and the mandibular angle. It is of suitable caliber for grafting defects of < 10 cm and, if dissected superiorly, can supply two to three branches for grafting several facial nerve branches. Donor morbidity is minimal. The greater auricular nerve's main disadvantage is its relatively short length in comparison to the sural nerve. The sural nerve is found posterior to the lateral malleolus, close to the lesser saphenous vein in the lower leg. It can be harvested in lengths of 20 to 30 cm and yields multiple branches for simultaneous grafting. Regardless of which nerve is used, tension-free epineurial coaptation is performed by using sufficient length for the graft to lie in a relaxed configuration.

If multiple branches are disrupted, the zygomatic and buccal divisions are preferentially grafted to provide eye closure and elevation of the oral commissure.

Planned postoperative radiation therapy does not contraindicate the use of nerve grafts, although controversy exists regarding its effect on graft success. Previous radiation or other scarring of the recipient bed negatively affects the survival of the grafts and subsequent chances of functional success.

Nerve Transfer

A nerve transfer is indicated in cases of complete paralysis of 2 to 3 years' duration, where a proximal facial nerve stump is not available for grafting or repair. The most likely patient scenario for this is the patient who has undergone resection of a cerebellopontine angle tumor, such as a vestibular nerve schwannoma or a facial nerve schwannoma. The requirements for success of this procedure are an intact extracranial facial nerve, an intact facial mimetic musculature, an intact hypoglossal nerve, and a patient who can tolerate sacrifice of this cranial nerve. Patients at risk for other cranial nerve deficits (CN IX, X) are considered poor candidates, because the speech and deglutition deficits would be compounded. Splitting the hypoglossal nerve can be effective and can avoid some of the disability associated with complete division of the nerve.

Patients with congenital facial nerve paralysis often lack a sufficient population of extracranial facial nerve fibers and facial muscles capable of accepting reanimation and thus are not candidates for this procedure.

Nerve transfer involves isolation and sectioning of the hypoglossal nerve close to its entrance into the tongue musculature. The paralyzed facial nerve is transected close to the stylomastoid foramen, and the cut ends of these cranial nerves are coapted without tension. Improved facial tone and symmetry occur within 4 to 12 months, and voluntary facial movements improve over the next 18 months. As with all the rehabilitative techniques, with the exception of cross-face nerve grafting, true spontaneous reflexive function is not expected.

Cross-Face Nerve Grafting

Cross-face nerve grafting uses a cable graft, typically from the sural nerve, to provide input from the facial nerve branches on the unaffected side. Typically the buccal branches are used on both sides. A sural nerve graft is usually required due to the distance involved. The graft is tunneled across the upper lip. Spontaneous expression is possible with this technique, and it is commonly used along with free microvascular muscle transfer in patients with congenital or longstanding facial paralysis.

Muscle Transfers

Muscle transfers should be reserved for patients who are not candidates for cable nerve grafts or hypoglossal nerve transpositions. The three most common procedures in this group are the temporalis transposition, masseter transposition, and microvascular free muscle transfers.

Temporalis and Masseter Transpositions

The temporalis and masseter transpositions require an intact ipsilateral trigeminal nerve and are both now used selectively to reanimate the lower face. In the traditional approach, the middle third of the temporalis muscle is turned inferiorly through a tunnel over the zygomatic arch and sutured to the oral commissure and upper lip.

More recently, orthodromic temporalis muscle transfer has been advocated. In this technique the approach is either intraoral or through an incision along the melolabial fold to expose the temporalis tendon and muscle as it attaches to the coronoid process of the mandible. The coronoid process is transected and mobilized to attach to the oral commissure and orbicularis oris using either native tendon or fascia lata. The masseter may likewise be detached from its insertion along the lower border of the mandible and transposed to the oral commissure and lower lip. These muscles can be used in combination as they exert different vectors of pull.

Deliberate overcorrection of each area is performed, because gravity and tissue relaxation will inevitably reduce the surgical effect.

Postoperatively, the patients are trained to effect facial movement by activating the transposed muscles (biting, chewing, etc.) with the aid of biofeedback, videotaping, and mirror feedback. Reanimation of the eyelid by muscle slips of the temporalis has been replaced by the lid loading and lower lid repositioning procedures previously discussed.

Microvascular Free Muscle Transfers

The use of free microvascular innervated muscle transfer has developed into the treatment of choice for many longstanding or congenital facial paralysis patients who otherwise would be candidates for temporalis and masseter transpositions. Conceptually, this involves a two-stage procedure using a cross-facial nerve graft followed by a free muscle transfer.

Initially the peripheral branches of the facial nerve on the nonparalyzed side are exposed, and several fascicles of the buccal division are transected. Sural nerve grafts are sutured to these normal branches and tunneled subcutaneously to the paralyzed side. A "babysitter" split hypoglossal nerve graft may also be used to speed neurotization.

Six to 9 months later, the second procedure is performed. This consists of harvesting the gracilis muscle (most commonly, although others have been used) from the medial upper leg, transferring it to the paralyzed face, and revascularizing it by microvascular anastomoses with the facial vessels. The nerves to the gracilis muscle are then anastomosed with the previously placed cross-facial nerve grafts. Tone, symmetry at rest, and varying degrees of movement have been obtained in large series.

The importance of free tissue transfer is most profound when rehabilitating patients with congenital paralyses. In patients with unilateral paralysis, the procedure is as outlined above; in those with bilateral deficits (Möbius syndrome), other cranial nerves are being used to innervate the transplanted muscle. Further delineation of the role for these procedures is evolving. Eyelid reanimation is still best accomplished as previously described.

Adjunctive Procedures and Management

Commonly applied physical therapy techniques used to treat facial palsy include electrical stimulation, exercise, and massage. None of these treatment modalities has successfully prevailed over the others. However, there is now scientifically valid evidence that supports the use of EMG biofeedback and mirror feedback in conjunction with a structured home rehabilitation program to improve function in patients with longstanding facial paralysis. Retraining before synkinesis and hyperkinesis have developed is more successful than treating established aberrant movements. The selective use of botulinum toxin can be very helpful in reducing both synkinesis and activity of the normal side to create symmetry. The information supplied by the feedback training substitutes for absent or diminished sensory input involved in voluntary movements. The use of these techniques after muscle transfer is also helpful.

In patients who are candidates for muscle transposition surgery but who are unable or unwilling to undergo the procedure, static sling operations may have some benefit. The purpose of these procedures is to provide symmetry at rest. Permanent sutures, fascia lata, and Gore-Tex strips (W.L. Gore and Associates, Inc., Newark, DE) have all been used to provide good static suspension. The material of choice may be sutured to the malar periosteum or temporalis fascia and tunneled to the oral commissure and upper lip. Once again, overcorrection is necessary because relapse is common. These techniques may improve facial symmetry and oral competence but are not as aesthetically effective as some of the previously described techniques. Their attraction lies in their relatively simple nature and short procedure time, as compared with the other techniques.

Contouring and tightening of the facial skin with a modified mini-facelift, excision of redundant nasolabial folds, and placement of alloplastic implants to lift sagging tissues can all be used to improve the aesthetic appearance. Upper-lid blepharoplasty and browlift, although often considered cosmetic, may improve the function of a lid load by reducing the resistance to closure and improving the visual field deficit from brow ptosis and dermatochalasia.

■ Practice Guidelines, Consensus Statements, and Measures

Grogan PM, Gronseth GS. Practice parameter: steroids, acyclovir, and surgery for Bell's palsy (an evidence-based review): report of the Quality Standards Subcommittee of the American Academy of Neurology. Neurology 2001;56(7):830–836

■ Suggested Reading

Azuma T, Nakamura K, Takahashi M, et al. Mirror biofeedback rehabilitation after administration of single-dose botulinum toxin for treatment of facial synkinesis. Otolaryngol Head Neck Surg 2012;146(1):40–45

Boahene KD, Farrag TY, Ishii L, Byrne PJ. Minimally invasive temporalis tendon transposition. Arch Facial Plast Surg 2011;13(1): 8–13

Coulson SE, Croxson GR, Adams RD, O'Dwyer NJ. Reliability of the "Sydney," "Sunnybrook," and "House Brackmann" facial grading systems to assess voluntary movement and synkinesis after facial nerve paralysis. Otolaryngol Head Neck Surg 2005;132(4):543–549

Gidley PW, Herrera SJ, Hanasono MM, et al. The impact of radiotherapy on facial nerve repair. Laryngoscope 2010;120(10): 1985–1989

Ishii L, Godoy A, Encarnacion CO, Byrne PJ, Boahene KDO, Ishii M. Not just another face in the crowd: society's perceptions of facial paralysis. Laryngoscope 2012;122(3):533–538

Ishii LE, Godoy A, Encarnacion CO, Byrne PJ, Boahene KDO, Ishii M. What faces reveal: impaired affect display in facial paralysis. Laryngoscope 2011;121(6):1138–1143

May M, Schaitkin B, eds. Facial Paralysis: Rehabilitation Techniques. New York, NY: Thieme; 2002

Ross B, Nedzelski JM, McLean JA. Efficacy of feedback training in long-standing facial nerve paresis. Laryngoscope 1991;101(7 Pt 1): 744–750

Seiff SR, Chang J. Management of ophthalmic complications of facial nerve palsy. Otolaryngol Clin North Am 1992;25(3):669–690

Shindo ML, Ed. Rehabilitation of facial paralysis. Facial Plast Surg Clin North Am 1997;5(3)

Shipchandler TZ, Seth R, Alam DS. Split hypoglossal-facial nerve neurorrhaphy for treatment of the paralyzed face. Am J Otolaryngol 2011;32(6):511–516

Sidle DM, Fishman AJ. Modification of the orthodromic temporalis tendon transfer technique for reanimation of the paralyzed face. Otolaryngol Head Neck Surg 2011;145(1):18–23

Sunderland S. Factors influencing the course of regeneration and the quality of the recovery after nerve suture. Brain 1952; 75(1):19–54

Sunderland S. Nerve Injuries and Their Repair. New York, NY: Churchill Livingstone; 1991:82–83

Terzis JK, Anesti K. Developmental facial paralysis: a review. J Plast Reconstr Aesthet Surg 2011;64(10):1318–1333

Terzis JK, Anesti K. Experience with developmental facial paralysis, II: Outcomes of reconstruction. Plast Reconstr Surg 2012; 129(1):66e–80e

100 Orthognathic Surgery

Introduction

Successful treatment of patients with dentofacial deformities is a complex process that involves careful analysis of the patient's occlusion, facial skeleton, and associated soft tissues. The decision to treat a given dentofacial deformity with orthodontics only, or with combined orthodontics and orthognathic surgery, should be made prior to initiating therapy. Patient evaluation should include a team approach, involving a general dentist, an orthodontist, and an orthognathic surgeon. Patient expectations, treatment goals, and length of treatment time must be communicated before therapy is started. If properly planned and executed, surgical treatment of dentofacial deformities can dramatically improve functional occlusion and facial aesthetics.

Orthognathic Evaluation

To achieve balanced proportion of facial features, the facial plastic surgeon must have a concept of aesthetic ideals, a method to analyze deformities, and the ability to apply specific techniques to given deformities. Complete evaluation of facial deformities should include detailed dental, skeletal, and soft tissue analyses. Dental and skeletal analyses involve observation of the patient's occlusion and review of panographic and frontal and lateral cephalometric radiographs. Soft tissue analysis is performed by focused physical examination and confirmed by reproducible frontal and lateral photographs. After completing the evaluation, a detailed pretreatment database can be compiled, providing the basis for a specific plan of treatment of the dentofacial deformity.

Dental Analysis

Balanced proportion of facial features requires good dental occlusion. The Angle classification system defines normal and abnormal dental occlusion according to the relationship of the maxillary and mandibular first molar teeth. Each molar tooth has four grinding surfaces called cusps and adjacent surfaces called grooves, which are anatomically defined by the terms *lingual, buccal, mesial,* and *distal.* Surfaces adjacent to the tongue are called lingual, whereas those adjacent to the cheek are referred to as buccal. Dental surfaces located anteriorly, or toward the midline, are termed mesial, and those situated posteriorly, or away from the midline, are called distal.

The Angle classification uses the first molar teeth as a reference point and allows description of anterior-posterior and transverse molar relationships. In class I occlusion, the mesial buccal cusp of the first maxillary molar fits in the buccal groove of the first mandibular molar tooth. In class II malocclusion, the mesial buccal cusp of the first maxillary molar is anterior, or mesial, to the buccal groove of the mandibular first molar. Class III malocclusion describes a molar relationship, with the mesial buccal cusp of the first maxillary molar being posterior, or distal, to the buccal groove of the first mandibular molar tooth.

In addition to anterior-posterior malocclusions, abnormal molar relations can occur in a medial-to-lateral, or transverse, dimension. The ideal relationship occurs when the buccal cusps of the maxillary first molar teeth are just buccal to the corresponding mandibular buccal cusps. If the first maxillary buccal cusps are lingual to their mandibular counterparts, or if the first maxillary and mandibular molar cusps are end-to-end, a lingual crossbite is present. A buccal crossbite is defined when the maxillary first molar teeth are lateral or buccal to their ideal position.

The Angle classification system has some limitations. The most significant is that this system describes the relationship of only the maxillary and mandibular first molar teeth. It does not identify the relative positions of the remaining teeth. In many instances, a normal or class I molar relationship may be associated with a less-than-ideal relationship between the anterior maxillary and mandibular teeth.

Dental malocclusion may result from either dental or skeletal abnormalities or from a combination of both. The etiology of the malocclusion may be congenital or traumatic. Suboptimal occlusion may have both aesthetic and functional consequences, including temporomandibular joint (TMJ) dysfunction and difficulty in chewing and swallowing. It is important to determine whether the occlusal deformity will require orthodontics only, or whether optimal therapy will involve both orthodontics and orthognathic surgery.

Skeletal Analysis

Achieving balanced facial proportions requires accurate skeletal analysis. Evaluation should occur in all three planes of space, including the vertical (superoinferior), horizontal (anteroposterior), and transverse facial dimensions. To identify and quantitate facial skeletal deformities, skeletal reference points must be defined and measured. The cephalometric radiograph, first described in the 1930s, is a standardized radiograph taken with the head held in a fixed and reproducible position. The lateral cephalometric radiograph provides a two-dimensional outline of the craniofacial skeleton and soft tissue profile. Tracing this lateral radiograph allows identification of important bony and soft tissue landmarks.

Cephalometric analyses allow description of various abnormal relationships of the facial skeleton. Vertical maxillary discrepancies play a significant role in affecting the position of the lips and teeth. Vertical maxillary excess is characterized by a short upper lip and excessive maxillary incisor display rest. Vertical maxillary deficiency results in an apparent excess of upper lip length, with a lack of incisor display at rest.

Abnormal anterior-posterior relationships of the maxilla and mandible can also be diagnosed. A class II facial skeletal relationship may result either from maxillary prognathism or mandibular retrognathism, or from a combination of both. Retrognathism, or mandibular deficiency, describes a condition in which the mandible is small or retruded.

A class III facial skeletal relationship may occur either with maxillary retrusion or with mandibular prognathism, or with a combination of both conditions. It is important to determine the relative maxillary versus mandibular contribution to the skeletal abnormality. Transverse discrepancies of the upper and lower jaws also exist. The most common transverse abnormality is maxillary constriction. This condition is commonly seen in patients with congenital cleft deformities.

Soft Tissue Analysis

Although dental and skeletal analyses are important in evaluating the relationship of the teeth and facial skeleton, these methods alone are inadequate in evaluating and predicting facial form. Assessment of the soft tissues is important in preoperative facial analysis and in analyzing postoperative facial appearance.

Soft tissue analysis is the final determinant in evaluating the overall attractiveness of the face. Comparing a patient to an ideal standard can provide the basis for treatment objectives. A commonly used analysis of vertical facial heights allows the face to be divided into three relatively equal thirds (trichion–nasion, nasion–subnasale, and subnasale–menton). An increase in the ratio of the middle to lower thirds may indicate vertical maxillary excess, foreshortening of the lower third of the face, or a combination of these elements. A vertical height ratio of < 1 (between middle and lower facial thirds) signifies vertical maxillary deficiency or elongation of the chin.

To accurately correct dentofacial deformities, the facial plastic surgeon must understand the amount of soft tissue change produced by a given bony alteration. Soft tissue responses vary with different procedures and in different facial anatomical regions. It is the accurate prediction of soft tissue responses that dictates success in facial skeletal surgery.

■ Management

Philosophy and Timing

Orthognathic surgery is an involved and lengthy process that requires complex treatment planning. A detailed discussion with the patient, family, orthodontist, and orthognathic surgeon should include patient expectations, treatment goals, and possible limitations. Cosmetic as well as functional considerations should be discussed. Treatment requires a motivated patient, because complete treatment often requires 18 to 24 months.

Combined orthodontic–orthognathic surgery is usually not initiated until the upper and lower jaws are fully grown. Determination of full growth requires serial dental models and cephalometric radiographs. It is important that therapy not be initiated prior to complete mandibular development, to prevent postoperative relapse.

All routine dental care, including treatment of dental caries, periapical abscesses, or other periodontal disease, should be completed prior to beginning orthodontic therapy. Treatment of TMJ dysfunction should also be completed before initiating therapy. Pretreatment of these problems allows better evaluation of the patient's functional occlusion and facilitates accurate treatment planning. After completing a pretreatment evaluation and compiling a database, a detailed treatment plan is formulated.

Preoperative Orthodontic Treatment

In most dentofacial deformities complex enough to require surgery, preoperative orthodontic treatment is necessary to align the dental arches. Although the goal of orthodontic therapy is to alleviate dental malrotation and improve dental spacing, treatment with braces may "decompensate" the occlusion and worsen the horizontal occlusal discrepancy. For this reason, it is crucial that the orthodontist and orthognathic surgeon work closely in outlining the total treatment plan. Orthodonture usually requires 6 to 18 months in preparation for orthognathic surgery.

At the end of presurgical orthodontic treatment, plaster dental progress models are constructed. The models are placed on an articulator, and model surgery is performed. This will allow the surgeon to determine whether optimal preoperative occlusion has been obtained.

Surgical Procedures

After preoperative occlusal relationships are obtained, the plaster models are remounted, and an acrylic, interocclusal wafer splint is fashioned. This splint provides an intraoperative template, which will determine the exact horizontal and transverse movements of the maxilla and mandible. If two-jaw surgery is planned, two splints (intermediate and final) are made to determine each jaw's movement independently. If the preoperative plan requires parasagittal splitting of the maxilla (multiple-piece Le Fort osteotomy), an intraoperative splint is fabricated with full palatal coverage.

Mandibular Surgery

The vertical-subcondylar osteotomy may be performed intraorally or extraorally and is typically used for mandibular setback in patients with significant mandibular prognathism. The major advantage of the vertical-subcondylar osteotomy is avoiding injury to the inferior alveolar nerve. The external (cervical) approach has the disadvantage of an external scar and potential injury to the marginal mandibular branch of the facial nerve. However, because it allows good exposure, it is the preferred approach for mandibular setbacks ≥ 10 mm.

The sagittal-split ramus osteotomy is a versatile procedure for mandibular deformities because it can be used for both mandibular setback and advancement. The procedure is done intraorally with a horizontal osteotomy on the lingual surface (above the level of the inferior alveolar nerve). A vertical osteotomy is made through the lateral cortex in the region of the second molar tooth. The osteotomies are connected along the oblique line, with man-dibular split being accomplished with heavy chisels. After the contralateral osteotomy is performed, the mesial (tooth-bearing) mandibular segment may be retruded, advanced, or rotated.

Maxillary Surgery

The Le Fort I maxillary osteotomy is the most commonly used procedure to correct maxillary deformities and allows advancement in the anteroposterior direction, or shortening or lengthening in the vertical dimension. Impaction of the maxilla is often used to close an open-bite deformity (apertognathia), and involves removal of a predetermined amount of bone to shorten the maxilla. Vertical lengthening of the maxilla can also be achieved and requires interpositional bone grafting. Downgrafting of the maxilla is usually accomplished with autogenous iliac crest or calvarial bone, or with allogeneic preserved bone.

Transverse deformities of the maxilla can also be corrected with variations of the Le Fort I osteotomy. If narrowing (constriction) of the maxilla is present, surgical widening can be achieved with a midpalatal split. If the maxilla is excessively wide preoperatively, a multiple-piece osteotomy with removal of bone (ostectomy) can be performed to narrow the maxilla. Correction of maxillary deformities in all three planes of space is possible with appropriate preoperative planning.

The Le Fort I maxillary osteotomy is performed under general anesthesia administered via a nasotracheal tube. A sublabial incision and subperiosteal dissection provide access to the maxilla. Horizontal maxillary osteotomy is performed with a reciprocating saw above the level of the tooth roots. This osteotomy is joined to bilateral vertical osteotomies anterior to the pterygoid plates. The maxilla is then downfractured.

An interdental wafer splint is placed to establish the anterior-posterior and transverse positions of the maxillary dental arch. This splint is securely wired into position with maxillomandibular fixation (MMF). Four low-profile miniplates are used to rigidly fix the maxilla into its new position. If mandibular surgery is also planned, the MMF and wafer splint are removed prior to mandibular osteotomies and movement. A final splint is then used to establish the three-dimensional position of both dental arches.

Genioplasty

Horizontal mandibular sliding osteotomy is a versatile procedure that enables the surgeon to correct most chin deformities. It is performed intraorally and does not involve the tooth-bearing portion of the mandible. Correction of microgenia, macrogenia, and rotational transverse asymmetries of the chin is possible.

The sliding genioplasty is performed in a subperiosteal dissection plane through a lower gingivolabial incision. The mental nerves are identified and preserved. The skeletal midline of the chin is scored, and horizontal osteotomy is accomplished with a reciprocating saw. The distal segment of the chin is downfractured and moved, and the chin is then fixated with a rigid miniplate. If chin shortening is required, bony ostectomy is performed. If chin lengthening is required, interpositional bone grafting is performed.

Sliding genioplasty is more versatile than placement of an alloplast. Bony genioplasty allows for reduction of the chin as well as correction of chin asymmetries. Although horizontal osteotomy of the mandible presents a slight increased risk of damage to the mental nerves, it provides natural correction in patients with significant microgenia.

Fixation in Orthognathic Surgery

Fixation of the maxilla after Le Fort midfacial osteotomies is usually rigid with L-shaped miniplates. Mandibular fixation is more controversial. Although the trend in mandibular surgery is for rigid fixation with two to three positional screws placed through a transbuccal delivery system, many reports have suggested that condylar resorption and TMJ dysfunction may be associated with rigid fixation of the mandible in orthognathic surgery. If interosseous (inferior border) wire fixation is used for mandibular fixation, dental and skeletal fixation are usually also used for stability. Dental and skeletal fixation cause less resorption of the TMJ but require 6 to 8 weeks of intermaxillary fixation for stability.

■ Summary

The goal of orthognathic surgery is to establish a stable, functional occlusion and to balance facial aesthetics. To successfully treat dentofacial deformities, a systematic evaluation, including dental, skeletal, and soft tissue analysis, must be performed. A detailed treatment plan is then established. A close relationship with the treating orthodontist is important for planning and for postsurgical orthodontic finishing. If carefully planned and executed, treatment of dentofacial deformities often dramatically improves the form and function of the patient.

■ Suggested Reading

Angle EH. Classification of malocclusion. Dent Cosmos 1899; 41:248–264

Bell WH, Dann JJ. Correction of dentofacial deformities by surgery in the anterior part of the jaws. Am J Orthod 1973;64:162–187

Burstone CJ, James RB, Legan H, Murphy GA, Norton LA. Cephalometrics for orthognathic surgery. J Oral Surg 1978;36(4):269–277

Cangemi CF Jr. Administration of general anesthesia for outpatient orthognathic surgical procedures. J Oral Maxillofac Surg 2011; 69(3):798–807

Cascone P, Di Paolo C, Leonardi R, Pedullà E. Temporomandibular disorders and orthognathic surgery. J Craniofac Surg 2008; 19(3):687–692

Gonzáles-Ulloa M, Stevens E. The role of chin correction in profileplasty. Plast Reconstr Surg 1968;41(5):477–486

Joss CU, Joss-Vassalli IM, Kiliaridis S, Kuijpers-Jagtman AM. Soft tissue profile changes after bilateral sagittal split osteotomy for mandibular advancement: a systematic review. J Oral Maxillofac Surg 2010;68(6):1260–1269

Lehman JA Jr. Soft-tissue manifestations of aesthetic defects of the jaws: diagnosis and treatment. Clin Plast Surg 1987;14(4): 767–783

Ricketts RM. Divine proportion in facial esthetics. Clin Plast Surg 1982;9(4):401–422

Sabri R. Orthodontic objectives in orthognathic surgery: state of the art today. World J Orthod 2006;7(2):177–191

Steel BJ, Cope MR. Unusual and rare complications of orthognathic surgery: a literature review. J Oral Maxillofac Surg 2012; 70(7):1678–1691

Sykes JM, Donald PJ. Orthognathic surgery. Fac Plast Reconstruct Surg 1992;27:233–248

Sykes JM, Rotas N. Orthognathic surgery in the cleft lip and palate patient, surgery of cleft lip and palate deformities. Facial Plast Clin North Am 1996;4:361–375

Trauner R, Obwegeser HL. The surgical correction of mandibular prognathism and retrognathia with consideration of genioplasty, II. Operating methods for microgenia and distoclusion. Oral Surg Oral Med Oral Pathol 1957;10(8):787–792

West RA. Vertical maxillary dysplasia: diagnosis, treatment planning, and treatment response. Atlas Oral Maxillofac Surg Clin North Am 1990;2:11

Worms FW, Isaacson RJ, Speidel TM. Surgical orthodontic treatment planning: profile analysis and mandibular surgery. Angle Orthod 1976;46(1):1–25

Zenga J, Nussenbaum B. Adjunctive use of medical modeling for head and neck reconstruction. Curr Opin Otolaryngol Head Neck Surg 2013;21(4):335–343

101 Local Flaps for Head and Neck Reconstruction

■ Introduction

The face can be divided into the following aesthetic facial units: forehead, cheeks, eyelids, nose, lips, and auricles. The scalp may also be included as a separate aesthetic unit. Techniques for local flaps vary according to the aesthetic unit.

■ Management

Classification of Local Flaps

Local cutaneous flaps use tissue immediately adjacent to or near the location of the defect. Flaps may be classified by the arrangement of their blood supply (e.g., random vs. arterial), by configuration (e.g., rhomboid, bilobe), by location (e.g., local, regional, distant), and by the method of transferring the flap (e.g., pivotal, advancement, and hinged; **Table 101.1**). Most local flaps are moved through a combination of pivoting and advancement. For example, most pivotal flaps use the intrinsic elasticity of the flap through stretching or advancement (i.e., "advancement rotation flap"). For classification purposes, however, the major mechanism of tissue transfer should dictate the description of a particular flap unless both mechanisms are of approximately equal importance, in which case the terms describing both mechanisms should be used.

Pivotal Flaps

The three types of pivotal flaps are rotation, transposition, and interpolation. All pivotal flaps are moved toward the defect by rotating the base of the flap around a pivotal point. Except with island axial flaps, which have been skeletonized to the level of the nutrient vessels, the greater the degree of pivot, the shorter is the effective length of the flap. This is because the pivotal point is fixed in position, and the

Table 101.1 Local flaps classified by tissue movement

Pivotal flaps
Rotation
Transposition
Interpolation
Advancement flaps
Single pedicle
Bipedicle
V-Y
Y-V
Hinged flap

base of the flap is restricted in pivoting around this point. The redundant tissue at the base is known as a standing cutaneous deformity (dog-ear flap). Pivotal flaps must be designed to account for this reduction in effective length as they move through the pivotal arch. The effective length of a pivotal flap moving through an arc of 180 degrees is reduced by 40%.

Rotation Flaps

Rotation flaps are pivotal flaps that have a curvilinear configuration. They are designed immediately adjacent to the defect and are best used to close triangular defects. The triangular defect uses a portion of the standing cutaneous deformity, thus facilitating the pivotal movement of the flap. Rotation flaps are usually random in their vascularity, but they may be axial, depending on the position of the base of the flap. Because a rotation flap has a broad base, its vascularity tends to be reliable. When possible, the flap should be designed so that it is inferiorly based, which promotes lymphatic drainage and reduces flap edema. Rotation flaps are useful in repairing medial cheek defects located near the alar facial sulcus or nasal sidewall. The curvilinear border of the flap can often be positioned along the infraorbital rim, which represents an important border of aesthetic units (eyelid and cheek). Positioning the incision for the flap along this border enhances scar camouflage.

Large rotation flaps are particularly useful for reconstruction of sizable posterior cheek and upper neck defects. Large medial, inferiorly based rotation flaps are a flexible means of transferring large amounts of tissue from the remaining cheek and upper cervical regions. Chin reconstruction can be readily accomplished with rotation flaps, using two flaps to optimize the use of the aesthetic border of the submental crease to camouflage incisions. Because pivotal flaps in general, and rotation flaps specifically, do not depend on tissue elasticity for movement, rotation flaps are particularly useful for scalp defects due to the inelasticity of scalp tissue. The curvilinear configuration of rotation flaps adapts well to the spherical cranium. A rotation scalp flap must be quite large relative to the size of the defect, with the length of the perimeter (arch) of the flap being at least four times the width of the defect.

Disadvantages of rotation flaps are relatively few. The defect itself must be somewhat triangular or must be modified by removing additional tissue to create a triangular defect. As with all pivotal flaps, rotation flaps develop standing cutaneous deformities at their base that may not be easily removed without compromising the vascularity of the flap. Thus a second-stage removal of the deformity is necessary.

Transposition Flaps

In contrast to rotation flaps, which have a curvilinear configuration, transposition flaps have a straight linear axis. Both are pivotal flaps moving around a pivotal point, and their effective length decreases as they pivot. Like rotation flaps, a transposition flap can be designed so that a border of the flap is also a border of the defect. However, it may also be designed with borders that are removed from the defect, with only the base of the flap contiguous with the defect.

The ability to construct a flap at some distance from the defect with an axis that is independent of the linear axis of the defect is one of the great advantages of transposition flaps. This allows the surgeon to recruit skin at variable distances from the defect, selecting areas of greater skin elasticity or redundancy. In addition, the ability to select variable sites for harvesting a flap ensures that the donor site scar can be optimally camouflaged.

Transposition is the most common method of moving local flaps into skin defects of the head and neck. Transposition flaps, elevated in a multitude of sizes, shapes, and orientations, are usually random cutaneous flaps but may occasionally be axial or compound. A transposition flap is a reconstructive option for small to medium-sized defects in almost any conceivable configuration or location, thus making it the most useful of local flaps in head and neck reconstruction.

Although it is recommended that the length of random cutaneous transposition flaps should not exceed three times their width, this is not very applicable to such flaps designed on the face and scalp. The abundant vascularity of the skin of the face and scalp often enables the development of flaps that exceed the 3:1 ratio. More important than this ratio is the location and specific orientation of the transposition flap. An example is the inferiorly or superiorly based melolabial (nasolabial) transposition flap, because its linear axis is directly above and parallel to the linear axis of the angular artery. Although the flap is rarely elevated as a true axial flap incorporating the angular artery, many small peripheral branches of the artery are included in the base of the flap, accounting for its dependability.

Rhombic Flaps

Rhombic flaps are a type of transposition-advancement flap. This flap is useful when the defect has a shape of a rhombus with angles approximating 120 degrees and 60 degrees. Success of the flap depends on adjacent areas of redundant skin. These areas should lie adjacent to the 120-degree angle of the rhombus. The flap is designed by making an extension line of the diagonal of the rhombus straight out from the point of the 120-degree angle of the rhombus. The length of this line should equal the length of the side of the rhombus. At the end of this line, a second line is extended parallel to the side of the defect and is of the same length. The flap is dissected in the subcutaneous plane and requires wide undermining of the entire area of the flap and defect. The flap is transposed and sutured into position. The donor site is closed primarily and represents the area of greatest wound closure tension. Usually a standing cutaneous deformity must be excised to complete the repair.

Bilobe Flaps

A bilobe flap represents a double transposition flap that has a single pivotal point; it is useful in repairing many types of defects. The two lobes recruit redundant tissue from independent locations to assist in wound repair. The axes of the two lobes are dependent on where this resource of tissue is located and, accordingly, may be separated by a few degrees up to 180 degrees. The greater the separation, the greater the standing cutaneous deformity between the two lobes. Smaller bilobe flaps are very useful for repair of nasal tip and supratip defects and can find uses in many other locations. Large bilobe flaps are useful for repair of central and lateral cheek defects recruiting tissue from the remaining preauricular and infra-auricular areas.

Depending on the location of the defect, the first lobe is designed the same size as the defect if no secondary movement is desired. It may be made progressively smaller than the defect according to the degree of secondary tissue movement possible or desirable. Likewise, the second lobe, which is used to repair the donor site of the first lobe, is usually constructed smaller than the first lobe to the degree that secondary tissue movement will allow wound repair.

The major advantage of a bilobe flap in general is the ability to recruit redundant tissue from two independent areas to assist in the repair of the defect. The major disadvantage of the flap is the extensive undermining that is required and the double-standing cutaneous deformity that develops from use of a double transposition flap. Much of the incision lines required to harvest the flap do not fall in the relaxed skin tension lines; thus scars may be less favorable. Bilobe flaps for repair of cheek defects should be based inferiorly, and the standing cutaneous deformities should be excised in such a way that the resulting scars are parallel to, or lie within, natural skin creases.

Interpolation Flaps

The interpolation flap is a pivotal flap that, like transposition flaps, has a linear configuration. However, it differs from transposition flaps in that its base is located at some distance from the defect. Thus the pedicle must pass over or under intervening tissue. If the pedicle passes over intervening tissue, the flap must subsequently be detached in a second surgical procedure. This is perhaps the greatest disadvantage of such flaps. On occasion, the pedicle can be deepithelialized or reduced to subcutaneous tissue only and can be brought under the intervening skin to allow a single-stage reconstruction.

A common interpolation flap is the vertically oriented midforehead flap, which includes the median and paramedian flap. These flaps are highly effective in reconstruction of the midface because of their excellent vascularity and their superb skin color and texture match with the skin of the nose. Their high success rate, reliability, and popularity are primarily the result of the dependable axial blood supply (i.e., the supratrochlear artery and its anastomoses to surrounding vessels). Modern use of the midforehead flap has been expanded beyond nasal reconstruction to include any soft tissue defect of the midface that the flap can be designed to reach (e.g., the medial canthal region, upper and lower eyelids, medial cheek, melolabial region, and upper lip). These flaps may also be used in combination with other flaps for reconstruction of complex facial defects (e.g., a midforehead flap can be combined with a scalping flap for total nasal reconstruction).

Advancement Flaps

Advancement flaps have a linear configuration and are moved into a defect by stretching. They depend on the elasticity of the tissues of the flap (primary movement) and tissue adjacent to the defect (secondary movement) to achieve wound closure. Tissue transfer is achieved by moving the flap and its pedicle in a single vector. Advancement flaps can be categorized as bipedicle, single-pedicle, V-Y, and Y-V flaps.

Bipedicle Advancement Flaps

Bipedicle advancement flaps are used primarily for repair of large defects of the scalp. The flap is designed adjacent to the defect and advanced at right angles to the linear axis of the flap. This leaves a secondary defect, which must be repaired with a split-thickness skin graft. As a consequence, bipedicle flaps are rarely used for reconstruction of the face and neck.

Single-Pedicle Advancement Flaps

A single-pedicle advancement flap is created by parallel incisions that allow a sliding movement of the tissue in a single vector into the defect. The flap must be developed adjacent to the defect, and one border of the defect becomes a border of the flap. Repair with an advancement flap involves both primary and secondary tissue movement. In primary movement, the incised flap is pushed or is pulled forward by stretching the skin. Secondary movement of surrounding skin and soft tissue immediately adjacent to the defect occurs in a direction opposite the direction of movement of the advancing edge of the flap. This secondary movement, while providing less wound closure tension, may be detrimental by displacing free margins of facial structures. Complete undermining of the advancement flap, as well as skin and soft tissue around the pedicle, is important to enhance tissue movement.

Standing cutaneous deformities are created with all single-pedicle advancement flaps and may require excision. The two deformities that develop may be excised anywhere along the length of the flap and not necessarily near the base. The optimal site for excision of the standing cutaneous deformities is dependent on placing the incisions in relaxed skin tension lines or along aesthetic borders. Bilateral Z-plasties performed at the base of the flap often eliminate or reduce the need for excision of standing cutaneous deformities. Occasionally, if the flap is sufficiently long, standing cutaneous deformities can be subdivided into multiple smaller puckers of tissue that need not be excised, but can merely be "sewn out" by sequentially suturing the flap lengths in half.

In certain locations on the face, single-pedicle advancement flaps work particularly well: the forehead (particularly in the vicinity of the eyebrow), helical rim, upper and lower lips, and medial cheek. Bilateral advancement flaps are commonly combined to close various defects. The two flaps harvested from either side of the defect do not necessarily have to be of the same length. The length of each flap is determined primarily by the elasticity and redundancy of the donor resource.

A special type of single-pedicle advancement flap is the island advancement flap. A segment of skin is isolated as an island disconnected from the peripheral epidermal and dermal attachments. The only connection with the face that is left intact is the underlying subcutaneous tissue. Although all local flaps can theoretically be based on only a subcutaneous pedicle, single-pedicle advancement flaps most often use this method of design. The geometric shape of the cutaneous island may vary but is usually triangular. As the flap advances toward the recipient site, the donor area is closed in a simple V-Y manner. This flap is particularly useful in repair of medium-sized defects of the medial cheek near the alar base.

V-Y Advancement Flaps

The V-Y advancement flap is unique in that the v-shaped flap achieves its advancement by recoil or by being pushed, rather than being pulled or "stretched," toward the recipient site. Thus the flap is allowed to move into the recipient site without any wound closure tension. The secondary triangular donor defect is then repaired by advancing the two edges of the remaining donor site wound toward each other. In so doing, the wound closure suture line assumes a y configuration, with the common limb of the y representing the suture line resulting from closure of the secondary defect.

V-Y advancement is useful when a structure or region requires lengthening or release from a contracted state. The technique is particularly effective in lengthening the columella in the repair of cleft-lip nasal deformities in which a portion or all of the columella is underdeveloped. A V-Y advancement flap is elevated, recruiting skin from the midportion of the lip between the philtral ridges. The length of the columella is augmented by advancing the flap upward into the base of the columella. The secondary donor defect is approximated by advancing the remaining lip skin together in the midline.

V-Y advancement is also helpful in releasing contracted scars that are distorting adjacent structures, such as the eyelid or vermilion. An example is the correction of an ectropion of the vermilion caused by scarring. The segment of distorted vermilion is incor-

porated into the v-shaped flap and advanced toward the lip to restore the natural topography of the vermilion–cutaneous junction. The skin edges on both sides of the secondary defect are then advanced toward each other and sutured. The suture line becomes the vertical or common limb of the y configuration.

Y-V Advancement Flaps

In contrast to the V-Y design, where the v-shaped flap is allowed to recoil or is pushed toward the area for supplementation, in the Y-V design, the flap is pulled or stretched toward the area for supplementation. The Y-V flap augments the surface area of the recipient site but is also responsible for repairing the donor site, whereas in the V-Y design, the donor site for the flap is closed by movement of adjacent skin. Y-V advancement flaps are indicated in circumstances where the surgeon intends to reduce the length or redundancy of an area by moving tissue away from the site. On occasion, it may also be useful in relocating a free margin of a facial structure to improve symmetry with its counterpart.

Hinge Flap

Cutaneous hinge flaps, sometimes referred to as trap-door, turn-in, or turn-down flaps, have a unique method of tissue movement. Hinge flaps may be designed in a linear or curvilinear shape, with the pedicle based on one border of the defect. The flap is dissected in the subcutaneous plane and turned over onto the defect (like a page in a book). The epithelial surface of the flap is turned downward to provide internal lining for a facial defect that requires both external and internal lining surfaces. The exposed subcutaneous surface of the hinge flap is covered by a second flap. Thus hinge flaps are always used in conjunction with another flap or graft that provides the external coverage of the defect.

The vascular supply for hinge flaps is derived from the soft tissue border of the defect that it is designed to repair; as a consequence, such flaps have limited and often restricted vascularity. Survival of hinge flaps can be improved if they are used in situations where the wound margin of the defect is well healed, rather than freshly created. Because the pedicle of the hinge flap is along a border of the defect, the flap should be elevated in such a way that as flap dissection proceeds toward the base of the flap, the plane of dissection becomes deeper; thus the base is thicker than the distal portion of the flap. This technique enhances the vascularity of the flap by increasing the likelihood of including within the pedicle a greater number of nutrient vessels.

Hinge flaps are commonly used for repair of full-thickness nasal defects in which there is sufficient remaining adjacent nasal skin to develop a hinge flap for internal nasal lining. Hinge flaps may also be used to close mature sinofacial and salivary fistulas anywhere in the upper aerodigestive tract. Hinge flaps consisting of subcutaneous tissue, and sometimes muscle without overlying skin, can be used to fill in contour deficits.

Local Flaps for Reconstruction by Anatomical Area

Local Flaps for Repair of the Nose

Skin cancer occurs most frequently on the nose. As a consequence, reconstructive surgeons must be familiar with several methods for repairing nasal defects using local flaps. Over the last decade, reconstructive rhinoplasty has been advanced to a higher level by emphasizing certain concepts, such as the importance of replacing deficient nasal tissue with like tissue. For example, defects of the internal nasal lining are replaced with hinged or bipedicle advancement mucosal flaps harvested from the remaining nasal interior. Missing cartilage or fibrofatty tissue giving contour to the nose is replaced with septal or conchal cartilage, positioned and sculpted to replicate as closely as possible the missing skeletal support. Great emphasis must be placed on thinning and contouring the cartilage grafts, so that they replicate the exact topography of the contralateral cartilage, if present, or the form one might expect in an ideally shaped nose.

Another important modern concept is the isolation of a nasal defect as a separate entity from any extension of the defect onto the cheek or lip, repairing the portion of the defect of each aesthetic unit with independent flaps. This maintains scars in borders between major aesthetic units and prevents distortion or obliteration of these borders while maximizing scar camouflage. Parallel to this concept is division of the nasal aesthetic unit into smaller topographic regions or subunits, which include the dorsum, nasal sidewalls, ala, tip, and columella. Each of these distinct regions is separated from adjacent regions by convexities or concavities, which cast shadows that serve to better camouflage scars. When a surface defect involves > 50% of the surface area of a given subunit, resurfacing the entire subunit with a flap usually provides a better aesthetic result by hiding scars in these shadows.

Smaller defects of the nasal dorsum, tip, and supratip can be repaired with a wide variety of local flaps. For very small defects, primary closure may be possible without distorting surrounding landmarks, but commonly a flap will provide optimal reconstruction. For small defects in the lateral supra-alar groove and above, the "note" type of advancement flap can be very useful. This flap is designed by making a vertical incision from one margin of the defect along the nasal sidewall and undermining the lateral nasal sidewall skin, which is then advanced inferiorly to fill the defect. This flap is most useful in patients with a fair amount of skin laxity and defects < 1 cm.

Somewhat larger defects of the tip and medial supratip region are most often repaired using the Zitelli modification of the bilobed flap. Although this flap is most commonly based inferiorly over the supra-alar groove, it can be based superiorly. The dorsal aesthetic unit flap may be used for larger defects of the supratip and lateral supra-alar region up to 2 cm. This flap is a rotation flap based on branches from the angular artery and is very hardy. The flap is a modification of the miter or Rieger type of glabellar flap, with the difference being that all of the incisions are confined to the nasal dorsum to avoid the glabellar scar. It takes advantage of the lax skin of the nasofrontal recess and lower glabella. The incisions curve along the lateral nasal sidewall, crossing the radix onto the opposite side, leaving a skin and subcutaneous pedicle of ~ 2 cm. Extensive undermining in the preperiosteal plane is possible and can lead to significant flap mobility. Care should be taken not to damage the vascular pedicle as dissection is carried down along the nasal sidewall beneath the pedicle.

The nasal ala is a common site of nasal defects resulting from removal of skin cancers. If not repaired properly, distortion of the alar margin and partial collapse of the external nasal valve occur, with compromise of the airway. Often the alar facial sulcus and nasal alar crease are violated by transposition flaps harvested from the medial cheek to repair alar defects. When this occurs, a completely natural appearing border between the cheek and the ala and nasal sidewall is extremely difficult to restore. For this reason, the use of interpolation flaps from the cheek—the pedicle of which crosses over but not through the alar facial sulcus—is recommended for resurfacing the ala. The pedicle may consist of skin or subcutaneous tissue only and is detached from the cheek 3 weeks following the initial transfer. Although 3 weeks is a long time for a patient to endure the deformity caused by the flap, this interval allows the surgeon to aggressively defat and sculpt the distal flap both at the time of flap transfer, and again at the time of pedicle detachment and flap inset. Upon detachment of the flap, the patient has a completely natural appearing alar facial sulcus and nasal alar crease (provided the defect does not extend into the crease) because no incisions or dissections have been made in these regions. Usually resurfacing of the entire ala is preferred, removing any remaining skin.

Full-thickness defects are reconstructed by restoring the internal nasal lining deficit with a vascularized vestibular skin or mucosal flap. Full-thickness defects of the ala with a vertical height ≤ 1.5 cm can use a bipedicle skin flap for internal lining. The flap is created by making an extended intercartilaginous incision from the nasal dome to the lateral floor of the vestibule. The vestibular skin is mobilized inferiorly, and the inferior edge is sutured to the inferior border of the nasal vestibular skin defect. If the vestibular skin defect extends to the alar rim, then the inferior aspect of the flap is sutured to the edge of the cutaneous flap used to provide external coverage of the defect. The flap is attached to the overlying cartilage grafts used to provide structural support by horizontal mattress sutures placed through the cartilage and bipedicle flap. The donor site for the flap is repaired with a thin full-thickness skin graft harvested from the standing cutaneous deformity removed from closing the donor site of the interpolated cheek flap.

Following reconstruction of the internal nasal lining defect with a bipedicle vestibular skin mucosal flap, the next step is to completely replace all missing nasal cartilage with free cartilage grafts harvested from the nasal septum or, preferably, from the auricle. If the inferior edge of the lateral crura has been removed, the missing cartilage must be replaced with a free cartilage graft, and additional grafts should be placed along the alar margin inferior to the position of the original lateral crus. This prevents notching and/or upward contraction of the alar rim. Likewise, when the fibrofatty tissue of the lateral portion of the ala is missing, it should also be replaced with free cartilage grafts, because this tissue, although not rigid, provides structural support and contour to the ala. If the surgeon depends strictly on a skin flap to replace the fibrofatty tissue in the ala, less structural support is provided, and scar contracture causes an unnatural appearance to the restoration, usually with some notching of the alar rim and partial collapse of the external nasal valve.

Once the structural support to the ala has been secured, a cheek flap is planned to resurface the ala and cover the restored skeletal support. A template is fashioned to exactly represent the size and shape of the surface defect. This template is then used to design a superiorly based melolabial interpolation flap. The flap should be designed so that the medial border falls in the melolabial sulcus. The flap is elevated in a subcutaneous plane and may be lifted on a skin and subcutaneous fat pedicle or based on a subcutaneous pedicle only.

The flap donor site is closed primarily by undermining the skin of the cheek. The standing cutaneous deformity that occurs with advancement of the cheek skin medially is excised, and a portion of this is used as a full-thickness skin graft to cover the donor site of the intranasal bipedicle vestibular skin flap, when used. The interpolation flap is transposed over the alar facial sulcus, and the distal portion of the flap is thinned appropriately so that the flap will drape over the cartilage grafts in a manner that will replicate the contour of the ala and alar nasal crease. This may require thinning of the flap to the level of the dermis in the area along the alar rim to restore the delicate topography of the rim. In instances where the defect involves the alar rim and internal nasal vestibular skin, the inferior border of the flap is sutured to the inferior border of the bipedicle skin flap developed to replace the missing internal nasal lining. The proximal portion of the interpolation flap is left with an ample amount of subcutaneous tissue to enhance flap vascularity. At the time of pedicle detachment, the proximal portion of the flap to be inset is defatted and contoured.

The main advantage of the melolabial interpolation flap is that it does not violate the aesthetically important alar facial sulcus. It also minimizes distortion of the melolabial fold because the majority of skin removed from the cheek is skin located at the inferior aspect of the fold where there is greater skin redundancy. When using a subcutaneous pedicle, only a small amount of skin from the upper melolabial fold is discarded as a result of a small standing cutaneous deformity that forms in that area during closure of the donor site.

When nasal defects extend into the alar facial sulcus, the task of restoring this area of complex topography to its natural appearance, identically symmetrical to its counterpart, is a particularly difficult challenge. When one is confronted with this problem, it is often preferable to reconstruct the medial cheek and alar facial sulcus component of the defect with an advancement cheek flap and to reconstruct the ala with either a separate cheek or a forehead interpolation flap. This allows separate flaps to reconstruct the independent aesthetic units of the nose and cheek and places the junction of the borders of the two flaps along the restored alar facial sulcus. When such defects are reconstructed with a single transposition cheek flap, partial or complete obliteration of the alar facial sulcus will occur, and it must be restored through additional operations. This usually involves multiple surgical procedures and only limited success.

Surface defects ≥ 2 cm on the nasal tip, columella, sidewalls, and dorsum are best repaired with paramedian forehead flaps, although partial loss of the columella may be repaired with a single or bilateral superiorly based melolabial interpolation flap. If the defect involves > 50% of the surface area of the aesthetic subunit, then the remaining skin is removed and the entire subunit of the nose is resurfaced. Similar to the principles of reconstructing the ala, all missing cartilage must be completely replaced. Auricular cartilage is most useful for replacing upper and lower lateral cartilage.

Full-thickness defects of the nasal tip require either single or bilateral hinge septal mucosal flaps for repair of the internal lining. The entire mucosal lining of the nasal septum can be mobilized as a hinge flap based anteriorly on the caudal septum and nourished by the septal branch of the labial artery. The hinge flap is turned laterally across the nasal passage to provide lining to the lateral nasal wall.

When greater lining deficits are present, such as the entire length of the sidewall, a second mucosal hinge flap from the contralateral side is developed by removing intervening septal cartilage and swinging the flap across to the defect. In contrast to the ipsilateral flap, the contralateral flap is hinged on the dorsal septum and is nourished by the anterior ethmoid artery. Thus the lining for a heminasal defect is supplied inferiorly by an ipsilateral hinge septal mucosal flap based on the superior labial artery and superiorly by a contralateral septal mucosal hinge flap based on the anterior ethmoid artery. A permanent septal fistula remains. Although crusting may occur for several months, the large septal fistula is rarely symptomatic.

The ipsilateral mucosal flap crosses the nasal passage in a way that blocks the airway, and thus must be detached from the caudal septum to restore a patent nasal passage. The maneuver is accomplished using local anesthesia 3 weeks following initial transfer. The excellent vascular supply of these mucosal flaps provides a well-vascularized recipient site to support free cartilage grafts of all sizes. The grafts are sandwiched between the mucosal flap internally and the interpolated forehead or cheek flap externally and thus have a dual source of revascularization.

In repair of full-thickness central nasal defects of the tip or dorsum, a composite turnout flap consisting of septal cartilage with attached mucosa on either side is developed. Its base is centered in the region of the nasal spine and upper lip and contains both septal branches of the superior labial arteries. A flap of appropriate dimensions is outlined and incised with a right-angle knife or scissors. Such flaps may include bone and extend from the nasal floor inferiorly to the medial canthi cephalically and posteriorly, to include portions of the perpendicular plate. To allow rotation, the septal leaves are separated from the septal cartilage near the nasal spine, and a triangular piece of septal cartilage at the level of the inferior septal angle is removed. This maneuver permits the flap to turn up and out to reach the tip and dorsum. The flap is designed overly wide and long to create an excess of mucosa and cartilage. As the flap pivots into position, its distal end passes over the exposed remnant of the nasal bones or dorsal septum and locks into position. The extra lining is peeled downward as bilateral hinge flaps, which extend laterally to line the middle nasal vault and tip. Cartilage grafts are then placed on top of these flaps to restore missing dome cartilage in the case of central tip defects, or nasal bridge in the case of dorsal defects. A para-

median forehead flap provides the external surface cover to complete the reconstruction.

Paramedian forehead flaps are the preferred local flap for resurfacing most large cutaneous nasal defects. The flap may be dissected under local or general anesthesia. The base of the pedicle is placed in the glabellar region centered over the supratrochlear artery on the same side as the majority of the nasal defect. The origin of the supratrochlear artery is consistently found to be 1.7 to 2.2 cm lateral to the midline and usually corresponds to a vertical tangent of the medial aspect of the brow. The vessel exits the orbit by piercing the orbital septum and passing under the orbicularis oculi muscle and over the corrugator supercilii muscle. At the level of the eyebrow, the artery passes through the orbicularis and frontalis muscles and continues upward in a vertical direction in a subcutaneous plane. The pedicle of the flap may be as narrow as 1.2 cm. With a narrower pedicle, there is a greater effective length to the flap and less standing cutaneous deformity as the flap pivots. An exact template of the defect is used to design the paramedian forehead flap, which is centered over the vertical axis of a single supratrochlear artery. The length of the flap is determined by measurement. If adequate length necessitates extending the flap into hair-bearing scalp, the flap may be angled horizontally along the hairline to prevent transfer of hair-bearing skin to the nose. The flap is elevated in a subfascial plane just superficial to the periosteum of the frontal bone.

To avoid injury to the arterial pedicle, blunt dissection is used near the brow to separate the corrugator muscles from the flap and facilitate mobility. Incisions can be extended below the brow if necessary to enhance the length of the flap. Adequate flap mobilization usually requires complete sectioning of the corrugator supercilii muscle to achieve free movement of the flap. Prior to inset, the flap is sculpted and contoured to properly fill the depth of the defect by removal of all or some of the muscle and subcutaneous tissues from the distal portion of the flap. When necessary, all but 1 mm of fat beneath the dermis may be removed. It is sometimes even necessary to resect a portion of the dermis along the edge of the flap so that the thickness of the skin of the flap matches that of the adjacent nasal skin. Only the distal three-fourths of the flap required for reconstruction is sculpted; the proximal one-fourth is left thick and is debulked at the time of the pedicle detachment 3 weeks later.

Donor site closure is accomplished by undermining the forehead skin in the subfascial plane from the anterior border of one temporalis muscle to the other. Several parallel vertical fasciotomies 2 to 3 cm apart may be necessary to achieve primary closure of the wound. Any portion of the donor site that cannot be closed primarily should be left to heal by second intention, keeping the open wound moist at all times. Healing by second intention usually results in an acceptable scar but may take several weeks for complete healing.

Three weeks following the initial flap transfer, the pedicle is separated under local anesthesia. The skin superiorly surrounding the defect is undermined for ~ 1 cm. The portion of the skin flap to remain attached to the recipient site and not thinned at the time of initial flap transfer is now thinned appropriately. In the case of reconstruction of skin-only nasal defects that extend to the rhinion, the flap must be aggressively thinned to the level of the dermis to reduplicate the thin skin that is normally found in this area. Deep-layer closure is not necessary, because the wound should not be under any closure tension. The base of the pedicle is returned to the donor site in a way that creates the normal inter-eyebrow distance. Care should be taken to maintain the muscular component of the proximal pedicle that is returned so that a depression between the brows does not result. Any excess pedicle should be discarded, rather than returned to the forehead above the level of the brow.

Local Flaps for Repair of the Lip

The lips play a key role in deglutition, formation of speech, and facial expressions. Their reconstruction offers a unique challenge to the surgeon. Over the last several years, there has been an emphasis on reconstructing lip defects with flaps contained within the aesthetic units of the lip or even the aesthetic subunits, which, for the upper lip, are the filtrum and the lip lateral to the filtrum. This principle can be applied in repairing smaller-sized defects of the lip and obviates the need to borrow tissue from the cheek and thus distort the melolabial sulcus.

Surgical procedures for reconstructing the lip may be classified as follows:

- Those that use remaining lip tissue
- Those that borrow tissue from the opposite lip
- Those that use adjacent cheek tissue
- Those that use distant flaps

The first two categories enable the reconstruction to remain within the aesthetic units of the lips and, when possible, are the preferred method of surgical management. The algorithms displayed in **Figs. 101.1** and **101.2** provide a helpful approach to reconstructing the lip for defects that are full thickness or represent loss of skin and muscle. This approach categorizes the size of lip defects into those less than half of the width of the lip, defects between one-half and two-thirds of the lip, and defects greater than two-thirds of the entire lip width. Defects of less than half of the lip width can usually be managed by primary wound closure or smaller local flaps confined to an aesthetic subunit of the lip. In the lower lip, conversion of the defect into a w-shaped configuration may be preferred. In its simplest form, this configuration is usually adequate for primary closure, though modification to include lateral advancement flaps may be required when the defect base is broad. The w-shaped configuration maximizes conservation of tissue and prevents an unsightly pointed chin when it is necessary to extend the incision beyond the mental crease.

Primary closure should be in four layers: mucosa, muscle, deep dermal, and skin. Care is taken to perform a precise approximation of the "white line" at the vermilion border on either side of the defect. Primary wound closure of defects in the midline of the upper lip can be facilitated by excising a crescent of cheek skin in the perialar region. Perialar skin excision allows advancement of the remaining lip segments medially and lessens wound closure tension.

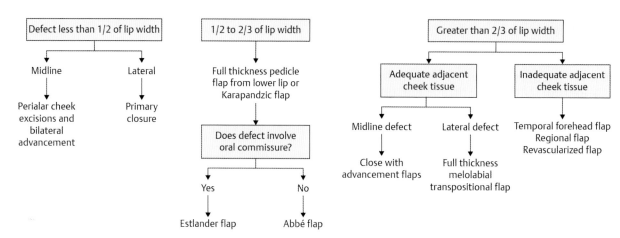

Fig. 101.1 Algorithm for upper lip reconstruction.

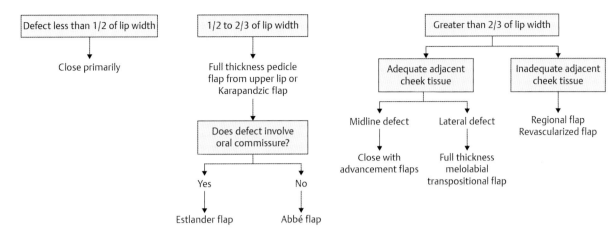

Fig. 101.2   Algorithm for lower lip reconstruction.

Reconstruction of defects of one-half to two-thirds of the width of the lip usually requires lip augmentation procedures. Closure can be most readily achieved by a full-thickness pedicle flap from the opposite lip (lip-switch flap) or from the adjacent cheek. The Karapandzic flap may also be effective in closing medium-sized defects of the lip and, in some instances, may provide better functional results than denervated flaps. This technique consists of circumoral incisions through the skin and subcutaneous tissue, encompassing the remaining portions of the upper and lower lips. The orbicularis oris is mobilized and remains pedicled bilaterally on the superior and inferior labial arteries. Adequate mobilization enables closure of the defect by rotating the bilateral musculocutaneous lip flaps into the defect. The advantage of Karapandzic flaps is that they restore a continuous circle of functioning orbicularis muscle, which maintains oral competence. However, because no new tissue is recruited to aid in the reconstruction of the lip, microstomia may be a problem. Patients in the sixth decade of life or older will often develop laxity of the oral stoma following a Karapandzic flap and will not require commissuroplasties to correct the microstomia.

Local flaps are preferable to regional flaps for closing defects of less than two-thirds of the lip width because of their close skin color and texture match and the availability of mucous membrane for lining. Defects located away from the commissure are best closed with an Abbé flap consisting of a full-thickness flap from the opposite lip pedicled on the vermilion border and containing the labial artery. The Estlander flap is a compound flap (skin, muscle, mucosa) like the éé flap and is designed similarly, but it is used for closure of lip defects near the commissure of the mouth. Since the original descriptions of the Abbé and Estlander flaps, the operations have been modified in many ways to accommodate surgical defects located anywhere in the upper or lower lip.

The Abbé and Estlander flaps should be constructed so that the height of the flap equals the height of the defect. The width of the flap should be approximately half that of the defect to be reconstructed. However, when the entire filtrum is missing, the width of this segment should be completely replaced with the Abbé flap. This will restore the total aesthetic subunit, which is preferable from the standpoint of cosmesis, as well as function. The pedicle should be made narrow to facilitate transposition and should be positioned near the center line of the recipient site. The secondary defect should be closed in four layers, with accurate approximation of the vermilion border.

The superiorly based Estlander flap is designed so that it lies medial to the melolabial sulcus. This provides better scar camouflage of the donor site and at the same time allows easy rotation of the flap into the lower-lip defect. Oral commissure distortion is caused by the Estlander flap. This distortion, and microstomia, may be corrected with a secondary commissuroplasty when desired.

The pedicle of the Abbé flap crosses the oral stoma and may be severed in 2 to 3 weeks. During the interval between transfer of the flap and division of the pedicle, the patient is maintained on a liquid or soft diet that does not require excessive chewing. It is essential that precise approximation of the vermilion border be ensured at the time of pedicle severance.

Defects greater than two-thirds of the width of the entire lip and some smaller lateral defects are best reconstructed by using adjacent cheek flaps in the form of advancement or transposition flaps. Massive or total lip defects are best reconstructed by using regional or distant flaps or vascularized microsurgical flaps. Large defects of the upper lip may be reconstructed by excising crescent-shaped perialar cheek tissue and advancing bilateral cheek flaps medially. If wound closure tension is excessive, an

Abbé flap harvested from the lower lip may be added in the midline.

Similarly, midline lower-lip defects may be closed by full-thickness advancement flaps. These techniques may require excision of additional triangles in the melolabial sulcus to allow advancement of the cheek flaps. Triangular excision should follow the lines of the sulcus and should include only skin and subcutaneous tissues. The underlying muscle is mobilized to form a new commissure. The mucous membrane is separated from the muscle and advanced outward to provide a vermilion border. Incisions are made in the gingival buccal sulcus as far posterior as the last molar tooth, if necessary, to allow proper approximation of the remaining lip segments without excessive wound closure tension.

Melolabial transposition flaps consisting of skin and subcutaneous tissue only or full-thickness advancement flaps consisting of skin, subcutaneous tissue, muscle, and mucosa can be useful in reconstructing lip defects as large as three-fourths of the width of the lip. Large skin-only defects of the lateral lip are repaired nicely with melolabial flaps. However, in keeping with the principles of maintaining borders between aesthetic units, it is usually preferable to repair defects that extend from the lip onto the cheek with two separate flaps. A large rotation flap from the opposite lip is used for repairing the defect of the lip, whereas the cheek component of the defect is repaired by a separate transposition or advancement cheek flap. This places nearly all the scars in the melolabial sulcus while maintaining the integrity of the border between the lip and cheek aesthetic units.

Adjacent cheek tissue may not be applicable or sufficient for reconstruction of near total defects of the lip. In such cases, regional flaps may be used for reconstruction. Excisions of the lower lip, chin, and anterior section of the mandible for carcinoma often require such flaps for reconstruction.

The temporal forehead flap, designed as a bipedicle advancement or unipedicle interpolation flap, may be used for total upper-lip reconstruction, but the unsightly secondary deformity precludes its common use. The flap may be lined with a split-thickness skin or mucosal graft. In males, hair-bearing scalp may be incorporated to provide hair growth for scar camouflage.

Local Flaps for Repair of the Cheek

Relative to the nose and lip, repair of cheek defects is less complex; they are usually best repaired with transposition or advancement flaps. Rhombic and other transposition flaps are very versatile and can be used anywhere in the cheek for small to medium-sized defects (< 6 cm in maximum dimension). Par-

ticular attention must be given to designing flaps for repair of defects near the lips or eyelids. For rhombic flaps, the orientation must be designed so that the area of greatest wound closure tension is away from these structures, so as not to cause distortion or ectropion. As previously mentioned, V-Y advancement flaps are very useful for medium-sized medial cheek defects, whereas larger medial and lateral cheek defects are more readily repaired using inferiorly based rotation or bilobed flaps that can recruit cervical or postauricular skin.

Rotation flaps are useful for repairing medial cheek defects located superiorly in the vicinity of the border between the nasal sidewall and the cheek. The curvilinear border of the flap can often be positioned along the infraorbital rim, which represents an important aesthetic boundary. By positioning the incision for the flap along this border, the surgeon can enhance scar camouflage. When possible, the margin of the rotation flap should extend above the level of the lateral canthus to assist in the prevention of lower lid retraction. It may also be helpful to suspend the flap to the periosteum of the lateral orbital rim.

Despite these precautions, lower lid retraction is not an uncommon sequela when a rotation flap is used to repair large medial cheek defects in elderly patients, who frequently have lax lower eyelids. Large rotation flaps are particularly useful for reconstruction of sizable defects of the posterior cheek and upper neck. Large medial inferiorly based rotation flaps provide a flexible means for transfer of large amounts of skin from the remaining cheek and upper cervical skin. Incisions for the flap are placed in a preauricular crease and along the anterior border of the trapezius muscle as far as the clavicle, or below to facilitate rotation of the upper cervical skin toward the posterior cheek area. To enhance vascularity to such flaps, it is advantageous to dissect the flap beneath the submuscular aponeurotic system (SMAS) in the cheek and beneath the platysmal muscle in the neck. A sub-SMAS dissection in the face allows the placement of a great deal of tension on the flap without compromise of the skin vascularity. Care must be taken, however, below the level of the mandible so as not to injure the mandible branch of the facial nerve.

Advancement flaps are dependent on the elasticity of the skin for successful repair and are used less frequently than pivotal flaps in the cheek. They have the disadvantage of being able to cover only relatively small defects and thus are best suited for use in older individuals with greater skin laxity. Advancement flaps should be designed so that the incisions fall into natural skin creases of the cheek. To follow this principle, incisions used to form the border of the flap usually must diverge slightly, rather than remain completely parallel. It is usually necessary to remove bilateral standing cutaneous deformities near the base of the flap. This should be accomplished in such a way that the resulting scar lies within relaxed skin tension lines. An alternative to this is performing bilateral Z-plasties at the base of the flap to reduce or eliminate the standing cutaneous deformities.

Advancement flaps work well for small to medium-sized central cheek defects (maximum dimension 6 cm). V-Y subcutaneous base advancement flaps are particularly useful flaps for repair of small and medium-sized skin defects of the medial cheek near the alar facial sulcus. This technique is indicated for younger patients who lack redundant facial skin and in patients who have considerable subcutaneous facial fat (chipmunk cheeks). The flap is designed in a triangular configuration, and the surface area of the flap should be 1.5 to 2 times the surface area of the defect. The skin of the flap is isolated on a subcutaneous pedicle by incisions around the perimeter of the flap. Incisions should be made through the fat down to the level of the facial musculature. This deep dissection provides the mobility of the flap, enabling it to be advanced 2 to 3 cm. This mobility is enhanced by undermining the proximal and distal one-fourth of the flap just deep to the skin. The peripheral margins of the donor and recipient sites should also be undermined for a distance of 2 cm in the subcutaneous plane to provide for secondary tissue movement and easy closure of the donor site. The flap is advanced and sutured in the recipient site first, followed by layered closure of the donor site.

The disadvantage of the V-Y subcutaneous advancement flap is that not all of the incisions used to harvest the flap fall in natural, relaxed skin tension lines. However, when appropriately selected, the flap has many advantages. A major advantage is the limited dissection, compared with other techniques required to close similar-sized wounds. Thus there is minimal dead space, with concomitant reduced risk of the development of hematomas and seromas. Another major advantage is that no standing cutaneous deformity develops so no tissue is discarded. The flap is harvested from the jowl area, where facial skin is most redundant. As a consequence, there is less deformity of the melolabial fold and sulcus than would be seen with a transposition flap.

Local Flaps for Repair of Forehead Defects

Reconstruction of forehead defects should have the following goals:

- Preservation of motor function of the frontalis muscle
- Preservation of sensation of the forehead skin
- Placement of scars in aesthetic borders or within the horizontal furrows of the forehead

The forehead aesthetic unit is defined by junctional, lines with the frontal scalp superiorly, which may or may not be bordered by hair, temporal scalp, and temple laterally, and with eyebrows and glabella inferiorly. The forehead can be divided into aesthetic subunits, which include median, paramedian, and lateral temporal areas. The median is the area 2 cm on either side of the midline of the forehead. The paramedian extends from the lateral border of the median unit to a line that is on a vertical axis with the pupil. The lateral temple unit extends from the paramedian border to a lateral line that is approximately horizontal with the superior palpebral crease. The aesthetic goals of repair of forehead defects include the following:

- Maintenance of brow symmetry
- Maintenance of natural-appearing temporal and frontal hairlines
- Concealment of scars, when possible, along hairlines or eyebrows
- Creation of transverse, instead of vertical, scars whenever possible (except in the midline forehead), and avoidance of diagonal scars

Primary wound repair of defects of forehead skin is often possible in older individuals and patients with solar-damaged skin. Deep horizontal furrows may provide extra skin for reconstruction. When primary closure is not possible, the use of single or multiple local flaps is preferred over skin grafts because of the poor aesthetic result with the use of skin grafts. For this reason, when a local flap is not possible, healing by second intention rather than the use of skin grafts is preferred because the resulting scar is often less deforming. For midline forehead defects, healing by second intention often produces a very acceptable aesthetic result, particularly when the defect is located in the superior aspect of the forehead. This is why donor sites for median and paramedian forehead flaps do not necessarily require complete wound closure.

In spite of a wound closure scar that is perpendicular to relaxed skin tension lines, defects of the central third of the forehead can be repaired in a vertically oriented axis with a predictably pleasant aesthetic result. This is probably due to the natural dehiscence or attenuation of the frontalis muscle in this portion of the forehead. Larger midline defects closed in a vertical orientation frequently result in large standing cutaneous deformities, which may be excised with use of a W-plasty inferiorly, if feasible, in the glabellar creases. An M-plasty superiorly may also be necessary at times to eliminate a standing cutaneous deformity at the hairline. M-plasty and W-plasty techniques reduce the overall vertical height of the wound closure scar. Primary wound closure usually requires extensive undermining in the subfascial plane to facilitate closure without compromise of motor or sensory function of the forehead.

Like the midline, defects of the paramedian zone of the forehead can be closed primarily with a vertical scar orientation and result in an acceptable result. However, wounds are best repaired with primary closure oriented in a horizontal axis or with flaps that have a horizontal orientation to facilitate scar camouflage. Vertical scars in the paramedian and lateral zones of the forehead may be quite noticeable because they are perpendicular to the horizontal furrows of the forehead, and their appearance is accentuated by movement of the frontalis muscle. Extrapolated to specific defects, this means vertically oriented primary repairs, rotation flaps, and transposition flaps are to be avoided. Median and paramedian forehead defects can frequently be reconstructed with unilateral or bilateral advancement flaps, keeping most of the resulting scars oriented horizontally.

The lateral forehead represents a transition in topography from the convexity of the median and paramedian forehead to a flat lateral forehead, which continues into a slightly concave temple. The slightly concave nature of the temple makes this region of the forehead a particularly good area for healing by second intention. The enhanced elasticity of lateral forehead skin compared with more centrally located skin allows a larger number of reconstructive options with various flaps. Primary wound closure is also often feasible with orientation of the repair parallel to the forehead skin creases, which become curvilinear as they arc downward toward the cheek. These lines present excellent locations for placement of incisions. The constraints of the location of the temporal hairline and the brow dictate the orientation and size of advancement, rotation, and transposition flaps, which are the types of flaps most frequently used in this area.

The surgeon must take particular care in the lateral forehead area when dissecting such flaps because of the vulnerability of the frontal branch of the facial nerve due to its superficial location. Advancement and advancement rotation flaps are perhaps the most useful of flaps for repair of lateral forehead defects. Usually bilateral advancement flaps are preferred over single flaps, with the greatest advancement achieved from the more elastic laterally based flap.

A variation of the standard advancement flap for repair of medium-sized defects of both the lateral and the paramedian forehead is the O-T or A-T repair. This method consists of making horizontal incisions on opposite sides of the base of the defect in the relaxed skin tension lines or along the border of the brow or temporal hairline. The two flaps are usually dissected in the subcutaneous plane and advanced and slightly rotated toward the triangular-shaped (A) or circular-shaped (O) defect. Standing cutaneous deformities are resected along the brow or eliminated by the rule of halving the wound closure. If necessary, the standing cutaneous deformity that results from the pivotal portion of the flap movement is removed by enlarging the defect itself. The final wound closure takes the configuration of a t-shaped repair. Thus circular defects closed by this method are referred to as O-T repairs, and triangular defects are referred to as A-T repairs.

O-T and A-T repairs are useful in other locations where there is a linear anatomical landmark, such as the mentolabial crease. These techniques allow scar camouflage of all but the central vertical wound closure line.

Rotation flaps are very useful in reconstructing medium and large lateral forehead defects. A unilateral rotation flap based inferiorly and laterally and designed so that its curvilinear incision follows the margin of the temporal hairline is an excellent method for reconstructing lateral forehead defects that are in the proximity of the hairline. The curvilinear incision can be designed to incorporate hair-bearing scalp as necessary to bring hair into the reconstructed area if some of the temporal tufts have been lost. The standing cutaneous deformity that inevitably forms with such a flap can be removed inferiorly in the crow's feet, when possible, to camouflage the scar, or at least as a W-plasty to prevent entering the brow or upper eyelid.

■ Suggested Reading

Baker SR. Local Flaps in Facial Reconstruction. 2nd ed. St Louis, MO: Mosby–Year Book; 2007

Baker SR. Transposition flaps. In: Baker SR. Local Flaps in Facial Reconstruction. 2nd ed. St Louis, MO: Mosby–Year Book; 2007:133–156

Baker SR, Johnson TM, Nelson BR. The importance of maintaining the alar-facial sulcus in nasal reconstruction. Arch Otolaryngol Head Neck Surg 1995;121(6):617–622

Baker SR, Krause CJ. Pedicle flaps in reconstruction of the lip. Facial Plast Surg 1984;1(1):61–68

Burget GC, Menick FJ. Aesthetic Reconstruction of the Nose. St. Louis: Mosby–Year Book; 1993

Hoffman JF. Reconstruction of the scalp. In: Baker SR. Local Flaps in Facial Reconstruction. 2nd ed. St. Louis, MO: Mosby–Year Book; 2007:637–664

Johnson TM, Baker S, Brown MD, Nelson BR. Utility of the subcutaneous hinge flap in nasal reconstruction. J Am Acad Dermatol 1994;30(3):459–466

Karapandzic M. Reconstruction of lip defects by local arterial flaps. Br J Plast Surg 1974;27(1):93–97

Rohrich RJ, Griffin JR, Ansari M, Beran SJ, Potter JK. Nasal reconstruction—beyond aesthetic subunits: a 15-year review of 1334 cases. Plast Reconstr Surg 2004;114(6):1405–1416, discussion 1417–1419

Siegle RJ. Reconstruction of the forehead. In Baker SR. Local Flaps in Facial Reconstruction. 2nd ed. St. Louis, MO: Mosby–Year Book; 2007:557–580

102 Laser Therapy of Cutaneous Vascular Lesions

Introduction

Recent developments in laser therapy of cutaneous vascular lesions have made a variety of new laser techniques available to surgeons and their patients. This chapter briefly summarizes the types of vascular lesions, properties of the most thoroughly evaluated laser therapies, and laser treatment of the most laser-responsive vascular lesions.

Classification of Cutaneous Vascular Lesions

Vascular lesions have been classified according to anatomical structure and biological behavior into two major categories: vascular malformations and hemangiomas. Most vascular malformations are present at birth. They increase in size as a patient grows, exhibit a normal rate of endothelial cell growth, and over time often become darker in color as their surface thickens. These lesions are composed of large ectatic vessels that lack the endothelial hyperplasia seen in hemangiomas. For pediatric subjects, the International Society for the Study of Vascular Anomalies (ISSVA) further subdivided vascular malformations into low-flow (capillary, venous, and lymphatic malformations) and high-flow (arteriovenous malformations and arteriovenous fistulae) lesions in 1996. Mixed lesions were also acknowledged as commonly occurring.

Capillary, venous, and lymphatic malformations, or low-flow lesions by ISSVA criteria, are responsive to laser treatment. Various laser modalities, especially pulsed-dye lasers (PDLs), are very effective in the treatment of capillary lesions, also referred to as port-wine stains (PWSs). Laser utility in venous malformations is predominantly limited to superficial cutaneous lesions or the mucocutaneous portions of more complex lesions, because sclerotherapy or surgical resection for well-circumscribed lesions offers the most definitive treatment. Carbon dioxide (CO_2) laser resurfacing has proven efficacious in the treatment of mucosal microcystic lymphatic malformations, but the majority of other lymphatic malformation subtypes are usually treated with sclerotherapy, surgical resection, or combination therapy. Telangiectasias, another vascular lesion commonly seen in adults, are primarily treated with laser or light therapy.

Hemangiomas biologically behave more like true neoplasms than like vascular malformations. Congenital hemangiomas are fully formed at birth and do not undergo a proliferative growth phase. However, infantile hemangiomas typically appear within the first few weeks of life and undergo a proliferative phase of rapid growth lasting 4 to 6 months in most cases, but proliferation can last up to a year. The proliferative phase is typically followed by a slow involutional phase, which can last for several years. Infantile hemangiomas are the most common vascular tumors occurring in infancy. As such, unlike vascular malformations, most hemangiomas are usually not present at birth. They also differ from vascular malformations in that they display endothelial hyperplasia in their component vessels.

Laser Therapy Options

Laser therapy of cutaneous vascular lesions historically relied primarily on the use of the CO_2 and argon lasers. However, various additional lasers and light therapies are now available for use in treating these lesions. These include the neodymium:yttrium-aluminum-garnet (Nd:YAG) laser; the potassium-titanyl-phosphate (KTP) laser; and the yellow-wavelength lasers, including the PDL, the copper vapor laser, and the continuous-wave yellow-dye lasers. Intense pulsed light (IPL) has also proven useful in the treatment of select vascular lesions.

Carbon Dioxide Laser

The CO_2 laser is the most commonly used laser in otolaryngology. Using CO_2 gas as its medium, the laser has a wavelength of 10,600 nanometers (nm), an invisible wavelength that is in the far-infrared range of electromagnetic radiation. Thus the surgeon must use a helium-neon laser-aiming beam to visualize the intended area of impact. Light at this wavelength is readily absorbed by water, making the CO_2 laser an ideal tool for incising or vaporizing any tissue with a high water content. The effects of the CO_2 laser are superficial because of its high absorption and minimal scatter. Lack of specificity for vascular tissues makes CO_2 lasers suboptimal for many vascular lesions in comparison with other available laser treatment modalities. However, favorable results are still reported for use of the CO_2 laser with mucosal microcystic lymphatic malformations.

Currently, the laser beam can be delivered only through mirrors and specialized lenses placed in an articulated arm. Such an arm may be attached to a microscope to allow for microscopic vision and precision, or the beam may be delivered through a focusing handpiece attached to the articulated arm.

Argon Laser

Cutaneous vascular lesions respond well to the argon laser because of the high rate of absorption of argon by hemoglobin. The argon laser employs a visible wavelength of 488 to 514 nm, and the delivery system is via fiberoptic carriers. Because of the makeup of the resonating chamber and the molecular structure of argon, the laser produces a band of wavelengths, rather than just a single wavelength. The laser's scattering effect is intermediate, between that of the CO_2 and the Nd:YAG laser. Although hemoglobin is the primary chromophore for argon lasers, it is also significantly absorbed by melanin, which can limit its depth of penetration and predispose patients to undesirable scabbing and scarring, particularly in the treatment of PWSs.

Neodymium:Yttrium-Aluminum-Garnet Laser

The wavelength of the Nd:YAG laser is 1,064 nm and is in the near-infrared spectral region. Because this region is not visible to the human eye, the Nd:YAG laser, like the CO_2 laser, requires a helium-neon laser-aiming beam. Although most tissues in the body do not absorb this wavelength well, pigmented tissues absorb it better than do tissues without pigment. Laser energy is transmitted through the superficial layers of most tissues and scattered into the deeper layers.

The scatter of the Nd:YAG laser is considerably greater than that of the CO_2 laser. Therefore, the depth of penetration is greater, making the ND:YAG laser well suited for coagulating deeper vessels. Good results have been reported in the use of the Nd:YAG laser for the treatment of perioral deep capillary and cavernous lesions, and it has also been used successfully in laser photocoagulation of hemangiomas, lymphangiomas, venous, and arteriovenous malformations. However, the increased depth of penetration and nonselective destruction characteristic of this laser also predispose patients to increased postoperative scarring. Clinically, scarring is minimized by using conservative power settings and a pointillistic approach to the lesion, and by using the laser in areas of thick skin. Although use of the Nd:YAG for PWSs has been virtually replaced by the yellow-wavelength lasers, it remains useful as an adjuvant laser for patients with thicker, nodular PWSs.

The physics and absorption properties of the Nd:YAG laser are drastically altered when the laser is used in the contact mode. When the sapphire or quartz contact tip is attached to the end of the laser fiber and directly applied to tissue, it functions as a thermal scalpel because the laser is used only to heat the contact tip.

Potassium-Titanyl-Phosphate Laser

The KTP laser is an Nd:YAG laser whose frequency is doubled (wavelength halved) by passing the laser beam through the KTP crystal. This results in a green light with a wavelength of 532 nm, corresponding to an absorption peak of hemoglobin. Its tissue penetration, scatter, and delivery mode are similar to that of the argon laser. In the noncontact mode, the laser vaporizes and coagulates. In the semicontact mode, the tip of the fiber barely touches the tissue, and the laser behaves like a cutting instrument. The higher the energy setting used, the more the laser behaves like a hot knife, analogous to the CO_2 laser. Lower energy settings are used primarily to coagulate blood in the target vessel.

Yellow-Wavelength Lasers

Three types of yellow-wavelength lasers have been developed, primarily for the treatment of benign vascular lesions of the face. These are the flashlamp-excited dye laser, or PDL; the copper vapor laser; and the continuous-wave, yellow-dye laser. The use of yellow lasers to treat vascular lesions is based on the principle called selective photothermolysis, which holds that the selective destruction of a vascular lesion is dependent on two factors: (1) the preferential light absorption and subsequent heat production in the target vessel, and (2) the localization of the heat through adjustment in the amount of exposure time.

The surgeon's goal is to heat the blood within an ectatic vessel until it coagulates and conducts the heat to the endothelial lining. The proper exposure time is critical to localize the thermal effect to the vessel and spare the surrounding dermis and overlying epidermis. Yellow-wavelength lasers are designed to produce yellow light in the range of 577 to 595 nm, because the third absorption peak of oxyhemoglobin occurs at 577 nm. Using this wavelength range results in more laser energy being absorbed by hemoglobin and less energy being absorbed by the competing chromophore, melanin. Also, the amount of tissue scatter of the laser light at this wavelength is decreased in comparison to the other visible wavelength lasers, such as the KTP and argon lasers.

Flashlamp-Excited Dye Laser, or PDL

The flashlamp-excited dye laser, or PDL, was the first medical laser specifically designed to treat benign vascular cutaneous lesions. It is a visible-light laser with a wavelength of 585 or 595 nm. As stated before, the close coincidence between this wavelength and the third absorption peak of oxyhemoglobin allows for preferential absorption of the laser by hemoglobin. It has been shown that there is increased tissue penetration with the PDL without loss of vascular selectivity when the wavelength is increased from 577 to 585 or 595 nm. With deeper penetration, there is faster clearing of the lesion. Currently, PDL is considered the mainstay of treatment for most PWSs.

The PDL uses as its medium a rhodamine dye that is excited optically by a flashlamp, and the delivery system is a fiberoptic carrier. The handpiece of the PDL has interchangeable lens systems that permit use of a 2, 5, 7, or 10 mm spot size. The PDL's fixed 450 ms pulse width was selected based on the thermal relaxation time of ectatic vessels found within benign vascular cutaneous lesions.

Copper Vapor Laser

The copper vapor laser is a visible-wavelength laser that produces two separate wavelengths, a pulsed green wavelength at 511 nm, and a pulsed yellow light at 578 nm. The laser medium, copper, is excited (vaporized) electrically. The yellow light of the copper vapor laser is used in treating benign vascular lesions of the face. The green wavelength may be used to treat pigmented lesions, such as freckles, nevi, and keratoses of the face.

The copper vapor laser may be used with a fiberoptic system that delivers the beam to a handpiece that is equipped with variable spot sizes ranging from 150 to 1,000 μm. The exposure time is variable,

ranging from 0.075 s to continuous operation. A Hexascan-type delivery system also may be used with the copper vapor laser. With the Hexascan (Lihtan Technologies, San Rafael, CA), a hexagonal area of tissue is systematically covered as the laser fires and coagulates tissue and then moves to a predetermined point away from the previously treated spot, allowing for tissue cooling.

Continuous-Wave, Yellow-Dye Laser

The continuous-wave, yellow-dye laser is a visible-wavelength laser that produces yellow light at 577 nm. Like the PDL and copper vapor laser, it is ideally suited for treating benign vascular lesions of the face. Like the PDL, it can be tuned by changing the dye within the activation chamber of the laser. The dye is excited by an argon laser. The delivery system for this laser, again like the PDL, is a fiberoptic cable that may be focused to variable spot sizes. The laser light may be pulsed by mechanical shutters, or a Hexascan handpiece can be used at the end of the fiberoptic system.

Intense Pulsed Light

IPL instruments emit polychromatic light in a broad-wavelength spectrum, typically between 500 and 1,400 nm. Filters attached to IPL devices can be applied to define a wavelength band targeting specific soft tissue structures under the skin surface. Depending on the attached filter, deep or superficial vessels may be targeted. Pigmented lesions and unwanted hair follicular units can also be targeted, adding to the versatility of these units. However, the bulkiness of IPL handpieces and typically large spot sizes are disadvantages of IPL in the treatment of small, concave facial areas. Currently, IPL devices are used to treat superficial PWSs, superficial hemangiomas, diffuse telangiectasias (often associated with rosacea), and poikiloderma of Civatte.

■ Treatment of Specific Lesions

Port-Wine Stains (PWSs)

Laser Selection

More correctly called congenital capillary vascular malformations, PWSs are benign vascular lesions that commonly involve the face and neck. Approximately 5% of PWSs are associated with Sturge–Weber syndrome and Klippel–Trénaunay syndrome. These flat, pink-to-red lesions are usually apparent at birth. As the patient ages, the lesions often become darker in color and develop a thickness and nodularity of their surface.

In the past, the CO_2 laser has been used to treat PWSs. However, eradicating the vessels within the dermis required vaporizing the overlying epidermis and a portion of the dermis. This commonly led to scarring and hypopigmentation. The argon laser has also been used extensively for the treatment of PWSs, because its blue-green light in the 488 to 514 nm range is absorbed by oxyhemoglobin, but hypertrophic scarring became a recurrent, troublesome complication. The KTP and Nd:YAG lasers have also been used in treating PWSs with varying degrees of success. Some promising results have been reported with the use of the Hexascan with the argon or KTP laser, but PWS treatment with the yellow-wavelength lasers, particularly the PDLs, has provided a breakthrough in the treatment of PWSs. PDL treatment, usually with an epidermal cooling unit, is currently considered the most established treatment for PWSs.

Treatment

When the PDL is used to treat a facial PWS, the first step is to determine the correct laser energy. This can be done by performing a purpuric threshold determination on normal skin of the volar aspect of the patient's forearm. Beginning at 2 J/cm² and increasing by 0.5 J/cm², successive pulses of laser energy are applied until the entire area of the spot is purple. The energy level at which this purpuric lesion appears is the patient's threshold level. This value is then multiplied by 1.5 or 2 to obtain the energy density to be used for a test area.

The test area is created by placing 10 to 20 slightly overlapping spots in a representative area of the patient's lesion. The test area is assessed at 6 weeks posttreatment, and adjustments in the energy density depend on the patient's response. Crusting or blistering indicates the need to decrease the energy density. An irregular pattern of clearance indicates the need for increasing the energy density. Once the correct energy density is determined, the lesion is treated in aesthetic units. Patients with darker skin color may require increases in energy density. Lesions involving the eyelids, upper lip, mucosa, and neck often require less energy. The same area may be treated every 6 weeks. The number of treatments necessary to clear a facial PWS varies according to the size, color, and location of the lesion, but multiple treatments are usually required.

Telangiectasias

Telangiectasias of the face are small ectatic vessels within the dermis. Various types occur, including linear, arborizing, reticular, punctate, and spider telangiectasias. Spider telangiectasias are commonly called spider nevi or spider angioma. These acquired vascular marks commonly appear on young children's faces or women during pregnancy, most frequently appearing in the second trimester and enlarging until delivery. Estrogen is thought to have a role in their formation.

Telangiectatic lesions have also been noted after nasal surgery. Other patients seem to have a hereditary predisposition for facial telangiectasias; these lesions are classified as essential hereditary telangiectasias.

Laser Selection and Treatment

PDLs and the other yellow-dye laser types (copper vapor and continuous-wave yellow lasers), as well as KTP lasers, can be used to treat facial telangiectasias. Treatment techniques with all of these lasers are similar. The surgeon chooses a spot size that is adequate to obliterate the dilated vessel (0.1–0.2 mm) and then traces the vessel with the laser beam until the vessel disappears. The smallest spot size and lowest power are used to minimize damage to the surrounding normal tissue and reduce scarring. When using the PDL for facial telangiectasias, the 2 mm spot size is usually selected to treat individual vessels and the 5 mm spot is selected to treat vessels that have associated erythema. The laser spots are placed in a contiguous or slightly overlapping pattern over the vessel. When treating spider telangiectasias with the PDL, as with the other yellow lasers, the radial vessels are obliterated from the periphery moving toward the center, and then the central vessel is treated.

The energy densities used for treating telangiectasias are usually lower than those for treating PWSs and are often in the range of 5.5 to 6 J/cm². Retreatment with yellow-wavelength lasers can usually be safely performed 6 to 8 weeks after the previous treatment. Favorable results have also been reported for treatment of diffuse telangiectasias with IPL treatment. As with other laser modalities, most optimal results for IPL telangiectasia treatment are usually achieved through a series of treatments, rather than a single treatment session.

Hereditary Hemorrhagic Telangiectasia (HHT)

Hereditary hemorrhagic telangiectasia (HHT), or Rendu–Osler–Weber syndrome, is an inherited autosomal-dominant disease manifested by multiple telangiectatic lesions that appear on the skin and mucosal membranes. Epistaxis, caused by bleeding from the nasal lesions, is the most common presenting symptom. Bleeding from lesions of the lips, gingiva, tongue, buccal mucosa, or hard palate may also occur. Histologically, ectatic vessels with incomplete surrounding muscular layers are observed.

Nonlaser therapies continue to be used in treating HHT. Patients with severe epistaxis have been treated successfully using septal dermoplasty. However, recurrent telangiectasias may appear at the edges of the graft or, in some cases, in the graft itself. Estrogen therapy has been advocated for the treatment of HHT. It is thought to work by reducing squamous metaplasia of the nasal mucosa and thereby reducing the incidence of bleeding.

Laser Selection

The CO_2, argon, Nd:YAG, and KTP lasers have all been used to photocoagulate the nasal and oral telangiectasias found in HHT. Fiber-directed lasers (Nd:YAG, KTP, and argon) have the advantage of accessibility to lateral and posterior nasal sites, and hemoglobin absorption offers the theoretic advantage of vascular selectivity. Dedicated nasal instruments available with the KTP laser facilitate its usage in the constricted nasal cavity. Although the Nd:YAG laser is not preferentially absorbed by oxyhemoglobin, its deeper penetration makes it extremely effective in coagulating these lesions.

Treatment

Regardless of the laser chosen, the free fiber is held above the mucosal surface, and the individual vessels are treated in a rosette fashion by first encircling the central portion of the lesion with pulses of laser energy and then coagulating the central lesion. For the Nd:YAG laser, power settings usually range from 10 to 25 W, the exposure time used is 0.5 s, and the beam is used in a slightly defocused mode. The laser energy should be applied perpendicular to the mucosal surface, making this treatment modality more difficult to achieve for lesions deeper in the nasal cavity.

Hemangiomas

Laser Selection and Treatment

Indications for laser treatment of infantile hemangiomas are evolving with the advent of oral propranolol for inducing hemangioma regression. Nevertheless, lasers still play a central role in the treatment of these vascular tumors. Treatment of capillary or cavernous hemangiomas has been performed with CO_2, Nd:YAG, argon, PDL, and KTP lasers. The vascular specificity of the PDL, KTP, and argon lasers enhances the selectivity of the photocoagulation and can minimize the risk for undesirable scarring. However, the shallow depth of penetration with these laser modalities limits their efficacy in thicker, nodular lesions. The Nd:YAG laser is useful when a greater depth of treatment is desired and can be used in conjunction with the PDL for lesions with both a superficial and a deep component, or alone when a greater depth of coagulation is desired. Excision of large hemangiomas of the nasal cavity and paranasal sinuses is facilitated by the KTP laser or contact-tip Nd:YAG lasers, both of which complement traditional surgical approaches.

■ Summary

Improvements in laser technology will continue to evolve, as will the role of specific lasers in the treatment of various cutaneous vascular lesions. Photodynamic therapy involving light activation of a photosensitizer to generate cytotoxic reactive oxygen species is currently under investigation and shows promise in the treatment of several vascular lesions, including PWS, venous malformations, and arteriovenous malformations. Various laser and light therapies, such as IPL, are now available to treat vascular cutaneous lesions. No single laser is best suited for the treatment of all lesions. In choosing the appropriate laser treatment, the surgeon must understand the specific wavelength of the laser, laser–tissue interactions, and the differences among targeted lesions undergoing treatment.

■ Suggested Reading

Anderson RR, Parrish JA. Selective photothermolysis: precise microsurgery by selective absorption of pulsed radiation. Science 1983;220(4596):524–527

Apfelberg DB, Bailin P, Rosenberg H. Preliminary investigation of KTP/532 laser light in the treatment of hemangiomas and tattoos. Lasers Surg Med 1986;6(1):38–42, 56–57

Athavale SM, Ries WR, Carniol PJ. Laser treatment of cutaneous vascular tumors and malformations. Facial Plast Surg Clin North Am 2011;19(2):303–312

Burns AJ, Navarro JA. Role of laser therapy in pediatric patients. Plast Reconstr Surg 2009;124(1, Suppl)82e–92e

Channual J, Choi B, Osann K, Pattanachinda D, Lotfi J, Kelly KM. Vascular effects of photodynamic and pulsed dye laser therapy protocols. Lasers Surg Med 2008;40(9):644–650

Galeckas KJ. Update on lasers and light devices for the treatment of vascular lesions. Semin Cutan Med Surg 2008;27(4):276–284

Glade RS, Buckmiller LM. CO2 laser resurfacing of intraoral lymphatic malformations: a 10-year experience. Int J Pediatr Otorhinolaryngol 2009;73(10):1358–1361

Hochman M, Adams DM, Reeves TD. Current knowledge and management of vascular anomalies: I. Hemangiomas. Arch Facial Plast Surg 2011;13(3):145–151

Kelly KM, Choi B, McFarlane S, et al. Description and analysis of treatments for port-wine stain birthmarks. Arch Facial Plast Surg 2005;7(5):287–294

Mulliken JB, Glowacki J. Hemangiomas and vascular malformations in infants and children: a classification based on endothelial characteristics. Plast Reconstr Surg 1982;69(3):412–422

Patel AM, Chou EL, Findeiss L, Kelly KM. The horizon for treating cutaneous vascular lesions. Semin Cutan Med Surg 2012;31(2):98–104

Puttgen KB, Pearl M, Tekes A, Mitchell SE. Update on pediatric extracranial vascular anomalies of the head and neck. Childs Nerv Syst 2010;26(10):1417–1433

Rosenfeld H, Wellisz T, Reinisch JF, Sherman R. The treatment of cutaneous vascular lesions with the Nd:YAG laser. Ann Plast Surg 1988;21(3):223–230

103 Otoplasty

■ Introduction

Cosmetic otoplasty to correct ear protrusion refers to a variety of surgical procedures designed to create a "natural" relationship of the auricle and its component parts with the head. The parameters of the aesthetically ideal ear include pinna position, size, and degree of protrusion. The surgeon must recognize that "normal" ears are often asymmetrical in these parameters, without producing a cosmetically unsatisfactory appearance. The cosmetically ideal degree of pinna protrusion is delineated by an auriculocephalic angle of 25 to 35 degrees. The cephaloconchal angle should be > 45 degrees, and the scaphaconchal angle should be < 90 degrees. The fossa triangularis should face laterally.

The distance of the helical rim from the mastoid skin should be 15 to 20 mm. A helical rim-to-mastoid skin distance < 10 mm gives a "stuck to the head" appearance. A relative protrusion of the middle third of the helical rim is permissible and adds a gentle, natural-appearing curve to the helical rim contour. Specific ideal measurements of helical rim distance to mastoid skin are 10 to 12 mm at the superior pole, 16 to 18 mm at the middle third of the helical rim, and 20 to 22 mm at the level of the cauda helix.

Incidence and Causes of Deformities

The incidence of abnormally protruding ears is ~ 5% in Caucasians. This deformity is inherited as an autosomal-dominant trait with incomplete penetrance. The incidence and risk of subsequent children inheriting the deformity are important issues to discuss in affected families.

A careful assessment of the ear reveals the precise anatomical features causing the deformity. The most common defect is lack of development of the normal antihelical and superior crural folds. An abnormally unfurled antihelix occurs in ~ 66% of cases, producing a noticeable outward projection of the superior anterior helix. A wide, protruding conchal wall is the second most common deformity and occurs in ~ 33% of cases. This may occur alone or in combination with antihelical unfurling. Other deformities include underdevelopment of the inferior crus, earlobe protrusion, prominence of the antitragus, and a deficient helical roll.

Syndromes refer to several types of overlapping auricular deformities. The lop ear is an acute downfolding of the superior pole of the ear, usually at the auricular tubercle, due to the faulty development of the helix, scapha, and antihelix. The ear appears smaller than normal, and its cartilage often lacks resiliency, which contributes to the limpness of the pinna and cupping of the conchal wall. The protruding ear refers to the unfurling of the body of the antihelix and superior crus. Excessive conchal cartilage may be partly or totally responsible for the deformity. The cup ear has characteristics of both lop ear and protruding ear deformities. The concha is overdeveloped, deep, and concave. A poorly developed superior pole of the ear and antihelical crura, a short helix, and cupping of the lobule may also be present. The vertical length of the auricle is usually smaller than normal. Unlike the lop ear, the cartilage in the cup ear deformity is often thick and unresilient, making correction more difficult to maintain. Infrequently occurring syndromes include the shell, satyr, Machiavellian, and Stahl ears.

Microtia combines atresia of the external auditory canal with underdevelopment of the entire pinna. The degree of the pinna and external auditory canal deformity is variable. The surgical management of the pinna deformity in microtia is beyond the scope of this chapter.

■ Evaluation

Indications

The optimal age for correction of ear deformities is at the completion of cartilaginous growth, which is 80 to 90% complete at ~ 5 years of age. Prior to this age, the cartilage lacks stiffness, and surgical correction is technically difficult. If the pinna appears smaller than normal, the procedure may be delayed until age 6 or 7. Correction of the ear deformity prior to enrollment in school can spare the child emotional trauma. Because the pliability of cartilage decreases with increasing age, surgical weakening of cartilage may be necessary in adults.

Contraindications

It is important to determine what, precisely, patients dislike about their ears. The specific goals and limitations of otoplasty should be discussed preoperatively to fully inform patients or their parents. If the patients have unrealistic expectations and cannot be brought to a more realistic view, they are not candidates for cosmetic surgery. If the psychological concern is disproportionate to the deformity, referral for counseling is indicated. There is no specific contraindication to delaying surgery, even to adulthood. Assessment of a patient's medical history should rule out coexisting anomalies, bleeding diathesis, and a tendency for keloid formation or hypertrophic scarring.

Assessment

Preoperatively, the position, size, and proportion of the ears to the facial features and head should be carefully assessed, along with a thorough evaluation of the specific anatomical features to be surgically corrected. The ears should be manipulated to a medialized position to assess the resilience of the cartilaginous framework and the redundancy of the postauricular skin. Helical rim to mastoid skin distances should be measured at the superior pole, middle third, and cauda helix. The presence of coexisting anomalies, such as aural atresia or craniofacial complex anomalies, must be determined. Preference regarding hairstyle should be noted.

■ Surgical Management

Goals

Otoplasty seeks to reestablish normal aesthetic parameters and proportions of the individual components of the ear, and to reinstate symmetry of the ears and their balance with facial features. A natural-appearing auricle, free of surgical stigmata, is the optimal result. Mallen has summarized the following guidelines for the otoplastic surgeon (the following

list summarizes Mallen's guidelines for the otoplastic surgeon):

- Protrusion of the upper third of the ear must be corrected. Some protrusion of the lower ear may be acceptable, but only if the superior aspect of the auricle has been corrected.
- The helical rim should not be seen beyond the antihelix from the frontal view, at least down to the mid-ear.
- There must be symmetry of protrusion of the ears to within 3 mm, as well as symmetry of shape. To achieve symmetry, a bilateral procedure is usually indicated. The closer the auricle is to the head, the less noticeable any postoperative asymmetry.
- The postauricular sulcus should be maintained.
- The helix should arch backward smoothly from its crus. It should be furled at its superior aspect and should gently lead into the lobule. The antihelix should curve forward into the superior crus and should be smoothly rounded.
- The distance of the helical rim from the mastoid skin should be 10 to 12 mm at the superior pole, 16 to 18 mm at the middle third, and 20 to 22 mm at the level of the cauda helix. The proper auriculocephalic angle is 25 to 35 degrees.
- All visible surfaces should be smooth, without buckles, puckering, scars, or ridges.

Surgical Technique

Early methods of otoplasty involved excision of skin and/or perichondrium in the postauricular sulcus or medial aspect of the desired antihelical fold. This technique transferred the tension of the medialized cartilage to the soft tissues of the line of closure. Hypertrophic scarring, obliteration of the postauricular sulcus, and wound complications resulted from the increased tension at the line of closure. Current surgical techniques to correct prominauris are divided into cartilage-cutting and cartilage-sparing techniques.

Cartilage-Cutting Techniques

Cartilage-cutting techniques involve resculpting the cartilage by altering its intrinsic tension. These methods may entail any combination of the following procedures:

- Incisions on the anterior or posterior surface of the auricle without extension through the full thickness of the cartilage

- Excision of cartilage to mobilize components of the auricular framework
- Scoring, abrading, or rasping the anterior surface of the auricle

The cartilage-scoring and -incision techniques are based on the principle of cartilage bending away from the side of the scored perichondrium.

Stenstrom developed the technique of disruption of the perichondrium along the line of the proposed antihelical fold. The lateral skin of the pinna was undermined, and incisions were made in the lateral perichondrium to allow folding at the antihelical line. Farrior formed the new antihelix by removing longitudinal cartilaginous wedges from the posterior surface of the pinna on either side of the antihelix. This produced a convex antihelix, which was stabilized with horizontal mattress sutures. Various methods of cartilage excision have been used for enlarged auricles to reduce scaphal size.

Cartilage-cutting techniques may be indicated when thick, inflexible cartilage or large anatomical deformities are present. Care must be used when these methods are performed, due to the risk of producing cartilage surface irregularities, ridges at the site of incision or excision, apparent reduction in pinna size, and scarring.

Cartilage-Sparing Techniques

Cartilage-sparing techniques, developed by Mustardé and later refined by Furnas, Webster, and others, revolutionized otoplastic surgery through their simplicity, ease of execution, and the maintenance of auricular cartilage integrity. These techniques set cartilage position and contour with permanent mattress sutures to provide a more natural shape with minimal cartilage irregularities. The position of the suture may be changed without permanent damage to the cartilage. The suture may be assessed, the auricular correction controlled, and the knot then completed.

Mustardé used multiple permanent scaphaconchal horizontal mattress sutures to modify the antihelical fold and scapha-fossa triangularis sutures to modify the superior crus. Furnas used permanent horizontal mattress sutures from the conchal bowl to the mastoid periosteum and from the fossa triangularis to the temporalis fascia to correct excessive conchal height or cupping. The auricle may be displaced in the cephalad or caudad direction with use of the conchamastoid sutures. The lobule can be medialized through either caudaconchal or caudasubcutaneous sutures. Webster used cartilage suturing techniques, along with excision of postauricular soft tissues and tangential shaving of conchal cartilage, to effect "setback" of the auricle.

The Graduated Approach

The graduated approach, advocated by Adamson, involves a detailed assessment of the patient's deformity, which allows precise correction of each specific deformity in a stepwise, logical fashion.

After infiltrative anesthesia is provided in combination with either intravenous sedation or general anesthesia, an eccentric fusiform incision is marked in the postauricular sulcus. The ear is manipulated to the desired medial position, and the redundant skin is assessed. The eccentric fusiform incision is placed so that more skin is excised from the posterior aspect of the pinna, rather than from the mastoid. This allows the final scar to lie in the sulcus. A releasing incision is placed at the superior pole to enhance positioning of the scapha-fossa triangularis and fossa triangularis-temporalis fascia sutures. The excision should terminate at least 1 cm from the superior and inferior aspects of the sulcus to prevent its anterior visualization.

A variable amount of postauricular sulcal soft tissue is excised in continuity with the overlying skin, depending on the degree of conchal wall protrusion present. This excision allows the conchal cartilage to be retropositioned, decreasing its lateral and anterior prominence. Dissection should be kept 1 cm from the external auditory canal to prevent entry into it. The conchal setback is effected with approximately three permanent Furnas-type, horizontal mattress, conchamastoid sutures. A 4–0 white synthetic permanent suture, such as Mersilene (Ethicon, Somerville, N) and/or nylon, is used to engage the full thickness of cartilage and anterior perichondrium laterally, and the mastoid periosteum medially. The suture should be white to prevent it from showing through the anterior pinna skin. The three sutures can be placed as follows: (1) superior conchal bowl (fossa triangularis); (2) inferior conchal bowl (cavum concha); and (3) mid-bowl (cymba concha). The vector of pull on the conchal bowl is superior and posterior to prevent stenosis of the external auditory canal as the sutures are tightened.

An excessively deep conchal bowl occasionally requires tangential (or shave) excision of the ponticulus, triangular, and conchal eminences to allow the concha to be positioned deeper in the sulcus. Care is taken to prevent overcorrection with the conchalmastoid sutures in the middle third of the ear or overresection of sulcal soft tissues. Overcorrection, especially with middle suture placement too high on the conchal wall, will cause cupping of the bowl and a "telephone ear" deformity.

The antihelical correction is performed after adequate positioning of the concha, since the degree of antihelical correction required is often less than initially anticipated because of the conchal setback. The antihelix is furled using 1 to 4 permanent 4–0 white Mustardé-type, horizontal mattress sutures. These sutures should transfix the full thickness of cartilage and anterior perichondrium, but not the overlying skin. The suture "bite" should be ~ 4 to 6 mm; larger bites may cause the cartilage to buckle. The desired antihelical fold is simulated by using gentle pressure on the helix. Superior crus and antihelical furling are effected with sutures placed from the superior scapha to the fossa triangularis, the mid-scapha to the concha, and the inferior antihelix to the concha. All sutures are placed first and then tightened in the same order to achieve the desired antihelical contour. The superior pole is slightly overcorrected in anticipation of postoperative cartilage recoil. A mid-auricle measurement of 15 to 18 mm is ideal. Thick, unresilient cartilage occasionally requires anterior cartilage scoring or anterior antihelical rasping to facilitate flexibility and reduce the tension placed on the Mustardé sutures.

An excessively large auricle may require reduction of the scapha and the helical rim circumference. Various techniques have been described in the literature. However, by just setting the ear back, its apparent size will be diminished. Minor degrees of lobule protrusion can be corrected by further fusiform tailoring of the initial postauricular excision. Generally, skin excision is not effective for correction of lobule protrusion. A permanent horizontal mattress suture from the cauda helix to the concha is effective for lobule medialization. This is preferable to excision of the cauda helix and possible loss of structural support.

Skin closure is effected with interrupted inverted dissolvable suture, such as 4–0 chromic gut, to allow egress of blood. A soft, molded dressing (e.g., cotton, mineral oil, and hydrogen peroxide) is placed. The dressing is removed on day 1 to inspect the wounds and, in children, is replaced for another 4 days. After removal of the dressing, a headband is worn for 2 weeks continuously and then at night for another 2 weeks to prevent accidental lateralization of the ear.

Potential problems with the graduated approach include suture extrusion, with or without loss of correction. After several months, correction is maintained primarily by the development of scar tissue. Resilient cartilage, especially if not scored, thinned, or excised, may lose some of its correction. This is most likely at the superior pole.

Incisionless Otoplasty

More recently, Fritsch introduced a technique involving the percutaneous insertion of retention sutures. This procedure entails the serial placement of percutaneous retention sutures to re-create the antihelical fold and medialize the conchal bowl to the mastoid periosteum.

The retention suture is a white 3–0 braided polyester suture on a cutting needle. The sutures are placed from the scapha to the triangular fossa, and the scapha to the conchal wall. The needle is inserted through the postauricular skin and cartilage and is exited on the anterior aspect of the pinna. The needle is regrasped, reinserted in exactly the same exit site, and advanced subcutaneously to a new skin exit point. These steps are repeated to return the suture to the initial insertion site on the posterior aspect of the pinna. The final knots are thrown after all the sutures are adequately positioned. The suture must remain subcutaneous in its final placement, to prevent epithelial inclusion cyst formation, suture extrusion, and chronic infection. A skin hook can be used to pull skin over an exposed knot, and a 6–0 mild chromic catgut suture can be used to close the skin and prevent suture exposure. Medialization of the concha can be effected with conchamastoid periosteum retention sutures.

Improper placement of sutures in the superficial plane can lead to skin dimpling. Other postoperative surgical concerns include suture extrusion, loss of correction from suture breakage, epithelial inclusion cyst formation, and postauricular suture banding. Excessively thick, unresilient cartilage and overly large or absent auricular features are contraindications for incisionless otoplasty. Long-term results are needed to reveal the ability of retention sutures to maintain the surgically corrected cartilage shape.

Complications

The complication rate of otoplasty is reported to range from 7.1 to 11.4%, regardless of surgical technique. Complications usually manifest themselves within 6 months postoperatively. Early complications include bleeding, infection, and necrosis. The incidence of hematoma formation is ~ 3%, but higher rates occur in cartilage-cutting techniques. Causes include dissection outside of tissue planes, inadequate hemostasis, and inadequate pressure dressing. Hypertension, rebound vasodilation after local vasoconstrictor injection, and trauma may be factors. Use of interrupted sutures allows egress of blood and prevents the occurrence of an expanding hematoma. An unevacuated hematoma may lead to infection, perichondritis, chondritis, and subsequent cosmetic deformity.

Wound infection may occur from a break in sterile technique or may present chronically as the result of an infected suture. Infection can result in cellulitis and ultimately perichondritis in 1% of cases. *Staphylococcus aureus, Escherichia coli,* and *Pseudomonas aeruginosa* have been reported in 2% of cases and usually occur 5 days postoperatively. Progression of infection to chondritis results in cartilage necrosis and resorption, which can yield profound auricular deformities. Treatment consists of empirical *Pseudomonas* coverage pending culture results, and irrigation with antibiotic solution. If infection persists, removal of permanent sutures in the affected area and debridement may be necessary. The risk of infection can be minimized by the use of a single, preincision, intravenous dose of a broad-spectrum antibiotic, such as clindamycin. The wounds can be irrigated with an antibiotic solution just prior to closure.

Late complications occur in the weeks to months following surgery. These include suture complications, cartilage irregularities, deformity recurrence, hypertrophic scarring and keloid formation, paresthesias, and aesthetic complications. Suture complications from permanent synthetic sutures include granuloma formation (8%), and suture extrusion. Excessive recoil of the ear may result from pull-through of one or more sutures, use of too few sutures, unusually thick cartilage, or trauma. Loss of correction in suture techniques occurs in up to 40% of cases. Recurrence can be minimized by using an adequate number of permanent cartilage-securing sutures, using cartilage-weakening procedures on inflexible cartilage, and using a postoperative headband.

Hypertrophic scarring occurs within the confines of the original scar and may result from increased tension on the postauricular closure. Young patients, patients with darker skin, and patients with a history of scarring are at greater risk. Keloid formation is rare. Keloids extend outside the boundaries of the original scar and tend to occur in African American and Asian patients. Conservative treatment includes weekly triamcinolone acetonide injections. Scar excision and closure without tension are possible in some cases.

Rarely, damage to the postauricular nerves may occur during excision of deeper tissue for the conchal setback, resulting in pain or numbness. This complication usually resolves over weeks to months without treatment. Disturbance of the auricular blood supply most likely explains the increased rate of frostbite in ears that have undergone otoplasty.

Commonly witnessed aesthetic deformities after otoplasty include the following:

- Telephone ear deformity
- Conchal deformity
- Antihelical deformity
- Vertical post deformity
- Overcorrection
- Undercorrection
- Hidden helix
- Asymmetry

Telephone Ear Deformity

Telephone ear deformity occurs when there has been excessive conchal setback or reduction of the middle third of the ear. It can also result with excessive exci-

sion of postoperative skin, failure to medialize a protruding cauda helix, or insufficient correction of the superior crus.

Conchal Deformity

A relative conchal prominence with respect to the upper and lower poles may occur when conchal hypertrophy is not addressed and the concha is repositioned with a conchal setback procedure. Buckling of the concha with impingement on the external auditory canal may occur with improper positioning of the concha.

Antihelical Deformity

Cartilage-cutting techniques have a higher risk than cartilage-sparing techniques of ridges and irregular contours along the new antihelix. Anterior cartilage scoring and rasping may produce a roughened, irregular scaphal surface. Puckering along the antihelical fold can result from taking large cartilage bites when placing Mustardé sutures, especially with improper placement of sutures or in thin cartilage.

Vertical Post Deformity

An overcorrected superior antihelix can result in an exaggerated vertical fold in the scapha. This fold can extend to the helix, causing helical buckling.

Overcorrection

The appearance of the ear being "stuck to the head" results from medializing the auricle with excessive antihelical fold correction while not addressing conchal bowl prominence, or by concomitant overcorrection of the conchal bowl and antihelical fold.

Undercorrection

A persistently protruding ear results from failure to correct a markedly protruding superior pole.

Hidden Helix

Excessive surgical folding of the antihelix may cause it to protrude laterally more than the helix. If conchal setback is performed first, the degree of antihelical folding needed will often be less than originally estimated. Antitragal prominence uncommonly requires reduction by excision after conchal setback.

Asymmetry

Symmetry of shape and protrusion is difficult to achieve surgically, especially when preoperative deformities are asymmetric. Both ears will usually require surgical alteration to maintain symmetry.

Preoperative discussion regarding realistic postoperative results is imperative before otoplasty. If any surgically correctable deformity is present postoperatively, it should be revised at an appropriate time. Reassurance is necessary if the result is not correctable.

■ Controversies

As should be evident from the discussion in this section, the major area of controversy in otoplasty is that of the so-called cartilage-sparing versus the cartilage-cutting techniques. Proponents of the cartilage-sparing techniques point to the potential for deformities induced by the cartilage-cutting techniques and the difficulty in correcting these deformities. Those surgeons who prefer cartilage-cutting techniques feel that they have less problems with recurrence of the deformity and that cartilage-cutting techniques are more useful in ears with very firm cartilage that may not be readily correctable with the cartilage-sparing techniques. As is often the case when a dichotomy of techniques is espoused, skillful surgeons will have both techniques in their armamentarium and apply them on an individualized basis.

■ Conclusion

Surgical correction of auricular deformities requires careful preoperative assessment of the contributing anatomical deformities. Cartilage scoring, shaving, incision, and excision may be required in cases of extreme deformity or unusually stiff cartilage. Many aesthetic problems associated with otoplasty can be avoided by identifying and correcting the specific causes of the deformity, placing sutures meticulously, excising minimal skin, and continuously reevaluating the contour and position of the ear throughout the procedure. If expectations are realistic, highly satisfactory results are usually achievable.

■ Suggested Reading

Adamson PA, Litner JA. Otoplasty technique. Facial Plast Surg Clin North Am 2006;14(2):79–87, v

Farrior RT. Otoplasty for children. Otolaryngol Clin North Am 1970;3(2):365–374

Mustarde JC. The correction of prominent ears using simple mattress sutures. Br J Plast Surg 1963;16:170–178

Nachlas NE. Otoplasty. In: Papel ID, ed. Facial Plastic and Reconstructive Surgery. New York: Thieme; 2009:421–434

Scharer SA, Farrior EH, Farrior RT. Retrospective analysis of the Farrior technique for otoplasty. Arch Facial Plast Surg 2007;9(3):167–173

104 Rhinoplasty

Introduction

Rhinoplasty is arguably the most challenging facial plastic surgery procedure. Many capable surgeons find this procedure highly fulfilling but constantly vexing; tolerances of < 1 mm can render the ultimate surgical outcome ideal or disappointing. Rhinoplasty surgeons must learn not only to execute the procedure but also to become skilled at accurately predicting further changes that will occur during the postoperative healing process. These skills are not developed rapidly, but are accumulated with experience as surgeons observe, study, and modify their surgical outcomes.

Patients with relatively minor deformities are almost always the best candidates for ideal rhinoplasty outcomes because less surgery is necessary to achieve the desired improvements. However, patients with minor deformities expect and demand perfection because of the minimal nature of the problem. Patients with deformities that demonstrate a significant departure from the aesthetic ideal (e.g., a large hump, an elongated drooping nose, a twisted nose) may be more likely to tolerate possible minor imperfections when the overall improvement is significant.

The final result of a rhinoplasty procedure is limited by both a patient's anatomy and the surgeon's skill. Accurately assessing the possibilities and limitations inherent in each patient is an absolute prerequisite to achieving consistently outstanding results while avoiding complications. No standard procedure suffices to reconstruct every nose perfectly. However, if the surgeon accurately analyzes the patient preoperatively and selectively applies fundamental techniques, rhinoplasty can be performed safely and effectively.

Diagnosis and Preoperative Evaluation

From the outset of the evaluation process, a patient's motivations and expectations must be clear. Cosmetic rhinoplasty patients should be capable of pointing out *exactly* what is disliked or in need of surgical alteration. Surgical possibilities and limitations are discussed with the patient. If anatomy restricts what is surgically achievable or the surgeon does not understand the problem, rhinoplasty is probably best not undertaken.

An orderly and instinctive visual evaluation of the nose and proportions of the surrounding facial features is essential. Balance and proportion combine to create the aesthetically pleasing face. Although no set of mechanical measurements may be used to define beauty, the rhinoplasty surgeon must possess the inner vision of the "ideal normal" when planning facial and nasal improvement.

Subsequent determination of what can be surgically achieved as limited by infinite variations in anatomy characterizes the experienced surgeon. The hallmarks of the nasal examination are inspection and palpation. It is helpful to conceive of the nose as being composed of a series of interrelated nasal anatomical components, which include the covering epithelium, the bony pyramid (maxillary ascending process, nasal bones, and bony septum), the cartilaginous pyramid (the quadrangular cartilage and attached upper lateral cartilages), and the mobile nasal tip (paired lower lateral cartilages and surrounding soft tissues). Topographic subunits within the nasal tip or base include the infratip lobule, the alae, and the columella.

Quality and thickness of the skin–subcutaneous complex contribute significantly to the eventual surgical outcome. Extremely thick skin that is rich in sebaceous glands and subcutaneous tissue may intrinsically provide nasal valve support, but it is the least ideal skin for achieving desirable refinement and definition. Thin skin with sparse subcutaneous tissue, although ideal for achieving critical definition, provides almost no cushion to hide even the most minute of skeletal irregularities or contour imperfections. The ideal skin type falls somewhere between these two extremes, being neither too thick and oily nor too thin and delicate. Evaluation of skin type is made by inspection and palpation, rolling the skin over the nasal skeleton and gently pinching it between the examining fingers.

Systematic analysis of the nose then begins cephalically. The length of the nasal bones may be palpably determined with relative ease. Step-offs or a depression may be palpable along the nasal bones if a previous fracture has occurred. When a hump is present, the bony-to-cartilaginous ratio can be estimated. Conversely, a saddle nose or inverted V deformity may be present when there is middle vault collapse or detachment of the upper lateral cartilages from the undersurface of the nasal bones. Middle vault width and symmetry are assessed as well.

In the lower third of the nose, it is essential to evaluate the critical factors relating to the inherent strength and support of the nasal tip. Finger depression of the tip toward the upper lip provides a quick and reliable test of the ability of the mobile tip structures to spring back into position. The size, shape, attitude, symmetry, and resilience of the lower lateral cartilages are estimated by both visualization and palpation. The adequacy and patency of the external nasal valve (bordered laterally by the alar rim and lateral crus of the lower lateral cartilage and medially by the septum) are assessed by palpation, as well as by observing for collapse during nasal inspiration. During this assessment, the surgeon makes the all-important decision on the need to surgically enhance, reduce, or carefully preserve the tip projection and lower lateral cartilages. Finally, the relationship of the nose to the remainder of the facial features and landmarks is evaluated. Specifically, the position and inclination of the nasofrontal and nasolabial angles, nasal axis, nasal width, nasal length, and nasal projection are considered. Facial asymmetries and adequacy of chin projection are noted as well.

The external inspection is supplemented by careful internal examination of the nasal cavities before and after shrinkage of the mucosa and turbinates. Once the nose is decongested, the surgeon can visualize subtle deflections of the nasal septum, mucosal abnormalities, the size and shape of the turbinates, and the condition of the nasal valves during quiet and forced inspiration. At the completion of the exam, the surgeon must make the patient aware of any and all limitations that his or her anatomy imposes on the desired surgical outcome.

Surgical Anatomy

Interpretation of a patient's individual surgical anatomy determines the ideal approach and technique. Reduction, augmentation, or reorientation of the individual anatomical components of the nose will produce the outcome of each surgical procedure. Conservative changes devoted to balancing the size and proportional relationships of these components during nasal surgery invariably lead to superior results.

Psychological Considerations

Critical to the successful outcome of any aesthetic operation is thorough communication between surgeon and patient. The surgeon must be assured that the patient's expectations about outcome are in fact realistic, that the motivations expressed are appropriate, and that the patient's anatomy is amenable to the desired changes. The patient, understandably anxious, must be reassured that a safe and relatively pain-free procedure can be performed, resulting in a natural and improved condition. Visual and written educational materials not only serve to inform and reassure patients, but also allow them to form a knowledge base from which may spring important questions in later discussions. Initially, the surgeon must be a good listener, drawing out the patient's concerns with open-ended and then more specific questions. It is critical both to learn why each individual seeks aesthetic surgical change and to understand what is expected.

■ Management

Anesthesia and Analgesia

Just as there exist multiple rhinoplasty techniques, there are varied approaches to nasal anesthesia and patient analgesia. Both general endotracheal and monitored intravenous analgesia with local topical and infiltration anesthesia are suitable for this operation. Adequate anesthesia will achieve the following goals during rhinoplasty: (1) a comfortable, relaxed, and responsive patient; (2) a bloodless operative field; and (3) minimal distortion of the nasal tissues.

Topical Decongestion

Before infiltration of local anesthesia, the nasal mucous membranes are decongested with 4% color-coded cocaine solution or 0.05% oxymetazoline, deposited in each nasal fossa on neurosurgical cottonoids. Although previously the topical agent of choice because of concurrent decongestant and anesthetic effects, cocaine is now used less frequently because of inherent risks of anesthetic complications and illicit diversion as well as decreased availability.

Infiltration Anesthesia

The goal of infiltration anesthesia is to render the nose completely anesthetic and intensely vasoconstricted, with the least possible distortion of normal anatomy. A 50:50 mix of 1% lidocaine and 0.25% bupivacaine with a 1:100,000 dilution of epinephrine, freshly mixed, is preferred for infiltration anesthesia. Except in unusual cases, a total of 5 to 8 mL of the solution, injected sparingly into the *proper surgical planes,* is sufficient to produce profound vasoconstriction and complete nasal anesthesia. No effort is made to block specific nerves. If septal reconstruction is to be performed, an additional 2 mL of the anesthetic is injected into the septal submucoperichondrial and subperiosteal planes to aid, by hydraulic dissection, the elevation of the septal flaps.

The infiltration of the local anesthetic is initiated by retracting the ala cephalically with thumb and forefinger, exposing the caudal edge of the upper lateral cartilage. A long 27-gauge needle is placed parallel to the long axis of the exposed upper lateral cartilage, and with a quick stabbing motion the needle penetrates the epithelium, usually with minimal sensation to the patient. Any sensation of the needlestick may be masqueraded by bluntly pinching the skin elsewhere in the face simultaneously, a technique referred to as "lateral inhibition." The needle is advanced along the lateral wall of the dorsum, hugging the perichondrium of the upper lateral cartilages and the periosteum of the nasal bones and remaining in the proper plane. Approximately 0.5 mL is deposited into this plane as the needle is withdrawn to, but not beyond, the point of initial penetration. The procedure is repeated over the dorsum and on the opposite side. Infiltration of the nasal base, columella, and tip follows. Anesthetic may now be deposited along the course of the lateral osteotomies, or if desired, may be delayed until later in the operation. The needle is inserted at the pyriform aperture near the insertion of the inferior turbinate and is advanced lateral and medial to the ascending process, depositing 0.5 mL on either side. A vasoconstricted pathway for the lateral osteotomy is thus established. Infiltration of the nasal septum follows.

Following infiltration anesthesia, it is critical to wait 10 to 15 minutes before proceeding with the operation, allowing vasoconstriction to reach its maximal effectiveness. This method of infiltration anesthesia ensures patient comfort, provides for constant patient monitoring, limits the number of needle penetrations, minimizes the amount of anesthetic required, and avoids tissue distortion. In the vast majority of operations, little if any bleeding occurs during the procedure, and postoperative ecchymosis is minimal or nonexistent. All of these factors help to permit the precise, bloodless dissection of nasal structures that is essential for the carefully controlled rhinoplasty operation.

General Anesthesia

Modern general endotracheal anesthesia is safe and preferable to conscious sedation for performance of most rhinoplasties. A cuffed endotracheal tube protects the airway from potential hemorrhage when concurrently performing septal or turbinate work. When compared with primarily reductive rhinoplasty performed in past decades, contemporary rhinoplasty favors techniques that maintain and reinforce cartilage structure; such techniques inevitably increase operative time. Grafting needs frequently demand cartilage harvest from a second site (e.g., ear, rib). General anesthesia seems most appropriate for these longer procedures involving multiple operative sites.

Operative Technique

Topographic Landmark Identification

Before infiltrating the nose with local anesthesia that may distort landmarks, sketching the topography of the nasal skeleton on the nasal surface to indicate key landmarks is especially helpful for the neophyte surgeon. It reinforces a thoughtful preview, through palpation and inspection, of the location and size of the individual nasal anatomical components to be modified. Critical decisions about planned tissue excision, augmentation, and reorientation of nasal structures can thereby be supported visually on the nose itself.

Nasal Tip

Experienced surgeons regard surgery of the nasal tip as the most challenging and exacting aspect of rhinoplasty. The surgeon is confronted by nasal anatomical components essentially bilateral (demanding symmetrical surgical technique and healing), animate, and mobile. These may require reduction, enhancement, or simply preservation of existing structure.

Surgeons have gradually come to understand that radical excision, division, and extensive sacrifice of alar cartilages and other tip support mechanisms all too frequently result in unpredictable healing, unnatural results, and the potential for airway compromise. No routine tip procedure can be applied to all patients. Instead, techniques are tailored to the tip anatomy of each individual patient. It is important to assess several factors prior to selecting the appropriate tip procedure. The surgeon must determine whether the tip requires any of the following:

- A change in the attitude and orientation of the alar cartilages
- A change in tip projection
- A change in tip rotation

Tip Support Mechanisms

Alteration of the nasal tip cannot be successfully undertaken, let alone mastered, until one appreciates the major and minor tip support mechanisms. In the majority of patients, the *major tip support mechanisms* consist of the following:

- Size, shape, and thickness of the lower lateral cartilages
- Attachment of the medial crural footplates to the caudal septum
- Attachment of the upper lateral cartilages to the lower lateral cartilages

Compensatory reestablishment of stable tip support with grafting must occur during the operation if any or all of these major tip support mechanisms are significantly compromised.

Minor tip support mechanisms—which in certain anatomical and ethnic configurations may assume a *major* support role—include the following:

- Dorsal cartilaginous septum
- Interdomal ligament
- Membranous septum
- Nasal spine
- Investing skin and soft tissues
- Alar sidewalls

A graduated, incremental, and anatomical approach to tip surgery with a focus on maintenance (and, when necessary, reconstruction) of support mechanisms is prudent to achieve consistent results. Conservative reduction of the volume of the cephalic margin of the lateral crus is a time-tested and simple technique that will decrease bulbosity and tip size. This technique alone may be the preferred operation in individuals in whom nasal tip changes need not be profound. As the tip deformity encountered becomes more abnormal, more aggressive techniques are required, from vertical dome division to lateral crural strut grafts that alter the tip and alar contour.

Rhinoplasty incisions and approaches are planned that will provide the minimum exposure needed to execute the selected tip refinement technique and also *preserve as many tip supports as possible.* In nasal tips where only very conservative volume reduc-

tion is indicated, endonasal nondelivery approaches allow the surgeon to make subtle changes with minimal disturbance of normal structures. The two endonasal nondelivery approaches are transcartilaginous and retrograde. Delivery approaches, both endonasal and external (i.e., open), offer greater access to the lower lateral cartilages but are more disruptive of tip support mechanisms. All approaches are performed in the relatively avascular subsuperficial musculoaponeurotic system (SMAS) plane over the lower lateral cartilages.

Endonasal Transcartilaginous Approach

Because of its atraumatic simplicity and ease of employment, the transcartilaginous approach is preferred when conservative tip refinement is indicated. This approach is useful in patients whose tip anatomy is fundamentally satisfactory, requiring only volume reduction to accomplish a thinning sculpture of the cephalic-medial margin of the lateral crus, preserving a generous residual complete strip. The initial incision penetrates only the vestibular skin underlying the lateral crus; the skin flap is easily dissected and preserved before continuing the incision through the alar cartilage.

Endonasal Retrograde Approach

This conservative, atraumatic approach is similar to the transcartilaginous approach, except that an intercartilaginous incision is used, dissecting beneath the vestibular skin flap in retrograde fashion to expose and reduce the size of the alar cartilage.

Endonasal Alar Cartilage Delivery Approach

Delivering the alar cartilages as individual bipedicled chondrocutaneous, or "bucket handle," flaps allows more exposure of the anatomy when the tip cartilages are asymmetric or in need of more significant alterations. Although more refinement is possible with this approach, it is also more traumatic. Delivering the alar cartilages is useful when nasal tip bulbosity or bifidity exists, when the paired domal angles are excessively broad, and when alar cartilage asymmetry exists. Performed through intercartilaginous and marginal incisions, delivery of the alar cartilages provides a binocular view of the tip anatomy and affords the added ease of bimanual surgical modification. If on frontal and basal views the alar cartilages flare or diverge unpleasantly, if tip triangularity is unsatisfactory, or if the tip appears too amorphous and bulbous, a delivery approach should be considered. Transdomal suture narrowing of broad domes as well as vertical dome division can be performed through the endonasal delivery approach.

External (Open) Approach

The external or open approach to the nasal tip is in reality a more aggressive form of the delivery approach, requiring an external incision across the waist of the columella. It is the approach of choice for more significant nasal tip deformities. The anatomical view is unparalleled through this approach, affording the surgeon diagnostic information unavailable through traditional closed approaches. These technical virtues must be balanced with the potential disadvantages of an external scar, delayed healing with prolonged tip edema, and increased operative time. The open approach is facilitated by bilateral marginal incisions that are carried down the columella along the caudal aspects of the intermediate and medial crura to the site of the external columellar incision. The open approach facilitates the suturing of cartilage grafts to the tip and dorsum and allows unparalleled assessment and correction of tip asymmetries. The external approach is also invaluable for difficult revision surgery.

Tip Sculpting Techniques

The choice of technique for modifying the alar cartilages and the relationship of the nasal tip to the remaining nasal structures should be based entirely on the anatomy encountered and the predicted result desired as defined from the known dynamics of long-term healing. The astonishing diversity of tip anatomy encountered demands a broad diversification of surgical planning and execution.

Five categories of nasal tip sculpturing procedures may be identified. Although additional subtle technical variations exist, these include the following:

1. Volume reduction (i.e., cephalic trim) with residual complete strip
2. Suture techniques (e.g., interdomal and intradomal)
3. Vertical dome division with interrupted (e.g., Goldman technique) or reestablished strip
4. Lateral crural grafting (e.g., lateral crural strut grafts)
5. Tip grafting (e.g., shield and Peck grafts)

Each of these techniques can be used alone or, more frequently, in combination with other techniques.

Cephalic Trim

A conservative cephalic trim that preserves an adequate intact residual alar cartilage strip is always preferred over more aggressive techniques to achieve subtle volume reduction. A cephalic trim can be performed via either a nondelivery or a delivery approach. A portion (typically 2–3 mm) of the cephalic margin

of the lateral crus and dome is excised, ideally leaving an intact strip 8 mm or greater in width and preserving the underlying vestibular skin. The normal contour and shape of the cartilage are retained, while its overall size is reduced. If a delivery approach is used, this technique is frequently combined with interdomal suturing that will further refine the tip and maintain tip projection.

Interdomal and Intradomal Sutures

Suture techniques can refine nasal tips with broad domal angles and bifidity of the intermediate crura that impart a bulky, trapezoidal configuration to the tip shape. Separate intradomal horizontal mattress sutures that span each dome will narrow the tip-defining points and decrease convexity in the lateral crurae. Care must be taken to ensure that lateral crural concavity does not result when performing this maneuver. Such concavity will create shadows between the tip and alar subunits, giving the tip the undesirable appearance of a ball. Additionally, external valve compromise may occur. A trans- or interdomal suture is then placed, which will provide narrowing and some tip support. Some surgeons advocate a single complex horizontal mattress suture that spans both domes and brings them together in one step. This is more likely to produce concavity and deformation of the lateral crurae and should be avoided.

Vertical Dome Division

The integrity of the residual complete strip cannot always be maintained due to more profound abnormalities and asymmetries encountered in certain unusual tip configurations, including marked overprojection, severe underprojection, and/or asymmetry. In these instances, the alar cartilage must be interrupted in a vertical fashion somewhere along its extent to achieve maximal refinement, decrease projection, and increase or reduce tip rotation. Early surgeons who performed dome division left the strip interrupted, but more contemporary techniques involve division, modification, and reestablishment of strip continuity.

Vertical dome division must be performed through a delivery approach. The risks of asymmetric healing are greater when interrupted strips are created, and initial loss of tip support occurs immediately. Via a delivery approach, the alar cartilages are presented and an initial cephalic trim is typically performed. Vertical division of the strip is performed at the medial, intermediate, or lateral crus, depending on desired impact. Shortening the strip by either overlapping or removing a vertical segment and reapproximating end to end will effect changes that can be anticipated based on the tripod concept.

Division and shortening of the medial crus result in decreased tip projection and rotation. Intermediate crus division and shortening narrow the tip-defining point and may decrease projection. Lateral crus division and shortening increase tip rotation and may decrease projection. Vestibular skin is meticulously preserved. Stabilizing sutures effect final tip reconfiguration, and grafting (e.g., columellar strut) may be necessary to maintain the desired tip projection.

Lateral Crural Strut Grafting

Lateral crural strut grafting is a contemporary technique that can be used to more predictably control tip shape by flattening a convex lateral crus while maintaining adequate external nasal valve support. Cartilage graft size is based on what is necessary to make desired changes, but it averages 20 × 5 mm. Vestibular skin is dissected off of the medial surface of the lateral crurae, and a subcutaneous pocket is created under each alar crease. The grafts are inserted into the pockets and under the lateral crurae, keeping the caudal edge of the graft near the caudal border of the crurae. The medial end of the graft sits at the desired location of the tip-defining point under the dome. The graft is mattress sutured to the lateral crus. Intradomal sutures can then be placed to narrow the tip-defining point and flatten the lateral crus without creating concavity or external valve deficiency.

Tip Grafting

Tip grafts are onlay grafts designed to increase projection and narrow the nasal tip. These grafts are useful in patients with medium-thickness or thicker skin that will camouflage graft edges. Tip onlay grafts should be placed with great caution or avoided altogether in patients with thinner skin. Peck grafts are rectangular grafts placed over the domes and tip-defining points. Shield grafts are placed at the caudal border of the intermediate crurae and positioned vertically, with the wider protruding edge defining the tip.

Tip Rotation

Altering or maintaining rotation of the nasal tip is essential for patients undergoing rhinoplasty. Selecting the desired degree of tip rotation is dependent on the following factors:

- Length of the nose
- Length of the face
- Height of the patient
- Length of the upper lip
- Patient's aesthetic desires
- Surgeon's aesthetic judgment

The surgeon must understand the difference between tip projection and tip rotation. Both are best analyzed on profile view. Projection is the distance the tip extends anteriorly parallel to the Frankfort horizontal line from the anterior facial plane. Rotation is the location the tip rests along—an arc between the lip and nasal dorsum. The nasolabial angle is defined by the degree of rotation present. Increasing rotation implies cephalic movement along this arc, whereas decreasing rotation refers to caudal movement. Ideally, the nasolabial angle will be 95 to 105 degrees for women and 90 to 95 degrees for men. Taller patients are less tolerant of higher degrees of rotation than shorter patients. Tip rotation and projection are complementary to each other, and their proper achievement in individual patients is constantly interrelated. Certain tip-rotation techniques will result in concurrent changes in tip projection, whereas others will not.

Essentially no cephalic tip rotation results from minimal volume reduction alone because the complete strip tends to resist cephalic rotation. Overly aggressive cephalic reduction results in a greater tissue void that may produce cephalic rotation due to scarring during healing. When complete strip techniques are selected, increasing tip rotation depends on the addition of other techniques to achieve the desired tip rotation. Tip rotation can be increased with vertical dome division in the lateral crus, as previously described. Tip position can be reset to either decrease or increase rotation and projection by securing the medial crurae to the caudal border of either the native septum or a caudal septal extension graft (i.e., "tongue-in-groove technique"); in this situation, rotation and nasal length will be entirely dependent on the caudal length of the native or modified septum. A columellar strut will increase rotation to a lesser degree. Plumping grafts placed at the base of the columella will blunt the nasolabial angle and create a beneficial illusion of rotation in select patients.

Tip Projection

In addition to the creation of narrowing refinement and symmetry of the operated nasal tip, appropriate tip projection must be preserved or created anew to set the tip subtly but distinctly apart from the nasal supratip region. This is referred to as the supratip break. Columellar struts will increase or preserve tip projection and are placed between the medial crura in a pocket that extends to just short of the maxillary spine. Projection can be significantly increased or decreased by setting the medial crura onto the native or modified caudal septum with a tongue-in-groove technique. Onlay grafts, such as the previously described shield and Peck grafts, provide quantifiable increased tip projection and are suitable for patients with medium-thickness or thicker skin.

A nose that projects too far beyond the anterior facial plane results in significant facial disharmony. Preoperative analysis of chin projection is imperative to help make this determination. A deficient chin will make the nose appear more protrusive and may limit the potential outcome if left untreated. Accurate diagnosis leads to the development of a logical individualized strategy for correction that may include concurrent chin augmentation and rhinoplasty. In almost every instance, weakening or reducing normal tip support mechanisms is required to initiate retroprojection. A complete transfixion incision alone that divides the medial crural footplates from the caudal septum will decrease projection slightly. Vertical dome division of the medial and/or lateral crurae will typically reduce projection as well. Substantial retropositioning of the overprojected nose may lead to alar base flaring that will necessitate an alar base reduction procedure to normalize the appearance.

Nasal Dorsum

Comparable surgical access to the nasal dorsum can be gained through the transcartilaginous, intercartilaginous, or external approach. As mentioned, the approach is selected based primarily on the exposure needed for tip refinement. If an endonasal approach is used, the incision is extended around the anterior septal angle as a partial transfixion incision for a distance of 5 to 8 mm to provide full visualization of the nasal dorsum. Routine complete transfixion incisions are unnecessary. Elevation is continued deep to the SMAS over the middle vault, and then subperiosteal over the nasal bones. Elevation of the tissue flap in this relatively avascular plane preserves the thickest possible epithelial soft tissue covering to ultimately cushion the newly formed bony and cartilaginous profile. Only sufficient skin is elevated to gain access to the profile, avoiding more traditional wide lateral undermining techniques.

Profile Alignment

Three anatomical nasal components are responsible for the preoperative profile appearance: (1) the nasal bones, (2) the cartilaginous cartilages, and (3) the alar cartilages. Generally, all three must undergo modification to create a natural profile alignment. The surgeon visualizes in the mind's eye the ultimate intended profile extending from the nasofrontal angle to the tip-defining point. The extent of reduction of bone, cartilage, and soft tissue will always depend on and be guided by stable tip projection; thus positioning the projection of the tip at the outset of the operative procedure is beneficial.

Because the thickness of the investing soft tissues and skin varies at different areas of the profile and from patient to patient, dissimilar portions of cartilage and bone constituting the nasal hump must be removed to result ultimately in a straight profile line.

Either of two methods of profile alignment are preferred: incremental or en bloc. In the former method the cartilaginous dorsum is reduced by incremental shaving maneuvers of the cartilaginous profile until an ideal tip–supratip relationship is established, followed by sharp osteotome removal of the residual bony hump. If en bloc hump removal is contemplated, the knife is positioned caudal to the osseocartilaginous junction as distal as the anterior septal angle as indicated. The knife is then advanced toward the nasal bones, removing the desired amount of the cartilaginous dorsum. In a large cartilaginous profile reduction, a portion of the upper lateral cartilage attachment to the quadrangular cartilage will of necessity be removed with the dorsal septum, leaving these two cartilaginous components attached by the intact underlying mucoperichondrial bridge. A sharp Rubin osteotome (honed to razor sharpness at the operating table), seated in the opening made by the knife at the osseocartilaginous junction, is driven gently cephalically to remove the desired degree of bony hump in continuity with the cartilaginous hump. The hump is then removed en bloc as a single segment.

Any irregularities remaining are corrected under direct vision with a knife or sharp tungsten rasp. Palpating the skin of the dorsum with the examining finger moistened with peroxide will often provide clues to unseen irregularities, as will intranasal palpation of the newly created profile with the noncutting edge of the no. 15 blade.

In patients in whom the nasofrontal angle is very deep, augmentation with residual septal cartilage grafts or remnants of the excised alar cartilages provides a beneficial aesthetic refinement, raising the radix such that the dorsum does not have to be lowered excessively to achieve a straight profile.

Cartilage spreader grafts should be strongly considered in most cases following dorsal reduction to maintain the middle nasal vault appearance and integrity over time. The spreader grafts are either sutured or placed submucosally into tight pockets between the septum and upper lateral cartilages. In a crooked nose, asymmetric spreader graft placement may be necessary to help straighten the nose with thicker or multiple grafts placed on the deficient side.

Bony Pyramid

Osteotomies, the most traumatic of all surgical maneuvers during rhinoplasty, are best delayed until the final step in the planned surgical sequence, when vasoconstriction exerts its maximal influence and the nasal splint may be promptly positioned. Swelling and ecchymosis are thus diminished or avoided entirely.

During the typical reduction rhinoplasty, hump removal inevitably results in an excessive plateau-like width to the nasal dorsum, requiring narrowing of the bony and cartilaginous pyramids to restore a natural, more narrow frontal appearance to the operated nose.

The lateral bony sidewalls (consisting of the nasal bones and maxillary ascending processes), must be completely mobilized by nongreenstick fractures and moved medially (exceptions may exist in older patients with more fragile bones, in whom green-stick fractures may be acceptable, or even prefer-able, to prevent excessive instability of more brittle bones). The upper lateral cartilages are also moved medially because of their stable attachment cephali-cally to the undersurface of the nasal bones.

Medial Osteotomies

To facilitate atraumatic low lateral osteotomy execu-tion, medial-oblique osteotomies angled laterally 15 to 20 degrees from the vertical midline are preferred, unless the bones are very short or thin. By creating an osteotomy dehiscence at the intended cephalic apex of the lateral osteotomy, the surgeon exerts added control of the exact site of back fracture in the lateral bony sidewall during low lateral osteotomy.

A 2 to 3 mm unguarded sharp micro-osteotome is positioned intranasally at the cephalic extent of the removal of the bony hump. In some cases of substan-tial bony hump removal, a medial osteotomy may not be necessary at all. If there has been no nasal hump removal, the site of osteotome positioning is at the caudal extent of the nasal bones in the midline. The osteotome is driven cephalomedially to the intended osteotomy apex at an angle of 15 to 20 degrees, depending on the shape of the nasal bony sidewall. Little trauma results from medial-oblique osteoto-mies, which prevent the ever-present possibility of eccentric or asymmetrical surgical fractures devel-oping when lateral osteotomies alone are performed.

Lateral Osteotomies

Employing a small osteotome to accomplish the desired infracture of the lateral bony sidewalls results in a significant reduction of surgical trauma. Furthermore, there is no need for traditional eleva-tion of the periosteum along the pathway of the lat-eral fractures because the small osteotomes require little space for their cephalic progression. Appropri-ately, the intact periosteum stabilizes and internally splints the complete fractures, facilitating controlled and precise healing.

The high-low-high curved lateral osteotomy is initiated by pressing the sharp osteotome through the vestibular skin to encounter the bony margin of the pyriform aperture at or just above the inferior turbinate attachment. Beginning the osteotomy at this site preserves the bony sidewall width along the floor of the nose (where narrowing would achieve no favorable aesthetic improvement but might compro-mise the lower nasal airway without purpose). The osteotome is then driven in a slightly curved direc-tion, first toward the base of the maxilla, then curv-ing up along the nasomaxillary junction to encounter the previously created medial-oblique osteotomy. A complete, controlled, and atraumatic fracture of the bony sidewall is thus created, allowing infracture without excessively traumatic infracture pressure maneuvers. Immediate finger pressure is applied bilaterally over the lateral osteotomy sites to fore-stall any further extravasation of blood into the soft tissues. In reality, no bleeding ordinarily occurs dur-ing lateral osteotomy performance, because the soft tissues embracing the bony sidewalls remain essen-tially undamaged by the diminutive osteotomes.

In the majority of rhinoplasty procedures, con-trolled nasal fractures as the result of osteotomies should create definite mobility of the bony sidewalls, stabilized by the internal and external periosteum that bridges the nasal fragments on either side of the osteotomy pathway. Large guarded osteotomes destroy this vital periosteal sling, potentially render-ing the bony fragments unstable and susceptible to eccentric or asymmetric healing.

Intermediate Osteotomies

In deviated noses characterized by convex or concave bony asymmetries, or excessively wide or extremely thick bones (including certain revision rhinoplas-ties), an intermediate osteotomy may be necessary for improved mobilization and regularization of the nasal bony sidewalls. In such cases, the higher (more anterior) osteotomy cut should be accomplished prior to the lower lateral osteotomy.

Alar Reduction Techniques

Usually the final step in the sequence of surgi-cal steps in rhinoplasty, alar base reduction, and sculpturing must be considered when the alae flare excessively or are asymmetric. Alar wedge excisions of various geometric designs and dimensions are necessary to improve nasal balance and harmony. These excision dimensions are determined by the present and intended shape of the nostril aperture, the degree and attitude of the lateral alar flare, the width and shape of the nostril sill, and the thickness of the alae.

The incision should be sited 1 to 2 mm above the alar–facial crease, rather than placing the incision exactly within the crease. This allows improved suture repair and significantly diminishes the appearance of any suture marks following healing.

Nasal Toilette, Dressings, and Splint

These final maneuvers are effected with an assistant maintaining constant finger pressure over the lateral osteotomy sites to prevent even minimal oozing and intraoperative swelling.

All incisions are now closed completely with 4–0 or 5–0 chromic catgut sutures. The transcolumellar incisions used in the open approach require *meticulous* closure with 6–0 suture. Nasal dressings are immediately applied. No intranasal dressing or packing is necessary in routine rhinoplasty. If septoplasty has been an integral part of the operation, a folded strip of Telfa is placed into each nostril along the floor of the nose to absorb any drainage, and is removed prior to patient discharge.

The external splint consists of a layer of compressed Gelfoam (Pfizer, New York, NY) placed along the dorsum and stabilized in place with flesh-colored Micropore tape (3M, St. Paul, MN), extending over and laterally beyond the lateral osteotomy sites. A thermoplastic splint is then cut to size and placed gently over the nose. This can be covered with an additional layer of brown paper tape for camouflage if desired.

Postoperative Care

The patient is discharged the day of surgery and is instructed to keep the head elevated at least 30 degrees for at least 72 hours if possible. Ice packs can be applied around the eyes as needed for bruising and swelling during the first 48 hours. Routine incision care includes cleaning and application of petroleum jelly to the columella at least two to three times daily. All patients are instructed to begin using saline mist four times daily starting the day after surgery.

The first postoperative visit typically takes place 5 to 7 days after surgery. At this visit, the thermoplastic splint and columellar sutures are removed. The patient is reassured about postoperative swelling that may require weeks or months to subside. A return visit is scheduled within 2 to 4 weeks. If septal or turbinate work has been done, the patient is instructed to continue using saline mist in the nose three to four times daily until the next appointment.

Complications

Early complications following rhinoplasty are unusual but include hemorrhage and infection. Hematomas are most common beneath septal mucoperichondrial flaps and can typically be evacuated in the clinic. If infection is identified, it must be treated aggressively with antibiotics. Cultures are obtained of purulent drainage to rule out resistant bacteria. Surgical clean-out and debridement are required if symptoms do not rapidly improve.

Late complications of rhinoplasty typically fall into one of two categories: (1) airway obstruction or (2) aesthetic deformity. Because healing and resolution of edema occur slowly following rhinoplasty surgery, patients are asked to wait several months if surgical revision will be required. Most patients will accept this process and understand the necessity if the surgeon is empathic, informative, and responsive to their concerns.

■ Controversy

Although there are many potential areas of controversy in rhinoplasty surgery, perhaps none is greater and more persistent than that of the open versus closed approach. This incision has undoubtedly provoked more discussion than any other! There are some expert surgeons who will maintain that every nose can and should be done by one method or the other. The bottom line for most is that there are some noses that would best be done open and some closed, and that the surgeon should feel comfortable with either approach as needed.

■ Summary

Rhinoplasty surgery is challenging, but it will often have satisfactory results if performed after thoughtful analysis and careful application of the fundamental techniques described in this chapter. The most conservative approaches and techniques for achieving desired changes are always preferable to unnecessarily aggressive maneuvers, which are more likely to result in unpredictable healing and complications. When functional or aesthetic complications do arise, most properly counseled patients are accepting when the surgeon is responsive to their concerns. Acquiring experience with constant attention to one's own outcomes is essential to improving surgical results over time.

■ Suggested Reading

Adamson PA, Litner JA, Dahiya R. The M-Arch model: a new concept of nasal tip dynamics. Arch Facial Plast Surg 2006;8(1):16–25

Anderson JR, Ries WR, eds. Rhinoplasty: Emphasizing the External Approach. New York, NY: Thieme; 1986

Gunter JP, Friedman RM. Lateral crural strut graft: technique and clinical applications in rhinoplasty. Plast Reconstr Surg 1997; 99(4):943–952, discussion 953–955

Johnson CM, Toriumi DM, eds. Open Structure Rhinoplasty. Philadelphia, PA: WB Saunders; 1990

Sheen JH, Sheen A, eds. Aesthetic Rhinoplasty. 2nd ed. St. Louis, MO: Mosby–Year Book; 1998

Tardy ME. Rhinoplasty: The Art and the Science. Philadelphia, PA: WB Saunders; 1997

Tardy ME, Brown RJ, eds. Surgical Anatomy of the Nose. New York, NY: Raven; 1990

Toriumi DM. New concepts in nasal tip contouring. Arch Facial Plast Surg 2006;8(3):156–185

105 Implants for Facial Plastic Surgery

■ Introduction

In addition to the need to correct traumatic and congenital defects in the head and neck region, cosmetic volume enhancements have stimulated the development of biomaterials for aesthetic and reconstructive surgery of the face. Autogenous tissue has long been the gold standard for reconstruction in the head region. More recently, synthetic biomaterials have become more readily available and often provide an alternative to autogenous tissue. Each biomaterial contains unique properties that make it suitable for specific and varied applications within the head and neck region.

■ Evaluation

Preoperative Assessment

During the preoperative phase, several factors should be accounted for when considering the use of implants. For the patient seeking cosmetic improvements of the face, to enhance symmetry or add volume the surgeon must carefully examine all aspects of the patient's soft tissue envelope and underling bony structure. Close attention should be paid to areas of asymmetry. A working understanding of the general aesthetic of the area is necessary. Photo documentation is often helpful during this process. When implants are used for reconstructive indications, deficiencies in the bone may be best evaluated with the use of computed tomography (CT). Three-dimensional (3D) CT scans can also be used to assist with evaluating the extent of the defect in addition to manufacturing implants with specific dimensions.

When preparing to place implants in the head and neck area, the surgeon should fully assess the patient's capacity for proper wound healing. Patients with irradiated tissue at the recipient site are often poor candidates for implants due to changes in vascularity and fibrosis in irradiated tissue, increasing the likelihood of tissue breakdown and implant extrusion. Additionally, patients with diabetes, tobacco use, or immunosuppression are at increased risk for wound infection or implant extrusion. As a result, patients should be encouraged to eliminate tobacco use as well as medically optimize diabetes and autoimmune diseases to improve wound healing.

Preoperative Counseling

The importance of proper preoperative counseling cannot be overemphasized when planning for reconstructive or cosmetic surgery. The risks of implantation should be discussed, including infection, malposition, and extrusion of the implant.

■ Implant Materials

When one is deciding on the best implant material to use, the main issues to consider are biocompatibility, strength, and pliability. Biocompatibility is determined by the physical characteristics of the implant and subsequent interaction with the surrounding tissues. Biocompatibility is a key factor in implant degradation and extrusion. Strength is determined by the implant's ability to withstand mechanical stress. Pliability is important for implants placed in locations with exposure to varying directional forces.

Concepts of Biocompatibility

Biocompatibility is one of the most important concepts when choosing an implant. Within hours of placement, the implant becomes coated with a layer of host proteins. The amount and composition of these proteins contribute to the inflammatory reaction that results. Hydrophobic interactions with the absorbed proteins that have accumulated on the surface of the implant can trigger an inflammatory cascade. To increase an implant's biocompatibility, the surface can be modified to reduce adherence of proteins, and thereby reduce the inflammatory cascade.

Metals and Metal Alloys

Historically, the most common metals used for implants in the head and neck area have been gold, platinum, stainless steel, titanium, and high-alloyed versions.

Properties

Stainless steel and stainless steel alloys are not as commonly used due to their potential for in vivo corrosion, resulting in the formation of granulation tissue. On the other hand, titanium has properties that resist corrosion, placing it among the most biocompatible of metals in use today. Other beneficial properties of titanium include a very low mass and the potential for osseointegration, which makes it a popular choice for facial plating systems. The elasticity of titanium also corresponds most closely to that of bone, which prevents stress shielding. Gold is the most chemically inert of metal implants, but it is extremely pliable, which makes it less suitable for areas of high mechanical stress.

Indications

Metal and metal alloy implants are often used for wires, reconstruction bars, fracture plates and screws, orbital floor implants, and eyelid weights.

Advantages

The advantage of metal implants used in the head and neck is a good balance of strength and elasticity. Titanium, in particular, has elastic properties that are compatible with bone. Additionally, gold is chemically inert, which results in minimal tissue reactivity, and makes it favorable for implantation in sensitive areas, such as the eyelid.

Disadvantages

The disadvantages of metal implants include the risk of corrosion and implant failure due to mechanical stress. Stainless steel is particularly susceptible to fatigue and weakness, causing implant failure. Gold is very pliable and therefore not suitable for areas of high mechanical stress.

Polymers

Polymers are macromolecules made up of repeating and cross-linking monomeric units. The different degrees of cross-linking determine the characteristic of the polymer, varying from pliable to hard and brittle.

Properties

Polymers exist in both resorbable and nonresorbable forms. The resorbable polymers, mainly poly-L-lactic acid, are used in the form of resorbable plates and screws. Nonresorbable polymers include silicone and polyurethane, which are often used for soft tissue augmentation. Some polymers used for soft tissue augmentation, such as porous polyethylene (Medpor, Stryker, Kalamazoo, MI), have perforations that allow for vascular and bony ingrowth. Studies have shown vascular ingrowth after 1 week and bony ingrowth after 3 weeks. Vascular and bony ingrowth stabilizes the implant, thus minimizing the implant's potential for migration.

Indications

Resorbable polymer plates and screws are commonly used in pediatrics for the reconstruction of facial fractures. Silicone is commonly used for soft tissue augmentation for both cosmetic and reconstructive applications.

Advantages

An important advantage of polymer implants is that their shape can be easily modified intraoperatively to accommodate the patient's and surgeon's needs. Polymers can be more flexible than bone, which is advantageous in areas that experience multidirectional forces, such as the midface. More recent technology allows polymers to be prefabricated into desired shapes and dimensions. Another important property of polymers is excellent bioavailability, which reduces tissue reactivity.

Disadvantages

The main disadvantage of polymer implants is the risk that internal defects acquired during molding can weaken the implant, causing failure in the long term.

Ceramics

Properties

Glass ceramics are bioactive, meaning that they induce osteostimulation at the surface of the glass ceramic and bone interface, creating a strong bond between the implant and surrounding bone. Hydroxyapatite is the ceramic that is most commonly used within the head and neck because of its ability to bond to surrounding bone.

Indications

Hydroxyapatite is used in dental implants, as a bone substitute in genioplasty, and for alveolar ridge augmentation. Additionally, hydroxyapatite is commonly used as a semipermanent subcutaneous filler or volumizer.

Advantages

The most unique advantage of hydroxyapatite is that it is osteoconductive and can be used as a substrate for osteointegration.

Disadvantages

Glass ceramics are fragile and are inappropriate for implantation in load-bearing areas, because they are prone to fracture.

Bioactive Cements

Properties

Bioactive cements comprise various combinations of hydroxyapatite and calcium phosphates. Hydroxyapatite is found as a natural component of teeth and is therefore highly biocompatible. Calcium phosphates occur naturally in the body as a component of hydroxyapatite, so they do not cause any inflammatory response or foreign body reaction. They have also been shown to be osseoconductive, which allows for ingrowth of bone into the implantation site.

Indications

Hydroxyapatite cement is used as bone filler for cranioplasty. Due to its bone-stimulating properties, it can also be used for bone substitute in genioplasty and alveolar ridge augmentation.

Advantages

Hydroxyapatite cement can be constituted in the operating room, which allows for molding into the desired implant shape. This makes it an ideal material for contoured bony defects. Studies have shown that hydroxyapatite induces bone growth at the implant site.

Disadvantages

Hydroxyapatite has poor flexibility and can be brittle, so it is best chosen for areas of low mechanical stress.

Bone and Cartilage

Properties

Autologous and heterologous bone and cartilage are commonly used substrates in the head and neck region. They have complete biological integration and biocompatibility. Allograft bone is harvested from cadavers and implanted after it has been industrially sterilized and denatured, but it retains the matrix of bone. Xenograft bone is usually of bovine origin.

Indications

Cartilage is the graft material of choice in nasal reconstruction. It can also be used in multiple areas of the head and neck to add bulk and support.

Advantages

Both bone and cartilage have complete biointegration as well as the capacity for growth with the patient.

Disadvantages

The risks of using autologous bone and cartilage are complications at the donor site, limited graft available for harvest at the donor site, and potential for resorption. Due to this risk of resorption, autologous bone is not used in facial augmentation or reconstruction of large aesthetic defects.

■ Management

When considering placement of an implant into a specific area of the head or neck, one must consider the need to withstand mechanical stress, the necessity for flexibility or pliability, and the size of the defect that must be reconstructed. These factors will narrow the options one has to choose from when selecting an implant.

Skull

When considering reconstruction of skull defects, the options for reconstruction include autologous bone, split calvarial bone grafts, polymethyl methacrylate (PMMA), hydroxyapatite, expanded porous polyethylene, and polyetheretherketone (PEEK).

As previously discussed, the gold standard in reconstructing skull defects has been native autologous bone graft because of its potential for growth and integration with host cells, as well as a low risk of infection. The main disadvantages are complications at the donor site, resorption of the graft resulting in contour irregularities, and scarring. The use of calvarial bone is limited in pediatric patients because their calvarial bone is thin and lacks a diploic space necessary for safe graft harvest.

Porous polyethylene and PEEK are alloplastic implants that are commonly used for the reconstruction of large calvarial defects because of their ability for fibrous ingrowth, decreased risk of infection, and potential for excellent contouring. Fine-cut 3D CT scan is used to create an implant specific to the defect. The benefits of porous polyethylene include avoidance of donor site complications and excellent contouring. The risks include infection, implant extrusion, and restriction of calvarial growth in pediatric patients.

Ear and Temporal Bone

Trauma, ablative procedures, or congenital deformities are the most common indications for auricular reconstruction. Depending on the location and extent of the deformity, autologous cartilage (ear, septal, or costochondral) or synthetic implant materials can be used for reconstruction. The primary alternative to autologous materials is premolded porous polyethylene (Medpor) implants. The benefits of using Medpor are better definition and projection, congruency with the normal ear, no donor site morbidity, and the need for only one operation. The risks for using Medpor include infection, skin necrosis, and extrusion that can occur months or even years after completing the reconstruction.

Midface

Many autogenous implants are available for the midface, including fat grafts, cartilage, and bone. The benefits of autologous implants are biocompatibility and lack of inflammatory reaction. The disadvantages include donor site morbidity, resorption, and less precise contouring than prefabricated synthetic implants.

Moldable implants, such as silicone and porous polytetrafluoroethylene, are often used with good success. The most common approach for placement into the midface is through an intraoral incision through which a submalar space is created over the face of the maxilla. The implant can be secured using either screws or external fixation.

Nose

Autologous cartilage is the most common implant used in reconstruction of the nose. Cartilage can be harvested from the septum, concha, or rib. Autogenous cartilage can be used for a multitude of grafting materials. The advantages of autologous cartilage are abundant and include minimal inflammatory reaction, as well as good integration with surrounding tissue. The main disadvantage is donor site morbidity.

In patients who may be poor candidates or are unwilling to consider autologous grafts, alternative implant materials can be considered. Common choices for nasal implants include silicone, Medpor, and Gore-Tex (W.L. Gore and Associates, Inc., Newark, DE). Medpor implants are used as the main alternative to autologous cartilage. Medpor has good integration with host tissue due to its porous quality, and it has the potential to provide greater bulk than cartilage grafts. The main disadvantages are the risk of infection and implant extrusion.

Mandible

Segmental defects of the mandible can be reconstructed with titanium plates of varying size and strength, depending on the length and location of the defect.

The most common use for implants in the mandible is for genioplasty. For soft tissue defects or augmentation, the mandibular implant material of choice is Silastic (Dow Corning Corp., Midland, MI), which is a silicone elastomer rubber. Silastic provides flexibility and firmness, is inert, and allows for fibrous tissue ingrowth to further stabilize the implant. Once a specific size is chosen, the implant can be further trimmed and shaped to ideally fit the patient. The subperiosteal or supraperiosteal pocket can be made from an intraoral or submental approach.

Advances in Regenerative Implants

Scientists and surgeons continue to focus effort on the development of regenerative implants that can be used to reconstruct traumatic or congenital defects.

Stem Cells

Embryonic stem cells have created promise for the future of facial implants because of their pluripotency and ability to differentiate into all three germ cell lines. These cells have the potential for differentiation into multiple cell lines, including osteogenic, chondrogenic, adipogenic, and myogenic. Adipose-derived stem cells are desirable due to their ease of harvest and potential abundance. Cowan et al were able to show regeneration of a critical-sized calvarial defect using mouse adipose-derived stem cells. The immense potential of multipotent cell lines and

the ability to control the pluripotency of cell lines through gene expression open many avenues for regenerative products in the future.

■ Summary

The complete and broad picture must be considered when planning for an implant in the head and neck region, including the site of implantation, function and aesthetic requirements of the defect, biocompatibility of the implant, and long-term goals of the patient. The ideal implant is biocompatible and functions with elasticity and strength similar to those of the native tissue. An ideal synthetic implant does not exist, so it remains the surgeon's challenge to find the best combination of these traits to fit the patient's needs. **Tables 105.1** and **105.2** summarize the applications, advantages, and disadvantages of head and neck implants.

Table 105.1   Application of facial plastic and reconstructive surgery implants

Implant	Material	Application
Metal	Titanium	Fracture bars and plates, screws, orbital floor
	Gold	Eyelid weights
Polymers	Silicone	Soft tissue augmentation
	Porous polyethylene (Medpor[a])	Rhinoplasty
	Polymethyl methacrylate (PMMA)	Cranioplasty
	Expanded polytetrafluoroethylene	Orbital floor, soft tissue augmentation, rhinoplasty
	Polyetheretherketone (PEEK)	Cranioplasty, large soft tissue or bony defects of the midface or mandible
Ceramics	Hydroxyapatite	Bone augmentation
	Bioglass	Middle ear ossicles
Bioactive cement	Hydroxyapatite cement	Cranioplasty, bone augmentation
Bone and cartilage	Autologous bone	Cranioplasty
	Calvarial bone	Rhinoplasty
	Autologous cartilage	Rhinoplasty

[a] Stryker, Kalamazoo, MI.

Table 105.2 Advantages and disadvantages of facial plastic and reconstructive surgery implants

Implant	Advantages	Disadvantages
Titanium	Lightweight Osseointegration	Risk of extrusion
Gold	Chemically inert	Poor tensile strength
Silicone	Can cause chronic, mild inflammatory reaction	Can be dislodged due to poor integration
Porous polyethylene	Tissue fibrous integration with good stability Osseointegration	Risk of extrusion
Polymethyl methacrylate	Can be premolded or molded in situ Good strength and rigidity	Thermogenic reaction
Expanded polytetrafluoroethylene	Chemically inert	Mild foreign body reaction
Polyetheretherketone	Can be premolded with computed tomographic guidance Strong, nonmalleable	Risk of extrusion
Hydroxyapatite cement	Osteoconductive	Poor flexibility
Autologous bone/cartilage	Excellent bioavailability Integration with host tissue	Resorption Donor site morbidity
Calvarial bone	Excellent bioavailability Integration with host tissue	Potential for immunogenic reaction

■ Suggested Reading

Anderson JM, Rodriguez A, Chang DT. Foreign body reaction to biomaterials. Semin Immunol 2008;20(2):86–100

Chim H, Gosain AK. Biomaterials in craniofacial surgery: experimental studies and clinical application. J Craniofac Surg 2009;20(1):29–33

Cowan CM, Shi YY, Aalami OO, et al. Adipose-derived adult stromal cells heal critical-size mouse calvarial defects. Nat Biotechnol 2004;22(5):560–567

Duranti F, Salti G, Bovani B, Calandra M, Rosati ML. Injectable hyaluronic acid gel for soft tissue augmentation. A clinical and histological study. Dermatol Surg 1998;24(12):1317–1325

Gladstone HB, McDermott MW, Cooke DD. Implants for cranioplasty. Otolaryngol Clin North Am 1995;28(2):381–400

Kwan MD, Longaker MT. Advances in science and technology: impact on craniofacial surgery. J Craniofac Surg 2008;19(4):1136–1139

Lees JG, Lim SA, Croll T, et al. Transplantation of 3D scaffolds seeded with human embryonic stem cells: biological features of surrogate tissue and teratoma-forming potential. Regen Med 2007;2(3):289–300

Lin AY, Kinsella CR Jr, Rottgers SA, et al. Custom porous polyethylene implants for large-scale pediatric skull reconstruction: early outcomes. J Craniofac Surg 2012;23(1):67–70

Matic DB, Manson PN. Biomechanical analysis of hydroxyapatite cement cranioplasty. J Craniofac Surg 2004;15(3):415–422, discussion 422–423

Moreira-Gonzalez A, Jackson IT, Miyawaki T, Barakat K, DiNick V. Clinical outcome in cranioplasty: critical review in long-term follow-up. J Craniofac Surg 2003;14(2):144–153

Neovius E, Engstrand T. Craniofacial reconstruction with bone and biomaterials: review over the last 11 years. J Plast Reconstr Aesthet Surg 2010;63(10):1615–1623

Neumann A, Kevenhoerster K. Biomaterials for craniofacial reconstruction. GMS Curr Top Otorhinolaryngol Head Neck Surg 2009;8:Doc08

Redbord KP, Hanke CW. Expanded polytetrafluoroethylene implants for soft-tissue augmentation: 5-year follow-up and literature review. Dermatol Surg 2008;34(6):735–743, discussion 744

Reinisch JF, Lewin S. Ear reconstruction using a porous polyethylene framework and temporoparietal fascia flap. Facial Plast Surg 2009;25(3):181–189

Sahoo N, Roy ID, Desai AP, Gupta V. Comparative evaluation of autogenous calvarial bone graft and alloplastic materials for secondary reconstruction of cranial defects. J Craniofac Surg 2010;21(1):79–82

Takahashi K, Tanabe K, Ohnuki M, et al. Induction of pluripotent stem cells from adult human fibroblasts by defined factors. Cell 2007;131(5):861–872

Thevenot P, Hu W, Tang L. Surface chemistry influences implant biocompatibility. Curr Top Med Chem 2008;8(4):270–280

106 Management of Thyroid-Associated Ophthalmopathy

◼ Introduction

The incidence of thyroid disease in the United States is 0.4%. Of these patients with thyroid glandular disease, estimates of the prevalence of clinical symptoms of thyroid-associated orbitopathy (TAO) vary from 5 to 50%. Although Graves disease is the thyroid disorder seen in the majority of patients with orbitopathy, eye findings may also occur in patients with Hashimoto disease, primary hypothyroidism, thyroid cancer, or history of radiation treatment to the area of the thyroid gland.

Like Graves disease, thyroid eye disease (TED) is four times more common in women than men. The clinical manifestations of TED may be seen in any age group, but are most commonly diagnosed in the fourth and fifth decades of life.

The activity of the glandular disease and the orbital disease are associated but not directly related. TAO may occur in patients who are euthyroid, hypothyroid, or hyperthyroid. As with the glandular disorders, evidence links the orbitopathy to a disorder in the immune system, but the exact features of the autoimmune miscommunication have not been completely characterized. It may be initiated by a primary abnormality of immune surveillance or by an intrinsic cellular disorder with secondary autoimmune sequelae. Shared antigenicity between the orbital tissues and the thyroid gland may be the link between thyroiditis and TAO. The thyrotropin receptor on orbital fibroblasts is a proposed target of the autoimmune attack in TED. Also, elevated levels of insulin-like growth factor-1 receptor have been found in orbital fibroblasts as well as B and T cells from patients with Graves disease. These and other cell surface receptors may play a role in the origin of the inflammatory orbitopathy. The incited inflammatory process leads to lymphocytic infiltrates and deposition of glycosaminoglycans in the periocular tissues. Resultant osmotic changes and tissue edema lead to a discrepancy between orbital volume and space.

TED is a clinical diagnosis made in the presence of a constellation of orbital, ocular, and eyelid abnormalities. The clinical hallmarks of TED include eyelid retraction, proptosis, restrictive extraocular myopathy, dilated conjunctival blood vessels, temporal flare of the upper eyelids, dilated vascular loops over the lateral rectus muscle, elevation of intraocular pressure in upgaze, resistance to retropulsion of the eye, lacrimal gland enlargement, increased mass of the orbital fat pads resulting in protuberant eyelids, edema of the eyelids, prominence of the corrugator muscles, exposure keratopathy, and optic nerve dysfunction. Imaging of the orbit may confirm enlargement of the extraocular muscles, and abnormal results in thyroid laboratory tests are present in 90% of patients when the full spectrum of antibody tests as well as thyroid function tests are performed.

Patients with TAO can be divided into two broad clinical groups: mild (or noninfiltrative) orbitopathy, and severe (or infiltrative) orbitopathy. Patients in the first group tend to be younger with eyelid retraction, minimal inflammatory signs or discomfort, and little or no exophthalmos. The noninfiltrative category includes 90% of cases of TAO. The 10% of cases with infiltrative disease are typically older individuals with dilated conjunctival vessels, chemosis, swelling of the eyelids, double vision, proptosis, and compressive optic neuropathy. This second group is at higher risk for complications that result in visual loss. Visual complications in these patients occur as a result of corneal exposure or compressive optic neuropathy.

◼ Examination of the Patient

Patient History

A patient's history should include details regarding the nature and duration of symptoms. The symptoms frequently reported by patients with TED are a pressure sensation within the orbit, dryness, tearing, double vision, difficulty focusing, and blurring of vision. Disruption of lacrimal gland function may lead to either increased or decreased production of tears. In some cases, the dryness may be interpreted by the patient as tearing because the irritation from exposure gives rise to reflex epiphora.

Diplopia, when present, is worsened in certain positions of gaze and can be oblique, vertical, or horizontal. Diplopia occurs when the inflamed extraocular muscles create asymmetric restriction of ocular movements. The two eyes will not be pointed in the same direction, and two different images will be created at the retina, resulting in diplopia. The patient may describe difficulty "focusing" because convergence is required for near vision. Convergence depends on coordinated movement of the two globes toward midline, and restriction will sometimes require a stronger-than-usual contraction of the medial rectus muscles. Of the six extraocular muscles, the inferior rectus is the most likely to be affected by TAO. When the inferior rectus muscle is enlarged, the patient will have difficulty looking up. The patient reports difficulty reading, or "eye strain." In contrast to diplopia from restricted eye movement, blurring of vision may refer to decreased visual acuity, decreased color sensitivity, or visual field abnormalities. The physical exam and vision testing will identify many of these concerns, but inquiring about these problems during the exam focuses the testing needed to clarify abnormalities.

An inquiry into the patient's smoking history and thyroid status is also mandatory, because an association between smoking and the severity of the orbitopathy has been noted in male patients with TED. Therefore, smoking cessation is suggested for all patients. Information about patients' hormonal status and treatments they have undergone to control abnormal thyroid hormone levels should be obtained.

Physical Examination

Examination of patients with TED should include a visual acuity test with a Snellen-type chart, color vision testing, and assessment of the visual fields. Subtle anomalies in visual function will escape detection by visual acuity testing, and formal computerized visual fields are more sensitive than visual acuity testing when testing for disorder of the optic nerves. A simple but sensitive technique to screen for optic nerve function is to check for red desaturation. The patient is asked to look at a bright red object with each eye individually, and then is asked if the hue is different in the two eyes. A positive response may indicate problems with compressive optic neuropathy.

Pupillary examination is performed to check for an afferent pupillary defect, which is a sign that the sensory input on the ipsilateral side is decreased. In TED, this defect may be due to optic neuropathy. The test is performed by shining a light from one pupil to the other. Normally, there is an equal constriction of the pupils to light. When there is an afferent pupillary defect and a pen light is directed into the affected eye, the pupil constricts to some degree or remains immobile. When the light is swung to the contralateral normal eye, both pupils will show an additional degree of constriction. When the light returns to the affected eye, the pupil dilates. This is the Marcus Gunn pupil or an afferent pupillary defect. This physical finding is based on normal equal central efferent motor innervation to both iris sphincter muscles. If the optic nerve on one side is not functioning as well as the other, the pupils get a weaker signal to constrict when the same level of light is placed in the affected eye. When the light hits the "normal" eye, additional constriction occurs. The presence of a new afferent pupillary defect in a patient with TED is an indication of compressive optic neuropathy or other damage of the optic nerve.

The assessment continues with evaluation of the patient's periocular external exam. Exophthalmometry can be accomplished with a variety of techniques. The Hertel exophthalmometer (Bernell Corp., Mishikawa, IN), Luedde Exophthalmometer (Gulden Ophthalmics, Elkins Park, PA), and the Naugle exophthalmometer (Richmond Products, Inc., Albuquerque, NM) may be used to measure the millimeters of proptosis. The globes should be palpated for retropulsion. The resistance of the orbit to retropulsion of the globe is a crude measure of the intrinsic orbital pressure. The presence of protruding orbital fat or lacrimal gland prolapse is also noted in the course of the external inspection.

Eyelid edema is subjectively graded. The amount of lid retraction is also noted and is recorded by measuring the vertical palpebral fissures and the distance from the corneal limbus to the margins of the affected eyelid. Typically, the upper eyelid margin covers 1 to 2 mm of the cornea. In its normal position, the lower lid is even with the limbus or covers 1 mm of the inferior cornea. In TED, the sclera may be abnormally exposed above and below the cornea. This is noted as either upper eyelid scleral show or lower eyelid scleral show. In thyroid patients with upper eyelid ptosis, one should consider the possibility of ocular myasthenia. Patients with Graves disease have a higher incidence of other autoimmune diseases, including myasthenia gravis.

Additional eyelid measurements are made as the patient is asked to gently close the lids. The millimeters of separation between the lids are recorded as the amount of lagophthalmos. This is correlated to problems with corneal exposure. The "stare" or widened palpebral fissures of TED are caused by lid retraction, exophthalmos, or a combination of both. Several mechanisms are responsible for eyelid retraction in TED, including sympathetic stimulation of the Müller muscle, inferior rectus muscle fibrosis with compensatory overaction of the superior rectus/levator muscle complex, and/or localized changes in the levator muscle. Exophthalmos resulting from increased orbital soft tissue volume causes anterior displacement of the globe that will also result in eyelid retraction and scleral show. The extraocular movements should be assessed in all positions of gaze, and abnormalities of eye movement should be recorded. The degree of redness and edema of the conjunctiva is assessed and subjectively graded.

To definitively assess corneal exposure, a slit-lamp examination is necessary. To screen for corneal problems by observation in the office setting, assess the patient for failure of eyelid closure and the amount of accompanying conjunctival injection or chemosis. Chronic corneal exposure can lead to breakdown of the corneal epithelium and subsequent ulceration and scarring. Topical fluorescein placed in the tear film will stain areas of dry or ulcerated epithelium to help assess the degree of surface disruption. Symptoms of corneal exposure may include blurry vision, burning, foreign body sensation, irritation, and pain.

A funduscopic examination is next performed. The physician assesses the optic disc and the retinal vasculature. Increased orbital pressure may manifest itself with dilation of the retinal venous circulation. Compressive optic neuropathy may result in disc edema or optic atrophy. However, ~ 50% of patients with compressive optic neuropathy will have no funduscopic abnormality. The presence of a normal-appearing optic disc on ophthalmoscopic examination will not rule out compressive optic neuropathy.

Additional Testing

When the TAO is unilateral, computed tomography (CT) is helpful in identifying the presence of enlarged posterior extraocular muscles and ruling out an orbital neoplasm. The classic CT scan findings include increased size of the muscle bellies with normal tendon insertion sites. In patients with unilateral proptosis and thyroid disease, a CT scan is ordered to rule out other causes of proptosis.

When surgery is indicated, the CT is also important for preoperative surgical planning. Axial and coronal scans of the orbits and sinuses are ordered. If the scans are done for surgical planning, contrast is not necessary. When the scans are done to rule out other causes of proptosis, they should be ordered with and without intravenous contrast. A magnetic

resonance imaging scan will also identify changes in the extraocular muscles and orbital soft tissue, but is less helpful for surgical planning because it does not delineate the anatomy of the bone structure of the orbits and sinuses.

■ Management

Management of TED is directed toward management of the following:

- Compressive optic neuropathy
- Exposure keratopathy
- Diplopia
- Cosmetic deformity caused by proptosis and eyelid retraction
- Patient's subjective discomfort
- Education of the patient about TED

Compressive Optic Neuropathy

Approximately 5% of patients with TED develop compressive optic neuropathy. It is postulated that compressive optic neuropathy arises from massive enlargement of the extraocular muscles, particularly at their insertion sites at the annulus of Zinn in the orbital apex. Large muscles within a fixed space may cause compression and either vascular compromise or decrease in axonal transport. Regardless of the mechanism, this compression is mechanical in nature and caused by the inflamed extraocular tissues and the resultant space-to-volume discrepancy of the orbit.

Treatment modalities for compressive optic neuropathy include corticosteroids, radiation, and surgical decompression. Nonsurgical treatment can be accomplished either with radiation (~ 2,000 rads delivered in fractionated doses) or with oral steroids that are initiated with dosages of ~ 80 mg daily and then tapered while monitoring the parameters of visual acuity, pupillary response, color vision, and the visual field.

Corticosteroids

Initially, most patients (65–80%) will have a beneficial response to steroid therapy. In mild cases, corticosteroids alone may control the compressive optic neuropathy. However, most patients will have recurrence of the optic neuropathy when the dose is tapered, or will develop steroid-related side effects that prohibit continued treatment. Therefore, steroid maintenance is rarely practical for longer than 6 months. When optic neuropathy recurs during the steroid taper, consideration is given to adding the treatment modalities of radiation or surgical decompression.

Radiation

Radiation treatment has been used to treat TAO since 1913. Because the early treatments were directed toward the pituitary gland, it was only through inadvertent spillover to the orbits that these patients derived any benefits. The modern treatment protocol delivers ten 2 Gy fractions of radiation (total of 20 Gy or 2,000 rads) to the orbital tissues at angles to minimize radiation exposure to the lens of the eye. The success rate for radiation treatment for all indications related to TED is 65%.

Radiation is usually performed concomitantly with the administration of oral steroids until the desired stabilization of vision is achieved. Prednisone will typically have an effect within 24 to 48 hours, decreasing orbital inflammation and alleviating nerve compression. Radiation typically takes days to months to show its maximal benefits, so the vision is maintained on the steroids and tapered as the radiation effects take place. The side effects of radiation therapy may include earlier development of cataract and radiation retinopathy in predisposed patients with underlying vascular disease. The incidence of these side effects is extremely rare. When they do occur, they take years to develop and may be difficult to distinguish from coincident pathology. In determining treatment modality, one should consider a randomized, double-blinded study from 2004 that calls into question the value of radiation treatment for TED. Six months after radiation treatment of one side, the authors found no difference between treated and untreated eyes with respect to lid retraction, orbital soft tissue volume, or diplopia. However, in this study, patients with compressive optic neuropathy (the ones typically treated with radiation therapy) were excluded from the study.

Surgical Decompression

In some cases, compressive optic neuropathy will recur, even after steroid and radiation therapy, and surgical decompression will be necessary. In other cases, initial therapy with surgical decompression is indicated for severe compressive neuropathy when the delayed response of radiation treatment may not be timely enough to prevent permanent optic nerve damage. Surgical decompression is the most rapid technique for relieving optic nerve compression. Orbital decompression is also indicated for treatment of corneal exposure due to anterior displacement of the globe and also for cosmetically disfiguring exophthalmos. Transantral, transorbital, and transnasal approaches have all been used with success in the management of optic nerve compression.

The choice of surgical technique depends on the experience of the surgeon, but some generalizations may be made based on the goals of the surgery. In the patient with compressive optic neuropathy and minimal proptosis, decompression of the medical and inferior walls (a two-wall decompression) is typically adequate to relieve compression of the nerve and minimize side effects. When a reduction of exophthalmos > 4 mm is also a desired outcome of the procedure, a lateral wall decompression or lateral wall decompression/advancement may be combined with the inferior-medial wall removal (a three-wall decompression). For extreme exophthalmos, a four-wall decompression, including removal of the orbital roof, has also been described. The inferior wall and medial wall may be approached endonasally, externally, or transantrally. All three approaches have similar results with respect to control of compressive optic neuropathy (~ 70%), but the incidence of postoperative strabismus requiring secondary surgical intervention is higher with the transantral approach. Up to 70% of patients require muscle surgery after transantral decompression, compared with 15 to 50% of patients after an external lid approach.

All techniques for orbital decompression have a similar profile of side effects, including orbital hemorrhage, inadvertent disruption of the orbital contents, postoperative onset or worsening of diplopia, late development of mucocele, disruption of sinus outflow, cerebrospinal fluid leakage, and disruption of the lacrimal outflow system. Tragic complications with loss of vision may occur with orbital hemorrhage, infection, or injury to the optic nerve or globe.

Corneal Exposure

Management options for exposure keratopathy range from topical lubricants, such as artificial tears and ointments, to orbital decompression to recess the globes, so that eyelid closure is possible. Between these two extremes are medical therapy with corticosteroids, or radiation and surgical procedures for ocular rehabilitation with repositioning of the eyelids. Mild corneal exposure can often be controlled with lubricating eye drops and ointment, but resistant cases will require intervention to increase mechanical coverage of the globe by the lids. Recall that the eyelid retraction of TED is a combination of lid malposition and exophthalmos.

Alteration of the eyelid position can be accomplished by the following:

- Decreasing orbital inflammation (corticosteroids or radiation)
- Releasing the muscles in the eyelids
- Increasing orbital volume (decompression surgery)

When the problem is related to the retraction of the eyelids rather than the exophthalmos, eyelid procedures altering the position of the lids to cover the globe will be appropriate. The latter is usually the case in the noninfiltrative category of TED.

These procedures include the following:

- Recession of the levator aponeurosis of the upper eyelids to lessen scleral show and improve upper eyelid closure.
- Elevation of the lower eyelids using preserved sclera, fascia, autogenous hard palate, or cartilage. Because eye muscle surgery for diplopia can affect eyelid position, it is often useful to wait until after strabismus surgery is completed to perform cosmetic eyelid surgery.

When an orbital decompression is performed to decrease exophthalmos, the amount of reduction in exophthalmos can be correlated to the number of orbital walls that are altered. For mild degrees of exophthalmos, a transconjunctival approach with removal of the medial wall and medial orbital floor may be adequate. For moderate degrees of exophthalmos, an endoscopic medial wall and floor decompression balanced with a lateral wall decompression is performed. For more severe exophthalmos a lateral wall advancement may be added to the decompression. Intraoperative reduction of the orbital volume by removal of the orbital and intraconal fat may also decrease exophthalmos. In extreme cases, orbital roof removal has also been described. As a generalization, 2 mm reduction of exophthalmos is attributed to medial wall removal, 2 mm reduction is attributed to the orbital floor, 2 mm reduction is attributed to the lateral orbital wall, and up to 4 mm of change in the exophthalmometry reading may be obtained by advancing the lateral orbital rim.

Diplopia

Patients with diplopia are followed carefully until the inflammatory phase of TED has stabilized and the motility deviation is stable for 6 months to 1 year. Motility is assessed by measuring ocular versions and prism deviations. When the measurements stabilize, the patients are candidates for strabismus surgery. The extraocular muscles can be divided at their insertion and reattached to the globe at alternative positions or lengths to counter the restrictive changes of TED. Adjustable muscle sutures can be used to maximize the predictability of the eye muscle surgery. Suture tension is adjusted in the early postoperative period to maximize ocular realignment. Because of the propensity for orbital decompression to give rise

to an alteration in ocular motility, if orbital decompression is contemplated, it should be performed prior to extraocular muscle surgery.

Cosmetic or Appearance Rehabilitation

Like eye muscle surgery, cosmetic rehabilitation is not undertaken until the inflammatory component of TAO is acquiescent and stable. Cosmetic surgery to improve exophthalmos uses the same orbital decompression techniques that are used for functional problems. Again, because orbital decompression may alter the relationship between the globe and the eyelids, when necessary, decompression is the first step. Additional cosmetic orbital decompression can be obtained through expansion of the lateral and superior orbital walls using a contour-type bur to remove bone from the orbital walls. The lateral orbital rim can also be advanced to increase orbital volume and to reposition the lateral canthus more anteriorly. This helps to camouflage the exophthalmic position of the globe by altering the lateral attachments of the upper and lower eyelids. In some cases, the exophthalmos is mild or nonexistent, and the rehabilitation proceeds directly to eye muscle or eyelid surgery. The techniques used to cosmetically reposition the eyelids are the same techniques described to correct eyelid retraction for corneal exposure. At the time of eyelid surgery, consideration can also be given to removal of excess orbital fat and to the resuspension of prolapsed lacrimal glands. Removal of the fat and soft tissue will decrease the puffiness of the upper and lower eyelids. TAO may be very disfiguring, and both the patient and the surgeon are gratified when the appearance is normalized.

◼ Summary

TAO remains a poorly understood disease. It appears to be related to the immunologic alteration that is central to the development of autoimmune thyroid disorders, but the nature of these relationships is poorly delineated. Clinicians can recognize the disease and try to prevent disease sequelae, but current medical and surgical treatments do not change the underlying disease process. TAO is a frustrating disease to observe and manage because of limited understanding and the resultant constraints on clinicians' ability to improve their patients' condition. Lubrication, steroids, radiation, and surgery are used to minimize patient discomfort, prevent visual loss, and rehabilitate patient appearance.

■ Suggested Reading

Chang M, Baek S, Lee TS. Long-term outcomes of unilateral orbital fat decompression for thyroid eye disease. Graefes Arch Clin Exp Ophthalmol 2013;251(3):935–939

Eing F, Abbud CM, Velasco e Cruz AA. Cosmetic orbital inferomedial decompression: quantifying the risk of diplopia associated with extraocular muscle dimensions. Ophthal Plast Reconstr Surg 2012;28(3):204–207

Feldon SE, Levin L. Graves' ophthalmopathy: V. Aetiology of upper eyelid retraction in Graves' ophthalmopathy. Br J Ophthalmol 1990;74(8):484–485

Garrity JA, Fatourechi V, Bergstralh EJ, et al. Results of transantral orbital decompression in 428 patients with severe Graves' ophthalmopathy. Am J Ophthalmol 1993;116(5):533–547

Gorman CA, Garrity JA, Fatourechi V, et al. A prospective, randomized, double-blind, placebo-controlled study of orbital radiotherapy for Graves' ophthalmopathy. Ophthalmology 2001; 108(9):1523–1534

Kennedy DW, Goodstein ML, Miller NR, Zinreich SJ. Endoscopic transnasal orbital decompression. Arch Otolaryngol Head Neck Surg 1990;116(3):275–282

Lucarelli MJ, Shore JW. Management of thyroid optic neuropathy. Int Ophthalmol Clin 1996;36(1):179–193

Stan MN, Garrity JA, Bahn RS. The evaluation and treatment of graves ophthalmopathy. Med Clin North Am 2012;96(2):311–328

Wulc AE, Popp JC, Bartlett SP. Lateral wall advancement in orbital decompression. Ophthalmology 1990;97(10):1358–1369

Yip J, Lang BH, Lo CY. Changing trend in surgical indication and management for Graves' disease. Am J Surg 2012;203(2):162–167

X

Trauma

107 Contemporary Management of Facial Fractures

■ Introduction

The management of facial fractures has been advanced by imaging, virtual planning, and exposure and fixation of the fracture segments. As a result, today the general management of facial fractures is completely different from that of the mid-1980s. This chapter focuses on the currently accepted methods of evaluating and managing facial fractures.

Organization of the Facial Skeleton

For many years little thought was given to the nuances of the facial skeleton, particularly the underlying organizational pattern of the bony framework. However, it is now recognized that the facial skeleton is organized to provide support for orbits and means of distributing the forces generated by the muscles of mastication. The facial skeleton, which is not of uniform thickness throughout its various regions, is primarily composed of thin cortical bone surrounding the paranasal sinuses and orbits. Within these sheets of thin cortical bone are areas where the bone condenses into thicker structures, referred to as buttresses. These buttresses provide strength and form to the midface. Their restoration and stabilization is the primary focus of modern-day facial fracture management.

Facial Buttresses

Three buttresses are responsible for maintaining the position of the maxilla in relation to the cranial base above the mandible below (**Fig. 107.1**):

1. The *medial* or *nasomaxillary* buttress extends from the anterior maxillary alveolus along the nasal piriform aperture and the nasal process of the maxilla to the frontal cranial attachment.

2. The *lateral* buttress, commonly referred to as the *zygomaticomaxillary* (ZM) buttress, extends from the lateral maxillary alveolus to the zygomatic process of the frontal bone and laterally to the zygomatic arch.

3. The *posterior* buttress, also referred to as the *pterygomaxillary* buttress, is responsible for attaching the maxilla posteriorly to the pterygoid plate of the sphenoid.

With midface trauma, fractures tend to cross these buttresses at right angles. If the fractured buttresses are accurately reduced and rigidly stabilized, the entire maxilla will be in its correct position. The posterior buttress does not need to be reconstructed; by realigning the anterior buttresses, the posterior buttress will be realigned and stabilized.

■ Evaluation and Imaging

A key advance in the management of facial trauma has been the ready availability of high-resolution computed tomographic (CT) scanning capabilities in most hospitals. These imaging techniques have significantly enhanced a surgeon's ability to accurately assess a patient's injuries preoperatively. In contrast, before CT was available, the facial skeleton had to be explored to determine the extent and site of fractures.

High-resolution coronal and axial CT scans with 5 mm cuts are now standard for management of midface fractures. With the detailed information available from CT imaging, a surgeon can formulate a detailed operative plan. In particular, with high-resolution CT scans, the surgeon can accurately determine the status of the orbital floor and whether an orbital floor exploration is indicated (**Fig. 107.2**). Virtual planning programs are now available that allow the surgeon to preoperatively estimate the extent of the remaining orbital floor after trauma, thus guiding implant specifications (**Fig. 107.3**).

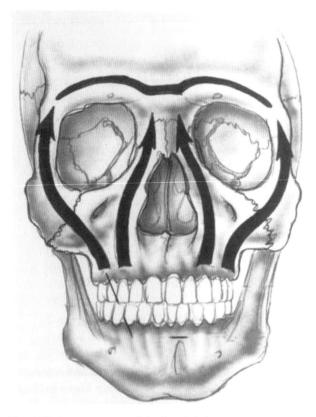

Fig. 107.1 Buttresses of the facial skeleton.

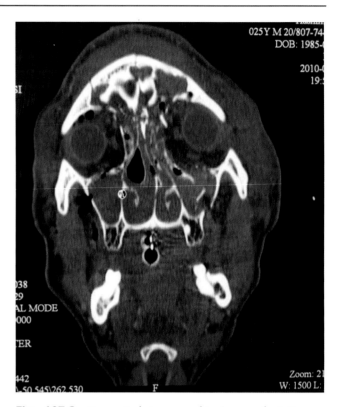

Fig. 107.2 Computed tomographic image depicting an orbital blowout fracture.

For assessment of possible mandibular fractures the standard study is a panogram (Panorex) study with plain films (right and left oblique, posteroanterior, and lateral skull) as indicated. For evaluation of fractures of the ramus and, in particular, the condyles, coronal CT scans give excellent visualization and will document displaced segments more accurately than Panorex or plain films (**Fig. 107.4**).

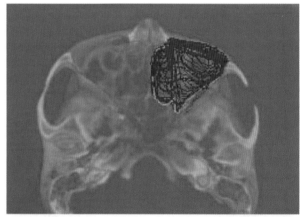

■ Management

Surgical Approaches to the Facial Skeleton

Until relatively recently, the open reduction and internal fixation of facial fractures represented a balancing act of making the smallest possible external incisions while providing adequate exposure for fracture reduction and fixation. A major advance in the management of facial trauma has been the development of the so-called extended-access/internal approaches to the facial skeleton. These extended-access approaches are performed in a subperiosteal plan and elevated under muscles, nerves, lymphatics, and blood vessels, thereby avoiding injury to these structures.

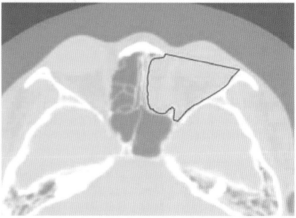

Fig. 107.3 Virtual planning estimation of orbital volume on computed tomographic scan.

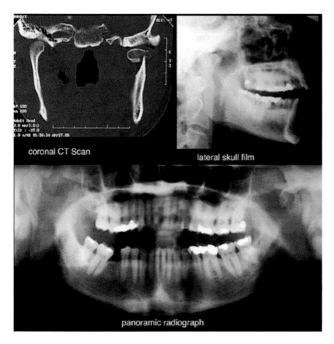

coronal CT Scan

lateral skull film

panoramic radiograph

Fig. 107.4 Computed tomography and Panorex depicting mandibular trauma.

Extended Access

The facial skeleton can be divided into four major regions, each of which has an extended-access approach that provides optimal exposure while minimizing external scars:

1. The *upper third* of the facial skeleton, including the zygomatic arches, lateral orbital rims, supraorbital rims, medial orbital rims, medial canthi, and frontonasal/ethmoid region, are approached through hemicoronal (unilaterally) or coronal (for bilateral or midline) incisions.
2. The *inferior orbital rim, orbital floor,* and *upper maxilla* are exposed with transconjunctival incisions.
3. The *lower two-thirds* of the maxilla (including the important ZM buttress) are exposed with either unilateral or bilateral sublabial incisions.
4. The *anterior two-thirds* of the mandible is approached intraorally through a gingival buccal incision. The posterior third of the mandible may also be managed with an intraoral approach, but there is no question that working on the posterior mandible through an intraoral approach requires additional expertise and instrumentation. It is generally recommended that experience be gained with the anterior approaches before attempting reduction and plating of posterior

body and angle fractures. Most surgeons still prefer the standard external approach through a neck skin crease as the preferred method for angle and posterior body fractures.

Fixation of Facial Fractures

For 2,000 years, facial fractures were stabilized with simple external bandages and splints with resulting malunions and nonunions. For most of the past 50 years, facial fractures have been managed with interfragment wiring, suspension wires, intermaxillary fixation, or a combination of all three. Although an improvement over external splints and bandages, these older methods of fracture fixation, based on wires, still have significant limitations.

Interfragment Wiring

Interfragment wiring is deficient in several respects:

- Wire fixation derives its stabilizing action by compressing the bone edges when the wire is tightened. The wire only contacts that portion of the drill hole closest to the fracture, leaving the remaining segment without support. This allows the fracture to pivot around the wire.
- When bone is compressed, its first response is to resorb, which happens at the bony interface as well as at the site where the wire is in contact with the bone. This resorption will eventually lead to loosening of the wires.
- If there are areas of comminution, multiple segments or loss of bone using a wire to span this gap will result in displacement of the fracture segments from their normal anatomical position.

Suspension Wires

To stabilize the midface, suspension wires are placed from a stable portion of the skull to arch bars on the teeth, and are tightened until the midface no longer moves. Suspension wires do not use anatomical fracture reduction; instead, they achieve stabilization by impacting the maxilla on itself. This impaction leads to loss of vertical height and usually, due to the pull of the wires, posterior displacement of the maxilla. Intermaxillary fixation with arch bars and wiring of the mandible together for 6 weeks will stabilize simple fractures but will not be suitable for more complicated fractures. Additionally, if the patient has poor dentition or is edentulous, then splints must be fabricated and secured in some fashion to the mandible or maxilla.

Plate and Screw Fixation

Contemporary management of facial fractures employs open-reduction and internal-fixation techniques. The use of plates and screws has almost totally replaced interfragment wiring for stabilization of facial fractures. A wide variety of plating systems are available, with sizes ranging from < 1 mm thickness and screw diameter to 2.7 mm screw diameters. The plates come in a variety of shapes.

Advantages

Plate and screw fixation offers several advantages. The plates and screws are composed of highly biocompatible materials, such as titanium, and can actually become osseointegrated (something stainless steel wire will not do). The screw thread engages the entire 360 degrees of the drill hole and gives solid fixation without rocking or pivoting. Plates can be used to span areas of bone loss or comminution without the need for displacing the remaining bone segments. With plates and screws it is possible to achieve rigid fixation of fracture segments with virtually no movement of the bone components. This makes primary bone healing (with minimal callous formation and bone resorption) possible and nonunion less likely.

Disadvantages

The major disadvantage of using plates and screws for fracture fixation is that to place them with two or three holes on either side of the fracture, more exposure than interfragment wiring is required. This problem is overcome in large part by using the extended-access approaches already discussed. Another potential disadvantage to the use of plates and screws relates to the implantation of foreign bodies. When plates and screws for fracture fixation were first introduced, most companies recommended removal of all hardware when the fractures were healed. However, experience has shown that the titanium implants, when properly placed, are exceptionally well tolerated and thus are only removed if they become symptomatic.

Management of Facial Fractures

Contemporary management of facial fractures integrates the three previously mentioned modalities into a comprehensive treatment plan. The surgeon uses high-resolution CT scans with physical examination to direct the procedure to the key fracture segments and buttresses. The fractures are exposed using extended-access approaches and are anatomically reduced. Once the fractures are in their pre-trauma position, they are rigidly fixated with plates and screws. This treatment method is a significant advance over the previous management methods, which relied on plain films (or tomograms) and physical examination, both of which are notoriously unreliable for making the diagnosis. Fractures were exposed through keyhole incisions, which provided limited exposure of the fractures and left external scars. The fractures were then often inadequately reduced and incompletely stabilized with wires. The current approach as already outlined provides superior fracture reduction and fixation with decreased morbidity, and avoids prolonged intermaxillary fixation.

Zygomaticomaxillary Complex (ZMC) Fractures

Fractures of the zygoma's articulations were previously referred to as tripod fractures. The term *tripod* referred to the mistaken belief that there were only three fracture sites (zygomaticofrontal (ZF) suture, orbital rim, and zygomatic arch). However, it is now recognized that there are at least four fracture sites (adding the ZM buttress, as well as a fracture along the sphenoid on the lateral orbital wall). Thus many surgeons now believe that *ZMC fracture* is a more descriptive term (**Fig. 107.5**). (Of course, this may cause confusion when describing a "complex" zygomatic fracture.)

Present-day management of ZMC fractures relies on an understanding of the facial buttresses and accurate CT scans to allow the surgeon to direct the surgery to the site of pathology. In almost all ZMC fractures, the key determinant for restoring the malar eminence is the ZM buttress. This buttress is approached through a sublabial incision, is reduced as anatomically as possible, and is then plated with a 1.5 or 2 mm diameter plate. Management of the remaining fracture sites (orbital rim and floor, ZF suture, and arch) is based on the CT scan findings and physical exam. In 45 to 50% of ZMC fractures, all that is required is accurate reduction and fixation of the ZM buttress. In the remaining cases, which are more complex, the orbital rim and floor are explored, realigned, and fixated. In very displaced fractures, a hemicoronal flap is used to expose the zygomatic arch, body, and ascending ramus of the zygoma for maximal exposure and accuracy of reduction.

Orbital Blowout Fractures

Blowout fractures of the orbital floor are specific fractures that, by definition, involve only the floor, sparing the rims. Rarely, a blowout fracture of the medial orbital wall can occur with entrapment of the medial rectus muscle. The presumed mechanism of

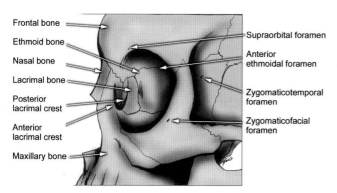

Fig. 107.5 Configuration of the zygomaticomaxillary buttress.

blowout fractures is increased intraorbital pressure, which puts pressure on the thin orbital floor, which then fractures into the maxillary sinus.

The management of orbital floor blowout fractures has changed significantly over the past 15 years. It is now recognized that not all fractures involving the floor need to be treated. Criteria have been developed to identify fractures that have a significant chance of having adverse sequelae (diplopia, enophthalmos, or muscle entrapment). These criteria are based on physical exam and CT scan findings. The following are indications for exploration and repair:

- Enophthalmos on physical exam
- Diplopia with associated evidence of muscle entrapment on forced duction testing
- CT scan evidence of muscle entrapment with associated diplopia

- CT scan evidence of significant orbital fat herniation into the maxillary sinus or orbital floor disruption, either of which could be expected to result in enophthalmos as the edema resolves

Patients with an orbital floor fracture who do not have one of these findings present are managed conservatively with simple observation. If enophthalmos or diplopia develops, then the fractures are explored and specific causes of symptoms are addressed.

Midface Fractures

Le Fort fractures of the midface are fractures that pass at right angles to the previously mentioned buttresses and disrupt the dental occlusion (**Fig. 107.6**). The three levels of midface fractures, as described by the French surgeon René Le Fort, are classified as follows:

- *LeFort I* (also known as the Guyren fracture) crosses the lower third of the maxilla, passing through the ZM buttress, the piriform aperture, the base of the nasal septum, and the pterygoid plates.
- *LeFort II* (also known as the pyramidal fracture) again crosses the ZM buttress, extends superiorly and medially across the orbital rim, and then crosses the nasal dorsum to follow a similar course on the opposite side.
- *LeFort III* (also known as cranial facial dysjunction) basically separates the facial skeleton from the skull base by passing superiorly across the root of the nose, medial orbit, orbital floor, lateral orbital wall, and zygomatic arch and passing posteriorly through the pterygoid plate.

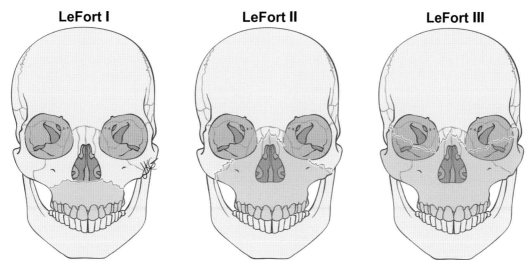

Fig. 107.6 Le Fort fracture patterns. (Used with permission from Sclafani AP, ed. Total Otolaryngology—Head and Neck Surgery. New York, NY: Thieme; 2015.)

Although René Le Fort described these fractures as distinct entities, it is rare to see a pure Le Fort fracture, especially with contemporary high-speed motor vehicle accidents. Today, the most common scenario is to have fractures involving a combination of Le Fort levels that may vary from side to side.

Sequelae of Midface Fractures

There are two main considerations in treating Le Fort fractures: functional and aesthetic. The functional components relate primarily to mastication (and occlusion) and vision. With any Le Fort fracture, there will be a component that passes through the pterygoids with posteroinferior displacement of the teeth-bearing maxilla, which will produce the classic open bite seen with midface fractures. With Le Fort II and III, a component of the fracture passes through the portion of the orbit with the potential for all of the sequelae of orbital fractures, such as enophthalmos and muscle entrapment. Additionally, with LeFort III, there is the distinct possibility of the fracture passing across the orbital apex and causing blindness.

The aesthetic issues relate to changes in facial appearance due to fracture displacement of facial bones. This may take the form of loss of anterior projection and increased facial width due to posterior displacement of the maxilla and splaying of the zygomatic arches. Changes in the appearance of the nose and globe positioning may also occur.

Management of Midface Fractures

Previously, management of midface fractures was directed at trying to simply attain midface stability, with little attention to accurate reduction of the fracture segments. Stability was achieved by placing arch bars on both the mandibular and the maxillary teeth and placing the patient into intermaxillary fixation. Suspension wires from a stable point on the cranium were then passed to the arch bars on the maxillary teeth. To achieve stability, the suspension wires were tightened, with the maxilla being drawn superiorly and impacted upon itself. The patient remained in intermaxillary fixation for 6 weeks. The frequent result of the use of suspension wires was malreduced fractures, with an external "dishpan"-appearing face and malocclusion.

Modern-day management of midface fractures consists of accurate reduction of the fractured segments with rigid fixation. This is achieved by making an accurate diagnosis of the site of pathology with high-resolution CT scans. Arch bars are placed on the maxillary and mandibular teeth, and the patient is placed in occlusion with intermaxillary wires. The fractures are then widely exposed by using extended-access approaches to the involved skeletal sites, and are anatomically reduced. The fractures are rigidly fixated with plates and screws, and the patient is released from intermaxillary fixation at the end of the procedure.

Mandibular Fractures

Perhaps the most significant change in the treatment of facial trauma is in the management of mandibular fractures. The treatment of mandibular fractures previously relied heavily on arch bar application to the teeth, with intermaxillary fixation for 6 weeks. Open reduction and interfragment wiring were performed through external incisions on comminuted or complicated fractures. For very complicated or unstable fractures, percutaneous pins were placed in the mandible and then connected by metal rods or bars of methyl methacrylate. However, intermaxillary fixation and interfragment wiring have two disadvantages:

1. Intermaxillary fixation and wiring do not provide rigid fixation of the bone segments. This means there will be some movement, and the fracture will heal by callous formation. Bone healing by callous formation takes at least 6 weeks and has a greater incidence of fibrous union and nonunion.
2. Six weeks of intermaxillary fixation is severely disruptive to a patient's lifestyle. Dentition is not very stable. The result of prolonged intermaxillary fixation is often significant gingival disease, dental caries, significant weight loss, and nonunion or fibrous union.

Current management of mandibular fractures consists of reestablishing the occlusion by arch bars and intermaxillary fixation. The fracture is then exposed and reduced with an intraoral approach whenever possible. The intraoral approach is almost always possible for symphyseal, parasymphyseal, and anterior body fractures. Angle fractures may be managed via an intraoral approach but require additional expertise and instrumentation (**Fig. 107.7**). Contrary to what might be expected, the incidence of wound infections and complications is significantly less with intraoral approaches than with external approaches (provided the fracture has been reduced and stabilized).

Plates and screws for rigid fixation of mandibular fractures were introduced for facial fractures several decades ago and have replaced fixation with stainless steel wires. The original plates were quite thick (2.7 mm diameter) and were made of stainless steel. At present, the most commonly employed plates are 2.4 mm diameter titanium plates, although 2 mm plates have been employed recently in the repair of most fractures. A useful feature of many mandibular plates is their ability to generate compression across the fracture line. The degree of rigidity achieved with modern plating systems is such that arch bars

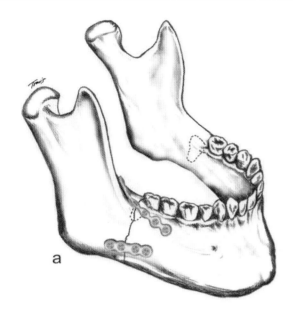

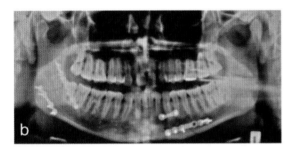

Fig. 107.7 **(a, b)** Mandibular angle fracture repaired with the Champ technique with two plates.

and intermaxillary fixation are used only to establish occlusion, and when the mandibular plate has been applied, the intermaxillary wires are cut. The patient is then placed on a soft diet and is spared the discomfort of prolonged intermaxillary fixation.

■ Controversial Issues

There exists little controversy in the management of nondisplaced mandible fractures in sites other than the mandibular condyle. For these fractures, open reduction and internal fixation (ORIF) of fractures is warranted due to the expected load and translation associated with occlusal forces. However, the mandibular condyle when nondisplaced warrants a conservative approach. According to Spiessl and Schroll classification of condylar fractures, classes II to V are displaced and dislocated fractures, whereas classes I and VI are nondisplaced, nondislocated fractures. The latter can be treated conservatively. Class I consists

of nondisplaced condylar fractures with an intact capsule, whereas class VI fractures are ones that are nondisplaced but that have a diacapitular fracture pattern. In these fractures, success rates of 75% versus 78% were attained for ORIF versus closed treatment. Early mobilization and conservative osteofixation using minimally invasive treatment of class VI fractures is preferential due to condyle remodeling and translational forces acting on these fractures.

The management of severely comminuted mandible fractures has improved with the advancement of osteosynthesis using miniplate and locking reconstruction plates. Whereas symphyseal and parasymphyseal comminuted fractures benefit from locking reconstruction osteofixation, external fixation devices have been less used. For nonunion and significant malunion where bone loss is an issue, an external fixation device is warranted. External fixation of mandible fractures is a useful technique when an open treatment is contraindicated because of extensive comminution, bone or soft tissue loss, and infection.

Management of panfacial fractures (PFF) warrants a "bottom up, outside in" approach. The goal for establishing a base and facial height commensurate with the preinjury state is paramount. In these patients, the most common sites of mandibular fractures in PFFs were the symphysis and condyle. The most common type of fracture was the isolated linear fracture. Repair of symphyseal and condylar fractures are the mainstay of our goal for symmetry in terms of width and height. After judicious repair of the mandible, approaches to the midface should concentrate on the zygomaticofrontal suture first, thus establishing height in the midface. Next ORIF of the zygomaticomaxillary and nasomaxillary buttresses should be obtained. A top-down, inside-out approach would not allow the surgeon to meet the goals of restoring the preinjury state. Although PFFs are difficult to treat, beginning with the end in mind with the goal of establishing width, height, and base offers a more feasible approach.

■ Conclusion

At present, facial fractures are managed with the goals of restoring the facial skeleton to its original three-dimensional configuration with rigid fixation of the fractures, while imparting minimal morbidity. These goals are achieved by using high-resolution CT scans to diagnose the sites of body disruption, extended-access/internal approaches to expose the fractures, and rigid fixation with plates and screws. Combined, these modalities allow surgeons to restore the facial form and function to trauma patients with few adverse sequelae.

■ Suggested Reading

Braidy HF, Ziccardi VB. External fixation for mandible fractures. Atlas Oral Maxillofac Surg Clin North Am 2009;17(1):45–53

Ellis E III, Kittidumkerng W. Analysis of treatment for isolated zygomaticomaxillary complex fractures. J Oral Maxillofac Surg 1996;54(4):386–400, discussion 400–401

Gilbard SM, Mafee MF, Lagouros PA, Langer BG. Orbital blowout fractures. The prognostic significance of computed tomography. Ophthalmology 1985;92(11):1523–1528

Gruss JS, Van Wyck L, Phillips JH, Antonyshyn O. The importance of the zygomatic arch in complex midfacial fracture repair and correction of posttraumatic orbitozygomatic deformities. Plast Reconstr Surg 1990;85(6):878–890

Gruss JS, Mackinnon SE. Complex maxillary fractures: role of buttress reconstruction and immediate bone grafts. Plast Reconstr Surg 1986;78(1):9–22

Klotch DW, Gilliland R. Internal fixation vs. conventional therapy in midface fractures. J Trauma 1987;27(10):1136–1145

Kwon J, Barrera JE, Jung TY, Most SP. Measurements of orbital volume change using computed tomography in isolated orbital blowout fractures. Arch Facial Plast Surg 2009;11(6):395–398

Kwon J, Barrera JE, Most SP. Comparative computation of orbital volume from axial and coronal CT using three-dimensional image analysis. Ophthal Plast Reconstr Surg 2010;26(1):26–29

Landes CA, Day K, Lipphardt R, Sader R. Closed versus open operative treatment of nondisplaced diacapitular (Class VI) fractures. J Oral Maxillofac Surg 2008;66(8):1586–1594

LeFort R. Étude expérimentale sur les fractures de la mâchoire inferieure. Parts I, II, III. Rev Chir Paris 1901;23:208–360

Manson PN, Markowitz B, Mirvis S, Dunham M, Yaremchuk M. Toward CT-based facial fracture treatment. Plast Reconstr Surg 1990;85(2):202–212, discussion 213–214

Millman AL, Della Rocca RC, Spector S, Leibeskind AL, Messina A. Steroids and orbital blowout fractures—a new systematic concept in medical management and surgical decision-making. Adv Ophthalmic Plast Reconstr Surg 1987;6:291–300

Shumrick KA, Kersten RC, Kulwin DR, Sinha PK, Smith TL. Extended access/internal approaches for the management of facial trauma. Arch Otolaryngol Head Neck Surg 1992;118(10):1105–1112, discussion 1113–1114

Shumrick KA, Kersten RC, Kulwin DR, Smith CP. Criteria for selective management of the orbital rim and floor in zygomatic complex and midface fractures. Arch Otolaryngol Head Neck Surg 1997;123(4):378–384

Yang R, Zhang C, Liu Y, Li Z, Li Z. Why should we start from mandibular fractures in the treatment of panfacial fractures? J Oral Maxillofac Surg 2012;70(6):1386–1392

108 Temporal Bone Trauma

■ Introduction

Temporal bone fractures result in a spectrum of injuries ranging from minor self-limited injuries to extremely complex injuries associated with high morbidity and mortality. Because of the structures within the temporal bone, many fractures result in complex diagnostic and therapeutic challenges. The extent of the injuries, based on examination, imaging studies, and audiometric findings, will determine the urgency and type(s) of surgical interventions required.

The management of temporal bone fractures is generally aimed at restoring functional deficits rather than reduction and fixation of bone fragments. Injuries resulting in hearing loss, facial nerve dysfunction, and cerebrospinal fluid (CSF) leaks are the types that most often require surgical intervention. Fractures involving the seventh cranial nerve may cause devastating cosmetic and functional injury.

The mechanism of injury can be divided into blunt trauma, with motor vehicle accidents accounting for the majority, and penetrating trauma, which is far less common but often more severe. Blunt temporal bone trauma requires a large amount of force. These fractures rarely occur in isolation, and 5% of patients with significant head trauma will sustain temporal bone fractures. Most injuries associated with temporal bone trauma can be managed in a delayed manner; however, high-velocity gunshot wounds can result in massive vascular and neurological injury that may require urgent intervention.

Anatomy of the Temporal Bone and Facial Nerve

The temporal bone is a complex association of bones with variable characteristics (resulting from structural variation and the presence of sutures, aerated spaces, and foramen) that contain several critical sensory and neurovascular structures (**Table 108.1**; **Figs. 108.1** and **108.2**). Sequelae of temporal bone fractures are related to injury of structures within or adjacent to the temporal bone, which include the cochlea, vestibular system, ossicles, tympanic membrane (TM), facial nerve, petrous carotid artery, sigmoid sinus, and meninges. Although cranial nerves (CN) IX, X, and XI have a close association with the temporal bone and exit the jugular foramen, they are rarely involved in temporal bone fractures.

The facial nerve innervates the muscles of facial expression. Microscopically, the nerve consists of myelinated axons surrounded by endoneurium. The axons are gathered into groups of fascicles surrounded by perineurium. The epineurium surrounds the fascicles and condenses into an external nerve sheath.

The nerve travels through a tunnel consisting of the internal auditory canal (IAC) and facial (fallopian) canal. The course of the nerve is irregular and has been divided into the IAC, labyrinthine, geniculate, tympanic, and mastoid segments. The narrowest portion of the canal is the meatal foramen (located at the lateral aspect of the IAC it is the junction between the IAC and labyrinthine facial nerve segments), through which the labyrinthine portion passes, and is thought to be a frequent site of compression injury. Furthermore, the nerve is tethered at various points. The most important is the perigeniculate region, where the nerve is tethered by the genu and the greater superficial petrosal branch. This complex anatomy and narrow bony pathway make the facial nerve highly susceptible to injury from compression, shearing, traction, or disruption.

Classification of Temporal Bone Fractures

Several systems for classifying temporal bond fractures have been proposed, each with advantages and disadvantages. They are generally complementary and help clarify the anatomical pathway and functional sequelae of a fracture.

Table 108.1 Components of the temporal bone and important relationships

Squamous	Adjacent to the temporal lobe comprising lateral wall of middle cranial fossa; extends anteriorly, forming the linea temporalis and the posterior aspect of the zygomatic arch
Tympanic	An incomplete ring of bone that comprises the majority of the external auditory canal (EAC) and frequently is involved in the fracture path
Mastoid	Comprises most of the aerated portion of the mastoid and middle ear and houses portions of the fallopian canal, sigmoid sinus, and ossicles; adjacent to the middle cranial fossa (superior) and posterior cranial fossa (posterior) and may be a pathway for cerebrospinal fluid leakage.
Petrous	Comprises the medial aspect and houses several critical structures, including the otic capsule (cochlea, vestibule, semicircular canals); the internal auditory canal; portions of the seventh cranial nerve, including the meatal (narrowest), labyrinthine, and perigeniculate region (the most commonly injured); and petrous carotid artery

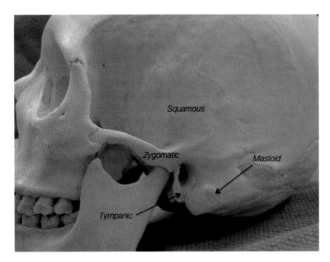

Fig. 108.1 Lateral view of the left temporal bone showing the squamous, mastoid, and tympanic portions in relation to surrounding structures. The petrous portion is not visible from this view.

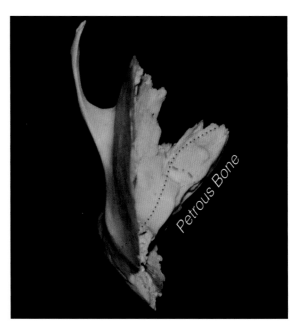

Fig. 108.2 Superior view of the left temporal bone in isolation. The image illustrates the long axis of the temporal bone and the course of longitudinal (*red dotted line*) and transverse (*blue dashed line*) patterns of fractures. The petrous portion of the temporal bone is seen best in this view. It houses the otic capsule, internal auditory canal, petrous carotid artery, and portions of the facial nerve and forms the petrous apex.

Longitudinal versus Transverse

Although this classification system is based on the anatomical pathway of the fracture, it is also useful for predicting sequelae. The system uses the long axis of the petrous apex as a reference and classifies fractures as longitudinal or transverse. Although this system is simple and easy to understand, many fractures have mixed patterns limiting the system's utility.

Longitudinal injuries are much more common and account for 70 to 90% of fractures. They follow a course through the external auditory canal (EAC) and TM progressing along the axis of the petrous apex following the path of least resistance, which often involves aerated regions, foramina, and/or suture lines. Longitudinal injuries classically result from a blow to the temporal parietal region, are associated with a conductive hearing loss (CHL), and may have an associated facial nerve injury in the perigenicu-late region. **Fig. 108.2** illustrates the path of a longitudinal and transverse fracture relative to the long axis of the petrous bone. **Fig. 108.3** represents the radiological appearance of a longitudinal fracture. This patient sustained a fracture in a motor vehicle accident and had a complete facial paralysis, requiring decompression.

Transverse fractures cross the petrous ridge and have a higher incidence of otic capsule involvement. These fractures require more force and classically result from a blow to the occipital region. Transverse fractures are more often associated with inner ear injury, resulting in sensorineural hearing loss (SNHL), and have a higher incidence of facial nerve injury.

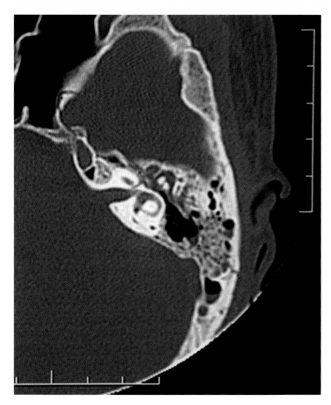

Fig. 108.3 Axial view of the left temporal bone with a longitudinal fracture (*dashed red line*) extending through the petrous apex into the sphenoid sinus.

Fig. 108.4 demonstrates the radiological appearance of a transverse fracture. This patient sustained his fracture in a motor vehicle accident as well; he had normal facial nerve function but severe SNHL.

Otic Capsule Sparing or Otic Capsule Involving

This classification system is based on the presence or absence of involvement of the otic capsule. This system was introduced to emphasize the functional sequelae of the fracture. Results from two series proposing this classification scheme indicate that 2.5 to 5.8% of fractures involve the otic capsule. **Fig. 108.3** illustrates an otic capsule–sparing fracture, whereas **Fig. 108.4** illustrates an otic capsule–involving fracture.

■ Evaluation

Clinical Findings

Medical History

Multitrauma patients with temporal bone trauma are initially evaluated by a trauma team that stabilizes the patient and manages life-threatening injuries.

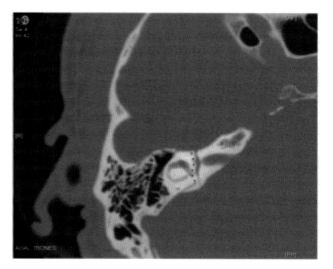

Fig. 108.4 Axial view of the right temporal bone with a transverse fracture (*dashed red line*) crossing the petrous bone and involving the lateral aspect of the internal auditory canal.

The evaluation includes a medical history and physical examination, but in severely injured patients a history may not be obtainable, and immediate management of life-threatening injuries becomes the primary objective. Multiple traumatic injuries and the occult nature of temporal bone injuries may result in an incomplete or delayed evaluation of temporal bone fractures. However, most temporal bone fractures are identified early because of patient symptoms, exam findings, or imaging results.

Symptoms associated with a temporal bone fracture include the following:

- Hearing loss
- Vertigo/imbalance
- Tinnitus
- Autophony (hearing one's own speech and internal noises more prominently)
- Aural fullness/pressure
- Facial weakness
- Drainage from the ear

Physical Examination

Physical evaluation allows assessment of the auricle, EAC, TM, middle ear, hearing, balance, and facial nerve function. Otoscopic examination is an excellent screening exam that usually indicates evidence of a temporal bone injury and can guide additional diagnostic testing. In all patients, evaluation of the facial nerve is critically important. Establishing baseline facial nerve function can aid in the prognosis and guide the decision to surgically manage the facial nerve. Physical examination should be performed to identify the injuries, as described in the following subsections.

Ecchymosis, Lacerations, and Hematoma

The soft tissue exam may demonstrate bruising, lacerations, or hematomas and can suggest temporal bone injury. Postauricular ecchymosis (Battle sign) can be an indicator of a basilar skull fracture, as well as ecchymosis around the eyes (raccoon eyes). Soft tissue should be inspected for lacerations, abrasions, or hematomas, which should be cleaned and treated.

Injury to the Outer and Middle Ear

Otoscopic examination may reveal a step-off in the bony ear canal, soft tissue trauma (blebs, ecchymosis, or lacerations), tympanic membrane rupture, middle ear effusion, or hemotympanum.

Hearing Loss

Hearing loss is one of the most common findings associated with temporal bone fractures. It can result from damage to the inner ear or middle ear, or from a combination, and is categorized as SNHL, CHL, or a mixed loss. Most fractures lead to a CHL resulting from injury of the TM, ossicular subluxation or discontinuity, hemotympanum, or any combination of these. Hearing loss is effectively screened at the bedside with a tuning fork examination.

Hemotympanum

Injury to the temporal bone and mucosa of the middle ear and mastoid frequently leads to accumulation of frank blood or serosanguinous fluid in the middle ear space. The volume of blood or fluid in the middle ear reflects the extent of injury and function of the eustachian tube. If the injury is severe enough, or if drainage through the eustachian tube is impaired, the entire middle ear may be filled with blood. This results in dark discoloration of the TM.

Otorrhea

When a TM perforation is present, fluid that accumulates in the middle ear space may pass through the perforation and produce otorrhea. The fluid may be hemorrhage, exudates from trauma, CSF, or a combination. CSF may also drain down the eustachian tube and manifest as rhinorrhea.

Imbalance

A neurological and/or vestibular injury may be associated with temporal bone fractures. Balance and vestibular function are challenging to evaluate acutely at the bedside and often require periodic reassessment. Neurological injuries include concussion and injuries to the brainstem and vestibular/cerebellar pathways and may coexist with inner ear injuries. The evaluation of a patient with dizziness should include a detailed neurological evaluation and a bedside vestibular evaluation. Further testing with audiography and vestibular function tests is useful, but such tests are frequently difficult and unnecessary to obtain acutely.

In trauma patients, a cervical spine injury should be ruled out before performing the vestibular evaluation. Bedside assessment of the peripheral vestibular system should include evaluation for spontaneous or gaze-evoked nystagmus, gait abnormalities, positive fistula test, Dix–Hallpike positioning to evaluate for benign paroxysmal positional vertigo, head thrust looking for refixation saccades, and an assessment for post-head-shaking nystagmus. A fracture of the otic capsule generally results in a severe vestibular injury, but injuries can occur in the absence of a fracture.

Facial Nerve Dysfunction (Paralysis or Paresis)

Early assessment of the facial nerve is very important. Therefore, baseline motor function should be established as soon as possible. Temporal bone fractures involve the intratemporal nerve rather than the peripheral branches, producing generalized hemifacial weakness and asymmetric movement. Asking patients to raise their eyebrows, close their eyes, smile, snarl, or grimace allows comparison of volitional movement that will highlight asymmetry. Marked edema limits facial expression and can give the impression of reduced facial movement. Furthermore, highly expressive movement on the normal side will cause some passive movement on the paralyzed side near the midline.

A patient with paralysis may appear to have limited function that is actually passive movement resulting from the uninjured side. When this is suspected, the clinician should restrict movement on the normal side by pressing on the facial soft tissue and reassess for any movement on the injured side. Different grading scales are available, but the important factor is to assess if there is paralysis (no movement) or paresis (weakness) of facial motor function. Sometimes terms like complete paralysis (indicating no movement) and incomplete paralysis (meaning weakness or paresis) are used. Although temporal fractures produce hemifacial involvement, it is best to record function for all five distal regions (forehead, eye closure, midface, mouth, and neck) because there may be some variation in the degree of dysfunction.

Any patient with residual motor function is likely to have a good long-term outcome with conservative management. Attention to eye closure is also important because incomplete eye closure requires careful management to avoid exposure keratitis. Often the facial nerve cannot be evaluated accurately because patients are uncooperative, unconscious, or sedated.

In an uncooperative patient, one method of stimulating facial movement is to induce pain with a sternal rub, or place a cotton-tipped applicator or instrument in the nose and stimulate the septum. This usually generates a grimace, which can allow comparison of right and left facial function.

Special Investigations

Radiological Evaluation

Imaging studies are indicated in patients with temporal bone injuries, and computed tomography (CT) is the modality of choice. Frequently the trauma team performs a head CT, but it is important to assess the temporal bone and skull base with a dedicated fine-cut CT reformatted in various planes. CT windowed for bone allows identification of the fracture path and involved structures and enables fracture classification. The CT should be reviewed in detail to assess for involvement of the facial nerve, carotid artery, and EAC; intracranial injury; displacement of the ossicles; and potential epithelial entrapment. **Figs. 108.3** and **108.4** are examples of otic capsule–sparing and –involving fractures. These images also demonstrate the longitudinal and transverse fracture patterns.

Penetrating temporal bone injuries are usually more complex, with greater involvement of regional structures. Penetrating injuries have a greater incidence of facial nerve, vascular, and intracranial injury. **Figs. 108.5** and **108.6** demonstrate the radiological appearance of penetrating injuries of the temporal bone from a gunshot wound and shrapnel injury. **Fig. 108.5** is of a patient who sustained a gunshot wound to the temporal bone. The trajectory of the projectile passed adjacent to the carotid artery, which was not fortunately injured; however, the

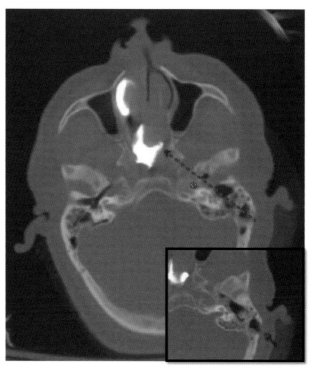

Fig. 108.5   Axial view demonstrating the path of a gunshot wound through the left temporal bone (*red dashed line*) and the proximity of the projectile path to the carotid artery (*red star*). Fragments from the projectile are seen in the nasopharynx and palate. This patient sustained facial nerve paralysis, but remarkably his carotid artery was uninvolved. The inset image is from a slightly more superior level and shows the entry point in the mastoid bone (*red solid arrow*).

facial nerve was involved. Additional radiological imaging with magnetic resonance imaging (MRI), arterial imaging, or interventional studies may be necessary with penetrating trauma.

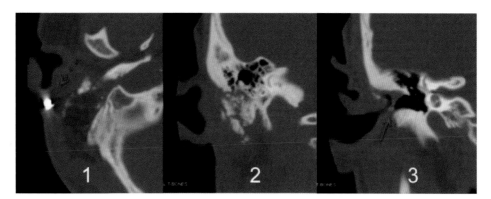

Fig. 108.6   Composite of images from penetrating shrapnel injury of the right temporal bone. Panel 1 is an axial view demonstrating a residual fragment of shrapnel (*dashed red arrow*) and injury to the mastoid tip. Panel 2 is a coronal view of the highly comminuted mastoid fracture. Panel 3 is a coronal view through the external auditory canal (EAC), demonstrating soft tissue stenosis (*solid red arrow*). This patient developed late complications of entrapment cholesteatoma and EAC stenosis. The fracture did not involve the otic capsule; however, the patient developed a profound sensorineural hearing loss.

Hearing Evaluation

Bedside evaluation with a 512 Hz tuning fork is a reliable method to screen for a CHL or SNHL. A CHL is indicated by a combination of a Weber test that lateralizes to the involved ear and a negative Rinne test (bone conduction perceived louder than air conduction). If a tuning fork is not available and the patient is cooperative, the clinician should ask the patient to hum strongly for several seconds and to specify in which ear the sound seems more intense. The hum will sound louder on the injured side when a significant conductive component is present. If a CHL is present, an audiogram can be obtained when the patient is stable and should be repeated prior to ossiculoplasty or tympanoplasty to determine residual hearing loss.

Tuning fork findings in a patient with SNHL can vary widely. A Weber test that lateralizes away from the involved ear suggests SNHL. The Rinne test is usually positive unless there is a profound SNHL loss. A fracture involving the otic capsule generally results in a profound SNHL. This may be manifested by severe tinnitus and vestibular signs; if so, an audiogram should be obtained as soon as possible.

Audiological testing is essential to quantify hearing deficits, confirm the clinical assessment, and allow for future comparison. The hearing status can also influence the surgical approach for facial nerve exposure. The timing of audiometry is dependent on the patient condition and type of suspected hearing loss.

Vestibular Evaluation

Imbalance or vertigo may be present acutely or chronically in patients with temporal bone trauma resulting from inner ear injury or neurological injury. Formal vestibular evaluation is not indicated acutely, but it can be useful in patients with persistent symptoms or signs of incomplete compensation. The evaluation typically includes ocular testing, which helps establish if there is central involvement; caloric testing, which assesses vestibular function in the horizontal canal and can be used to determine hypofunction; rotary chair testing, which is especially useful in diagnosing bilateral injury; and posturography, which can be a useful tool for monitoring vestibular compensation.

Facial Nerve Evaluation

Facial nerve injuries range from mild to severe. Although we frequently use the House–Brackmann scale to classify clinical function, it is also important to understand the Sunderland classification of nerve pathophysiology:

- First-degree injury, or neuropraxia, is the most limited injury. It results in a conduction blockade in an otherwise anatomically intact nerve. These lesions tend to recover completely.
- Second-degree injury, or axonotmesis, results in axonal injury, but the endoneurium is intact. These injuries have good recovery.
- Third-degree injury results in axon and endoneurium injury, but the perineurium is preserved. Aberrant regeneration occurs and can leave patients with some weakness and synkinesis.
- Fourth-degree injury indicates severe nerve trunk injury, but the epineurial sheath remains intact.
- Fifth-degree injuries completely transect the entire nerve trunk and epineurium.

Third-, fourth-, and fifth-degree injuries are all termed neurotmesis. Although this classification system helps clinicians predict recovery, injuries rarely conform to just one category.

A partial facial nerve injury can progress to a complete paralysis over the course of a few days. Increased swelling leads to compression of the nerve in the fallopian canal. A patient who presents with paresis and then progresses to complete paralysis generally has a good prognosis for spontaneous recovery.

Patients who present immediately with a complete facial paralysis generally fall into a poor prognostic category. They typically have much more severe facial nerve injuries and are more likely to benefit from facial nerve exploration and repair. This is why early clinical evaluation to establish baseline facial nerve function is so important.

Sometimes a patient's condition prevents initial facial nerve evaluation, which presents a diagnostic challenge when the patient is later found to have complete facial paralysis. In this scenario, the clinician does not know if an initial paresis in the patient progressed to paralysis, or if the patient had paralysis immediately after the injury. The patient's management is determined by the electrophysiological testing and guided by the radiological interpretation and clinical features of the injury.

Electrophysiological testing can provide prognostic information in a patient with complete facial paralysis. This testing is of very little value when a patient retains some movement. There are several tests available. The two most commonly used tests are electromyography (EMG), a volitional test, and electroneurography (ENOG), an evoked test. These tests help differentiate a neuropraxic injury from a neural degenerative injury and assess the proportion of degenerated axons.

Electromyography

EMG is performed by intramuscular-recording electrodes to assess for voluntary action potentials, which correlate with a good prognosis. EMG patterns can also include fibrillation potentials (indicating degeneration) and polyphasic potentials (indicating recovery).

Electroneurography

ENOG is an evoked test that compares the compound action potential of the two sides of the face to determine the percentage of degeneration on the affected side. Wallerian degeneration, which is progressive nerve degeneration distal to the site of injury, occurs 3 to 5 days postinjury. Early testing may produce erroneous results if Wallerian degeneration is incomplete. This is why serial electrophysiological testing is performed. Controversy still exists regarding the electrophysiological criteria for facial nerve decompression, and data regarding prognostic ENOG use are incomplete. Chang and Cass reviewed the data on facial nerve injury in temporal bone trauma and recommend that decompression be offered to patients with > 95% degeneration within 14 days of injury. **Fig. 108.7** presents an algorithm for evaluating and managing patients with facial nerve injury.

Cerebrospinal Fluid Leak Evaluation

CSF leaks result from disruption of the meninges in the IAC and middle or posterior fossa and occur in 17% of temporal bone fractures. A CSF leak can result in middle ear effusion, rhinorrhea, or otorrhea, depending on the integrity of the TM and eustachian tube. A persistent CSF leak places the patient at risk for meningitis.

Copious clear fluid is suggestive of a CSF leak, but the presentation is often not that obvious. Detection and localization of a subtle CSF leak can be challenging. Although the halo sign (a clear ring of fluid surrounding a bloody spot on filter paper) is quick and easy to identify and may suggest a CSF leak, it has a high false-positive rate. Otorrhea can be tested to examine the glucose, protein, and electrolyte content; however, this test is also unreliable. b2-Transferrin is the preferred test and is highly sensitive and specific for CSF, but it requires a discrete volume for analysis.

High-resolution CT imaging with intrathecal contrast is an effective way to detect and localize a CSF

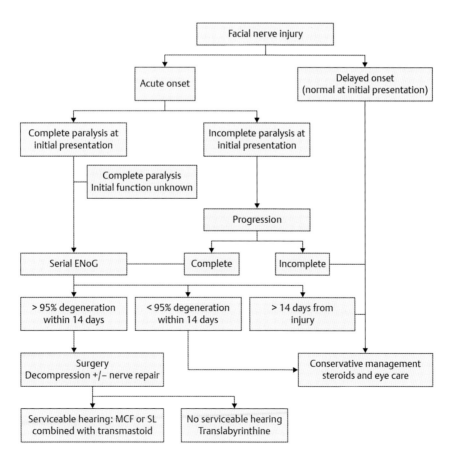

Fig. 108.7 Facial nerve evaluation and management algorithm. Adapted with permission from Chang CYJ, Cass SP. Management of facial nerve injury due to temporal bone trauma. Am J Otol 1999;20(1):96–114.

leak. If that fails, intraoperative localization with fluorescein is an alternative. A lumbar puncture is required and dilute intrathecal fluorescein is administered to stain the CSF. Otorrhea or rhinorrhea can be assessed for gross discoloration or can be collected on a pledget and evaluated with a Wood lamp to detect fluorescein staining. Appropriate counseling is required because rare but serious complications such as seizure can occur.

■ Management

Nonsurgical Management

Many sequelae of temporal bone fractures are self-limited or managed nonsurgically. Sometimes it is difficult to determine if the sequelae will require surgery, and initial conservative management is frequently the best course of action.

Antibiotic Therapy

In a large review of temporal bone fractures, the incidence of meningitis in patients without a CSF leak was 1%. The authors concluded that systemic prophylactic antibiotics were not indicated in the absence of a CSF leak. Conflicting data exist regarding prophylactic antibiotic use in patients with a suspected or known CSF leak. The vast majority of patients with a CSF leak will resolve with conservative measures, and antibiotics may not provide any benefit. However, patients who have a persistent CSF leak have a significantly higher risk of meningitis, so patients who have failed conservative therapy for a CSF leak may benefit from systemic prophylactic antibiotics.

Conductive Hearing Loss

Traumatic CHL can result from an ossicular injury, effusion, tympanic membrane injury, or a combination of these. CHL resulting from serous effusion or hemotympanum will generally resolve with time. Likewise, the majority of traumatic tympanic membrane perforations close spontaneously. Observation and serial audiometry will clarify persistent hearing loss. Amplification is an effective alternative to surgery for residual CHL.

Sensorineural Hearing Loss

SNHL may result with or without radiological evidence of otic capsule involvement. Acute management with steroids is reasonable, based on the use of steroids in other types of SNHL. Data on the management of SNHL associated with temporal bone fractures are very limited. Persistent serviceable SNHL should be managed with amplification. A contralateral routing of signal (CROS) hearing aid trial should be conducted for single-sided deafness, especially before any surgically implanted bone conduction device is considered.

Cerebrospinal Fluid Leak

With rare exceptions, the initial management of a CSF leak should be conservative. This should begin with a trial of bed rest, head-of-bed elevation, and stool softeners. If the leak persists despite these measures, 3 to 5 days of active CSF diversion with a lumbar drain is often successful. The majority of CSF leaks will resolve with these measures.

Facial Nerve Injury

Nonsurgical management of facial nerve dysfunction may include observation, eye protection, and steroids. Establishing baseline facial motor function is important and can provide prognostic information. Patients with incomplete facial paralysis, even if they progress to complete paralysis, rarely require facial nerve surgery. Those patients have a good prognosis and should be observed. Steroids are frequently used in patients with complete paralysis and may be considered in patients with paresis that show signs of progressive dysfunction (level 4 evidence).

Impaired or incomplete eye closure, following facial nerve injury, can cause exposure keratitis. Early management of the eye includes aggressive eye protection with lubricants, moisture chambers, nightly taping, and possibly tarsorrhaphy. Synkinesis of the orbicularis oculi muscle is a late sequela and can be managed with Botox (Allergan, Irvine, CA) injections.

Surgical Management

Surgery for temporal bone fractures is performed to restore function or manage complications. Immediate surgery is rarely indicated, the exception being severe vascular injury. Early surgery may be appropriate for severe facial nerve injury or persistent CSF leak. Sequelae are otherwise managed in a delayed manner. Most data related to the management of temporal bone trauma consist of case series and expert opinions and thus are level 4 or 5 evidence.

Indications for Surgery

- Persistent CHL (TM or ossicular injury)
- Complete facial paralysis with poor prognosis

- Persistent CSF leakage
- Injury requiring debridement or risking entrapment cholesteatoma
- EAC stenosis
- Development of meningocele or encephalocele

Tympanic Membrane Repair and Ossicular Reconstruction

Multiple techniques exist to repair the TM. Most involve the use of autologous tissue. Medial and lateral graft tympanoplasty are the two most common techniques, but many other variations exist. In patients with an intact TM and CHL, a middle ear exploration is performed to identify the cause of CHL, which is repaired through an ossiculoplasty.

There are many ossiculoplasty materials and techniques. The basic techniques use autologous tissue or a synthetic prosthesis to restore a functional ossicular chain and couple the TM to the stapes. Results of this surgery are generally better than similar surgery for chronic otitis media. A recent review, specifically evaluating surgical rehabilitation of CHL resulting from trauma, reported a significant improvement in hearing after surgery.

Facial Nerve Repair

Patients with immediate complete paralysis, radiological evidence of severe facial nerve injury, and evidence of severe degeneration on ENOG generally fall into a poor prognostic category and may benefit from facial nerve surgery. The majority of explorations reveal an intact nerve with a focal injury secondary to compression or traction. The geniculate is the most commonly injured region. Most surgery involves wide decompression of the nerve, removing any impinging bone. The nerve is infrequently transected. Explorations that reveal severe segmental injury or frank nerve disruption are managed by rerouting the nerve or interposition grafting. Regardless of the repair technique, a tensionless closure is critical. The proximal portion of the nerve is usually available, so options such as 12–7 interposition are generally not necessary.

Many questions remain regarding the role of surgery in traumatic facial paralysis. These include the indications for surgery, the benefit of surgery versus natural history, the timing of surgery, the extent of decompression, and the best surgical approach. The approaches to the facial nerve are described later in the chapter. A recent systematic review attempted to clarify the issue but found that existing studies were uniformly level 4 evidence, thus limiting the ability to make definitive conclusions.

Cerebrospinal Fluid Leaks

Persistent CSF leaks increase the risk of meningitis and require surgical exploration for closure. The exact location of a CSF fistula can be challenging to identify. Intrathecal fluorescein is a useful adjunct during exploration. Small leaks may be treated with autologous tissue, such as fascia, pericranium, fat, bone pâté, or processed or synthetic materials, such as dural substitutes, glues, or hydroxyapatite formulations.

Most leaks are approached via the mastoid. CSF leaks associated with large tegmental defects are approached with a combined mastoid and middle cranial fossa technique. Depending on the size of the leak and strength of the repair, continued lumbar drainage may not be necessary. Larger leaks may require tympanomastoid obliteration, which involves transection of the EAC, plugging of the eustachian tube, and obliteration of the mastoid and middle ear with abdominal fat. This is an excellent method in patients with profound hearing loss. This technique will result in CHL in patients with residual hearing, but it may be necessary for large or multiple leaks.

Cholesteatoma and External Auditory Canal Injury

Epithelial entrapment can occur with blunt trauma, but it is more likely with penetrating trauma. A small fragment of epithelium buried in soft tissue can, over time, lead to a cholesteatoma. Unless a patient has gross evidence of epithelial entrapment, it is difficult to identify who is at risk for this. Any patient with penetrating injury or severe injury of the EAC is at some risk. Patients with obvious entrapment should undergo surgical debridement to remove the epithelium. Serial monitoring by examination or CT is indicated in high-risk patients to detect late development of entrapment cholesteatoma.

Extensive injury to the EAC may result in stenosis. Once the patient is stable and hearing has been evaluated, a canalplasty and split-thickness skin graft can be considered. **Fig. 108.6** is a series of radiographs from a soldier with a penetrating shrapnel injury of the right temporal bone. He sustained a comminuted fracture of the mastoid tip and EAC and later developed entrapment cholesteatoma and EAC stenosis. Although his fracture did not involve the otic capsule, he developed a profound SNHL on the right side.

Late Meningocele and/or Encephalocele Development

Severe injury of the tegmen can result in delayed development of a meningocele or encephalocele. These usually present as a late CSF leak, meningitis, or CHL. Diagnosis is confirmed on CT when there is a tegmen defect and nondependent soft tissue. MRI is also indicated and can demonstrate disruption of the meninges and clarify if tissue is granulation or neural. Surgical management consists of a combined middle cranial fossa and transmastoid repair. The efficacy of combined repair of mastoid encephaloceles and CSF leaks (mixed etiology: traumatic, iatrogenic, spontaneous, and infectious) shows excellent success.

Surgical Approaches

There are multiple surgical approaches to the middle ear, TM, mastoid, and segments of the facial nerve. Frequently, more than one approach is required, and selection depends on the extent of the injuries and the goals of treatment.

Mastoidectomy

Mastoidectomy is an osseous approach with several variations, but the basic approach allows access to the mastoid air cell system, antrum, epitympanum, and mesotympanum (if the facial recess is opened). It also allows extended access to various structures housed in the temporal bone, such as the semicircular canals, IAC, and portions of the facial nerve. Mastoidectomy is indicated in cases requiring debridement of entrapped skin, facial nerve decompression, and CSF leak exploration/repair and when maximal access to the middle ear is required. The portions of the facial nerve accessible through a basic mastoidectomy approach include the majority of the tympanic and mastoid segments.

Combined Middle Cranial Fossa and Transmastoid Approach

A combined middle cranial fossa/transmastoid approach is used when facial nerve decompression/repair is required and hearing is serviceable. The middle cranial fossa approach provides access to the IAC, labyrinthine, and geniculate segments of the facial nerve. The procedure involves a craniotomy, extradural elevation of the temporal lobe, and bone removal from the petrous ridge to expose the facial nerve.

This is a technically challenging procedure. It is combined with a mastoidectomy for access to the tympanic and mastoid segments of the facial nerve. In a patient with an intact ossicular chain, the incus will have to be removed to allow access to the tympanic segment. Evidence suggests that decompression should include the meatal foramen and labyrinthine segment because a nerve injury results in retrograde degeneration and edema, and these are the narrowest portions of the fallopian canal.

Translabyrinthine Approach

A translabyrinthine approach is used for decompression of the facial nerve when hearing is not serviceable. The translabyrinthine approach provides excellent access to all portions of the facial nerve. Its advantages over the combined middle cranial fossa/transmastoid approach include a more direct approach, less brain retraction, and improved access.

Supralabyrinthine Approach

A supralabyrinthine approach is used for decompression of the facial nerve when hearing is serviceable and the mastoid is well aerated. The technique involves a mastoidectomy with extensive exposure of the epitympanum. Bone is removed to identify the superior semicircular canal and expose the labyrinthine and geniculate portions of the facial nerve. This approach allows access to the labyrinthine portion of the facial nerve, and may allow for decompression. However, this technically challenging approach does not provide sufficient exposure if nerve repair is indicated in the IAC or labyrinthine segment.

■ Controversial Issues

Facial Nerve Decompression

The role of surgical management of traumatic facial nerve paralysis continues to be an area of uncertainty and controversy. Most clinicians agree that a small subset of patients will benefit from surgery. The difficulty is accurately identifying patients who will benefit from surgery and those who will not. Additional uncertainty exists regarding the timing of repair and the extent of decompression. The meatal foramen is the narrowest portion of the facial nerve. Many clinicians advocate decompression of the meatal foramen and labyrinthine segment, regardless of the site of injury, because of the possibility of retrograde degeneration. Exposure of this region is technically challenging and may increase the risk of damage to the inner ear or further damage to the facial nerve.

Carotid Artery Injuries

The petrous carotid artery may be involved with temporal bone fractures. The artery may be injured within its canal, or at the entrance or exit of the petrous bone. Blunt head trauma may result in a variety of carotid injuries: laceration, occlusion, thrombosis, aneurysm, arteriovenous fistula, intimal tear, and dissection. Limited data exist regarding carotid injury in blunt temporal bone trauma, but it is assumed that a fracture of the carotid canal increases the risk of injury. It is not uncommon for the fracture to run adjacent to the carotid canal. In the absence of neurological findings, it is unclear which patients require additional studies to assess for occult carotid injury. Patients with fractures involving the carotid pathway and central neurological findings should definitely have additional imaging studies.

■ Suggested Reading

Brodie HA, Thompson TC. Management of complications from 820 temporal bone fractures. Am J Otol 1997;18(2):188–197

Cannon CR, Jahrsdoerfer RA. Temporal bone fractures: review of 90 cases. Arch Otolaryngol 1983;109(5):285–288

Chang CYJ, Cass SP. Management of facial nerve injury due to temporal bone trauma. Am J Otol 1999;20(1):96–114

Conoyer JM, Kaylie DM, Jackson CG. Otologic surgery following ear trauma. Otolaryngol Head Neck Surg 2007;137(5):757–761

Dahiya R, Keller JD, Litofsky NS, Bankey PE, Bonassar LJ, Megerian CA. Temporal bone fractures: otic capsule sparing versus otic capsule violating clinical and radiographic considerations. J Trauma 1999;47(6):1079–1083

Kari E, Mattox DE. Transtemporal management of temporal bone encephaloceles and CSF leaks: review of 56 consecutive patients. Acta Otolaryngol 2011;131(4):391–394

Nash JJ, Friedland DR, Boorsma KJ, Rhee JS. Management and outcomes of facial paralysis from intratemporal blunt trauma: a systematic review. Laryngoscope 2010;120(7):1397–1404

Nosan DK, Benecke JE Jr, Murr AH. Current perspective on temporal bone trauma. Otolaryngol Head Neck Surg 1997;117(1): 67–71

109 Penetrating and Blunt Neck Trauma

■ Penetrating Neck Trauma

Introduction

Penetrating neck trauma has historically carried a high mortality rate, ranging as high as 16% during World War I, when nonsurgical management was performed. During World War II, when mandatory neck exploration was instituted, the mortality fell to 7% and remained between 4 and 7% during the Vietnam War. Surgical management has evolved over the last 2 decades based on the advent of advanced radiographic studies and endoscopic techniques. Most civilian centers currently practice selective neck exploration, with mortality rates ranging between 3 and 6% for low-velocity penetrating neck trauma (LVPNT). Most recently, U.S. military surgeons have treated high-velocity penetrating neck trauma (HVPNT) patients in Iraq and Afghanistan with selective neck exploration and have reported mortality rates equivalent to the 3 to 6% civilian mortality rates for LVPNT.

Projectiles, Ballistics, and Mechanisms of Injury

Different types of projectiles are associated with different ballistics and mechanisms of injury because the severity of projectile injury is directly related to the kinetic energy that the missile imparts to the target tissue (**Table 109.1**).

Table 109.1 Formula for the relationship between projectile injury and kinetic energy imparted to target tissue

$KE = \frac{1}{2} M (V1 - V2)^2$
KE = kinetic energy of the missile
M = missile mass
V1 = entering velocity
V2 = exiting velocity

The Most Lethal Missiles

The most lethal missiles are high-velocity projectiles that impart all of their energy into the tissues without exiting (V2 = 0). These types of projectiles include tumbling missiles, expanding bullets, and explosive bullets.

Temporary and Permanent Bullet Cavities

Given the foregoing understanding of kinetic energy of missiles, a single projectile will form two bullet cavities upon tissue impact: a permanent and a temporary cavity. The permanent cavity follows the injury tract due to the direct disruption of tissue from the missile. The temporary cavity is proportional to the kinetic energy of the missile and may be up to 30 times the cross-section of the missile along the injury tract.

Historical Categorization, Types, and Treatment of Penetrating Neck Wounds

High-velocity projectiles cause significantly more damage and tissue destruction when compared with low-velocity projectiles. **Table 109.2** presents the categories of missiles resulting in penetrating neck trauma and the types of wounds they cause. Historically, these seven wound types have been divided into low- and high-velocity trauma.

Historical Treatment of Penetrating Neck Wounds

Since World War II, surgeons stratified management of penetrating neck trauma based on mortality rates and the rates of pathology discovered during neck exploration. LVPNT was typically managed with selective neck dissection because the overall mortality rate was 3 to 6%, with < 50% of patients having major pathology found on neck exploration. On the other hand, HVPNT was historically treated with mandatory neck exploration because those patients had mortality rates > 50%, with 90 to 100% major

Table 109.2 Historical categories of missiles and types of penetrating neck wounds

Categories of missiles resulting in penetrating neck wounds	Types of penetrating neck wounds	
	Low velocity (< 610 m/s)	**High Velocity (> 610 m/s)**
Knives	• Stab wounds	• Close-range (< 5 m victim-to-weapon range) birdshot wounds
Single projectiles	• Handgun wounds	• Close-range buckshot wounds
• Handguns	• Long-range (> 5 m victim-to-weapon range) birdshot wounds	• Rifle wounds
• Rifles	• Long-range buckshot wounds	• Wounds from bombs, mortars, IEDs, grenades, mortars, and rockets
Multiple projectiles		
• Shotgun pellets		
• Improvised explosive devices (IEDs)		
• Grenades		
• Mortars		
• Rocket		

pathology found on neck exploration due to the tremendous amount of kinetic energy (up to 3,000 foot-pounds) imparted to the tissue. However, as previously discussed, combat surgeons are currently using selective neck dissection to treat HVPNT in Iraq and Afghanistan, with resulting low morbidity and mortality similar to rates seen in civilian trauma centers managing LVPNT.

Evaluation

Initial orderly assessment using the Advanced Trauma Life Support protocol as developed by the American College of Surgeons is appropriate in any trauma. This protocol includes rapid assessment of the "A, B, Cs" of trauma. Accordingly, airway management is the first priority in penetrating neck trauma.

Approximately 10% of patients present with airway compromise, with larynx or trachea injury. Although endotracheal intubation may be performed in these patients, nasotracheal intubation, cricothyroidotomy, or tracheostomy may be required in the presence of spinal instability. To avoid air embolism, the patient should be supine or in the Trendelenburg position. Direct pressure without indiscriminate clamping should be used to control active hemorrhage in the neck. Deeply probing open neck wounds below the platysma muscle should be avoided in the emergency room because this may lead to clot dislodgment and subsequent hemorrhage. Two large-bore intravenous lines should be placed to establish access for fluid resuscitation. Subclavian vein injuries should be suspected in zone I injuries (to be discussed), and intravenous access should be placed on the contralateral side of the penetrating injury to avoid extravasation of fluids. Spinal stabilization should be maintained until cleared clinically and/or radiographically. Tetanus toxoid should be administered if the patient's status is unknown or outdated. If possible, initial radiographic survey in the trauma

bay should include chest X-ray and cervical spine X-rays. Prophylactic antibiotics and nasogastric tube suction placement may also be considered.

Anatomy

Vital Structures in the Neck

To organize primary assessment, secondary survey, and surgical approaches to penetrating neck injuries, four types of vital structures in the neck must be considered: (1) airway (pharynx, larynx, trachea, lung); (2) blood vessels (carotid arteries, innominate artery, aortic arch vessels, jugular veins, subclavian veins); (3) nerves (spinal cord, brachial plexus, cranial nerves, peripheral nerves); and (4) gastrointestinal tract (pharynx, esophagus).

Skeletal Anatomy

Skeletal anatomy (mandible, hyoid, styloid process, and cervical spine) should be considered as well.

Muscular Landmarks

Muscular landmarks are also important. Penetration of the platysma muscle defines a deep injury in contrast to a superficial injury. The sternocleidomastoid muscle also serves as a valuable landmark because this large obliquely oriented muscle divides each side of the neck into anterior and posterior triangles. The anterior triangle contains airway, major vasculature, nerves, and gastrointestinal structures, whereas the posterior triangle contains the spine and muscle.

Neck Zones

The neck is commonly divided into three distinct zones, which facilitates initial assessment and management based on the limitations associated with surgical exploration and hemorrhage control unique to each zone (**Fig. 109.1**).

- Zone 1, the most caudal anatomical zone, is defined inferiorly by the clavicle/sternal notch and superiorly by the horizontal plane passing through the cricoid cartilage. Structures within this zone include the proximal common carotid arteries; vertebral and subclavian arteries; subclavian, innominate, and jugular veins; trachea; recurrent laryngeal and vagus nerves; esophagus; and thoracic duct. Vascular injury management is challenging in zone 1, and mortality is high. Due to the sternum, surgical access to zone I may require sternotomy or thoracotomy to control hemorrhage.
- Zone 2, the middle anatomical zone, is between the horizontal plane passing through the cricoid cartilage and the horizontal plane passing through the angle of the mandible. Vertically or horizontally oriented neck exploration incisions provide straightforward surgical access to this zone, which contains the carotid arteries; jugular and vertebral veins; pharynx, and larynx; proximal trachea; recurrent laryngeal and vagal nerves; and spinal cord.
- Zone 3, the most cephalad anatomical zone, lies between the horizontal plane passing through the angle of the mandible and the skull base. Anatomical structures within zone 3 include the extracranial carotid and vertebral arteries, jugular veins, spinal cord, cranial nerves IX through XII, and sympathetic trunk. Because of the craniofacial skeleton, surgical access to zone 3 is difficult, making surgical management of vascular injuries challenging with a high associated mortality at the skull base. Surgical access to zone 3 may require craniotomy as well as mandibulotomy or maneuvers to anteriorly displace the mandible.

Vascular Injuries

The incidence of vascular injuries is higher in zone 1 and zone 3 penetrating neck trauma injuries. This occurs because the vessels are fixed to bony structures, larger feeding vessels, and muscles at the thoracic inlet and the skull base. Consequently, when the primary and temporary cavities are damaged, these vessels are less able to be displaced by the concussive force from the penetrating missile. However, in zone 2, the vessels are not fixed; therefore, they are more easily displaced by concussive forces, and the rate of vascular injury is lower.

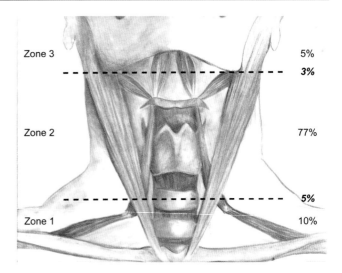

Fig. 109.1 The neck is divided into zones 1, 2, and 3.

Also, in zone 1, the esophagus is at risk for injury. Missed esophageal injuries occur because up to 25% of penetrating esophageal injuries are occult and asymptomatic. These missed esophageal injuries may be devastating, with reported mortality rates approaching 25%. Therefore, for zone 1 and for some zone 2 penetrating neck injuries, it is imperative that esophageal injuries be ruled out with endoscopic examination and, possibly, swallow studies.

Diagnostic Evaluation and Management

Selective Neck Exploration Criteria

Selective neck exploration may be used to manage penetrating neck trauma when two important conditions are present at the trauma facility: reliable diagnostic tests that exclude injury and appropriate personnel to provide active observation. In the setting of these two conditions, contemporary penetrating neck trauma management is selective neck exploration.

The decision whether to explore the penetrating neck wound is determined based on the patient's symptoms at presentation, regardless of the missile velocity. Symptomatic patients are explored in the operating room. If symptomatic patients are stable, computed tomographic angiography (CTA) may be obtained before exploration because this study may better define anatomical approaches to zones 1 and 3 of the neck. Asymptomatic patients are evaluated with diagnostic studies and, if there are pathological findings during this workup, are taken to the operating room for neck exploration (**Fig. 109.2**). If asymptomatic patients have a negative diagnostic workup showing no neck pathology, they will be observed.

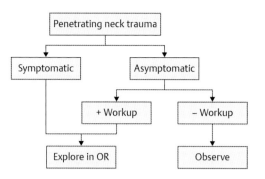

Fig. 109.2 Management algorithm based on symptoms if computed tomographic angiography, panendoscopy, and appropriate personnel are available.

Significant symptoms from penetrating neck trauma will occur depending on which of the four groups of vital structures in the neck are injured.

- Vascular injury may result in active hemorrhage, expanding hematoma, vascular bruit, and pulse deficit.
- Airway injury may cause subcutaneous emphysema, hoarseness, stridor, and respiratory distress.
- Esophageal injury is often asymptomatic and may result in leakage of saliva, subcutaneous emphysema, bleeding from the esophageal inlet, and ultimately neck or mediastinal abscess.
- Nerve injury may result in cranial nerve deficits or hemiparesis. These fixed neurological deficits may not require immediate neck exploration in an otherwise stable patient.

If appropriate diagnostic testing and personnel are not available, then penetrating neck trauma patients should undergo mandatory neck exploration, or if stable, should be immediately transferred to a facility with those capabilities.

Computed Tomographic Angiography

CTA is generally considered the initial procedure of choice to evaluate cervical vasculature in asymptomatic penetrating neck trauma. In the past, formal neck angiography via groin catheters was the procedure of choice. However, because CTA has a sensitivity ranging between 90 and 100%, along with a specificity ranging between 93 and 100%, this procedure is currently used to evaluate neck vessels.

Signs of probable injury on CTA include hematoma, subcutaneous air adjacent to the carotid sheath, intravenous contrast extravasation, and mis-

sile tracts in close proximity to vital structures. CTA may have a 1.2 to 2.2% incidence of nondiagnostic studies due to the artifact from bullet fragments and metallic foreign bodies. CTA is also useful in evaluating the trajectory of the missile tract and may help select patients who will benefit from further workup of the aerodigestive tract.

Evaluation of Aerodigestive Tract Injuries

Aerodigestive tract injuries, especially those involving the cervical esophagus, should be identified and repaired within 12 to 24 hours of injury to minimize associated morbidity and mortality. Evaluation of asymptomatic aerodigestive tract injuries includes contrast swallow studies and endoscopy (rigid and flexible esophagoscopy, bronchoscopy, and laryngoscopy).

Endoscopy is more reliable than contrast swallow studies to identify injuries to the hypopharynx and cervical esophagus. Several authors have demonstrated that endoscopy will identify 100% of digestive tract injuries, whereas contrast swallow studies are less sensitive, especially for hypopharyngeal injuries. Rigid and flexible esophagoscopy, rigid and flexible bronchoscopy, and rigid direct laryngoscopy are performed in the operating room under general anesthesia. It is recommended that both rigid and flexible esophagoscopy be performed to rule out occult esophageal injuries. Rigid esophagoscopy may provide a better view of the proximal esophagus near the cricopharyngeal muscle, whereas flexible esophagoscopy, with its magnification on the viewing screen and ability to insufflate, gives excellent visualization of more distal esophageal anatomy.

Finally, swallow studies with either Gastrografin (Bracco Diagnostics, Inc., Monroe Township, NJ) or barium may not be available in the austere environments to rule out occult esophageal injuries and, as already noted, are less accurate than endoscopy. Missed esophageal injuries, which may be occult in 25% of patients, can be devastating, with mortality rates ranging up to 25%.

Summary

Penetrating neck trauma patients can be divided into two categories on presentation: symptomatic and asymptomatic. Symptomatic patients are taken to the operating room for neck exploration. Asymptomatic patients undergo workup with CTA, panendoscopy, and possibly swallow studies. If the workup shows occult neck pathology, those patients are taken to the operating room for neck exploration. Asymptomatic patients with a negative diagnostic workup are simply observed.

■ Blunt Neck Trauma

Introduction

Although the same anatomical structures described in penetrating neck trauma (airway, vascular structures, nerves, and gastrointestinal tract) may be impacted during blunt neck trauma, the laryngotracheal airway and cervical spine are the most clinically susceptible to injury. Vascular injuries are potentially devastating but are uncommon overall, occurring in 0.08 to 1.5% of blunt neck trauma, depending on how aggressively asymptomatic patients are screened. Despite the widespread use of advanced safety mechanisms, such as shoulder harness seatbelts and airbags, motor vehicle collisions remain the most common etiology for blunt neck trauma. Other mechanisms include blunt object impact sustained in assault, and sports injuries, crush injuries, and hanging or clothesline trauma.

Evaluation

As in penetrating neck trauma, the presenting signs and symptoms of blunt neck trauma injuries are based on the dysfunction of the anatomical structures in the neck. Therefore, evaluation of the blunt neck trauma patient should follow the rapid, orderly process of trauma assessment, starting with the airway.

Initial Diagnostic Airway Evaluation

Initial diagnostic airway evaluation with flexible laryngoscopy is helpful in documenting endolaryngeal findings as well as postinjury changes given that significant edema may occur during the first 12 to 24 hours. Computed tomographic imaging may be considered for surgical planning in symptomatic patients or in asymptomatic patients with suspected laryngeal injury. Securing the airway is advocated in the setting of acute airway symptoms, such as stridor or respiratory distress, prior to considering imaging.

Hemodynamic Instability or Signs of Vascular Injury

Hemodynamic instability or signs of vascular injury, such as bruit, expanding/pulsating hematoma, hemorrhage, or loss of pulse warrant, surgical exploration, as described earlier in the discussion of penetrating neck trauma.

Hemodynamically Stable Patients Showing Risk Factors

Hemodynamically stable patients should undergo initial diagnostic imaging with CTA if at-risk factors are present, including severe cervical injury, anoxic brain injury from hanging, closed-head injury with diffuse axonal injury, midface or complex mandibular fractures, marked neck soft tissue swelling injury, high-risk cervical spine fractures (such as vertebral body subluxation, C1–C3 vertebral body fracture, and any fracture extending into the transverse foramen), or basilar skull fractures involving the carotid canal.

Cervical Spine Injury Assessment

After clinical examination, cervical spine injury assessment should include initial lateral and anteroposterior plain X-ray films, if possible. Further evaluation with imaging should be based on the individual patient's musculoskeletal and neurological complaints, as well as physical exam findings.

Controversial Issues

1. Mandatory versus selective neck exploration for penetrating neck trauma
   a. *Pro* Mandatory exploration identifies asymptomatic injuries.
   b. *Con* Mandatory exploration carries unnecessary morbidity for patients with negative findings.
   c. *Pro* Selective exploration avoids unnecessary morbidity for asymptomatic patients with negative diagnostic studies.
   d. *Con* Selective exploration requires appropriate diagnostic testing and experienced personnel.
2. Workup/diagnostic studies for penetrating neck trauma
   a. *Pro* Imaging and endoscopy are valuable tools for selective management of penetrating neck trauma.
   b. *Con* Diagnostic studies require significant resources.
3. Treatment of high-velocity versus low-velocity penetrating neck trauma
   a. HVPNT is traditionally managed with mandatory neck exploration due to significant morbidity and mortality associated with this mechanism of injury. The tissue destruction is greater with HVPNT than with LVPNT, and major pathology is found on neck exploration with the majority of neck explorations for HVPNT.
   b. If appropriate diagnostic testing and experienced personnel are available, then selective management of both HVPNT and LVPNT results in similarly low morbidity and mortality rates.

■ Suggested Reading

Ahmed N, Massier C, Tassie J, Whalen J, Chung R. Diagnosis of penetrating injuries of the pharynx and esophagus in the severely injured patient. J Trauma 2009;67(1):152–154

Armstrong WB, Detar TR, Stanley RB. Diagnosis and management of external penetrating cervical esophageal injuries. Ann Otol Rhinol Laryngol 1994;103(11):863–871

Biffl WL, Moore EE, Rehse DH, Offner PJ, Franciose RJ, Burch JM. Selective management of penetrating neck trauma based on cervical level of injury. Am J Surg 1997;174(6):678–682

Brennan J, Gibbons MD, Lopez M, et al. Traumatic airway management in Operation Iraqi Freedom. Otolaryngol Head Neck Surg 2011;144(3):376–380

Brennan J, Lopez M, Gibbons MD, et al. Penetrating neck trauma in Operation Iraqi Freedom. Otolaryngol Head Neck Surg 2011;144(2):180–185

Brennan JA, Meyers AD, Jafek BW. Penetrating neck trauma: a 5-year review of the literature, 1983 to 1988. Am J Otolaryngol 1990;11(3):191–197

Carducci B, Lowe RA, Dalsey W. Penetrating neck trauma: consensus and controversies. Ann Emerg Med 1986;15(2):208–215

Davis JW, Holbrook TL, Hoyt DB, Mackersie RC, Field TO Jr, Shackford SR. Blunt carotid artery dissection: incidence, associated injuries, screening, and treatment. J Trauma 1990;30(12):1514–1517

Holt GR, Kostohryz G Jr. Wound ballistics of gunshot injuries to the head and neck. Arch Otolaryngol 1983;109(5):313–318

Inaba K, Munera F, McKenney M, et al. Prospective evaluation of screening multislice helical computed tomographic angiography in the initial evaluation of penetrating neck injuries. J Trauma 2006; 61(1):144–149

Jurkovich GJ, Zingarelli W, Wallace J, Curreri PW. Penetrating neck trauma: diagnostic studies in the asymptomatic patient. J Trauma 1985;25(9):819–822

Kerwin AJ, Bynoe RP, Murray J, et al. Liberalized screening for blunt carotid and vertebral artery injuries is justified. J Trauma 2001; 51(2):308–314

Mazolewski PJ, Curry JD, Browder T, Fildes J. Computed tomographic scan can be used for surgical decision making in zone II penetrating neck injuries. J Trauma 2001;51(2):315–319

McConnell DB, Trunkey DD. Management of penetrating trauma to the neck. Adv Surg 1994;27:97–127

Munera F, Danton G, Rivas LA, Henry RP, Ferrari MG. Multidetector row computed tomography in the management of penetrating neck injuries. Semin Ultrasound CT MR 2009;30(3):195–204

Obeid FN, Haddad GS, Horst HM, Bivins BA. A critical reappraisal of a mandatory exploration policy for penetrating wounds of the neck. Surg Gynecol Obstet 1985;160(6):517–522

Ordog GJ, Albin D, Wasserberger J, Balasubramanium S. Shotgun 'birdshot' wounds to the neck. J Trauma 1988;28(4):491–497

Osborn TM, Bell RB, Qaisi W, Long WB. Computed tomographic angiography as an aid to clinical decision making in the selective management of penetrating injuries to the neck: a reduction in the need for operative exploration. J Trauma 2008;64(6):1466–1471

Schroeder JW, Baskaran V, Aygun N. Imaging of traumatic arterial injuries in the neck with an emphasis on CTA. Emerg Radiol 2010;17(2):109–122

Shama DM, Odell J. Penetrating neck trauma with tracheal and oesophageal injuries. Br J Surg 1984;71(7):534–536

Stanley RB Jr, Hanson DG. Manual strangulation injuries of the larynx. Arch Otolaryngol 1983;109(5):344–347

110 Dentoalveolar Trauma

■ Introduction

Anatomy

The dental alveolus is the tooth-bearing portion of the maxilla and mandible. It is highly vascular, consisting of a buccal and lingual, or palatal, cortical plate with trabecular bone between. The tooth sockets are within the alveolar process and are lined with the periodontal ligament, which attaches the teeth to the alveolus. The tooth root consists predominantly of dentin with an outer lining of cementum, which attaches to the periodontal ligament. The crown of the tooth is composed of the inner, sensate dentin and the outer, harder enamel. Sensitivity of a tooth is transmitted through dentinal tubules to the pulp within the tooth. The pulp is a vital neurovascular bundle that supplies nutrition to the living dentin of the tooth.

Etiology

The most common injuries to permanent teeth occur secondary to falls, followed by traffic accidents, violence, and sports.

Pathology

Trauma to the alveolus can disrupt the blood supply to the pulp of the tooth or the periodontal ligament. In the mature permanent tooth, the vascular supply to the dental pulp enters through a small apical foramen. Without collateral blood supply, a disruption of that source usually results in the necrosis of the pulp. If the tooth sustains a hard enough blow to cause inflammation within the pulp, the consequent edema can restrict blood flow to the pulp, resulting in pulpal necrosis. Because pulpal necrosis can occur in the absence of obvious external injury to the tooth, any tooth that sustains trauma sufficient to cause its

loosening should be evaluated by a dentist and followed for up to a year to ensure that necrosis does not occur.

Injuries to the periodontal ligament can result in periodontal defects that collect bacterial plaques. The resulting periodontitis can slowly weaken the support for the tooth, resulting in tooth loss months to years after the trauma.

■ Evaluation

Clinical Findings

History

Dentoalveolar trauma usually occurs in the context of more complex facial trauma. The history should be directed to elicit evidence of other visible and occult injuries to the head, face, and neck, to include loss of consciousness.

A standard full medical history should be elicited as well. Ask if the patient has hepatitis or human immunodeficiency virus (HIV), since manipulating the fractures can subject the practitioner to needlestick injury. A history of a bleeding diathesis can complicate treatment, and aspirin or nonsteroidal medications can interfere with clotting. The social history can help determine if the patient is reliable for follow-up. This is an important discriminator in the treatment that is chosen because maintenance of luxated or fractured teeth can be time consuming and expensive for the patient.

Isolated dentoalveolar trauma is characterized by a loose tooth or loose segment of teeth, malocclusion, and tenderness to palpation of the associated teeth. Patients may report that their "bite feels off."

Determine if patients have any removable dental prosthetics, such as a full denture or a partial denture, and ask if they have any fixed dental prosthesis, such as a fixed bridge or implant-supported bridge.

Physical Examination

Examine the face and lips for lacerations, ecchymosis, and edema, and conduct a cranial nerve exam. The oral cavity is best examined with a bright headlight. Use gloves and a dental mirror or tongue blade to examine the oral cavity and get a general assessment of the health of the patient's dentition and the quality of dental hygiene. A patient with gross caries and periodontal disease is not a good candidate for salvaging extruded teeth, and the disease can compromise healing. Examine the buccal mucosa and palpate the alveolus, maxilla, and mandible for step-offs, mobile segments, or crepitus. Ecchymosis in the buccal or lingual vestibule is often a sign of an underlying fracture. Lacerations of the attached gingiva are also strong predictors of an underlying fracture. Examine the teeth, looking for mobility, cracked enamel, missing crown structure, and evidence of exposed dentin or bleeding exposed dental pulp. Have the patient close into maximal intercuspation, and look for evidence of a pathological crossbite or open bite, being aware that some patients will have those abnormalities in their premorbid occlusion.

Special Investigations

Clinical Laboratory Studies

Blood Tests

There are no specific laboratory blood tests indicated to help in the diagnosis or treatment of dentoalveolar trauma.

Imaging

Panoramic Dental X-Ray (Panorex, Orthopantomogram)

A panoramic dental X-ray is a two-dimensional radiograph of the upper and lower jaw and is very useful for diagnosing dental and dentoalveolar injury. Periapical radiographs taken at 90 degrees to the long axis of the tooth give the most detailed view of an individual tooth. However, these types of radiographs are often not available in the typical emergency room. If the hospital is associated with an oral and maxillofacial surgery service, panoramic and periapical films are usually available there during normal hours of operation.

Computed Tomographic Scan

A computed tomographic (CT) scan of the face is very helpful for facial fractures and dentoalveolar fractures, but some of the fine detail of dental root fractures may be obscured.

Differential Diagnosis

When examining the trauma patient for dental and dentoalveolar injury, it is important to understand the variety of injuries that occur to the teeth and alveoli and the indications for treatment and referral.

Alveolar Bone Fractures

Alveolar bone fractures include the following:

- Comminution of the alveolar socket, resulting from intrusive luxation injuries that produce a crushing injury
- Fractures of the buccal or lingual plates of the alveolar process
- Fractures of the alveolar process, resulting in mobility of an entire segment of teeth and bone
- Fractures of the mandible and maxilla. These fractures are covered in the module on facial fractures. They can be accompanied by fractures of the crowns or roots of the associated teeth. A fractured tooth within a mobile segment can complicate the treatment plan for that segment.

Luxation

- *Subluxation:* Loosening of the tooth without displacement
- *Lateral luxation:* Displacement of the tooth in any direction, except axially
- *Intrusion:* Apical displacement into the alveolar bone
- *Extrusion:* Partial avulsion

Avulsed Teeth

The tooth is completely displaced from the socket, tearing the periodontal ligament and possibly fracturing the socket.

Fractured Teeth Concisely

- Enamel fractures
- Enamel and dentin fractures, but no exposure of the dental pulp
- Enamel and dentin fractures with an exposed dental pulp
- Fractures of the crown and root
- Root fractures

■ Management

Alveolar Bone Fractures

Comminution of the Alveolar Socket

Comminution of the alveolar socket requires no treatment other than referring the patient to a dentist and stabilizing the tooth if it is loose.

Fractures of the Buccal and Lingual Plates

Fractures of the buccal and lingual plates should be repositioned, the gingival lacerations should be sutured, and the loose teeth should be stabilized for 2 weeks with a flexible splint.

Fractured Alveolar Segment

When an alveolar segment is fractured, resulting in mobility of an entire segment, the segment should be stabilized for 4 weeks. Fractured teeth within the fractured alveolus should be evaluated and treated by a dentist. Teeth with root fractures or coronal fractures that extend into the pulp will need endodontic therapy.

Luxation

Subluxation and Intrusion

Subluxation and intrusion typically require no treatment. If the intrusion is > 7 mm, the tooth may require surgical or orthodontic repositioning by a dentist. Refer these patients to the dentist for follow-up to monitor for necrosis of the pulp.

Lateral Luxation and Extrusion

Lateral luxation and extrusion are treated with repositioning and splinting. The lateral luxated tooth will require repositioning of the alveolar plate in most cases and should be splinted for 4 weeks. The extruded tooth can be splinted with a flexible splint for up to 2 weeks.

Avulsed Teeth

Avulsed Primary Teeth

Avulsed primary teeth should not be replanted.

Avulsed Permanent Teeth

Avulsed permanent teeth fall under three categories of management when presenting to the practitioner.

- A tooth that was immediately replaced by the patient or parent should be checked for normal positioning. If properly positioned, the tooth should be left in place. Suture any gingival lacerations, and apply a flexible splint for up to 2 weeks. Prescribe oral tetracycline if there are no developing permanent teeth; otherwise prescribe penicillin, such as amoxicillin. Check the patient's tetanus status, and refer the patient to a dentist for root canal treatment within 7 to 10 days.
- A tooth that has been transported in an appropriate medium and has been out of the socket for less than 1 hour should be cleaned with a stream of saline and soaked in saline. Administer local anesthetic and clean the socket with saline, removing any clot. Reposition any fractured segments of the socket, and gently replace the tooth. Confirm normal position clinically, and apply a flexible splint for up to 2 weeks. The postoperative treatment is the same as above. Suitable transport media are saline, milk, saliva, tissue culture medium, cell transport media, and Hank's balanced salt solution.
- If a tooth has been out of the socket for longer than 1 hour, the chances for a successful replantation are significantly diminished. The expected eventual outcome is ankylosis and resorption of the root, and the tooth will be lost eventually. To replant these teeth, clean the nonviable attached soft tissue with gauze. A root canal can be performed prior to replantation or within 7 to 10 days of injury; otherwise, treat the tooth in the same manner as described above.

Although most isolated dental injury will be managed by a dentist, this information can be useful to otolaryngologists–head and neck surgeons when evaluating patients who present with these types of injuries in conjunction with other facial injuries.

Fractured Teeth

Refer isolated fractured teeth to a dentist for evaluation and treatment. Most fractured teeth can be preserved; including those with fractures of the roots. A fracture that extends into the pulp of the tooth will require endodontic treatment, such as a root canal. Even teeth with fractured roots can be preserved with the application of a flexible splint and close follow-up by the dentist to watch for evidence of pulpal necrosis.

▪ Controversial Issues

Indications for Tooth Removal during Mandible Fracture Repair

There is concern that leaving a tooth in the line of fracture can predispose to infection, malunion, or nonunion. Leaving the tooth in the line of fracture often helps restore the premorbid bony alignment and occlusion, making reduction and fixation of the fracture easier. There are studies that demonstrate an increase in infection with retention of the tooth in the line of fracture, and studies that demonstrate a decrease in infection or no difference in the rate of infection. A high percentage (87%) of teeth in the line of fracture can be saved, but many (38%) require endodontics in the postoperative period, especially if the patient is older and the fracture runs through the apex of the tooth root. Postoperative occlusal interferences can be found in 38% of teeth in the line of fracture. Most of the literature concludes with the caveat that the decision to retain a tooth in the line of fracture is a clinical decision best made at the time of repair.

▪ Practice Guidelines, Consensus Statements, and Measures

American Academy of Pediatric Dentistry. Guideline on the Management of Acute Dental Trauma. Chicago, IL: American Academy of Pediatric Dentistry; 2011. http://www.aapd.org/media/Policies_Guidelines/G_Trauma.pdf

▪ Suggested Reading

Andersson L, Andreasen JO, Day P, et al; International Association of Dental Traumatology. International Association of Dental Traumatology guidelines for the management of traumatic dental injuries: 2. Avulsion of permanent teeth. Dent Traumatol 2012;28(2):88–96

Casey RP, Bensadigh BM, Lake MT, Thaller SR. Dentoalveolar trauma in the pediatric population. J Craniofac Surg 2010;21(4):1305–1309

Cvek M, Mejàre I, Andreasen JO. Healing and prognosis of teeth with intra-alveolar fractures involving the cervical part of the root. Dent Traumatol 2002;18(2):57–65

Day P, Duggal M. Interventions for treating traumatised permanent front teeth: avulsed (knocked out) and replanted. Cochrane Database Syst Rev 2010;1(1):CD006542 http://www.thecochranelibrary.com

Diangelis AJ, Andreasen JO, Ebeleseder KA, et al; International Association of Dental Traumatology. International Association of Dental Traumatology guidelines for the management of traumatic dental injuries: 1. Fractures and luxations of permanent teeth. Dent Traumatol 2012;28(1):2–12

Granger T, Gunn A, Welbury R. Tooth replantation: a worthwhile exercise? Acta Stomatol Croat 2011;45(2):75–85

Oikarinen K, Lahti J, Raustia AM. Prognosis of permanent teeth in the line of mandibular fractures. Endod Dent Traumatol 1990;6(4):177–182

Oikarinen K, Raustia AM. Occlusal interferences in association with teeth left in the line of mandibular fractures. Endod Dent Traumatol 1993;9(2):57–60

Rai S, Pradhan R. Tooth in the line of fracture: its prognosis and its effects on healing. Indian J Dent Res 2011;22(3):495–496

Yadavalli G, Hema M, Shetty J. Clinical evaluation of mandibular angle fractures with teeth in fracture line, treated with stable internal fixation. Indian J Stomatol 2011;2(4):216–221

Index

Note: Page numbers followed by *f* or *t* indicate figures or tables, respectively.

A

ABCDE mnemonic, for cutaneous melanoma, 149
ABC mnemonic, for trauma assessment, 731
Ablative skin resurfacing, laser for, 83–85
ABO incompatibility, and blood transfusion, 47
ABR. *See* Auditory brainstem response (ABR)
Abscess
- brain, 397, 398*f*
- with deep neck infection, 90, 92
-- dysphagia caused by, 383
- parapharyngeal, 93
- peritonsillar, 529
- prevertebral, 93
- retropharyngeal, 93
- with sialadenitis, 122
- temporal lobe, 398*f*
ACA (Affordable Care Act). *See* Patient Protection and Affordable Care Act
ACAD. *See* Atherosclerotic carotid artery disease
Accessory meningeal artery, 137
Accountability, of office staff, 26
Accountable care organizations, 5*t*, 11, 19
Accounts payable, 20, 26
Accounts receivable, 20
Accreditation Council for Graduate Medical Education (ACGME), core competencies, 71–73
Acetaminophen
- adverse effects and side effects of, 39
- in combination regimen, 40
-- for acute/postoperative pain, 39
ACGME. *See* Accreditation Council for Graduate Medical Education (ACGME)
Achalasia, 312, 314–315
- clinical presentation of, 314
- epidemiology of, 314
- etiology of, 314
- treatment of, 314–315
Achondroplasia, 484*t*
Acinic cell carcinoma, of salivary glands, 201*t*
Acneiform eruptions, after chemical peel, 631
Acne scars
- dermabrasion for, 629
- laser resurfacing for, 643
ACOs. *See* Accountable care organizations
Acoustic assessment, of voice, 335, 347
Acoustic neuroma(s). *See also* Schwannoma, vestibular
- and facial nerve paralysis, 458
- MRI characteristics of, 406*t*
- and tinnitus, 432, 436

Acoustic reflex
- testing, 390
- threshold, 390
-- elevated or absent, and site of lesion, 390
Acronyms, in health care quality and safety, 5*t*
Acrylic polymers, as implant materials, 647
ACS. *See* Anterior cricoid split
ACS-NSQIP. *See* American College of Surgeons National Surgical Quality Improvement Program
Actinic keratoses, and cutaneous squamous cell carcinoma, 155
Acupuncture, to control drooling, 515
Acyclovir, for respiratory papillomatosis, 372
Adenocarcinoma
- of ear canal, 419
- of middle ear and mastoid, 419
- of salivary glands
-- basal cell, 201*t*
-- mucinous, 201*t*
-- not otherwise specified, 201*t*
-- polymorphous low-grade, 201*t*
- sinonasal
-- classification of, 603
-- epidemiology of, 603
-- intestinal, 603
-- non-intestinal, 603
-- risk factors for, 602
-- treatment of, 603
Adenoid(s)
- anatomy of, 526
- hypertrophy, 529
- physiology of, 526
- recurrent infections, and adenotonsillectomy, 528
- surgical removal, indications for, 528–529
Adenoid cystic carcinoma
- of ear canal, 419
- of salivary glands, 201*t*
- sinonasal, 602–603
-- cribriform, 602
-- outcomes with, 602–603
-- solid, 602
-- treatment of, 602–603
-- tubular, 602
Adenoidectomy, velopharyngeal insufficiency after, 522–523
Adenolymphoma, of salivary glands. *See* Warthin tumors
Adenoma. *See also* Papillary adenoma of endolymphatic sac
- basal cell, of salivary glands, 201*t*, 202
- mucosal, of middle ear and mastoid, 419
Adenotonsillar hypertrophy, 527–528
Adenotonsillectomy
- clinical practice guidelines for, 531
- complications of, 530–531

- contraindications to, 529–530
- controversies about, 530
- evaluation for, 529
- indications for, 528–529
- outpatient, 530
- postoperative care, 530–531
- preoperative management, 529–530
- surgical technique for, 530
Adenovirus
- dysphagia caused by, 383
- nasopharyngeal infection, 526
- pharyngotonsillar infection, 526
Advertising, ethical considerations with, 33
Aerodigestive tract injury, in penetrating neck trauma, 731, 732, 733
Aerodynamic assessment, in clinical voice laboratory, 334–335
Aesthetic surgery. *See also* Blepharoplasty; Endoscopic forehead lift; Rhytidectomy
- endoscopic, 615–619
Afferent pupillary defect, in thyroid eye disease, 704
Affordable Care Act. *See* Patient Protection and Affordable Care Act
Agency for Health Care Policy and Research, 5. *See also* Agency for Healthcare Research and Quality
- Patient Outcomes Research Teams (PORTs), 63
Agency for Healthcare Research and Quality, 3, 4*t*, 5–6, 10
- cancer pain management guidelines, 42
Agger nasi (cell), 543, 553*t*, 554–555, 554*f*
Aging
- disequilibrium of, 451
-- rehabilitative strategies for, 470
- and olfactory decline, 560
AHI. *See* Apnea/hypopnea index
AHRQ. *See* Agency for Healthcare Research and Quality
AI. *See* Apnea index (AI)
AIDS (acquired immunodeficiency syndrome). *See also* HIV-infected (AIDS) patients
- otologic manifestations of, 453–454
Air–bone gap, 389
Air cell(s)
- of petrous apex, trapped fluid in, 409, 410*f*, 410*t*
- posterior nasal septal, 566
Air-conduction thresholds, 389–390
Airway
- evaluation
-- in blunt neck trauma, 734
-- in penetrating neck trauma, 731
- Fujita classification of, 116
- obstruction
-- after adenotonsillectomy, 531

-- with deep neck infection, 91–92
-- and sleep-disordered breathing, 115–116
- upper, obstruction, and adenotonsillectomy, 528
Albinism, 484*t*
Albuterol, for anaphylaxis, 60*t*
Alcohol, and bleeding time, 580
Alcoholism, esophageal dysmotility in, 317
ALDs. *See* Assistive listening devices
Alexander's law, 468
Allergen(s), 535
- avoidance of, 538
- environmental control measures against, 538
Allergic rhinitis
- clinical features of, 535–536
- diagnosis of, 535–536
- epidemiology of, 535
- in HIV-infected (AIDS) patients, 77
- immunotherapy for, 539–541
- intermittent, management of, 539*f*
- management of, 538–541, 538*f*
-- clinical practice guidelines for, 541
- pathogenesis of, 535
- pathophysiology of, 535
- persistent, management of, 539*f*
- pharmacotherapy for, 538–539
- signs and symptoms, 535
Allergic shiner, 535
Allergy
- definition of, 535
- diagnosis of, 535–538
- epidemiology of, 535
- immunotherapy for, 539–541
- management of, 538–541
- pharmacotherapy for, 538–539
- skin testing for, 536–537
- stomatitis caused by, 99
Alopecia
- androgenic
-- evaluation, 636–637
-- inheritance of, 635
- autoimmune diseases causing, 636, 638*t*
- causes of, 636–637
- dermatologic causes of, 636
- differential diagnosis, 636
- endocrine causes of, 636, 638*t*
- evaluation, 637–638
- inheritance of, 635
- iron depletion and, 636, 638*t*
- laboratory investigation in, 636, 648*t*
- medical management of, 639
- pressure, 636
- punch biopsy in, 637, 638*t*
- surgical management of, 639–640
- syphilis and, 636, 638*t*
- tests for, 636–637, 638*t*
- toxic, 636
- traction, 636
- traumatic, 636
- vitamin D and, 638*t*

741